THE NEXT STEP

Medical Coding
from Classroom to Practice

A Worktext

THE NEXT STEP

Medical Coding
from Classroom to Practice

A Worktext

CAROL J. BUCK, MS, CPC, CPC-H, CCS-P
Program Director, Retired
Medical Secretary Programs
Northwest Technical College
East Grand Forks, Minnesota

with 109 illustrations

SAUNDERS
ELSEVIER

SAUNDERS
ELSEVIER

11830 Westline Industrial Drive
St. Louis, Missouri 63146

THE NEXT STEP: MEDICAL CODING FROM
CLASSROOM TO PRACTICE, A WORKTEXT

ISBN-13: 978-1-4160-2321-0
ISBN-10: 1-4160-2321-6

Notice

Neither the Publisher nor the Author assume any responsibility for any loss or injury and/or damage to persons or property arising out of or related to any use of the material contained in this book. It is the responsibility of the treating practitioner, relying on independent expertise and knowledge of the patient, to determine the best treatment and method of application for the patient.

The Publisher

ISBN-13: 978-1-4160-2321-0
ISBN-10: 1-4160-2321-6

Acquisitions Editor: Susan Cole
Developmental Editor: Colin Odell
Publishing Services Manager: Pat Joiner
Project Manager: Gena Magouirk
Design Direction: Kathi Gosche

Printed in USA.
Last digit is the print number: 9 8 7 6 5 4 3 2 1

To all the students, whose abilities to surmount tremendous obstacles to achieve their goals have been a source of unending inspiration.

To the teachers, who give of their talent, time, and knowledge to help the students who enter their classrooms, may this work make your load just a little lighter as we travel the same road, toward the same goal.

To Ray Cross, an educational leader with the vision to see the future of an institution and the drive to make it happen.

To my husband, Dennis, for understanding the mission, supporting the journey, and keeping the faith.

To my dear friend, Chang Lee, your memory and lessons will last a lifetime.

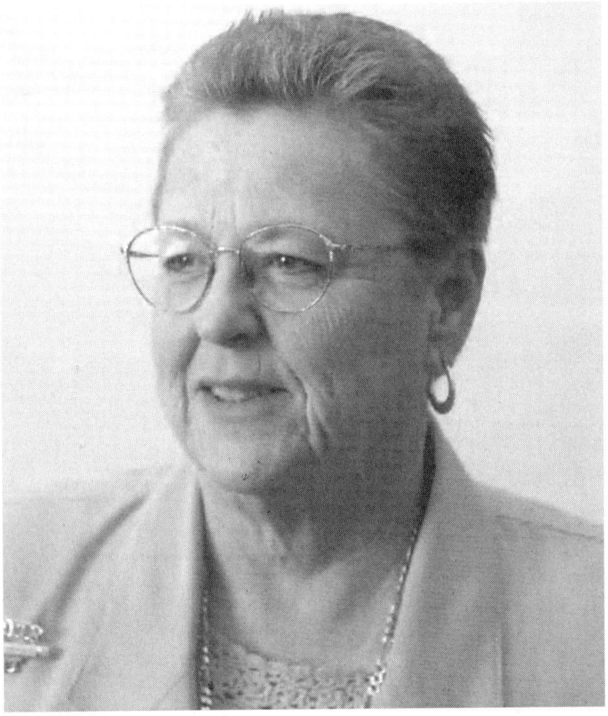

Carol J. Buck

Collaborators and Reviewers

Technical Collaborators

Jacqueline Klitz Grass, CPC, MA
Coding and Reimbursement Specialist
Altru Clinic
Grand Forks, North Dakota

Jody L. Klitz
Coding and Reimbursement Specialist
Grand Forks, North Dakota

Senior Reviewer

Karen Lockyer, BA, RHIT
Adjunct Professor
Montgomery College, Takoma Park
Southlake, Texas

Reviewers

Sharon Parr, CPC
Patients Accounts Supervisor
Cardiology Specialists, Inc.
St. Louis, Missouri

Kathleen C. Pride, AS, CPC, CCS-P
Training Manager
QuadraMed Corporation
Port St. Lucie, Florida

Debora Neville, RHIA, CCS-P, CPC
Financial Analyst
Rochester, Minnesota

Judy Breuker, CPC, CCS-P, CHCC, CHBME, ACS-GS
President
Medical Educational Services, Inc.
Jenison, Michigan

Marilyn Rasmussen, RHIA, CPC
Coding Supervisor
Albert Lee, Minnesota

Jana Hensche
Inpatient Hospital Coder
Austin Medical Services
Alden, Minnesota

Brenda J. Dombkowski, CPC
Certified Professional Coder
Obstetric Gynecology & Infertility Group, PC
Woodbridge, Connecticut

Cynthia L. Stahl, CPC, CCS-P
President
Central Indiana Chapter of AAPC
Lebanon, Indiana

Karla R. Lovaasen, RHIA, CCS, CCS-P
President
Coding and Consulting Services
Wahpeton, North Dakota

Carlene Harrison, MPA, CMA
Chair, Allied Health Programs
International College
Naples, Florida

Sandra Hertkorn
Adviser,
Program Medical Office Careers
Techskills Sacramento
North Highlands, California

Cynthia Zumbrun, RHIT
Instructor
Allegany College of Maryland
LaVale, Maryland

Lori Warren, MA, RN, CPC, CCP, CLNC
Medical Department Co-Director,
Medical Coding Program
Spencerian College
Louisville, Kentucky

Deborah Cross, RHIA, CCS
Adjunct Instructor
Lamar Institute of Technology
Beaumont, Texas

Wendy Ryder, CPC, CPC-H
President
Ryder Medical Coding & Consulting
Hilliard, Ohio

Julie Orloff, CPC, CMA, RMA, CPT
National Program Director
CEC, Miami Operations
Miami, Florida

Letitia Patterson, MPA, CPC, CCS-P
Medical Coder
Illinois College of Optometry
Chicago, Illinois

Contents

Preface

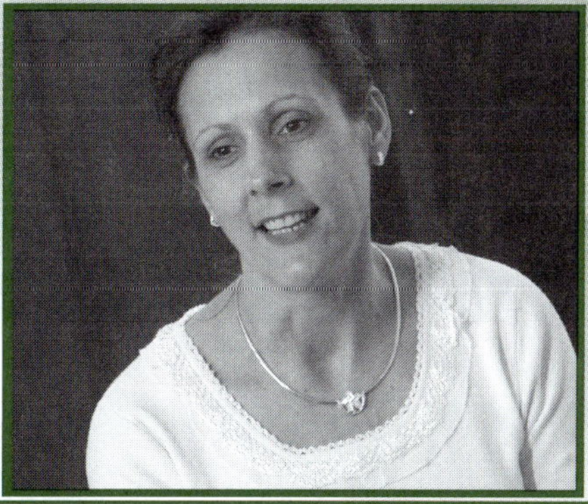

Debra Fields, CPC
Collections Representative
Women's Health Alliance, DBA
Chapel Hill OB/GYN
Chapel Hill, North Carolina

Types of Codes

This worktext presents cases that are to be coded with **service codes** (CPT and HCPCS) and **diagnosis codes** (ICD-9-CM) in the outpatient settings of the clinic and outpatient departments of the hospital for both the physician (professional) and the facility (hospital) services.

Appendix E of this worktext displays the 1995 and 1997 Documentation Guidelines for Evaluation and Management Services. Each medical facility chooses one of the documentation guidelines and submits all Medicare and Medicaid E/M charges using that specific set of guidelines. This worktext has been developed using the 1995 guidelines, as that tends to be the more popular version. Even though the private third-party payers (not Medicare, Medicaid, or any other government program) may not require adherence to a specific set of E/M documentation guidelines, the facility-chosen guidelines are usually applied to all E/M services.

Unlike the inpatient coder, who has all the documentation from a hospital stay available when assigning diagnoses codes, the outpatient coder reports diagnoses based on the information present in the one report being coded. In this worktext, a case may contain numerous reports that chronicle the patient's care. When coding each of the reports in the case, the coder is to consider only the diagnoses information present in that report, because this is the way the reports are coded in outpatient settings. For example, a physician admits a patient to the hospital for possible pneumonia with chief complaint of shortness of breath and wheezing. The coder reporting the physician's admit service would report the symptoms of shortness of breath and wheezing, even though on a subsequent report within that case the physician does diagnose the patient's condition as pneumonia. One exception to this rule would be when coding an operative report in which a specimen was sent to the pathology department for analysis. The pathologist's diagnosis would be used as the diagnosis when coding the operative report, because the findings are usually more current and definitive than the diagnosis stated by the surgeon.

Clarification regarding the reporting guidelines for diagnostic tests, such as pathology reports, is located in AB-01-144. The Centers for Medicare and Medicaid, Program Memorandum (PM), Transmittal AB-01-144 is displayed in **Appendix B** of the worktext and outlines current coding guidelines for reporting the diagnosis for diagnostic tests. The PM provides direction on coding diagnostic tests and coordinates with the Official Guidelines for Coding and Reporting. An excerpt from the PM is as follows:

A. Determining the Appropriate Primary ICD-9-CM Diagnosis Code for Diagnostic Tests Ordered Due to Signs and/or Symptoms

1. If the physician has confirmed a diagnosis based on the results of the diagnostic test, the physician interpreting the test should code that diagnosis. The signs and/or symptoms that prompted ordering the test may be reported as additional diagnoses if they are not fully explained or related to the confirmed diagnosis.

Example 1: A surgical specimen is sent to a pathologist with a diagnosis of "mole". The pathologist personally reviews the slides made from the specimen and makes a diagnosis of "malignant melanoma". The pathologist should report a diagnosis of "malignant melanoma" as the primary diagnosis.

Example 2: A patient is referred to a radiologist for an abdominal CT scan with a diagnosis of abdominal pain. The CT scan reveals the presence of an abscess. The radiologist should report a diagnosis of "intra-abdominal abscess."

The PM is an important document to read before beginning to use this text as it outlines the guidelines used when this text was developed. The coder is introduced to this document in Chapter 1 of the worktext under the heading Diagnosis Coding. This document is foundational information that must be carefully read and thoroughly understood by the coder prior to assigning diagnosis codes. The Official Guidelines for Coding and Reporting are also displayed in **Appendix C** and are the rules for diagnosis coding.

A **List of Physicians** is located in **Appendix F** of the text and contains the names of the physicians that provide services to the patients in this worktext. The list is displayed in alphabetic order by physician last name and by specialty. There are two physicians that are employed by the hospital (Dr. Hart and Dr. Sutton), and the remaining physicians are employed at the local clinic. The coder will be assigning codes for all the physicians.

Select **abbreviations** and **acronyms** used in the cases in the chapter are displayed at the beginning of the chapter. **Appendix D** contains a compilation of these abbreviations and acronyms.

Content

This book is a text and workbook in one volume (a worktext). The following are the chapters of the worktext:

1. Evaluation and Management
2. Medicine
3. Radiology
4. Pathology and Laboratory
5. Integumentary System
6. Cardiovascular System
7. Digestive System, Hemic/Lymphatic System, and Mediastinum/Diaphragm
8. Musculoskeletal System
9. Respiratory System
10. Urinary, Male Genital, and Endocrine Systems
11. Female Genital System and Maternity Care/Delivery
12. Nervous System
13. Eye and Auditory Systems
14. Anesthesia

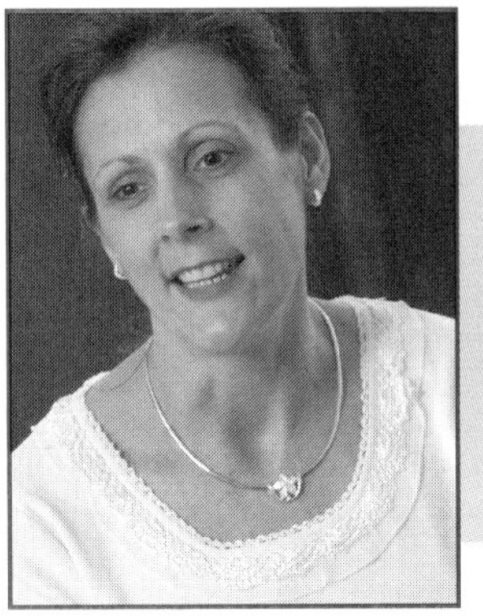

FROM THE TRENCHES

Debra

"You have to be a private investigator . . . You always have to be able to look at something and say 'What is wrong with this? Why didn't the insurance company pay on it?' You have to be able to figure out what the problem is."

The number of cases in each chapter was determined by the complexity of coding the most common services in the specialty. For example, Chapter 6, Cardiovascular System, is quite lengthy as this is a very complex area to code and many of the basic cardiovascular services are commonly provided in most outpatient settings, such as ECG and Holter monitor. There are many coding challenges in cardiology, such as coronary artery bypass graft, and only through repeated cases can the coder gain understanding and then confidence in his/her cardiology coding skill.

Case Numbering System

The cases are numbered by chapter, case, and report. For example, in 7-15A, the "7" indicates the case appears within Chapter 7. The "15" indicates the case is the 15th case in Chapter 7. The "A" indicates that the report is the first report in the case. Subsequent reports within 7-15 are identified by B, C, etc.

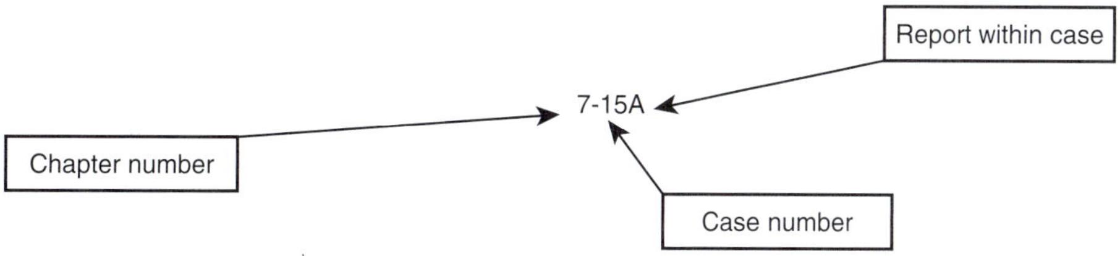

Tests are identified by a "T" preceding the case. For example, T7-1A indicates the test (T) is from Chapter 7 and is the first case (1) and first report (A) in the case. The web cases are numbered in the same way, but with a "W" preceding the case. For example, W7-1A indicates this is a web case from Chapter 7 and is the first case (1) and first report (A) in the case. Each chapter has an outline that lists all the cases and reports at the beginning of the chapter, as illustrated in the following:

Evaluation and Management Services

CASE 6-1

6-1A Cardiothoracic Surgery Consultation

Cardiac Artery Bypass Grafts

CASE 6-2

6-2A Coronary Artery Bypass

Pacemaker

CASE 6-3

6-3A Cardiology Follow-up Note

CASE 6-7

6-7A Cardiology Consultation
6-7B Hospital Service
6-7C Radiography Report, Chest
6-7D Cardiothoracic Surgical Consultation
6-7E Radiography Report, Chest

CASE 6-8

6-8A Echo Doppler Report

CASE 6-9

6-9A Cardiology Consultation

6-12C Radiology Report, Chest
6-12D Cardiac Catheterization Report
6-12E Radiology Report, GI

Miscellaneous Reports

Cardioversion

CASE 6-13

6-13A Cardioversion

CASE 6-14

6-14A Transesophageal Echocardiogram Report

In Chapter 1, Evaluation and Management, the coder is introduced to the following audit form:

CHAPTER 6, CASE 6-7D

HISTORY ELEMENTS	Documented
HISTORY OF PRESENT ILLNESS (HPI)	
1. Location (site on body)	✗
2. Quality (characteristic: throbbing, sharp)	
3. Severity (1/10 or how intense)	
4. Duration (how long for problem or episode)	✗
5. Timing (when it occurs)	✗
6. Context (under what circumstances does it occur)	
7. Modifying factors (what makes it better or worse)	✗
8. Associated signs and symptoms (what else is happening when it occurs)	✗
TOTAL	5
LEVEL	4
REVIEW OF SYSTEMS (ROS)	Documented
1. Constitutional (e.g., weight loss, fever)	✗
2. Ophthalmologic (eyes)	
3. Otolaryngologic (ears, nose, mouth, throat)	
4. Cardiovascular	✗
5. Respiratory	✗
6. Gastrointestinal	✗
7. Genitourinary	✗
8. Musculoskeletal	✗
9. Integumentary (skin and/or breasts)	✗
10. Neurologic	✗
11. Psychiatric	
12. Endocrine	✗
13. Hematologic/Lymphatic	✗
14. Allergic/Immunologic	
TOTAL	10
LEVEL	4
PAST, FAMILY, AND/OR SOCIAL HISTORY (PFSH)	Documented
1. Past illness, operations, injuries, treatments, and current medications	✗
2. Family medical history for heredity and risk	✗
3. Social activities, both past and present	✗
TOTAL	3
LEVEL	4

History Level	1	2	3	4
	Problem Focused	Expanded Problem Focused	Detailed	Comprehensive
HPI	Brief 1-3	Brief 1-3	Extended 4+	Extended 4+
ROS		Problem Pertinent	Extended 2-9	Complete 10+
PFSH			Pertinent 1	Complete 2-3
			HISTORY LEVEL	4

EXAMINATION ELEMENTS	Documented
CONSTITUTIONAL	
1. Blood pressure, sitting	✗
2. Blood pressure, lying	
3. Pulse	✗
4. Respirations	✗
5. Temperature	
6. Height	
7. Weight	
8. General appearance	✗
NUMBER	1
BODY AREAS (BA)	Documented
1. Head (including face)	✗
2. Neck	✗
3. Chest (including breasts and axillae)	
4. Abdomen	✗
5. Genitalia, groin, buttocks	
6. Back (including spine)	
7. Each extremity	
NUMBER	3
ORGAN SYSTEMS (OS)	Documented
1. Ophthalmologic (eyes)	✗
2. Otolaryngologic (ears, nose, mouth, throat)	✗
3. Cardiovascular	✗
4. Respiratory	✗
5. Gastrointestinal	✗
6. Genitourinary	
7. Musculoskeletal	✗
8. Integumentary	
9. Neurologic	✗
10. Psychiatric	
11. Hematologic/Lymphatic/Immunologic	
NUMBER	7
TOTAL BA/OS	11

Exam Level	1	2	3	4
	Problem Focused	Expanded Problem Focused	Detailed	Comprehensive
	Limited to affected BA/OS	Limited to affected BA/OS & other related OSs	Extended of affected BA & other related OSs	General multi-system or complete single OS
# of OS or BA	1	2-7 limited	2-7 extended	8+ or 1 complete single system
			EXAMINATION LEVEL	4

MDM ELEMENTS	Documented
# OF DIAGNOSIS/MANAGEMENT OPTIONS	
1. Minimal	
2. Limited	
3. Multiple	✗
4. Extensive	
LEVEL	3
AMOUNT OR COMPLEXITY OF DATA TO REVIEW	Documented
1. Minimal/None	
2. Limited	
3. Moderate	✗
4. Extensive	
LEVEL	3
RISK OF COMPLICATION OR DEATH IF NOT TREATED	Documented
1. Minimal	
2. Low	
3. Moderate	✗
4. High	
LEVEL	3

MDC*	1	2	3	4
	Straightforward	Low	Moderate	High
Number of DX or management options	Minimal	Limited	Multiple	Extensive
Amount or complexity of data	Minimal/None	Limited	Moderate	Extensive
Risks	Minimal	Low	Moderate	High
			MDM LEVEL	3

*To qualify for a given type of MDM complexity, 2 of 3 elements in the table must be met or exceeded.

History: Comprehensive
Examination: Comprehensive
MDM: Moderate

Number of Key Components: 3 of 3

Code: 99254

Each of the elements of the history, examination, and medical decision making complexity is reviewed in the chapter in detail. The coder will then complete an audit form for each of the E/M cases.

The E/M audit form is located in **Appendix A** of the worktext. The coder is to photocopy the audit form for each E/M case in the worktext and for the tests that contain E/M cases. A blank copy of the form is located on the companion web page.

Report Format

Information is provided regarding a coding concept, such as pacemaker implantation:

Pacemaker

A pacemaker is an electrical device that is inserted into the body to shock the heart electrically into regular rhythm. The two parts of a pacemaker are the battery and the electrode. The *electrode* is the device that emits the electrical charge. The electrode is also called the *lead* and is a flexible, thin tube. The battery is also called a *pulse generator.* Some generators are programmable and have a wide range of programming options. The pulse generator is placed into a pocket either under the clavicle, as illustrated in **Figure 6-4,** or under the muscle of the abdomen, below the rib cage.

Either an epicardial or transvenous approach can be used to implant the electrode portion of the pacemaker. The epicardial approach involves opening the chest to the view of the surgeon and the device being placed on the heart. The transvenous approach is most commonly used because it is the least traumatic to the patient and involves inserting a needle with a wire attached (guide wire) into a vein. The guide wire then directs the placement electrode into the heart while the surgeon views the progression using a fluoroscope. The electrode is then attached to the pulse generator.

The pacemaker can be a single- or dual-chamber unit. A single-chamber pacemaker uses one pulse generator and one electrode that is placed in either the atrium or the ventricle. A dual-chamber pacemaker uses a pulse generator and two electrodes—one placed in the atrium and the other placed in the ventricle.

Pacemakers can be permanent or temporary. A temporary pacemaker can be used when the heart needs only short-term pacing support, for example, an adverse drug reaction, waiting for placement of a permanent pacemaker, or postsurgical cardiac instability. After the pacemaker is placed, the physician will test the device to ensure that it is operating correctly.

As the text progresses, the coder is assigned more complex cases with less directive and less information to ensure the development of the ability to transfer previously learned knowledge, thereby strengthening confidence in his/her coding abilities. The **goal of this text** is to present the coder with a wide array of cases from across the major medical specialties. These reports are the "real thing" from clinics and hospitals. The reports were selected to give you a realistic picture of the type and scope of reports you will be coding on the job.

The format of the worktext is two columns to save space and contain the cost of production. Although the coder will not see a two-column report on the job, it is the documentation that is important, in whatever format that information is presented in. For example, the pathology reports may be in the front of the medical record at one facility, and at another facility, the reports may be in the back of the record. Or the coder may work exclusively with on-line records and never use the printed format.

The coder assigns the service and diagnosis codes to reports. The following is an example of a report from the worktext:

6-5C OPERATIVE REPORT, PACEMAKER IMPLANTATION

LOCATION: Hospital Outpatient

PATIENT: Herbert Gillford

SURGEON: Dr. Marvin Elhart

PROCEDURE PERFORMED: Dual-chamber pacemaker implantation

INDICATION: Bradyarrhythmia

BRIEF HISTORY: This patient has been experiencing recurrent syncope. He was evaluated in the last year or so. Because of the presence of first-degree AV block, sinus bradycardia, and bundle-branch block, the cause for his syncope most likely is his bradyarrhythmia; for that reason, a dual-chamber pacemaker implantation was recommended after discussion with his cousin, who consented to the procedure. The cousin was informed of all the potential complications, including infection, hematoma, pneumothorax, hemothorax, myocardial infarction, and even death. He agreed to proceed.

PROCEDURE: The patient was brought to the cardiac catheterization laboratory. He was placed on the catheterization table, where he was prepped and draped in the usual fashion. The procedure was extremely difficult to perform as a result of the patient's agitation despite adequate sedation. With reasonable hemostasis, the pacemaker pocket was performed in the left infraclavicular area after anesthetizing the area with 0.5 cc of Xylocaine. Hemostasis was secured with cautery. The patient had excessive venous oozing from Valsalva and straining, and that was controlled with pressure. A single stick was performed because of the patient's agitation. Using a 9 French peel-away sheath, we introduced an atrial and a ventricular lead and placed them in an excellent position.

Thresholds were obtained adequately. The leads were sutured using 0 silk over their sleeves and secured. The pulse generator was connected. The pacemaker pocket was flushed with antibiotic solution. The pacemaker and leads were placed in the pocket and the pocket closed in two layers.

COMPLICATION: None

EQUIPMENT USED: Pulse generator was Medtronic model 7960 Thera DRI, serial B4328H. The ventricular lead was Medtronic serial LAR420V, model 4524 Link. The atrial lead was Medtronic 4024-58, serial LJ326V.

The following parameters were obtained after implantation: Pacing threshold in the atrium was excellent at 0.5 msec and 0.5 V, and impedance was 445 ohms and sensing 2.1 mV. In the ventricle, 0.5 msec and 0.3 V with R wave of 19.9 mV and impedance 668.

The following parameters were left at implantation: DDDR with lower rate limit of 70 and an upper rate limit of 120. The amplitude was 3.5 V in the atrium at 0.4 msec with a sensitivity of 0.5 mV. The ventricle was 3.5 V and 0.4 msec at 2.8-mV sensitivity.

CONCLUSION: Successful implantation of dual-chamber pacemaker without immediate complications.

PLAN: Patient to return to recovery unit and to be discharged late this evening to the nursing home with routine post pacemaker care.

6-5C:

SERVICE CODE(S):______________________

DX CODE(S):______________________

Multiple Modifiers

Multiple modifiers are added to codes by placing the numbers first in ascending order followed by the lettered modifiers in alphabetic order. For example, if the code were to be reported with -55 and –RT, the -55 would be placed first followed by the –RT. Or as an another example, if the code were to be reported with -50 and -52, the -50 would be placed first followed by the -52. This is the format that is followed in this text.

Use of Modifier -26 and –TC

- Modifier -26 requests payment from the third-party payer for the professional component percentage of the fee only.
- Modifier –TC requests payment for the technical component percentage of the fee only.

These modifiers are usually used with radiology and pathology services. An example is an independent radiology facility that takes the x-rays (technical component) and sends them to a private radiologist who reads the x-rays and writes a report of the findings (professional component). The independent radiology facility would report the service with the x-ray code with modifier –TC added to indicate only the technical component was provided. The physician's services would be reported with modifier -26 added to the x-ray code to indicate that only the professional component of the x-ray service was provided. If both the technical and professional services of the x-ray were provided at the same place, such as the clinic, no modifiers would be added since both components of the service were provided at the same place and reporting the x-ray code without a modifier requests the full fee from the carrier.

For the purposes of this worktext, the radiologist and pathologists are employed by the facility unless specifically stated otherwise.

Pathology and Laboratory

Chapter 4, Pathology and Laboratory, information guides the coder in the use of a standard laboratory requisition or superbill as illustrated on the following page.

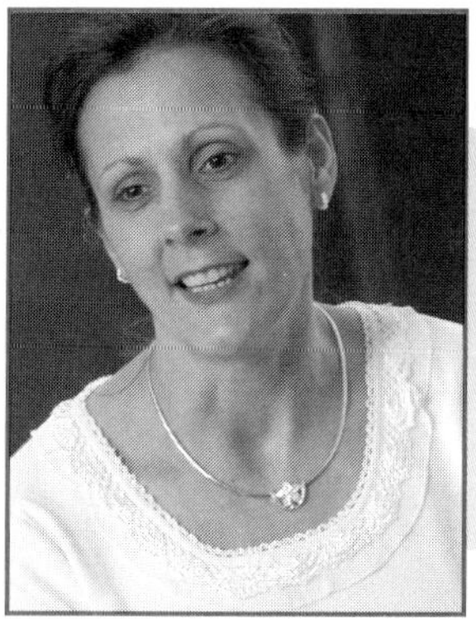

FROM THE TRENCHES

Debra

"If you don't have everything coded to the highest level, then you're not necessarily going to get paid. The claim is either going to come back rejected or you many not get the reimbursement that you deserve."

General Laboratory Requisition

Order Date: ______________ Order Time: ______________

PRIORITY (Routine unless otherwise specified)
☐ ASAP ☐ STAT All tests: ☐ Yes ☐ No
If No, Specify Tests: ______________

☐ **RECURRING ORDER** (not to exceed 12 months)
Frequency: ________ Start Date: ________ End Date: ________

SPECIAL INSTRUCTIONS

FOR PHYSICIAN OFFICE COLLECTION ONLY:
Collected: Date: ________ Time: ________ By: ________

FOR LAB COLLECTION ONLY:
Collected: Date: ________ Time: ________ By: ________

	Code	CHEMISTRY	DX
	82040	Albumin/Serum	
	84075	Alkaline phosphatase	
	84460	ALT/SGPT	
	82150	Amylase	
	82803	Arterial Blood Gas	
	84450	AST/SGOT	
	82248	Bilirubin, direct	
	82247	Bilirubin, total	
	84520	BUN, Quant	
	82310	Calcium, total	
	82374	Carbon dioxide (CO_2)	
	82378	CEA	
	82435	Chloride, blood	
	82465	Cholesterol, serum	
	82550	CK (creatine kinase)	
	82565	Creatinine, blood	
	83001	FSH	
	82728	Ferritin	
	82746	Folic Acid (Folate), blood	
	82977	GGT	
	82947	Glucose, blood non-reag	
	83036	Glycated Hgb (Hgb A1C)	
	84703	HCG-Qualitative	
	84702	HCG-Quantitative	
	83718	HDL Cholesterol	
	86334-90	Immun. Electrophoresis	
	83540	Iron	
	83550	Iron Binding Capacity	
	NC	% saturation requires iron & IBC to be ordered	
	83615	LDH (lactate dehydrogenase)	
	83002	LH (luteinizing hormone)	
	83735	Magnesium	
	84100	Phosphorus, blood	
	84132	Potassium, blood	
	84146	Prolactin, blood	
	84155	Protein, total	
	84165-90	Protein Electrophoresis, serum	
	84153	PSA, total	
	84295	Sodium, serum	
	84439	T4, free (thyroxine)	
	84443	TSH	
	84478	Triglycerides	
	84550	Uric Acid, blood	
	82607	Vitamin B12	
		CALCULATIONS	
	NC	LDL requires Chol & HDL to be ordered	
	NC	CHOL/HDL requires Chol & HDL to be ordered	

	Code	TOXICOLOGY/ THERAPEUTIC DRUGS	DX
Last Dose:			
	80156	Carbamazepine	
	80162	Digoxin	
	80178	Lithium	
	80184	Phenobarbital	
	80185	Phenytoin (Dilantin)	
	80196	Salicylate	
	80164	Valproic Acid	
	80198	Theophylline	

	Code	IMMUNOLOGY (Blood)	DX
	86038	ANA (FANA) Screen if ANA positive, 86039 titer performed, if titer >1:160 cascade performed (anti-ds DNA, ENA I & ENA II)	
	86225	Anti-ds DNA	
	86235x2	ENA I (Sm, RNP)	
	86235x2	ENA II (SSA, SSB)	
	86063	ASO screen (ASO titer if screen positive 86060)	
	86430	Rheumatoid factor (qual)	
	86593	RPR (Syphilis Serology), quant	
	86157	Cold Agglutinin titer	
	87340	Hep B surface antigen	
	87340-90	Hep B surface antigen OB (PHL)	
	86701-90	HIV	
	86308	Mono test	
	86762	Rubella Antibody	

	Code	PANELS	DX
	80051	Electrolytes CO_2, Cl, K Na	
	80048	Basic metabolic Ca, CO_2, Cl, Creat, Glu, K, Na, BUN	
	80053	Comprehensive metabolic Alb, Bili tot, Ca, Cl, Creat, Glu, Alk phos, K, Prot tot, Na, AST, ALT, BUN, CO_2	
	80076	Hepatic Function Alb, Bili tot and dir, Alk phos, AST, ALT, Prot tot	
	80061	Lipid Chol tot, HDL, Trig., calc, LDL, Chol/HDL ratio	
	80050	Gen health, Comp met, CBC, TSH	

	Code	HEMATOLOGY	DX
	85004	Hemogram WBC, auto WBC diff	
	85007	Hemogram micro exam, WBC diff	
	85008	Hemogram micro exam, w/o diff	
	85009	Hemogram manual WBC diff, buffy	
	85014	Hematocrit	
	85018	Hemoglobin	
	85049	Platelet count, auto	
	85044	Reticulocyte count, manual	
	85652	Sedimentation Rate, auto	
	85048	WBC, automated	
	85025	CBC, with diff Hgb, Hct, RBC, WBC, Platelet	
	85027	CBC, w/o diff Hgb, Hct, RBC, WBC, Platelet	

	Code	COAGULATION	DX
	☐ Coumadin ☐ Heparin		
	85730	APTT	
	85610	Prothrombin time	
	85002	Bleeding time	

	Code	OFFICE TESTING	DX
	81002	UA, Dipstick in Office	

	Code	URINE/STOOL	DX
	81003	UA, Routine	
		UA SAVE (for possible urine culture if requested)	
	81001	UA with microscopic	
	81002	Urinalysis, Dipstick, Lab	
	82270	Occult Blood	
	81025	Urine HCG	
	81003	Diabetic urine cascade	

	Code	TIMED URINE	DX
Hours:			
	82575	Creatinine Clearance	
	82340	Calcium, Urine, Quant.	
	84560	Uric acid	

	Code	BODY FLUID	DX
Fluid Source:			
	89051	Cell Count w/ Diff	
	84154	Protein	
	82945	Glucose	
	89300	Semen Analysis	
	89320	Semen Analysis, Comp	

	Code	IMMUNOHEMATOLOGY	DX
	86900	Blood type ABO, Rh(D)	
	86901	Weak D performed if Rh negative	
	86850	Antibody Screen Identification, if positive, titer if indicated	
	86880	Direct Coombs additional testing if positive	

WRITE-IN TESTS	DX	Lab Use

Medical Necessity Statement: Tests ordered on Medicare patients must follow CMS rules regarding medical necessity and FDA approval guidelines and must include diagnosis, symptoms, or reason for testing as indicated on the medical record. For any patient of any payor (including Medicare and Medicaid) that has a medical necessity requirement, order only those tests which are medically necessary for the diagnosis and treatment of the patient.

DX	ICD-9 CODE	WRITTEN INDICATION/DIAGNOSIS (Match Diagnosis # to Test)
1		
2		
3		
4		

LAB USE ONLY

	Code	
	36600	Arterial Puncture
	36415	Venipuncture
	G0001	Venipuncture MC/MA
	99000	Handling Fee
	81050	Urine Volume Measurement
	84030-90	PKU

Chart #: ______________ Date: ________
Name: ______________ M/F
DOB: ______________
Physician: ______________

Medicare #: ______________ Medicaid #: ______________
☐ No ABN needed ☐ Patient refused to sign ABN
Nursing Home Part A Medicare: ☐ Yes ☐ No
Worker's Comp: ☐ Yes ☐ No
Company Account: ______________

General Laboratory Requisition Form.

When the coders have finished the activities within the chapter, they will have a completed laboratory requisition that contains the codes for the tests listed. The coder will then be familiar with the most frequently ordered laboratory tests.

Glossary

Terms are bolded in the worktext to indicate an important concept, and other words are in color to indicate that the term is defined in the Chapter Glossary. There is a main **glossary** of defined terms that is a compilation of the words in the chapter glossaries.

Evaluation

The tests contain at least two reports that are similar to ones that appeared in the chapter.

Web

The text has an accompanying web site located at http://evolve.elsevier.com/Buck/next/Classroom/.

A Special Note

Coders are a very special group of individuals. They have keen minds and tend to be those individuals gifted with great patience for the detail-oriented process of medical coding. They have immense professionalism and seek to do an exemplary job of the most difficult task of translating services and diagnoses into codes and ensuring appropriate reimbursement. They are exemplified by a statement made many years ago by Orison Swett Marden:

> *People who have accomplished work worthwhile have had a very high sense of the way to do things. They have not been content with mediocrity. They have not confined themselves to the beaten tracks; they have never been satisfied to do things just as others do them, but always a little better. They always pushed things that came to their hands a little higher up, a little farther on. It is this little higher up, this little farther on, that counts in the quality of life's work. It is the constant effort to be first class in everything one attempts that conquers the heights of excellence.*

Medical coding is a fine profession that has the ability to intrigue and captivate you for a lifetime. Practice your craft carefully, with due diligence, patience for the process, and always the highest ethical standards.

Carol J. Buck, MS, CPC, CPC-H, CCS-P

The Top 10 List for Coders

Contributed by Karen Lockyer

10. Abstracting is getting the essence of the relevant facts.
9. When in doubt, ASK—don't assume anything.
8. Never be afraid to question a doctor.
7. Work with good reference books.
6. Always use current code books.
5. Make notes in your coding manuals—it saves time later on.
4. Good coders are always learning.
3. Speed of record reading comes with practice; never sacrifice accuracy.
2. If it isn't documented, it didn't happen.
1. **NEVER CODE DIRECTLY FROM THE INDEX!**

Acknowledgments

This worktext was developed through a team effort. Each member of the team was vital to complete this volume of work. Each person shared the vision for an advanced coding text that would enable the learner to be better prepared to meet the exciting challenge presented by medical coding.

Special thanks goes to the team of wonderful people at Elsevier. Your professionalism, amazing skill, and genuine desire to assist in the educational process by providing high-quality texts are readily apparent and greatly appreciated.

Sally Schrefer, Executive Vice President, Nursing and Health Professions, with her keen insights, ingenuity, and excellent problem-solving ablities, makes the process work.

Andrew Allen, Publishing Director, Health Professions, with his mild manner, wit, and patience, helps keep the team focused on the ultimate goal.

Michael Ledbetter, Publisher, for always holding fast to the course with his unflagging devotion to producing innovative educational materials.

Susan Cole, Acquisitions Editor, for her enthusiasm for medical coding and talent that guided this work to completion.

Beth LoGiudice, Developmental Editor, for having the patience of a saint and the talent to match, and for using ample supplies of both in this long process of the development of this text.

Jackie Grass, who cares deeply about students and is always willing to share her skill in accomplishment of the most formidable tasks for them, and without whose effort this text would have been an impossible task.

Karen Lockyer, who spent hours reviewing each and every word in this worktext with the greatest of dedication. Her expertise had a major impact on this work.

Jody Klitz, Coding Specialist, who used her great skill and spent innumerable hours checking this work.

The Publisher would like to acknowledge and thank the following people:

Lynn Anderanin, Ruth Brockmann, Christy Conway, Patricia Feldner, Debra Fields, Joan Gilhooly, Charlene Smith Isaacs, Betty Johnson, Terence Johnson, Deepa Malhotra, Sharon Parr, Letitia Patterson, Jeanice Porta, Kathleen Pride, Dorothy Steed, and Maryann Ward for their enthusiasm for coding and dedication to the profession.

Jack Foley of Jack Foley Photography for his talent, patience, and photographs.

Sherry Pokaka'a at the Hawaii Convention Center for her sense of humor, flexibility, and outstanding managerial skill.

The Next Step

MEDICAL CODING

FROM CLASSROOM TO PRACTICE

A Worktext

Chapter 1
Evaluation and Management Services

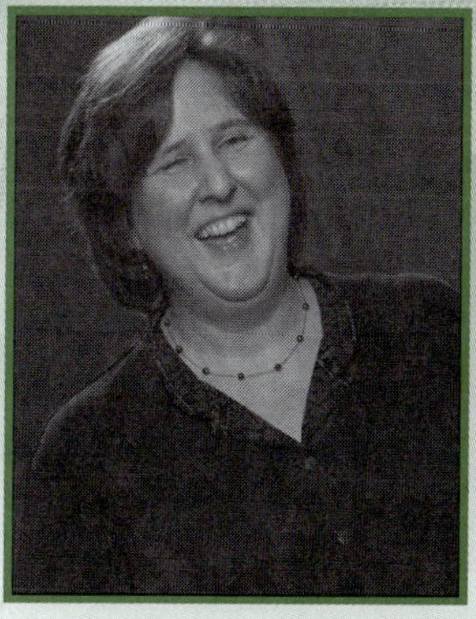

Kathy Pride, CPC, CCS-P
Quadramed, Inc.
Port St. Lucie, Florida

ABBREVIATIONS

ABG arterial blood gases
ACLS Advanced Cardiac Life Support
AIC amino-imidazole carboxamide, anti-inflammatory corticoid
ALT alanine transaminase (formerly SGPT)
ARDS acute or adult respiratory distress syndrome
AST aspartate amino-transferase (formerly SGOT)
ATN acute tubular necrosis
AV arteriovenous
b.i.d. twice a day
BOOP *Bronchiolitis obliterans* organizing pneumonia
BSO bilateral salpingo-oophorectomy
BUN blood urea nitrogen
CABG coronary artery bypass graft
CBC complete blood count
CEA carcinoembryonic antigen
CHF congestive heart failure
CK creatine kinase
COPD chronic obstructive pulmonary disease
CPK creatine phosphokinase
CT computerized tomography
CVA cardiovascular accident
D5 dextrose 5% water
D deciliter
ENT ear, nose, throat
EOMs extraocular movements
FI forced inspiration
GERD gastroesophageal reflux
GI gastrointestinal
GU genitourinary
h hour
H&H hematocrit and hemoglobin, also stated HH
H_2 histamine-2
HEENT head, ears, eyes, nose, throat
Hs at bedtime
I&O intake and outputs
IM intramuscular
INR International Normalized Ratio
IV intravenous
JP jugular process, jugular pulse
JVD jugular vein distention
LMP last menstrual period
MAP mean aortic pressure, mean arterial pressure
MB methylene blue, mesio-buccal
MDM medical decision making
mEq milliequivalent
mg milligram
MI myocardial infarction
mL milliliter
mm millimeter
neb nebula, a spray
NG nasogastric, nitroglycerin
n.p.o nothing by mouth
O_2 oxygen
OBT occult blood test
OP outpatient
OPC outpatient clinic
OPD outpatient department
OPS outpatient surgery
OPV oral poliovirus vaccine
OR operating room
OTC over-the-counter
OURQ outer upper-right quadrant
OV office visit
PCO_2 partial pressure of carbon dioxide
PEEP positive end expiration pressure
pH potential of hydrogen
p.o. by mouth
p.r.n. as needed
PT prothrombin time
PTH parathyroid hormone, posttransfusional hepatitis
q every
q.2wk every 2 weeks
q.3h every 3 hours
q.4h every 4 hours
q.4wk every 4 weeks
q.a.m. every morning
q.d. every day
q.d.s. four times a day
q.h. every hour
q.h.s. each bedtime
q.i.d. four times a day
q.m. every morning
q.o.d. every other day
q.os. as needed
q.p.m. every afternoon or every evening
q.q.h. every fourth hour
q.s. quantity sufficient
qq. each, every
qq.h every hour
QRS Q-wave R-wave S-wave
RLQ right lower quadrant
s *sans* (without), *sigma* (sign, mark), *semis* (half)
S1 first heart sound
S2 second heart sound
S3 third heart sound
S4 fourth heart sound
SBE subacute bacterial endocarditis
SIMV synchronized intermittent mandatory ventilation
T_4 thyroxine
TMJ temporomandibular joint
URI upper respiratory infection

The most often used codes in the CPT manual are those in the Evaluation and Management (E/M) section. These codes can also be the most troublesome for the new coder to assign because there are so many variables; but once you learn all the intricacies of E/M coding, you will be able to assign E/M codes with complete confidence that you have assigned the correct code. The first step is to review some of the basics of E/M code assignment. If you are comfortable with the basics of E/M code assignment and are familiar with an audit form, go right to Case 1-1 and begin applying E/M codes to physician services.

Within this worktext, the Centers for Medicare and Medicaid Services (CMS) *1995 Documentation Guidelines for Evaluation and Management Services* have been used when coding E/M services. A copy of the guidelines is located in Appendix E of this worktext. The discussion that follows about documentation of E/M services has been developed based on these guidelines.

The audit form is only one of many ways a facility could choose to assess E/M services provided to the patients of the facility. For the purposes of this text, the audit form that you are going to learn about is how E/M services are to be assessed throughout this text. Let us begin with some basics.

E/M Review—The Basics

Three Factors of E/M Code

The codes in the E/M section are based on three factors:

1. Place of service
2. Type of service
3. Patient status

Place of Service The first step to choose the correct E/M code is to identify the place or setting in which the service was provided. Codes vary based on the place of service. For example, there are different codes for **outpatient** and **inpatient** settings.

Type of Service The second step in choosing the correct E/M code is to identify the type of service. The type of service is the kind of service. Examples of types of service are **consultation,** hospital **admission,** or an **office visit.** Codes are divided based on the type of service.

Patient Status The third step in choosing the correct E/M code is to identify the patient status correctly. There are four types of patient status:

1. **New patient**—has not received professional services from the physician or another physician of the same specialty in the same group practice within the past 3 years.
2. **Established patient**—has received professional services from the physician or another physician of the same specialty in the same group practice within the past 3 years.
3. **Outpatient**—has not been formally admitted to a health care facility.
4. **Inpatient**—has been formally admitted to a health care facility.

Key Components

Once you have identified the place of service, type of service, and patient status, you are ready to locate the information in the medical record that identifies the **key components** of the service. The three key components are the history, examination, and medical decision-making complexity.

History

The history is the subjective (patient provided) information that the physician elicits regarding the chief complaint. There are four elements of a history:

- Chief Complaint (CC)
- History of Present Illness (HPI)
- Review of Systems (ROS)
- Past, Family, and Social History (PFSH)

Chief Complaint The **CC** is a concise statement describing the symptom, problem, condition, diagnosis, physician-recommended return, or other factor that is the reason for the encounter/visit, usually in the patient's words.

All encounters have a CC or reason for the visit. The patient's medical record will state the CC, most often at the beginning of the report with a title, such as CC, indications, reason for consultation, reason for admission, or similar wording. Sometimes the physician will simply place the CC within the report with no title.

History of Present Illness The HPI is a chronological description of the development of the patient's present illness from the first sign and/or symptom or from the previous encounter to the present. The HPI may include the following:

- Location (site on the body)
- Quality (characteristics, such as throbbing, sharp)
- Severity (how intense or on a scale of 1/10)
- Duration (how long for this problem or episode)
- Timing (when does it occur)
- Context (under what circumstances does it occur)
- Modifying factors (what makes it better or worse)
- Associated signs and symptoms (what else is happening when it occurs)

The physician documents the HPI in the medical record. The following is an example of an HPI containing each of the elements:

> The patient presents with a radiating (**quality**) pain in the right arm (**location**). He states that the pain is a 5 on a scale of 1/10 (**severity**). He states that the pain began last Monday (**duration**) when he was bending over (**context**) shoeing his horse in the barn, and he has experienced the same pain several times throughout the week (**timing**). He tried icing the area on his arm several times and that did provide him with a bit of relief (**modifying factor**). There has been some dizziness during these episodes (**associated signs and symptoms**).

Often the coder has a copy of the encounter report to use when coding services so the coder can write directly on the copy to identify elements in the report. For example, the HPI as it would appear on the coder's copy of the report with eight elements of the HPI marked by the coder:

> The patient presents with a radiating[1] pain in the right arm.[2] He states that the pain is a 5 on a scale of 1/10.[3] He states that the pain began last Monday[4] when he was bending over[5] shoeing his horse in the barn, and that he has experienced the same pain several times throughout the week.[6] He tried icing the area on his arm several times, and that did provide him with a bit of relief.[7] There has been some dizziness during these episodes.[8]

The coder might also use an audit form to check off the information if the facility policy does not allow for an additional copy of the report. The coder must work directly from the original report in these circumstances and place check marks on the audit form rather than on the record.

The HPI area of the audit form is illustrated in **Figure 1-1**.

HPI elements

HISTORY ELEMENTS	Documented
HISTORY OF PRESENT ILLNESS (HPI)	
1. Location (site on body)	X
2. Quality (characteristic: throbbing, sharp)	X
3. Severity (1/10 or how intense)	X
4. Duration (how long for problem or episode)	X
5. Timing (when it occurs)	X
6. Context (under what circumstances does it occur)	X
7. Modifying factors (what makes it better or worse)	X
8. Associated signs and symptoms (what else is happening when it occurs)	X
TOTAL	8
LEVEL	

FIGURE 1-1 History of Present Illness (HPI) section on an audit form.

The extent of the HPI as problem focused, expanded problem focused, detailed, or comprehensive is based on the physician's professional judgment, depending on the needs of the patient. The two levels of HPI are brief (1–3 elements) and extended (4+ elements). The problem-focused and expanded problem-focused HPI contain a brief review. The detailed and comprehensive level of HPI contains an extended review of the HPI elements. HPI levels are illustrated in **Figure 1-2.**

Review of Systems The ROS is an inventory of the body systems obtained through a series of questions seeking to identify signs or symptoms that the patient may be experiencing or has experienced. The ROS may be asked by the physician or nurse or by means of a questionnaire filled out by the patient or ancillary personnel. Regardless of how the information is obtained, before the information can qualify as an ROS, the physician must review the information and document the review in the medical record. The ROS may include the following information or elements:

- Constitutional (e.g., weight loss, fever)
- Ophthalmologic (eyes)
- Otolaryngologic (ears, nose, mouth, throat)
- Cardiovascular
- Respiratory

History Level	1	2	3	4
	Problem Focused	Expanded Problem Focused	Detailed	Comprehensive
HPI	Brief 1-3	Brief 1-3	Extended 4+	Extended 4+
ROS		Problem pertinent	Extended 2-9	Complete 10+
PFSH			Pertinent 1	Complete 2-3
			HISTORY LEVEL	4

HPI levels

FIGURE 1-2 History of Present Illness (HPI) levels.

- Gastrointestinal
- Genitourinary
- Musculoskeletal
- Integumentary (skin and/or breasts)
- Neurologic
- Psychiatric
- Endocrine
- Hematologic/Lymphatic
- Allergic/Immunologic

An ROS example from a medical record is as follows:

REVIEW OF SYSTEMS Eyes: Blurred double vision (**ophthalmologic**). Ears: Hearing is okay (**otolaryngologic**). GI: As noted above (**gastrointestinal**). GU: Negative (**genitourinary**). Chest: No complaints of dyspnea (**respiratory**). Neurologic: Negative (**neurologic**). Psychiatric: Negative. Sleep pattern has been off in the past, and he has been treated with amitriptyline. This has not been such a significant problem of late (**psychiatric**).

The coder may identify each of these seven ROS elements directly on the copy of the report as follows:

REVIEW OF SYSTEMS Eyes: Blurred double vision.[1] Ears: Hearing is okay.[2] GI: As noted above.[3] GU: Negative.[4] Chest: No complaints of dyspnea.[5] Neurologic Negative.[6] Psychiatric: Negative. Sleep pattern has been off in the past, and he has been treated with amitriptyline. This has not been such a significant problem of late.[7]

If an audit form were used, the ROS area of the audit form would be as illustrated in **Figure 1-3**.

There are four levels of ROS: none, problem pertinent (1 element), extended (2–9 elements), and complete (10+ elements). There are times that an ROS is not necessary, such as a simple recheck of ears. The **problem pertinent** ROS is a review that is focused on the organ system (OS) involved in the complaint, such as a fractured finger in which the musculoskeletal system is the center of the review. The **extended** ROS includes not only the system directly involved in the complaint, but up to nine other systems. For example, a complaint of left-sided chest pain would focus primarily on the cardiovascular system but could also include the respiratory system and gastrointestinal system. The **complete** ROS includes at least 10 of the 14 OSs. The coder counts the number of systems reviewed as documented in the medical record and enters that number on the audit form.

Not all physicians indicate the OS being reviewed with "Neurologic" or "Gastrointestinal," which makes it necessary for the coder to be able to identify the OS by the terminology used in the report. For example, rather than labeling the section "psychiatric," the physician may state, "Sleep pattern has been off in the past, and he has been treated with amitriptyline. This has not been such a

ROS elements

REVIEW OF SYSTEMS (ROS)	**Documented**
1. Constitutional (e.g., weight loss, fever)	
2. Ophthalmologic (eyes)	X
3. Otolaryngologic (ears, nose, mouth, throat)	X
4. Cardiovascular	
5. Respiratory	X
6. Gastrointestinal	X
7. Genitourinary	X
8. Musculoskeletal	
9. Integumentary (skin and/or breasts)	
10. Neurologic	X
11. Psychiatric	X
12. Endocrine	
13. Hematologic/Lymphatic	
14. Allergic/Immunologic	
TOTAL	7
LEVEL	

FIGURE 1-3 Review of Systems (ROS) section on an audit form.

According to Huffman's *Health Information Management*,* the following systems are recognized for the ROS:

- Constitutional symptoms
  Usual weight, recent weight changes, fever, weakness, fatigue
- Eyes (Ophthalmologic)
  Glasses or contact lenses, last eye examination, visual glaucoma, cataracts, eyestrain, pain, diplopia, redness, lacrimation, inflammation, blurring
- Ears, Nose, Mouth, Throat (Otolaryngologic)
  Ears: hearing, discharge, tinnitus, dizziness, pain
  Nose: head colds, epistaxis, discharges, obstruction, postnasal drip, sinus pain
  Mouth and Throat: condition of teeth and gums, last dental examination, soreness, redness, hoarseness, difficulty in swallowing
- Cardiovascular
  Chest pain, rheumatic fever, tachycardia, palpitation, high blood pressure, edema, vertigo, faintness, varicose veins, thrombophlebitis
- Respiratory
  Chest pain, wheezing, cough, dyspnea, sputum (color and quantity), hemoptysis, asthma, bronchitis, emphysema, pneumonia, tuberculosis, pleurisy, last chest radiograph

*Definitions from Huffman E: *Health information management*, ed 10. Revised by the American Medical Records Association. Berwyn, IL, Physician's Record Company, 1994, pp. 57-62.

- Gastrointestinal
  Appetite, thirst, nausea, vomiting, hematemesis, rectal bleeding, change in bowel habits, diarrhea, constipation, indigestion, food intolerance, flatus, hemorrhoids, jaundice
- Genitourinary
  - Urinary: frequent or painful urination, nocturia, pyuria, hematuria, incontinence, urinary infection.
  - Genitoreproductive:
    Male—venereal disease, sores, discharge from penis, hernias, testicular pain or masses
    Female—age at menstruation (frequency, type, dura tion, dysmenorrhea, menorrhagia; symptoms of menopause), contraception, pregnancies, deliveries, abortions, last Papanicolaou smear
- Musculoskeletal
  Joint pain or stiffness, arthritis, gout, backache, muscle pain, cramps, swelling, redness, limitation in motor activity
- Integumentary (skin or breast)
  Rashes, eruptions, dryness, cyanosis, jaundice, changes in skin, hair, or nails
- Neurologic
  Faintness, blackouts, seizures, paralysis, tingling, tremors, memory loss
- Psychiatric
  Personality type, nervousness, mood, insomnia, headache, nightmares, depression
- Endocrine
  Thyroid trouble, heat or cold intolerance, excessive sweating, thirst, hunger, or urination
- Hematologic/Lymphatic
  Anemia, easy bruising or bleeding, past transfusions
- Allergic/Immunologic

  Sneezing, itching eyes, rhinorrhea, nasal obstruction, or recurrent infections
  Environmental allergies, such as dust, mold, or latex

According to the CPT manual,* the following are the items that indicate a past, family, or social history:

- **Past history** is the patient's past experience with illnesses, operations, injuries, and treatments; specifically:
  Prior major illnesses and injuries
  Prior operations
  Prior hospitalizations
  Current medications
  Allergies (e.g., drug, food, latex)
  Age-appropriate immunization status
  Age-appropriate feeding/dietary status

- **Family history** is a review of medical events in the patient's family that includes significant information about the following:
  The health status or cause of death of parents, siblings, and children
  Specific diseases related to problems identified in the CC or HPI, or ROS
  Diseases of family members, which may be hereditary or place the patient at risk

- **Social history** is an age-appropriate review of past and current activities that includes significant information about the following:
  Marital status and/or living arrangements
  Current employment
  Occupational history
  Use of drugs, alcohol, and tobacco
  Level of education
  Sexual history
  Other relevant social factors
  Exercise habits or other activities

Three of the elements of a history (HPI, ROS, and PFSH) are included to varying degrees in all patient encounters. The degree or level of HPI, ROS, and PFSH is determined by the CC or presenting problem of the patient.

* Definitions from 2002 CPT, *Evaluation and Management Guidelines,* pp. 3–4. CPT codes, descriptions, and materials only are © 2002 American Medical Association.

significant problem of late." As the coder, you must know that the sleep pattern would be part of a psychiatric ROS.

The following is an example of the PFSH from a medical record:

The ROS area on an audit form is illustrated in **Figure 1-4.**

History Level	1	2	3	4
	Problem Focused	Expanded Problem Focused	Detailed	Comprehensive
HPI	Brief 1-3	Brief 1-3	Extended 4+	Extended 4+
ROS		**Problem pertinent**	**Extended 2-9**	**Complete 10+**
PFSH			Pertinent 1	Complete 2-3
			HISTORY LEVEL	

ROS levels

FIGURE 1-4 Review of Systems (ROS) section on an audit form.

Past, Family, Social History The **PFSH** is a review of the past, family, and social history of the patient. Some encounters do not include any PFSH elements, whereas other encounters contain an extensive review of all elements. The physician decides the extent of the PFSH based on the needs of the patient.

PAST MEDICAL HISTORY

1. Diabetes mellitus
2. Sinusitis
3. Asthma

MEDICATIONS

1. Humalog 7 units in the morning, noon, and q.h.s.
2. Ultralente 14 units q.a.m. and 14 units q.p.m.
3. Elavil 100 mg p.o. q.hs.s.

FAMILY HISTORY Neither of her parents has diabetes mellitus; however, there is a history of diabetes in that her brothers and an uncle all have it. There is also a history of CVAs, myocardial infarctions, and cancer.

SOCIAL HISTORY The patient states she consumed alcohol in the past. She smokes three to five cigarettes daily. She is otherwise a normal, healthy high-school senior.

The coder would enter each of these elements onto an audit form as documented in the medical record and illustrated in **Figure 1-5.**

The three levels of PFSH are none, pertinent (1), and complete (2–3). The problem focused and expanded problem focused history do not require any PFSH elements. The detailed history requires one element of the PFSH. For example, if the patient's CC is an allergic rash, the physician would certainly inquire about the patient's past history of allergies—drug, food, and inhaled allergies. The complete PFSH includes at least two of the three elements. For example, if the patient had intermittent chest pains, the physician would want to know the family history to identify family members with a history of heart disease and the social history to identify the relevant factor that would contribute to heart disease, such as use of tobacco and diet. The audit form indicates the PFSH as illustrated in **Figure 1-6.**

PFSH elements

PAST, FAMILY, AND/OR SOCIAL HISTORY (PFSH)	Documented
1. Past illness, operations, injuries, treatments, and current medications	X
2. Family medical history for heredity and risk	X
3. Social activities, both past and present	X
TOTAL	3
LEVEL	

FIGURE 1-5 Past, Family, and Social History (PFSH) section on an audit form.

There are four levels of histories; the level is based on the extent of the history during the history-taking portion of the physician/patient encounter.

History Levels The level is based on the extent of the history. The following are the four history levels:

1. Problem focused
2. Expanded problem focused
3. Detailed
4. Comprehensive

Problem Focused The physician focuses on the CC and a brief history of the present problem of a patient.

- A brief history includes a review of the history regarding pertinent information about the present problem or CC. Brief history information centers around the severity, duration, and symptoms of the problem or complaint. The brief history does not have to include the PFSH or ROS.

Expanded Problem Focused The physician focuses on a CC, obtains a brief history of the present problem, and also performs a problem-pertinent review of systems. The expanded problem-focused history does not have to include the PFSH.

History Level	1	2	3	4
	Problem Focused	Expanded Problem Focused	Detailed	Comprehensive
HPI	Brief 1-3	Brief 1-3	Extended 4+	Extended 4+
ROS		Problem pertinent (1)	Extended 2-9	Complete 10+
PFSH			**Pertinent 1**	**Complete 2-3**
			HISTORY LEVEL	

PFSH levels

FIGURE 1-6 Past, Family, and Social History (PFSH) levels on an audit form.

- This history would center around specific questions regarding the system involved in the presenting problem or CC. The ROS for this history would cover the OS most closely related to the CC or presenting problem and any related or associated OS. For example, if the presenting problem or CC is a red, swollen knee, the system reviewed would be the musculoskeletal system.

Detailed The physician focuses on a CC, and obtains an extended history of the present problem, an extended ROS, and a pertinent PFSH.

- The system review is "extended," which means that positive responses and pertinent negative responses relating to multiple OSs should be documented in the medical record.

Comprehensive This is the most complex of the history types. The physician documents the CC, obtains an extented history of the present problem, does a complete ROS, and obtains a complete PFSH.

- Some third-party payers have established standards for the number of elements that must be documented in the medical record to qualify for a given level of service. For example, a third-party payer may state that to qualify as a comprehensive history, the medical record must document that an extended HPI was conducted and that it included four of the eight elements (e.g., location, quality, severity, duration), a complete ROS that included a review of at least 10 of the 14 OSs, and a complete review of all three areas of the PFSH.

The four elements (CC, HPI, ROS, and PFSH) are the basis of the history portion of the E/M service. **Figure 1-7** illustrates a completed audit form for a level 4 or comprehensive history.

To assign a given history level, all three levels must be at the level or higher; for example, if the HPI was 4 or comprehensive, the ROS was 3 or detailed, and the PFSH was a level 4 or comprehensive, the history would be a level 3. The history level can be a level 4 only if the HPI was 4 or comprehensive, the ROS was 4 or comprehensive, and the MDM (medical decision making) was 4.

Examination

The *history* is the subjective information the patient provides the physician, and the *examination* is the objective information the physician gathers. The examination is the findings that the physician observes during the encounter. The physician documents the examination in the medical record, and the coder uses this documentation to code the service.

Elements of the examination include various body areas (BAs) and OSs as well as an assessment of a patient's general condition, which is indicated by such items as the patient's general appearance, vital signs, or level of distress. The three elements—general (constitutional), BAs, and OSs—are as follows.

General (Constitutional)

- Blood pressure, sitting*
- Blood pressure, lying*
- Pulse
- Respiration
- Temperature†
- Height
- Weight
- General appearance

Body Areas

- Head (including face)
- Neck
- Chest (including breasts and axillae)
- Abdomen
- Genitalia, groin, buttocks
- Back
- Each extremity

Organ Systems

- Ophthalmologic (eyes)
- Otolaryngologic (ears, nose, mouth, throat)
- Cardiovascular
- Respiratory
- Gastrointestinal
- Genitourinary
- Musculoskeletal
- Integumentary (skin)
- Neurologic
- Psychiatric
- Hematologic/Lymphatic/Immunologic

Note: For purposes of the examination, the endocrine system is not listed as an OS in the CPT manual, although the endocrine system is listed as an OS in the ROS of the history.

*Two blood pressures, sitting and lying, are included because the patient's blood pressure may be taken twice—once in the sitting position and once in the lying position. Each blood pressure reading counts as a constitutional element.

†The statement of afebrile without an indication of a degree does not count as a temperature reading.

HISTORY ELEMENTS HISTORY OF PRESENT ILLNESS (HPI)	Documented	
1. Location (site on body)	X	
2. Quality (characteristic: throbbing, sharp)	X	
3. Severity (1/10 or how intense)	X	
4. Duration (how long for problem or episode)	X	
5. Timing (when it occurs)	X	
6. Context (under what circumstances does it occur)	X	
7. Modifying factors (what makes it better or worse)	X	
8. Associated signs and symptoms (what else is happening when it occurs)	X	
TOTAL	8	
LEVEL	4	← HPI level
REVIEW OF SYSTEMS (ROS)	**Documented**	
1. Constitutional (e.g., weight loss, fever)		
2. Ophthalmologic (eyes)	X	
3. Otolaryngologic (ears, nose, mouth, throat)	X	
4. Cardiovascular		
5. Respiratory	X	
6. Gastrointestinal	X	
7. Genitourinary	X	
8. Musculoskeletal		
9. Integumentary (skin and/or breasts)	X	
10. Neurologic	X	
11. Psychiatric	X	
12. Endocrine	X	
13. Hematologic/Lymphatic	X	
14. Allergic/Immunologic		
TOTAL	10	
LEVEL	4	← ROS level
PAST, FAMILY, AND/OR SOCIAL HISTORY (PFSH)	**Documented**	
1. Past illness, operations, injuries, treatments, and current medications	X	
2. Family medical history for heredity and risk	X	
3. Social activities, both past and present	X	
TOTAL	3	
LEVEL	4	← PFSH level

History Level	1	2	3	4	
	Problem Focused	**Expanded Problem Focused**	**Detailed**	**Comprehensive**	
HPI	Brief 1-3	Brief 1-3	Extended 4+	Extended 4+	
ROS		Problem pertinent	Extended 2-9	Complete 10+	
PFSH			Pertinent 1	Complete 2-3	
			HISTORY LEVEL	4	← History level

FIGURE 1-7 History section on an audit form.

The examination elements may be placed on an audit form. An example of an examination with 4 constitutional, 2 BAs, and 9 OSs is as follows:

PHYSICAL EXAMINATION The patient is very sluggish,[1(general appearance/constitutional)] although he does answer questions. Blood pressure 96/76,[(constitutional)] pulse 130, and regular [(constitutional)] respirations 22.[(constitutional)] Eyes: Sunken significantly. Fundi are not visualized.[(OS/ophthalmologic)] Ears: Negative.[(OS/otolaryngologic)] Carotids are 4/4 without bruits.[(OS/cardiovascular)] Neck: supple,[(BA/neck)] nodes are negative. Thyroid is normal to palpitation. Axillary nodes negative.[(OS/lymphatic)] Chest: Clear to auscultation.[(OS/respiratory)] Heart: Tachycardic but no extra heart sounds heard. No murmur is appreciated.[(OS/cardiovascular)] Abdomen: Some minimal tenderness in the right mid abdomen and left upper abdomen.[(BA/abdomen)] Genital/Rectal: Not performed. Peripheral extremities reveal good pulses in the legs with no edema.[(OS/also cardiovascular)] Respiratory: Negative.[(OS/respiratory)] GI: Negative.[(OS/gastrointestinal)]

References to extremities that indicate a visual assessment, such as "no clubbing," "digits intact," "arthritic changes," or reference to the abdomen, such as "no masses," "nontender," or "soft," are recorded as a BA. References to extremity pulses, such as "pedal" or "peripheral," are recorded as the cardiovascular system. One element in the constitutional area equals 1 BA/OS whether all 8 elements are checked or only 1 element is checked. If there is more than 1 part of the BA or OS checked in the BA/OS area (such as otolaryngologic, ears, nose, mouth, throat), there is still only 1 check placed on that line on the audit form. An exception to this is the extremities, in which case the extremities are referenced and 4 checks are placed on the extremity line on the form (unless a specific number of extremities is specified).

Figure 1-8 illustrates the audit form with examination elements recorded.

The reports in the medical record are transcribed in a variety of locations by many transcriptionists. Although most facilities have an established report format, not all facilities have the same report format, and even if they have a format, not every physician or transcriptionist follows the format completely. As such, you need to be able to work with a variety of report formats, and you will not like all of them equally. For example, you will learn to appreciate a report in which the examination elements are in capital letters, but remember that format is no substitution for reading the entire report. Within this text, you will see an assortment of report formats that represent real-world medical reports.

The following are the four levels of examination based on the extent of the examination:

- Problem focused
- Expanded problem focused
- Detailed
- Comprehensive

1. **Problem focused:** Examination is limited to the affected BA or OS identified by the CC.
2. **Expanded problem focused:** A limited examination of the affected BA or OS and other related BAs or OSs.
3. **Detailed:** An extended examination of the affected BAs or related OSs.
4. **Comprehensive:** This is the most extensive examination; it encompasses a complete single-specialty examination or a complete multisystem examination.

The elements required for each level of examination are illustrated in **Figure 1-9**.

Note that the expanded and detailed examinations contain 2 to 7 BAs or OSs. The difference is that the expanded problem focused examination is focused on the BA/OS of the CC and other directly related BAs/OSs, whereas the detailed examination covers not only the BA/OS of the CC but also other BAs/OSs not directly related to the CC.

Medical Decision Making Complexity

The key component of MDM is based on the complexity of the decision the physician must make regarding the patient's diagnosis and care. Complexity of decision making is based on three elements:

1. Number of diagnoses or **management options.** The options can be minimal, limited, multiple, or extensive.
2. Amount or complexity of **data to review.** The data can be minimal or none, limited, moderate, or extensive.
3. **Risk** of complication or death if the condition goes untreated. Risk can be minimal, low, moderate, or high.

Although the level of the MDM is the most subjective element in establishing the level of E/M services, characteristics of the MDM can indicate complexity. The information that follows will provide you with foundational information regarding the MDM.

Management Options Some basic guidelines for documentation of management options in the medical record are as follows:

1. For each encounter, an assessment, clinical impression, or diagnosis should be documented. It may be explicitly stated or implied in documented decisions regarding management plans or further evaluation.
   - For a **presenting problem** with an established diagnosis, the record should reflect whether the problem is (a) improved, well-controlled, resolving, or resolved; or (b) inadequately controlled, worsening, or failing to respond as expected.

EXAMINATION ELEMENTS	Documented
CONSTITUTIONAL	
1. Blood pressure, sitting	X
2. Blood pressure, lying	
3. Pulse	X
4. Respirations	X
5. Temperature	
6. Height	
7. Weight	
8. General appearance	X
NUMBER	1
BODY AREAS (BA)	**Documented**
1. Head (including face)	
2. Neck	X
3. Chest (including breasts and axillae)	
4. Abdomen	X
5. Genitalia, groin, buttocks	
6. Back (including spine)	
7. Each extremity 4 checks	
NUMBER	2
ORGAN SYSTEMS (OS)	**Documented**
1. Ophthalmologic (eyes)	X
2. Otolaryngologic (ears, nose, mouth, throat)	X
3. Cardiovascular	X
4. Respiratory	X
5. Gastrointestinal	X
6. Genitourinary	
7. Musculoskeletal	
8. Integumentary	
9. Neurologic	
10. Psychiatric	
11. Hematologic/Lymphatic/Immunologic	X
NUMBER	6
TOTAL BA/OS	9

← Total BA/OS

FIGURE 1-8 Examination elements on an audit form.

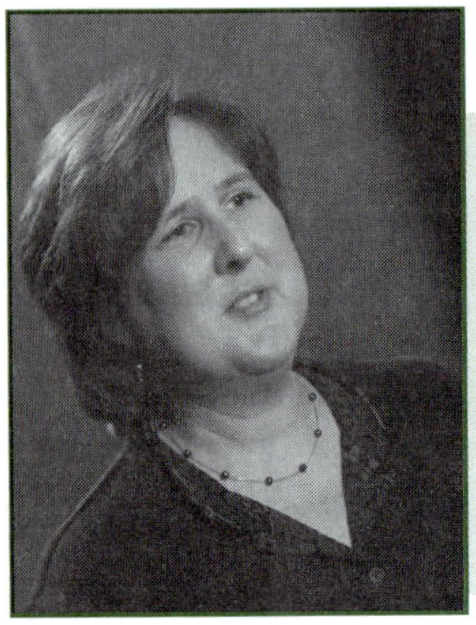

FROM THE TRENCHES

Kathy

"[Coding] is a very diverse field. People think that in order to be a coder you have to sit at a desk and code all day. It's not like that at all... I always make a point of telling people about all the different types of jobs that are out there in the coding field. There are probably things I haven't even thought of yet!"

Exam Level	1	2	3	4
	Problem Focused	**Expanded Problem Focused**	**Detailed**	**Comprehensive**
	Limited to affected BA/OS	Limited to affected BA/OS & other related OSs	Extended of affected BA & other related OSs	General multi-system or complete single OS
# of OS or BA	1	2-7 limited	2-7 extended	8+ or 1 complete single system
			EXAMINATION LEVEL	4

Examination level

FIGURE 1-9 Examination levels.

- For a presenting problem without an established diagnosis, the assessment or clinical impression may be stated in the form of differential diagnoses or as a "possible," "probable," or "rule out" (R/O) diagnosis.

2. The initiation of, or changes in, treatment should be documented. Treatment includes a wide range of management options, including patient instructions, nursing instructions, therapies, and medications.
3. If referrals are made, consultations requested, or advice sought, the record should indicate to whom or where the referral or consultation is made or from whom the advice is requested.

Data to Be Reviewed The following are some basic documentation guidelines for the amount and complexity of data to be reviewed:

1. If a diagnostic service (test or procedure) is ordered, planned, scheduled, or performed at the time of the E/M encounter, the type of service (e.g., laboratory or radiology) should be documented.
2. The review of laboratory, radiology, or other diagnostic tests should be documented. An entry in a progress note such as "WBC elevated" or "chest x-ray unremarkable" is acceptable. Alternatively, the review may be documented by initializing and dating the report containing the test results.
3. A decision to obtain old records or to obtain additional history from the family, caregiver, or other source to supplement that obtained from the patient should be documented.
4. Relevant findings from the review of old records or the receipt of additional history from the family, caregiver, or other source should be documented. If there is no relevant information beyond that already obtained, that fact should be documented. A notation of "old records reviewed" or "additional history obtained from family" without elaboration is insufficient.
5. The results of discussion of laboratory, radiology, or other diagnostic tests with the physician who performed or interpreted the study should be documented.
6. The direct visualization and independent interpretation of an image, tracing, or specimen previously interpreted by another physician should be documented.

Risk Some basic documentation guidelines for risk of significant complications, morbidity, or mortality include the following:

1. Comorbidities, underlying diseases, or other factors that increase the complexity of MDM by increasing the risk of complications, morbidity, or mortality should be documented.
2. If a surgical or invasive diagnostic procedure is ordered, planned, or scheduled at the time of the E/M encounter, the type of procedure (e.g., laparoscopy) should be documented.
3. If a surgical or invasive diagnostic procedure is performed at the time of the E/M encounter, the specific procedure should be documented.
4. The referral for or decision to perform a surgical or invasive diagnostic procedure on an urgent basis should be documented or implied.

Examples of the levels of risk are found in Table 1-1.

The extent to which each of these elements is considered determines the levels of MDM complexity:

- Straightforward
- Low

TABLE 1-1 Examples of Levels of Risk

LEVELS OF RISK	PRESENTING PROBLEM OR PROBLEMS
Minimal Low	One self-limited or minor problem (e.g., insect bite, tinea corporis)
Low	Two or more self-limited or minor problems One stable, chronic illness (e.g., well-controlled hypertension or non-insulin dependent diabetes, cataract, benign prostatic hypertrophy) Acute, uncomplicated illness or injury (e.g., cystitis, allergic rhinitis, simple sprain)
Moderate	One or more chronic illnesses with mild exacerbation, progression, or side effects of treatment Two or more stable chronic illnesses Undiagnosed new problem with uncertain prognosis (e.g., lump in breast) Acute illness with systemic symptoms (e.g., pyelonephritis, pneumonitis, colitis) Acute complicated injury, e.g. head injury with brief loss of consciousness
High	One or more chronic illnesses with severe exacerbation, progression, or side effects of treatment Acute or chronic illnesses or injuries that pose a threat to life or body function (e.g., multiple trauma, acute myocardial infarction, pulmonary embolus, severe repository distress, progressive severe rheumatoid arthritis, psychiatric illness with potential threat to self or others, peritonitis, acute renal failure.) An abrupt change in neurologic status (e.g., seizure, transient ischemic attack, weakness, or sensory loss)

- Moderate
- High

1. **Straightforward decision making:** Minimal diagnosis and management options, minimal or none for the amount and complexity of data to be reviewed, and minimal risk to the patient of complications or death if untreated.
2. **Low-complexity decision making:** Limited number of diagnoses and management options, limited data to be reviewed, and low risk to the patient of complications or death if untreated.
3. **Moderate-complexity decision making:** Multiple diagnoses and management options, moderate amount and complexity of data to be reviewed, and moderate risk to the patient of complications or death if untreated.
4. **High-complexity decision making:** Extensive diagnoses and management options, extensive amount and complexity of data to be reviewed, and high risk to the patient for complications or death if the problem is untreated.

When you select one of the four types of MDM complexity—straightforward, low, moderate, or high—the documentation in the medical record must support the selection in terms of the number of diagnoses or management options, amount or complexity of data to be reviewed, and risks.

Given the information in the medical record, you would consider the information in the context of the complexity of the diagnosis and management options, data to be reviewed, and risks to the patient to choose the complexity of MDM. The MDM portion of an audit report would be as illustrated in **Figure 1-10.** To qualify for a given level of MDM complexity, two or three elements must be met or exceeded. This differs from the history where all three elements must be of the same or greater level.

Figure 1-11 illustrates the levels of MDM complexity on the audit form and the MDM location.

MDM ELEMENTS	Documented
# OF DIAGNOSES/MANAGEMENT OPTIONS	
1. Minimal	
2. Limited	
3. Multiple	X
4. Extensive	
LEVEL	3
AMOUNT OR COMPLEXITY OF DATA TO REVIEW	Documented
1. Minimal/None	
2. Limited	
3. Moderate	X
4. Extensive	
LEVEL	3
RISK OF COMPLICATION OR DEATH IF NOT TREATED	Documented
1. Minimal	
2. Low	
3. Moderate	X
4. High	
LEVEL	3

FIGURE 1-10 Medical Decision Making (MDM) section on an audit form.

MDC*	1	2	3	4
	Straightforward	**Low**	**Moderate**	**High**
Number of DX or management options	Minimal	Limited	Multiple	Extensive
Amount or complexity of data	Minimal/None	Limited	Moderate	Extensive
Risks	Minimal	Low	Moderate	High
			MDM LEVEL	**3**
*To qualify for a given type of MDM complexity, 2 of 3 elements in the table must be met or exceeded.				

← Levels of MDM (pointing to the Straightforward/Low/Moderate/High row)

← MDM level (pointing to the MDM LEVEL row)

FIGURE 1-11 Medical Decision Making (MDM) levels of complexity and location.

Audit Form with All Key Components Figure 1-12 illustrates a completed audit form. With this information, you can correctly identify the code, depending on the place, type of service, and patient status. For example, if a comprehensive history, comprehensive examination, and a moderate complexity of MDM were provided in an office consultation, the correct code would be 99244, Office or other Outpatient Consultation. If the same level of service were provided to an inpatient at the initial service, the code would be 99254, Initial Inpatient Consultation.

You also need to know about the **contributing factors** that could affect the correct code selection.

Contributing Factors

The four contributing factors are counseling, coordination of care, the nature of the presenting problem, and time. Contributing factors are those conditions that help the physician to determine the extent of history, examination, and decision making (key components) necessary to treat the patient. The contributing factors may or may not be considered in every patient case and are the following:

- Counseling
- Coordination of care
- Nature of the presenting problem
- Time

Counseling Counseling is a service that physicians provide to patients and their families. It involves discussion of diagnostic results, impressions, and recommended diagnostic studies; prognosis; risks and benefits of treatment; instructions for treatment; importance of compliance with treatment; risk factor reduction; and patient and family education. Some form of counseling usually takes place in all physician and patient encounters, and this was factored into the codes when they were developed by the American Medical Association (AMA). Only when counseling is the reason for the encounter or consumes most of the visit time (more than 50% of the total time) is counseling considered a component of code assignment. The following statement is made often within the codes in the E/M section:

Counseling and/or coordination of care with other providers or agencies are provided consistent with the nature of the problem(s) and the patient's and/or family's needs.

You will know when to factor in the counseling because the physician must indicate the additional time in the medical record.

Coordination of Care Coordination of care with other health care providers or agencies may be necessary for the care of a patient. In coordination of care, a physician might arrange for other services to be provided to the patient, such as arrangements for admittance to a long-term nursing facility.

Nature of the Presenting Problem The presenting problem is the patient's CC or the situation that leads the physician into determining the level of care necessary to diagnose and treat the patient. The CPT describes the **presenting problem** as a disease, condition, illness, injury, symptom, sign, finding, complaint, or other reason for the encounter, with or without a diagnosis being established at the time of the encounter. There are five types of presenting problems:

- Minimal
- Self-limited
- Low severity
- Moderate severity
- High severity

1. **Minimal:** A problem may not require the presence of the physician, but service is provided under the physician's supervision. A minimal problem is a blood pressure reading, a dressing change, or another service that can be performed without the physician being immediately present.
2. **Self-limited:** Also called a minor presenting problem, a self-limited problem runs a definite and prescribed course, is transient (it comes and goes), and is not likely to alter health status permanently, or the presenting problem has a good prognosis with management and compliance.
3. **Low severity:** The risk of complete sickness (morbidity) without treatment is low, there is little or

CHAPTER 1, CASE EXAMPLE	
HISTORY ELEMENTS	**Documented**
HISTORY OF PRESENT ILLNESS (HPI)	
1. Location (site on body)	X
2. Quality (characteristic: throbbing, sharp)	X
3. Severity (1/10 or how intense)	X
4. Duration (how long for problem or episode)	X
5. Timing (when it occurs)	X
6. Context (under what circumstances does it occur)	X
7. Modifying factors (what makes it better or worse)	X
8. Associated signs and symptoms (what else is happening when it occurs)	X
TOTAL	8
LEVEL	4
REVIEW OF SYSTEMS (ROS)	**Documented**
1. Constitutional (e.g., weight loss, fever)	
2. Ophthalmologic (eyes)	X
3. Otolaryngologic (ears, nose, mouth, throat)	X
4. Cardiovascular	
5. Respiratory	X
6. Gastrointestinal	X
7. Genitourinary	X
8. Musculoskeletal	
9. Integumentary (skin and/or breasts)	X
10. Neurologic	X
11. Psychiatric	X
12. Endocrine	X
13. Hematologic/Lymphatic	X
14. Allergic/Immunologic	
TOTAL	10
LEVEL	4 ~~3~~
PAST, FAMILY, AND/OR SOCIAL HISTORY (PFSH)	**Documented**
1. Past illness, operations, injuries, treatments, and current medications	X
2. Family medical history for heredity and risk	X
3. Social activities, both past and present	X
TOTAL	3
LEVEL	4

(X)

History Level	1	2	3	4
	Problem Focused	**Expanded Problem Focused**	**Detailed**	**Comprehensive**
HPI	Brief 1-3	Brief 1-3	Extended 4+	Extended 4+
ROS		Problem pertinent	Extended 2-9	Complete 10+
PFSH			Pertinent 1	Complete 2-3
			HISTORY LEVEL	4

all have to be 4

EXAMINATION ELEMENTS	Documented
CONSTITUTIONAL	
1. Blood pressure, sitting	X
2. Blood pressure, lying	
3. Pulse	X
4. Respirations	X
5. Temperature	
6. Height	
7. Weight	X
8. General appearance	
NUMBER	1
BODY AREAS (BA)	**Documented**
1. Head (including face)	
2. Neck	X
3. Chest (including breasts and axillae)	
4. Abdomen	
5. Genitalia, groin, buttocks	
6. Back (including spine)	
7. Each extremity	
NUMBER	1
ORGAN SYSTEMS (OS)	**Documented**
1. Ophthalmologic (eyes)	X
2. Otolaryngologic (ears, nose, mouth, throat)	X
3. Cardiovascular	X
4. Respiratory	X
5. Gastrointestinal	X
6. Genitourinary	
7. Musculoskeletal	
8. Integumentary	
9. Neurologic	
10. Psychiatric	
11. Hematologic/Lymphatic/Immunologic	X
NUMBER	6
TOTAL BA/OS	8

Exam Level	1	2	3	4
	Problem Focused	**Expanded Problem Focused**	**Detailed**	**Comprehensive**
	Limited to affected BA/OS	Limited to affected BA/OS & other related OSs	Extended of affected BA & other related OSs	General multi-system or complete single OS
# of OS or BA	1	2-7 limited	2-7 extended	8+ or 1 complete single system
			EXAMINATION LEVEL	4

MDM ELEMENTS	Documented
# OF DIAGNOSES/MANAGEMENT OPTIONS	
1. Minimal	
2. Limited	
3. Multiple	X
4. Extensive	
LEVEL	3
AMOUNT OR COMPLEXITY OF DATA TO REVIEW	**Documented**
1. Minimal/None	
2. Limited	
3. Moderate	X
4. Extensive	
LEVEL	3
RISK OF COMPLICATION OR DEATH IF NOT TREATED	**Documented**
1. Minimal	
2. Low	
3. Moderate	X
4. High	
LEVEL	3

MDC*	1	2	3	4
	Straightforward	**Low**	**Moderate**	**High**
Number of DX or management options	Minimal	Limited	Multiple	Extensive
Amount or complexity of data	Minimal/None	Limited	Moderate	Extensive
Risks	Minimal	Low	Moderate	High
			MDM LEVEL	3

*To qualify for a given type of MDM complexity, 2 of 3 elements in the table must be met or exceeded.

History: Comprehensive
Examination: Comprehensive
MDM: Moderate

Number of Key Components: 3 of 3

99244

FIGURE 1-12 Completed audit form.

no risk of death without treatment, and full recovery without impairment is expected.

4. **Moderate severity:** The risk of complete sickness (morbidity) without treatment is moderate, there is moderate risk of death without treatment, and an uncertain prognosis or increased probability of impairment exists.
5. **High severity:** The risk of complete sickness (morbidity) without treatment is high to extreme, there is a moderate to high risk of death without treatment, or there is a strong probability of severe, prolonged functional impairment.

The patient's medical record should contain the physician's **observation** of the complexity of the presenting problem(s).

Time Time was not included in the CPT manual before 1992 but was incorporated to assist with selection of the most appropriate level of E/M services. The times indicated with the codes are only averages and represent a simple estimate of the possible duration of a service.

Direct face-to-face time and **unit/floor time** are two measures of time. Outpatient visits are measured as direct face-to-face time. Direct face-to-face time is the time a physician spends directly with a patient during an office visit obtaining the history, performing an examination, and discussing results. Inpatient time is measured as unit/floor time and is used to describe the time a physician spends in the hospital setting dealing with the patient's care. Unit/floor time includes care given to the patient at the bedside face-to-face as well as the physician working on behalf of the patient within other settings on the unit or floor (e.g., the nursing station). It is often said that physicians get paid a great deal of money just for stopping in to visit a hospitalized patient quickly; however, what is not realized is that the physician spends additional time reviewing the patient's records, writing orders for the patient's care, and directing the care of the patient.

Time in the E/M section is referred to in statements such as this one, which is located with code 99203:

> Usually, the presenting problem(s) is (are) of moderate severity. Physicians typically spend **30 minutes** face-to-face with the patient and/or family.

These statements concerning time are used when counseling or coordination of care represents more than 50 percent of the time spent with a patient. The times referred to in these statements are then considered in the selection of the correct E/M code. For example, an established patient returns for an office visit to get results of previous tests. The physician spends 25 minutes with the patient, with 20 minutes of the time spent in counseling regarding the unfavorable results of the tests. The physician discusses various treatment options, the prognosis, and the risks of treatment and of treatment refusal. The code for the service is 99214, in which the time statement is, "Physician typically spends 25 minutes face-to-face with the patient and/or family."

It is important to note that the physician's documentation must prove that more than 50 percent of the visit was spent in counseling or coordination of care. For example, the physician may state, "I spent 25 minutes with this patient and 20 minutes of that was counseling regarding pain management options" or "The greatest majority of the 25 minutes of the visit was spent discussing his diabetic nutrition management." An example of coordination of care documentation is, "I spent 25 minutes coordinating care for this patient with her visiting nurse agency, physical therapist, and social worker. This included medication and treatment orders, as well as options for living arrangements."

You can assign a code based on the time the physician spends if the medical documentation supports the exact time the physician spent face-to-face, counseling, or coordinating care with or on behalf of the patient. For example, if the physician provided a problem-focused interval history, a problem focused examination, during a subsequent service in which the MDM was low, you would assign 99231. If, however, the physician notes in the medical record that rather than the 15 minutes usually spent in this service, the physician spent 20 minutes, you could move the case to 99232. Usually, the physician would have to provide an extended problem-focused interval history and an expanded problem-focused examination with an MDM of moderate complexity. However, because the time was more than 50% of the stated time for 99231, you can move the case up to 99232. Watch for reports that indicate the time the physician spent with the patient. However, just because time is documented, it does not mean that the time is in excess of any given code. Some physicians always document the time spent with a patient in the medical record; so you cannot assume the indication of time calls for an increase in code assignment. You need to check the time statements in the codes to ensure that it is appropriate to assign a higher-level code.

Having reviewed the key components and the contributing factors used to assess the level of E/M services, it is time to review Hospital Inpatient Services and then put the information to practice by coding reports.

Hospital Inpatient Services

Hospital Inpatient Services codes (99221–99239) are used to indicate a patient's status as an inpatient in a hospital or partial hospital setting; therefore, these codes are used to identify the hospital setting as the place where the physician renders service to the patient. An inpatient is one who has been formally admitted to an acute health care facility.

Note that within the subsection Hospital Inpatient Services, all the subheadings except Hospital Discharge Services are divided primarily on the basis of the 3 key components of history, examination, and MDM complexity. **Discharge** services are based on time. The Initial Hospital Care codes require 3 of the 3 key components, and the Subsequent Hospital Care codes require 2 of the 3 key components to be at the level described in the code. For example, the key components for code 99222 are a comprehensive history, a comprehensive examination, and a moderate level of MDM complexity. If the case you are coding has a comprehensive history and a comprehensive examination but a low MDM complexity, you cannot assign code 99222; instead, you would assign a lower-level code, 99221.

The subsection of Hospital Inpatient Services is divided into three subheadings:

1. Initial Hospital Care
2. Subsequent Hospital Care
3. Hospital Discharge Services

Initial Hospital Care

Initial Hospital Care codes are used to report the initial service of admission to the hospital by the admitting physician. Only the admitting physician can use the Initial Hospital Care codes. These codes reflect not only the admission but the services in any setting (office, emergency department, nursing home) provided in conjunction with the admission. For example, if the patient is seen in the office and is immediately admitted to the hospital, the office visit is bundled into the initial hospital care service and not reported separately. These services provided in the office may be taken into account when selecting the appropriate level of hospital admission. The hospital admission includes the patient admitting diagnosis, history, physical, and orders directing the nursing and ancillary staff regarding the patient's care.

Subsequent Hospital Care

Subsequent Hospital Care (99231–99233) is the second subheading of codes in the Hospital Inpatient Services subsection. The Subsequent Hospital Care codes are used by physicians to report daily hospital visits while the patient is hospitalized.

The first Subsequent Hospital Care code is 99231, and it typically implies that the patient is in stable condition and responding well to treatment. Codes in the subsection indicate the status of the patient (in the "Usually, the patient" area), such as stable/unstable or recovering/unresponsive.

> Usually, the patient is stable, recovering, or improving. Physicians typically spend 15 minutes at the bedside and on the patient's hospital floor or unit.

More than one physician can use the subsequent care codes on the same day. This is called **concurrent care.** Concurrent care is being provided when more than one physician provides service to a patient on the same day for different conditions. An example of concurrent care is a circumstance in which physician A, a cardiologist, treats a patient for a heart condition, and at the same time physician B, an oncologist, treats the patient for a cancer condition. The patient's **attending physician** maintains the primary responsibility for the overall care of the patient, no matter how many other physicians are providing services to the patient, unless a formal transfer of care has occurred.

An **attending physician** is a physician who, on the basis of education, training, and experience, is granted medical staff membership and clinical privileges by a health care organization to perform diagnostic or therapeutic procedures. An attending physician is legally responsible for the care and treatment provided to a patient. The attending physician may be a patient's personal physician or may be a physician assigned to a patient who has been admitted to a hospital through the emergency department or another physician who assumed responsibility for the patient. The attending physician is usually a provider of primary care, such as a family practitioner, internist, or pediatrician, but may also be a surgeon or other type of specialist. In an academic medical center, the attending physician may be a member of the academic or medical school staff who is responsible for the supervision of medical residents, interns, and students and oversees the care these individuals provide to patients.

There is no comprehensive history or comprehensive examination level in the codes in the Subsequent Hospital Care subheading because the comprehensive level of service would have been provided at the time of admission.

Hospital Discharge Services

Inpatient Hospital Discharge Services are reported on the final day of services for a multiple-day stay in a hospital setting. The service reflects the final examination of the patient as appropriate, follow-up instructions to the patient, and arrangements for discharge, including completion of discharge records. The Hospital Discharge Services codes are based on the time spent by the physician in handling the final discharge of the patient as 99238 for 30 minutes or less and 99239 for more than 30 minutes.

The Hospital Discharge Services codes are not used if the physician is a **consultant.** If a consulting physician is seeing the patient for a separate condition, those services would require a subsequent hospital care code. Only the attending physician is responsible for completion of the final examination, follow-up instructions, and arrangements for discharge and discharge records, and therefore only the attending physician can report services using the discharge codes.

Diagnosis Coding

The ICD-9-CM *Official Guidelines for Coding and Reporting* are displayed in **Appendix C** of this text. These guidelines assist the coder in assignment of ICD-9-CM codes. Review the *Guidelines* if you need a refresher on code assignment and to ensure that you are up-to-date on the changes that have taken place within the *Guidelines*. In October 2002, the new and extensively revised *Guidelines* were introduced in a more user-friendly format.

As with all diagnosis coding, the coder is to report the most definitive diagnosis available at the time of the report. However, before assigning a code, the coder must identify the correct diagnosis to ensure coding the correct diagnostic statement. It is always tempting to code what you know about the patient from previous documentation in the medical record, but it is important to remember that you must not use information from any other area of the chart except the report you are coding (except in operative reports, for which the pathology report is considered). In the first case you are going to code the CC of the patient, which is recurrent nausea and vomiting that would be reported with 787.01. On reading the report, however, you find that the physician indicated the patient has nausea and vomiting due to early diabetic ketoacidosis. The first-listed (primary) diagnosis would not then be the symptoms of nausea and vomiting but would be the diabetic ketoacidosis, which is the most definitive diagnosis.

Another area of challenge is the coding of diagnostic tests. The *Program Memorandum* from the Centers for Medicare and Medicaid Services (CMS) dated September 26, 2001, (AB-01-44) addressed the issue of diagnostic testing and diagnosis (see box on p. 20).

The reason for the diagnostic test is to be documented in the patient's medical record by the physician ordering the test. This order is then faxed, mailed, delivered, e-mailed, or telephoned to the testing facility. This order would include the diagnostic information that indicates the **reason** the test was requested. This establishes medical necessity and is a very important concept for justification of the procedure.

Incidental findings are findings that were not the reason for the test. For example, a patient is sent to a radiologist for a chest x-ray because of wheezing. The chest x-ray is negative, but a degenerative joint disease of the spine is visualized on the examination. The radiologist would report the wheezing (symptom) as the primary diagnosis, and may then list the degenerative joint disease as a secondary diagnosis. This incidental finding is unrelated to the reason the test was ordered.

If a test is ordered for screening (no signs or symptom exists), an ICD-9-CM screening code, such as V70-V83, would be assigned as the reason for the test.

The coder is directed to report the diagnosis code that most precisely explains the **reason** the test was ordered. This is often referred to as the *greatest level of specificity*. What this means is that the diagnosis code should match the reason the test was ordered as closely as possible. For example, if you are reporting a chest x-ray for malignancy of the left lower lobe of the lung, 162.5 most closely matches the diagnosis or the reason for the test. It would be incorrect to assign 162.8 for other parts of the bronchus or lung or 162.9 for unspecified bronchus or lung. **The greatest level of specificity also means that all available fourth or fifth digits must be assigned for the code to be complete. If there is a four-digit code available, you cannot report a three-digit code; and if there is a five-digit code available, you cannot report a four-digit code.**

Any report that has been prepared or interpreted by a physician can be the basis of a diagnosis. This would include a radiology report and a pathology report because both are written and interpreted by physicians. A routine laboratory report is prepared by a laboratory technician and is not to be used for the diagnostic statement until a physician has interpreted the report. For example, the surgical specimen is sent to the pathology department for analysis. The diagnosis statement on the operative report indicates skin lesion. The pathology report is available at the time of code assignment with a diagnosis of basal cell carcinoma. The code assigned would indicate basal cell carcinoma, not skin lesion, because the pathologist is a physician and as such is qualified to make the assessment. If, however, a patient is sent to the laboratory for a urine analysis based on the CC of frequent urination and the analysis indicated a bacterial infection, the diagnosis of bacterial infection is not reported until a physician has interpreted the report, even if the report is available at the time of code assignment. This is because a laboratory technician, not a physician, performed the laboratory analysis.

Inpatient and Outpatient Coders

There is a difference between the medical record documentation available to the inpatient and outpatient coder at the time of code assignment. The **inpatient coder** reports the services provided to the patient at the end of the hospital stay and has all the medical documentation for that stay available at the time of code assignment. The diagnoses are

The following are excerpts from the Program Memorandum of the CMS:

"The ICD-9-CM Coding Guidelines for Outpatient Services (hospital-based and physician office) have instructed physicians to report diagnoses based on test results. The Coding Clinic for ICD-9-CM confirms this long-standing coding guideline. CMS agrees with these long-standing official coding and reporting guidelines.

"Following are instructions for contractors, physicians, hospitals, and other health care providers to use in determining the use of ICD-9-CM codes for coding diagnostic test results. The instructions below provide guidance on the appropriate assignment of ICD-9-CM diagnoses codes to simplify coding for diagnostic tests consistent with the ICD-9-CM Guidelines for Outpatient Services (hospital-based and physician office). Note for the accuracy of the information submitted on the bill.

A. Determining the Appropriate Primary ICD-9-CM Diagnosis Code for Diagnostic Tests Ordered Due to Signs and/or Symptoms.

1. If the physician has confirmed a diagnosis based on the results of the diagnostic test, the physician interpreting the test should code that diagnosis. The signs and/or symptoms that prompted ordering the test may be reported as additional diagnoses if they are not fully explained or related to the confirmed diagnosis.

   Example 1: A surgical specimen is sent to a pathologist with a diagnosis of "mole." The pathologist personally reviews the slides made from the specimen and makes a diagnosis of "malignant melanoma." The pathologist should report a diagnosis of as the primary diagnosis.

   Example 2: A patient is referred to a radiologist for an abdominal CT scan with a diagnosis of abdominal pain. The CT scan reveals the presence of an abscess. The radiologist should report a diagnosis of "intra-abdominal abscess."

   Example 3: A patient is referred to a radiologist for a chest x-ray with a diagnosis of "cough." The chest x-ray reveals a 3-mm peripheral pulmonary nodule. The radiologist should report a diagnosis of "pulmonary nodule" and may sequence "cough" as an additional diagnosis.

2. If the diagnostic test did not provide a diagnosis or was normal, the interpreting physician should code the sign(s) or symptom(s) that prompted the treating physician to order the study.

   Example 1: A patient is referred to a radiologist for a spine x-ray due to complaints of "back pain." The radiologist performs the x-ray, and the results are normal. The radiologist should report a diagnosis of "back pain" since this was the reason for performing the spine study.

   Example 2: A patient is seen in the ER for chest pain. EKG is normal, and the final diagnosis is chest pain due suspected gastroesophageal reflux disease (GERD). The patient was told to follow up with his primary care physician for further evaluation of the suspected GERD. The primary diagnosis code for the ECG should be chest pain. Although the ECG was normal, a definitive cause for the chest pain was not determined.

3. If the results of the diagnostic test are normal or nondiagnostic, and the referring physician records a diagnosis preceded by words that indicate uncertainty (e.g., probable, suspected, questionable, rule out, or working), the interpreting physician should not code the referring diagnosis. Rather, the interpreting physician should report the signs(s) or symptom(s) that prompted the study. Diagnoses labeled as uncertain are considered by the ICD-9-CM Coding Guidelines as unconfirmed and should not be reported. This is consistent with the requirement to code the diagnosis to the highest degree of certainty.

   Example: A patient is referred to a radiologist for a chest x-ray with a diagnosis of "rule out pneumonia." The radiologist performs a chest x-ray, and the results are normal. The radiologist should report the sign(s) or symptom(s) that prompted the test (e.g., cough)."

A copy of the full program memorandum is included as Appendix B and is also available on the companion web site for this work text.

based on all information compiled during the stay. The **outpatient coder** has only the latest service available at the time of code assignment. The services to that patient may or may not be concluded at the time of code assignment. For example, a patient presents to the physician's office with the symptom of wheezing. The physician examines the patient and orders a chest x-ray for the clinical indication of "wheezing." The results probably will not have been returned when the coder assigns a code for the physician's office visit service, and as such the diagnosis would be reported as "wheezing" (786.07). On a later date, the x-ray report for the patient comes back with the radiologist's diagnosis of "pneumonia" (486) based on the results of the x-ray. When the coder reports the radiologist's services, the diagnosis of pneumonia (486) would be reported. Upon reviewing the radiologist's report, the patient's physician orders a pathology examination of the patient's sputum to determine the organism responsible for the pneumonia.

The results are returned from the pathologist with a diagnosis of "streptococcus, type B" (482.32, pneumonia due to streptococcus, Group B). The coder would report the pathologist's services using 482.32, streptococcus Group B pneumonia. At each step in the process, the diagnosis for the patient became more definitive and the coder reported the most definitive diagnosis available at the time based on the documentation available in the report being coded. Had this wheezing patient been an inpatient, the inpatient coder would have had the final definitive diagnosis of pneumonia due to streptococcus, Group B, and would have assigned 482.32 as the diagnosis when reporting the services for that inpatient stay.

The medical coder employed by a hospital to assign codes to services provided in its outpatient departments, such as the ambulatory or same-day surgery center, reports those outpatient services provided by the facility. For example, a patient presents to the ambulatory surgery center at the hospital for a surgical procedure that is performed by a clinic-employed general surgeon. The clinic outpatient coder would report the service provided by the surgeon. The hospital outpatient coder would report the facility portion of the same service. Both coders report outpatient services, one employed by the clinic and the other employed by the hospital. The clinic coder reports the physician (professional) portion of the service on the CMS-1500 Universal Claim Form, and the hospital (facility) coder reports the facility portion of the service on the CMS-1450 (UB-92). Both coders assign codes based on the documentation available at the time of code assignment. All tissue removed during an operative procedure requires pathological examination, which becomes a specimen. The pathologist analyzes the tissue and prepares a written report of the findings. To ensure reporting of the most definitive diagnosis, the operative report service is not usually reported until the results of the pathological examination are known.

If you are a hospital coder and the hospital employs a physician, you report the physician's professional services on the CMS-1500. If you are a hospital coder reporting the hospital services provided to an inpatient, you report these facility services on a CMS-1450 after the patient is discharged. Again, as the inpatient coder, you have available all of the documentation compiled during the hospital stay and assign diagnoses codes based on the entire stay. You will not be assigning codes to inpatient services in this worktext.

When you are assigning diagnoses codes to the reports within this worktext, **you are functioning as the outpatient coder and will assume that you have only the current report available to you and on which you will assign a code for the diagnosis.** For example, if a case contains three reports and you are assigning a diagnosis code for the first report, you have only the first report available and on which to base code assignment. If you are assigning a diagnosis code for the second report, you will assume you have only the second report available and on which to assign the most precise code. If you are assigning a diagnosis code to the third of three reports, you will assume you have only the third report available and on which to base code assignment. Each report, in the outpatient setting, stands on its own, and the coding is based on the information in just that report. There are two major exceptions to this rule. The first exception is an operative report that indicates a specimen had been removed. The diagnosis for the operative report is reported only *after* reviewing the pathology report that indicates the results of the specimen analysis (because the result of benign or malignant will determine the code choice). Within this worktext each operative report will be followed by the pathology report, or a note at the end of the operative report will indicate "Pathology Report Later Indicated" followed by the pathology results. The second exception to the "each report stands on its own" rule is when the directions for the case indicate that you are to report the services in a particular way. For example, Case 1-16 requires you to report the critical care services that a physician provided to a patient during a 24-hour period. Because critical care services are reported once for each 24 hours, you will be using all three reports in that case when assigning a code.

Medical reports are printed as dictated by the physician and may contain typographical errors. Also, the physician gives direction on the format he or she wants used when the report is transcribed and as such report formats vary. For example, some physicians want each major element of an examination in capital letters, such as ENDOCRINE, CARDIOVASCULAR, and RESPIRATORY. Therefore, the coder should anticipate that the formats within this text vary to reflect the real world of coding.

Time to Code!

You will find one blank audit form in Appendix A of this text. Make copies of the form to be used with the E/M cases in this text.

You will be assigning ICD-9-CM codes, and as a review of diagnosis coding, the *Official Guidelines for Coding and Reporting* are presented in **Appendix C** of this text.

The most important thing about abstracting a medical record, whether it is an operative report or inpatient/outpatient record, is knowing what you are looking for and understanding what you are reading. As you work through this worktext, read with a highlighter in your hand and a medical dictionary close by. The following steps were submitted by Karen Lockyer and contain excellent advice to help you build your coding skill.

Steps to Building Your Coding Skills

Step 1 Read the record for the first time for content and the second time for understanding.

Step 2 During the second reading, highlight important words that may apply to either the diagnosis (acute, chronic, malignant, etc.) or procedure (with or without, internal, external). Words a physician or surgeon uses to further document relevant aspects of the procedure may necessitate the use of modifiers. Look for words and phrases, such as "heavily obstructed" or "severely impacted."

Step 3 This is a fundamental skill coders build upon by practice. For example, there is a big difference between nephrectomy and nephrostomy, and the difference affects the code choice.

Step 4 When tips are given in this worktext, consider transferring them to your coding manual for instant reference when you are coding service or diagnosis in the future.

Now, let's put the information that you have just learned about coding E/M services to work by coding Hospital Services using CPT, ICD-9-CM, and HCPCS codes.

CASE 1-1A DISCUSSION

Let's do this one together. First, read the report carefully.

It is customary to assign the diagnoses codes before assigning the CPT code. Assign the diagnosis code(s), then return to review the diagnosis information that follows:

Diabetic Ketoacidosis

The physician indicates in the Impression section of the report that the symptoms of nausea and vomiting are due to the diabetic ketoacidosis (accumulation of acid in the blood). Ketoacidosis is very serious if left untreated, and there is a high risk of death. In the Index of the ICD-9-CM, when you locate "Diabetes, with ketoacidosis," you are referred to 250.1. When the Tabular is referenced, the fifth digit 1 is added to indicate type 1 (250.11, Note that the fifth digit 1 is chosen rather than 3 because even though both are type 1, the fifth digit 1 indicates "not stated as uncontrolled" and the fifth digit 3 is "uncontrolled." This patient has diabetic ketoacidosis, which means the diabetes is uncontrolled; however, unless the physician's diagnostic statement specifically indicates "uncontrolled," you cannot report uncontrolled.) You could also locate this code under the main term "Ketoacidosis, diabetes." As always, there are many ways to locate codes in the Index of the ICD-9-CM. The symptoms of nausea and vomiting are not reported as the etiology (cause) is identified as the diabetic ketoacidosis. The second statement under the Impression section is "Diabetes mellitus type 1 with a history of recurrent ketoacidosis," and this is not reported separately as it is included in the 250.11.

Asthma

Asthma is also indicated as a diagnosis. Asthma is a disease of the airways in which the airways are hypersensitive. The typical manifestations of an acute asthma attack are wheezing, rapid and labored breathing, and cough with marked dyspnea. In the Index under the main term "Asthma," the coder is directed to 493.9. A note is also present in the Index to direct the coder to assign a fifth digit to indicate if the type of episode is unspecified (0); with status asthmaticus (1); or with acute exacerbation (2). Status asthmaticus is the most severe form of asthma attack and may last for days or weeks. The medical record may indicate severe airway obstruction that does not respond to bronchodilators or other terms that mean status asthmaticus, such as intractable, prolonged, or refractory asthma. Report 1-1A does not indicate that there is any current exacerbation of the asthma, so the correct fifth digit is 0 (unspecified), and the correct code is **493.90**.

Assignment of E/M Code

Label the blank E/M audit form that you copied from Appendix A Case 1-1A. It is now time to identify the level of history, examination, and MDM complexity.

History Level

Identify the elements of the HPI, then return to review the elements below.

There are four elements:

- The **location** is stomach because that is the area of complaint.
- The **duration** is indicated by "since 5 A.M." located in the first paragraph of the HPI.
- There are also **associated signs and symptoms** (often the hardest to spot in the HPI) of confused, cramping in legs, sore throat, and abdominal discomfort. The presence of any one of the S&S (signs and symptoms) would allow you to check off that element on the audit form.
- The **modifying factors** would be the Humalog and Ultralente (insulins).

The following highlight the elements of the HPI:

HISTORY OF PRESENT ILLNESS: The patient is a 17-year-old female with type 1 diabetes mellitus who in the past has had several admissions for ketoacidosis. The patient indicates that she was feeling quite good last night and ate her evening meal without problems. She had a blood sugar of about 168 mg% sometime yesterday. This morning she woke about 5:00 A.M. [**DURATION**] and had sugar that was over 500 mg%. This was associated with emesis, which has continued on a recurrent basis since that time. The patient did take Humalog 10 units, Ultralente 14 units [**MODIFYING FACTORS**] when she awoke with the high sugar. She also apparently took an additional dose of possibly 20 units of Humalog around 9:00 this morning. Because of the persistence of vomiting, [**LOCATION IS STOMACH**] her mother called in at noon and was advised to bring her in. She does indicate that the daughter has been a little bit confused. In addition, she states that the daughter is having some abdominal discomfort [**ASSOCIATED SIGNS AND SYMPTOMS**] ongoing nausea, and cramping in her legs [**ASSOCIATED SIGNS AND SYMPTOMS**]. The patient's mother indicates she has been very good with her diet and has not had any recent problems with skipped shots or high sugars. She has been testing anywhere from two to four times per day. The patient denies that she has had any cough, although she has had a slightly sore throat [**ASSOCIATED SIGNS AND SYMPTOMS**] today. No other symptoms, such as diarrhea, have been noted.

Your audit form should now have these four elements checked. This HPI is a level 4 or comprehensive HPI.

Now, on to the Review of System (ROS). Review the report to identify the ROS elements, and check them off on your form. Then return here to review the elements identified below.

There are 10 elements in this ROS, as follows:

- Ophthalmologic (eyes)
- Otolaryngologic (ears and mouth)
- Cardiovascular (cardiac)
- Respiratory (chest)
- Immunologic (infectious disease)
- Gastrourinary
- Musculoskeletal
- Neurologic
- Psychiatric
- Hematologic

The following highlight the ROS elements:

REVIEW OF SYSTEMS: Eyes: [**OPHTHALMOLOGIC**] Negative. Ears: Negative. Mouth: As noted above. [**OTOLARYNGOLOGIC**] Chest: As noted above. [**RESPIRATORY** and noted above was "The patient denies that she had any cough, although she has had a slightly sore throat today."] Cardiac: [**CARDIOVASCULAR**] As noted above. Hematologic: [**HEMATOLOGIC**] Negative. Infectious disease: [**IMMUNOLOGIC**] Negative. Neurologic: [**NEUROLOGIC**] Negative. Psychiatric: [**PSYCHIATRIC**] As noted above. Musculoskeletal: [**MUSCULOSKELETAL**] Negative. GU: [**GASTROURINARY**] The patient generally has nocturia.

Your audit form should have these 10 elements checked off to qualify this ROS for a level 4 or comprehensive HPI.

The Past, Family, and Social History (PFSH) includes all three elements identified in paragraphs within the report. This PFSH is a level 4 or comprehensive PFSH.

The following highlight the PFSH elements:

PAST MEDICAL HISTORY

SURGICAL: None.

MEDICAL:

1. Diabetes mellitus type 1 with history of recurrent ketoacidosis.
2. Asthma, p.r.n. albuterol.

SOCIAL HISTORY: The patient lives with her parents. She has two brothers, both of whom now have type 1 diabetes. Her oldest brother was recently diagnosed with diabetes. She is going into the senior grade in high school. She states that she does not smoke or use drugs.

FAMILY HISTORY: Strongly positive for diabetes in a cousin and an uncle. There is also a history of coronary artery disease and stroke.

Because the HPI, ROS, and PFSH are all at a 4 or comprehensive level, this history is a level 4.

Examination

Now it's time to work on the examination. Complete the examination portion of the audit form, then return to review the elements identified in the examination portion of the report.

The examination elements include 4 constitutional items which equals 1 OS:

- Blood pressure
- Pulse
- Respiration
- General appearance (sluggish)

There were 2 BAs:

- Neck
- Chest (symmetrical).

There were 6 OSs:

- Ophthalmologic (eyes)
- Otolaryngologic (ears, mouth)
- Respiratory (clear to auscultation)
- Cardiovascular (heart and good pulses)
- Lymphatic (axillary nodes)
- Gastrointestinal (abdomen, some tenderness)

The following highlight the element of the examination: PHYSICAL EXAMINATION: The patient is very sluggish, [CONSTITUTIONAL, GENERAL APPEARANCE] although she does answer questions. Blood pressure [CONSTITUTIONAL, BLOOD PRESSURE] 97/76, pulse [CONSTITUTIONAL, PULSE] 130 regular, respirations [CONSTITUTIONAL, RESPIRATIONS] normal. EYES: [ORGAN SYSTEM, OPHTHALAMOLOGIC] Sunken significantly. Fundi are not visualized. EARS: [ORGAN SYSTEM, OTOLARYNGOLOGIC] Negative. MOUTH: [ORGAN SYSTEM, OTOLARYNGOLOGIC] Tongue is dry and throat looked all right. Carotids are 4/4 without bruits. Thyroid is normal to palpation. NECK [BODY AREA] supple, nodes are negative. Axillary nodes [ORGAN SYSTEM, LYMPHATIC] negative. CHEST: [BODY AREA] Symmetrical. Clear to auscultation. [ORGAN SYSTEM, RESPIRATORY] HEART: [ORGAN SYSTEM, CARDIOVASCULAR] Tachycardic but no extra sounds heard. No murmur is appreciated. ABDOMEN: Some minimal tenderness in the right midabdomen and left upper abdomen. [ORGAN SYSTEM, GASTROINTESTINAL] GENITAL/RECTAL: Not performed. Peripheral extremities reveal good pulses [ORGAN SYSTEM, CARDIOVASCULAR] in the legs with no edema.

There was a total of 9 BAs/OSs reviewed, placing this examination at a level 4 or comprehensive physical examination.

Medical Decision Making Complexity (MDM)

In the opinion of many coders, the identification of MDM level is the most difficult part of E/M coding. This is because it is the most abstract, which means the coder can't just check off a list and add the items to arrive at the level. Rather, the coder must assess the complexity, which takes time and practice to learn. Think about the report in total, identify the level of MDM, and then return here.

Level of Diagnoses/Management Options

Here are some questions you need to ask yourself to assess the level of diagnoses/management options for this case:

- Was there an established diagnosis when the patient presented? (*At this time the patient presents with nausea and vomiting, cause unknown at presentation.*)
- Does the report reflect whether the problem was improved, well controlled, resolving, or resolved or was the problem inadequately controlled, worsening, or was the patient failing to respond? (*This patient's problem was inadequately controlled; without care it would have continued to worsen.*)
- Could there be multiple causes of nausea and vomiting? (*Yes, there could be; and the physician will have to identify the cause from a wide range of possibilities in a patient with known multiple health problems.*)

This is an example of extensive diagnoses and management options, or a level 4.

Level of Data to Review

Did the physician review data? (*There was no indication that data from old records were called for or reviewed, and if it is not documented it didn't happen. So, there was no data reviewed, except the fingerstick indicated before the Impression section of the report.*)

This is a minimal/none level of data review or a level 1.

Level of Risk

Does the patient have other conditions that could affect the management and treatment of the condition? (*Yes, the patient is a diabetic with reoccurring ketoacidosis and in addition has asthma. The report indicates ketoacidosis in the diagnosis section of the report.*)

There is a high level of risk of death or complication for this patient or a level 4.

The MDM level is based on 2 of 3. You do not need all 3 elements of the MDM to be at the same level to assign that level, as you must for the history. There are two elements at a level 4, so this is a level 4 MDM.

This report contained a comprehensive history, comprehensive examination, and high MDM complexity. This is an initial hospital care service, which requires 3 of 3 key components to be at the same or higher level before assigning a code from this category. 99223 requires a comprehensive history, comprehensive examination, and high MDM complexity, which matches the levels of this report and is therefore assigned.

CASE 1-1
1-1A Initial Hospital Care
1-1B Discharge Summary

CASE 1-1

Report Dr. Alanda's professional services for Sally Jacobson's initial hospital care.

1-1A INITIAL HOSPITAL CARE

LOCATION: Inpatient Hospital

PATIENT: Sally Jacobson

PHYSICIAN: Leslie Alanda, M.D.

CHIEF COMPLAINT: Recurrent nausea and vomiting.

HISTORY OF PRESENT ILLNESS: The patient is a 17-year-old female with type 1 diabetes mellitus who has had several admissions for ketoacidosis. The patient indicates that she was feeling quite good last night and ate her evening meal without problems. She had a blood sugar of about 168 mg% sometime yesterday. This morning she woke about 5:00 A.M and had sugar that was over 500 mg%. This was associated with emesis, which has continued on a recurrent basis since that time. The patient did take Humalog 10 units and Ultralente 14 units when she awoke with the high sugar. She also apparently took an additional dose of possibly 20 units of Humalog around 9:00 A.M.

Because of the persistence of vomiting, her mother called in at noon and was advised to bring her in. She indicates that the daughter has been a little bit confused. In addition, she states that the daughter is having some abdominal discomfort ongoing nausea, and cramping in her legs.

The patient's mother indicates she has been very good with her diet and has not had any recent problems with skipped shots or high sugars. She has been testing anywhere from two to four times per day. The patient denies that she has had any cough, although she has had a slightly sore throat today. No other symptoms, such as diarrhea, have been noted.

MEDICATIONS:
1. Humalog 7 units, Ultralente 14 units at breakfast and suppertime, and Humalog 7 units at noon.
2. Albuterol nebulizer treatments p.r.n.

ALLERGIES: None.

PAST MEDICAL HISTORY:

SURGICAL: None.

MEDICAL:
1. Diabetes mellitus type 1 with history of recurrent ketoacidosis.
2. Asthma, p.r.n albuterol.

SOCIAL HISTORY: The patient lives with her parents. She has two brothers, both of whom now have type 1 diabetes. Her oldest brother was recently diagnosed with diabetes. She is going into the senior grade in high school. She states that she does not smoke or use drugs.

FAMILY HISTORY: Strongly positive for diabetes in a cousin and an uncle. There is also a history of coronary artery disease and stroke.

REVIEW OF SYSTEMS: Eyes: Negative. Ears: Negative. Mouth: As noted above. Chest: As noted above. Cardiac: As noted above. Hematologic: Negative. Infectious disease: Negative. Neurologic: Negative. Psychiatric: As noted above. Musculoskeletal: Negative. GU: The patient generally has nocturia.

PHYSICAL EXAMINATION: The patient is very sluggish, although she does answer questions. Blood pressure 96/76, pulse 130 and regular, respirations normal. EYES: Sunken significantly. Fundi are not visualized. EARS: Negative. MOUTH: Tongue is dry and throat looked all right. Carotids are 4/4 without bruits. Thyroid is normal to palpation. NECK: supple, nodes are negative. Axillary nodes negative. CHEST: Symmetrical. Clear to auscultation. HEART: Tachycardic but no extra heart sounds heard. No murmur is appreciated. ABDOMEN: Some minimal tenderness in the right midabdomen and left upper abdomen. GENITAL/RECTAL: Not performed. Peripheral extremities reveal good pulses in the legs with no edema.

Fingerstick in the office was 110 mg%.

IMPRESSION:
1. Nausea and vomiting due to diabetic ketoacidosis.
2. Diabetes mellitus type 1 with a history of recurrent ketoacidosis.
3. Asthma.

PLAN: The patient will need intravenous fluids and low doses of insulin along with intravenous glucose for her rehydration. She has been sluggish in the past when hospitalized, so I suspect she will have a slow recovery time but should be able to go home tomorrow.

There is no apparent etiology for the onset of the acidosis.

The situation has been discussed frankly with the patient's mother, and she understands the objectives and our treatment plan.

1-1A:

SERVICE CODE(S): ____________________

DX CODE(S): ____________________

HOSPITAL DISCHARGE SERVICES

The hospital discharge services are based on the time the physician spends in the final discharge of the patient. The service may or may not include an examination of the patient. If the physician does not indicate the time spent in discharge of the patient, the lowest level of discharge would be reported (99238). Physician education about documentation is very important to ensure appropriate reimbursement since only if the physician records the amount of time, can the coder assign a discharge code for a higher level discharge service. The time must be documented in the medical record with the beginning and ending time and the time does not have to be consecutive. The physician may spend time on preparation of the final discharge and then return and spend additional time on the discharge documentation.

At the time of discharge, the physician will indicate the discharge diagnoses usually in a "Discharge Diagnosis" section of the report. However, the full report must be carefully read to ensure that other diagnoses pertinent to the service provided are also reported.

Recall that you do not code symptoms when there is a more definitive diagnosis available, but note that in report 1-1B the discharge diagnosis indicates "Vomiting with dehydration, secondary to early diabetic ketoacidosis." The vomiting is a symptom of the ketoacidosis, but the dehydration is not a symptom of the ketoacidosis but a separate, distinct condition and is therefore assigned a code. Although there is a combination code for vomiting with nausea, there is no combination code for vomiting with dehydration.

1-1B DISCHARGE SUMMARY (99238-99239)

Report Dr. Alanda's professional services for Sally's discharge from the hospital.

LOCATION: Inpatient Hospital

PATIENT: Sally Jacobson

PHYSICIAN: Leslie Alanda, M.D.

DISCHARGE DIAGNOSES:

1. Vomiting with dehydration, secondary to early diabetic ketoacidosis.
2. Diabetes mellitus type 1.
3. Asthma.

HOSPITAL COURSE: The patient was admitted with recurrent vomiting and clinical evidence for dehydration. Earlier the day of admission, the patient had sugar over 500 mg% but was able to get this down to about 120 mg% around the time of admission. Nonetheless, she was also confused on admission, and with rehydration and intravenous insulin, she gradually rehydrated and returned to her normal status. It is unclear why the patient developed this problem because there was no other evidence for any gastroenteritis or intestinal problems. The patient's measured bicarbonate level on admission was 22.2, which is slightly low. Blood sugars while hospitalized ranged from 77–328 mg%.

DISCHARGE ACTIVITY: Regular.

DISCHARGE DIET: 2400 calories ADA.

DISCHARGE FOLLOW-UP: The patient will see me in one week's time at the clinic. She is to continue testing her sugars four times a day and taking regular meals.

LABORATORY STUDIES: Hemoglobin 15.9 with an MCV of 78. Platelet count was 491,000. White count was 12,550. BUN was 27, bicarb 22.2, and glucose 154 on admission.

DISCHARGE CONDITION: The patient is eating, ambulatory, and alert.

DISCHARGE MEDICATION: Ultralente 14 units, Humalog 7 units at breakfast and supper, and Humalog 7 units at noon, albuterol, p.r.n.

1-1B:

SERVICE CODE(S): ____________________

DX CODE(S): ____________________

CASE 1-1B DISCUSSION

The physician made no note of the length of time spent providing the discharge service, so the lowest level discharge service is reported (99238). The diagnoses are type 1 diabetes with ketoacidosis (250.11), dehydration (276.51 is a separate, distinct condition), and asthma without mention of the status (493.90).

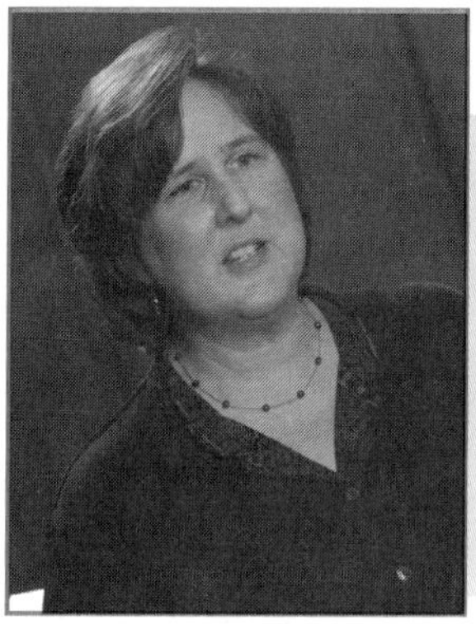

FROM THE TRENCHES

Kathy

"Coding isn't something you can learn in a classroom and have all the knowledge you need. On the job training is just as important as the classroom training...You need that structured training, [but] you can't just learn it all in a classroom."

Chest (some cough)

CASE 1-2

1-2A Emergency Department Services

CASE 1-2

The patient in Case 1-2 is the same patient in Case 1-1. The patient presents to the emergency department with nausea and recurrent vomiting.

(99281–99288)

1-2A EMERGENCY DEPARTMENT SERVICES

LOCATION: Hospital Emergency Department

PATIENT: Sally Jacobson

PHYSICIAN: Paul Sutton, M.D.

CHIEF COMPLAINT: Nausea and recurrent vomiting with dehydration.

HISTORY OF PRESENT ILLNESS: The patient is a 17-year-old with type 1 diabetes mellitus since age 11 who has had pharyngitis for about the past 5 days. She was seen by her regular internist 2 days ago, and throat culture was negative. The feeling was she had a viral pharyngitis because her brother had similar symptoms. The patient indicates that she has had nausea with some vomiting for the past 3 days and has really not eaten anything for the past 2 days. For the past day, she has had some diarrhea. She also indicates she has had some fever and chills and some cough. Generally, she feels poorly and indicates that she has been running to the bathroom quite frequently. She does indicate that she has taken all of her insulin shots as noted below, but she has not been able to eat. She does indicate that she has had an associated headache but no other symptoms. Blood sugar at noon today was about 190 by Accu-Chek.

ALLERGIES: None known.

MEDICATIONS:

1. Ultralente 16 units, morning and evening.
2. Humalog 14 units in the morning, 7 units at noon, and 14 units at supper.
3. Albuterol nebulizer treatments p.r.n.

PAST MEDICAL HISTORY: Asthma, presently albuterol p.r.n. Diabetes mellitus type 1 with several admissions for ketoacidosis.

PAST SURGICAL HISTORY: None.

FAMILY HISTORY: Positive in two brothers with type 1 diabetes mellitus. She also has a cousin and uncle with diabetes. There is also positive family history for coronary artery disease. An uncle has lung cancer.

SOCIAL HISTORY: The patient is a senior in high school.

REVIEW OF SYSTEMS: Eyes: Blurred double vision. Ears: Hearing is okay. GI: As noted above. GU: Negative. Cardiac: Negative. Chest: As noted above. She has had no shortness of breath (SOB) or heavy breathing. Hematologic: Negative. Infectious disease: As noted above. Neurologic: Negative. Psychiatric: Negative. Sleep pattern has been off in the past, and she has been treated with amitriptyline. This has not been such a significant problem of late.

EXAMINATION: The patient appears dehydrated with sunken eyeballs and a flushed face. Blood pressure 102/70, pulse 120 and regular, and temperature 97.8. Tongue is mildly dry. Eyes: Good range of motion of the eyes, but the eyeballs are sunken. Neck: Supple. Nodes are negative. Carotids are 4/4 without bruits. Thyroid is normal to palpation. Chest: Clear to auscultation. Heart: Tachycardia is present, but no murmurs or extra sounds appreciated. No Kussmaul breathing is noted. Abdomen: Soft, nontender without palpable masses. Genitorectal: Not performed. Peripheral extremities reveal good pulses and normal reflexes. No edema is present.

IMPRESSION: 2

1. Dehydration secondary to #2 with possible ketoacidosis.
2. 3 Viral pharyngitis with what appears to be a gastroenteritis component.
3. Diabetes mellitus type 1, six years without complication.
4. 4 Asthma, presently stable.

PLAN: The patient will be treated with intravenous fluids and insulin as indicated. Once she is able to eat and is ambulatory, she will be able to go home.

1-2A:

SERVICE CODE(S): ________________

DX CODE(S): ________________

CASE 1-3
1-3A Initial Hospital Service
1-3B Consultation
1-3C Radiology Report
1-3D Radiology Report

CASE 1-3

The patient in Cases 1-1 and 1-2 is again admitted, at a later time, to the hospital, this time for abdominal pain.

1-3A INITIAL HOSPITAL SERVICE

LOCATION: Inpatient Hospital

PATIENT: Sally Jacobson

ATTENDING PHYSICIAN: Leslie Alanda, M.D.

CHIEF COMPLAINT: Abdominal pain for 48 hours.

HISTORY OF PRESENT ILLNESS: This is a 17-year-old female who presents with a 24- to 48-hour history of right lower-quadrant abdominal pain. The patient has a history of diabetes mellitus. The patient states that nothing has made it better and nothing has made the pain any more tolerable. She states that the pain is becoming gradually worse. She states she has taken Advil to no avail. The patient does have positive nausea with no vomiting. No diarrhea and no constipation. No dysuria. The patient states that she has eaten very little today because of the pain and is not hungry at this time.

PAST MEDICAL HISTORY:
1. Diabetes mellitus.
2. Sinusitis.
3. Asthma.

MEDICATIONS:
1. Humalog 7 units in the morning, noon, and q.h.s.
2. Ultralente 14 units q.a.m. and 14 units q.p.m.
3. Elavil 100 mg p.o. q.h.s.

ALLERGIES: None.

SOCIAL HISTORY: The patient now states that she has drunk in the past. She does smoke three to five cigarettes daily. She is otherwise a normal healthy senior high school student.

FAMILY HISTORY: Neither of her parents has diabetes mellitus; however, there is a history of diabetes in that her two brothers have it and that a cousin and uncle have it. There is also a history of CVAs, myocardial infarctions, and cancer.

REVIEW OF SYSTEMS: General: The patient states she has been in good health other than the right abdominal pain. HEENT: The patient denies any headache, diplopia, blurred vision, eye pain, redness, cataracts, glaucoma, loss of vision, hearing loss, tinnitus, or epistaxis. Cardiovascular: The patient denies any chest pain, chest pressure, orthopnea, or PND. Respiratory: The patient denies any coughing, wheezing, and hemoptysis. She does complain of the history of asthma as stated in the past medical history. She does not take medications for that. GI: The patient complains of right lower-quadrant pain and nausea but denies vomiting, constipation, or diarrhea. GU: The patient denies dysuria, hematuria, nocturia, or changes in frequency. Extremities: The patient has a good range of motion and states that she has no complications of gait. Neurologic: The patient denies any paresthesias or paralysis complications. Psychiatric: She denies any agitation, increased depression, or personality disorders.

PHYSICAL EXAMINATION: Vitals: Blood pressure 123/67, pulse 115, respirations 20, and temperature 35.0. HEENT: Head is normocephalic with no contusion or abrasions. Eyes: EOMS are intact. Ears: Tympanic membranes are visualized with no erythema. Nose: Nares are patent. Mucosa pink and moist. Throat: Mucosa pink and moist. Tongue and uvula midline. Cardiovascular: S1 and S2 with a regular rate and rhythm. No murmurs are audible. No bruits evident on examination. Respiratory: Lungs are clear to auscultation bilaterally. No wheezing or rhonchi. Abdomen: There are positive bowel sounds. There is right lower-quadrant pain, which she rates 8/10. There is also positive Rovsing's sign and negative rebound tenderness. There are no masses palpable on examination. Extremities: The patient has good range of motion and peripheral pulses are intact.

LABORATORY: White cell count of 5.46, with a hemoglobin of 14.0 and a hematocrit of 40.9.

ASSESSMENT:
1. Rule out appendicitis.
2. Diabetes mellitus, type I.
3. Sinusitis, acute.
4. Asthma.

PLAN: Admit the patient to the hospital. The patient will be n.p.o. Will get her vitals q.4h. Will start IV fluids of D5 LR 125 cc per hour. Will give Accu-Cheks q.i.d. Will get a CBC and basic metabolic panel in the morning. We will continue the patient on her regular insulin regimen. We will also give her Demerol for pain, and we will re-evaluate in the morning. We will hold the Demerol at 4 A.M. so that our evaluation in the morning is adequate.

1-3A:

SERVICE CODE(S): ____________________

DX CODE(S): ____________________

CASE 1-3A DISCUSSION

The outpatient coder reports the reason for the service or encounter as presented in the report that is being coded, not on diagnoses stated previously in the patient record. You will have only the report you are currently coding to reference.

Rule Out Diagnosis

There were many diagnoses referred to in the 1-3A report of initial hospital services. In the HPI section of the report, the "right lower-quadrant abdominal pain" is stated. In the Assessment section of the report, "rule out appendicitis" is stated. Because outpatient coders do not report "rule out" statements, you report the symptom of abdominal pain rather than the appendicitis. Note that in the HPI section the statement is made that the patient has nausea. Some coders consider the nausea to be an integral part of the abdominal pain and would not report the nausea separately; however, other coders would report the nausea with a separate code (787.02).

The type 1 diabetes mellitus and asthma would need to be reported as these conditions would have implications for the medications and treatment ordered for the patient. The acute sinusitis should probably be reported as it may be significant in the care of an asthmatic patient (although in the Physical Examination section of the report, there is no mention of the symptoms of sinusitis). The physician should be queried as to the sinusitis. On the CMS-1500, there is space for 4 diagnoses. The diagnoses for this report are abdominal pain (789.03), diabetes (250.01), sinusitis (461.9), and asthma (493.90).

1-3B CONSULTATION (99251-99255)

You will find detailed information regarding coding a consultation in the information that follows Case 1-9. You will begin to code an assortment of consultative services there. Dr. Alanda requested a consultation from Dr. Jayco, an endocrinologist, prior to the planned appendectomy. Report the professional consultation services of Dr. Jayco.

LOCATION: Inpatient Hospital

PATIENT: Sally Jacobson

ATTENDING PHYSICIAN: Leslie Alanda, M.D.

CONSULTANT: Gordon Jayco, M.D.

REASON FOR CONSULTATION: Preoperative diabetes management.

HISTORY: The patient is a 17-year-old girl with type 1 diabetes, history of asthma, sinusitis, and migraine headache. She was in good health until approximately 1 to 2 days ago, when she developed right lower-quadrant pain with decreased appetite. She states that the intensity of the pain is 6/10. She had no change in bowel habits and no fevers or chills. No other viral symptoms. She was admitted to the hospital with a concern of possible acute appendicitis. She was kept n.p.o., and admission blood sugar was approximately 270. I had been asked to manage her diabetes. The patient normally is on a basal bolus insulin regimen at home with 14 Ultralente b.i.d. and 7 units Humalog with meals. Her past level of glycemic control has been fair with her hemoglobin A1C's ranging from about 8.5 to 10%. She did have a mild degree of microalbuminuria when last tested but no other diabetes complications.

PAST MEDICAL HISTORY:
1. Type 1 diabetes as discussed above.
2. History of asthma.
3. History of sinusitis.
4. History of migraine headaches.

ALLERGIES: None.

HABITS: The patient does occasionally smoke. No alcohol use.

CURRENT MEDICATIONS:
1. Ultralente 14 units b.i.d. and 7 units Humalog with meals.
2. Elavil 100 mg p.o. q.h.s.

FAMILY HISTORY: She has two brothers with type 1 diabetes as well as a cousin and uncle. Father's side of family has coronary artery disease. Another uncle had lung cancer.

SOCIAL HISTORY: The patient is a senior in high school.

REVIEW OF SYSTEMS: As discussed above.

PHYSICAL EXAMINATION: The patient is in no acute distress. Weight is 151 pounds. Height 5 feet 3 inches. Vital signs are stable. She was afebrile. Lungs are clear to auscultation. Cardiac exam shows a regular rate and rhythm with a normal S1 and S2 without murmurs. Abdomen is notable for some mild hypertrophy. There is some tenderness in the right lower quadrant. No guarding or rebound. Bowel sounds are present. Extremities are unremarkable.

LABORATORY STUDIES: Admission blood sugar was 276. White count was normal.

ASSESSMENT AND PLAN:
1. Type 1 diabetes. The patient admitted with presumptive diagnosis of acute appendicitis, now n.p.o. with hyperglycemia. I recommend continuing dextrose-containing IV fluids, but we will add 15 units of insulin per liter. Total fluids to run at 125 cc per hour. We will monitor blood sugars q.4h. and q.1h. perioperatively with a target range of 100 to 200. Once her diet is resumed, we will get her back on her usual outpatient insulin regimen.
2. Abdominal pain. Plans for monitoring and possible exploratory surgery per surgical team.

1-3B:

SERVICE CODE(S): ____________________

DX CODE(S): ____________________

CASE 1-3B DISCUSSION

The reason for this service is the first-listed (primary) diagnosis, and in this case the diabetes management is the primary reason Dr. Jayco is providing a consultation. In the Assessment and Plan section of the report, the physician also indicates the abdominal pain and discusses this pain in the History section of the report; therefore, the abdominal pain is listed second. The asthma, sinusitis, and migraine headaches mentioned in the Past Medical History section of the report would not usually be reported. If you were to report any of the "History of" (H/O) conditions, the asthma would be the most significant and would, therefore, be reported.

1-3C RADIOLOGY REPORT (76700–76705)

Report Dr. Monson's radiology service.

LOCATION: Inpatient Hospital

PATIENT: Sally Jacobson

ATTENDING PHYSICIAN: Leslie Alanda, M.D.

RADIOLOGIST: Morton Monson, M.D.

ULTRASOUND OF RIGHT LOWER QUADRANT: The patient has right lower-quadrant pain and a normal white blood count. Ultrasound views of the right lower quadrant are submitted. We do image a tubular structure. This tubular structure is, however, compressible, and that is not the usual case with an appendix that is inflamed. This could be a loop of bowel, but the technologist indicates that this area did not show peristalsis throughout the examination. This tubular structure measures 1.4 cm × 7.6 mm. In cross-section, it does not show the typical target sign. There are no fluid collections. There is no free fluid. Technologist indicates that the patient was tender over this tubular structure.

IMPRESSION:

1. We do demonstrate a tubular structure in the right lower quadrant that is tender when the technologist presses on it.
2. This tubular structure is, however, compressible, which would not be the usual case in an inflamed appendix.
3. It could be that we are dealing with very early appendicitis. It could also be that the structure we are seeing is simply a loop of bowel, which did not happen to peristalses during the course of the evaluation. Overall, this does not demonstrate a structure that fits all the criteria of inflamed appendix.
4. No free fluid or fluid collections.

1-3C:

SERVICE CODE(S): ______________________

DX CODE(S): ______________________

CASE 1-3C DISCUSSION

Interpreting Physician

Recall that in the Program Memorandum (PM) from the CMS on page 20 of this worktext, if the diagnostic test did not provide a diagnosis or was normal, the interpreting physician (in this case the radiologist) should code the sign(s) and symptom(s) that prompted the treating physician to order the study. The first example in the PM was "A patient is referred to a radiologist for a spine x-ray due to complaints of "back pain." Since the result of the x-ray was normal, the radiologist should report a diagnosis of "back pain" since this was the reason for performing the spine study." In Case 1-3C, Dr. Alanda referred Sally to the radiologist, Dr. Monson, for right lower-quadrant pain with a normal white blood count. (The reason the normal white blood count is stated is the physician would have expected the white blood count to be elevated indicating infection, which would be expected in an appendicitis.) However, based on the results of the x-ray, the radiologist provided no more definitive (specific) diagnosis, so the presenting symptom of abdominal pain is reported as the diagnosis.

1-3D RADIOLOGY REPORT (71010 – 71035)

Report Dr. Monson's radiology service.

LOCATION: Inpatient Hospital

PATIENT: Sally Jacobson

ATTENDING PHYSICIAN: Leslie Alanda, M.D.

RADIOLOGIST: Morton Monson, M.D.

INDICATIONS: Cough and fever

PA & LATERAL CHEST, 9:15 A.M.: The previous film is from last month. There is no pneumonia. The lung fields are clear. There are no effusions. The heart and vascular markings are normal. Bony structures are unremarkable.

IMPRESSION: Normal chest x-ray.

1-3D:

SERVICE CODE(S): ______________________

DX CODE(S): ______________________

CASE 1-3D DISCUSSION

In 1-3A, Dr. Alanda again requests radiology services for Sally because of her cough and fever. Again, no more definitive diagnosis is stated, and as such the presenting symptoms of cough and fever are reported as the diagnoses.

CASE 1-4

The patient in Case 1-4 is a 32-year-old male who is seen by his physician, Dr. Green, at the outpatient clinic. Dr. Green immediately admitted the patient to the hospital. Report Dr. Green's service.

1-4A INITIAL HOSPITAL CARE

LOCATION: Inpatient Hospital

PATIENT: Jonathan Harley

ATTENDING PHYSICIAN: Ronald Green, M.D.

The patient along with his wife comes in today as he relates issues with worsening of his dyspepsia/GERD. He relates that his medications are not working as previously noted to be since he has been removed from a proton pump inhibitor, Prevacid, to the Protonix secondary to insurance issues. He also relates to me issues of his worsening shortness of breath beyond his chronic status. This is more predominant with exertion. He has had worsening of daytime somnolence and sleep issues. He has had persisting fatigue over the course of the past 2 months as well as mild fluid gain.

SURGICAL HISTORY: The patient's past surgical history is positive for an appendectomy as a youth.

MEDICAL HISTORY:

1. Hypertension that has been under good control currently.
2. Asthma that is under fair control; the asthma is of chronic obstructive nature.
3. Chronic back pain, treated with a TENS unit.
4. Diverticulosis.
5. Dysphagia.

CURRENT MEDICATIONS:

1. Albuterol inhaler 4 puffs q.i.d.
2. Allegra 180 mg q.d.
3. Aspirin 325 mg, 6 tablets q.d. on a p.r.n. basis.
4. Flovent inhaler 4 puffs b.i.d.
5. Labetalol 300 mg b.i.d.
6. Nasacort AQ 2 sprays b.i.d.
7. Norvasc 5 mg q.d.
8. Protonix 40 mg 1 tablet per day. He has been using 2 recently.
9. Serevent inhaler 2 puffs q.i.d.

ALLERGIES: Ultram.

FAMILY HISTORY: Positive for emphysema in his father, who died at a young age from an accident. Mother is age 67, has had abdominal issues and surgery from noncarcinoma issues, about which he is nonspecific. The patient is the second of five children, having three brothers and one sister, all of whom are in good health.

SOCIAL HISTORY: The patient is disabled secondary to his chronic back pain. He is married. He relates eating a non–heart-healthy diet, high in fatty products. He is a nonsmoker. He averages 4 to 5 glasses of wine and 10 to 12 beers a week in alcohol intake. He has very limited exercise, including any active walking, secondary to his chronic back pain.

REVIEW OF SYSTEMS: No worsening of his headache issues. No change in mentation. Hearing is gone in the right ear and diminished some in the left. His vision has been intact. Appetite has been good. He shows positive weight gain. He has no difficulty swallowing. He relates his dyspepsia/GERD has been worsening with some abdominal discomfort, postprandial specifically. He has had a nontender lower abdomen, predominantly the upper bothering him more. This radiates upward somewhat, specifically in his sleep. His sleep pattern has been disturbed. He relates chronic fatigue issues in the past month and has had worsening of the dyspepsia and GERD despite the use of proton pump inhibitor. No constipation; regular bowel movements. No dysuria or polyuria. Occasional nocturia. No aches or pains in the extremities but notes slight swelling of his legs. He has had some shortness of breath on exertion, specifically on stairways, but denies any type of chest pain of a cardiac nature. He relates immobility issues secondary to chronic pain as well as worsening shortness of breath.

PHYSICAL EXAMINATION: His examination today shows he is age 32 and is in no apparent distress. Slightly pale in color. Weight is 202 pounds. Height is 5 feet 5 inches. Blood pressure is 118/78. Pulse is 80 and regular. Respiratory rate is 20. He is afebrile at 96.4 degrees. HEENT: Negative for discharge or deformity. The right tympanic membrane is severely scarred. The left shows a bolus-type effusion. No tenderness to the tragus, auricle, or mastoid process. Pupils are equal, round, and light accommodating. Nondilated funduscopy reveals no nicking or scarring. No tenderness of sinuses. Nasal and oral mucosa is pink and moist. There is extreme gag reflex elicited on attempt to view the posterior oropharynx. Neck is soft and supple. No lymphadenopathy. No supraclavicular nodes are noted. There are no carotid bruits. Cranial nerves II–XII are grossly intact. Lateralization Weber to the left as well as air-to-bone conduction being normal on the left and extremely reduced hearing on the right. Thorax: Scattered wheezes throughout; no crackles are noted. Cardiac: S1 and S2 with a 1/6 systolic murmur, best heard at the base on the right side of the sternum at the second and third intercostal space. This does not seem to change during inhalation, exhalation, or positioning. Abdomen is round, obese, with tenderness of the upper right quadrant with palpation as well as the epigastric region, which promotes some issue of reflux to the esophagus on deep palpation. The lower part of the abdomen is nontender. No rebound tenderness. Bowel sounds are present throughout. Normal-appearing male genitalia. Negative for inguinal hernia. Rectal exam reveals sphincter tone intact. Prostate is firm, mildly tender but more of a pressure sensation. Stool is guaiac negative for occult blood. There is edema of the lower extremities, +2. Skin is warm and dry. Sensation is intact.

LABORATORY DATA: Laboratory analysis conducted at this time for an amylase, lipase, comprehensive metabolic panel, CBC, TSH, T4, lipid panel, PSA for screening, and *H. pylori.* Results at this time show his triglycerides to be 1410, total cholesterol 266. His hepatic panel shows his bilirubin total at 0.4. His AST is 69 with ALT of 75. Total protein is 7.4. BUN is 18, sodium 137, chloride 102, creatinine 0.8, glucose mildly elevated at 117. His albumin is 3.7, alkaline phosphatase 79. Amylase is 40. WBC 4.67, hemoglobin 14.6, hematocrit 42.2; monocytes elevated at 12.8. He is negative for *H. pylori* antibody.

PLAN: The patient will be admitted to general medical, with pancreatitis and shortness of breath with exertion. Vital signs will be q.4h. times three, then q. shift. He will have bathroom privileges. The patient will be n.p.o. Will establish an IV of D5 half normal saline at 100 cc per hour. He will have sequentials on while in bed. I&Os will be done with daily weights on his chart. Will obtain an echocardiogram for Dr. Elhart to read and obtain a 1-day stress test if possible, and if the patient is in stable condition secondary to his shortness of breath on Monday or Tuesday at the time of his discharge. He will be on O_2 on a p.r.n. basis per nasal cannula to keep saturations greater than 90%. He will receive albuterol nebs q.i.d. and p.r.n.; Flovent inhaler 4 puffs b.i.d.; Serevent inhaler 2 puffs b.i.d. We will place him on Labetalol 20 mg IV b.i.d.; Nasacort AQ 2 sprays b.i.d.; and Protonix 40 mg IV q.d. Consideration for implementation of Tricor 160 mg as soon as the amylase and lipase are both showing negative.

Secondary to the patient's intense gag reflex, we will refrain from placing an NG or Cor-Flo at this time and see whether adequate hydration and n.p.o. status will help resolve.

Chest x-ray was obtained via the dictation line, showing a stable appearance from the previous film, which had been done here in the clinic, free of any acute infiltrates.

His right upper quadrant underwent ultrasound, which was negative for cholelithiasis or cholecystitis, and the head of the pancreas appeared to be near normal from what was able to be visualized with the rest obscured secondary to bowel gas.

The patient will be admitted to the hospital. Discussion in the event of blood and blood products that the patient has no religious beliefs contraindicating the aspect of the blood transfusion. The risks and benefits were explained, including transfusion reaction, hepatitis, HIV, incompatibility, and other risks. The patient does agree to this, and I explained to him that unless it was an emergent situation that discussion would be held again at the time if something did arise where he required blood, that there would be a further explanation discussing the risks and benefits of that being held. Both he and his wife agreed with this. He will be admitted at this time to the floor as a code level I.

1-4A:

SERVICE CODE(S): ______________________

DX CODE(S): ______________________

CASE 1-4A DISCUSSION

Pancreatitis

In the Plan section of the report, the physician indicates that he is admitting the patient with "pancreatitis and shortness of breath with exertion." Pancreatitis is an inflammation of the pancreas and can be either in an acute (577.0) or chronic form (577.1). The ultrasound was performed to determine the status of the pancreas. The shortness of breath on exertion is often a symptom of a problem with the heart, and the physician ordered a stress test be conducted by Dr. Elhart (under the Plan section). A chest x-ray was also done to assist in the diagnosis as to the origin of the shortness of breath. Code shortness of breath 786.05 is used to substantiate the medical necessity for the stress test.

This patient has numerous other conditions, such as hypertension, asthma, chronic back pain, diverticulosis, and dysphagia. These were not the primary reasons the service was provided, nor is there an indication that tests are going to be done regarding these additional diagnoses. The physician did order medications for some of these conditions, such as the patient's asthma (albuterol, Flovent, Serevent, Nasacort), hypertension (labetalol), and GERD (gastroesophageal reflex disease, Protonix); additionally the physician has ordered Tricor after laboratory workup. Tricor is prescribed for patients with primary hypercholesterolemia (excess cholesterol in the blood). In the inpatient setting, all of these conditions would be reported; but in the outpatient setting, we focus on reporting the condition(s) that prompted the encounter, which are pancreatitis and shortness of breath.

CASE 1-5
1-5A Initial Hospital Care
1-5B Progress Report

CASE 1-5

The patient in Case 1-5 is an 87-year-old female who is to be admitted by her nephrologist, Dr. Pleasant, after the patient had been seen in Dr. Pleasant's office that morning and comes to the emergency department to care for the patient.

1-5A INITIAL HOSPITAL CARE

LOCATION: Inpatient Hospital

PATIENT: Rosie Hovett

ATTENDING PHYSICIAN: Timothy L. Pleasant, M.D.

I am admitting this patient primarily because of symptomatic bradycardia secondary to medications. The patient is an 87-year-old woman who was recently discharged from the hospital after being diagnosed to new-onset atrial fibrillation with rapid ventricular response. The patient was started on medications with digoxin, labetalol, Cardizem, and metoprolol.

Since discharge from the hospital back on May 20, the patient has related that she has had some episodes of weakness. There were also some episodes when she was noted to be significantly hypotensive and feeling generally weak with some diaphoresis. Because these symptoms persisted, the patient then decided to come into the emergency room, where she was found to be in bradycardia, with a heart rate in the 40s to 50s. I think this is primarily brought about by the combination of digoxin, labetalol, Cardizem, and metoprolol. Therefore, at this time, the plan is to admit the patient to the telemetry unit and rule her out for MI because she is also at risk for that problem. At this time, I am going to hold the digoxin, labetalol, Cardizem, and metoprolol. Obviously we cannot hold the clonidine patch because this may lead to rebound hypertension. I will continue the rest of her medications except for the ones that I have mentioned above.

We will also check her cardiac enzymes to rule out MI.

The patient has a past medical and past surgical history that consists of the following:

1. Hypertension.
2. New-onset atrial fibrillation.
3. Thoracic abdominal aortic aneurysm.
4. Hyperthyroidism. I am not exactly sure which one she has—hyperthyroidism or hypothyroidism—because the discharge summary indicates the presence of hypothyroidism, whereas the admission history and physical per Dr. Green indicated hyperthyroidism. Nevertheless, she is not on any thyroid supplements. If she indeed is hypothyroid, this certainly could contribute to her present situation as well. We need to review her old medical records for this particular issue.

SOCIAL HISTORY: The patient is currently retired. She does have family here in town. She is widowed and lives on her own. She has an 86-pack-year smoking history. She denies any current or previous use of alcohol or intravenous or recreational drugs.

FAMILY HISTORY is positive for cancer and diabetes and negative for heart disease, hypertension, stroke, kidney disease, bleeding disorder, or dyscrasia. A sister has been diagnosed with breast cancer, and her two other sisters have been diagnosed with uterine cancer. There is a strong family history of diabetes in the immediate family.

MEDICATIONS currently being taken at home include the following:

1. Clonidine patch.
2. Digoxin 0.125 mg q.d.
3. Diltiazem CD 240 mg q.d.
4. Vasotec 10 mg q.d.
5. Labetalol 200 mg b.i.d.
6. Maalox extra strength 15 ml q.h.s.
7. Metoprolol 25 mg q.h.s.
8. Nitroglycerin sublingual 0.4 mg p.r.n.

ALLERGIES: No known drug allergies.

Latest laboratory results are as follows: Hemogram shows an H&H of 10.6/31.4, WBC 7.5, normochromic/normocytic indices, platelets 182. There is no left shift as neutrophils are only 63.6%. Chemistries are as follows: sodium 141, potassium 4.3, chloride 105, CO_2 27.2, BUN and creatinine 19.1/1, glucose 146, calcium 9.1. Digoxin level is 0.3, which is low. Magnesium level is 1.6. Cardiac enzymes are essentially unremarkable, as troponin is less than 0.3 and CK-MB is less than 1 and total CPK is 36. Thyroid function tests done on previous admission were well within normal limits, as TSH was measured to be 4.53.

REVIEW OF SYSTEMS: Constitutional: No fever or chills. No recent weight change. She appears to be fairly weak. No night sweats. Skin: No skin lesions. No active dermatosis. Eyes: No eye discharge. No eye itching. No visual changes. No diplopia. ENT: No ear discharge. No hearing difficulty. No pharyngeal hyperemia, congestion, or exudates. Lymph nodes: No lymphadenopathy in the neck, axillary, or groin.

Neurologic: Positive headaches. Positive gait instability. No falls. No seizures. Psychiatric: No behavioral changes. Neck: No thyromegaly. Respiratory: Positive cough. No colds. No hemoptysis. Positive for shortness of breath with strenuous exertion only. No colds. No hemoptysis. Cardiovascular: No chest pain. Positive palpitations. No orthopnea. No paroxysmal nocturnal dyspnea. Gastrointestinal: Positive anorexia. No nausea, vomiting, dysphagia, odynophagia, constipation, or diarrhea. No abdominal pain. No fecal incontinence. No hematemesis. No hematochezia. No melena. Genitourinary: No urgency, frequency, dysuria, hematuria, urinary incontinence, nocturia, vaginal discharge, vaginal lesions, or vaginal bleeding. Musculoskeletal: Positive joint pains. Positive occasional muscle pains/weaknesses. Hematologic: No bleeding tendencies. No purpura. No petechiae. No ecchymosis. Endocrinologic: No heat or cold intolerance.

PHYSICAL EXAMINATION: Vital signs are stable. Blood pressure is 117/80. Heart rate is in the 50s. Respirations 20. She is afebrile. Normocephalic, atraumatic. Pink palpebral conjunctivae, anicteric sclerae. No nasal or aural discharge. Moist tongue and buccal mucosa. No pharyngeal hyperemia, congestion, or exudate. Supple neck. No lymphadenopathy. Symmetrical chest expansion. No retractions. Positive rhonchi. A few bibasilar crackles. No wheezes. S1 and S2 are distinct. No S3 or S4. Regular rate and rhythm. Abdomen: Positive bowel sounds. Soft, nontender. Both upper and lower extremities reveal arthritic changes. Pulses are fair.

ASSESSMENT/PLAN:

1. Symptomatic bradycardia secondary to medications, namely, digoxin, labetalol, Cardizem, and metoprolol. Admit to telemetry. Check cardiac enzymes to rule out MI. Start enteric-coated aspirin 325 mg q.d.

Please note this patient also had a recent 2-D echocardiogram performed by Dr. Monson showing a normal overall LV systolic function, 3+ mitral insufficiency, 1–2+ aortic insufficiency, 2–3+ tricuspid insufficiency, 1+ pulmonic valve insufficiency, and moderate pulmonary hypertension.

2. Anemia, questionable etiology. Would need to review old medical records to see whether this has been worked up already. Anemia in this elderly age group needs to be evaluated more closely because the possibility of malignancy runs high on the list.
3. History of hypothyroidism, stable. She is not requiring thyroid supplements. As noted above, the latest TSH level was well within normal limits.
4. Thoracic abdominal aortic aneurysm, stable.
5. Hypertension. Blood pressure right now is well controlled with a systolic blood pressure ranging from 117 to 120. There may be a possibility of her blood pressure going up because we are withholding three of her blood pressure medications, namely, labetalol, Cardizem, and metoprolol. At this time, we just have to continue to observe the patient, and if blood pressure goes up to higher levels, then we may consider starting the patient on either labetalol or Norvasc.
6. Atrial fibrillation. I am wondering why this patient was not placed on anticoagulation. We will check PT and INR. We will discuss with Dr. Green on Monday whether or not the patient needs to be anticoagulated or whether there is a contraindication that was noted in the past.

We will continue to follow up on this patient from the critical care standpoint.

I-5A:

SERVICE CODE(S): ______________________

DX CODE(S): ______________________

CASE I-5A DISCUSSION

Well-Controlled or Stable Conditions

This report is an excellent example of how you can identify the most important and therefore, reportable diagnoses. Note that under the Assessment/Plan section of the report there are 6 diagnoses stated and 3 are stated to be well controlled or stable. These controlled or stable conditions are not usually reported in the outpatient setting—hypothyroidism, aortic aneurysm, and hypertension. This leaves the bradycardia, anemia, and atrial fibrillation as the reason this service was provided.

Cardiac Dysrhythmia

The cardiac dysrhythmia (427) of bradycardia (427.89) is also known as bradyarrhythmia and is defined as fewer than 60 beats per minute. (Tachyarrhythmia or tachycardia is a condition in which the heart beats in excess of 100 per minute.) Bradycardia can have many origins, such as central nervous system disease, infectious disease, or vascular disease. The bradycardia in this report is a symptom of a condition yet to be identified.

Another cardiac dysrhythmia is fibrillation. Fibrillation is an involuntary contraction of a muscle. Atrial fibrillation (427.31) is a cardiac dysrhythmia of the atrial myocardium in which the atria quivers continuously in an irregular pattern. This is also known as AFib or AF. A Vfib or VF is a ventricular fibrillation (427.41) involving the ventricular muscle of the heart. Note that the codes are different for A/V fibrillation or flutter. These are two different conditions.

Anemia

Anemia is a reduction in number of erythrocytes or decrease in quality of hemoglobin. There are many types of anemia such as:

- Iron-deficiency anemia (280)
- Other deficiency anemias (281, pernicious, vitamin B_{12}, folate deficiency, etc.)
- Hereditary hemolytic anemias (282, thalassemias, sickle-cell, etc.)
- Acquired hemolytic anemias (283, autoimmune, non-autoimmune, hemoglobinuria, etc.)
- Aplastic anemia (284, constitutional, other specified, unspecified)
- Other and unspecified anemias (285, in chronic illness)

I-5B PROGRESS REPORT (99231–99233)

Dr. Pleasant, as the attending physician, continues to monitor Rosie Hovett's progress while she is in the hospital. Report his services.

LOCATION: Inpatient Hospital

PATIENT: Rosie Hovett

ATTENDING PHYSICIAN: Timothy L. Pleasant, M.D.

She states she feels much better today compared with yesterday, although she has some nausea. The patient was seen and examined and chart reviewed. The patient appears to be hemodynamically stable, not in any form of respiratory distress or compromise. No specific complaints. No chest pain. No shortness of breath. No diaphoresis. No nausea or vomiting. No palpitations. No diarrhea or constipation. No frequency, urgency, or dysuria.

PHYSICAL EXAMINATION: Vital signs are stable. Blood pressure is 133/54. Heart rate is 59. Respirations 20. She is saturating 96% on 2 liters O_2 nasal cannula. Temperature is 36.2°C. Normocephalic, atraumatic. Pink palpebral conjunctivae, anicteric sclerae. No nasal or aural discharge. Moist tongue and buccal mucosa. No pharyngeal hyperemia, congestion, or exudate. Supple neck. No lymphadenopathy. Symmetrical chest expansion. No retractions. Positive rhonchi. No crackles. No wheezes. S1 and S2 are indistinct. Regular rate and irregular rhythm. Abdomen: Positive bowel sounds. Soft, nontender. Both upper and lower extremities reveal arthritic changes. Pulses are fair.

Latest laboratory tests are as follows: sodium 144, potassium 4.9, chloride 107, CO_2 31.2, BUN and creatinine 15/0.8, glucose 94, calcium 8.8. Hemogram shows H&H of 10.7/32.2, WBC 7.28, normochromic/normocytic indices, and platelets 174. Cardiac enzymes have remained negative in the past 16 hours. Latest PT and INR are 12.5 and 1.1, respectively. It must be noted that this patient was discharged home and was not sent home on Coumadin. I am suspecting that this has something to do with her thoracic aortic aneurysm. I think this patient would still benefit, however, from anticoagulation because of her underlying atrial fibrillation. Her anemia is improving. (3)

IMPRESSION/PLAN: (2)

(1)
1. Symptomatic bradycardia secondary to medications, namely, labetalol, Cardizem, digoxin, and metoprolol. Cardiac enzymes remain negative, suggesting MI has been ruled out. Will check 12-lead ECG. Her blood pressure right now appears to be well controlled with the Clonidine patch, Vasotec 10 mg q.d., and nitroglycerin sublingual p.r.n. At this time, she does not require initiation of the other antihypertensive medications, which were held at the time of admission.

Await cardiology consult. I did speak with Dr. Elhart from cardiology yesterday, who feels that because most of the recent clinical scenario resulted from overzealous use of heart rate allowing medications, it is worthwhile to keep this medication on hold before reconsidering the issue of pacemaker.

I-5B:

SERVICE CODE(S): ______________________

DX CODE(S): ______________________

CASE I-5B DISCUSSION

Report 1-5B is a good example of the type of report that does not contain all of the diagnoses within the Impression/Plan section of the report. Again, you must focus on the primary reason the service is being provided to this patient. Remember, that you only have this one progress report available to you when the service is coded. According to the Impression/Plan section, the patient has bradycardia due to previously prescribed medications. It is not until the entire report is read that the additional diagnoses of atrial fibrillation (second to last sentence of Physical Examination section) and "Her anemia is improving" (last sentence of Physical Examination section) are noted. Both the atrial fibrillation and anemia are reported. There is mention of nausea in the first line of the report, which could be reported with (787.02), although the physician made no mention of a treatment for the condition nor correlated it to any current condition.

CASE 1-6
1-6A Progress Report

CASE 1-6

Dr. Pleasant has been the attending physician for the patient in Case 1-6 while the patient's physician, Dr. Alanda, was out of town on a personal emergency. Dr. Pleasant is providing the last service to the patient because Dr. Alanda is returning this evening from out of town and will assume responsibility for the patient. Report Dr. Pleasant's service.

1-6A PROGRESS REPORT (99231—99233)

LOCATION: Inpatient Hospital

PATIENT: Kyle Ottegard

ATTENDING PHYSICIAN: Timothy L. Pleasant, M.D.

The patient was seen and examined and chart reviewed. The patient appears to be hemodynamically stable, not in any form of respiratory distress or compromise. No abdominal pain today and no dyspepsia noted. One of other complaints he had on admission is that of left otalgia pain. Since we started him on empiric antibiotic coverage with IV Claforan, this has not been bothering him anymore. We are still awaiting ENT consultation at this time.

PHYSICAL EXAMINATION: Vital signs are stable. Blood pressure is 143/82. Heart rate is 82. Respirations 24. Saturating 97% on room air. Temperature is 36.6°∞C. Normocephalic, atraumatic. Pink palpebral conjunctivae, anicteric sclerae. No nasal or aural discharge. Moist tongue and buccal mucosa. No pharyngeal hyperemia, congestion, or exudate. Supple neck. No JVD. No lymphadenopathy. No bruits. Symmetrical chest expansion. No retractions. No rhonchi. No crackles. No wheezes. S1 and S2 are distinct. No S3 or S4. Regular rate and irregular rhythm. Abdomen: Positive bowel sounds. Soft, nontender, obese. Both upper and lower extremities reveal no gross deformities or edema. Pulses are full and equal.

ASSESSMENT/PLAN:

1. Abdominal pain. Pancreatitis, ruled out. Severe hypertriglyceridemia of 1410 mg/dl. Continue low-fat, low-cholesterol diet. Continue Tricor 160 mg q.d. with meals.
2. Left ear infection, questionable. The patient has been started on IV Claforan and has been clinically responsive to that medication.

At this time, we are awaiting the ENT consultation. It is hoped that the patient can be discharged by Dr. Alanda's service and be followed up in 6 weeks for recheck of his cholesterol and triglyceride profile.

Dr. Alanda will reassume care tomorrow.

1-6A:

SERVICE CODE(S): ______________________

DX CODE(S): ______________________

CASE 1-6A DISCUSSION

Hypertriglyceridemia

The first numbered item of the Assessment/Plan section of the report indicates diagnoses of abdominal pain and hypertriglyceridemia. Hypertriglyceridemia is a condition in which there are excessive triglycerides and very low-density lipoproteins in the blood. A lipoprotein is a protein wrapped around cholesterol (272.0), lipids (272.2), or triglycerides (272.1).

- High-density lipoproteins (HDL, mostly phospholipids and protein) are the "good" cholesterol.
- Low-density lipoproteins (LDL, mostly cholesterol and protein) are the "bad" cholesterol.
- Very low-density lipoproteins (VLDL, primarily triglyceride and protein) are the "very bad" cholesterol.

Pancreatitis has been "ruled out" as a diagnosis and, as such, will not be reported in the outpatient setting. The ear infection is only "suspected" and not confirmed, so as such cannot be reported. The ear pain (otalgia 388.70) can be reported as it is mentioned.

"Rule out" means the condition is *going to be* either proven to exist or not to exist. "Ruled out" means that the diagnosis *has already been* proven not to exist.

CASE 1-7

Dr. Pleasant is the attending physician for Arnold Gonzalez. Report Dr. Pleasant's service.

1-7A PROGRESS REPORT

LOCATION: Inpatient Hospital

PATIENT: Arnold Gonzalez

ATTENDING PHYSICIAN: Timothy L. Pleasant, M.D.

The patient was seen and the chart reviewed. The patient appears to be hemodynamically stable, not in respiratory distress or compromise.

PHYSICAL EXAMINATION: Vital signs are stable. Blood pressure is 132/72. Heart rate is 108. Respirations 20s. Saturating 94% on room air. Input and output in the last 24 hours is 3796/1925. Normocephalic, atraumatic. Pink palpebral conjunctivae, anicteric sclerae. Symmetrical chest expansion. Positive rhonchi. Positive crackles. No wheezes. S1 and S2 are indistinct. No S3 or S4. Irregular rhythm, tachycardiac rate, no rubs. Abdomen: Decreased bowel sounds, soft and nontender. Both upper and lower extremities reveal arthritic changes. Pulses are fair.

Latest labs are as follows: Sodium 141, potassium 4.6, chloride 115, CO_2 17.4, BUN and creatinine 50/1.4, glucose 112, calcium and phosphorus are 8.1 and 2.2, respectively, magnesium 1.4, and albumin 1.1. Digoxin level is 2.4. Latest hemogram shows H&H of 10.5/33.2, WBC 13.32, platelets 108. PT and INR are 13 and 1.2, respectively.

ASSESSMENT/PLAN:

1. Acute renal failure/chronic renal failure. The patient has had improved urine output.
2. Status post ruptured appendix with cecectomy.
   a. Nutrition. After reviewing patient's electrolytes, I would recommend resuming the same tube feedings except with additives of 10 mEq potassium phosphate/L and 10 mEq sodium plus citrate/L. Recommend checking chemistries again in the morning.
3. Status post tracheostomy. Continue inhaler treatments.
4. Anemia of chronic illness/chronic renal disease.
5. Questionable small bowel obstruction.
6. New onset atrial fibrillation. The patient is now day two of Coumadin 5 mg q.d. Target INR is 2–3. It was decided not to heparinize this patient anymore but to proceed with Coumadin anticoagulation outright.

Yesterday afternoon I was called in because the patient was due to receive a fourth dose of 0.25 mg digoxin IV push, but his heart rate was already in the 80s. Therefore, I recommended decreasing the dose to 0.125 instead of the previously ordered 0.25 mg. This morning his digoxin level turned out to be 2.4; therefore, we are going to hold the digoxin today. His heart rate, however, remains in the 90s to 100 range.

1-7A:

SERVICE CODE(S): ____________________

DX CODE(S): ____________________

CASE 1-7A DISCUSSION

Renal Failure

Acute renal failure (584.X) is sudden onset of renal failure. It can be caused by trauma, infection, inflammation, or exposure to a toxic substance (toxicity). There are several types of acute renal failure:

- Prerenal
  - Associated with poor systemic perfusion
  - Decreased renal blood flow
    - Such as with congestive heart failure
- Intrarenal
  - Associated with renal parenchyma disease (functional tissue of kidney)
    - Such as acute interstitial nephritis
- Postrenal
  - Resulting from urine flow obstruction out of kidney

The symptoms of acute renal failure are uremia (excess of urea in the blood), oliguria (decreased output) or anuria (no output), hyperkalemia (high potassium in the blood), and pulmonary edema. Treatment involves resolution of the underlying condition, dialysis, and monitoring the patient's fluid and electrolyte balance. Acute renal failure is usually a reversible condition.

Chronic renal failure (585.X) is a gradual loss of function that involves progressively more severe renal insufficiency until the end stage of end-stage renal disease (ESRD) or irreversible kidney failure is reached. The cause is often exposure to nephrotoxins. The symptoms are polyuria, nausea or anorexia, dehydration, and neurological manifestations.

Unspecified renal failure (586) is renal failure that is not documented as acute or chronic.

Chronic kidney disease is referred to as a specific stage (I, II, III, IV, V), end-stage, or unspecified chronic kidney disease. The stages are based on the glomerular filtration rate (GFR). In Stage I the kidney is damaged, but the GFR is normal or near normal. In Stage II there is a mild decrease in the GFR; in Stage III there is a moderate decrease in the GFR; in the Stage IV there is a severe decrease in the GFR; and in Stage 5 there is kidney failure or the patient is on dialysis. In each of the stages, the patient may recover kidney function, but in end-stage renal disease the patient will not recover without a kidney transplant. If the stage is documented, report the diagnosis that corresponds to that stage (585.1-585.5). If the documentation indicates end-stage renal disease or end-stage kidney disease, assign 585.6. If the documentation indicates nonspecific diagnostic statements such as "chronic renal disease" or "chronic renal insufficiency," report 585.9.

According to the *Official Guidelines for Coding and Reporting,* Section 1.10., the coder is to report both an acute and chronic condition if there are separate subentries in the Alphabetic Index of the ICD-9-CM at the same indentation level. The acute condition is sequenced first, and the chronic condition is sequenced second.

Circumstances of the Encounter

In Case 1-5B, you were presented information about anemia, and the anemia in this case is that in a chronic illness. The code for the anemia is reported in conjunction with the code(s) that describe the underlying chronic illness and are sequenced according to the circumstances of the encounter. If the patient encounter is primarily for the anemia in end-stage renal disease, the anemia code would be reported first, but if the anemia is not the primary reason for the encounter, it is not reported first.

Again, questionable, probable, suspected, ruled out, or rule out are not reported by outpatient coders.

CASE 1-8
1-8A Progress Report

CASE 1-8

Dr. Pleasant provides a follow-up service to a patient he admitted to the hospital to rule out pancreatitis.

1-8A PROGRESS REPORT

LOCATION: Inpatient Hospital

PATIENT: Corrbet Zornomba

ATTENDING PHYSICIAN: Timothy L. Pleasant, M.D.

The patient was seen and examined and chart reviewed. The patient appears to be hemodynamically stable, not in any form of respiratory distress or compromise. No specific complaints. No abdominal pain or dyspepsia since admission to the hospital.

Amylase and lipase values have been obtained, and both are within normal limits.

PHYSICAL EXAMINATION: Vital signs are stable. Blood pressure is 126/61. Heart rate is 63. Respirations 18. Saturating 96% on room air. Temperature is 35.7° C.

Normocephalic, atraumatic. Pink palpebral conjunctivae, anicteric sclerae. No nasal or aural discharge. Moist tongue and buccal mucosa. No pharyngeal hyperemia, congestion, or exudate. Supple neck. No JVD. No lymphadenopathy. No bruits. Symmetrical chest expansion. No retractions. No rhonchi. No crackles. No wheezes. S1 and S2 are distinct. No S3 or S4. Regular rate and rhythm. Abdomen: Positive bowel sounds. Soft and nontender. Both upper and lower extremities reveal no gross deformities or edema. Pulses are full and equal.

ASSESSMENT/PLAN:

1. Abdominal pain. Pancreatitis ruled out. Severe hypertriglyceridemia at 1410 mg/dl. The plan right now is to start him on clear liquids and then to advance his feedings as tolerated to a low-fat, low-cholesterol diet. We will start him on Tricor 160 mg daily with his evening meal.
2. Hypothyroidism. We will restart Synthroid p.o. May discontinue IV Synthroid.
3. Hypertension, fairly controlled. We will start Labetalol and Norvasc p.o.
4. We will discontinue all IV medications at this time as he is going to be started on oral feedings.

At this time, we will continue to monitor the patient's progress and plan for discharge sometime on Monday with subsequent follow-up with Dr. Alanda.

We will continue to follow this patient from the critical care standpoint.

1-8A:

SERVICE CODE(S): ____________________

DX CODE(S): ____________________

CASE 1-8A DISCUSSION

In the Assessment/Plan section of the report, the diagnoses listed are abdominal pain, hypertriglyceridemia, hypothyroidism, and hypertension, and these conditions are being treated. Note that pancreatitis was ruled out and would therefore not be reported.

CASE 1-9
1-9A Discharge Summary

CASE 1-9

Today, Dr. Pleasant is discharging the patient. Report Dr. Pleasant's service.

1-9A DISCHARGE SUMMARY (99238–99239)

LOCATION: Inpatient Hospital

PATIENT: Corrbet Zornomba

ATTENDING PHYSICIAN: Timothy L. Pleasant, M.D.

REASON FOR ADMISSION: Chronic duodenal ulcer

SUMMARY OF HOSPITAL COURSE: The patient is a 60-year-old female with a history of ulcer disease that failed medical management. She was subsequently referred to Dr. Friendly for partial duodenectomy. On Monday, the patient was admitted and taken to the operating room, where she underwent exploratory laparotomy with partial duodenectomy. All pathology reports were benign. The patient tolerated the procedure well. She had an epidural in place following this, and she was transferred to the ICU for observation postoperatively. (The epidural was "in place" in her back for pain control.)

The patient did well in the ICU, and by Thursday the patient was ready for transfer to the floor. By Saturday, her ileus was resolving, her NG discontinued, and she was started on a diet. By Monday, the patient was tolerating a regular diet. Her Jackson-Pratts were removed. She was afebrile with stable vital signs and was ready for discharge home.

DISCHARGE INSTRUCTIONS: Activity as tolerated. Diet as tolerated.

DISCHARGE MEDICATIONS: Tylenol no. 3, 1 or 2 tablets p.o. q.4h. p.r.n. pain.

FOLLOW-UP: The patient is to call for an appointment with Dr. Friendly.

CONDITION ON DISCHARGE: Improved.

DISCHARGE DIAGNOSIS:
1. Chronic duodenal ulcer

PROCEDURE PERFORMED: Duodenectomy

1-9A:

SERVICE CODE(S): ______________________

DX CODE(S): ______________________

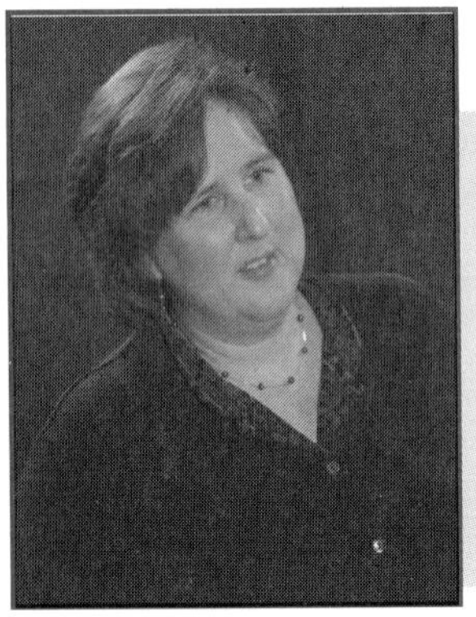

FROM THE TRENCHES

Kathy

"You can be the best physician in the world–the most brilliant, compassionate physician of all time–but if you're not bringing the money in, the doors will not stay open and the lights will not stay on for very long. Your coding is very important because that's what keeps you in business. Doctors have to see that there are two sides to their practice... they can't do one without the other."

Consultations, Prolonged Services, Physician Standby, and Critical Care Services

Consultation Services

When physicians need opinions and advice, they ask another physician for an opinion or advice on the treatment, diagnosis, or management of a patient. The physician asking for the advice or opinion is making a **request for consultation** and is the **requesting physician.** The physician giving the advice is providing a consultation and is the **consultant.** Consultations can be done for both outpatients and inpatients. The CPT manual has different codes for each of the two types of patient consultation–*outpatient* and *inpatient.*

"Request for consultation" used to be termed "referral"; making a referral meant that the referring physician was asking for the advice or opinion of another physician (a consultation). Some third-party payers have chosen to define "referral" to mean a total transfer of the care of a patient. In other words, if a patient is referred by physician A to physician B, physician A is expecting physician B to evaluate and treat the patient for the condition for which the patient is being referred. The services of physician B would *not* be reported using consultation codes. On the other hand, if physician A makes a request for a consultation to physician B, it is expected that physician B will provide physician A with his or her advice or opinion and that the patient will return to physician A for any necessary treatment. Physician B would then report his or her services using consultation codes. Although these semantics (uses of words) may seem unimportant, they make a difference in the codes you use to report the services.

In the Consultation subsection, the two subheadings of consultations are:

1. Office or Other Outpatient Consultations (99241–99245)
2. Initial Inpatient Consultations (99251–99255)

Office or Other Outpatient Consultations and Initial Inpatient Consultations define the location in which the service is rendered; the patient is either an outpatient or an inpatient. Both subheadings are for new or established patients.

Only one initial consultation is reported by a consultant for the patient on each admission, and any subsequent service is reported using codes from the Subsequent Hospital Care codes (99231–99233).

A **consultation** is a service provided by a physician whose opinion or advice regarding the management or diagnosis of a *specific problem* has been requested. The consultant provides a written report of the opinion or advice to the attending physician and documents the opinion and services provided in the medical record; the care of the patient is thus complete. Sometimes the attending physician will request the consultant to assume responsibility for a specific area of the patient's care. For example, a consultant may be asked by the attending physician to see an inpatient regarding the care of the patient's diabetes while the patient is hospitalized for gallbladder surgery. After the initial consultation, the attending physician may ask the consultant to continue to monitor the patient's diabetic condition. The consultant assumes responsibility for management of the patient in the specific area of diabetes. Subsequent visits made by the consultant would then be coded using the codes from the subheading Subsequent Hospital Care.

Documentation in the medical record for a consultation must show a request from the attending physician for an opinion or the advice of a consultant on a specific condition. Findings and treatments rendered during the consultation must be documented in the medical record by the consultant and communicated to the attending physician. A consultant can order tests and services for an inpatient, but the medical necessity of all tests and services must be indicated in the medical record.

Office or Other Outpatient Consultations The Office or Other Outpatient Consultations codes (99241–99245) are used to code consultative services provided a patient in an office or other ambulatory patient setting, including hospital observation services, home services, custodial care, and services that are provided in a domiciliary, rest home, or emergency department. Outpatient consultations include consultations provided in the emergency department because the patient is considered an outpatient in the emergency department setting. The codes are for both new and established patients and are of increasing complexity, based on the three key components and any contributing factors.

Initial Inpatient Consultations The codes in the Initial Inpatient Consultations subheading (99251–99255) are used to report services by physicians in inpatient settings. This subheading is used for both new and established patients and can be reported only one time per patient admission per consulting physician. After the initial consultation report, the subsequent hospital visit codes would be used to report services.

A patient may have more than one concurrent (at the same time) consultant during an admission. For example, the attending physician may request a consultant, an endocrinologist, to render an opinion on a patient's diabetes, while at the same time another consultant, a cardiologist, is rendering an opinion on the patient's heart murmur.

Critical Care Services

Critical Care Services codes are used to identify services that are provided during medical emergencies to patients who are either critically ill or injured. These service codes require the physician to be constantly available to the patient and provide services exclusively to that patient. For example, a patient who is in shock or cardiac arrest would require the physician to provide bedside critical care services. Critical care is often, but not required to be, provided in an acute care setting of a hospital. Acute care settings are intensive care units, coronary care units, emergency departments, pediatric intensive care units, and similar critical care units of a hospital. Codes in this subsection are listed according to the *time* the physician spends providing critical care to the patient.

The total critical care time, per day, the physician spends in care of the patient is stated in one amount of time, even if the time was not concurrent. Code 99291 is used only once a day. As an example, if a physician sees a critical care patient for 74 minutes and then leaves and returns for 30 minutes of critical care at a later time in the same day, the coding would be for 104 minutes of care. The coding for 104 minutes would be:

99291 for the 74 minutes
99292 for the additional 30 minutes

The physician must document the times in the medical record. Code 99291 is reported for the first 30 to 74 minutes of critical care, and code 99292 is used for the time beyond 74 minutes. If the critical care is less than 30 minutes, an E/M code would be used to report the service.

There are service codes that are bundled into the Critical Care Services codes. These services are normally provided to stabilize the patient. An example of this bundling is as follows: A physician starts ventilation management (94656) while providing critical care services to a patient in the intensive care unit of a hospital. The ventilator management is not reported separately but, instead, is considered to be bundled into the Critical Care Services code. The notes preceding the critical care codes in the CPT manual list the services and procedures bundled into the codes. If the physician provided a service at the same time as critical care and that service is not bundled into the code, the service could be reported separately. You will know what is bundled into the codes because this information is listed either in the extensive description of the code or in the notes preceding the code. Be certain to read these notes, as they contain many exclusions and inclusions for these codes.

If the patient is in a critical care unit but is stable, you report the services using codes from the Hospital Inpatient Services subsection, Subsequent Hospital Care subheading or from the Consultations subsection, Inpatient or Follow-up Inpatient subheadings.

Prolonged Physician Services

In the Prolonged Services subsection there are three subheadings:

- Prolonged Physician Services with Direct (Face-to-Face) Patient Contact
- Prolonged Physician Services without Direct (Face-to-Face) Patient Contact
- Physician Standby Services

Prolonged Physician Services codes are all add-on codes, except for the codes in the Physician Standby Services subheading. Note the plus symbol (+) beside all codes in the range 99354 to 99359. Because add-on codes can be used only with another code, all Prolonged Physician Services codes are intended to be used only in addition to other codes to show an addition to some other service. The following example illustrates the use of these codes.

> ***EXAMPLE:*** An established patient with a history of asthma presents, in an office visit, with acute bronchospasm and moderate respiratory distress. The physician conducts a problem focused history followed by a problem focused examination, which shows a respiratory rate of 30, and labored breathing and wheezing are heard in all lung fields. Office treatment is initiated; it includes intermittent bronchial dilation and subcutaneous epinephrine. The service requires the physician to have intermittent face-to-face contact with the patient over a 2-hour period. The MDM complexity is low.

The office visit service would be reported using the office visit code 99212, but the additional time the physician spent providing service to the patient over and above that which is indicated in code 99212 would have to be coded using a prolonged services code. As the notes indicate, the first 30 minutes of prolonged services are not counted but are considered part of the initial service. So you cannot use a prolonged services code until after the first 30 minutes of the prolonged services have been provided. The physician, therefore, has to spend 60 minutes with the patient in prolonged services before it is possible to code for 30 minutes using code 99354. That takes care of 1 hour of our physician's time for the case above. Now what about the next hour?

Read the description for the indented code 99355. The description states that 99355 is to be used for each additional 30 minutes, but this is where the second-time rule applies. You can use 99355 only if the physician has spent at least 15 minutes providing service over and above the first 60 minutes. The physician in this example spent 1 hour beyond the first 60 minutes providing service, so you can report 99355 twice. The coding for the case is 99212 for the office visit, 99354 for the first hour of prolonged services, and 99355 ×2 for the next hour.

The time the physician spends providing the prolonged services does not have to be continuous, as is the situation in this example; the physician monitored the patient on an intermittent basis, coming into the room to check on the patient and then leaving the room. However, the time must be documented in the patient record.

Let's change this case a bit and see how the coding changes. If the physician spent 70 minutes with the patient, you could code only the first hour at 99354. The additional 10 minutes beyond the first 60 are not coded separately. Remember that you would need at least 15 minutes beyond the first hour to code for the time beyond the first hour. For help in applying these codes, note the table preceding the Critical Care codes; there you can locate the total time your physician spent with the patient and see an example of the correct coding.

Prolonged Physician Services with Direct (face-to-face) Patient Contact codes describe services that require the physician to have direct contact with the patient. However, the Prolonged Physician Services without Direct (Face-to-Face) Patient Contact codes describe services during which the physician is not in direct contact with the patient. For example, a physician evaluates an established patient, a 70-year-old female with dementia, in an office visit. The physician then spends an extensive amount of time discussing the patient's condition, her treatment plan, and other recommendations with the patient's daughter. The services are reported using an office visit code for the patient evaluation and the appropriate Prolonged Physician Services without Direct Patient Contact code for the time spent with the daughter.

Prolonged Physician Services codes are most often used with the higher level E/M codes, which themselves carry longer time frames.

Prolonged Physician Services with Direct Patient Contact codes are divided on the basis of whether the services were provided to an outpatient or an inpatient.

Physician Standby Services

The codes for Physician Standby Services are used when a physician, at the request of the attending physician, is standing by in case his or her services are needed. The standby physician cannot be rendering services to another patient during this time. The standby codes are reported in increments of 30 minutes. The 30-minute increments refer to the 1st to 30th minute and do not have any of the complicated rules for reporting time that exist for reporting prolonged or critical services. For example, a cardiac surgeon may "stand by" during a cardiac catheterization in case the procedure needs to be converted to open heart surgery. This standby time is reported for each increment of 30 minutes. If the surgeon must then perform an open heart surgery, the surgeon would not report the time spent in standby but would instead report the open heart procedure.

An important note concerning the standby codes is that these codes are used only when no service is performed and there is no face-to-face contact with the patient. These codes are *not* used when a standby status ends in the physician's providing a service to a patient. The service the physician provides is reported as any other service would be, even though it began as a physician standby service.

CASE 1-10
1-10A Consultation

CASE 1-10

Report Dr. Alanda's professional service.

I-10A CONSULTATION (99241-99245

LOCATION: Outpatient, Clinic

PATIENT: Gloria Freeman

PRIMARY CARE PHYSICIAN: Leslie Alanda, M.D.

CONSULTANT: Elmer Lauer, M.D.

The patient is a 37-year-old female I am asked to see by Dr. Alanda regarding painful varicose veins located on her lower left thigh posteriorly. These developed after her pregnancies. She works in a nursing home and does get rather severe pain when she is up on her feet for long periods. She does use support hose but has not used any Jobst support stockings. She has had no previous pelvic radiation. She has had no previous deep vein thrombosis. She has had a hysterectomy in July for endometriosis.

CURRENT MEDICATIONS: Premarin q.d.

PHYSICAL EXAMINATION: On examination there are no obvious varicosities involving the saphenous vein of either leg. The only area of varicosities is located in the posterior surface of the lower left thigh. These are small to moderate-sized veins.

We discussed in detail indications for vein stripping as well as sclerotherapy. I talked about the risks of sclerotherapy, including skin slough, induration, pigmentation, as well as recurrence. She wanted to have the veins injected. I explained to her that I have stopped injecting veins mainly because of patients' high expectations with venous sclerotherapy. The other problem is that at this time we are not able to get 3% sodium tetradecyl sulfate. Given the location of these veins in the upper leg, I think that if any injection were to be done, I would recommend using the 3% solution just because of the location. It is not known when this solution will become available again. We have been contacting the company periodically, and they are still not sure when they will have 3% solution on the market again.

We decided to give her a prescription for Jobst waist-high moderate support stockings to see if they work. I told her she could call us in 3 months to see whether we have gotten the solution.

I-10A:

SERVICE CODE(S): ______________________

DX CODE(S): ______________________

CASE I-10A DISCUSSION

This patient presents with the CC of varicose veins, which are veins in which blood has pooled. Usually varicose veins occur in the saphenous veins of the leg and become distended. People who stand for long periods of time, cross their legs at the knees, or wear constricting garments are more prone to developing varicose veins. Conservative treatment for varicose veins is antiembolism stockings (such as Jobst) and the avoidance of other contributory factors, such as standing and crossing of legs. If the conservative treatment is not effective, saphenous vein stripping would be considered. If left untreated, varicose veins can develop and lead to venous stasis ulcers, which are susceptible to infection. ICD-9-CM codes for varicose veins are divided based on the location of the vein; lower extremities (454) and other sites (456). There are specific codes for lower extremities when there is ulcer (454.0); inflammation (454.1); ulcer and inflammation (454.2); other complications, such as edema, pain, and swelling; and asymptomatic (454.9), which are those without any symptoms.

Note that category 455 is hemorrhoids, which technically are varicose veins of the anus.

Varicose veins of other sites (456) are specific as to the location, such as esophageal (456.0 with bleeding, 456.1 without bleeding), sublingual (456.3), scrotal (456.4), pelvic (456.6), and varices of other sites (456.8).

CASE 1-11

Report Dr. Alanda's professional service.

1-11A CONSULTATION

LOCATION: Outpatient, Clinic

PATIENT: Gilda Spellhurst

PHYSICIAN: Leslie Alanda, M.D.

CONSULTANT: Elmer Lauer, M.D.

I was asked to evaluate the patient by the patient's primary for preparation for pending gastric resection. The patient was examined and the chart reviewed.

HISTORY OF PRESENT ILLNESS: She has been having problems with recurrent peptic ulcer disease despite therapy with Zantac and Prilosec. She had undergone several endoscopies, which revealed a large ulcer that was reported to be benign. The patient was also noted to have a slightly elevated CEA of 11. On June 30, the patient underwent laparoscopy, which turned out to be normal as well and benign. There were no signs of any lymphadenopathy.

PAST SURGICAL HISTORY:
1. Hysterectomy.
2. Tubal ligation.

The patient never has problems with surgery or anesthesia.

SOCIAL HISTORY: Positive for smoking. The patient denies alcohol abuse. She smokes about a pack per day.

FAMILY HISTORY: Negative for colonic carcinoma, premature coronary artery disease, but positive for severe peptic ulcer disease in her mother.

ALLERGIES: NONE.

REVIEW OF SYSTEMS: Negative for melena, hematochezia, and hematemesis.

PHYSICAL EXAMINATION demonstrates a slender Hispanic female in no acute distress. She is uncomfortable, however, because of epigastric discomfort. Her neck is supple. There is no thyromegaly or regional lymphadenopathy. No subclavicular or supraclavicular lymph nodes. ENT is within normal limits. Eyes: Sclerae anicteric. Conjunctivae are pale. Funduscopic exam shows no AV nicking, hemorrhages, exudates, or papilledema. Chest is barrel-shaped without dullness to percussion but with rhonchi scattered throughout the lung fields. Prolonged expiratory phase was noted. Cardiac exam: Regular rhythm. Distant heart sounds, 1/6 systolic ejection murmur at the base. Abdomen is soft and tender to palpation. Epigastric area without rebound, tenderness, or guarding. Liver span is 7 cm; edge at right costal margin. Aorta diameter is normal. Extremities: Upper and lower show no edema, cyanosis, or clubbing. Neurologic exam is nonfocal.

REVIEW OF LABORATORY ANALYSIS revealed hypercalcemia of 10.3, which is probably exaggerated by a low albumin and likely is to be more significant than that. Creatinine is 0.5. AST is 15. Cancer embryonic antigen is 11.5. *H. pylori* is 4.8.

IMPRESSION/PLAN: Nonhealing peptic ulcer disease. Patient's doctor increased her Prilosec to 2 a day and continue Zantac at the present dose. In fact, one might increase it to 300 mg b.i.d. if necessary. There is certainly a need to rule out Zollinger-Ellison and hyperparathyroidism as the source of the patient's nonhealing ulcer. C-terminal PTH will be checked along with ionized calcium. One might plan parahyperthyroidectomy simultaneous with gastrectomy if patient has high PTH, which I suspect will be the case, although in the case of treatment with H_2 blockers and Prilosec, a gastrin level might be elevated. Anyhow, we will check it and make sure that it is not extreme. If the gastrin level is high, one might consider complete gastrectomy rather than a partial one on the presumption of Z-E syndrome. The patient will be re-evaluated after results of the aforementioned tests are available and scheduled for surgery. Elevated CEA is bothersome. She has not had colonoscopy for some time and should it again be elevated, one might consider colonoscopy simultaneous during the same admission. The patient will be sent to Dr. Dawson. I am concerned with her pulmonary status. She is advised to curtail her cigarette consumption to as low as possible and switch to low-tar nicotine cigarettes in the interim. Once she is admitted, therapy with beta agonists and Atrovent will be immediately initiated, and the patient will be started on incentive spirometry.

Thank you for letting me see this interesting case. We discussed the aforementioned problem with the patient's primary, who will hold surgery for 1 week until all laboratory analyses are completed. A total of 80 minutes was spent with patient, and 55 minutes was spent going over the data in the patient's medical record.

1-11A:

SERVICE CODE(S): ____________________

DX CODE(S): ____________________

CASE 1-11A DISCUSSION

Ulcer

An ulcer is an erosive area or a break. The term *peptic* pertains to pepsin or to digestion. A peptic ulcer occurs on the mucosal lining of the stomach (531) or duodenum (532) that results in the submucosal areas being exposed to gastric secretions. The site may be unspecified (533) in the medical record. All three categories also have fourth digit subcategories for acute or chronic, with or without hemorrhage, and/or perforation. These categories have a fifth digit available to indicate those without mention of obstruction (0) and with mention of obstruction (1).

Tobacco Dependence

In Case 1-11A, note that the physician indicates her concern for the patient's pulmonary status and has advised the patient to stop her cigarette consumption or to keep the number of cigarettes smoked as low as possible. She also indicated that once the patient was admitted, pulmonary therapy was to be initiated (beta agonists, Atrovent, incentive spirometry). Given these statements in the medical documentation, the patient's dependency on tobacco will have to be reported (305.1).

CASE 1-12
1-12A Consultation
1-12B Progress Report
1-12C Progress Report

CASE 1-12

Report Dr. Pleasant's service.

1-12A CONSULTATION

LOCATION: Hospital Inpatient

PATIENT: Gladys Hanson

ATTENDING PHYSICIAN: Alma Naraquist, M.D.

CONSULTANT: Timothy L. Pleasant, M.D.

I am being consulted to see this patient primarily because of azotemia.

The patient is a 74-year-old white woman who had been admitted primarily because of right-sided hemiparesis secondary to a presumed cerebrovascular accident.

The patient has been followed up in the hospital by Dr. Naraquist.

She had laboratory work done recently, which showed the following results: sodium 139, potassium 4.8, chloride 108, CO_2 21.3, BUN and creatinine 89/4.6 (71/4.1 yesterday; 46/2.4 on April 6, creatinine baseline of 0.8 to 1.2 as far back as October), glucose 162, calcium 9. Hemogram shows H&H of 10.9/33.2, WBC 15.99, normochromic/normocytic indices, and platelets 384.

This patient has also been seen by Dr. Green over the weekend while covering for Dr. Naraquist and has been given a working diagnosis of acute renal failure secondary to severe intravascular volume depletion. Postrenal causes have likewise been ruled out by ultrasound, which did not reveal any hydronephrosis but did reveal an unobstructing calculus 4 mm in the left renal system. Review of the patient's medical record does not really reveal any obvious culprit as far as her underlying renal failure is concerned, but gentamicin/aminoglycoside nephrotoxicity seems to be an attractive consideration. Eosinophils were also checked because of the possibility of an acute interstitial nephritis, but this turned out to be negative. Nevertheless, the patient has been placed on a course of intravenous steroids.

The patient has a past medical and past surgical history that consists of the following:

1. Hypertension.
2. Hyperlipidemia.
3. Degenerative joint disease; questionable osteoporosis.
4. Coronary artery disease, congestive heart failure.
5. Cerebrovascular accident.
6. History of gastric ulcer/duodenal bulb, complicated by anemia.
7. History of Sjögren syndrome.

SOCIAL HISTORY: She is married and retired. She lives with her husband and is accompanied by her husband during hospital visit today. She denies any current use of alcohol, tobacco, IV or recreational drugs.

FAMILY HISTORY: Noncontributory.

LABORATORY RESULTS: As noted above.

REVIEW OF SYSTEMS: Constitutional: No fever or chills. Positive recent weight loss. She appears to be fairly well nourished. No night sweats. Skin: No skin lesions. No active dermatosis. Eyes: No eye discharge or itching. No visual changes or diplopia. ENT: No ear discharge. No difficulty hearing. No pharyngeal hyperemia, congestion, or exudates. Lymph nodes: No lymphadenopathy in the neck, axillary, or groin. Neurological: Positive occasional headache. Positive gait instability. No recent falls. No seizures. Psychiatric: No behavior changes. Neck: No thyromegaly. Respiratory: Positive occasional cough. No cold. No hemoptysis. No shortness of breath. Cardiovascular: No chest pain. No palpitations. No orthopnea. No paroxysmal nocturnal dyspnea. Gastrointestinal: Positive anorexia. Positive nausea. No vomiting. No dysphagia. No odynophagia. No constipation or diarrhea. No abdominal pain. No fecal incontinence. No hematemesis, hematochezia, or melena. Genitourinary: No urgency, frequency, or dysuria. No hematuria. No urinary incontinence. No nocturia. No vaginal discharge. No vaginal lesion. No vaginal bleeding. Musculoskeletal: Positive joint pain. Positive muscle weakness/pain. Hematologic: No bleeding tendencies. No purpura. No petechiae. No ecchymosis. Endocrine: No heat or cold intolerance.

CURRENT MEDICATIONS:

1. Iron sulfate
2. Vasotec 10 mg q.h.s., 20 mg q.a.m.
3. Lacrisert eye drops
4. Synthroid 0.125 q.d.
5. Tegretol 200 t.i.d.
6. Plavix 75 mg q.d.
7. Digoxin 0.125 q.d.

ALLERGIES: TETRACYCLINE.

PHYSICAL EXAMINATION: Vitals sign stable. Blood pressure 137/76, heart rate 81, respirations 20, and saturating 93% on room air. Input and output in the last 24 hours is 2969/1479. Pink palpebral conjunctivae and anicteric sclerae. Positive weakness of the right extraocular muscles. No pharyngeal hyperemia, congestion, or exudates. Somewhat dry tongue and buccal mucosa related to mouth breathing. Supple neck. No lymphadenopathy. Symmetrical chest expansion. Poor inspiratory effort with decreased breath sounds in both lung fields. Occasional rhonchi. No crackles. No wheezes. S1 and S2 are distinct. No S3 or S4. Regular rate and rhythm. Positive 3/6 systolic murmur over the apex radiating to the carotid, most likely suggestive of an aortic stenosis. Abdomen obese. Positive bowel sounds, soft and nontender. No abdominal bruits. Both upper and lower extremities reveal arthritic changes. Pulses are fair.

ASSESSMENT/PLAN:

1. Acute renal failure (baseline creatinine is 0.8–1.2 past-four months), secondary to the following:
   A. Intravascular volume depletion brought about by decreased p.o. intake/decreased IV fluids.
   B. Nephrotoxic ATN/aminoglycoside/gentamicin.
   C. Acute interstitial nephritis probably related to cephalosporin antibiotics. The patient is on IV steroids per Dr. Naraquist.

At this time, patient continues to make a fair amount of urine output even though she is off diuretic medications. Assuming that this is primarily secondary to nephrotoxic effects of aminoglycoside antibiotics, one should expect full to partial recovery of renal function in this particular lady. Per chart notes, the patient and her husband vehemently have expressed their lack of desire to pursue any dialysis treatment if it is ever required.

Today I had a brief discussion with the patient's husband, and I explained to him that I think her renal failure is primarily acute in nature, although the possibility of a chronic renal failure cannot be undermined despite a normal baseline creatinine, considering her significant hypoalbuminemia. Nevertheless, because she continues to make an excellent amount of urine output, and the possible culprit medications have been withdrawn, one should expect her creatinine to plateau and stabilization followed by a subsequent declining trend, which should be observed within at least the next 3 weeks.

At this point, the patient does not require dialysis or any form of renal replacement therapy. If the time comes that she would, however, we will discuss these options again with the patient and her husband and proceed from there on.

At this time, I am going to continue with the patient as requested by Dr. Naraquist.

1-12A:

SERVICE CODE(S): ______________________

DX CODE(S): ______________________

CASE 1-12A DISCUSSION

Dr. Pleasant is providing an initial consultation for Gladys Hanson because of azotemia. Azotemia, also known as uremia, is an excess of urea or other nitrogenous wastes in the blood, and is a symptom of renal dysfunction. In the Assessment/Plan section of the report, Dr. Pleasant states a diagnosis of acute renal failure. (For information regarding renal failure, refer to the information following Case 1-7.)

The dehydration, ATN (acute tubular necrosis) and nephritis are not reported because the physician states that each of these conditions is caused by (secondary to) the acute renal failure.

The attending physician, Dr. Naraquist, has requested that Dr. Pleasant continue treating the patient, so Dr. Pleasant's future visits would be either follow-up consultations or subsequent hospital care, based on the circumstances and documentation.

1-12B PROGRESS REPORT

Report Dr. Pleasant's service.

LOCATION: Hospital Inpatient

PATIENT: Gladys Hanson

ATTENDING PHYSICIAN: Alma Naraquist, M.D.

CONSULTANT: Timothy L. Pleasant, M.D.

The patient is seen and examined, chart reviewed.

I have had a lengthy discussion with the patient and her husband today regarding issues pertaining to renal functioning.

Latest labs performed on April 9: Sodium 138, potassium of 4.6, chloride of 107, CO_2 f 19.6, BUN and creatinine 107/5.4, glucose 138, calcium 9.3. Hemogram shows an H&H of 9.6/29.2, WBC 19.84, normochromic/normocytic indices. Platelets are 380. There is a significant left shift of 90% neutrophils. Magnesium is 2.3. Phosphorus is 4.5.

Several issues have been brought forth this morning. Because the patient's renal functioning is worsening, the issue of renal replacement therapy in the form of dialysis has been brought forth again.

According to the chart notes, it has been assumed that this patient's acute renal failure is secondary to nephrotoxic acute tubular necrosis secondary to aminoglycoside/gentamicin nephrotoxicity. There are, however, some components of this patient's clinical scenario that may or may not be consistent with either nephrotoxic ATN or even acute interstitial nephritis. Because of this, the issue of performing a renal biopsy was considered. In my opinion, a renal biopsy would be a good definitive way of determining her diagnosis. As far as the interstitial nephritis is concerned, it may not yield significant findings primarily because of the patient being on at least 5 to 7 days of steroid therapy. On the other hand, if it turns out to be a vasculitis or one of those glomerular diseases, it must be noted that this patient has already been on steroids, and she should show some form of response already. Finally, I do not believe that the patient would eventually be a candidate for any form of cytotoxic therapy with cyclophosphamide or chlorambucil or the like. Therefore, renal biopsy may not be an option at this point.

On the other hand, what is clear from this present examination is that the patient does require renal replacement therapy or dialysis. The patient's husband has expressed concern that because of her other comorbid illnesses pertaining to her cardiac status, he has expressed reservation about proceeding with dialysis. I have spent a great deal of time explaining to him and the patient that if the patient's kidney function continues to decline and dialysis is not chosen as an option, then she will certainly die from the complications of uremia. If we choose to proceed with intermittent hemodialysis, however, if it turns out that her underlying renal disease is secondary to nephrotoxic causes, then we should see at least some improvement in renal function.

PHYSICAL EXAMINATION: On examination, vital signs are stable. Blood pressure is 145/69, heart rate 106, respirations 20, and saturations 93%. Temperature is 36.4° C. Pink palpebral conjunctivae and anicteric sclerae. No nasal or aural discharge. Moist tongue and buccal mucosa. No pharyngeal hyperemia, congestion, or exudates. Supple neck. No lymphadenopathy. Symmetrical chest expansion. Decreased breath sounds in both lung fields related to poor inspiratory effort. Positive rhonchi. No crackles. No wheezes. S1 and S2 are distinct. No S3 or S4. Regular rate and rhythm. Abdomen: Positive bowel sounds, soft and nontender. Both upper and lower extremities reveal arthritic changes. Pulses are fair.

ASSESSMENT/PLAN:

1. Acute renal failure (baseline creatinine was 0.8-1.2 since October), secondary to the following:
   A. Intravascular volume depletion brought about by decreased p.o. intake/decreased fluids.
   B. Nephrotoxic ATN/aminoglycoside/gentamicin.
   C. Acute interstitial nephritis, probably related to cephalosporins.
   D. Questionable glomerular/vascular disorder.

Please refer to the above for more detailed discussion.

I am going to schedule the patient for a tentative hemodialysis catheter placement tomorrow morning and eventual dialysis. If the patient's family decides not to proceed with dialysis, then my recommendation is to proceed with possible do-not-resuscitate status or code III.

I have spent a total of 60 minutes evaluating and reviewing this patient's medical record. I have spent an additional 20 minutes discussing the case with the patient and her husband. The counseling of the patient took over 50% of the time of this service.

1-12B:

SERVICE CODE(S): ______________________

DX CODE(S): ______________________

1-12C PROGRESS REPORT

Report Dr. Pleasant's service.

LOCATION: Hospital Inpatient

PATIENT: Gladys Hanson

ATTENDING PHYSICIAN: Alma Naraquist, M.D.

CONSULTANT: Timothy L. Pleasant, M.D.

The patient is seen and examined, chart reviewed. Today I had a discussion with the patient's husband, and it has been finally decided that the patient not be subjected to any form of renal replacement therapy or dialysis. The pros and cons of this decision have been discussed once again, and the patient's husband understands.

Latest labs are as follows: Hemogram: Hemoglobin 9.3, hematocrit 28.7, WBC 17.67, normochromic/normocytic indices, and platelets 411. There is a significant left shift of 90% neutrophils. The rest of the chemistries are as follows: Sodium 141, potassium 5.1, chloride 108, CO_2 18.8, BUN 114, and creatinine 6 (89 and 4.6 yesterday; 71 and 4.1 on April 7), glucose 115, and calcium 9.3.

EXAMINATION: Vital signs are stable. Blood pressure 130s/50s. Heart rate is in the 90s. Respirations 20s. She is febrile. HEENT: Normocephalic and atraumatic. Pink palpebral conjunctivae and anicteric sclerae. No nasal or aural discharge. Moist tongue and buccal mucosa. No pharyngeal hyperemia, congestion, or exudates. Supple neck. No lymphadenopathy. Symmetrical chest expansion. Decreased breath sounds in both lung fields related to poor inspiratory effort. Positive rhonchi. No crackles. No wheezes. S1 and S2 are distinct. No S3 or S4. Regular rate and rhythm. Abdomen: Positive bowel sounds, soft and nontender. Both upper and lower extremities reveal arthritic changes. Pulses are fair.

ASSESSMENT/PLAN:

1. Acute renal failure (baseline creatinine 0.8 and 0.2 since November), secondary to the following:
   A. Intravascular volume depletion brought about by decreased p.o. intake.
   B. Nephrotoxicity ATN/aminoglycoside/gentamicin.
   C. Acute interstitial nephritis, probably related to cephalosporins.
   D. Questionable glomerular/vascular disorder.

Please refer to my progress note from yesterday for more details.

At this time, because it has been decided not to consider dialysis, I am going to withdraw from this case. I have informed the husband as well. At the same time, I would recommend that the patient be considered a code III level status/palliative/comfort care. Dr. Naraquist is taking over the case from here on.

1-12C:

SERVICE CODE(S): ______________________

DX CODE(S): ______________________

CASE 1-13

The physician in this case is being requested to provide a consultation for the tachypnea (excessive, rapid breathing) as indicated in the first paragraph by the statement "The main reason for consultation is that of possible mechanical ventilation primarily for airway protection due to tachypnea." Report Dr. Dawson's service.

1-13A CRITICAL CARE

LOCATION: Hospital Inpatient

PATIENT: Peter Gluzinski

ATTENDING PHYSICIAN: Ronald Green, M.D.

CONSULTANT: Gregory Dawson, M.D.

I am being consulted by Dr. Green to see this patient from the critical care standpoint because the patient is in acute alcohol intoxication. The main reason for consultation is that of possible mechanical ventilation primarily for airway protection due to tachypnea.

The patient is a 62-year-old white man who has had multiple admissions in the past for multiple acute alcohol intoxications/detoxifications.

The patient was initially brought to the emergency room, where patient was noted to be significantly intoxicated. His blood alcohol level is 400 mg/dl, and this was drawn at 4 o'clock this morning.

The patient was then placed on intermittent dosing of Ativan with no success. And so Dr. Green decided to contact me, and we have agreed to have the anesthesia service intubate the patient.

The patient is being placed on an initial mechanical ventilation setup consisting of FiO_2 of 100%, SIMV of 14, tidal volume of 600, PEEP of 5, pressure support of 10. Blood gases are to be drawn in 30 minutes, and chest x-rays are to be done to reassess placement of the endotracheal tube.

Latest laboratory tests performed on this patient are as follows: Sodium 141, potassium 3.9, chloride 100, CO_2 25.4, BUN and creatinine 10/1, glucose 113, calcium 8.5, ALT 54. Alcohol level is 400 mg/dl as noted above.

Hemogram shows H&H of 16/45.2, WBC 7.46, normochromic/normocytic indices, and platelets 202. There is no left shift, as neutrophils are only 46.7%.

PAST MEDICAL/SURGICAL HISTORY:

1. Hypertension.
2. Nicotine dependence.
3. Alcohol abuse/dependence with multiple admissions for acute intoxications; alcohol withdrawal/alcohol withdrawal seizures; alcohol rehabilitation/detoxifications.
4. Questionable coronary artery disease (per medical records).

FAMILY HISTORY: According to the medical records, it is positive for diabetes. Negative for hypertension, stroke, kidney disease, bleeding disorder/dyscrasia.

SOCIAL HISTORY: He works at the local automobile factory, and he smokes two packs per day. As noted above, he does have a history of significant alcohol binges. He denies any previous or current use of intravenous or recreational drugs. His daughter has terminal liver disease/illness.

MEDICATIONS: Lotensin 10 mg q.d.

ALLERGIES: No known drug allergies.

LABORATORY RESULTS: As noted above.

REVIEW OF SYSTEMS: Unobtainable at this time as patient is intubated, mechanically ventilated (96 hours), and sedated with an Ativan drip.

PHYSICAL EXAMINATION: On examination, vital signs are stable. Blood pressure 137/69, heart rate 89, respirations 16, and saturation 94%. Latest blood gases are as follows: 7.34/45.7/92.4/24.1/97.6% on setting of FiO_2 of 80%, SIMV of 14, tidal volume of 600, PEEP of 5, and pressure support of 10. Normocephalic and atraumatic. Pink palpebral conjunctivae and anicteric sclerae. Intubated and mechanically ventilated. Supple neck. No lymphadenopathy. Symmetrical chest expansion. No retractions. No rhonchi. No crackles. No wheezes. S1 and S2 are distinct. No S3 or S4. Regular rate and rhythm. Abdomen: Obese. Positive bowel sounds, soft and nontender. No abdominal bruits appreciated. Both upper and lower extremities reveal arthritic changes. No edema on both lower extremities. Pulses are fair.

ASSESSMENT/PLAN:

1. Acute alcohol intoxication. It must be noted that the toxicity of ethanol is dose-related but tolerance has a wide variation. In this case, with levels in excess of 400 mg/dl, respiratory depression is common and death is possible from such problem; hence, the patient has been intubated and mechanically ventilated. At this time, the plan is as follows:
   a. Admit to medical ICU.
   b. Monitor vital signs q.4h.
   c. Monitor daily weights, inputs, and outputs.

d. Nasogastric tube, Foley catheter.
e. IV fluids D5½ normal saline with 100% thiamine plus multivitamin 1 ampule plus folic acid 1 mg at a rate of 150 ml/hour followed by D5¼ normal saline to infuse at a maintenance IV fluid rate of 150 ml/hour.

I do not believe that charcoal would be helpful at this time because of rapid absorption of alcohol from the stomach. At this time, he does not really require hemodialysis yet. Based on my clinical examination and evaluation of this patient, there is indeed presence of alcohol intoxication; however, there does not seem to be any underlying illness or significant alcoholic ketoacidosis. At this time, we will continue ventilatory support as required and also will continue to observe him until he is sober, that is, until blood alcohol level is less than 100 mg/dl, at which time he can be transferred to the medical floor. At that time, I would recommend consultation with psychiatry and an alcohol guidance counselor.

After reviewing his blood gases, I would recommend that we try to wean his oxygen down while maintaining a saturation of greater than or equal to 90%. Likewise, I am going to recommend to increase SIMV to 16. Blood gases will be repeated in the morning.

2. Hypertension, fairly controlled. At this time, blood pressure appears to be relatively well-controlled. If he does develop a hypertensive crisis in relation to alcohol withdrawal, my recommendation would be to place him on either atenolol or clonidine for blood pressure control.
3. History of tobacco abuse; questionable chronic obstructive pulmonary disease.
4. Psychiatric issues.

I will continue to follow up on this patient from the critical care standpoint, and Dr. Green will take over in the morning as far as management of his ventilation is concerned. I spent a total of 90 minutes evaluating and reviewing this patient's medical record. I spent another 10 minutes discussing the case with Dr. Green.

1-13A:

SERVICE CODE(S): ____________________

DX CODE(S): ____________________

CASE 1-13A DISCUSSION

Acute Alcohol Intoxication

You did a fine job if you reported the tachypnea, acute alcohol intoxication, and hypertension. The hypertension is reported because the report indicated that it was "fairly controlled," and as such, is a consideration in treatment. In Point 2 in the Assessment/Plan section of the report, the physician indicates that he is concerned that the patient may develop a hypertensive crisis in relation to the alcohol withdrawal. The report indicates that the patient was admitted many times for acute alcohol intoxications/detoxifications. When an alcohol-dependent patient is acutely intoxicated and presents for care, you would code 303.0X, Acute alcoholic intoxication, with a fifth digit to indicate the episode of care as:

0	unspecified
1	continuous
2	episodic
3	in remission

The fifth digit 2 is assigned, as this is an episode of intoxication since the medical record confirms he has had previous episodes.

The COPD was questionable and as such would not be reported in an outpatient setting. The history of tobacco abuse and psychiatric issues do not seem to have a direct involvement in the service being provided, so they are not reported.

Cerebral Hemorrhage

The three protective membranes that surround the brain and spinal cord are the dura mater, arachnoid, and pia mater (as illustrated in **Figure 1-13**). Intracranial hemorrhage can be extradural (outside the dura), subdural (between the dura and arachnoid), subarachnoid (between the arachnoid and pia mater), or cerebral (parenchymatous or within the tissues of the brain).

In the Index of the ICD-9-CM, locate the main term "Hemorrhage," subterm "brain (miliary), (nontraumatic)." ("Miliary" means resembling a small seed and is an area of minute lesion.) You are directed to 431 within the Tabular for **nontraumatic** hemorrhage. 431 is the code for **intracerebral** hemorrhage of various anatomical areas, such as ventricular and cerebellar (See Figure 1-13) Nontraumatic intracerebral hemorrhage can be caused by any number of conditions such as leukemia, hemophilia, liver disease, or hypertension.

Subarachnoid hemorrhage is reported with 430 and includes congenital cerebral aneurysm and berry aneurysm. (An aneurysm is a sac formed by dilatation of a vessel wall.) A berry aneurysm is one that forms in the cerebral artery, usually at a junction of a vessel. It is termed a berry aneurysm because the neck of the aneurysm is smaller than the body of the aneurysm. It is also known as a cerebral aneurysm.

Nontraumatic **subdural** hemorrhage is reported with 432.1, nontraumatic extradural hemorrhage is reported with 432.0, and unspecified intracranial hemorrhage that is not further specified is reported with 432.9.

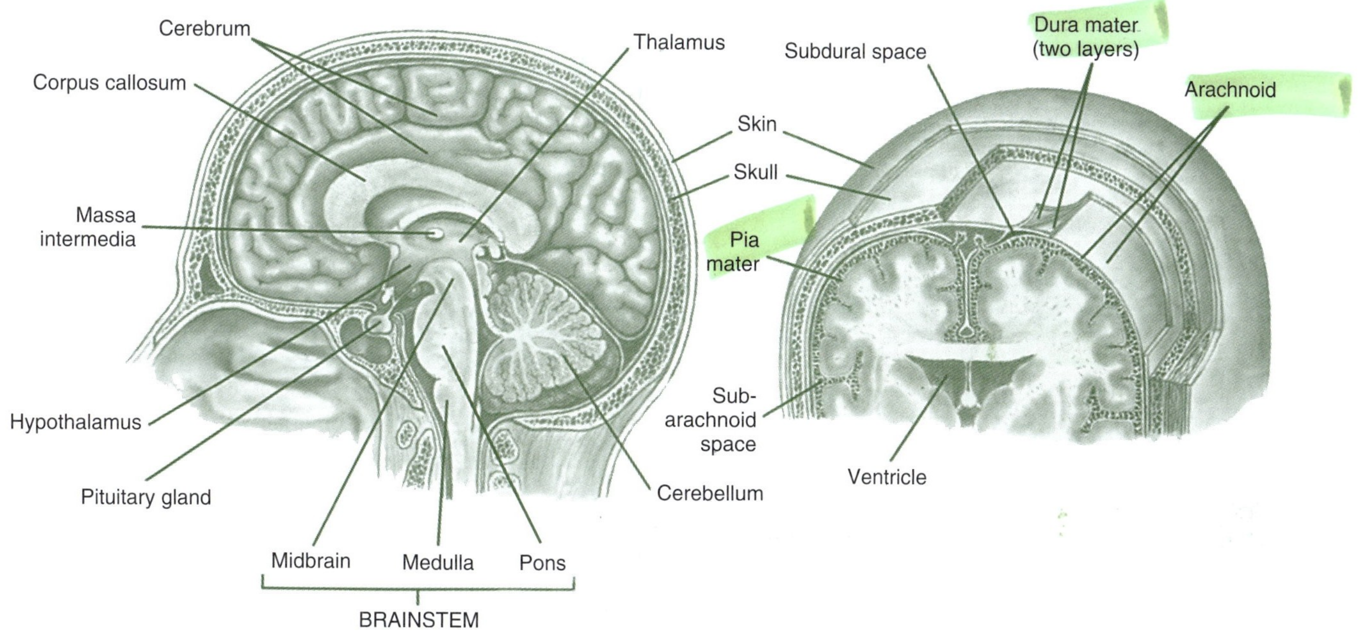

FIGURE 1-13 Meninges of the brain. (From Thompson JM et al: *Mosby's Clinical Nursing,* ed 5, St. Louis, 2002, Mosby.)

0	unspecified state of consciousness
1	with no loss of consciousness
2	with brief [less than one hour] loss of consciousness
3	with moderate [1–24 hours] loss of consciousness
4	with prolonged [more than 24 hours] loss of con sciousness and return to pre-existing conscious level
5	with prolonged [more than 24 hours] loss of consciousness and without return to pre-existing conscious level Use fifth-digit 5 to designate when a patient is unconscious and dies before regaining conscious ness, regardless of the duration of the loss of consciousness
6	with loss of concussioness of unspecified duration
9	with concussion, unspecified

If the hemorrhage was caused by a trauma, the condition is reported with a code from 851–854. A fifth digit is added to indicate if the trauma resulted from a loss of consciousness.

Locate the main term "Hemorrhage," subterm "brain," and subterm "traumatic" in the Index of the ICD-9-CM. It is under the subterm "traumatic" that you will locate the Tabular locations for the types of traumatic hemorrhage, such as extradural (852.4X), subarachnoid (852.0X), and subdural (852.2X). The Tabular will further define the specifics of the code includes those injuries with an open intracranial wound and those without mention of an open intracranial wound.

Open **wounds** of the head without intracranial injury are reported with 873.XX. Skull **fractures** are reported with 800.XX (fracture of vault of skull), 801.XX (fracture of base of skull), 803.XX (other and unqualified skull fractures), and 804.XX (multiple fractures involving skull or face). E codes are reported with traumatic injury if the facility policy directs the collection of E code data.

Subdural and cerebral hemorrhage of a fetus or newborn caused by birth trauma is reported with 767.0. If known, an additional code is used to identify the cause. Intraventricular hemorrhage is reported with 772.1X with a fifth digit to indicate the grade of bleeding, such as Grade II (into the ventricle) or Grade IV (into the cerebral cortex).

CASE 1-14
1-14A ICU Report

CASE 1-14

Report Dr. Naraquist's service.

1-14A ICU REPORT

LOCATION: Hospital Inpatient

PATIENT: Morley Overmoe

ATTENDING PHYSICIAN: Alma Naraquist, M.D.

I am admitting this patient to the medical ICU because of a recent hemorrhagic stroke involving the left frontal area.

The patient is a 49-year-old white obese known hypertensive patient who was found to be unresponsive in his home. The history of present illness started a few hours before admission this morning when he stated to have acute onset of headache involving the right temporal area. He started becoming weak afterward, and he self-medicated with two enteric-coated aspirins, 81 mg per day. The patient did not have any seizure episodes, but was later noted on by his wife to manifest suddenly a staggering gait and then later followed by unresponsiveness.

The patient then was brought to the hospital, where subsequent CT scan showed a significant large left frontal lobe hemorrhage.

The patient was evaluated in the emergency room and was noted to have 2-mm pupils, nonreactive, positive cornealis, with no appreciable spontaneous breaths, at least during my examination.

LABORATORY TESTS that were performed in the hospital include the following: Electrocardiogram primary shows sinus bradycardia with first-degree AV block, rate of 51 beats per minute, no ST or T wave changes. Hemogram shows an H&H of 16.5/48.8, WBC of 11.8, normochromic/normocytic indices, and platelets 252. Sodium is 127, potassium 3.1, chloride 102, CO_2 28, BUN and creatinine 18/1.2, glucose 251, and calcium is 9.1.

In the hospital, the patient is also intubated and mechanically ventilated. Latest blood gases prior to intubation are as follows: 7.37/47.3/115/27/29/98% Venti mask.

PAST MEDICAL/SURGICAL HISTORY:
1. Hypertension.
2. Obesity.
3. Questionable congestive heart failure.

MEDICATIONS taken at home including the following:
1. Atenolol 75 mg q.d.
2. Norvasc 5 mg q.d.
3. Digoxin 0.25 mg q.d.
4. Quinapril 40 mg q.d.
5. Doxazosin 4 mg q.d.
6. Aspirin 1tab q.d.
7. Hydrochlorothiazide 25 mg q.d.

ALLERGIES: Penicillin.

FAMILY HISTORY: Positive for hypertension and cancer. Father and mother have been afflicted with hypertension and heart disease. Negative history of diabetes, stroke, kidney disease, bleeding disorder, or dyscrasia.

SOCIAL HISTORY: According to the wife, the patient has not had any usage of alcohol, tobacco, or intravenous or recreational drugs.

REVIEW OF SYSTEMS: Unobtainable.

NEUROLOGICAL EXAMINATION: Please refer to Sutton's note for more details.

PHYSICAL EXAMINATION: On examination, vital signs are stable. Blood pressure is 180s/80s. Heart rate is in the 60s to 70s. Respirations are 12. He is afebrile. Normocephalic and atraumatic. Pink palpebral conjunctivae, anicteric sclerae. Supple neck. No lymphadenopathy. Intubated and mechanically ventilated. Symmetrical chest expansion. No retractions. Positive rhonchi. No crackles or wheezes. S1 and S2 are distinct. No S3 or S4. Regular rate and rhythm. Abdomen is obese. Positive bowel sounds. Soft and nontender. No abdominal bruits. Both upper and lower extremities reveal no gross deformities; positive arthritic changes. Pulses are fair.

ASSESSMENT/PLAN: Left frontal lobe hemorrhage. A neurosurgeon, Dr. Hodgson, has been consulted. The patient's poor prognosis has been discussed with the patient's wife. The patient is actually a code level III according to the wife.

PLAN right now is to render conservative medical management with antihypertensive regimen consisting of nitroprusside drip. Dr. Pleasant also has suggested giving the patient a dose of mannitol. We will continue to monitor the patient's daily weights, inputs, and outputs.

We will try to do neuro checks on an hourly basis. We will also check the patient's lab values. I am also going to order cardiac enzymes on this patient.

Target systolic blood pressure is 140s to 160s, so that we do not precipitate any ischemic deficit as a result of overzealous antihypertensive medication use.

A lengthy discussion with the patient's wife was held, during which it was explained that surgery is an option; however, the results may not necessarily be encouraging. The wife has expressed her understanding and appreciation of our explanations.

The patient is going to be admitted to medical ICU and monitored with re-evaluate in the morning.

I spent a total of 60 minutes evaluating and reviewing this patient's medical records.

1-14A:

SERVICE CODE(S): ____________________

DX CODE(S): ____________________

CASE 1-14A DISCUSSION

Code Levels

Hospitals have pre-established resuscitation levels. These levels specify the conditions under which a patient is or is not to be resuscitated. The patient has agreed to the conditions of this level, usually stated in terms such as "Code 1," "Code 2," etc. The higher the level, the more conditions that have to be met before the patient is resuscitated should that situation arise. Note that this patient is a code level 3, which means that the patient or his wife have recognized the severity of the patient's condition and have chosen a code level that is less likely to result in resuscitation.

Critical Care

The physician has indicated the time he spent with this patient providing critical care service, which is necessary to accurately report the service. If the physician does not indicate the time, you can only report the lowest level critical care service. It is important to educate the physician regarding the need for indicating time on the medical record in order to correctly report critical care services.

Remember that critical care is the *type* of service rendered, not necessarily the place (e.g., the critical care unit) it was provided.

CASE 1-15

Report Dr. Naraquist's service.

1-15A CRITICAL CARE

LOCATION: Hospital Inpatient

PATIENT: Sebastian Gunther

ATTENDING PHYSICIAN: Alma Naraquist, M.D.

CONSULTANT: Gregory Dawson, M.D.

I am being consulted primarily because of acute onset of hypotension.

The patient is a 76-year-old white, obese man who had been admitted to his hometown hospital around 2 days ago, primarily because of mild degree of shortness of breath. The patient has had a long-standing history of alcohol abuse in the past and continues to abuse alcohol on a regular basis.

On admission, he was started on diuretic medications in the form of Bumex for what I suppose is pulmonary congestion/fluid overload, questionable. The patient was likewise empirically started on Levaquin for a questionable pneumonia.

In the past 24 hours, the patient has been stable; however, he has had some episodes of hypotension earlier today. This evening, he once again had an episode of hypotension, with the systolic blood pressure running in the 60s to 70s range. He was likewise noted to be somewhat obtunded. On further review of the patient's medical records, the patient continues to receive Bumex and lisinopril as well as Ativan on a continuous basis, and I think this can probably account for the patient's hypotension. With regard to the alleged pneumonia, I do not think based on my clinical examination that the patient is actually septic. Nevertheless, the patient is already empirically started on Levaquin, which was later changed to moxifloxacin/Avelox.

At this time, with the patient's hypotension, the plan is to admit the patient to the medical ICU with cultures to be drawn, namely, blood culture times two, urinalysis, urine culture, sputum culture, and Gram stain. We will check a CBC with manual differential count, basic metabolic panel, phosphorus, magnesium, and albumin.

A blood gas was performed this evening, which showed the following results: 7.442/40.4/56.6/27/98.6% on 2 liters O_2 nasal cannula.

I will also change the patient's IV fluids to D5 half normal saline with incorporations of multivitamins 1 ampule, thiamine 100 mg, and folic acid 1 mg on a daily basis followed by a maintenance fluid of D5 normal saline infusing at a rate of 65 ml/hour. The reason why we are going to start off with a low intravenous fluid rate is primarily because the patient may have some degree of congestive heart failure and is the reason why he was receiving Bumex earlier on. If he has any bouts of hypotension in the next few hours, plan would be either to increase IV fluids rate or change them to 0.9% normal saline/isotonic solution and/or start the patient on dopamine infusion. At this point, these measures do not seem to be necessary; hence we are going to hold off on them.

I still believe that a significant contribution to this patient's hypotensive episode is that of the combination of medications, namely Bumex, lisinopril, and Ativan.

The patient has a past medical history and past surgical history that consists of the following:

1. Alcoholic cardiomyopathy, congestive heart failure, history of atrial fibrillation, status postatrial fibrillation.
2. Pulmonary hypertension/chronic obstructive pulmonary disease.
3. Alcohol abuse.
4. Hypertension.
5. Chronic renal insufficiency, questionable, probably related to long-standing cardiac history as well as hypertension.
6. Depression.

He continues to drink alcohol on a regular basis. He claims to have not drunk any alcohol in the past four days before admission. He denies any use of tobacco or intravenous or recreational drugs.

FAMILY HISTORY: Negative for heart disease, hypertension, diabetes, stroke, cancer, kidney disease, bleeding disorder, or dyscrasia.

Although the patient denies significant history of tobacco, according to medical records, he has a history of smoking a cigar on a daily basis as well.

MEDICATIONS:
1. Aspirin.
2. Lisinopril 40 q.d.
3. Atrovent and albuterol metered dose inhaler.
4. Bumex.
5. Protonix.

I think the patient was on Lasix at home, but when he was admitted this was changed to Bumex.

Past laboratory tests on this patient are as follows: Sodium 132, potassium 4.4, chloride 94, CO_2 32.9, BUN and creatinine 75/1.2, glucose 94, and calcium 8. Hemogram shows an H&H of 12.1/36.5, WBC 5.82, normochromic/normocytic indices, and platelets 88. There is a slight left shift of neutrophils measured at 78.2%.

Latest blood gases are as noted above.

REVIEW OF SYSTEMS: (Primarily based on patient's medical records as the patient is quite confused and disoriented at this time): Constitutional: No fever or chills. No recent weight change. He appears to be fairly disheveled. No night sweats. Skin: No skin lesions. No active dermatosis. Eyes: No eye discharge. No eye itching. No visual changes. No diplopia. ENT: No ear discharge. No hearing difficulty. No pharyngeal hyperemia, congestion, or exudates. Lymph nodes: No lymphadenopathy in the neck, axillae, or groin. Neurologic: No headaches. Positive gait instability. No falls. No seizures. Psychiatric: No behavioral changes. Neck: No thyromegaly. Respiratory: Positive cough. No colds. No hemoptysis. Positive shortness of breath. Cardiovascular: No chest pain, questionable palpitations. No orthopnea. No paroxysmal nocturnal dyspnea. Gastrointestinal: Positive anorexia. Positive nausea. No vomiting. No dysphagia. No odynophagia. No constipation. No diarrhea. No abdominal pain or fecal incontinence. No hematemesis, hematochezia, or melena. Genitourinary: No urgency, frequency, dysuria, or hematuria. No urinary incontinence. No nocturia. No penile discharge. No penile lesions. Musculoskeletal: Positive joint pains. Positive muscle pains/weaknesses. Hematologic: No bleeding tendencies. No purpura. No petechiae. No ecchymosis. Endocrinologic: No heat or cold intolerance.

PHYSICAL EXAMINATION: Vital signs are stable. Blood pressure 120s/70s. Heart rate is in the 70s. Respirations 20s. He is afebrile. As soon as the patient was brought to the medical ICU, his blood pressure has been in the 120s to 130s systolic. Normocephalic and atraumatic. Pink palpebral conjunctivae. Anicteric sclerae. No nasal or aural discharge. Somewhat dry tongue and buccal mucosa. Supple neck. No lymphadenopathy. No obvious JVD. Symmetrical chest expansion. No retractions. Positive rhonchi. A few basilar crackles. No wheezes. S1 and S2 are distinct. No S3 or S4. A 3/6 systolic murmur heard throughout the precordium. Abdomen: Positive bowel sounds; soft and nontender. No abdominal bruits. Morbidly obese. Both upper and lower extremities reveal arthritic changes. Positive edema on both lower extremities. Positive retrosacral edema. Pulses are fair.

ASSESSMENT/PLAN:

1. Alcoholic cardiomyopathy.
2. Congestive heart failure.
3. Pulmonary hypertension.
4. Chronic renal insufficiency.

1/2/3/4

At this time, the plan is as dictated above. Admit to medical ICU. Hold lisinopril and Bumex until further orders. Monitor daily weights, inputs, and outputs. Follow-up plan cultures. Continue empiric antibiotic coverage.

I am also going to check for cardiac enzymes primarily to rule out the possibility of an acute myocardial infarction, which may have had some temporal relation with the hypotensive episode.

If the patient remains stable and all the labs are satisfactory, the patient could probably be transferred to the medical floor for subsequent management by primary service/family practice teaching service.

Code-level issues have apparently been addressed by the primary physician with the patient's relatives and the patient, and this patient is currently code level I. I would also recommend that long-term plans be made for this patient. Apparently this patient lives alone, but the way things are going, I think he is probably better off living in an assisted-living situation, such as a nursing home or the like.

Would also consider the possibility of rehabilitation medicine, physical therapy/occupational therapy following up on this patient's care.

Tomorrow, we are also going to check for the patient's CBC and manual differential, basic metabolic panel, and chest x-ray. We may also need to check blood gases if he continues to show signs of respiratory compromise.

As noted above, I have recommended holding off the diuretics because I think this is significantly contributing to the patient's intravascular volume depletion/hypotension.

I have spent a total of 90 minutes evaluating and reviewing this patient's medical records. Again, this is a critical care consultation note.

1-15A:

SERVICE CODE(S): ____________________

DX CODE(S): ____________________

CASE 1-15A DISCUSSION

This is a long and complicated report that must be carefully read. The physician who prepared this report did two things that assist the coder in accurate coding: She listed the complete diagnoses in the Assessment/Plan section of the report, and she indicated the time for her critical care services. If all physicians were this careful in their documentation, it would greatly help the coders.

Cardiomyopathy

This patient has alcoholic cardiomyopathy, which is thought to be brought on by the toxic effect of alcohol, nutritional deficiencies, and the toxic effect of the additives in alcohol (such as cobalt). Cardiomyopathy affects the myocardium and is categorized as dilated, hypertropic, restrictive, or obliterative, depending on the effects. Alcoholic cardiomyopathy is a dilated type that is characterized by ventricular dilation and impaired systolic function. This means the heart does not contract sufficiently and therefore does not eject blood with the force it should.

Congestive Heart Failure

Congestive heart failure is a condition, in which the heart is unable to generate adequate output. When the heart has lost its ability to pump effectively, blood may back up into other organs, such as the liver or lungs. When the organs do not get a sufficient blood supply, they can be damaged and lose their ability to function properly. In the Index of the ICD-9-CM, one way to locate the code is under the entry "Failure, heart, congestive." You are then directed to the Tabular to read the full description and all notes regarding the code.

Pulmonary Hypertension

Pulmonary hypertension occurs when the blood pressure in the arteries of the lungs is too high. The arteries narrow, which increases the resistance to blood flow. This makes the heart work harder to pump, and eventually the right side of the heart becomes enlarged for the additional workload. There is no known cure, only treatment of the symptoms, such as shortness of breath. Pulmonary hypertension is also known as primary pulmonary hypertension, idiopathic (unknown cause) pulmonary arteriosclerosis, and essential pulmonary hypertension.

Chronic Renal Insufficiency

Chronic renal insufficiency is a progressive condition in which the renal tissue is destroyed through sclerosis and loss of nephrons over time. The designation as chronic renal insufficiency is assessed by the glomerular filtration rate (GFR) that progressively decreases with the loss of nephrons. **Chronic renal failure** is the term used for patients whose GFR is less than 30 cc/min. **Chronic renal insufficiency** is the preferred term for patients with mild-to-moderate renal impairment, those whose GFR falls at 30–70 cc/min. **End-stage renal disease** (ESRD), is often associated with uremia, and is the term used for patients whose GFR has declined to levels of less than 10 cc/min.

See Assessment / Plan
1.
2. } Same as Report
3.
4

CASE 1-16

The services in 1-16A, B, and C were all provided on the same day. You will report services for Dr. Orbitz's based on all three reports within this case.

1-16A CRITICAL CARE

Report Dr. Orbitz's service.

LOCATION: Hospital Inpatient

PATIENT: Ann Danube

ATTENDING PHYSICIAN: George Orbitz, M.D.

The emergency room physician called me in primarily because this patient was transferred from Anytown after being noted to have gone into a cardiopulmonary arrest. I was informed that advanced cardiac support measures were rendered, and the patient was revived; hence, the patient was transferred here.

The patient is a 56-year-old white woman who is well known to me because she is one of my chronic renal failure patients whom I had last seen last year. The patient apparently had a recent episode of congestive heart failure/fluid overload, during which time the patient was noted to have severe mitral valve disease. The patient was then subjected to a mitral valve replacement surgery per cardiothoracic surgery.

The patient was discharged improved 90 days ago. According to the patient's daughters, she was not doing well; she had significant limitation in her activities because she would easily get short of breath since the time of discharge. Furthermore, they noticed she has been having significant fluid retention/worsening edema since that time. On the day of admission, the patient was noted to have gone into a state of cardiopulmonary arrest and was subjected to ACLS measures by EMS team, and the patient was brought into the emergency room, already intubated and Ambu-bagged.

During my evaluation, the patient was subjected to a transthoracic echocardiogram, which confirmed the presence of some fluid in the pericardium but was not consistent with that of a pericardial tamponade. This issue was actually discussed by the echocardiogram technician and Dr. Monson as well as Dr. Sutton. Furthermore, Dr. Monson's opinion was also obtained by the ER physician.

At this time, the patient appears to be hemodynamically stable, and she is intubated and mechanically ventilated. My plan right now is to admit her to medical ICU and stabilize her. We will work her up for a rule-out myocardial infarction. Her blood pressure right now is stable at 110 to 120 systolic. I have also discussed the issue of putting her on heparin with Dr. Elhart of cardiology, and he agreed.

The patient has a past medical history and past surgical history that consists of the following:

1. Coronary artery disease, congestive heart failure, bilateral pleural effusions with severe mitral regurgitation/stenosis, status post mitral valve replacement, aortic insufficiency, and hypertension.
2. Chronic renal insufficiency–latest creatinine clearance is 93 ml/min. with a creatinine of 0.8, total volume of 2550 ml with undetermined proteinuria performed, most likely secondary to the following:
   a. Hypertension.
   b. Type 2 diabetes.
   c. History of bilateral renal artery stenosis, status post bilateral stent placements in April.
   d. Coronary artery disease. See note above.
3. Chronic obstructive pulmonary disease/pulmonary hypertension/? cor pulmonale.
4. Anxiety/depression.
5. Hyperlipidemia.
6. Degenerative joint disease.
7. Peptic ulcer disease.
8. Status post previous cataract surgery (questionable retinopathy).
9. Status post previous finger amputation (questionable related to diabetic vascular neuropathies).

SOCIAL HISTORY: The patient smoked one to two packs of cigarettes per day for at least 40 to 50 years. She occasionally drank alcohol but denies any current use of tobacco, alcohol, intravenous or recreational drugs.

FAMILY HISTORY: Positive for diabetes and heart disease. Negative history for stroke, cancer, kidney disease, bleeding disorder, or dyscrasia. Her mother died at age 76 because of diabetes complications. Her father died at age 65 because of cardiac complications.

ALLERGIES: She has no known drug allergies.

CURRENT MEDICATIONS:

1. Albuterol metered dose inhaler 2 puffs b.i.d.
2. Combivent metered dose inhaler 2 puffs q.i.d.

3. Bumex 1mg b.i.d.
4. Calcium carbonate 650 mg 1 tablet q.d.
5. Diltiazem CD 180 mg b.i.d.
6. Sodium docusate 100 mg b.i.d.
7. Amitriptyline 10 mg at bedtime.
8. Lorazepam 1 mg q.8h. p.r.n. anxiety.
9. Propoxyphene 1–2 tablets q.3–4h. p.r.n.
10. Novolin NPH 15 units b.i.d.
11. Regular Novolin R as directed.
12. Lisinopril 10 mg q.d.
13. Metoprolol 25 b.i.d.
14. Coumadin 2 mg q.d.

REVIEW OF SYSTEMS: Unobtainable because the patient is intubated and mechanically ventilated.

EXAMINATION: Vital signs are stable. Blood pressure is 120s/60s. Heart rate is in the 70s. Respirations are 20s. Saturating 95%. Normocephalic and atraumatic. Pink palpebral conjunctivae. Anicteric sclerae. Intubated and mechanically ventilated. Symmetrical chest expansion. Positive rhonchi. Positive basilar crackles. No wheezes. S1 and S2 are distinct. No S3 or S4. Regular rate and rhythm. Positive history of pacemaker placement? Abdomen is obese. Positive bowel sounds. Soft and nontender. No abdominal bruits appreciated at this time. Both upper and lower extremities reveal arthritic changes. Positive edema on both lower extremities. Positive retrosacral edema. Pulses are fair.

ASSESSMENT/PLAN:

1. Status post cardiopulmonary arrest. Rule out myocardial infarction. Admit to medical ICU. Mechanical ventilation as ordered. Heparin as ordered. Cardiology consultation by Dr. Elhart. Cardiothoracic consultation by Dr. Barton. Check chemistries, CBC, PT, INR, 12-lead ECG, chest x-ray, and cardiac enzymes q.8h. times three. Monitor I's and O's, daily weights. NGT. Foley catheter. Aspirin 325 p.o. now and then q.d.
2. Respiratory failure, intubated and on ventilator. We will check the chest x-ray to see if this patient has any evidence of congestive heart failure/fluid overload, which may necessitate the use of intravenous diuretics for preload reduction.
3. Acute renal failure (latest creatinine clearance is 93 ml/min with a creatinine of 0.8, total volume 2550 ml/min, and undetermined proteinuria previously performed), secondary to the following:
   a. Hypertension, fairly controlled. Hold blood pressure medications right now because her blood pressure is tethering from 100 to 120 systolic range.
   b. Type 2 diabetes mellitus, fairly controlled. Novolin R sliding scale as ordered. Check blood sugars every 6 hours.
   c. History of bilateral renal artery stenosis, status post bilateral renal artery stent placement.
   d. Coronary artery disease. See note above.
4. Chronic obstructive pulmonary disease/pulmonary hypertension/? cor pulmonale. Mechanical ventilation setup FiO_2 100%, SIMV 14, tidal volume 500, PEEP of 5, and pressure support of 10. Dr. Dawson will follow up from the pulmonary/critical care standpoint starting tomorrow. Albuterol/Atrovent nebulization treatments q.4h. p.r.n. Check ABGs.
5. Anxiety disorder/depression.
6. Hyperlipidemia.
7. Degenerative joint disease.

LATEST LABORATORY TESTS PERFORMED AS FOLLOWS: Hemogram shows an H&H of 9.1/29.9, WBC 11.11, hyperchromic indices, and platelets of 283. There is a left shift of 93.4 neutrophils. Chemistries are as follows: Sodium 138, potassium 6.2, chloride 98, CO_2 22.2, BUN and creatinine 41/1.6 (24/0.9 two months ago), glucose 213, and calcium 8.4. PT and INR are 14.6 and 1.5, respectively, suggesting undercoagulation. The latest blood gases are as follows: 7.573/32.4/306.8/29.2, and this is while the patient is being Ambu-bagged. First set of cardiac enzymes are as follows: Troponin less than 0.04, CK-MB 5, and total CPK of 72.

I have spent a total of 90 minutes evaluating and reviewing this patient's medical record and formulating the treatment strategy.

I-16B PROGRESS REPORT—SAME DAY AS CASE I-16A

Report Dr. Orbitz's service.

LOCATION: Hospital Inpatient

PATIENT: Ann Danube

ATTENDING PHYSICIAN: George Orbitz, M.D.

Review of the labs reveals several abnormalities, the most important of which is that of an acute renal failure, most likely superimposed on top of an underlying chronic renal insufficiency. Evidence of this is the acute rise in BUN and creatinine, 41/1.6 (from 24/0.9), and accompanying hyperkalemia of 6.2. This is most likely explained by the recent cardiopulmonary arrest/decreased myocardial pump function, which leads to renal underperfusion and manifested by azotemia.

At this time, I am going to order 30 g of Kayexalate to be given per nasogastric tube to decrease the patient's potassium. I am also going to order for around-the-clock albuterol nebulization treatments, which may help in shifting potassium levels in between cells.

One has to be very cautious in the overzealous use of diuretics in this patient as the patient may be pushed into a state of intravascular volume depletion, especially now that there is some semblance of prerenal state. The patient is also significantly anemic, and this has to be monitored closely.

We will continue to follow this patient from the critical care standpoint.

I have spent an additional 40 minutes re-evaluating and reassessing this patient's labs and making adjustments in the medications.

1-16C PROGRESS REPORT—SAME DAY AS CASE 1-16A AND 1-16B

Report Dr. Orbitz's service.

LOCATION: Hospital Inpatient

PATIENT: Ann Danube

ATTENDING PHYSICIAN: George Orbitz, M.D.

I am re-evaluating the patient for hypotension with systolic blood pressure in the 60s range.

At this time the plan is to:

1. Start her on dopamine 5 mg/kg per minute.
2. We are going to bolus her with 1 liter of normal saline now.
3. Withhold intravenous diuretic as ordered earlier.

I have also obtained the patient's latest blood gases as follows: 7.341/56.5/110.4/96.% on setting of FiO_2 of 50%, SIMV of 14, tidal volume of 500, PEEP of 5, and pressure support of 10.

PLAN:

1. Decreased SIMV to 12.
2. Decreased FiO_2 to 40%.

A few minutes since starting the dopamine and giving her around 250 ml of normal saline, the patient's blood pressure was noted to have recovered to 160–170 systolic. At this time, we are going to try to cut down on the dopamine to titrate MAP to greater than or equal to 60. I am also going to cut down on her normal saline infusion to 100 ml/hour.

Again, for her hyperkalemia, I have ordered 30 mg of Kayexalate p.o. as well as albuterol nebulization treatments q.2h × four.

At this time, I have spent another 45 minutes re-evaluating and reassessing the situation and formulating the above treatment plan. During this examination also, there was some concern brought about that she had some ecchymosis noted on her lower abdominal area. I spoke with the family concerning this particular problem, but they relay to me this has been there since her recent hospitalization when she had her mitral valve replacement surgery. Therefore, I think it is okay to start her on heparin anticoagulation at this time.

Another issue noted is that of some abdominal distention. I suspect the patient may have had a misintubation in the field such that there was some abdominal distention brought by the Ambu bagging of the gastrointestinal tract. Based on the patient's clinical situation right now and her latest blood gases as well as review of the patient's portable chest x-ray performed in the emergency room, I am pretty sure that the endotracheal tube is in the right place, that is in the airway. I am also going to drop a nasogastric tube for decompression purposes. We will also use this for administration of the 30 g of Kayexalate.

The patient has had a 225 ml urine output from the emergency room. We will send a sample of this urine sodium and urine creatinine.

1-16A, 1-16B, 1-16C:

SERVICE CODE(S): ______________________

DX CODE(S): ______________________

CASE 1-16 DISCUSSION

This is a very challenging set of reports, but they are the types of reports that you need to know how to code. Let's go through this one step at a time and analyze how these services and diagnoses are reported.

Critical Care Services

Read each report carefully with your attention on the diagnoses and indications of time spent in care of the patient, as these are all critical care reports. The three reports in 1-16 are considered together for reporting purposes because they are all critical care services. Do not complete an E/M audit form for critical care services, as it is assumed the patient is in a life-threatening situation with a high risk for death. The services provided involved a very high level of complexity to assess, manipulate, and support the patient's vital functions. This patient had multiple vital OS failure (heart, respiratory, kidneys). Time spent with the patient must be recorded in the critical care note. In this case, add together the time indicated on each report, and report the total time with critical care codes 99291 and 99292, based on the total time of 175 minutes.

Cardiac Arrest

The diagnoses reported for this critical care service (1-16A, B, and C) are considered together. When there are many diagnoses stated in the reports, it is difficult to identify which ones should be reported. Dr. Orbitz, the nephrologist, treated the patient last year. In the Assessment/Plan section of the report, Dr. Orbitz indicates in point 1 that the patient has experienced cardiac arrest (the heart stopped beating). The patient was mechanically resuscitated (as mentioned in paragraph 1 of 1-16A). When referencing the term "Arrest, cardiac" in the Index of the ICD-9-CM, the coder is referred to 427.5. Read the full description of the code in the Tabular.

Respiratory Failure

In 1-16A, point 2 indicates respiratory failure. The underlying reason for the failure has yet to be determined. If the underlying reason had been indicated to be, for example, the congestive heart failure, the respiratory failure would be considered a symptom of the diagnosis of congestive heart failure and would not be reported separately. In this case, however, the physician is considering multiple diagnoses that could be the cause of the respiratory failure, so the condition that is reported is acute respiratory failure NOS (not otherwise specified). Reference "Failure, respiratory, acute" in the Index of the ICD-9-CM, and review the code information in the Tabular to assign a code to this second diagnosis.

Chronic Renal Failure

In 1-16A, point 3 indicates acute renal failure. Previously, information regarding reporting renal failure was presented (after 1-7A). There is mention in paragraph 2 of 1-16A that this patient was "…well known to me because she is one of my chronic renal failure patients…" Chronic renal failure is a permanent condition that worsens over time, which means that this patient currently has CRF and it is a diagnosis that must be reported. The physician should have stated that the patient had CRF in the Assessment/Plan section of the report. Remember to sequence the acute and chronic renal failure according to Section 1.10. of the *Guidelines*.

Questionable Diagnosis

In 1-16A, point 4 indicates "Chronic obstructive pulmonary disease/pulmonary hypertension/? cor pulmonale." This cor pulmonale is a chronic heart disease characterized by hypertrophy that is also known as chronic pulmonary heart disease (There is also an acute cor pulmonale). This condition is secondary to pulmonary hypertension caused by a disorder of the chest wall or lungs. The "?" before cor pulmonale indicates questionable diagnoses that the physician is considering at the time the report was dictated, and as such, is not reported in the outpatient setting. The COPD was treated and is therefore reported.

Diagnoses Not Reported

In 1-16A, points 5, 6, and 7, the physician indicates that the patient has anxiety disorder/depression, hyperlipidemia (excess fat in the blood), and degenerative joint disease; but at this time these conditions are not affecting care, nor were there treatments undertaken. These diagnoses are, therefore, not reported.

Hyperkalemia

In 1-16B, paragraph 1, the physician discusses the rise in some of the laboratory values. In an effort to decrease the level of calcium in the patient's urine, the physician orders Kayexalate, which is an antihyperkalemic medication. Because the physician diagnosed and treated the hyperkalemia, the diagnosis is reported. The physician reports that the patient is "significantly anemic," but since no treatment was undertaken, this diagnosis is not reported.

Hypotension

In 1-16C, the physician states that he is re-evaluating the patient for hypotension (low blood pressure) and orders medication and treatment for the condition, so the diagnosis is reported.

How was that for a complex case! You can see that if you analyze the case, one line and one report at a time, you will arrive at a reason for the inclusion or exclusion of each diagnosis. This is a time-consuming process at the beginning, but it goes more quickly as you work through the various reports.

1. Cardiac Arrest
2. Respiratory Failure (acute NOS)
3. acute renal failure
4. chronic renal failure
5. COPD
6. hyperkalemia
7. hypotension

CASE 1-17

Report Dr. Dawson's service.

1-17A CRITICAL CARE ADMISSION

LOCATION: Hospital Inpatient

PATIENT: Theodore Wilson

ATTENDING PHYSICIAN: Gregory Dawson, M.D.

The patient is being admitted primarily because of hypotension/respiratory failure.

The patient is a 75-year-old white man who is visiting from Texas. Today he had some strenuous exertion when he lifted heavy luggage on their way back to Texas; however, while at the airport, his wife noticed that he was having some diaphoresis and he did not feel well. This prompted him to be brought to the emergency room where he was noted to be in CHF/fluid overload with chest x-rays. He was initially placed on BiPAP, but he continues to desaturate. Eventually, he was intubated and mechanically ventilated.

He was also given a dose of Lasix 80 mg IV push and a p.o. dose of Lasix 60 mg. Accordingly, in the emergency room, his blood pressure has been in the 120s to 140s systolic; however, as soon as he hit the medical ICU, his blood pressure was noted to start trending down, as it was in the 60s/40s. At this time, I have recommended starting the patient on dopamine drip, discontinued the nitroglycerin drip, and discontinued normal saline infusion. The patient's blood pressure started to improve to MAP of 60s to 70s.

I had a lengthy discussion with the patient's wife regarding the rest of his history. See note below. I have also consulted Dr. Elhart in cardiology for his expertise.

The patient has a past medical history and past surgical history that consists of the following:

1. Coronary artery disease, status post five-vessel CABG; multiple stent/plasties in the past with most recent myocardial infarction requiring two stent placements.
2. Hypertension.
3. Type 2 diabetes (he was on Glucophage, but this was discontinued as his blood sugars were fairly controlled in the 110–120 range).
4. Degenerative joint disease.

MEDICATIONS:

1. Toprol 50 b.i.d.
2. Aspirin.
3. Plavix 75 q.d.
4. Lasix 80 b.i.d.
5. Imdur 60 q.d.
6. Lotensin 40 b.i.d.
7. Potassium chloride 20 mEq.
8. Zocor 20 q.d.

SOCIAL HISTORY: He has not been using any tobacco or intravenous or recreational drugs currently. He used to smoke heavily in the past, one pack per day for at least 25+ years, but he is noted to have quit smoking for at least 25 years also. He drinks a couple of beers on a daily basis regularly.

FAMILY HISTORY: Positive for heart disease, hypertension, and stroke. Negative for kidney disease, cancer, bleeding disorder, or dyscrasia. Both parents died of heart disease complications.

REVIEW OF SYSTEMS: Unobtainable as the patient is intubated, mechanically ventilated, and sedated.

Latest LABS are as follows: Hemogram shows an H&H of 15.8/46, WBC 13.29, normochromic/normocytic indices. Platelets 196. There is no left shift as neutrophils are only 70.9%. Sodium 136, potassium 3.7, chloride 100, CO_2 25.7, BUN and creatinine 38/2.2, glucose 287, calcium is 8, and magnesium is 1.9.

The latest blood gases prior to intubation are 7.116/61.1/53.9/19.2/71.3% on 100% nonrebreather.

PHYSICAL EXAMINATION: Vital signs are stable. Blood pressure is 101/40s, MAP in the 70s, respirations 20s. He is afebrile. Heart rate in the 50s. He has a pacemaker also. Normocephalic, atraumatic. Pink palpebral conjunctivae, anicteric sclerae. Intubated and mechanically ventilated. Supple neck. No lymphadenopathy. Symmetrical chest expansion. Positive rhonchi, positive crackles. No wheezes. S1 and S2 are noted. Positive pacemaker. No rubs appreciated. Abdomen: Positive bowel sounds. Soft, nontender. No abdominal bruits. Both upper and lower extremities reveal arthritic changes. Pulses are fair.

ASSESSMENT/PLAN:

1. Rule out myocardial infarction. Check cardiac enzymes. Cardiology consult. Check 12-lead ECG.
2. Congestive heart failure, fluid overload/pulmonary edema secondary to #1. Follow-up daily chest x-rays.
3. Acute renal failure, most likely superimposed on top of underlying chronic renal failure secondary to the following:
   A. Congestive heart failure/overload.
   B. Hypertension.
   C. History of type 2 diabetes.

4. Check blood sugars q.6h. We will also check urine sodium and urine creatinine. I suspect this patient has some degree of prerenal failure brought about by decreased renal perfusion secondary to cardiac pump dysfunction. At this time, we are going to continue the dopamine drip as ordered. We are will waiting input from Dr. Elhart from a cardiology standpoint.
5. Code level I per discussion with the patient's wife.
6. Will continue to follow this patient from the critical care standpoint.

I have spent a total of 120 minutes evaluating and reviewing this patient's medical record, from 9 A.M to 11 A.M

1-17A:

SERVICE CODE(S): ______________________

DX CODE(S): ______________________

1. hypotension
2. Respiratory failure
3. Congestive heart failure
4. acute renal failure

OFFICE AND OTHER OUTPATIENT SERVICES

You will recall that a new patient is defined as one who has not seen the physician or another physician with the same specialty in the same group practice within the past 3 years. A physician must spend more time with a new patient–obtaining the history, conducting the examination, and considering the data–than with an established patient. Consider that the established patient is probably known to the physician and the person's medical records are available.

For these reasons, the cost of a new patient office visit is higher, so third-party payers reimburse the physician at a higher rate for new patient services than for the same type of service when it is provided to an established patient. An established patient is one who has received professional services from the physician or another physician of the same specialty in the same group practice within the past 3 years. The medical record of the patient is available to the physician.

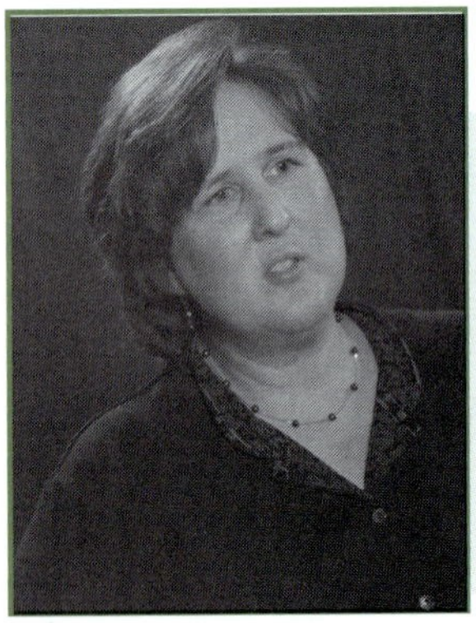

FROM THE TRENCHES

Kathy

"Get your foot in the door any way you can. You have to prove to someone that you can do the job"

CASE 1-18

Report Dr. Naraquist's services for this case.

1-18A OFFICE VISIT

LOCATION: Outpatient, Clinic

PATIENT: Susan Oyez

PRIMARY CARE PHYSICIAN: Alma Naraquist, M.D.

CHIEF COMPLAINT: Dizziness.

SUBJECTIVE: This established patient is a 32-year-old female who reports she was feeling well until yesterday, when she developed some dizziness, which has persisted. She also feels like pills and food have been "sticking" in her throat. She is concerned that she may have a thyroid problem. She has a history of hypothyroidism for which she is on Synthroid 0.125 mg q.d. Her last TSH level was done in March, and at that time was normal at 0.57.

OBJECTIVE: White female who appears to be in general good health. Her blood pressure is 118/82. Afebrile. HEENT is unremarkable. Neck is supple. No masses. No palpable thyromegaly, nodules, or tenderness. TSH level is elevated at 11.77.

ASSESSMENT: Hypothyroidism.

PLAN: We will increase Synthroid to 0.15 mg q.d. Recommend follow-up TSH level in 3 months.

1-18A:

SERVICE CODE(S): ______________________

DX CODE(S): ______________________

1. Hypothyroidism

CASE 1-19
1-19A Office Visit
1-19B Office Visit
1-19C Clinic Progress Note

CASE 1-19

1-19A OFFICE VISIT

LOCATION: Outpatient, Clinic

PATIENT: Sally Lin

PRIMARY CARE PHYSICIAN: Alma Naraquist, M.D.

This new patient is a $2^1/_2$-year-old child seen today because of swelling on the right side of the neck. Nothing she has tried has reduced the swelling. It is the first time the patient has been seen here at the clinic. Mother has noticed this lump in her neck for the last week. She has had a little bit of an upper respiratory infection. They also have a dog at home, which the patient plays with infrequently.

PAST MEDICAL HISTORY: Pregnancy was probably complicated by gestational diabetes. It was a term, normal spontaneous vaginal delivery birth. No problems with jaundice. The patient has been developing normally. She sat at 6 months. Walked a little before a year. The patient is developing normally. Past history is complicated by a recurrent otitis. The patient had PE tubes placed at 11 months of age.

ALLERGIC to SULFA–developed a rash. Currently, no medications.

Immunizations are up to date.

FAMILY HISTORY: Mother is 32. Dad is 35. Mother is 5 feet 5 inches, and father is 6 feet 2 inches. Both in good health. They have a 5-year-old daughter, a 1-year-old son, and the patient, who is $2^1/_2$ years old. There is a family history of lung disease and also diabetes. Otherwise negative for renal, cystic fibrosis, asthma, Crohn's, ulcerative colitis, or childhood deaths.

REVIEW OF SYSTEMS: HEENT is otherwise negative other than the recurrent otitis. Lungs: Negative. Heart: Negative. GI: Negative. Neurologic: Negative.

PHYSICAL EXAMINATION: Happy, alert $2^1/_2$-year-old child in no acute distress. Afebrile. Weight is 23 pounds. Length is $33^3/_4$ inches. Both at just below the 5th percentile. Mother states this is where she has been tracking for the last year and a half or so. HEENT: Head, nontraumatic. TMs: Both tubes are out, but they are clear. Pupils are equal and reactive to light and accommodation. Extraocular movements are intact. Nose with some mild congestion. Throat mildly erythematous. Neck supple, with some shotty anterior cervical adenopathy. On the left side, there is a lymph node of about 0.8 mm. No erythema. Easily movable. No supraclavicular nodes. No axillary nodes are felt. Lungs are clear. Cardiovascular: Regular rate and rhythm. Intermittent vibratory 1/6 murmur, left sternal border. Abdomen: Bowel sounds are positive. No hepatosplenomegaly. No masses. Nontender. GUR: Normal Tanner I female. Spine is straight. Neurologically intact.

IMPRESSION: Lymphadenopathy, secondary to URI.

PLAN: Will go ahead and screen her with a CBC and diff. We will also do a throat culture. Will begin Augmentin 125/5, 1 teaspoon p.o. t.i.d. for 10 days. Recheck in 2 weeks.

1-19A:

SERVICE CODE(S): ______________________

DX CODE(S): ______________________

1-19B OFFICE VISIT

LOCATION: Outpatient, Clinic

PATIENT: Sally Lin

PRIMARY CARE PHYSICIAN: Alma Naraquist, M.D.

The patient comes in for a 2-week follow-up visit for lymphadenitis, which was treated with **augmentin.** Mother states that the lump that was on the right side of her neck is still there; however, it is not sore, and she will allow them to check it with no problems. She did get some diarrhea with the antibiotic. She has not had any cold symptoms with congestion since finishing her antibiotics. The mother states that the patient has returned to herself being playful and eating well and being more interactive.

PHYSICAL EXAMINATION: HEENT: TMs have good landmarks and are pearly gray bilaterally. Sinus mucosa is pink and moist. Pharynx is unremarkable. There is some shotty lymphadenopathy on the left side of the neck. There is a small, 0.5-cm enlarged lymph node underneath the right mandible. There is also a small, approximately 0.5-cm lymph node on the right side of the neck. Chest is clear to auscultation bilaterally. The heart has a regular sinus rhythm without clicks, rubs, or murmurs. Abdomen is soft with no organomegaly or masses.

IMPRESSION: Resolving lymphadenitis.

PLAN: We will not put the patient on antibiotics at this time; however, we will have her return to the clinic in 1 month to make sure the lymph node continues to get smaller. If there are any problems with high fever or increased cough or other health problems before the 1-month time, she is instructed to bring the patient in for evaluation.

1-19B:

SERVICE CODE(S): ____________________

DX CODE(S): ____________________

1-19C CLINIC PROGRESS NOTE

LOCATION: Outpatient, Clinic

PATIENT: Sally Lin

PRIMARY CARE PHYSICIAN: Alma Naraquist, M.D.

HISTORY: This established patient came in with complaints of cold symptoms for the past couple of days. She had a couple of episodes of emesis this morning, however, nothing for the past 6 hours now. She has drunk fluids and eaten a little bit since then without difficulty. She has had a little bit of a low-grade temperature and occasional cough. She has also complained intermittently of a sore throat. No diarrhea. She is otherwise healthy, and her immunizations are up-to-date, according to Mom.

EXAMINATION: She is alert and in no distress. She is afebrile. Eyes are clear. Tympanic membranes are clear with good landmarks. Nose reveals some crusting to the nares. Mucous membranes are moist, and her pharynx shows some mild erythema but no exudate. Neck is supple without significant lymphadenopathy. Lungs are clear to auscultation. Heart has a regular rate and rhythm without murmur. GI is benign.

IMPRESSION: Upper respiratory infection with a little bit of pharyngitis.

PLAN: Symptomatic care is discussed. The possibility of this evolving into more of a gastroenteritis picture was discussed. If she starts vomiting more, they should place her on clear liquids and avoid dairy products. Push fluids, small amounts frequently. We will go ahead and get a throat culture, and if it comes back positive, we will start her on antibiotics. Otherwise, continue symptomatic care. They should return if her condition worsens or if they have other concerns.

1-19C:

SERVICE CODE(S): ____________________

DX CODE(S): ____________________

Hospital Observation Services

The codes in the Hospital Observation subsection are used to identify initial observation care or observation discharge services. The services in the observation subsection are for patients who are in a hospital on observation status.

Observation is a status used for the classification of a patient who does not have an illness severe enough to meet acute inpatient criteria and does not require resources as intensive as an inpatient but does require hospitalization for a short period. Patients are also admitted to observation so further information can be obtained about the severity of the condition, and so it can be determined whether the patient can be treated on an outpatient basis. In some parts of the country, observation status is conducted in the temporary care unit (TCU).

The observation codes are for new or established patients. There are no time components with observation codes because codes are based on the level of service.

If a patient is admitted to the hospital as an inpatient after having been admitted earlier the same day as an observation patient, *do not* report the observation status separately. Services provided during observation become part of (are bundled into) the initial inpatient hospital admission code.

Observation Care Discharge Services

The Observation Care Discharge Services code includes the final examination of the patient on discharge from observation status. Discussion of the hospital stay, instructions for continued care, and preparation of discharge records are also bundled into the Observation Care Discharge Services code. The code is used only with patients who are discharged on a day that follows the first day of observation.

Initial Observation Care

Initial Observation Care codes (99218–99220) are used to designate the beginning of observation status in a hospital. The hospital does not need to have a formal observation area because the designation of observation status is dependent on the severity of illness of the patient. The codes also include development of a care plan for the patient and periodic reassessment while on observation status. Observation admission can be reported only for the first day of the service. If the patient is admitted and discharged on the same day, a code from the range 99234–99236, Observation or Inpatient Care Services, is used to report the service. If the patient is in the hospital overnight but remains there for a period that is *less than 48 hours,* the first day's service is coded with a code from 99218–99220, Initial Observation Care, and the second day's service is coded 99217, Observation Care Discharge Services. If the patient is on observation status for *longer than 48 hours,* the first day is coded with 99218–99220, Initial Observation Care; the second day is coded with 99211–99215, Established Office or Other Outpatient Services; and the third day is coded with 99217.

Observation Care Discharge Services

Services performed in sites other than the observation area (e.g., clinic, nursing home, emergency department) and that precede admission to observation status are bundled into the Initial Observation Care codes and are not coded separately.

For example, an established patient was seen in the physician's office for frequent fainting of unknown origin. The history and examination were comprehensive, and the MDM complexity was moderate. The code for the office visit is 99215, but the physician decided to admit the patient immediately on observation status until a further determination could be made as to the origin of the fainting. You would choose a code from the Hospital Inpatient Services subsection, Initial Observation Care subheading, in order to report the physician's service of admission on observation status (99219) and would not separately report the office visit.

If a patient is admitted to observation status and then becomes ill enough to be admitted to the hospital, an initial hospital care code (99221–99223), not an observation code, is used to report services.

CASE 1-20

Report Dr. Narquist's service.

I-20A OBSERVATION

LOCATION: Hospital Observation Unit

PATIENT: Missy Lunde

ATTENDING PHYSICIAN: Alma Naraquist, M.D.

REASON FOR ADMISSION: Acute diarrhea and volume depletion.

HISTORY OF PRESENT ILLNESS: The patient is a 52-year-old white female who is known to have chronic renal failure, presumed to be related to lupus nephritis, who was vacationing in Jamaica and came back last night. She went out and had dinner at Mable's Castle here in town. Since 8:00 P.M. last night, she has been having diarrhea at least four times an hour. Her diarrhea increased to 6:00 in the morning. I received a call from her husband in the early morning, and I advised them to come to the emergency room. She was thought to be dehydrated in the ER and was admitted.

Her diarrhea is mostly loose. It does not seem to be explosive; minimal mucus, and no blood. It is associated with some cramping, especially after she passes a bowel movement. She denies any fever or chills. She has no night sweats. This seems all to be acute and she did not have any problems with diarrhea before.

She has no heartburn, nausea, or vomiting.

She has seen a physician in Jamaica, who added to her medications, Mavik 4 mg q.d. and Catapres to treat her uncontrolled hypertension.

The patient seemed frustrated with her care because she is taking five medications for high blood pressure, and she has been compliant with diet, but her blood pressure does not seem to be controlled.

PAST MEDICAL HISTORY: Significant for the following:

1. Systemic lupus erythematosus, which seems to be inactive.
2. Chronic renal failure requiring dialysis for a few weeks and then recovery of her renal function documented with a creatinine clearance of 23 ml/min with a serum creatinine of 2.9 and urine creatinine of 76 mg/dl last month. She continues to have a right IJ tunneled dialysis catheter, but she has not been on dialysis for 3 weeks. The patient has been feeling good about that. She has been seen at the Jamaican Clinic and was started on CellCept 1g b.i.d.
3. Also, the patient had a kidney biopsy done here under CT guidance. Unfortunately, no glomeruli were noted. Most of the two pieces of tissue submitted contained medulla. The patient had proteinuria up to 6 g in 24 hours. This is at the time when she had her kidney biopsy. She had only one kidney biopsy, and this has never been followed up. We do not have any diagnosis, unfortunately, at this time, and she has been treated empirically.
4. Uncontrolled hypertension with multiple medications and regimens back and forth for the past few months without any benefit. The patient still runs 160–180 systolic over 90–100 diastolic.
5. History of BOOP in the past, status post thoracotomy.
6. Restrictive lung disease.
7. Chronic dry cough.
8. Chronic dry mouth.
9. Chronic anemia of kidney disease and probably of chronic disease.
10. History of bilateral flank pain of unclear etiology while she was on dialysis. It has never been worked up.
11. Multiple compression fractures with osteoporosis.
12. Hyperlipidemia.

ALLERGIES: AMOXICILLIN.

CURRENT MEDICATIONS:

1. Prednisone 10 mg q.d.
2. CellCept 500 mg 2 b.i.d.
3. Cozaar 50 mg 2 b.i.d.
4. Epogen 15,000 subcutaneously twice a week.
5. Nephrocaps 1 q.d.
6. Renagel 1 t.i.d with meals.
7. Norvasc 10 mg q.d.
8. Metoprolol XL 100 mg b.i.d.
9. Catapres patch 0.1 mg 2 patches once a week.
10. Tylenol PM.
11. Lasix 40 mg b.i.d.
12. Protonix 40 mg 1 q.d.
13. Mavik 4 mg 1 q.d. for the past week.

SOCIAL HISTORY: The patient is a nonsmoker and nondrinker. She lives with her husband.

FAMILY HISTORY: She has 2 sisters and 1 brother, and most of them are hypertensive. Otherwise, her family history is noncontributory.

REVIEW OF SYSTEMS: General: No fever, chills, night sweats, or recent weight change. ENT: Dryness in her mouth and nose, which is chronic. Eyes: Status post cataract surgeries. Neurologic: No numbness, tingling, headaches, or fainting spells. Respiratory: Chronic cough, occasional sputum production. No orthopnea or PNDs. Occasional leg edema. Cardiac: No chest pain, orthopnea, PNDs, leg edema, or claudication. GI: As mentioned in the HPI. GU: No frequency, urgency, hematuria, or nocturia. Skin: No recent rashes or itching. Endocrine: No diabetes or thyroid problems, but she has been on chronic steroid therapy.

PHYSICAL EXAMINATION: On examination, the patient is lying in bed. She looks dry. She is not in any distress. Blood pressure is 180s/90s. She is afebrile. Respiratory rate is 16 per minute. Saturations are maintained on room air in the mid 90s. She has no increased jugular venous pressure. She has right IJ tunnel dialysis catheter. No cervical lymphadenopathy other than dry mucous membranes. ENT is negative. Lungs: Good air entry bilaterally without crackles. No sacral edema. 1+ leg edema bilaterally. Abdomen is very soft and nontender. I cannot hear any renal bruits. Cardiac exam: Regular S1 and S2 without any murmurs or friction rubs. Neurologic: The patient is awake, alert, and oriented. Cranial nerves II–XII seem to be intact. Motor power is 5/5 bilaterally with normal gait. Spine straight.

LABORATORY STUDIES: Sodium 144, potassium 4.5, chloride 117, bicarb 13.3, glucose 94, creatinine 2.3, calcium 8.3, and BUN 46.

Hemoglobin is 9.5, white count 7.1 thousand, and platelets were 111,000.

Her last bicarb last month was 25.1. At that time her last platelet count was 188,000.

Urinalysis showed no white or red cells. Rare hyaline casts, pH of 6.0, protein more than 300, and specific gravity of 1.020.

Stool was negative for PMNs.

Abdominal x-rays were negative.

IMPRESSION:

1. Acute diarrhea, probably infectious in etiology, and so far she does not have any loose stools since she has been admitted.
2. I do not know what her renal function is like. I suppose that her kidney function will improve with hydration.
3. Metabolic acidosis secondary to diarrhea.
4. Chronic renal failure, related to lupus nephritis, but no tissue diagnosis unfortunately in this relatively young woman.
5. Very uncontrolled hypertension with multiple medications.

PLAN:

1. The patient was admitted for observation.
2. We will give her D5W, 3 amp of bicarb at 150 cc an hour for a total of 3 liters.
3. We will repeat her labs in the morning.
4. After she gets fluids, I will check aldosterone and renin levels in the morning.
5. I will obtain a renal ultrasound.
6. I will hold her Cozaar and Mavik at this time.
7. I will hold her furosemide.
8. I will hold her CellCept and Protonix at this time.
9. We will continue with metoprolol and Norvasc for blood pressure.
10. I will check a phosphorus level on her and repeat labs in the morning.
11. I will check and also recheck her platelets in the morning.

I had a long discussion with the patient. I spent 60 minutes out of 85 minutes with the patient and her husband counseling on her kidney disease and uncontrolled hypertension. We also discussed her acute problem with diarrhea. We have discussed the possibilities of secondary causes of hypertension. She has been on chronic steroid therapy, but renal stenosis has never been pursued. She has never had an ultrasound of her kidneys. We do not have even a tissue diagnosis on her renal failure. This is all unfortunate. The patient needs to be followed up more closely, and we need to try and evaluate for possible treatable causes of hypertension.

I will probably discharge the patient by tomorrow if she is feeling better and her diarrhea has resolved. I will schedule her to have an MRA next week. I would also schedule her to have a kidney biopsy by myself under real time ultrasound guidance.

The patient is a candidate for kidney transplant if her kidney function is going to deteriorate and stays in the mid-20s; however, we need to look at her tissue, look at her glomeruli and interstitium, and see whether there is any possibility for reversibility.

All the above was discussed with the patient and her husband. They both seem to understand and agree with the above plan. I also have stressed to them that only one physician should follow her blood pressure and manage it.

Both the patient and her husband seem to be satisfied and agreeable with the above plan.

I-20A:

SERVICE CODE(S): ____________________

DX CODE(S): ____________________

CASE 1-20A DISCUSSION

This report contained several diagnoses, so check with your instructor on the correct codes for this case. In addition to the other codes, the following are two coding situations that you may not have encountered. Section I.C7.3 of the *Guidelines* directs the coder to assign codes from category 403 (hypertensive renal disease) when a condition classified to 585–587 (chronic renal failure, unspecified renal failure, unspecified renal stenosis) is present. This means that if hypertension is present along with the renal failure or stenosis, you report only a hypertensive renal disease code (403). The diagnoses of chronic renal failure and hypertension become the one diagnosis of hypertensive renal disease.

Lupus Nephritis

In the Impression section of the report, the physician stated the CRF is related to lupus nephritis. Lupus nephritis is inflammation of the kidney caused by systemic lupus erythematosus (SLE), a disease of the immune system. When referencing "Lupus, nephritis" in the Index of the ICD-9-CM, the coder is directed to report the etiology (cause), which in this case is lupus, and the manifestation (symptom), which in this case is nephritis. The Index displays the order in which the codes should be reported, with the lupus code placed before the nephritis code.

Neonatal Care Services

A neonate is a newly born infant. Two groups of codes are used to report neonatal care services: Inpatient Neonatal Intensive Care (NIC) (99295–99298) and **Newborn Care** (99431–99440). Newborn Care codes are to report the services to a normal newborn, and Inpatient Neonatal Intensive Care codes are used to report services when the newborn needs additional services. Neonatal coding is a bit more complex then other E/M services because not only does the neonate have a separate set of intensive care codes, but also separate history and examination codes (Newborn Care) when the service is provided in the hospital setting. In addition to using these two groups of codes to report neonate services, you also must also use codes from throughout the CPT manual to report accurately report the services provided to the neonate.

When coding neonatal services, the status of the newborn, location in which the service was provided, and the type of service must first be considered.

The first consideration is the **status** of the newborn:

- Services for a critically ill neonate who weighs less than 1500 g and is less than 30 days of age can be reported with Inpatient Neonatal Critical Care codes.
- Services for a neonate that is no longer critically ill, weighs more than 1500 g, and/or is more than 30 days old cannot be reported with Inpatient Neonatal Critical Care codes.

The second consideration is the **location** of the service:

- If the location of initial service was newborn care in the **hospital** setting, you would report 99431 (history and examination of normal newborn infant, initiation of diagnostic and treatment programs, and preparation of hospital records) and service on a subsequent day with 99433 (Subsequent hospital care, for the evaluation and management of a normal newborn, per day).
- If the initial newborn service is provided in the office or other **outpatient** setting, the established patient codes 99201–99205 (New patient, Office or Other Outpatient Service) are used to report the service as you would for any new patient.

The third consideration is the **type** of service:

- If an infant is seen in the hospital by a pediatrician for the newborn's initial pediatric service, report the service with an **Initial Hospital Care** code (99221–99223) as you would for any patient.
- If the first service was an outpatient **preventive medicine service,** use 99381 to report an initial comprehensive preventive medicine service provided to an infant (under 1 year).

With these three considerations in mind, let's take a closer look at the specifics of the Neonatal Intensive Care codes and the Newborn Care codes.

Neonatal Intensive Care (NIC)

The name of the intensive care unit does not matter in the application of NIC codes. The services can be provided in a pediatric intensive care unit, neonatal critical care unit, or any of the many names that these types of intensive care units have. What is important in the use of NIC codes is that the neonate:

- is less than 30 days old
- has a weight of less than 1500 g (very low birth weight, VLBW), or
- is critically ill

NIC codes (99295–99298) are critical care codes for neonates, and the medical record must contain documentation that indicates that the neonate is in an acute life-threatening situation. The codes from the NIC subsection are reported only once in every 24-hour period (same day). There are no hourly service codes as there are in other critical care codes. If an infant older than 30 days is admitted to an intensive care unit and is critically ill, the services would be reported using the Critical Care Service codes 99291 and 99292, which are based on hourly service.

Bundled into the NIC codes are many services you would anticipate would be used in the support of a critically ill neonate, for example, umbilical arterial catheters, nasogastric tube placement, endotracheal intubation, and invasive electronic monitoring of vital signs. The extensive notes preceding the NIC codes list bundled services. As you code NIC services, you will need to refer back to the list of services and codes that are bundled into the codes in this subsection. If the physician performed a service not listed in the notes, you would report for the service separately. Other notes indicating bundled services appear in the code descriptions. Locate and read the description for code 99295, and you will see that the description indicates that cardiac and/or respiratory support, as well as many other services, are bundled into the code. *You must carefully read all notes, parenthetical information, and code descriptions to accurately assign these codes.*

The NIC codes are divided based on the status of the neonate as being critically ill, critically ill and unstable, or critically ill and stable. The physician will indicate the status of the infant in the medical record.

If the physician provides physician standby (99360), attendance at delivery (99436), or resuscitation (99440) in addition to NIC services, these services are reported in addition to the NIC codes.

Newborn Care (NCS)

The Newborn Care codes (99431–99440) are used to identify services provided to normal or high-risk newborns. Within the NCS are two history and examination codes; one is specifically for a newborn assessment and discharge from a hospital or birthing room on the same date (99435), and one is for birthing room deliveries (99431) without a discharge service on the day of birth. If the physician provides a discharge service to a newborn that is discharged subsequent to the admission date, choose a code from the Hospital Inpatient Services subsection, Hospital Discharge Services subheading (99238–99239) to report the service.

The obstetrician cares for the mother during delivery. Sometimes the obstetrician may request a pediatrician to be in attendance during delivery to stabilize and provide immediate care to the neonate. The pediatrician would report this service with 99436 (Attendance at delivery). If the pediatrician needs to resuscitate the newborn by means of chest compression or positive pressure ventilation (PPV), the resuscitation service would be reported with 99440 (Newborn resuscitation). A parenthetical note following the code description for 99436 (Attendance at delivery) indicates that 99436 and 99440 (Newborn resuscitation) cannot be reported at the same time. Because you can report only one of the services—either the attendance at delivery or the resuscitation—you should report the resuscitation (99440) because the resuscitation code has a higher reimbursement than the attendance code (99436).

When an infant is born, a slimy substance (mucilaginous material, meconium) is present in the esophagus, stomach, and intestines of the infant. This substance is a mixture of secretions from the liver, intestines, and amniotic fluid. It may be necessary for the pediatrician to suction this material from the trachea and stomach by **endotracheal intubation.** The intubation service would be reported separately with a Respiratory System code 31500 (Intubation, endotracheal, emergency procedure). The pediatrician in attendance may also need to **catheterize the umbilical vein** for blood sampling or administration of medication, and this service is reported separately with 36510 (Catheterization of umbilical vein).

When reporting services with the Neonatal Intensive Care codes, recall that there were many services bundled into the codes, and a list of the bundled services appears in the notes preceding the codes. With the Newborn Care codes, that is not the case. With the NCS codes, the services the physician provides are reported separately, such as central catheters (36510), peripheral vessel catheterization (36000), lumbar puncture (62270), bladder aspiration (51000), and so on. See the list of services that are bundled into the NIC codes for further examples of services that are not bundled into the NCS.

Newborn Diagnosis Coding

Reporting the Liveborn Infant

V30–V39 are used to report liveborn infants along with fourth-digit subdivisions of:

0 Born in hospital
1 Born before admission to hospital
2 Born outside hospital and not hospitalized

A fifth digit is also available for those born in the hospital (fourth digit 0):

0 Delivered without mention of cesarean delivery
1 Delivered by cesarean delivery

The codes identify single, twin, other multiple, or unspecified births. These codes are only assigned to the newborn record, not the mother's record. If the infant's medical record indicated other significant conditions, these conditions would be reported in addition to the V30–39 code.

Disorders Relating to Short Gestation and Low Birth Weight

The gestation of a fetus takes approximately 266 days or 40 weeks. Code 765 is used to report short gestation and low birth weight. There are fifth digits 0–9 for assignment, depending on the weight of the newborn in grams.

- **765.0X** is reported for **extreme immaturity,** which implies a birth weight of less than 1,000 grams. The fifth digit is assigned to indicate the weight range at birth. In addition to the extreme immaturity code, a code is reported for the weeks of gestation (765.2X).
- **765.1X** is reported for **other preterm infants,** which implies a birth weight of 1,000–2,499 grams. The fifth digit is assigned to indicate the weight range at birth. In addition to the preterm code, a code is reported for weeks of gestation (765.2X). Conversely, "late infant," "heavy for dates," and "exceptionally large" infants are coded to 766.X.

CASE 1-21

The newborn in Case 1-21 was a liveborn, full-term twin delivered by the obstetrician by means of cesarean section. You will code the services of Dr. Ortez, the pediatrician, which will include the daily services (1-1 through 1-4, a procedure, and a discharge service) based on the information in the Progress Notes section of the form. The first day, 1/1, services are indicated on the check-off portion of the form.

1-21A NEWBORN CARE

LOCATION: Inpatient, Hospital

PATIENT: Anthony Marcello

ATTENDING PHYSICIAN: Roland Ortez, M.D.

1-21A:

SERVICE CODE(S): ______________________

DX CODE(S): ______________________

NEWBORN EXAM RECORD

	Normal	Abnormal	ADMISSION EXAM Date: 1/1	Normal	Abnormal	DISCHARGE EXAM Date: 1/5
Head/Fontanels		✓	*1 cm area between fontanels and to (L) of*	✓		*Head healing well*
Eyes	✓		*sagittal suture of no skin*	✓		
Ears/Nose/Throat	✓		✓			
Heart	✓		✓			
Lungs	✓		✓			
Abdomen	✓		✓			
Trunk/Spine	✓		✓			
Anus	✓		✓			
Genitalia	✓		✓			
Negative Barlow Test	✓		✓			
Negative Ortolani Test	✓		✓			
Extremities/Clavicles	✓		✓			
Skin	✓		✓			
Neurological/Tone	✓		✓			

PROGRESS NOTES:

1/2 Exam on 1x top of head, which is clean and dry. Color good. Wt down 2.5%. Nursing poorly. GJH	
1/3 Exam: head healing well. Color good. Nursing better. Wt down 6.8%. Circumcised per parent request. GJH	
1/4 Exam: wt down 8.9%. Nursing poorly. Color good. GJH	
1/5 Exam: wt down 9.2%. Nursingpoorly. Discharge from the hospital and I will see on Monday in the office. GJH	
	Hearing Exam: Passed *AZ*

FIGURE 1-14 Newborn examination record.

CASE 1-22

Report Dr. Ortez's services for Case 22, which includes both the delivery and the NICU care.

1-22A HOSPITAL SERVICES

LOCATION: Hospital Inpatient, Delivery Room and Neonatal Intensive Care Unit

PATIENT: Robert Zimmerman

ATTENDING PHYSICIAN: Roland Ortez, M.D.

CHIEF COMPLAINT: Prematurity with respiratory difficulty.

HISTORY: This is a 30-week gestation male infant with a birth weight of 1808g. Mom is a 27-year-old gravida 3, now para 3 mom. Her blood type is B, antibody negative, RPR nonreactive, rubella immune, hepatitis B surface antigen negative, HIV negative, GC negative, *Chlamydia* negative, group B strep status unknown. No neural tube defect. No amniocentesis performed. She was on prenatal vitamins.

First pregnancy went without complications. She is doing well at 3 years of age; however, she does have Noonan syndrome. Mom presented with questionable rupture of membranes in preterm labor 4 weeks ago. It was found that her membranes were intact, and she continued throughout the rest of her pregnancy to have a high AFI. Preterm labor was stopped with magnesium sulfate. Mom's magnesium level today is 7.5. She was also on penicillin G 1/2 48 hours. She received two doses of betamethasone.

Mom was noted to have increased urinary frequency today, and labs were obtained, which showed elevation of her AST and ALT into the 300s. Also, elevation of her bilirubin to 2.6 with concerns for her developing fatty liver of pregnancy. Her platelet count was 178,000 today and hemoglobin 11.6. Coagulation studies were normal on the mom. Because of concern for fatty liver of pregnancy, an emergent cesarean section was performed

I did attend the delivery, and the infant was delivered at 2:01 P.M. today. Spontaneous cry noted and Apgar scores were 7 at 1 minute with points off for color, tone, and grimace. Then at 5 minutes, an Apgar score of 8 with points off for grimace and tone. The infant was brought back to the NICU for further management.

The infant's face does look somewhat dysmorphic with concerns of Noonan syndrome. A very small posterior pharyngeal space was noted with difficult intubation, and after several attempts, anesthesia was called and came up and intubated the infant. Throughout the intubation attempts, standard procedure was followed, and the infant tolerated the attempts very well. The intubation was performed because of concerns of hypoventilation noted on exam with decreased breath sounds bilaterally as well as increased work of breathing.

Umbilical artery catheter was also placed without difficulty. First blood sugar did come back at 23, and a peripheral IV was placed promptly and 2 cc/kilo of D10 was given along with placing the infant on D10 at 80 cc/kilo. Second blood sugar has come back elevated.

Chest x-ray is obtained as well as abdominal films and shows good placement of the UAC at T7, and the endotracheal tube is also in good placement and is 3.02. The OG has been advanced. The lung fields do show significant granularity present. No pneumothorax. No cardiomegaly. Blood gas is 7.32, PCO_2 of 50, PO_2 of 100, and that is on a setting of 22/4, rate of 60, and 80% FiO_2.

PHYSICAL EXAMINATION: Currently is intubated. His weight is 1808 g. His OFC is 30.5 cm. Length is 39.4 cm. Heart rate is in the 130s to 140s. Respiratory rate is 60 on the ventilator. O_2 saturation is in the mid 90s. Blood pressure in right arm 67/34 with a mean of 46 and right leg 67/32 with a mean of 44.

Mild splitting of the cranial sutures is noted along with open posterior and anterior fontanel. Red reflex times two. The eyes appear to be hypertelorism present and questionable epicanthal folds along with some down-slanting palpebral fissures. Ears appear to be low set and posteriorly rotated. Palate is intact. Small retropharyngeal space. Clavicles are intact. I do not appreciate any webbing on the neck. Nipples questionably mildly wide-spaced. Lungs at this time are clear to auscultation. He has good symmetric aeration, minimal chest rise noted. Prior to that, lungs were remarkable for decreased aeration with crackles. Heart is regular rate and rhythm; no murmurs noted. Femoral pulses palpable. Capillary refill less than 2 seconds. Abdomen without hepatosplenomegaly. Three-vessel cord. Genitourinary: Normal external male. Testes are not descended. Extremities: Adequate range of motion. No contractures or hip abnormalities noted. The skin is ruddy in complexion. Neurologic exam: Hypotonia diffusely.

Developmental assessment: No breast buds. Soft pinna with minimal recoil. No creases on the feet. No rugae on the testes. All consistent with a 30-week preterm infant.

IMPRESSION:
1. Premature male infant.
2. Respiratory distress consistent with hyaline membrane disease as well as a component of hypoventilation secondary to maternal elevated magnesium.
3. Observation for sepsis.
4. Maternal hypermagnesemia with elevated magnesium in the infant as well.

PLAN: Admission to the NICU. Intubation has been performed, and he is on mechanical ventilation. Will go ahead with the surfactant therapy per protocol. Close cardiorespiratory monitoring and monitoring of blood gases and chest x-rays. NPO status, and he will be on D10 with 0.94 mEq of calcium gluconate added to run at 80 cc/kilo per day. Ampicillin and gentamicin per protocol. Blood cultures have been obtained as well as a CBC, magnesium level, and further glucose monitoring. He will also need chromosomal testing, and that will be drawn in the near future. Also head ultrasound at 6 days of life will need to be performed. I have not talked with the mother. Her condition has deteriorated post cesarean section and is not available at this time. I have talked in detail with the father in regard to the above, including the possibility of further deterioration, prompting transfer to another facility. All his questions were answered.

1-22A:

SERVICE CODE(S): ____________________

DX CODE(S): ____________________

CASE 1-22A DISCUSSION

Hyaline Membrane Disease

The primary reason this service is being provided is the newborn has hyaline membrane disease, which is a respiratory syndrome of a newborn. As such, this is the first-listed diagnosis.

Gestation and Birth Weight

This is a premature infant, so you will need to assign two codes, one for the gestation and one for the birth weight (refer back to the information before case 1-21A).

Observation

Note that in this report the physician indicated that the newborn was being placed on observation for sepsis. Sepsis is a condition in which pathogenic microorganisms and/or their toxins are in the blood. This status of "observation" is reported with a V code to indicate observation for a condition in a newborn for an infectious disease.

Hypermagnesemia

In point 4 of the Impression section of this report, the physician indicated that the infant has hypermagnesemia, which is a high level of magnesium in the blood.

1-22B NICU PROGRESS REPORT

On a subsequent day, Dr. Zimmerman provided the following service.

LOCATION: Hospital Inpatient, Neonatal Intensive Care Unit

PATIENT: Robert Zimmerman

ATTENDING PHYSICIAN: Roland Ortez, M.D.

SUBJECTIVE: Baby boy is slightly under 24 hours old.

OBJECTIVE: Weight today is 1.851 kg (increased 43 g over birth weight). OFC is 30.5 cm (unchanged). Intake and output from yesterday do appear adequate, although it is less than 24 hours. He has had no stool since birth. Vital signs reveal his temperature to be acceptable while being maintained on an open radiant warmer. Heart rate is generally in the 110s to 140s. Respiratory rate is generally equal to the IMV (60). Mean blood pressures had decreased last night to the low 30s but are now in the low to mid 40s while on dopamine infusion.

PHYSICAL EXAMINATION: In general, he is pink on current ventilator settings. He does appear slightly dysmorphic with eyes wide set and slightly down-slanting palpebral fissures. Ears appear low-set and posteriorly rotated. Endotracheal tube is in place. Chest reveals symmetric expansion, and the lungs are clear to auscultation on current ventilator settings. Cardiac exam reveals a regular rate without murmur or click. Peripheral pulses are 2+ and symmetric. Abdominal exam reveals an umbilical arterial catheter in place. Liver is palpable 1 cm below the right costal margin. No splenomegaly or masses are noted. Genital examination reveals normal male; testes are not palpable. Extremity examination reveals no fixed decreased range of motion, deformity, or joint abnormality. Neurologic exam reveals diffuse hypotonia. No focal deficits are appreciated.

CURRENT MEDICATIONS:
1. Ampicillin 90.4 mg IV q.12h.
2. Gentamicin 5.4 mg IV q.18h.
3. Morphine sulfate 0.18 mg IV q.6h and q.1h p.r.n.
4. Dopamine 5 mcg/kg per minute.
5. Vecuronium 0.18 mg IV q.1-2h. p.r.n.

LABORATORY STUDIES: Last arterial blood gas was obtained on ventilator settings of IMV 60, pressure 22/4, and FiO_2 0.53 and revealed pH 7.3, PCO_2 46.6, PO_2 52.7, and bicarbonate 22.7. Chemistry panel this A.M. revealed sodium 123, potassium 5.7, chloride 93, glucose 66, BUN 12, creatinine 0.9, calcium 7.3, magnesium 5.4, phosphorus 6.8, bilirubin 4.4, alkaline phosphatase 200, ALT 14, AST 38, albumin 1.7, and total protein 3.6. Electrolytes were repeated and were unchanged. CBC with differential this A.M. revealed a white count of 8230 with 7 bands, 46 neutrophils, 33 lymphocytes, 8 monocytes, and 6 eosinophils. H&H was 20.7 and 61.8 with an MCV of 113. Platelet count was 98,000. Chest x-ray continues to show significant evidence of hyaline membrane disease.

IMPRESSIONS/RECOMMENDATIONS:

1. Less than 24-hour-old infant who was born at 30 weeks gestation. Based on clinical examination, he may have Noonan syndrome.
2. RESPIRATORY: He has evidence of hyaline membrane disease with respiratory distress. He has received two doses of surfactant and will receive a third dose soon. We will adjust his ventilator setting based on serial clinical examinations, pulse oximetry, arterial blood gas determinations, and chest x-rays. Will continue sedation and paralysis at this time. Would recommend a short course of steroids because of the intubation attempts when he is extubated.
3. CARDIOVASCULAR: Cardiovascular status is acceptable at this time while on dopamine 5 mcg/kg per minute. Blood pressure has improved on echocardiography to evaluated PDA, depending on his clinical course.
4. GASTROINTESTINAL: Abdominal exam remains benign. He is NPO. He has mild hyperbilirubinemia, and Mom is noted to have O positive blood and Rh. We are going to obtain a direct antibody test. Will follow with serial bilirubin determinations.
5. HEMATOLOGIC: He has developed a mild thrombocytopenia, will monitor.
6. INFECTIOUS DISEASE: Blood culture remains negative. He is on ampicillin and gentamicin. We will check closely.
7. NEUROLOGIC: Neurologic exam remains acceptable given his extreme prematurity. He will require screening intracranial ultrasounds and long-term neurodevelopmental follow-up.
8. RENAL/METABOLIC: Urine output remains adequate at this time. Metabolic parameters were acceptable. Will monitor closely.
9. FLUID/ELECTROLYTE/NUTRITION: He has gained some weight since birth. Multiple electrolyte dysfunctions are noted. This is partially due to dilution. We have restricted fluid somewhat and added various electrolytes/minerals to his TPN. We will monitor with serial chemistry panels.
10. APNEA/BRADYCARDIA: None since birth.
11. HEALTH CARE MAINTENANCE: None yet.
12. SOCIAL: Mom and Dad have been kept up-to-date in regards to their son's condition. Their questions have been answered, and they are in agreement with the outlined management plan.

I-22B:

SERVICE CODE(S): ____________________

DX CODE(S): ____________________

I-22C NICU PROGRESS REPORT

LOCATION: Inpatient Hospital, Neonatal Intensive Care Unit

PATIENT: Robert Zimmerman

ATTENDING PHYSICIAN: Roland Ortez, M.D.

SUBJECTIVE: Baby Boy is currently 2 days old, slightly under 48 hours.

OBJECTIVE: Weight today is 1.716 kg (decreased to 135 g). He is down 5.1% of his weight since birth. OFC is 30 cm (decreased 0.5 cm). Intake yesterday was 152 cc, 82 cc/kg per day. Output was 170 cc, 3.8 cc/kg per hour. He has had no stools since birth. Vital signs reveal his temperature to be acceptable while on an open, radiant warmer. Heart rate is generally in the 110s 120s. Respiratory rate is generally equal to the IMV (60). Mean blood pressures have generally been in the 40s to 50s. Oxygen saturations have remained in the high 90s.

PHYSICAL EXAMINATION: In general, he is pink on current ventilator settings. Endotracheal tube is in place. Neck is without masses. Chest reveals symmetric expansion, and the lungs are clear to auscultation on current ventilator settings. Cardiac exam reveals a regular rate without murmur or click. Peripheral pulses are 2+ and symmetric. Abdominal exam reveals an umbilical arterial catheter in place. Liver is palpable 1 cm below the right costal margin. No splenomegaly or masses are noted. Genital examination reveals a normal male; testes are not palpable. Extremity examination reveals no fixed decreased range of motion, deformity, or joint abnormality. Neurologic exam reveals mild diffuse hypotonia. No focal deficits are appreciated.

CURRENT MEDICATIONS:

1. Ampicillin 90.4 mg IV q.12h.
2. Gentamicin 5.4 mg IV q.18h.
3. Morphine sulfate 0.18 mg IV q.6h and q.1h p.r.n.
4. Dopamine 5 mcg/kg per minute.
5. Vecuronium 0.18 mg IV q.1-2h p.r.n.

LABORATORY STUDIES: Last arterial blood gas was obtained on ventilator settings of IMV 60, pressure 24/4, and FiO_2 0.5 and revealed pH 7.27, PCO_2 51.1, PO_2 66.5, and bicarbonate 22.5. Chemistry panel this A.M. revealed sodium 134, potassium 4.9, chloride 102, glucose 111, BUN 18, creatinine 1.0, calcium 7.5, magnesium 3.8, phosphorus 7.5, and bilirubin 7.8. CBC reveals a white count of 6190. H&H is 17.6 and 54.3. Platelet count was 98,000. Chest x-ray continues to show significant evidence of hyaline membrane disease. Endotracheal tube is near the carina and has been withdrawn somewhat.

IMPRESSIONS/RECOMMENDATIONS:

1. Two-day-old infant who was born at 30 weeks gestation. He does have clinical features suggestive of Noonan syndrome.
2. RESPIRATORY: Continues to show evidence of hyaline membrane disease with respiratory distress. He has received three doses of surfactant therapy. He does have echocardiographic evidence of PDA, and we will be treating this at this time. We will attempt to decrease his ventilator settings based on serial clinical examination, pulse oximetry, arterial blood gas determinations, and chest x-ray.
3. CARDIOVASCULAR: Cardiovascular status is acceptable at this time while on dopamine at 5 mcg/kg per minute. Echocardiogram shows a patent ductus arteriosus. There also appears to be a slight abnormality to the pulmonary valve, which could be associated with his possible Noonan syndrome. He is going to receive indomethacin therapy.
4. GASTROINTESTINAL: Abdominal exam remains benign. He is NPO. He does have mild hyperbilirubinemia. Direct antibody test was negative. We will begin phototherapy at this time.
5. HEMATOLOGIC: Serial CBCs have been acceptable except for mild thrombocytopenia. We will continue to monitor, especially in light of the indomethacin therapy. He has not required any blood product transfusions since birth.
6. INFECTIOUS DISEASE: Blood culture remains negative at this time. We have discontinued his gentamicin, and he is being placed on cefotaxime because of the indomethacin.
7. NEUROLOGIC: Neurologic exam remains acceptable given his extreme prematurity. He will require screening intracranial ultrasound and also long-term neurodevelopmental follow-up.
8. RENAL/METABOLIC: Urine output remains adequate, and renal function studies are acceptable. Previous metabolic parameters are acceptable. We will repeat in the a.m.
9. FLUIDS/ELECTROLYTES/NUTRITION: Weight loss is acceptable, and electrolytes are in the normal range today. We will adjust his TPN accordingly.
10. APNEA/BRADYCARDIA: None since birth.
11. HEALTH CARE MAINTENANCE: None yet.
12. SOCIAL: Their questions have been answered, and they are in agreement with the outlined management plan.

I-22C:

SERVICE CODE(S): ____________________

DX CODE(S): ____________________

CASE I-22C DISCUSSION

The primary condition of this newborn is that he is in respiratory distress, so this will be the first listed diagnosis.

Noonan Syndrome

Although the physician mentioned Noonan syndrome, both in the Laboratory Study and the Impression/Recommendations (point 1) sections of the report, there is no definitive diagnosis of this condition. The physician uses "significant evidence" and "suggestive of" statements, but no definitive diagnostic statement; therefore it cannot be coded. Noonan syndrome is a condition in which the features of the infant are down-slanting eyes and webbed neck, and in which 25% of the newborns are mentally retarded. Half of the newborns have congenital heart disease, and usually there are physical deformities. So, without being able to review the entire medical record or query the physician, this would not be coded as it is not definitively stated in the record or confirmed by a chromosomal report.

Converting Kilograms to Grams

The physician indicated that the patient was premature, which means you need to assign a premature gestation code with a fifth digit based on the weight of the newborn in grams. In the Objective section of the report, the physician refers to the weight of the newborn in kilograms. To calculate kilograms into grams, multiply the kilograms by 1000: (1.851 kg × 1000 = 1,851 g). You also need to report the weeks of gestation as stated in the report as 30 weeks.

Thrombocytopenia

In point 5 of the Impression/Recommendations section of the report, you can see that the physician diagnosed thrombocytopenia, which is a decrease in the number of platelets in the newborn's blood. A platelet transfusion was ordered.

Hyperbilirubinemia

In point 4 of the Impression/Recommendation section of the report, the physician indicated that the newborn has hyperbilirubinemia, which is excess bilirubin in the blood. The physician ordered phototherapy for the infant.

I-22D NICU PROGRESS REPORT

LOCATION: Hospital Inpatient, NICU

PATIENT: Robert Zimmerman

ATTENDING PHYSICIAN: Roland Ortez, M.D.

SUBJECTIVE: The patient is currently 4 days old.

OBJECTIVE: Weight today is 1.744 kg (decreased by 25 g). He is down 3.5% of his birth weight. OFC is 29 cm (no change from yesterday). Intake yesterday was 158 cc, 89.3 cc/kg per day. Output was 84 cc, 1.98 cc/kg per hour. He has had no stools since birth. Vital signs reveal his temperature to be acceptable while on the warmer. T-max 37.5 degrees and T-current 36.8 degrees. Heart has been in the 110s to 130s. Respiratory rate is equal to IMV of 60. Mean blood pressures have been 40s to 50s, mean values were noted to be 27 and 36 yesterday, a couple in the 60s and 71. O_2 saturations remain in the high 90s. He does have occasional episodes when being examined where he desaturates.

PHYSICAL EXAMINATION: In general, he is pink on ventilator settings. Endotracheal tube is in place. Neck is without masses. Chest reveals symmetrical expansion. Lungs reveal crackles bilaterally. Cardiac exam: Regular rate without murmur or click. Peripheral pulses are 2+ and symmetric. Abdominal exam reveals a UAC in place. Liver is palpable 1 cm below the right costal margin. No splenomegaly or masses noted. Genital examination reveals a normal male; testes nonpalpable. Extremity examination reveals no fixed decreased range of motion, deformity, or joint abnormality. Neurologic exam reveals a mild diffuse hypotonia. No focal deficits are appreciated.

CURRENT MEDICATIONS:
1. Ampicillin 90.4 mg IV q.12h.
2. Cefotaxime 85 mg IV q.12h.
3. Morphine sulfate 0.1 mg/kg q.1h p.r.n.
4. Dopamine 5 mcg/kg per minute.
5. Lasix 0.18 mg times one dose at 3 P.M. on the 5th.
6. Zantac 0.858 mg IV q.6h.

LABORATORY STUDIES: Arterial blood gas was obtained on ventilator settings of IMV 60, PIP 22, PEEP 4, and FiO_2 42%. The pH was 7.298, PCO_2 46.6, PO_2 91.4, and bicarbonate 22.1, base excess 3.3. Chemistry panel revealed sodium 139, potassium 4.0, chloride 105, CO_2 23.4, glucose 91, BUN 34, creatinine 1.3, calcium 8.9, magnesium 3.0, and phosphorus 5.1. Hematology showed a white count of 5.98, hemoglobin 15.9, hematocrit 50.8, and platelets 74.

Chest x-ray continued to show evidence of hyaline membrane disease; however, he was slightly more improved today, with heart borders appearing clearer. There was a question of an enlarging cardiothymic silhouette; however, this may be related to poor inspiration. Supportive apparatuses were in place.

IMPRESSIONS/RECOMMENDATIONS:
1. Four-day-old infant born at 30 weeks gestation does have clinical features of Noonan syndrome; chromosomal studies are pending.
2. RESPIRATORY: Patient continues to show evidence of hyaline membrane disease with respiratory distress. He has received three doses of surfactant therapy. He does have echocardiographic evidence of a small patent ductus arteriosus without a left-to-right shunt. We will continue to try to wean down on the ventilator settings based on serial clinical examination, pulse oximetry, arterial blood gas determinations, and chest x-rays.
3. CARDIOVASCULAR: We are continuing dopamine blood pressure support at 5 mcg/kg per minute. Mean blood pressures have slowly been rising, so we will continue to watch those. Echocardiogram showed a small patent ductus arteriosus without left-to-right shunt. The patient has been treated with indomethacin therapy times three doses. We will be repeating the echocardiogram today.
4. GASTROINTESTINAL: Abdominal exam remains benign. He is NPO. He does have mild hypobilirubinemia, which has improved with phototherapy. We will continue with treatment. Direct antibody test was negative.
5. HEMATOLOGIC: Serial CBCs have shown worsening thrombocytopenia today at 74,000. The patient will be transfused with one unit of platelets today, leukodepleted, and irradiated. Risks and benefits of transfusion were discussed with the mother, and an informed consent was obtained.
6. INFECTIOUS DISEASE: Blood cultures remain negative. We will continue with ampicillin and cefotaxime at this time.
7. NEUROLOGIC: Neurologic exam remains acceptable given his extreme prematurity. We will obtain screening intracranial ultrasound tomorrow. The patient will need long-term neurodevelopmental follow-up.
8. RENAL/METABOLIC: Renal output remains adequate, and renal function studies are acceptable. The patient received a dose of Lasix 0.18 mg times one yesterday with good diuresis. Metabolic parameters are acceptable.
9. FLUID/ELECTROLYTES/NUTRITION: Weight loss is currently 3.5% from birth weight. We would like to see more of a weight loss because there is concern with fluid overload in this patient. We will adjust the patient's TPN accordingly.
10. APNEA/BRADYCARDIA: None since birth.
11. HEALTH CARE MAINTENANCE: None yet.
12. SOCIAL: The mom and dad are up to date with regard to their son's condition.

I-22D:

SERVICE CODE(S): ________________________

DX CODE(S): ________________________

CASE 1-22D DISCUSSSION

Patient Ductus Arteriosis

All of the diagnoses in this report are ones that you have reported previously, except for the patent ductus arteriosus. **Patent ductus arteriosus** (PDA) is a heart defect in which the ductus arteriosus (blood vessel) does not close after birth as it usually would. This open channel allows blood to bypass the lungs. A large PDA will lead to respiratory distress and can flood the lungs with blood, resulting in congestive heart failure.

Preventive Medicine Services

Use Preventive Medicine Services codes to report the routine evaluation and management of a patient who is healthy and has no complaint or when the patient has a chronic condition or disease that is controlled but involves yearly routine physicals. The codes in this subsection would be used to report a routine physical examination done at the patient's request, such as a well-baby checkup. Preventive Medicine codes are intended to be used to identify comprehensive services, not a single-system examination, such as an annual gynecologic examination. The codes are used for infants, children, adolescents, and adults; they differ according to the age of the patient and whether the patient is a new or an established patient.

Note that in the code descriptions for both the New Patient and the Established Patient categories, the terms "comprehensive history" and "comprehensive examination" are used. These terms are not the same as the ones used with other E/M codes (99201–99350). Here, "comprehensive" means a complete history and a complete examination, as is conducted during an annual physical. The comprehensive examination performed as part of the preventive medicine E/M service is a multisystem examination, but the extent of the examination is determined by the age of the patient and the risk factors identified for that individual.

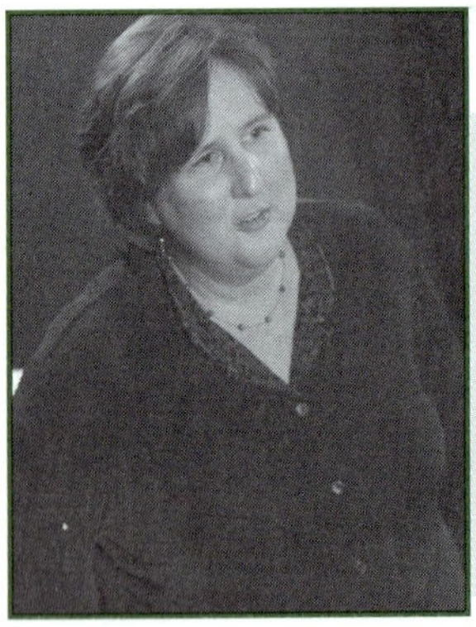

FROM THE TRENCHES

Kathy

"There is always something new to learn. I don't know anybody who knows it all. I learn something new every day, if not ten new things every day! I've been doing this for ten years, and I still learn something new. That's why I love it."

You have done a super job of working through this difficult chapter. You will find that the reports that follow are not quite as complex as the ones you have been working with. The next few reports are commonly provided office services.

V Codes

V codes from the *Supplementary Classification of Factors Influencing Health Status and Contact with Health Services* are found under such main term references as "admission," "examination," "history," "observation," and "problem." V codes are used under the following circumstances:

- When a person who is **not currently sick** encounters health services for a specific purpose, such as to act as a donor or receive a vaccination
- When a person with a **known disease or injury** presents for specific treatment of that condition—such as dialysis, chemotherapy, or cast change
- When a circumstance **may influence** a patient's health status
- To indicate the **birth status and outcome** of delivery of a newborn

The *Supplementary Classification* is located near the end of Volume 1, Tabular List, and contains three- or four-digit code numbers preceded by the letter *V*. The codes in this section are called V codes, and are used in these two ways:

1. When a person who is currently not sick encounters the health services for some specific purpose, such as to act as donor of an organ or tissue, to receive a preventive vaccination, or to discuss a problem that is in itself not a disease or injury. Occurrences such as these will be fairly rare among hospital inpatients but common among outpatients at health clinics. Examples are a kidney donor who is not sick but encounters health care (V59.4), a well child who receives a polio vaccination (V04.0), or a student who seeks health care to discuss a problem with school (V62.3)
2. When a circumstance or problem is present that influences the person's health status but is not in itself a current illness or injury. For example, a family history of malignant gastrointestinal neoplasms (V16.0) is significant to the patient's health care. The main term in this case is "History, **family**, malignant neoplasm, gastrointestinal tract." If, however, the diagnosis was a personal history of malignant neoplasm, the Index location would be History, **personal**, malignant, neoplasm, gastrointestinal tract, and the code would be V10.00.

CASE 1-23

I-23A OFFICE VISIT

Report Dr. Alanda's service.

LOCATION: Outpatient, Clinic

PATIENT: Annabel Goth

PRIMARY CARE PHYSICIAN: Leslie Alanda, M.D.

CHIEF COMPLAINT: Pap and physical.

SUBJECTIVE: This 30-year-old married white female is an established patient who presents for routine annual exam and Pap. No particular concerns.

PAST MEDICAL HISTORY: Generally healthy. She has been treated for hypothyroidism for the past 4 years. Recent TSH was normal at 1.30.

GYN HISTORY: Gravida 3, para 3. Daughters aged 15 months, 4 and 5 years. No history of abnormal Pap smears. Husband has had a vasectomy. Menses regular q. month. LMP: 3 weeks ago.

FAMILY HISTORY: Father—MI. Mother—high cholesterol and hypertension. Cancer, in grandparents.

SOCIAL/OCCUPATIONAL: She is a physical therapist working 3 days a week at the local rehabilitation hospital. Husband is a factory foreman at the local water treatment plant.

HABITS: Tobacco: None. Alcohol: Rare. Diet: Watches fat. She daily drinks 8 cups of coffee. She has started a walking program to facilitate weight loss. Sleep is fair. Seatbelts are used consistently.

REVIEW OF SYSTEMS: Essentially negative. She would like to lose 50 pounds over the next several months.

EXAMINATION: Weight refused. Blood pressure of 118/68. General: Well-developed, well-nourished female. Skin is negative. HEENT is unremarkable. Neck is supple with no palpable nodes. Thyroid easily palpable but not enlarged. Breasts are symmetric and nontender with no palpable mass or discharge. Lungs clear to auscultation. Heart: Regular rate; no murmur. Abdomen is mildly obese, soft, and nontender with no palpable mass. No CVA tenderness. Pelvic: Normal female genitalia. No odor or discharge. Cervix is clear. No uterine or adnexal mass or tenderness.

IMPRESSION:

1. Normal gynecologic exam.
2. Hypothyroidism, on replacement therapy.
3. Overweight.

PLAN: Pap; will notify. Reinforced monthly BSE and positive lifestyle behaviors. Encourage weight-loss program. Refill Levothroid 0.125 mg 1 q.d. for one year. Return to clinic annually and p.r.n.

I-23A:

SERVICE CODE(S): ____________________

DX CODE(S): ____________________

I-23B OFFICE VISIT

The patient returns to the clinic 1 year later. Report Dr. Alanda's service.

LOCATION: Outpatient, Clinic

PATIENT: Annabel Goth

PRIMARY CARE PHYSICIAN: Leslie Alanda, M.D.

CHIEF COMPLAINT: Checkup.

SUBJECTIVE: The patient is a 31-year-old married white female who is an established patient who presents today for her annual examination. She reports that she has been doing well except for some mild cold symptoms, which are now resolving. Over the past year, she has lost more than 50 pounds through an organized weight-loss program. She has been exercising on a regular basis. She is very pleased with the results and wishes to lose another 15 to 20 pounds.

PAST MEDICAL HISTORY: Significant for hypothyroidism for which she is on Synthroid 0.125 mg q.d. She has otherwise enjoyed very good health. She is gravida 3, para 3. She reports that her menstrual cycle is regular. Husband has had a vasectomy. No breast or pelvic complaints.

FAMILY HISTORY: Father—MI. Mother—high cholesterol and hypertension. Cancer, in grandparents.

SOCIAL HISTORY: The patient continues to work as a physical therapist at the local rehabilitation hospital. She is a nonsmoker. No alcohol problems.

OBJECTIVE: White female who appears to be in general good health. Her weight is down to 152 pounds. Blood pressure today somewhat elevated at 142/92. HEENT remarkable for a healing cold sore above her lips. Neck is supple; no masses. Lung fields are clear to auscultation. Heart is regular rate and rhythm; no audible murmurs. Breasts are symmetrical in size and shape. No masses, tenderness, or nipple discharge. Axillae negative. Abdomen is benign. Pelvic examination deferred due to menses. Extremities without edema. Skin is clear.

ASSESSMENT:
1. Healthy female.
2. History of hypothyroidism.
3. Obesity with weight loss of 50 pounds.

PLAN: Preventative health measures reviewed. The patient will have an annual TSH level today as well as a screening cholesterol level. She will return in 2 weeks to complete pelvic examination and Pap smear, at which time we will also recheck her blood pressure. At that time, we will review her lab results and refill her Synthroid as indicated.

1-23B:

SERVICE CODE(S): ____________________

DX CODE(S): ____________________

1-23C OFFICE VISIT

The patient returns to the clinic 2 weeks later. Report Dr. Alanda's service.

LOCATION: Outpatient, Clinic

PATIENT: Annabel Goth

PRIMARY CARE PHYSICIAN: Leslie Alanda, M.D.

CHIEF COMPLAINT: College physical.

SUBJECTIVE: The patient is a 32-year-old married white female who presents today for a college physical. She is also due for her annual GYN exam. She denies any particular concerns. No recent illnesses or injuries. She was seen earlier this month with complaints of dizziness. She has a history of hypothyroidism, and her TSH level is elevated at 11.77. Subsequently, her Synthroid has been increased to 0.15 mg q.d. The patient reports that she is feeling fine at this time.

PAST MEDICAL HISTORY: Otherwise significant only for pregnancy and delivery. She is gravida 3, para 3. No breast or pelvic complaints. Husband has had a vasectomy.

OBJECTIVE: White female who appears to be in general good health. Her weight is 151 pounds. Blood pressure is 100/70. HEENT: Within normal limits. Neck: Supple. No masses. Normal thyroid. Lung fields are clear. Heart: Regular rate and rhythm. No audible murmurs. Breasts are symmetrical in size and shape. No tenderness, masses, or nipple discharge. Axillae: Negative. Abdomen: Benign. Pelvic exam is within normal limits. Pap smear was done. Extremities: Normal. Skin: Clear.

ASSESSMENT:
1. Healthy female.
2. Normal gynecologic exam.
3. Hypothyroidism, which is under good control with Synthroid.

PLAN: Preventative health measures reviewed. College forms completed with copies enclosed in chart. Return clinic visit in one year and p.r.n.

1-23C:

SERVICE CODE(S): ____________________

DX CODE(S): ____________________

CASE 1-23 DISCUSSION

In 1-23A, you reported a preventive medicine service at which a pap was performed. If there are other conditions that the physician stated or treated, you would report the diagnosis codes for these conditions in addition to the V code for the gynecological examination. Note that when gynecological and physical examinations are completed at the same time, the physical examination does not require a separate diagnosis code, rather only the gynecological examination code is reported.

In 1-23B, the patient again presented for a preventive medicine service, this time without pap performed. A routine health examination is reported with a V code. Any additional conditions indicated in the report and treated would be reported.

In 1-23C, the patient presents for a college physical and there is a special V code for students. Any diagnosis noted and treated would be reported.

CASE 1-24
1-24A Office Visit

CASE 1-24

Report Dr. Alanda's service.

1-24A OFFICE VISIT

LOCATION: Outpatient, Clinic

PATIENT: Lionel VanDoran

PRIMARY CARE PHYSICIAN: Leslie Alanda, M.D.

The patient is in for his annual checkup and is a 54-year-old established patient.

For past medical history, please see assessment.

CURRENT MEDICATIONS: Lotrel 5/20, #100 per day. Also takes Tylenol and ibuprofen on a p.r.n. basis.

ALLERGIES to sulfa drugs and bees.

SOCIAL HISTORY: Two-pack-per-day smoker. He has not tried recently to quit smoking. Alcohol use has decreased from six to two beers per day. He works in the summertime as a pool cleaner and doing yardwork.

HEALTH MAINTENANCE: The last lipid panel was good. Cholesterol was 203. He wears a seatbelt all the time.

FAMILY HISTORY: Mother, father, one brother, four daughters are all in good health. Denies family history of colon or prostate cancer, diabetes, or glaucoma.

REVIEW OF SYSTEMS: Complains of a sore throat in the morning, worse in the winter months when it is dry. He is a loud snorer. His wife states that he has had some bouts of apneic spells but not that prominent.

OBJECTIVE: Weight is stable at 220 pounds. Blood pressure is decreased to 142/88. Pulse is 84.

PERRLA: Normal extraocular movements. Tympanic membranes are benign. Pharynx is erythematous. Nasal mucosa is erythematous, more so on the left. No areas that I can cauterize easily today. Neck is benign. Thyroid is not enlarged. Heart is S1 and S2. Lungs are clear. Abdomen is benign. There are no masses, tenderness, or organomegaly appreciated. There is no cervical, supraclavicular, axillary, or inguinal adenopathy appreciated. Reflexes are brisk. There is no pitting edema appreciated.

ASSESSMENT:
1. Physical examination.
2. Hypertension, under improved control on treatment.
3. Tobacco and alcohol use.
4. No hospitalizations, but did have foot injury in the past.
5. Sore throat in the morning. Question component of sleep apnea and loud snoring.

PLAN: Samples of Lotrel and prescription were given today. We will check a complete metabolic panel to check on his electrolytes, etc., and also his previous elevated liver enzymes. I discussed with him that we should reduce his alcohol use down to a maximum of two drinks per day because it is toxic to the heart and raises blood pressure. I also discussed again that smoking is definitely bad for his blood pressure as well, and he needs to quit. I discussed also increasing the humidity in the bedroom at nighttime and if he still has a sore throat after this, I would recommend an ENT referral. Health sheet was given along with standard recommendations. We will send a letter with his complete metabolic panel and cholesterol level return.

1-24A:

SERVICE CODE(S): ____________________

DX CODE(S): ____________________

CASE 1-25

Report Dr. Alanda's service.

1-25A OFFICE VISIT

LOCATION: Outpatient, Clinic

PATIENT: Tiffany Hopman

PRIMARY CARE PHYSICIAN: Leslie Alanda, M.D.

PRESENTING COMPLAINT: Checkup

This girl is in for a checkup. She is now 1 year of age and an established patient. She is doing very well. Her birthday was April 21. She is cruising around furniture, but not quite walking. She eats well and sleeps well. Has no difficulties.

I examined this young girl and filled out the form for 1 year. Please see same. She has four lower and four upper teeth. Can say hi; waves bye-bye. Cruises here in the office.

ASSESSMENT: Healthy 1-year-old female.

Mom has diabetes and is pregnant. She is due in May. At that time, the patient will get a new sibling. We are certain this one will be born early. Mom will be going in for prenatal steroids. I will see her back at 15 months or p.r.n.

1-25A:

SERVICE CODE(S): ____________________

DX CODE(S): ____________________

CASE 1-26
1-26A Office Visit

CASE 1-26

Report Dr. Alanda's service.

1-26A OFFICE VISIT

LOCATION: Outpatient, Clinic

PATIENT: Marissa Glendale

PRIMARY CARE PHYSICIAN: Leslie Alanda, M.D.

CHIEF COMPLAINT: Pelvic exam and Pap smear.

SUBJECTIVE: This is a 41-year-old married white female who presents today to complete her pelvic exam and Pap smear. She was seen 2 weeks ago for her annual checkup.

OBJECTIVE: Blood pressure today is normal at 118/68. Pelvic exam: Normal external genitalia. Vagina without discharge. Cervix: Multiparous, clear. Pap smear done. Bimanual exam unremarkable.

ASSESSMENT:
1. Normal blood pressure.
2. Normal pelvic exam.

PLAN: Return clinic visit in one year and p.r.n.

1-26A:

SERVICE CODE(S): ____________________

DX CODE(S): ____________________

Glossary

admission attention to an acute illness or injury resulting in admittance to a hospital.

attending physician the physician with the primary responsibility for care of the patient.

concurrent care the provision of similar services (e.g., hospital visits) to the same patient by more than one physician on the same day. Each physician provides services for a separate condition not reasonably expected to be managed by the attending physician. When concurrent care is provided, the diagnosis must reflect the medical necessity of different specialties.

confirmatory consultations type of consultations requested by patients, insurance companies, and/or third-party payers, as an additional opinion and diagnosis.

consultation includes those services rendered by a physician whose opinion or advice is requested by another physician or agency concerning the evaluation and/or treatment of a patient.

consultant the physician providing a consultation to a requesting physician; a consultant is not an attending physician.

contributing factors counseling, coordination of care, nature of the presenting problem, and time of E/M service.

direct face-to-face time time a physician spends directly with a patient during an office visit, which can include obtaining a history, performing an examination, and/or discussing results.

discharge release from a hospital.

incidental findings findings that were not the reason a diagnostic test was performed; may be unrelated to the reason the test was ordered.

inpatient one who has been formally admitted to a health care facility.

key components the history, examination, and MDM complexity of an E/M service; used to determine level of service.

newborn care the evaluation and determination of care management of a newborn infant.

observation the classification status of a patient that requires an inpatient stay for a short period to gather further information for diagnosis and treatment; the patient does not require acute inpatient care or intensive resources.

office visit a face-to-face encounter between a physician and a patient to allow for primary management of a patient's health care status.

outpatient a patient who receives services in an ambulatory health care facility and is currently not an inpatient.

presenting problem a disease, condition, illness, injury, symptom, sign, finding, complaint, or other reason for a patient encounter, with or without a diagnosis being established at the time of the visit.

requesting physician a physician who asks another physician for advice or opinion on the treatment, diagnosis, or management of a patient.

unit/floor time the time a physician spends in the hospital setting dealing with a patient's case. This can include bedside face-to-face time, or time spent working in other settings (e.g., the nursing station) on behalf of the patient.

Chapter 2
Medicine

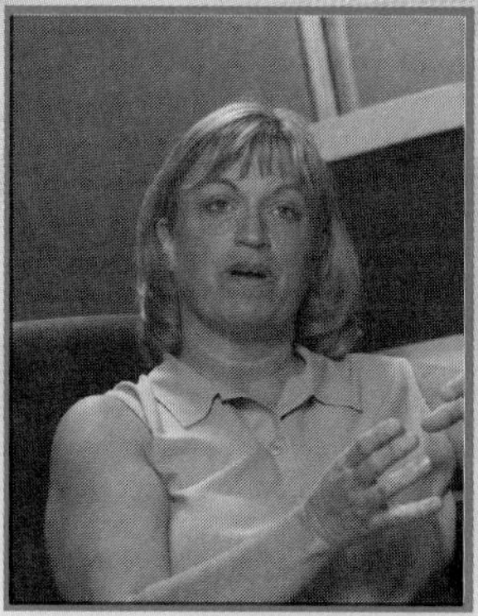

Joan Gilhooly, CPC, CHCC
President/Owner
Medical Business Resources, LLC
Deer Park, Illinois

ABBREVIATIONS

ARDS	adult respiratory distress syndrome
ASCVD	arteriosclerotic cardiovascular disease
ASHD	arteriosclerotic heart disease
bid	twice a day
BUN	blood urea nitrogen
C	Celsius
CABG	coronary artery bypass graft
CAPD	continuous ambulatory peritoneal dialysis
cc	cubic centimeter
CHF	congestive heart failure
CMT	chiropractic manipulative treatment
CNS	central nervous system
CO_2	carbon dioxide
CO × 2	cyclooxygenase-2 inhibitors
CVA	cardiovascular accident or costovertebral angle
CVD	cerebrovascular disease
CVP	central venous pressure
DC	doctor of chiropractic
DO	doctor of osteopathy
DVT	deep vein thrombosis
ECHO-C	echocardiogram
ESRD	end-stage renal disease
GYN	gynecology
H&H	hematocrit and hemoglobin
ICU	intensive care unit
IM	intramuscular
IV	intravenous
kg	kilogram
LVET	left ventricular ejection time
m/sec	millisecond
mc	millicurie
mcg	microgram
mg	milligram
MI	myocardial infarction
mL	milliliter
mm Hg	millimeters of mercury
MMPI	Minnesota Multiphasic Personality Inventory
MMRV	measles, mumps, rubella, varicella
OMT	osteopathic manipulative treatment
PAD	peripheral arterial disease
PD	peritoneal dialysis
PEEP	positive end expiratory pressure
PMI	point of maximal impulse
po	by mouth
prn	as needed
RV	right ventricle
Rx	medication
S_1	first heart sound
S_2	second heart sound
S_3	third heart sound
S_4	fourth heart sound
tid	three times a day
T_4	thyroxine
TCD	transcranial Doppler
TSH	thyroid-stimulating hormone
WBC	white blood cell (count)

The Medicine section has many subsections that encompass a broad range of services. Take a moment to review these subsections in the *CPT*, then review the Medicine Guidelines. The section contains diagnostic (determining nature of disease) and therapeutic (curative) services that are both invasive (entering the body) and noninvasive (not entering the body).

Immunizations

The two types of immunization are active and passive. **Active immunization** can be either a toxoid or a vaccine and is administered in anticipation that a patient will come into contact with a disease. Toxoids are the bacteria that cause the disease that have been made nontoxic. When the toxoid is injected, the body's immune system produces an immune response that builds protection from the disease. A vaccine is the injection of the actual virus in small doses to allow the body's immune system to produce an immune response. **Passive immunization** does not cause an immune response; rather, immune globulins (antibodies) are injected to protect the body from a specific disease. Within the Medicine section, the codes for active immunizations are Vaccines/Toxoids (90465–90749), and the codes for passive immunizations are Immune Globulins (90281–90399).

Whenever an immunization is administered, the substance (vaccine/toxoid or immune globulin) is reported along with an administration code (90465–90474). For example, an immunization of diphtheria antitoxin (90296) for a patient over 8 years of age, is reported as follows:

90296 Diphtheria antitoxin (substance)
90471 Administration, immunization (injection)

Codes 90465/90466 (under 8 years of age) and 90471/90472 report intradermal (ID), percutaneous (PERC), **subcutaneous (subcu),** or **intramuscular (IM)** administration, and 90467/90468 (under 8 years of age) and 90473/90474 report administration by intranasal or oral methods. It is the number of injections that is reported, not the number of substances being injected. For example, if the patient (over 8 years of age) received a tetanus toxoid, rubella virus, and diphtheria toxoid in three separate injections, the service would be reported as follows:

Substance (Drug Supply)	Administration (Service)
90703 Tetanus toxoid	90471 Administration, tetanus toxoid
90706 Rubella virus	90472 Administration, rubella virus
90719 Diphtheria toxoid	90472 Administration, diphtheria toxoid

If a combination of tetanus and diphtheria were injected in one syringe and the rubella in another syringe, the service would be reported as follows:

Substance (Drug Supply)	Administration (Service)
90702 Tetanus and diphtheria toxoids	90471 Administration, tetanus and diphtheria toxoids
90706 Rubella virus	90472 Administration, rubella virus

An E/M code is reported with an immunization service only when there is another separate, identifiable evaluation and management service provided and documented in the medical record. Report the E/M service with modifier -25 added to the code to indicate that the service was separate from the immunization service. If the only service provided was the injection, it is not appropriate to report an E/M service because administration of the injection is reported with the administration code (90465–90474). The substance injected is reported with the toxoid, vaccine, or immune globulin code, so it is not correct to report a supply code (e.g., 99070) unless some other supply was provided in conjunction with another separate service in addition to the immunization.

Two vaccinations that are commonly provided are influenza and pneumococcal. Report a code for the substance injected (vaccine) and a code for the administration of the vaccine. The third-party payer may require you to submit CPT codes or CPT with HCPCS codes for the service. The following identifies the codes that are usually reported for influenza and pneumococcal immunizations:

CPT influenza **vaccine** codes:

90657	Influenza virus vaccine split virus, for children age **6–35 months,** for intramuscular use
90658	Influenza virus vaccine, split virus, for use in individuals **age 3 years and older,** for intramuscular use

HCPCS code used to report the **administration** of an influenza vaccine to a Medicare patient:

G0008	Administration of influenza virus vaccine

CPT codes used to report the **administration** of the influenza vaccine:

90471	Intramuscular **administration,** one vaccine
90472	Intramuscular **administration,** each additional vaccine

V-code

The diagnosis code used when the only reason for the encounter is an influenza vaccine (flu shot) is V04.81, Influenza vaccination. The diagnosis and service codes must correlate.

CPT pneumococcal **vaccine** code:

90732	Pneumococcal polysaccharide **vaccine,** 23-valent, adult dosage (age 2 years and older), for either subcutaneous or intramuscular use

HCPCS code to report the **administration** of the pneumococcal vaccine to a Medicare patient:

G0009	**Administration** of pneumococcal vaccine

CPT codes used to report the **administration** of the influenza vaccine:

90471	Intramuscular **administration**, one vaccine
90472	Intramuscular **administration**, each additional vaccine

The diagnosis code used when the only reason for the encounter is a pneumococcal vaccine (pneumonia shot) is V03.82. The diagnosis and service codes must correlate.

V-code

Diagnoses Coding for Vaccinations

Vaccinations are reported with V codes because there is no sign, symptom, or disease actually present. In the Index of the ICD-9-CM, locate the term "Vaccination." The subterms are listed by type of vaccination, such as "measles (alone) V04.2." When the referencing the Tabular for V04.2, you will see that **V04** is for vaccination and inoculation for certain viral diseases. The Excludes note indicates that vaccines against a combination of diseases are reported with **V06.0–V06.9**. If measles, mumps, and rubella were administered in the same vaccination, V06.4 would be reported.

V03 codes are for vaccination and inoculation against a single bacterial disease, such as cholera (V03.0) and typhoid-paratyphoid alone (V03.1). If both cholera and typhoid-paratyphoid were administered in the same vaccination, V06.0 would be reported. V06.0 is a combination code (more than one condition represented by one code) for other combinations of vaccines.

V05 codes are for vaccination and inoculation against a single disease, such as viral hepatitis (V05.3) or varicella (chickenpox caused by the human herpesvirus; V05.4).

If one encounter included vaccination for measles, mumps, rubella, and varicella, report the combination code **V06.4** (measles, mumps, and rubella) in addition to the single code **V05.4** (varicella).

CASE 2-1
2-1A Chart Note

CASE 2-1

Mary Ann Roberts, a Medicare patient, presents for an influenza vaccination. A HCPCS administration code is used to report the vaccination of a Medicare patient.

2-1A CHART NOTE

LOCATION: Outpatient, Clinic

PATIENT: Mary Ann Roberts

PHYSICIAN: Alma Naraquist, M.D.

AGE: 72

COVERAGE: Medicare

Patient presents for administration of an IM injection of split virus influenza vaccine administered by her nurse.

2-1A:

SERVICE CODE(S): ______________________

DX CODE(S): ______________________

CASE 2-2

Gerald is a Medicare patient. Report the services provided by Dr. Naraquist's nurse.

2-2A CHART NOTE

LOCATION: Outpatient, Clinic

PATIENT: Gerald Parr

PHYSICIAN: Alma Naraquist, M.D.

AGE: 82

COVERAGE: Medicare

Patient presents for administration of an IM injection of split virus influenza vaccine and a 23-valent pneumococcal vaccination administered by Dr. Naraquist's nurse.

2-2A:

SERVICE CODE(S): ______________________

DX CODE(S): ______________________

CASE 2-3
2-3A Chart Note

CASE 2-3

Use the CPT code for the administration and injection service for this non-Medicare patient. A V code from the ICD-9-CM is assigned. There is a combination V code for MMR. There is only one administration; there are several substances in the one administration.

2-3A CHART NOTE

LOCATION: Outpatient, Clinic

PATIENT: Mindy O'Bright

PHYSICIAN: Rolando Ortez, M.D.

AGE: 10

Patient presents for administration of a subcutaneous injection of a combination injection of measles, mumps, rubella, and varicella (MMRV) that was ordered by Dr. Ortez and administered by Dr. Ortez's nurse.

2-3A:

SERVICE CODE(S): ____________________

DX CODE(S): ____________________

Hydration, Therapeutic, Prophylactic, and Diagnostic Injections and Infusions

Codes 90760-90776 are used to report the hydration, injection, and infusion services. The physician's work related to these services usually involves the oversight of the treatment plan and staff supervision. When the physician provides a significant, separately identifiable E/M service, report the service with an appropriate E/M code using modifier -25. Sometimes third-party payers will require any E/M service provided on the same day as a hydration, injection, or infusion to have a different diagnosis than the condition for which the hydration, injection, or infusion is being provided, but that is not the case for reporting E/M services with these codes. However, modifier -25 must be added to the E/M code, or the E/M service will be thought to be related to the physician's service for the hydration, injection, or infusion service.

Bundled into the hydration, injection, and infusion services are local anesthesia, placing the intravenous line, accessing an indwelling access line/catheter/port, flushing at the end of the infusion, and all standard supplies.

Hydration

Codes 90760-90761 are used to report an intravenous hydration infusion that includes the pre-packaged fluid and electrolytes (such as normal saline). The substance is considered incidental to the hydration service and is therefore not reported separately. If other than a pre-packaged substance is used, that substance would be reported separately. Included in these codes are the physician supervision and oversight of the staff providing the direct services. Code 90760 is reported for the first hour of intravenous infusion hydration service, and 90761 is used to report each additional hour, up to eight hours.

CASE 2-4

This is a Medicare patient.

2-4A CHART NOTE

LOCATION: Outpatient, Clinic

PATIENT: Connor Lunderquist

PHYSICIAN: Alma Naraquist, M.D.

AGE: 74

COVERAGE: Medicare

Therapeutic infusion of saline solution with pre-packaged 5% dextrose IV 500 mL for dehydration, lasting 50 minutes.

2-4A:

SERVICE CODE(S): ______________________

DX CODE(S): ______________________

Therapeutic, Prophylactic, and Diagnostic Injections and Infusions

Codes 90765-~~90799~~ 90779 are used to report the administration of a therapeutic, prophylactic, or diagnostic intravenous infusion or injection. Intravenous **infusions** are reported with 90765-90768 and are divided based on the time and type of infusion. The initial infusion is reported with 90765 (up to 1 hour) and each additional hour (up to 8 hours) with 90766. Sometimes one infusion is provided followed by another infusion (sequential infusions), in which case the initial infusion is listed first and then the additional sequential infusion (90767). There are times when more than one infusion is provided at the same time, in which case the initial infusion is listed first, and then the additional concurrent infusion is listed (90768).

Therapeutic, prophylactic, and diagnostic **injections** are divided based on the administration method. *Subcutaneous* and *intramuscular* injections are reported with 90772, along with a code to report the substance injected. For example, if the vaccine was a subcutaneous influenza virus, 90657 is reported for the substance, and 90772 is reported for the administration. The vaccines/toxoids are reported with 90465-90466 and 90471-90472. Code 90772 is not used to report chemotherapy administration (see 96401-96402). Injections for allergen immunotherapy are reported with 95115-95117, not with therapeutic, prophylactic, or diagnostic injection codes. *Intra-arterial* (90773) and *intravenous push* (90774-90775) are reported with therapeutic, prophylactic, and diagnostic injection codes.

CASE 2-5
2-5A Chart Note

CASE 2-5

Report the injection service for this Medicare patient using an HCPCS code to report the substance injected and a CPT code to report the intramuscular antibiotic injection.

2-5A CHART NOTE

LOCATION: Outpatient, Clinic

PATIENT: LuLu Busquet

PHYSICIAN: Alma Naraquist, M.D.

AGE: 81

COVERAGE: Medicare

Patient presents for an injection of tetracycline for an acute upper-respiratory infection. She was seen in the clinic on Friday and returns on Tuesday after talking with Dr. Naraquist, who instructed the patient to come to the office for an injection. Dr. Naraquist's nurse administers an IM injection of tetracycline, 200 mg.

2-5A:

SERVICE CODE(S): ____________________

DX CODE(S): ____________________

Psychiatry

Psychiatric diagnostic interview (90801) includes a history, mental status, and disposition. It may also include discussion with other informants, such as members of the family. Interactive psychiatric diagnostic interview (90802) involves the use of objects and nonverbal communication to assess the patient's status. Usually, interactive psychiatric interview is used with children who have not developed sufficient communications skills or have lost the ability to communicate.

Codes 90804–90815 report insight orientation, behavior modification, and supportive psychotherapy in addition to interactive psychotherapy on an outpatient basis. Codes 90816–90829 report the same types of services but provided on an inpatient, partial hospital, or resident care facility basis. Insight-oriented psychotherapy is the face-to-face time the physician spends with the patient in therapy and is based on time spent (20–30, 45–50, 75–80 minutes). If the physician also provides medical evaluation and management services to the patient during the session, psychiatry codes such as 90805 are available for that type of combination service.

Interactive psychotherapy is usually provided to children and uses physical aids and nonverbal communication—90810–90815 and 90823–90829. These codes are also based on time and whether or not additional services of medical evaluation or management services were provided.

The remainder of the codes in the subsection are for Other Psychotherapy (90845–90857) that describe individual, family, multiple-family, or group services and Other Psychiatric Services or Procedures (90862–90899) that describe medication management, electroconvulsive therapy, biofeedback, hypnotherapy, evaluation of hospital records, and other services.

When reporting psychotherapy, the code is assigned based on:

1. Type of therapy
2. Place of service
3. Face-to-face time spent with the patient
4. Other services furnished, such as E/M services

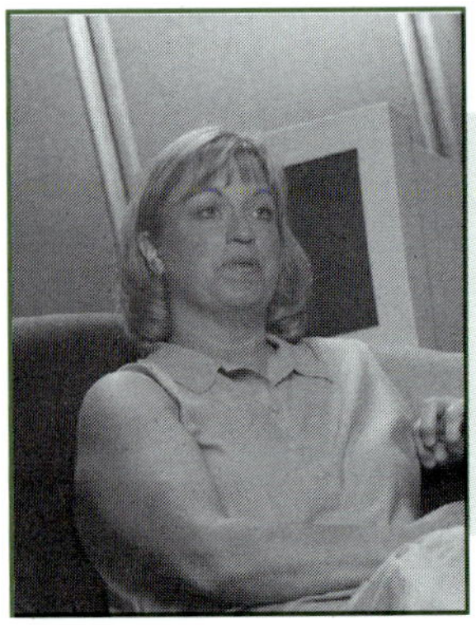

FROM THE TRENCHES

Joan

"The most interesting thing is taking ... complex clinical scenarios, pulling out the information, and putting it back together in a way that accurately paints a picture for the insurance carrier [of] what was done to the patient, why it was done, and why they should pay."

CASE 2-6
2-6A Psychological Evaluation

CASE 2-6

Joel Wall is an inpatient for whom Dr. Nelson provided an inpatient psychotherapy service. ***This is not a consultation.***

2-6A PSYCHOLOGICAL EVALUATION

LOCATION: Inpatient Hospital

PATIENT: Joel Wall

PHYSICIAN: Jerome Nelson, M.D.

REASON FOR VISIT: Joel Wall is a 50-year-old right-handed gentleman who was seen for 1 hour of interview and records review, in addition to 1.5 hours of testing, scoring, interpretation, and generation of documentation. He is being assessed primarily in regard to postconcussion syndrome.

HISTORY: The patient was involved in a motor vehicle accident on 04/07 of this year and sustained multiple injuries, including bilateral pulmonary contusions, bilateral pneumothorax, and multiple facial fractures, particularly on the left. He is currently on ventilation. The patient did have an alcohol level of .142 at the time of his admission. He has had some reactive depression. Reportedly, the patient has had several prior concussions and motor vehicle accidents. Previous medical history is also significant for chemical dependency treatment in 2000 and again in 2001. The patient had one prior hospitalization on the psychiatric unit last year with adjustment issues following the suicide of his daughter.

Previous medical history is also significant for rotator cuff repair 3 or 4 years ago. The patient is a chronic smoker at the rate of three packs a day. He has a history of borderline diabetes and hypertension. He has chronic arthritis and a history of peptic ulcer.

CURRENT MEDICATION: Mucomyst, albuterol, ipratropium, bacitracin, bisacodyl, Procrit, heparin, Mycostatin, PCS, morphine, Protonix, and Zosyn.

FAMILY HISTORY: Significant for heart disease in the patient's father who died at age 52; his mother died at age 65 from cardiovascular accident.

SOCIAL HISTORY: The patient lives in Manytown and is currently a widower. He has no surviving children, is a graduate of a 2-year vocational college in the East, and has completed military service.

INTERVIEW: The patient admits he feels somewhat reactively depressed; however, he states that this is nothing like the depression he had about 2 years ago. The patient states that this depression is primarily attributed to being laid off at his place of employment. He feels he is doing well with it. He does not have suicidal ideation. He states that several years ago he became a devoted Buddhist and that has been supportive for him during difficult times. He states that he could go home and stay with one of his nephews with whom he is close.

BEHAVIOR OBSERVATIONS: On interview, the patient is lying in his bed. He is on the ventilator and so has to communicate primarily by writing, which he does do quite efficiently. I do note, however, that the patient includes some extra letters or mis-sequences his letters at times. When asked about this, the patient attributes it to not having his reading glasses. The patient is able to tell me about his accident, although we asked when it happened, he writes that it occurred "July 4."; and when asked whether he is sure about this, he insists that it is true and that it happened after he had been to the local theater to see an adventure show he had been looking forward to. He insists it was on July 4th. He seems surprised and embarrassed when told that in fact it happened in April. The patient states that prior to the accident he was actively employed as a carpenter and, when he had time, worked in the evenings and weekends as a painter.

TESTING: On testing, the patient is found to be alert, motivated, and cooperative. Good rapport was easily established. The patient was confident, relaxed, and focused. Of note is the fact that the patient was wearing wrist restraints, which did interfere slightly with some of the testing. The patient did not appear bothered by this. He displayed no difficulty with the comprehension or retention of test instructions. He was careful and reflective in his approach to testing tasks. Test results are believed to be a valid reflection of his current abilities.

The patient proves to be well oriented today (8/8). He has an excellent fund of personal and current information (6/6). He has excellent performance on a test of foresight and planning (Porteus Maze Test: 121/121). Immediate verbal span of concentration is average at 6 forward and 5 backward (50th percentile). On verbal block-tapping span is better yet at 6 forward and 6 backward (91st percentile).

Copying of simple figures is performed well (14/14), as is matching simple figures (4/4). Immediate memory for simple designs is average (58th percentile). After a delay, however, he is noted to lose one of the designs and invert another one. His recollection of the other two is as it was initially. With recognition cueing, he does well (3/4).

Learning of a 9-word categorized list (California Verbal Learning Test) reveals an identifiable learning curve (4, 6, 8, 9, 9).

Introduction of a distractor list results in mild retroactive inhibitions (7/9), but the patient improves his performance with semantic cueing (8/9). After a delay he has retained this information. Semantic cueing is not helpful, but with recognition cueing, he is able to identify correctly all 9 of the 9 list items with no intrusive error.

The patient's response to the Beck Depression Inventory-II results in a score within the normal or nondepressed range (1/3). The patient relates only that he has less energy than he used to have. He denies feeling of dysphoria or sadness and denies any element of suicidal ideation.

IMPRESSION: Joel Wall was involved in a serious motor vehicle accident and received significant facial and upper-torso trauma; he also suffers from postconcussion syndrome. He has been on a ventilator and has had some reactive depression. Current testing would suggest that the patient is not experiencing significant depression at this time. From a cognitive standpoint, he seems to be doing quite well, and there is really minimal if any evidence of cognitive disfunction.

I will work with Joel to help him better understanding of the specific obstacles to his being discharged and any progress he might be making on these. When I spoke to him, he indicated that he had no idea of what the specific issues were and certainly had no sense of a timeline, which was a source of great frustration for him.

The patient also identifies that he has benefited from pastoral care from the local Buddhist monk, and hopefully they will be able to follow up with him on a regular basis to provide support.

2-6A:

SERVICE CODE(S): ____________________

DX CODE(S): ____________________

Dialysis

Dialysis, cleansing of the blood, can be temporary or permanent, depending on the needs of the patient. End-stage renal disease (ESRD) is a condition from which the patient will not recover without a kidney transplant, so these patients require permanent dialysis support. Non-ESRD is a condition from which the patient will recover and needs dialysis support only temporarily.

The End Stage Renal Diseases Services (90918–90925) are divided initially on a full month of service or a per-day service and then subdivided by the age of the patient. These codes are used to report the physician portion of the dialysis service. The **monthly service** codes (90918–90921) cover all physician visits to the hemodialysis laboratory during that month to assess the patient while receiving hemodialysis as well as the establishment of a treatment plan (dialyzing cycle) and management of the patient during the month. If less than a full month of service is provided to an ESRD patient in an outpatient setting, use 90922–90925 to report these per-day services.

The ESRD codes report only the physician portion of the dialysis services and do not include the actual hemodialysis treatment sessions. The treatment sessions are reported with 90935, 90937, 90945, or 90947. If the physician provides services that are non-ESRD related, those services are reported separately.

Patients can be trained in self-dialysis, which can be performed at home (peritoneal dialysis). Hemodialysis is performed at the hospital. The physician services are reported based on the **type** of dialysis the patient is receiving, the **complexity** of the service, and the **number** of visits the physician provides to the patient. As with all patients, dialysis patients must sometimes be admitted to the hospital for other medical problems, such as gallbladder, and while in the hospital must continue to receive dialysis treatments. When the physician provides an evaluation of the hemodialysis for an inpatient while the patient is receiving dialysis, you would report 90935 (single visit) or 90937 (multiple visits). The multiple visits are provided during the same dialysis session. Code 90937 may include a significant revision of the dialysis prescription. If a hospitalized patient receiving peritoneal dialysis is seen by the physician, the physician services are reported with 90945 (single visit) and 90947 (multiple visits). Code 90947 may include a significant revision of the dialysis prescription. Modifier -26 is not used on these codes to indicate that only the professional component of the service was provided, because the code descriptions already describe only the physician service to the dialysis patient.

When a patient does not receive a full month of dialysis in the outpatient setting because of a kidney transplant, relocation, or death, report the number of days that the patient received dialysis. For example, a 50-year-old patient receives peritoneal dialysis from March 1 through 10. On March 11, the patient receives a kidney transplant and no longer requires dialysis. The 10 days of service are reported with 90925 × 10.

CASE 2-7
2-7A Hemodialysis Progress Report

CASE 2-7

This is an admission to observation status, which is an outpatient unit. The facility and the physician report a V code as the principal/primary reason for encounter followed by the diagnosis(es) for that patient. The date of this service marks the 30th day of services provided to this ESRD patient by Dr. Orbitz. Report the monthly ESRD service code for this 32-year-old patient.

2-7A HEMODIALYSIS PROGRESS REPORT

LOCATION: Outpatient Hospital

PATIENT: Maryellen Menez

PHYSICIAN: George Orbitz, M.D.

This 32-year-old patient is seen, and I examined her hemodialysis chart. The patient appears to be hemodynamically stable and not in any form of respiratory distress or compromise. She is tolerating dialysis without any problems. Predialysis vital signs are noted. Blood pressure is 148/60, heart rate 58, respirations 16, temperature 36.3° C, and today she weighs 62.7 kg. Normocephalic and atraumatic. Pink palpebral conjunctivae, anicteric sclerae. No nasal or aural discharge. Moist tongue and buccal mucosa. No pharyngeal hyperemia, congestion, or exudate. Supple neck. No lymphadenopathy. Symmetrical chest. No retractions. No rhonchi, crackles, or wheezes. S1 and S2 are distinct. No S3 or S4. Regular rate and rhythm. Abdomen: Positive bowel sounds, soft and nontender. No laboratory tests are available today.

HEMODIALYSIS: Today we will dialyze her using her left-sided Perm-A-Cath for a total of 3 hours using an HP-150 dialyzer with a 2.0 potassium bath. Will give her a heparin loading dose of 2000 units and a maintenance dose of 1 mL per hour. Vital signs at present are stable. Blood pressure is 120/70, heart rate in the 70s, and she is tolerating a blood flow rate of 350 mL per minute.

ASSESSMENT/PLAN:

1. Chronic renal failure/end-stage renal disease (on maintenance hemodialysis Tuesday, Thursday, and Saturday), secondary to the following:
   a. Status post right-sided nephrectomy in 1996.
   b. Diabetes II.
   c. Diabetic nephropathy.
   d. Coronary artery disease.
2. Multiple electrolyte abnormalities related to problem chronic renal failure/end-stage renal disease.
   a. Hyperphosphatemia. Continue Renagel and Phoslo.
   b. Hypocalcemia.
3. Hypothyroidism. Continue Synthroid.
4. Nutrition.
5. Analgesia.
6. Deconditioning.

At the end of the dialysis, we will give her a dose of Zemplar.

2-7A:

SERVICE CODE(S): ______________________

DX CODE(S): ______________________

CASE 2-7A DISCUSSION

The physician provided 1 month of service to the patient. Codes 90918–90921 are reported only once for each month of physician service and include patient management services and evaluations during that month. This 32-year-old patient was provided services for an entire month, and as such the physician's service is reported with 90921.

Diagnoses

The reason for the encounter was dialysis, and this is the first-listed (primary) diagnosis (**V56.0**).

Hypertension and Chronic Renal Failure

The Assessment/Plan section of the report indicates that the other diagnosis is chronic renal failure due to hypertension. When hypertension is present with renal failure (585.X), the Guidelines direct the coder to assume a cause-and-effect relationship (the hypertension caused the kidney disease). Reference "Hypertension" in the Index of the ICD-9-CM under the subterm in the hypertension table "kidney, with renal failure." The statement that is located there indicates "(conditions classifiable to 585, 586)." This means that if a condition is present that is classifiable to 585 or 586 (in this case the patient has chronic renal failure classifiable to 585), the coder is to report the hypertension and renal failure with that one combination code (**403.91**).

Of special note is that Official Guideline C7, 3. indicates that the coder is to assign codes from category 403 when conditions classifiable to categories 585–587 are present—not 585–586 as indicated in the ICD-9-CM under the entry in the hypertension table "kidney, with renal failure." The Guidelines assist in assigning codes in the ICD-9-CM, and if there are discrepancies between the Guidelines and the ICD-9-CM, follow the directives in the ICD-9-CM.

Official Guidelines Coding and Reporting

C7, 3. **Hypertensive Renal Disease with Chronic Renal Failure.** Assign codes from category **403,** Hypertensive renal disease, when conditions classified to categories 585–587 are present *(Note: 585 is chronic kidney disease, 586 is unspecified renal failure, and 587 is unspecified renal sclerosis).* Unlike hypertension with heart disease, the ICD-9-CM presumes a cause-and-effect relationship and classifies renal failure with hypertension as hypertensive renal disease.

Electrolyte Imbalance

The electrolyte imbalance is reported with **276.9.**

Diabetes

The next diagnosis is the diabetes. When referencing the Index of the ICD-9-CM under the main term "Diabetes" subterm "nephropathy," the codes are listed as "250.4 [583.81]." This means that you would report **250.4X** and **583.81** to indicate diabetic nephropathy, and you would report the codes in the order indicated in the Index.

The patient previously had a kidney removed, which is significant for this episode of care and is reported with **V45.73.**

Peritoneal Dialysis

Peritoneal dialysis uses the **peritoneal cavity** as a filter. The dialysis fluid is introduced into the peritoneal cavity and left there for several hours as cleansing takes place and as illustrated in **Figure 2-1**. The fluid is then drained from the cavity. This dialysis service is reported on a per-day basis. Since patients can do this at home every day alone, there is usually no physician service involved unless physician evaluation is required. In that case, the patient most likely would come to the office or be admitted to the hospital.

One of the risks of peritoneal dialysis is *peritonitis,* an infection of the peritoneal cavity. The treatment for the infection usually involves introduction of antibiotics into the peritoneal fluid, as you will see in the following case.

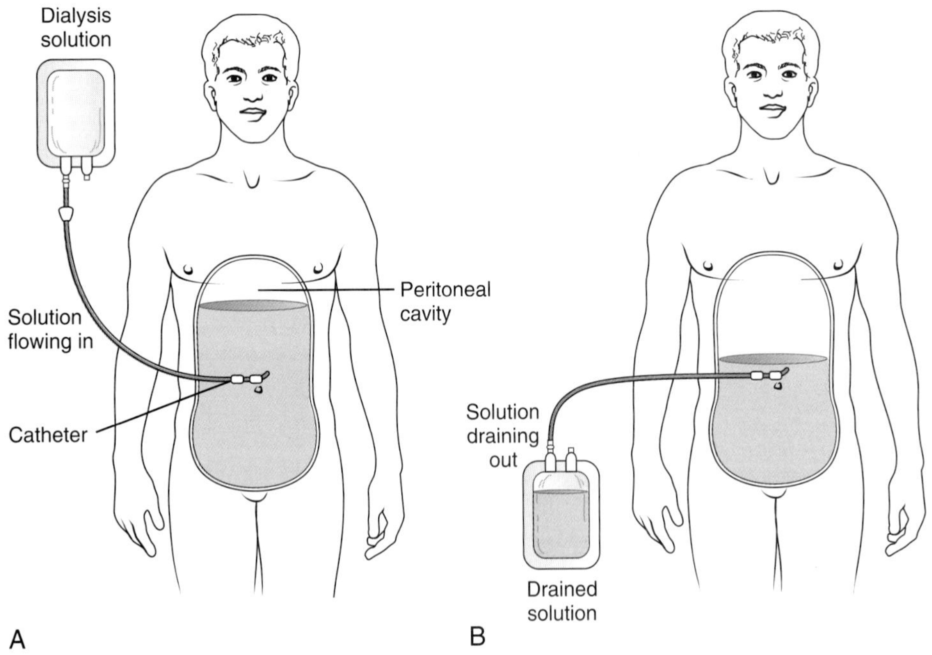

FIGURE 2-1 Peritoneal dialysis can be done by the patient. The dialysis solution enters the peritoneal cavity through a catheter. After the solution has remained within the patient for several hours, it is drained out through the catheter.

CASE 2-8
2-8A History and Physical Examination
2-8B CAPD Progress Note
2-8C Dialysis Progress Note
2-8D Thoracic Medicine and Critical Care Progress Note
2-8E Dialysis Progress Note
2-8F Dialysis Progress Note
2-8G Discharge Summary

CASE 2-8

This patient has been receiving ambulatory peritoneal dialysis for several years. She has encountered a complication and is admitted to the hospital by Dr. Orbitz for treatment for the complication. The complication is the primary reason for the treatment. This patient has hypertensive renal disease, so review C7.3 of the Official Guidelines for Coding and Reporting (Appendix C) before assigning the diagnoses for this case.

2-8A HISTORY AND PHYSICAL EXAMINATION

LOCATION: Inpatient Hospital

PATIENT: Grace Hargrove

PHYSICIAN: George Orbitz, M.D.

This 79-year-old woman is being admitted because of acute peritonitis due to peritoneal dialysis.

HISTORY OF PRESENT ILLNESS: This patient is a chronic ambulatory peritoneal dialysis patient who is currently on cycle PD for 10 hours at night. She was started on dialysis last year and has been a model patient having done superbly with no episodes of peritonitis prior to now. Her husband died 6 months ago. Since then, she has had increasing depression and failure to thrive with decreased nutrition and of late has been complaining of 2/10 abdominal discomfort and/or bloating for the past few days. Her ESRD is multifactorial and/or idiopathic. She has a long history of hypertension. She also has coronary artery disease and history of an MI, CABG 3 years ago, and remote history of recurrent CHF. She also has hyperlipidemia and 4 years ago had a parathyroidectomy. She had a CVA 2 years ago, anemia of chronic disease, and degenerative arthritis. She is attended by her son.

SOCIAL HISTORY: She used to be a factory worker, currently retired. Catholic. Tenth-grade education. She was married for 58 years. She is a nonuser of alcohol, tobacco, or other medications. She has a remote history of smoking, 40-pack-year total.

FAMILY HISTORY: Positive for cardiovascular disease and complications thereafter as well as cancer in the father with heart failure, who died at age 83.

MEDICATIONS: See Medications Admittance Record.

PHYSICAL EXAMINATION: Her lungs have decreased percussion note or dullness at the bases with decreased breath sounds. Some crackles, otherwise hyporesonant. PMI not well-felt. Probably diffuse. Heart regular. She has no significant murmur at this time, rub, or S3. Abdomen: Soft. Some discomfort diffusely. Fluid from the exit site looks okay. Extremities: No peripheral edema. No lateralizing neuro signs. Mental status normal. Skin: Normal. GYN, breasts, and rectal exams deferred.

Fluid exam shows evidence of peritonitis. Her current hemoglobin is 9.7 as a result of cessation temporarily of Epogen.

CLINICAL IMPRESSION: Acute peritonitis resulting from peritoneal dialysis, end-stage renal failure due to hypertension.

OTHER DIAGNOSES: As above, including failure to thrive, recent depression because of the death of her husband, malnutrition with hypoalbuminemia, atherosclerotic heart disease, ASCVD, etc.

2-8A:

SERVICE CODE(S): ____________________

DX CODE(S): ____________________

Complications

Complications of medical and surgical care that are not classified elsewhere are reported with 996–999. Routine conditions that occur after medical or surgical care are not considered complications. Complications of pregnancy, abortion, labor, or delivery are located in Chapter 11. Complications that affect multiple systems are usually reported with codes 996–999. Complications that are specific to a system are located in the chapter of the ICD-9-CM where the other codes for that system are located. You can locate the codes in the Index under the complication term, such as the following for location of "complication of intrauterine device":

Contraception
device (in situ) V45.59
causing menorrhagia 996.76

or

Complications
contraceptive device, intrauterine NEC 996.76

2-8B CAPD PROGRESS NOTE

The complication is now being managed by means of antibiotics in the peritoneal fluid; so the complication diagnosis is now listed second and the hypertensive renal disease is listed first.

LOCATION: Inpatient Hospital

PATIENT: Grace Hargrove

PHYSICIAN: George Orbitz, M.D.

CAPD PROGRESS NOTE: The patient was admitted and re-evaluated regarding her dialysis prescription. Because of her diagnosis of acute peritonitis due to peritoneal dialysis, the plan at this time is to use all of 1.5% Dianeal and 2-liter volumes and do CAPD instead of cycler. The initial bag will contain antibiotic. The gent bag is next. Cultures are pending. We will proceed from there. The patient was evaluated after admission. She is empty at this point, and we have yet to place the first bag. Her abdomen is a little tender, and she is bloated. There is no doubt in my mind that we are seeing a developing peritonitis. The concern, of course, is the fact that she has been constipated and the worry is that this may represent a more serious colonic perforation.

2-8B:

SERVICE CODE(S): ____________________

DX CODE(S): ____________________

2-8C DIALYSIS PROGRESS NOTE

The complication continues to be treated with antibiotics.

LOCATION: Inpatient Hospital

PATIENT: Grace Hargrove

PHYSICIAN: George Orbitz, M.D.

DIALYSIS PROGRESS NOTE: The patient continues to be on peritoneal dialysis. She is doing well with that. She is using 1.5%. No ultrafiltration. In fact, ultrafiltration is negative. Her peritonitis seems to be doing better since she has no pain. Her appetite is better, and she is not having any more diarrhea.

Her vital signs are stable except that her pressure is a little high, 180s/90s. Temperature is 37° C.

We will continue with antibiotic treatment and continue to watch her blood pressure. She has no edema right now and will continue to use 1.5%. We possibly could use 2.5% over the weekend.

The patient agrees with the plan. Will probably plan on discharging her on Monday.

2-8C:

SERVICE CODE(S): ____________________

DX CODE(S): ____________________

2-8D THORACIC MEDICINE AND CRITICAL CARE PROGRESS NOTE

The infection is now known to be streptococcal, and as such this diagnosis must be added to the list of diagnoses for this patient. Place the code for the streptococcal infection immediately after the peritonitis code.

LOCATION: Inpatient Hospital

PATIENT: Grace Hargrove

PHYSICIAN: George Orbitz, M.D.

THORACIC MEDICINE AND CRITICAL CARE PROGRESS NOTE: This is a CAPD/peritoneal dialysis note. The patient is admitted for acute peritonitis with group A, not group D, peritonitis. She is getting her dialysis performed while she is here. She gets five exchanges in a day. She gets Kefzol 500 mg in each dialyzing exchange. Also has gentamicin as dosed by pharmacy to each exchange, and she gets 2 liters of 1.5% five times a day. Abdomen today is still a little tender. She is, however, afebrile. We will make sure she has something for pain because she says it is somewhat uncomfortable. On reviewing her medications, she does not have anything ordered for pain, so I will make sure that she does.

2-8D:

SERVICE CODE(S): ____________________

DX CODE(S): ____________________

2-8E DIALYSIS PROGRESS NOTE

The patient continues to receive treatment for the complication.

LOCATION: Inpatient Hospital

PATIENT: Grace Hargrove

PHYSICIAN: George Orbitz, M.D.

THORACIC MEDICINE AND CRITICAL CARE PROGRESS NOTE: The patient is in with acute peritonitis, group A, and is undergoing peritoneal dialysis. The pain is less. She has only used 3 pain pills since yesterday. She remains afebrile. Abdomen is actually fairly benign on palpation today. The max temperature was 36.2° C in the last 24 hours. She has 5 exchanges in the day with CAPD, and we will not change that. We used a 2-liter volume 1.5%, added Kefzol 500 mg to each dialysis exchange, and then added gentamicin to be decided on by pharmacology. That will be done to each exchange. She has Tylenol no. 3 for pain, and it is controlling the pain fairly well.

No need to change anything at this point; dialysis is going fine. I do not need to change anything there. Her weight is stable, 129.3 pounds. It has been like that for 2 days now.

2-8E:

SERVICE CODE(S): ____________________

DX CODE(S): ____________________

2-8F DIALYSIS PROGRESS NOTE

The patient is discharged from the hospital. The first-listed diagnosis continues to be the complication for which the admission was made.

LOCATION: Inpatient Hospital

PATIENT: Grace Hargrove

PHYSICIAN: George Orbitz, M.D.

DIALYSIS PROGRESS NOTE: The patient had no more major events during the night. She has less pain. She is eating well. She denies any complaints. She is tolerating peritoneal dialysis very well with 1.5%. Her vital signs are stable. She is afebrile at 36.5° C. The plan is to send her home taking Kefzol. She will be discharged home today. Patient agrees with the plan.

2-8F:

CASE 3 HD>SERVICE CODE(S): ____________________

DX CODE(S): ____________________

Infection has resolved —

2-8G DISCHARGE SUMMARY

LOCATION: Inpatient Hospital

PATIENT: Grace Hargrove

PHYSICIAN: George Orbitz, M.D.

PRIMARY DIAGNOSIS: Acute peritonitis due to peritoneal dialysis.

SECONDARY DIAGNOSIS: End-stage renal disease, hypertensive, on chronic peritoneal dialysis for chronic renal failure.

HISTORY OF PRESENT ILLNESS: The patient is a 79-year-old white female who is known to have end-stage renal disease on CAPD.

HOSPITAL COURSE: She was admitted with abdominal pain and cloudy dialysate. She was found to have alpha streptococcal peritonitis. She was given vancomycin, gentamicin, and Kefzol. The Group A strep was sensitive to cephalosporins. She did well during her hospitalization and felt better.

DISCHARGE PLAN: The patient will be discharged home today. Mario, from dialysis, will teach her how to add antibiotics to her peritoneal dialysis bags.

The patient agrees with the plan. She was advised to call us back if she has any more problems.

2-8G:

SERVICE CODE(S): ____________________

DX CODE(S): ____________________

CASE 2-8G DISCUSSION

This is a short report, but contains considerable diagnoses coding. The reason the patient received this care is primarily the complication of an infection from a catheter. The dialysis complication is, therefore, the first-listed diagnosis. Next, the complication led to peritonitis due to a streptococcal infection. The peritonitis is listed next, followed by the causative/bacteria (streptococcal infection). The patient has hypertensive end-stage renal disease, which is why she is on CAPD. According to C7. 3. you are to assign a code from 403 (Hypertensive renal disease) when a condition classified to category 585–587 is present. Code 585 is chronic kidney disease, 586 is unspecified renal failure, and 587 is unspecified renal sclerosis.

Noninvasive Vascular Diagnostic Studies

Many of the codes in the Cardiovascular subsection (92950–93990) of Medicine are reviewed in Chapter 6, *Cardiovascular System* because these codes predominantly refer to diagnostic and therapeutic services for heart conditions such as coronary thrombolysis, electrocardiogram, electrocardiography, cardiac catheterization, and electrophysiology. Noninvasive Vascular Diagnostic Studies codes (93875–93990) are used to report extracranial (outside the cranium) vascular studies, as well as vascular studies of the extremities, viscera, penis, etc. Noninvasive Vascular Diagnostic Studies codes include the supervision, interpretation, and written report of the results. Vascular flow analysis is the determination of the blood flow within arteries and veins. One analysis method used is a **duplex scan,** which uses ultrasound that bounces off the vessel and produces a color picture on a monitor showing the blood flow within veins and arteries. The duplex scan uses real-time and color-flow Doppler imaging to view the blood flow. Most of the codes within the Noninvasive Vascular Diagnostic Studies subsection are used to report services using a duplex scan. These scans are helpful in diagnosing a wide range of vascular diseases, such as varicose veins of the leg, which is a chronic venous disease. The duplex scan allows for the identification of a specific area(s) of restriction or blockage. **Cerebrovascular disease** is blockage of the arteries of the brain, which increases the risk of stroke. Cerebrovascular disease can be detected with transcranial Doppler (TCD) or carotid artery duplex scan; this is reported with 93875–93888. Subheading codes indicate the area of study, for example, cerebrovascular, renal, the extent of the study as bilateral (e.g., 93880), unilateral (e.g., 93882), complete (e.g., 93975), or limited (e.g., 93976). The 3 subheadings of extremity study codes are arterial (93922–93931), venous (93965–93971), and arterial-venous hemodialysis access (93990).

Modifier -26 is added to the physician portion of these services to indicate that only the professional component of the service was provided.

CASE 2-9

The following arterial study was performed by a physician who specializes in vascular diseases for a 76-year-old female with suspected narrowing of the carotid artery, causing an increased heart rate.

2-9A DUPLEX CAROTID ARTERY STUDY

LOCATION: Outpatient, Hospital

PATIENT: Elizabeth McConnell

REQUESTING PHYSICIAN: Alma Naraquist, M.D.

PHYSICIAN: Leslie Alanda, M.D.

CLINICAL SYMPTOMS: Rapid ventricular rate

DUPLEX CAROTID ARTERY TEST: Real-time (imaging) analysis: On the right side, there is a little "hard plaque" in the posterior wall of the internal carotid. On the left side, there is some hard plaque in the distal common carotid in the posterior wall.

Doppler (flow) analysis is normal throughout both sides, indicating less than 50% stenosis. There is no spectral broadening, which if present, would indicate turbulence.

The vertebral arteries both show antegrade flow.

CONCLUSION: There is some atherosclerotic change, but it is not prominent.

2-9A:

SERVICE CODE(S): ______________________________

DX CODE(S): ______________________________

Late Effects

Late effects codes are not assigned to a separate chapter in the Tabular. Instead, you must first identify a case as a late effect and then code it as such. You use late effects codes when the acute phase of the illness or injury has passed but a residual remains. Sometimes an acute illness or injury leaves a patient with a residual health problem that remains after the illness or injury has resolved.

The residual is coded first, *and then* **the late effects code is assigned** to indicate the cause of the residual. An example would be scars (residual) that remain after a severe burn (cause).

The late effects code is accessed in the Index under the main term "Late." In most instances, two codes will be assigned—one code for the residual that is being treated and one code that indicates the late effect.

There is no time limit for the development of a residual. It may be evident at the time of the acute illness, or it may occur months after an injury. It is also possible that a patient may develop more than one residual. For example, a patient who has had a stroke may develop right-sided hemiparesis (paralysis of one side) and aphasia (loss of ability to communicate). A person cannot have a current hip fracture (820.8) and a late effect of hip fracture (905.3).

The code is either a current injury or a condition caused by a prior injury. It cannot be both at the same time. (The only exception to this rule is in category 438, Late effects of cerebrovascular disease, which is explained below.)

Official Guidelines for Coding and Reporting Section I, B, 12. Late Effects

A late effect is the residual effect (condition produced) after the acute phase of an illness or injury has terminated. There is no time limit on when a late effect code can be used. The residual may be apparent early, such as in cerebrovascular accident cases, or it may occur months or years later, such as that due to a previous injury. Coding of late effects generally requires two codes sequenced in the following order: The **condition or nature** of the late effect is sequenced first, and the **late effect code** is sequenced second. An exception to the above guidelines are instances in which the code for a late effect is followed by a manifestation code (identified in the Tabular List and title), or the late effect code has been expanded (at the fourth-and fifth-digit levels) to include the manifestation(s). The code for the acute phase of an illness or injury that led to the late effect is never used with a code for the late effect.

Official Coding and Reporting Guidelines Section I, C7, B. Late Effects of Cerebrovascular Disease

Category 438 is used to indicate conditions classifiable to categories 430–437 as the causes of late effects (neurologic deficits), which are themselves classified elsewhere. These "late effects" include neurologic deficits that persist after initial onset of conditions classifiable to 430–437. The neurologic deficits caused by cerebrovascular disease may be present from the onset or may arise at any time after the onset of the condition classifiable to 430–437. Codes from category 438 may be assigned on a health care record with codes from 430–437 if the patient has a current cerebrovascular accident (CVA) and deficits from an old CVA. Assign code V12.59 (not a code from category 438) as an additional code for history of cerebrovascular disease when no neurologic deficits are present.

For example:

Diagnosis:	Dysphagia due to a previous cerebrovascular accident
Residual:	Dysphagia (The dysphagia is a problem that remains following the acute illness of the cerebrovascular accident.)
Cause:	Cerebrovascular accident (This patient had a previous cerebrovascular accident.)
Terms to code:	Dysphagia [residual] Cerebrovascular accident [cause]. The late effect of cerebrovascular accident is reported with a combination code.

Locate the terms "Late, effect, cerebrovascular disease, with dysphagia," and you will be directed to 438.82, which includes both the residual and the cause in 1 code.

CASE 2-10

This patient has late effects (hemiparalysis and aphasia) of a cerebrovascular accident (stroke). These late effects are the reason for the encounter.

2-10A DUPLEX CAROTID ARTERY STUDY

LOCATION: Outpatient, Hospital

PATIENT: Larry Smith

EXAMINATION OF: Duplex carotid artery outpatient study

CLINICAL SYMPTOMS: Previous stroke with right hemiparesis and aphasia.

ORDERING PHYSICIAN: Ronald Green, M.D.

PHYSICIAN: James Noonar, M.D.

DUPLEX CAROTID ARTERY STUDY: The patient is a 30-year-old male who suffered a massive stroke 1 month ago and has resultant right hemiparesis and aphasia.

Real-time (imaging) analysis: On the right side, there is some soft plaque on the anterior wall of the distal bulb/proximal internal carotid. On the left side, there is soft plaque on the anterior wall of the bulb and on the anterior and posterior walls of the internal carotid.

stenosis (Narrowing, carotid) bilateral

Doppler (flow) analysis: On the right side, the peak systolic velocity of the internal carotid artery is 1.42 m/sec, indicating 50% to 75% stenosis. Peak diastolic velocity is 0.27, indicating a less than 50% stenosis, and the IC/CC ratio is 1.31. There is slight spectral broadening.

On the left side, we get extremely low velocities and then a "thud," indicating occlusion just downstream from the scanning area.

The vertebral arteries both show antegrade flow.

CONCLUSION: There is some stenosis on the right side. The left side implies occlusion distal to the area scanned. This would certainly fit with the above symptoms.

2-10A:

SERVICE CODE(S): ______________________

DX CODE(S): ______________________

CASE 2-11
2-11A Arterial Doppler Test

CASE 2-11

The patient is a diabetic with pain in the left leg. The physician orders a Doppler arterial analysis (not a duplex scan) in which ultrasound is used to analyze the vessels.

2-11A ARTERIAL DOPPLER TEST

LOCATION: Outpatient, Hospital

PATIENT: Gary Kettle

REQUESTING PHYSICIAN: Alma Naraquist, M.D.

PHYSICIAN: Leslie Alanda, M.D.

CLINICAL SYMPTOMS: Diabetes, pain in left leg

ARTERIAL DOPPLER TEST: The patient is a 72-year-old with diabetes and pain in the left leg.

The results of the study are abnormal. On the right side, despite normal ankle-to-brachial index at 1.22, the waveforms are monophasic. The digital pressure is only 70 for an index of 0.5. I believe there is disease in this leg throughout, but more distally than proximally.

In the left leg, the waveforms are even more abnormal. Again, an ankle-to-brachial index of 1.3 is erroneous due to calcified vessels. Waveforms are severely monophasic distally. The digital pressure is only 12 for an index of 0.09, which indicates severe ischemia.

CONCLUSION: I believe there is probably disease in both legs, but it is quite severe on the left, which would explain the pain. The disease level on the left would appear to be proximal to the popliteal and perhaps very proximal.

2-11A:

SERVICE CODE(S): ______________________

DX CODE(S): ______________________

CASE 2-12
2-12A Vascular Laboratory Report, Arterial Doppler Test

CASE 2-12

Report Dr. Noonar's service.

2-12A VASCULAR LABORATORY REPORT, ARTERIAL DOPPLER TEST

LOCATION: Outpatient, Hospital

PATIENT: Ilene Sogla

ORDERING PHSYCIAN: Ronald Green, M.D.

PHYSICIAN: James Noonar, M.D.

INDICATION: Leg pain

The patient is 65-year-old female with known coronary artery disease. She complains of some pain with walking. She exercised for 5 minutes at 2 miles an hour at 10% grade. The resting ankle-to-brachial index is 1.23 on the right and left. The brachial pressure went up from 115 to 130. The right ankle pressure dropped minimally from 142 to 132, and the left ankle pressure remains stable.

CONCLUSION: There may be trivial arterial insufficiency, but nothing impressive here.

2-12A:

SERVICE CODE(S): ____________________

DX CODE(S): ____________________

Cardioversion

Cardioversion is the restoration of the heart to normal rhythm. The electrical conversion of an arrhythmia may be done externally by placing the paddles on the chest or internally by opening the chest and exposing the heart to the view of the surgeon with paddles being placed directly on the heart. The cardioversion codes are designated "separate procedure" and are reported only when the cardioversion is the only procedure performed. A cardiologist usually performs an elective cardioversion as a treatment for arrhythmia. You will be coding another cardioversion case in Chapter 6, *Cardiovascular System.*

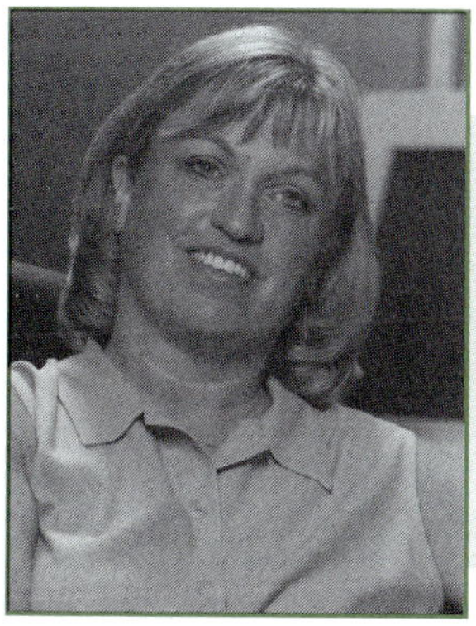

FROM THE TRENCHES

Joan

"One of the biggest changes I've seen in the industry in the last five or six years has been the increasing complexity in terms of following all the rules ... our coding is getting more and more important. Having people trained in the rules and trained to know exactly what the services are—and how they should be coded—is going to be more and more important."

CASE 2-13
2-13A Electrical Cardioversion

CASE 2-13

Report the cardioversion provided by Dr. Elhart.

2-13A ELECTRICAL CARDIOVERSION

LOCATION: Inpatient, Hospital

PATIENT: Rick Eck

PREOPERATIVE DIAGNOSIS: Atrial flutter

POSTOPERATIVE DIAGNOSIS: Atrial flutter

PROCEDURE PERFORMED: Electrical cardioversion

SURGEON: Gary Sanchez, M.D.

PRIMARY PHYSICIAN: Ronald Green, M.D.

CONSULTING PHYSICIAN: Marvin Elhart, M.D.

BRIEF HISTORY: This is a 59-year-old patient with respiratory failure and on a ventilator. He was noted to have supraventricular tachycardia in the form of atrial flutter. Cardioversion was recommended. The patient is already anticoagulated. He has a low risk for embolization. Indication for cardioversion is to improve his hemodynamics and control his rate. The procedure was explained to the wife, and she consents to it.

PROCEDURE: The patient was sedated with Versed and morphine. He was given a total of 5 mg Versed. He was cardioverted with 50 joules into sinus tachycardia.

The patient was given 20 mcg Cardizem IV push. His heart rate went down to 110s, and he was definitely in sinus tachycardia.

CONCLUSION: Successful electrical cardioversion of atrial flutter into sinus tachycardia.

PLAN: The patient will need to have his rate and blood pressure controlled. A Cardizem drip is an excellent choice until the patient can take p.o. He needs to have his TSH and T_4 levels assessed.

2-13A:

SERVICE CODE(S): ____________________

DX CODE(S): ____________________

Ultrasound

Diagnostic ultrasound is the use of high-frequency sound waves to image anatomic structures and to detect the cause of illness and disease. It is used by the physician in the diagnosis process. Ultrasound moves at different speeds through tissue, depending on the density of the tissue. Forms and outlines of organs can be identified by ultrasound as the sound waves move through or bounce back (echo) from the tissues.

The ultrasound codes for heart and vessels are in the Medicine section; all other ultrasound codes are in the Radiology section. Codes for ultrasound procedures are found in 3 locations:

- Radiology section, Diagnostic Ultrasound subsection, 76506–76886, divided on the basis of the anatomic location of the procedure (chest, pelvis)
- Medicine section, Non-Invasive Vascular Diagnostic Studies subsection, 93875–93990, divided on the basis of the anatomic location of the procedure (cerebrovascular, extremity)
- Medicine section, Echocardiography (ultrasound of the heart and great arteries), 93303–93350

CASE 2-14
2-14A Ultrasound, Lower Extremities

CASE 2-14

Report the ultrasound service provided by Dr. Monson.

2-14A ULTRASOUND, LOWER EXTREMITIES

LOCATION: Outpatient, Hospital

PATIENT: Dennis Hooperman

REQUESTING PHYSICIAN: Alma Naraquist, M.D.

PHYSICIAN: Morton Monson, M.D.

EXAMINATION OF: Ultrasound of both lower extremities

CLINICAL SYMPTOMS: Bilateral edema

ULTRASOUND OF BOTH LOWER EXTREMITIES: FINDINGS: Ultrasound examination of the deep venous system of the lower extremities shows no evidence of a deep venous thrombosis. Bilateral posterior tibial, greater saphenous, popliteal, and femoral veins are patent with no evidence of thrombus. The distal portion of both superficial femoral veins is not well seen because of patient body habitus but shows no gross evidence of DVT.

2-14A:

SERVICE CODE(S): ______________________

DX CODE(S): ______________________

Codes Reviewed Elsewhere

Many of the codes in the Medicine section are reviewed elsewhere in this text because the codes are best studied in the specialties within which they are most often used. As with all codes within the CPT, any physician can report any code, but most often the codes are applicable to specialty areas of practice, and therefore the following codes are presented in other chapters of the text as follows:

- Gastroenterology codes 91000–91299, Chapter 7, Digestive System, Hemic/Lymphatic System, and Mediastinum/Diaphragm
- Ophthalmology codes 92002–92499 and Special Otorhinolaryngologic Services 92502–92700, Chapter 13, Eye and Auditory Systems
- Pulmonary codes 94010–94799, Chapter 9, Respiratory System
- Endocrinology code 95250, Chapter 10, Urinary, Male Genital, and Endocrine Systems
- Neurology and Neuromuscular Procedures 95805–96004, Chapter 12, Nervous System
- Special Dermatological Procedures 96900–96999, Chapter 5, Integumentary System
- Qualifying Circumstances for Anesthesia and Sedation with or without Analgesia (Moderate [Conscious] Sedation) 99143–99150, Chapter 14, Anesthesia

Central Nervous System Assessments/Tests (e.g., Neurocognitive, Mental Status, Speech Testing)

The codes in the Central Nervous System Assessment/Tests (96103–96119) are used to identify psychological testing, speech/language assessments, developmental progress assessments, and thinking/reasoning status examination (neurobehavioral). The codes are reported based on a per-hour basis except for the basic developmental assessments. The physician or other health care provider would interpret the test results and provide a written report of the assessment.

Cognitive (thinking) processes are assessed with a variety of testing instruments, such as MMPI (Minnesota Multiphasic Personality Inventory), which is an assessment of personality types. The Rorschach is an assessment in which inkblots are shown to the patient, and the patient is asked to describe what he or she sees in the image.

Developmental testing is used to assess the psychomotor or cognitive abilities by means of assessment instruments such as the Early Language Milestone Screen or the Bayley Scales of Infant Development. Neurobehavioral status is an assessment of the thinking and reasoning abilities of the patient, for example, an elderly patient with Alzheimer's.

Dementia

Primary dementia is the most common type of dementia. It is a progressive disease that results in damage to neurons and is usually fatal within 3–20 years. There are many causes, such as infection, metabolic disorders, lesions, vascular disorders, toxins, and infarction. The symptoms are impaired memory, thinking, and behavior. There is no cure, only treatment of the symptoms. Secondary dementia (caused by another condition, and also known as nutritional degenerative disease) results from a deficiency of B vitamins, niacin, and pantothenic acid associated with alcoholism.

Code 294.1 has fifth-digits to identify those dementias with the presence or absence of behavior disturbances, for example, dementia in a patient with Alzheimer's without behavior disturbance. Locate the following in the Index of the ICD-9-CM:

Dementia
  due to or associated with condition(s) classified elsewhere
    Alzheimer's
      with behavioral disturbance 331.0 *[**294.11**]*
      without behavior disturbance 331.0 *[**294.10**]*

The Index directs the coder to reference 331.0 and 294.10 in the Tabular where the following is displayed:

331 **Other cerebral degenerations**
  311.0 Alzheimer's disease
294 **Other organic psychotic conditions (chronic)**
  Includes: organic psychotic brain syndromes (chronic) not elsewhere classified
  294.1 Dementia in conditions classified elsewhere
    Code first any underlying physical condition as:
      Dementia in:
        Alzheimer's disease
    294.10 Dementia in conditions classified elsewhere without behavior disturbance

Note that following 294.1, it is stated that the underlying physical condition is to be reported first. Both the Index and the Tabular direct the coder to report the physical condition first, 331.0 (Alzheimer's) and 294.10 (dementia).

If the dementia is stated without any underlying condition, such as "senile dementia," only the code for the dementia is reported (290.2X) with a fifth digit assigned based on if the dementia was with or without depression.

CASE 2-15

Report Dr. Shongo's service.

2-15A COGNITIVE FUNCTION ASSESSMENT

LOCATION: Outpatient, Clinic

Dr. Leslie Alanda refers Sam Kaiser, an 83-year-old male patient with suspected dementia, to Dr. Fred Shongo for an assessment. The physician administered a battery of written and oral neurobehavioral tests to assess Sam's memory (cognitive function) that took 2 hours to complete. The diagnosis was stated as senile dementia with depression.

2-15A:

SERVICE CODE(S): ____________________

DX CODE(S): ____________________

Health and Behavior Assessment/Intervention

The prevention, treatment, or management of a health problem that requires an assessment of psychological, behavioral, emotional, thinking, or social factors is reported with codes 96150–96155. An acute or chronic illness or prevention of an illness or maintenance of the patient's health is associated with the use of these codes. Codes 96150–96155 are for services provided to patients who have an established illness or symptom and do not have symptoms or an established diagnosis of mental illness. The Health and Behavior Assessment/Intervention codes are not used instead of Preventive Medicine Services, Counseling, and/or Risk Reduction Intervention (99401–99404) from the E/M section. The E/M codes are used to report services to a patient without symptoms or an established illness.

CASE 2-16
2-16A Behavior Assessment

CASE 2-16

Report Dr. Shongo's service.

2-16A BEHAVIOR ASSESSMENT

LOCATION: Outpatient, Clinic

Dr. Alma Naraquist referred Beth Roy, a 13-year-old female patient, to Dr. Fred Shongo, a psychiatrist, for a behavior assessment regarding her chronic nail biting. She bites the nails until they bleed and further aggravates the situation by picking at the cuticles. Dr. Naraquist has treated the chronic infection present on Beth's fingers and asks Dr. Shongo to assess Beth's behavioral condition. Dr. Shongo provides an initial assessment of 45 minutes and schedules Beth to return the following week.

2-16A:

SERVICE CODE(S): ____________________

DX CODE(S): ____________________

Chemotherapy Administration

Chemotherapy may be administered by several methods:

- **Subcutaneous** or **intramuscular** injection for a neoplasm or microbes.
- **Intralesional** or direct injection into a lesion.
- Intravenous or intra-arterial **push** (quick administration by forcing medication into the veins).
- Intravenous or intra-arterial **infusion** (administration over a long period, based on the time it takes to complete the infusion, e.g., 1, 2–8, or 9+ hours).
- Insertion into the **pleural cavity.**
- Insertion into the **peritoneal cavity.**
- **CNS** administration (e.g., intrathecal).
- **Subarachnoid** or **intraventricular** administration by means of a subcutaneous reservoir.

The medical record will indicate the method used for administration of the medicine, which will direct the choice of codes to report the service. Chemotherapy Administration codes (96401–96549) report only the **administration** and do not include an office service. If the patient requires a separate E/M code to report a significant office service in addition to the administration, the service is reported with modifier -25 (Significant, Separately Identifiable Evaluation and Management Service by the Same Physician on the Same Day of the Procedure or Other Service). The provision of the chemotherapy **agent** is reported separately with the appropriate HCPCS J code.

If the patient is given an additional medication such as an analgesic or antiemetic before or after chemotherapy, report the administration of the medication based on the method of administration and the drug(s) reported with a HCPCS J code (based on the type of medication).

The chemotherapy codes (96440–96549) are for services such as refilling and maintaining portable and implantable chemotherapy pumps or central nervous system and pleural peritoneal cavity administration.

Diagnosis Coding for Chemotherapy

There are also encounter codes for chemotherapy (V58.11) and radiotherapy (V58.0). When coding an encounter for chemotherapy or radiotherapy, code the V code first, followed by the active code for the malignant neoplasm, even if that neoplasm has already been removed. As long as the neoplasm is being treated with adjunctive therapy following a surgical removal of the cancer, you can code that neoplasm as if it still exists. You would not assign a "history of" V code, because the neoplasm is the reason for the treatment. Instead, the neoplasm is coded as a current or active disease.

CASE 2-17

2-17A INFUSION

LOCATION: Outpatient, Clinic

Pat Strand is a 40-year-old patient with multiple myeloma. She presents for 50 minutes of infusion of carmustine (100 mg) chemotherapy administration.

2-17A:

SERVICE CODE(S): ______________________

DX CODE(S): ______________________

Photodynamic Therapy

Photodynamic therapy (PDT) is a medical procedure in which a photosensitive (light-activated) drug is injected, infused, or applied to an area. The drug accumulates in the diseased tissue at a higher rate than the surrounding nondiseased tissue. Targeted irradiation of the tissue is then administered with laser.

Porfimer sodium (Photofrin®, J9600, 75 mg) is a light-sensitive drug that is used in PDT for esophageal cancer or lung cancer. The drug is administered in a two-stage process. In the first stage the drug is injected, and approximately 40 hours later the laser is applied. The second stage of the procedure is performed through an esophagoscopy tube for esophageal cancer and a bronchoscopy tube for lung cancer. The procedure would be reported separately with a code such as:

31641	Bronchoscopy, with destruction of tumor
J9600 × 2	Photosensitive drug (Porfimer sodium 150 mg)
96570	Endoscopic application of laser (96570 [first 30 minutes] and 96571 [each additional 15 minutes])

Verteporfin (Visudyne®, J3395, 15 mg) is a light-activated drug used to destroy lesions that occur as a result of age-related macular degeneration. Fluorescein angiogram is used to determine the extent of the degeneration and demonstrate the medical necessity of the photodynamic treatment(s). Verteporfin is intravenously injected, and laser light is directed into the patient's eye(s) for about 90 seconds. The injection of the drug is adequate for treatment of both eyes. The procedure is reported with a code such as 67221 (Destruction of choroid lesion).

Aminolevulinic acid HCL (Levulan® Kerastick®, J7308, 354 mg) is a photosensitive topical drug used to treat nonhyperkeratotic actinic keratosis. Nonhyperkeratotic actinic keratosis is a cutaneous growth that may develop into squamous cell carcinoma. It is caused by excessive exposure to the sun and usually occurs in the middle-aged or elderly, especially those with fair skin. As a treatment for this condition, the photosensitive drug is applied, then blue light is delivered to the area approximately 16 hours later. The service is reported with a code such as 96567 (PDT, external application). Both the drug and 96567 are reported for each PDT session.

CASE 2-18
2-18A Photodynamic Therapy

CASE 2-18

2-18A PHOTODYNAMIC THERAPY

LOCATION: Outpatient, Clinic

Dr. Barton provided service for Donna Sinne has actinic keratosis on her lip. The treatment provided entails 3 phototherapy exposures over the course of several weeks using a 354-mg single-unit dose of aminolevulinic acid HCL during each session. Report all 3 sessions.

2-18A:

SERVICE CODE(S): ______________________

DX CODE(S): ______________________

Physical Medicine and Rehabilitation

A physician or a therapist can report the Physical Medicine and Rehabilitation codes. Rehabilitation uses a variety of modalities for treatment (whirlpool, electrical stimulation). Services are usually reported based on the time spent in the session. Unit coding (i.e., code ± 2) is frequently used. For those services reported based on time, the time must be documented in the medical record.

Codes 97001 and 97002 are used to report a physical therapy evaluation or re-evaluation. The physician or physical therapist examines the patient and provides an assessment of the current status of the patient in the area or areas requested. This would include a prognosis and plan for interventional physical therapy that would improve the condition.

The codes in the Modalities category (97010–97028) specify that the provider does not need to be in constant attendance to report the service. For example, the provider may place hot packs (97010) on the patient's lower back and leave the treatment room to attend to other patients. The Constant Attendance category requires the provider to be in direct contact during the entire session. An example is a contrast bath (in which the patient is placed into a hot tub and then a cold tub for contrasting temperatures). For this service, the provider must be in attendance throughout the entire session. This is represented by codes 97032–97039.

Therapeutic Procedures (97110–97546) require direct patient contact and report services such as those performed to improve or develop strength, endurance, range of motion, and/or flexibility. Many of these services are exercises, neuromuscular reeducation, water therapy, gait training, massage, and manipulation. There are also codes to report the services of fitting and training of orthotic or prosthetic devices.

CASE 2-19

The patient presents for an after visit following musculoskeletal surgery; therefore, a V code will be the first-listed diagnosis.

2-19A PHYSICAL THERAPY EVALUATION

LOCATION: Outpatient, Rehabilitation Clinic

Nikki Fire is referred to the local rehabilitation center by her family physician for a physical therapy evaluation after a knee repair. Nikki has degenerative osteoarthritis. The rehabilitation physician provided the evaluation, and a written report was developed. Report the rehabilitation physician's evaluative services.

2-19A:

SERVICE CODE(S): ______________________

DX CODE(S): ______________________

CASE 2-20
2-20A Physical Therapy Evaluation
2-20B Physical Therapy Evaluation
2-20C Physical Therapy Evaluation

CASE 2-20

The following is a full-length physical therapy evaluation for which you are to report Dr. Barneswell's service. This is not a consultation, but a physical therapy evaluation. A V code for the physical therapy is reported as the first-listed diagnosis, because that is the primary reason the patient is being evaluated. Next listed would be the quadriplegia.

2-20A PHYSICAL THERAPY EVALUATION

LOCATION: Outpatient, Clinic

PATIENT: Terra Benson

REFERRING PHYSICIAN: Ronald Green, M.D.

PHYSICIAN: Mary Barneswell, M.D.

DIAGNOSIS: Congenital cerebral palsy spastic quadriplegia with intrathecal baclofen pump.

SUBJECTIVE: Terra is referred to Physical Therapy for evaluation for a session of intensive summer programming. The patient has participated in the summer programming in the past, and both the patient and her mother state that she has benefited from this programming, particularly in the area of balance. Terra states that at the time of her first summer session she was unable to sit independently on the toilet, and following the summer session, she has been able to sit independently on the toilet. The patient states that she uses both a power and manual wheelchair for transportation. Her mother states that they switch on and off which one they use. Her mother is with her quite a bit of the time to assist her with activities. The patient is a 10th grader this year at Mother of Hope school. The patient states that she is not receiving any physical therapy programming at school. They are also not performing any type of home exercise program at this time. Both the patient and her mother state that both sitting balance and tightness of the adductor musculature are their primary concerns at this time. Patient/Family goal: Both the patient and her mother state that they would like to increase Terra's sitting balance.

OBJECTIVE: Observation: Terra does demonstrate a windswept posture to the right, indicating weakness of the left gluteal musculature compared to the right.

Range-of-Motion: Ankle dorsiflexion on the left is to the neutral position. The patient does reports that she did have an injury to that leg a few weeks ago, which may be causing some decrease in the range of motion. On the right, ankle dorsiflexion is to 10 degrees. Straight leg raise bilaterally is 90 degrees. Internal and external rotation of the hips is within normal limits bilaterally. Abduction bilaterally is to 30 degrees passively.

Manual Muscle Testing: Strength of the lower extremities, including hip flexion, knee extension, and knee flexion is 2/5; the patient is not able to move her extremity through the full range of motion. Hip flexion on the right is at 1/5; the patient does elicit a muscle contraction but is not able to move the lower extremity against gravity.

Mobility: The patient transfers from her wheelchair to a mat with maximal assistance of her mother. It has been noted in the past that the patient was able to transfer from the wheelchair to the mat; however, she did require maximal assistance on this date. The patient is able to roll from supine to side-lying with minimal assistance. She transitions from a supine to sitting position with maximal assistance. She also transitions from sitting to standing with maximal assistance and with maximal assistance to remain standing.

Balance: The patient's balance was tested in a seated position. In short sitting, the patient is able to resist balance disturbances; however, she has some difficulty when trying to balance without the use of upper extremities for support. The patient particularly struggles with balance if an anterior balance disturbance is given. In long sitting, the patient is able to maintain the long-sit position with use of upper extremities for supports.

ASSESSMENT: The patient presents to physical therapy with decreased balance reactions, some decrease in range of motion of the lower extremities, and decrease in pelvic stabilization musculature, particularly on the left side. I believe this patient would benefit from a physical therapy program to adjust these issues. Goals for this patient include (1) that the patient's passive hip abduction will increase by 5 degrees for increased motion for daily activities; (2) that the patient will be able to maintain balance on a dynamic surface times 10 seconds without the use of upper extremities for increased balance; (3) that the patient's pelvic stability will be increased through activity such as tall kneeling and bridges, which will also help to improve her balance reaction; (4) that the patient will reach for rings while maintaining balance on a dynamic surface successfully on 8/10 trials.

PLAN: We will plan to see this patient two times a week for the summer programming utilization at dynamic surface to help encourage balance reactions. The patient may also be progressed into a home-exercise program for increased strengthening of the pelvic stabilizers. Thank you for this referral.

2-20A:

SERVICE CODE(S): ____________________

DX CODE(S): ____________________

2-20B PHYSICAL THERAPY EVALUATION

Terra presents to the Orthotics Department to be fitted with an ankle-foot orthotic. Report the orthotic fitting only.

LOCATION: Outpatient, Clinic

PATIENT: Terra Benson

REFERRING PHYSICIAN: Ronald Green, M.D.

PHYSICIAN: Mary Barneswell, M.D.

ORTHOTICS TECHNICIAN: Carl Enerson

DIAGNOSIS: Cerebral palsy with inversion tone, left ankle.

Terra was originally seen in our department 4 weeks ago on Tuesday, as per Dr. Barneswell's order for an AFO. At that time, a negative impression of Terra's lower-left leg was obtained for the fabrication of the brace. Terra returned today to get fit in her new AFO and appeared rather relaxed while casting, resulting in a neutral casting position. For optimal results, the brace is fabricated in 2 degrees of dorsiflexion and trimmed in a leaf-spring style posterior to the malleolus to afford a flexible brace. The foot portion of the brace terminates distal to her toes. The patient's leg was securely held in place with one proximal tibial Velcro strap. The patient's presenting footwear worked well in combination with the AFO. Overall fit was excellent.

The family is aware of the signs of skin irritation. Terra's improvement and function will be monitored through Dr. Barneswell. This fitting took 30 minutes. If any questions arise, please feel free to contact us at the Orthotics Department.

2-20B:

SERVICE CODE(S): ____________________

DX CODE(S): ____________________

2-20C PHYSICAL THERAPY EVALUATION

Dr. Green decides that Terra would benefit from a physical therapy program based on the initial assessment performed by Dr. Barneswell. Dr. Barneswell conducts a complete re-evaluation prior to the beginning of Terra's therapy program.

LOCATION: Outpatient, Clinic

PATIENT: Terra Benson

REFERRING PHYSICIAN: Ronald Green, M.D.

PHYSICIAN: Mary Barneswell, M.D.

SUBJECTIVE: Terra was referred for direct physical therapy on a twice-weekly basis to increase lower-extremity range of motion, and strength, and to increase weight-bearing tolerance, and for assisted transfer training. Programming should include therapeutic pool, if available. Terra recently underwent multiple orthopedic procedures at the Manytown Children's Hospital, including femoral derotation osteotomy on the left, bilateral rectus femoris lengthening, phenol injection, two left hip adductor tendons. She returned to see Dr. Almaz last Monday to have a recheck appointment, at which time all restrictions were lifted, including weight-bearing. Referral was written to begin physical therapy programming. Terra was accompanied today by her father, who lifted her from her manual wheelchair to the elevated mat for evaluation.

OBJECTIVE: Observation: Terra arrives seated in her manual wheelchair with her left hip in a position of internal rotation and adduction. Her right hip was in a neutral position. She stated that she has decreased endurance for lower-extremity weight-bearing because her left hip begins to hurt after approximately 10 minutes of standing in her stander.

Lower-Extremity Passive Range of Motion:

JOINT	RIGHT	LEFT
Hip flexion	120 degrees	107 degrees
Hip abduction	25 degrees	16 degrees
Straight leg raising	90 degrees	85 degrees
Excessive dorsiflexion	20>	10 degrees

Lower Extremity Strength:

Muscle Group		
Quadriceps	F–/F+	F–
Hip abductors	P–	P–
Hip flexion	F–	F–
Hamstrings	F–	P+
Hip extensors	P–	P–

Tone in the lower extremities is increased. Mobility: Terra requires maximum assistance for standing pivot transfer from wheelchair to elevated mat. She requires a moderate assist to roll over from supine to prone and minimal assistance to roll from prone to supine. Her main means of mobility is by way of her power wheelchair. Gross Motor Skills: Terra is dependent on her power wheelchair for mobility. Her mom and dad lift her from her wheelchair instead of allowing her to use transfer with moderate to maximum assistance. Terra stands in her stander, but is no longer able to walk. Adaptive Equipment: She uses her power wheelchair at school and has a stander for home use.

ASSESSMENT: Impression: Patient's legs are very deconditioned as a result of her recent surgery and recovery. All restrictions are lifted, and she is ready to take responsibility for her own transfers with assist as needed. Strengths: (1) Interacts well with others in her environment; (2) motivated and cooperative. Problem list: (1) Left hip resting position of internal rotation and adduction; (2) she is not actively involved in her own transfers; (3) leg spasms causing her sitting posture to be asymmetrical; (4) decreased hip abduction on left leg to migrate into windswept position to her right. Goals: (1) To improve sitting balance: Terra will sustain erect sitting posture with upper- and lower-extremity support while seated on the bench or elevated mat; (2) improved lower-extremity passive range of motion: increased left hip flexion to 120 degrees and left hip abduction to 25 degrees; (3) increased lower-extremity strength by a half to a full muscle grade; (4) improved sliding board transfers with standby assistance from wheelchair to elevated mat or bed or standing pivot transfer with minimal to moderate assistance.

PLAN/RECOMMENDATION: (1) Terra is ready to begin a program of direct physical therapy on a twice-weekly basis for 3 to 4 months. A portion of that programming will occur in the therapeutic pool. (2) Plan of treatment for physical therapy program is listed under goals. (3) Patient will be seen in the gym during one 1 session in the week and in the therapeutic pool for the other sessions to maximize her outcome. (4) Terra should place a towel roll between her knees when sitting in her wheelchair (to keep her hips in neutral alignment) to reduce her hip muscle spasms in her adductor muscle on the left. This will also promote body symmetry. (5) Her home exercise program should begin with standing in the stander on a daily basis for 10 to 30 minutes. She tolerated a 1-minute stand today and should increase her tolerance for standing gradually up to 30 minutes. Her home exercise program will be updated as needed. (6) Terra will return to the office for a recheck appointment in 4 months' time.

2-20C:

SERVICE CODE(S): ______________________

DX CODE(S): ______________________

Medical Nutrition Therapy

Medical Nutritional Therapy codes (97802–97804) are used to report medical nutritional therapy assessment or intervention services performed by a person other than a physician. The services are provided either individually or in a group. For example, a patient who the physician believes is not eating appropriately to maintain optimal health is referred to a dietitian for assessment and design of a more balanced eating plan. The dietitian's services are reported in increments of 15 minutes. If the dietitian spent 1 hour in an initial assessment with a patient, the services would be reported 97802 × 4, Medical nutritional therapy, initial assessment and intervention, individual, face-to-face with the patient, each 15 minutes.

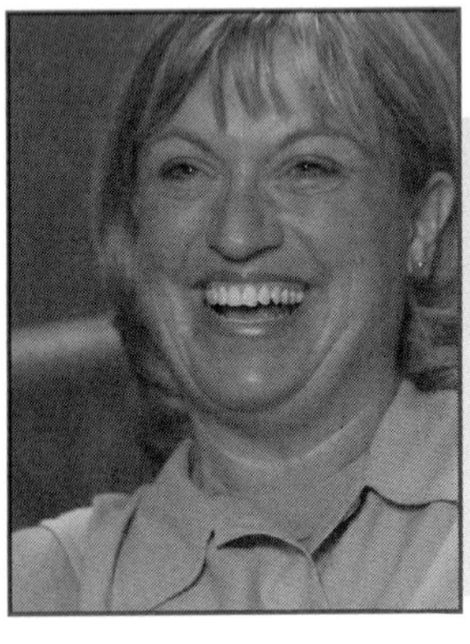

FROM THE TRENCHES

Joan

"Coding is very much a rules-based profession. I take pride in knowing those rules and how to apply [them] ...and being able to look at [coding] creatively, rather than in a very linear, straightforward fashion. I like being able to look at the whole picture and to put the information together in a way that meets the rules, but also provides the opportunity for the physician to get the most reimbursement for the services."

Osteopathic and Chiropractic Manipulative Treatment

A doctor of osteopathy (D.O.) or a doctor of chiropractic (D.C.) is a physician who uses alternative methods of treatment. Osteopathic Manipulative Treatment (OMT) codes (98925–98929) are used to report osteopathic manipulative treatment based on the number of body regions treated. Chiropractic Manipulative Treatment (CMT) codes (98940–98943) are used to report chiropractic manipulative treatment based on the number of spinal regions treated. Included in all these codes is a patient assessment and treatment. An E/M code is reported only if the physician provided a separate and distinct E/M service.

Special Services, Procedures, and Reports

This is the miscellaneous services section of the CPT for medical services. These codes reflect services rendered at unusual hours of the day or on holidays, in unusual locations, for unusual supplies or materials, for preoperative and postoperative visits included in the surgical package (bundled), and for other miscellaneous services. These codes are used throughout the reporting of all medical services, such as 99070 for supplies and materials. There are also codes within this subsection that are not used often, for example, medical testimony, 99075. Take time to review all codes and descriptions within this often-used subsection of the CPT.

HCPCS Level II Modifiers

The Healthcare Procedural Coding System (HCPCS) is used with CPT codes and HCPCS codes. The anatomical modifiers in this system are used to specify side, eyelid, thumb, finger/toe, and coronary artery.

-LT	Left side
-RT	Right side
-E1	Upper-left, eyelid
-E2	Lower-left, eyelid
-E3	Upper-right, eyelid
-E4	Lower-right, eyelid
-FA	Left hand, thumb
-F1	Left hand, second digit
-F2	Left hand, third digit
-F3	Left hand, fourth digit
-F4	Left hand, fifth digit
-F5	Right hand, thumb
-F6	Right hand, second digit
-F7	Right hand, third digit
-F8	Right hand, fourth digit
-F9	Right hand, fifth digit
-TA	Left foot, great toe
-T1	Left foot, second digit
-T2	Left foot, third digit
-T3	Left foot, fourth digit
-T4	Left foot, fifth digit
-T5	Right foot, great toe
-T6	Right foot, second digit
-T7	Right foot, third digit
-T8	Right foot, fourth digit
-T9	Right foot, fifth digit
-LC	Left circumflex, coronary artery
-LD	Left anterior descending coronary artery
-RC	Right coronary artery

Anatomical modifiers are not used with skin procedures, such as removal of skin tags from any area. The exception is with codes that indicate the skin of the feet, hands, fingers, legs, arms, and eyelids. A full list of HCPCS modifiers is located in the HCPCS coding manual.

CASE 2-21
2-21A Office Procedure
2-21B Clinic Progress Note

CASE 2-21

Sally Jones presented to Dr. Warner's office at the clinic for repair of a bilateral ingrown toenail of the great toe, which is a surgical procedure that can be performed in the physician's office using local anesthetic. Use HCPCS modifiers to indicate the digits repaired.

2-21A OFFICE PROCEDURE

LOCATION: Outpatient, Clinic

PATIENT: Sally Jones

PHYSICIAN: Alma Naraquist, M.D.

SURGEON: Samuel Warner, M.D.

PREOPERATIVE DIAGNOSIS: Ingrown lateral borders, great toes, bilateral.

POSTOPERATIVE DIAGNOSIS: Ingrown lateral borders, great toes, bilateral.

SURGICAL PROCEDURE: Nail resection with chemical destruction and nail matrix lateral borders, great toes bilateral.

PROCEDURE: The patient's right and left feet were prepped and draped in the usual aseptic manner. The great toes were then anesthetized with 50/50 mixture of 2% lidocaine plain and 0.5% Marcaine plain with a quantity of 2.5 cc into each great toe. She was first directed to the left great toe, where a mini-tourniquet was placed around the toe for hemostasis. The lateral border was then incised and excised in total. Phenol was then applied for 45 seconds, dry-swabbed, reapplied for 45 seconds, and dry-swabbed again. The area was then flushed with copious amounts of alcohol. The tourniquet was removed, and blood flow returned to normal. Sterile dressing with Neosporin cream was applied. Identical procedure then was performed on the right great toe lateral border. Following completion of both procedures, the dressings were taped in place. Stockinette was applied over the dressings, and surgical shoes were dispensed. The patient was given all verbal and written postoperative instructions. The patient is to use Extra-Strength Tylenol for pain. We will see the patient back in approximately 1 week's time for a checkup.

2-21A:

SERVICE CODE(S): ______________________

DX CODE(S): ______________________

2-21B CLINIC PROGRESS NOTE

This is a patient of Dr. Naraquist's who comes in for a routine postoperative checkup during the postoperative period. A V code would be reported for this follow-up examination, since the originally diagnosed condition of "ingrown toenail" no longer exists. Reference the Index of the ICD-9-CM under the terms "Examination, follow-up, specified surgery NEC." Also, note that other "follow-up examination" codes are specific to pap smear, chemotherapy, radiotherapy, etc.

LOCATION: Outpatient, Clinic

PATIENT: Sally Jones

PHYSICIAN: Alma Naraquist, M.D.

SURGEON: Samuel Warner, M.D.

The patient had phenol procedures performed to the lateral border on each great toe 6 days ago. She is doing well and presents without problems or complications.

EXAMINATION reveals a normal appearance from phenol procedure to the lateral border of each great toe. Mucous and granulation tissue was debrided from those margins.

She is encouraged to continue with soaks and return in 2 weeks for another postoperative check.

2-21B:

SERVICE CODE(S): ______________________

DX CODE(S): ______________________

Glossary

active immunization injection that can either be a toxoid or a vaccine; causes an immune response to protect the patient from later infection by a specific disease.

cardioversion electrical shock to the heart to restore normal rhythm.
cerebrovascular disease (CVD) blockage of arteries to the brain.

duplex scan one method of vascular flow analysis using sound waves and real-time/color-flow Doppler imaging to produce a color picture of the blood flow within the vessels.

hemodialysis mechanical cleansing of the blood; can be temporary or permanent.

infusion administration of medicine over a long time.
intralesional into a lesion.
intramuscular into a muscle.
intraventricular within a ventricle.

passive immunization injection of antibodies into the body to protect the patient from a specific disease; does *not* cause an immune response.
peritoneal cavity the space within the abdominal lining.
pleural cavity the body cavity containing the organs and membranes of the thoracic region.

subarachnoid between the arachnoid and the pia mater.
subcutaneous tissue below the dermis, primarily fat cells that insulate the body.

toxoids bacteria that cause a disease.

vaccine injection of a small dose of a virus into the body to produce an immune response that protects the patient from later infection by a specific disease.

Chapter 3
Radiology

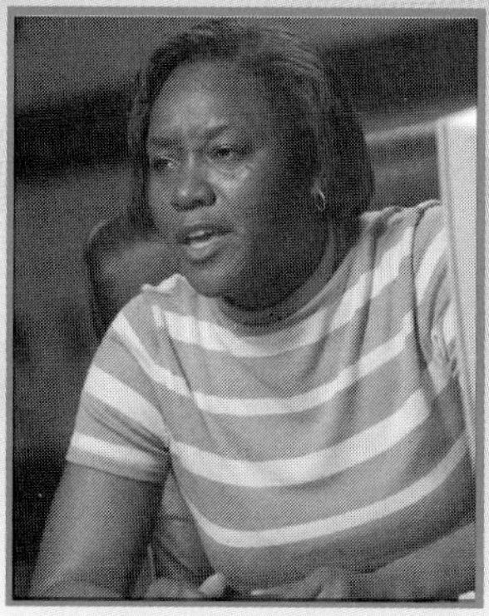

Letitia Patterson, CPC
Illinois College of Optometry
Chicago, Illinois

ABBREVIATIONS

AP	anterior posterior
ARDS	adult respiratory distress syndrome
ASVD	arteriosclerotic vascular disease
BUN	blood urea nitrogen
CABG	coronary artery bypass graft
cc	cubic centimeter
cm	centimeter
CT	computed tomography scan
DTPA	diethylene-triamine penta-acetic acid
DVT	deep vein thrombosis
FUO	fever of unknown origin
IV	intravenous
KUB	kidney, ureter, bladder
MAA	melanoma associated antigen
ml	milliliter
mm	millimeter
NG	nasogastric
PEG	percutaneous endoscopic gastrostomy
PICC	peripherally inserted central catheter
WES	wall echo shadow

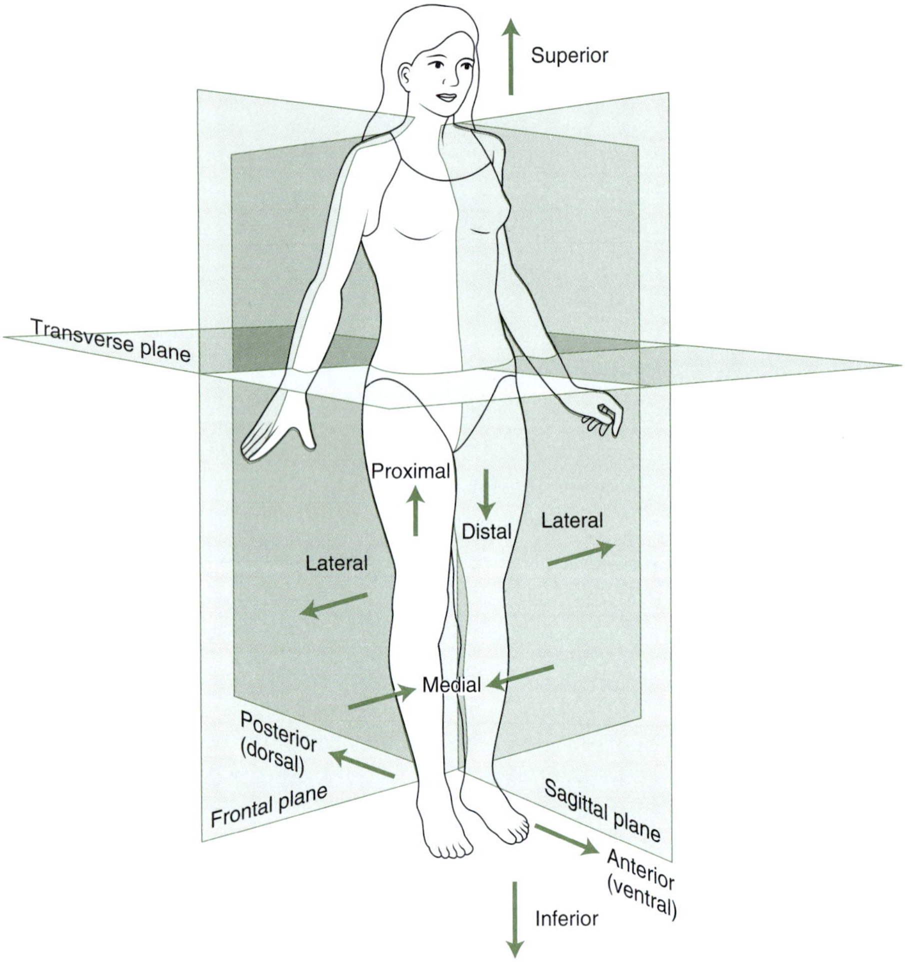

FIGURE 3-1 Planes of the body and terms of location and position of the body.

Radiology is the branch of medicine that uses radiant energy to diagnose and treat patients. The term originally referred to the use of x-rays to produce radiographs but is now commonly applied to all types of medical imaging. A physician who specializes in radiology is a **radiologist.** Radiologists can provide services to patients independent of or in conjunction with another physician of a different specialty. The Radiology section of the CPT manual is divided into the main subsections of Diagnostic Radiology, Diagnostic Ultrasound, Radiation Oncology, and Nuclear Medicine.

Positions and Placement

Terminology referring to planes of the body and positioning of the body is often used in the Radiology section. A **position** is how the patient is placed during the x-ray examination, and a **projection** is the path of the x-ray beam. **Figure 3-1** illustrates the major planes and the surfaces of the body that can be accessed by positioning the body.

Figure 3-2 shows proximal and distal directional body references that mean closest to (proximal) or farthest from (distal) the trunk of the body. These terms are relative,

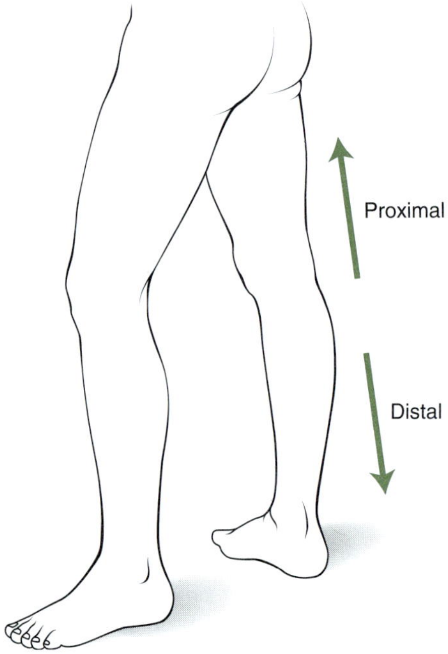

FIGURE 3-2 Proximal and distal.

FIGURE 3-3 Anteroposterior (AP) projection.

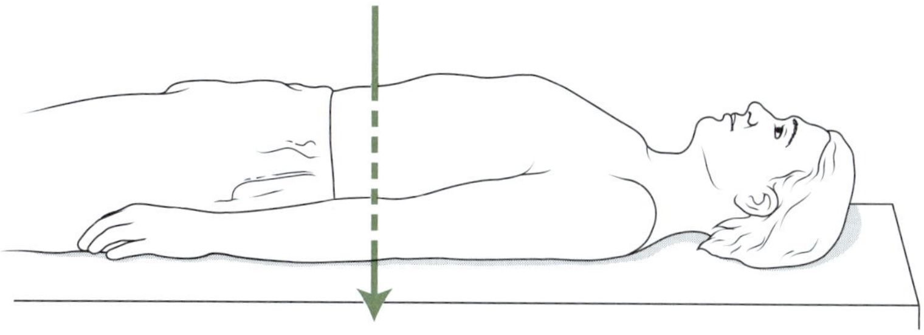

FIGURE 3-4 Posteroanterior (PA) projection.

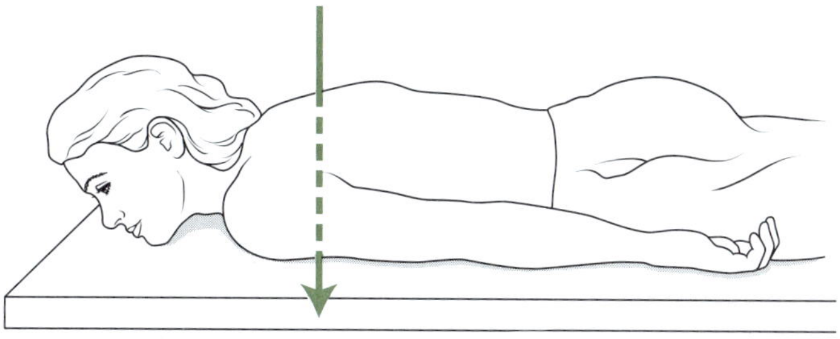

meaning they are used to describe the position of the part as compared with another part. Therefore, the term **proximal** describes a part as being closer to the body trunk than another part, and the term **distal** describes a part as being farther away from the body than another part. The knee would be described as being proximal to the ankle, and it would also be described as being distal to the thigh or hip.

Figure 3-3 illustrates the **anteroposterior** (AP) (front to back) position, in which the patient has his or her front (anterior) closest to the x-ray machine, and the x-ray travels through the patient from the front to the back. In **Figure 3-4**, the **posteroanterior (PA)** position, the patient has his or her back (posterior) located closest to the machine, and the beam travels through the patient from back to front.

Lateral positions are side positions. When the patient's right side is closest to the film, it is called *right lateral.* When the patient's left side is closest to the film, it is called *left lateral.* **Figure 3-5** shows a left lateral position, and **Figure 3-6** shows

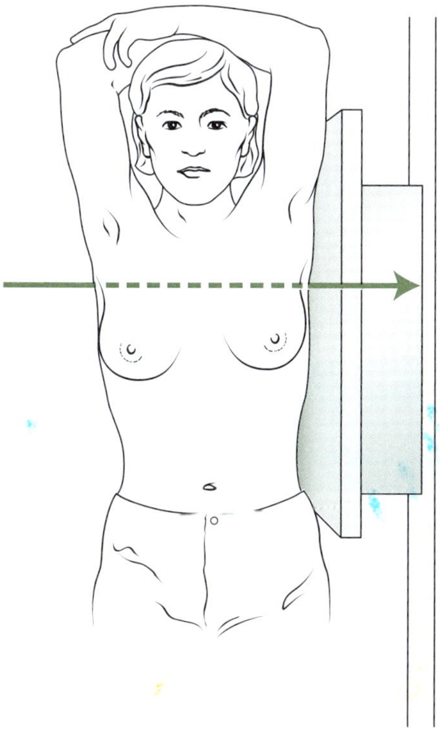

FIGURE 3-5 Left lateral position.

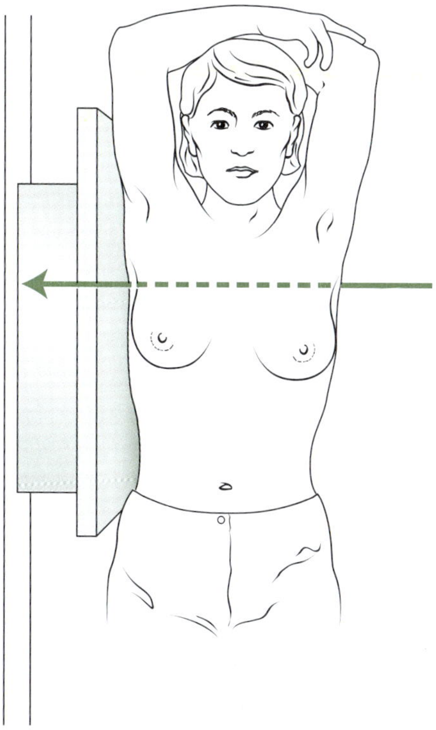

FIGURE 3-6 Right lateral position.

a right lateral position. The use of these various positions allows the physician to view the body from a variety of angles.

Dorsal, more commonly referred to as supine, means lying on the back (sUPine means lying on the back with the face UP); **ventral,** more commonly referred to as prone, means lying on the stomach; and **lateral** means lying on the side.

Decubitus positions are recumbent positions; the x-ray beam is placed horizontally. Ventral decubitus (prone) is the act of lying on the stomach (**Figure 3-7, *A***), and dorsal decubitus (supine) is the act of lying on the back (**Figure 3-7, *B***). The term *decubitus,* generally shortened to "decub," has a special meaning in radiology. The simple act of lying on one's back would be referred to as lying supine, but if a horizontal x-ray beam is used, the position becomes decubitus. The type of decubitus is determined by the body surface on which the patient is lying.

Recumbent means lying down. Thus, *right lateral recumbent* means the patient is lying on the right side (**Figure 3-7, *C***), and *left lateral recumbent* means the patient is lying on the left side (**Figure 3-7, *D***). In the ventral decubitus position, the patient is positioned prone, and the x-ray beam comes into the patient from the right side and exits on the left (**Figure 3-7, *E***).

In the **left lateral decubitus** position, the patient is lying on the left side with the beam coming from the front and passing through to the back (anteroposterior) (**Figure 3-7, *F***).

When the patient is positioned on his or her back (dorsal decubitus) and the x-ray beam comes into the left side of the patient, the positioning is *dorsal decubitus,* but the view obtained is a right lateral (because the right side is closest to the film) (**Figure 3-7, *G***).

Oblique views refer to those obtained while the body is rotated; so it is not in a full anteroposterior or posteroanterior position but is somewhat diagonal. Oblique views are termed according to the body surface on which the patient is lying. The *left anterior oblique* (LAO) position is depicted in **Figure 3-7, *H*,** with the patient's left side rotated forward toward the table. The patient is lying on the left anterior aspect of his or her body. The *right anterior oblique* (RAO) position has the patient on his or her right side rotated forward toward the table, as in **Figure 3-7, *I*.**

Two more oblique views are left posterior oblique and right posterior oblique. In the *left posterior oblique* (LPO) view, the patient is rotated so that the left posterior aspect of his or her body is against the table, as in **Figure 3-7, *J*.** The right posterior oblique (RPO) view has the patient on the right side rotated back, as in **Figure 3-7, *K*.**

Tangential is the patient position that allows the beam to skim the body part, which produces a profile of the structure of the body (**Figure 3-8, *A***). **Figure 3-8, *B*** illustrates the **axial projection,** which is any projection that allows the beam to pass through the body part lengthwise.

Odontoid is a view with the patient's mouth open. **Swimmers** is a position in which the arms are over the head.

Component Coding

Coding radiology services often includes component coding. The following are components:

1. **Professional:** describes the services of the physician, including the supervision of the taking of the x-ray film and the interpretation with report of the x-ray films
2. **Technical:** describes the services of the technologist as well as the cost of the equipment, film, and usual supplies
3. **Global:** describes the combination of the professional and technical components (1 and 2)

When only the professional (physician) component is provided, use modifier -26 after the code to indicate that the physician provided only the professional portion of the service, not the entire service. For example, a radiologist from the local clinic analyzes x-rays taken of a patient at the hospital radiology department. The radiologist prepares a written report of the findings and reports the service with a radiology code with modifier -26 added to indicate that the equipment, film, technical services, and supplies were NOT provided by the physician preparing the report at the time of this service.

Two billing forms are used in the hospital setting: CMS-1500 for professional services provided by professional employees of the hospital and the UB92 used to report facility (hospital) services. At times the hospital will employ a radiologist to provide professional services, such as mammography interpretation. Hospital-based physicians may also staff various departments of the hospital, such as the hospital-based radiology department. These physicians may work exclusively for the hospital or may be employed by both the clinic and hospital at the same time. When reporting the services of the physician portion of the service performed by a hospital-employed physician, you would report the professional service on the CMS-1500 with modifier-26. The technical component of the service is reported on the UB92. When reporting these technical components on the UB92, there is no need for the -TC modifier because the UB92 is used to report only the technical component of the services.

At the clinic, both the professional (physician) and the technical components are reported on the CMS-1500. If only the professional component is reported, modifier-26 is added to the code. If only the technical component is provided, -TC is added to the code. If both the professional and technical components are reported, known as *global services,* the radiology code is reported without a modifier.

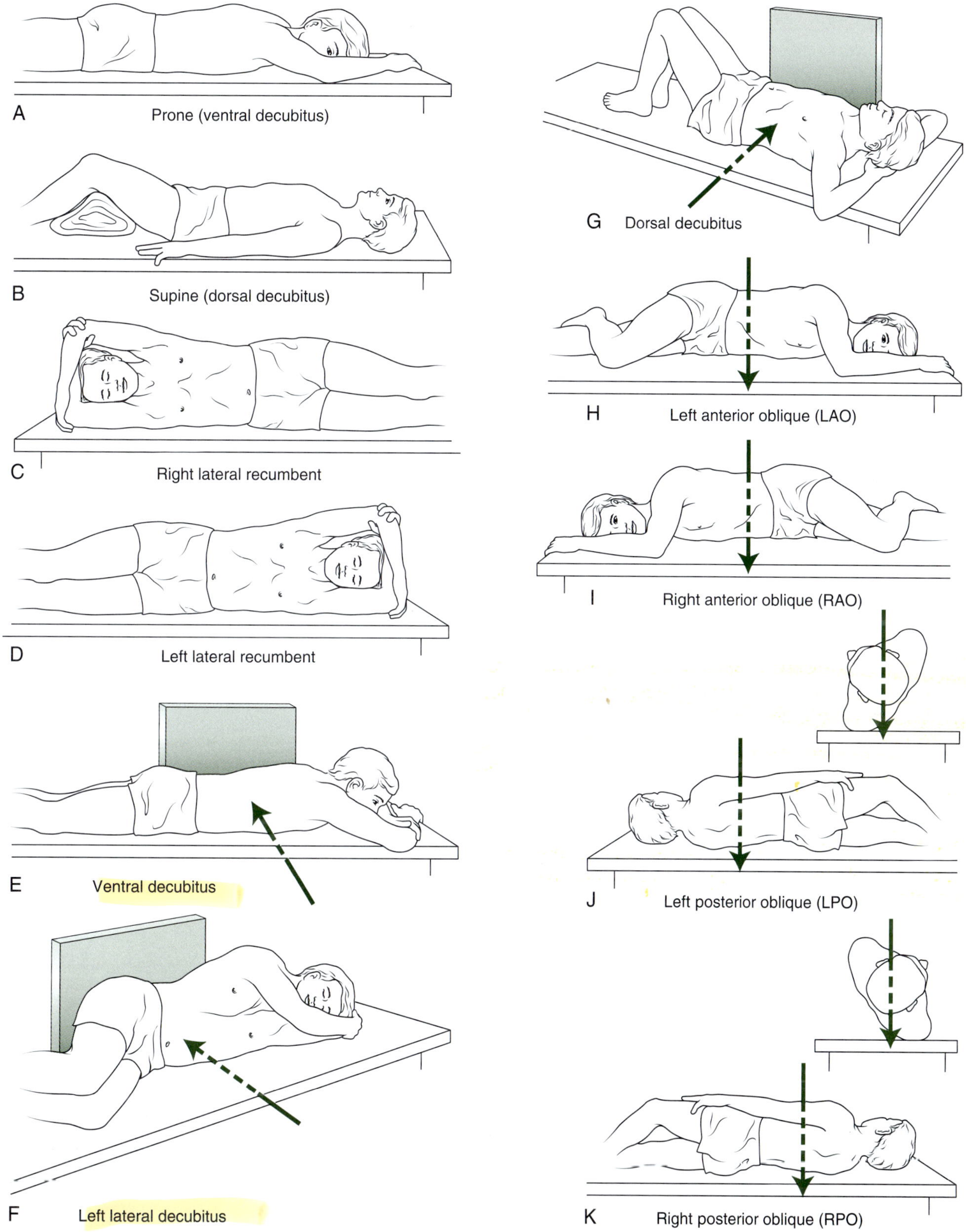

FIGURE 3-7 Radiographic positions. **A,** Prone (ventral decubitus). **B,** Supine (dorsal decubitus). **C,** Right lateral recumbent. **D,** Left lateral recumbent. **E,** Ventral decubitus. **F,** Left lateral decubitus. **G,** Dorsal decubitus. **H,** Left anterior oblique (LAO). **I,** Right anterior oblique (RAO). **J,** Left posterior oblique (LPO). **K,** Right posterior oblique (RPO).

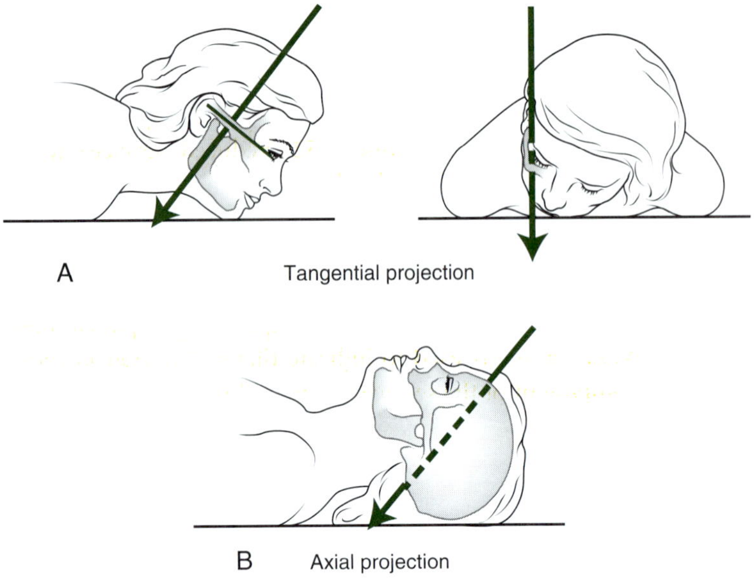

FIGURE 3-8 Radiographic projections. **A,** Tangential projection. **B,** Axial projection.

Contrast

Codes in the Radiology section describe only the radiology procedures, not the injections or placement of other materials necessary to provide the service; therefore, these would be reported in addition to the radiology service. For example, contrast material that is injected during a radiographic procedure is reported separately. The phrase "with contrast" in the CPT manual means contrast that was injected. Report the supply of the injected contrast material with Medicine section code 99070 or HCPCS code, such as A4643, Injection during MRI. If the procedure indicates that contrast was administered orally or rectally, the service is coded as "without contrast" because only intravascular contrast qualifies as "with contrast."

An **intra-articular** injection is one that is within a joint. An **intrathecal** injection is one that is placed through the theca (enclosing sheath) of the spinal cord into the subarachnoid space.

Contrast is typically administered in the following methods:

Does Not Qualify as with Contrast	Qualifies as with Contrast
• Oral: Mouth • Rectal: Rectum	• Intra-arterial: Injected into an artery • Intra-articular: Injected into a joint • Intravenously: Injected into a vein • Intrathecal: Injected into a subarachnoid/subdural space

Many **types** of contrast are often used with the various radiographic procedures. For example:

- Isovue ⇒ Nonionic CT
- Gadolinium ⇒ MRI
- Barium ⇒ Gastrointestinal
- Iodine ⇒ CT/IVP/arthrograms/angiograms

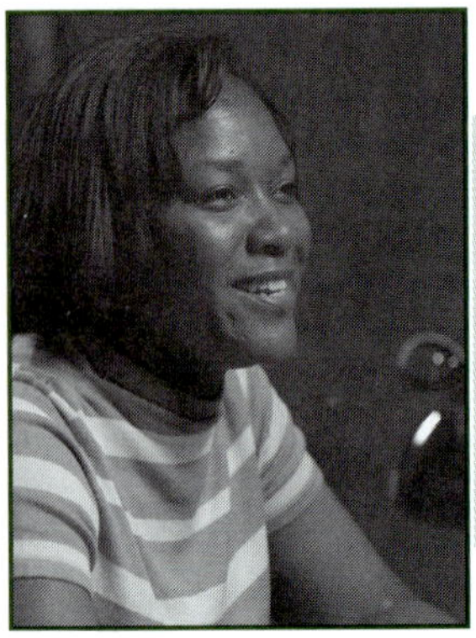

FROM THE TRENCHES

Letitia

"I take pride in learning new things. I take pride in being a resource to those that need the information…people can benefit from the information and knowledge that I have."

Facility Specifics

In the outpatient departments of the hospital, CPT codes for the radiologic examination are established by the facility *Chargemaster,* the computer software program used to process hospital billing. Many facilities have included modifiers programmed within the chargemaster software. The modifiers automatically are placed on the insurance claim form without any intervention by coding staff.

The main difference in ICD-9-CM coding for the hospital facility in the outpatient setting is the use of Volume 3 for the procedure codes. Chapter 16 of Volume 3, Miscellaneous Diagnostic and Therapeutic procedures (87-99), includes many procedures performed in a radiology department. For example, an x-ray of facial bones is assigned procedure code 87.16 from Volume 3.

Many facilities have specific policies designating which procedures performed within the facility will be assigned codes from Chapter 16. Policies vary between the inpatient and outpatient setting within a hospital facility. These policies are usually reviewed annually because of the rapid changes in technology and the more invasive and complicated procedures that are being performed in the radiology department. For the purposes of this text, most of the invasive radiology procedures (entering the body) are performed in the hospital radiology department. Routine procedures, such as x-rays, CTs, and ultrasounds, are usually performed in the clinic outpatient setting.

Diagnostic Radiology

Codes 70010-76999 are often used from the Radiology section. These codes describe diagnostic imaging, **computed axial tomography** (CAT, CT), **magnetic resonance imaging (MRI),** and magnetic resonance angiography (MRA). The codes are divided by x-ray, CAT/CT, MRI, and MRA throughout the subsection. For example, subheading Spine and Pelvis (72010-72295) includes the following:

- Radiographic examination (x-rays) of the spine (72010-72120)
- CT of the spine (72125-72133)
- MRI of the spine (72141-72159)

If fewer than the total number of views specified in the code are taken, modifier -52 (reduced service) would be used to indicate to the third-party payer that less of the procedure was performed than described by the code unless a code already exists for the smaller number of views.

X-ray is a common diagnostic radiology service. The service can be provided on an outpatient or inpatient basis. Modifier -26 is used to indicate that only the professional component of the service was provided.

Hemodialysis Catheter Placement

A hemodialysis catheter is used to access the blood for hemodialysis. The catheter has two joined lines. One line is used to pull blood from the patient's blood system for cleaning, and the other line is used to return the cleaned blood back to the blood system. The catheter can be temporary or permanent. A temporary catheter is placed in the neck, chest, or groin by a nephrologist. This type of catheter can stay in place for about 3 weeks. An x-ray will be taken to ensure that the catheter is in the correct location. Catheters are not ideal for permanent access. They can clog, become infected, or cause narrowing of the vessel into which the access catheter is placed. If the patient needs to start hemodialysis immediately, a catheter will suffice for several weeks while permanent access is developed. Catheters that will be needed for more than about 3 weeks are designed to be tunneled under the skin to increase comfort and reduce complications. A patient who needs dialysis for longer than 3 weeks or so will usually receive a permanent catheter. An x-ray is taken after placement to ensure that the catheter is in the correct location.

CASE 3-1
3-1A Radiology Report, Chest

CASE 3-1

Morris Lancer had a hemodialysis catheter placed. Report Dr. Monson's services for the follow-up x-ray done to ensure correct placement of the catheter. For the purpose of a diagnosis, this is an "Encounter for dialysis catheter fitting and adjustment, extracorporeal." In hemodialysis, blood is removed from the body and circulated through an extracorporeal fluid circuit (outside the body), where it is cleansed of wastes and then returned to the patient.

3-1A RADIOLOGY REPORT, CHEST

LOCATION: Outpatient, Hospital

PATIENT: Morris Lancer

PHYSICIAN: Ronald Green, M.D.

RADIOLOGIST: Morton Monson, M.D.

EXAMINATION OF: Portable chest x-ray

CLINICAL SYMPTOMS: Follow-up placement of hemo-catheter

PORTABLE 15-DEGREE UPRIGHT AP CHEST X-RAY, 5:00 A.M.: An endotracheal tube ending is located well above the carina. An NG tube is present, the tip of which is not seen in our field of view but goes below level of the left hemidiaphragm. A central line from left subclavian ends in the right atrial contour. Cardiomegaly is noted. Confluent change is seen in all lung fields, sparing only the left apex. The finding has increased compared with 1 week previously, suggesting it is fluid-overloaded failure pattern rather than pneumonia. Some atelectatic change is still seen at the right base. Partial collapse of left lung base is still present. These are stable findings. Effusions would not be seen on a 15-degree upright chest x-ray. No bony lesion of significance is seen.

IMPRESSION:
1. Support lines as mentioned.
2. Cardiomegaly with failure pattern. Failure pattern increasing since yesterday morning's x-ray.

Partial collapsed right lower lobe and left lower lobe. Those are stable findings.

3-1A:

SERVICE CODE(S): ______________________

DX CODE(S): ______________________

Types of Catheters

Many types of catheters are available, such as central venous catheters (for administration of fluids or medications), feeding tubes, or cardiac catheters (to obtain blood samples, intracardiac pressures, and for diagnostic purposes). Reference a medical dictionary under the term *catheter* to see all the various types of catheters. It is a common practice for an imaging service to be provided before and/or after a catheter placement.

CASE 3-2
3-2 A Radiology Report, Line Placement

CASE 3-2

In the following case, Dr. Sanchez, general surgeon, placed a catheter and has requested Dr. Monson to interpret the x-ray of the patient's chest to ensure that the catheter is correctly placed.

3-2A RADIOLOGY REPORT, LINE PLACEMENT

LOCATION: Outpatient, Hospital

PATIENT: George Barr

PHYSICIAN: Gary Sanchez, M.D.

RADIOLOGIST: Morton Monson, M.D.

EXAMINATION OF: Chest

CLINICAL SYMPTOMS: Congestive heart failure

CHEST, SINGLE VIEW: FINDINGS: No previous examination is available for comparison. A right internal jugular central venous catheter is present. The distal tip of the catheter overlies the expected location of the superior vena cava. The heart size appears at the upper limits of normal. The pulmonary vasculature markings also appear at the upper limits of normal. Abnormal focal density is present within the retrocardiac region of the left lung base. Increased markings are present in the right infrahilar region as well. These densities could be related to either atelectasis or infiltrate. Blunting of the left costophrenic angle is consistent with a left-sided pleural effusion. Definite pneumothorax is not identified on this examination.

IMPRESSION:

1. Status post placement of right internal jugular central venous catheter as described above.
2. The heart size and pulmonary vasculature markings appear at the upper limits of normal.
3. Focal density is present within both lung bases, which could be related to either atelectasis or infiltrate. Documentation of radiographic clearing is recommended to exclude underlying lesions.
4. Small left-sided pleural effusion.

3-2A:

SERVICE CODE(S): ______________________

DX CODE(S): ______________________

Nasogastric Tube

A nasogastric tube is placed through the nose and into the stomach. The tube is used to deliver nutrition to the patient. To ensure proper placement, an x-ray is taken after placement.

CASE 3-3
3-3A Radiology Report, Abdomen

CASE 3-3

Report Dr. Monson's professional service for an abdominal x-ray to check the placement of a nasogastric feeding tube. For the diagnoses for this patient, assign a V code for the encounter for adjustment of a nonvascular catheter, followed by the presenting symptom of abdominal pain.

3-3A RADIOLOGY REPORT, ABDOMEN

LOCATION: Outpatient, Hospital (Observation Care)

PATIENT: Jody Cornwallace

PHYSICIAN: Ronald Green, M.D.

RADIOLOGIST: Morton Monson, M.D.

EXAMINATION OF: Abdomen

CLINICAL SYMPTOMS: Cor-Flo placement due to abdominal pain.

SINGLE VIEW OF ABDOMEN: (-76 Comparison is made with the previous study of 11:00 A.M. this day.)

The nasogastric feeding tube is again identified. Its distal aspect lies at what appears to be the gastric antrum or possibly the first portion of the duodenum. This should be adequate for feeding the 3:00 P.M. study. The remainder of the abdomen is relatively unchanged.

CONCLUSION:

1. Interim repositioning of nasogastric feeding tube. Its distal aspect now lies at the gastric antrum or first portion of the duodenum. This should be adequate position for feeding.
2. The gastrointestinal air pattern is otherwise nonspecific.

3-3A:

SERVICE CODE(S): ____________________

DX CODE(S): ____________________

The following cases will provide you an opportunity to code a variety of routine x-ray services.

CASE 3-4
3-4A Radiology Report, Chest

CASE 3-4

Report Dr. Monson's professional service.

3-4A RADIOLOGY REPORT, CHEST

LOCATION: Outpatient, Hospital

PATIENT: Lorenz Miller

PHYSICIAN: Ronald Green, M.D.

RADIOLOGIST: Morton Monson, M.D.

EXAMINATION OF: Chest

CLINICAL SYMPTOMS: Primary, malignant neoplasm of the hilus of the lung

TWO-VIEW CHEST: Frontal and lateral views obtained of the chest. These are submitted on September 3 for interpretation. Comparison is made with a portable view of the chest, July 27. Blunting of the left posterior costophrenic sulcus suggests small pleural effusion on the left. Abnormal opacity, right perihilar/suprahilar region, is best seen on the frontal view. The patient has a history of lung cancer. Opacity was noted there previously. Previously noted bibasilar opacities appear essentially resolved. Oral contrast is noted within the abdomen.

IMPRESSION: Persistent opacity, right perihilar/suprahilar region, presumably reflecting the patient's clinical history of lung cancer. This was noted previously. Suspect small pleural effusion on the left. Basilar regions otherwise appear cleared since the prior study.

3-4A:

SERVICE CODE(S): ______________________

DX CODE(S): ______________________

CASE 3-5
3-5A Radiology Report, Femur

CASE 3-5

Code the professional component of the service. Use a HCPCS modifier to indicate the side of the body x-rayed.

3-5A RADIOLOGY REPORT, FEMUR

LOCATION: Outpatient, Hospital

PATIENT: Simon Fields

PHYSICIAN: Leslie Alanda, M.D.

RADIOLOGIST: Morton Monson, M.D.

CLINICAL SYMTPOMS: Leg pain

EXAMINATION OF: Left femur

TWO VIEWS, Left Femur: This examination is compared with an AP view of the femur dated 3 months previously from a skeletal survey. Again seen is a mixed sclerotic and lytic lesion within the distal diaphysis of the left femur. This is not significantly changed since the previous examination dated 3 months previously. This is seen to involve the posterior aspect of the left femur. Finding is highly suspicious for the presence of metastatic disease. Vascular calcifications and surgical clips are noted to be present.

IMPRESSION: Mixed lytic and sclerotic lesion involving the distal left femur. This is highly suspicious for the presence of metastatic disease.

3-5A:

SERVICE CODE(S): ____________________

DX CODE(S): ____________________

CASE 3-6

Report the global service for this x-ray that was performed at the clinic where Dr. Monson supervised the technician and then interpreted the results and wrote a report of the findings. When reporting an ICD-9-CM code for a fracture, unless the skin is broken, code the fracture as "closed." If the documentation does not indicate whether the fracture is closed or open, report closed fracture. Distal means lower or farthest from the point of origin, and proximal means higher or nearest to the point of origin.

3-6A RADIOLOGY REPORT, KNEE

LOCATION: Outpatient, Clinic

PATIENT: Jason Glassheim

PHYSICIAN: Leslie Alanda, M.D.

RADIOLOGIST: Morton Monson, M.D.

EXAMINATION OF: Two views, left knee

CLINICAL SYMPTOMS: Fracture of the distal femur

TWO VIEWS, LEFT KNEE: A comminuted fracture involves the distal femur. This is incompletely demonstrated on this study. Medial angulation of the distal femoral shaft fragment appears to be present. Multiple fracture fragments are present over the fracture site. There is also mild anterior angulation of the distal femoral shaft and overriding at the fracture site with the proximal portion of the shaft anteriorly displaced by approximately 1/4 to 1/3 shaft width.

IMPRESSION: Comminuted fracture, distal femur, incompletely demonstrated on these films.

3-6A:

SERVICE CODE(S): ______________________

DX CODE(S): ______________________

CASE 3-7
3-7A Radiology Report, Shoulder

CASE 3-7

Report Dr. Monson's professional service for an x-ray of the right shoulder.

3-7A RADIOLOGY REPORT, SHOULDER

LOCATION: Outpatient, Hospital

PATIENT: Nelda Cavazos

PHYSICIAN: Mohomad Almaz, M.D.

RADIOLOGIST: Morton Monson, M.D.

EXAMINATION OF: Right shoulder

CLINICAL SYMPTOMS: Right shoulder pain

These films are from 15 days previously just now submitted for interpretation having been with the orthopedist in the interval.

RIGHT SHOULDER: Two sets of films from 15 days previously done at 11:20 A.M. and another set done at 1:00 P.M. The three views are from 11:20 A.M. and three from 1:00 P.M. on the same day. Again, there is no change from 15 days prior. No fracturing is identified. Degenerative change is as described before.

IMPRESSION:

1. Degenerative change without fracture or dislocation.
2. Films are just now submitted for interpretation.

3-7A:

SERVICE CODE(S): ______________________

DX CODE(S): ______________________

CASE 3-8

This patient underwent an outpatient surgical procedure for placement of a feeding tube for dysphagia resulting from a cerebrovascular accident 3 weeks ago. Report the professional component of the x-ray. For the diagnosis, report only the primary purpose for this encounter with a V code, which in this case is adjustment of a nasogastric tube (non-vascular catheter).

3-8A KUB

LOCATION: Outpatient, Hospital

PATIENT: Sally Ozark

PHYSICIAN: Ronald Green, M.D.

RADIOLOGIST: Edward Riddle, M.D.

EXAMINATION OF: KUB, abdominal view

CLINICAL SYMPTOMS: Check Cor-Flo feeding tube placement

KUB, ONE FILM DONE PORTABLE SUPINE, 12:15 P.M. No prior film. There is degenerative change in bony structures. Bowel gas pattern is nonspecific. Mainly we see stomach and colon gas. No distended bowel loops. Feeding tube extends from esophagus down into stomach and ends in the anticipated location of the second portion of the C-loop. That position could be used as a feeding tube. No organomegaly or significant calcification is seen on field of view.

IMPRESSION: This was done to check feeding tube placement. It appears to end or have its tip in the anticipated location of the second portion of the C-loop.

3-8A:

SERVICE CODE(S): ______________________

DX CODE(S): ______________________

Cine-Pharyngoesophagram

Cine-pharyngoesophagram, also called *cineradiography* or a *video swallow*, is a serial (moving picture) x-ray of the digestive tract. It allows dynamic (with motion) visualization of the swallowing function as well as strictures and other abnormalities.

CASE 3-9
3-9A Video Swallow

CASE 3-9

Dr. Monson is a clinic physician who reviews a video swallow (swallowing evaluation) that was done at the local hospital outpatient department for a patient of Dr. Naraquist. Report Dr. Monson's service.

3-9A VIDEO SWALLOW

LOCATION: Outpatient, Hospital

PATIENT: Loren Zann

PHYSICIAN: Alma Naraquist, M.D.

RADIOLOGIST: Morton Monson, M.D.

EXAMINATION OF: Pharynx

CLINICAL SYMPTOMS: Dysphagia

VIDEO SWALLOW: FINDINGS: The patient's swallowing mechanism was examined using various liquid and solid barium consistencies. The patient demonstrated trace penetration on a single swallow with the nectar consistency barium by cup and also with the thin barium consistency by cup without and with chin tuck. No aspiration. Pooling of the liquid barium consistencies within the valleculae and piriform sinuses is seen.

3-9A:

SERVICE CODE(S): ______________________

DX CODE(S): ______________________

CAT/CT Scans

Computed axial tomography (CAT or CT) is a procedure by which selected planes of tissue are pinpointed through computer enhancement. The CAT is produced by means of a circular machine that takes pictures of the patient from many different angles. If needed, a three-dimensional image can be produced. The scan can be with or without contrast (remember that oral or rectal contrasts do not count as contrast). The scan can also be without and with contrast, which means that the scan would be conducted first without contrast and then repeated again with contrast. The codes are usually divided based on the statement of with or without contrast and then the extent of the study. The scan is located in the index of the CPT manual under the term "CT Scan" and further subdivided by "Without and with Contrast," "Without Contrast," and "With Contrast." Locate "CT Scan" in the index of the CPT manual, and note that these three divisions list the same or similar subterms, such as "Abdomen" in each division. The "Without and with Contrast" is when the CT scan is done without contrast first and then repeated with contrast. The "Without Contrast" is the use of no intravenous contrast. The "With Contrast" is with the use of injected contrast.

A technician, under the supervision of a radiologist, performs the scan, and the radiologist interprets the results and writes a report. No -TC is needed if the technical component is provided at the hospital because, as stated earlier, the UB92 does not require the use of the technical modifier. If the radiologist performs only the professional component of the service, modifier -26 is added to the code.

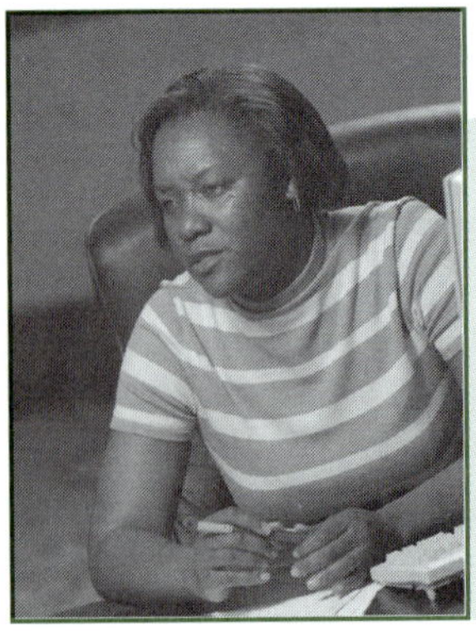

FROM THE TRENCHES

Letitia

"At our faculty meetings, we actually talk about coding. We talk about how it relates to the practice. [The physicians] want to know the steps to documentation, the steps to E/M, and what we have to do in order to code properly...It is an eye-opener for them and an eye-opener for me...I'm learning, they're learning. They take my position very seriously, and I think that is very important."

CASE 3-10
3-10A CT Scan, Brain

CASE 3-10

Report the radiologist's service for the following CT. For the diagnosis, report the presenting symptom as indicated "alteration of mental status" because there are so many questionable diagnoses in this report, that when all of these diagnoses are disregarded, the only diagnosis remaining is "alteration of mental status."

3-10A CT SCAN, BRAIN

LOCATION: Outpatient, Hospital

PATIENT: John Doe

PHYSICIAN: Ronald Green, M.D.

RADIOLOGIST: Morton Monson, M.D.

EXAMINATION OF: Brain CT

CLINICAL SYMPTOMS: Alteration of mental status

COMPUTED TOMOGRAPHIC EXAMINATION OF THE BRAIN was performed without contrast material. The study was performed in my absence and is presented for evaluation. There is movement in multiple images.

In image 11, there is questionable low density involving the superior surface of the left frontal lobe. Most probably, this is not real. Adjacent images do not show this low density; however, if the patient moved between images, there certainly would be misregistration.

I do believe there may be abnormal low density involving the base of the right frontal lobe. I believe this may represent encephalomalacia, most probably from an old injury of the right frontal lobe. There is a questionable very small amount of similar low density within the left frontal lobe on image 11.

There are patchy areas of low density within the white matter of both hemispheres. These are symmetric. Most probably, they represent areas of gliosis of indeterminate etiology.

Bilaterally, several small areas of decreased density of the subcortical white matter of the insular regions are present that might be representative of previous ischemic change. I do not believe this is acute.

There is no hemorrhage. No mass. No indication of raised intracranial pressure.

IMPRESSION: Possible encephalomalacia at the base of the right frontal lobe, most probably from an old injury. Questionable encephalomalacia changes of left frontal lobe. Questionable low density (most probably not real) of the superior margin of the left temporal lobe. If this were real, it might be recent ischemic change. Possible small lacunar-type infarctions of the brain parenchyma are subjacent to each insular region. No hemorrhage.

3-10A:

SERVICE CODE(S): ____________________

DXCODE(S): ____________________

Reconstruction

A CT scan is a small slice (cross sectional view) of a layer of the body. A **reconstruction** is when several of these cross-sectional views are put together (reconstructed) into a three-dimensional image. Reconstruction can be done with CT scans, **MRIs,** or other **tomography** (body-section radiography). The reconstruction service is reported in addition to the radiographic procedure (CT, MRI, or other tomography). The reconstruction service is located in the CPT manual under the procedure (CT, MRI, etc.) and then "Other Planes."

A *neuroradiologist* is a radiologist who specializes in radiographic procedures of the nervous system. Dr. Phillip Hart is a neuroradiologist employed by the hospital and is the head of the Radiology Department at the hospital. When radiographic service was provided in the hospital setting, thereby using the radiology equipment provided by the hospital, both the professional and technical portions of the radiology service were provided to the patient. The professional component is reported on the CMS-1500 with modifier -26, and the technical portion of the service is reported on the UB92 with no modifier because modifiers are not used on the UB92. You will be reporting services for Dr. Hart in the next three cases.

Congestive Heart Failure

Congestive heart failure (428) is a condition in which the heart is unable to generate adequate output. When the heart has lost its ability to pump effectively, blood may back up into other organs, such as the liver or lungs. When the organs do not get a sufficient blood supply, the oxygen level is decreased and the organ can be damaged and lose the ability to function properly.

Hypoxemia

Hypoxemia, also known as anoxia, is a deficiency in the level of oxygen in the arterial blood.

CASE 3-11
3-11A CT Scan, Sinuses

CASE 3-11

Report Dr. Hart's service.

3-11A CT SCAN, SINUSES

LOCATION: Inpatient, Hospital

PATIENT: Cheryl West

PHYSICIAN: Ronald Green, M.D.

RADIOLOGIST: Phillip Hart, M.D.

CLINICAL SYMPTOMS: Intubated due to congestive heart failure, hypoxemia.

COMPUTED TOMOGRAPHIC EXAMINATION OF THE PARANASAL SINUSES was performed using thin, overlapping images in the axial plane. The patient's condition did not allow direct coronal images. Coronal reconstructions (3D) were performed from the original data set and required an independent workstation.

Frontal, ethmoid, and sphenoid sinuses are virtually all filled with abnormal soft-tissue density. There is no bone erosion. The septations of the ethmoid complexes remain intact. Nasal cavity shows decreased aeration bilaterally.

Both maxillary sinuses show a considerable amount of abnormal soft-tissue density, but there is some aeration. There certainly could be fluid levels.

There is nasal intubation on the right.

IMPRESSION: Abnormal density almost filling all of the paranasal sinuses, as described above, without bone erosion. Certainly, this might be due to inflammation/infection; however, it is certainly not unusual for fluid to collect within paranasal sinuses when patients are intubated. The findings do need close clinical correlation.

3-11A:

SERVICE CODE(S): ______________________

DX CODE(S): ______________________

CASE 3-12
3-12A CT Scan, Sinuses

CASE 3-12

Report Dr. Hart's service. Remember to also assign a V code to report the "status, ventilator."

3-12A CT SCAN, SINUSES

LOCATION: Outpatient, Hospital

PATIENT: Lonny Barker

PHYSICIAN: Ronald Green, M.D.

RADIOLOGIST: Phillip Hart, M.D.

EXAMINATION OF: CT of sinuses

CLINICAL SYMPTOMS: FUO

COMPUTED TOMOGRAPHIC EXAMINATION OF THE PARANASAL SINUSES was performed with intravenous contrast in the axial plane, computed for high-resolution bone algorithm. The patient is on a ventilator. Direct coronal images could not be obtained.

The left maxillary sinus is almost completely filled with abnormal soft-tissue density. The right maxillary sinus also shows a considerable amount of abnormal soft-tissue density, and there is a bubble appearance. I believe there is fluid within both sinuses.

Most of the ethmoid sinuses are filled with abnormal soft-tissue density. Septations of the ethmoid complexes are intact. Right sphenoid sinus shows some aeration. There are also mural nodulations of soft tissue within the left sphenoid sinus, but there might be a fluid level.

Both frontal sinuses are well aerated, but there is a rim of mucosal thickening of each frontal sinus, and there may be fluid within the left frontal sinus inferiority.

IMPRESSION: All the paranasal sinuses show abnormalities as described above. Many of the air cells are filled with abnormal soft-tissue density. There is indication of fluid within at least the maxillary sinuses and perhaps the left sphenoid sinus. The findings can be consistent with a sinusitis condition; however, the patient is also on a ventilator. Patients with endotracheal intubation can have fluid in the sinuses without having a sinusitis condition.

3-12A:

SERVICE CODE(S): ____________________

DX CODE(S): ____________________

CASE 3-13
3-13A CT Scan, Chest

CASE 3-13

Amyloidosis is a group of conditions in which a protein (amyloid) collects in the tissues and organs of the body to the point where the function is compromised. The following CT scan is of the chest of a patient with clinical symptoms of amyloidosis, and the scan is being done to determine the extent of the disease. The elevated creatinine level, bilateral pleural effusions, adenopathy, degenerative osseous structures, and the lung opacity are all a part of the amyloidosis and therefore not reported separately.

3-13A CT SCAN, CHEST

LOCATION: Outpatient, Hospital

PATIENT: Jane Gallo

PHYSICIAN: Ronald Green, M.D.

RADIOLOGIST: Phillip Hart, M.D.

EXAMINATION OF: CT scan of the chest

CLINICAL SYMPTOMS: Amyloidosis

CT SCAN OF THE CHEST: Technique: Multiple computed axial tomograms were obtained from the thoracic inlet to ischial tuberosities following the administration of oral but not IV contrast. IV contrast was withheld secondary to the patient's elevated creatinine status. Small bilateral pleural effusions/pleural thickening are seen, the left greater than the right. There is linear opacity in the right apex consistent with subsegmental volume loss or scarring. There is a very small area of nonspecific opacity in the posteromedial left lung base, which may be related to scarring, but it could also represent a small focal area of infiltrate or even volume averaging with the adjacent vessel. A short-term 3-month follow-up is suggested to document stability. The osseous structures demonstrate degenerative change. Evaluation for adenopathy is limited by a lack of IV contrast. Atherosclerotic change involves the aorta and its branches, including the coronary arteries. Small nonspecific pretracheal lymph nodes are present, none of which appear enlarged by CT criteria.

IMPRESSION:
1. Bilateral pleural effusions, left greater than right.
2. Study limited for evaluation of adenopathy due to lack of IV contrast.
3. Very tiny patchy, nonspecific opacity, left medial lung base. Short-term follow-up in 3 months is suggested.
4. Minimal linear opacity, right apex, is consistent with subsegmental volume loss or scarring.

3-13A :

SERVICE CODE(S): ______________________________

DX CODE(S): ______________________________

In the previous three cases, the billing from the hospital would include charges for both the professional services (Dr. Hart) and the CT examination, unlike when an examination is done at the hospital and the radiologist is employed by the clinic. In that case, a billing would be sent from the hospital for the exam and from the clinic for the professional services.

Now, back to reporting Dr. Monson's services.

CASE 3-14
3-14A CT Scan, Abdomen and Pelvis

CASE 3-14

The patient in this case also has amyloidosis. Dr. Monson, the clinic physician, provides the professional service for the CT that was performed at the hospital outpatient department.

3-14A CT SCAN, ABDOMEN AND PELVIS

LOCATION: Outpatient, Hospital

PATIENT: Les Carlisle

PHYSICIAN: Ronald Green, M.D.

RADIOLOGIST: Morton Monson, M.D.

EXAMINATION OF: CT scan of abdomen and pelvis

CLINICAL SYMPTOMS: Amyloidosis

CT SCAN OF THE ABDOMEN AND PELVIS:

FINDINGS: Evaluation of visceral organs and adenopathy is limited by lack of IV contrast. The liver, spleen, adrenals, and kidneys have a normal noncontrasted CT appearance. Opacified portions of the bowel have a normal CT appearance. The pancreas demonstrates calcifications within the body and tail as well as a larger calcification seen in the region of the head of the pancreas. Clinical correlation regarding possible previous pancreatitis is suggested. On this study, there is also questionable prominence of the head of the pancreas, but it is immediately adjacent to the duodenum and difficult to separate without IV contrast. Ultrasound may be helpful for evaluation of the pancreas, although the pancreas is not always well visualized with ultrasound. Vascular calcifications are seen in the aorta and its branches. Degenerative change is seen in the spine. The noncontrasted bladder has a normal CT appearance.

IMPRESSION:

1. Calcifications within the pancreas. Clinical correlation regarding possibility of prior pancreatitis is suggested.
2. Questionable prominence to the head of the pancreas is immediately adjacent to the bowel, and it is uncertain whether this represents volume averaging within the bowel. Please see above comments regarding ultrasound.
3. Atherosclerotic change involves the aorta and its branches.

3-14A:

SERVICE CODE(S): ____________________

DX CODE(S): ____________________

CASE 3-15
3-15A CT Scan, Chest

CASE 3-15

Report Dr. Monson's service. The patient is status post mastectomy, which should be reported with a V code. Reference the Index of the ICD-9-CM under "Absence of breast, acquired" for the Tabular location of the code.

3-15A CT SCAN, CHEST

LOCATION: Outpatient, Hospital

PATIENT: Christina Saenz

PHYSICIAN: Gregory Dawson, M.D.

RADIOLOGIST: Morton Monson, M.D.

EXAMINATION OF: Chest CT

CLINICAL SYMPTOMS: Shortness of breath

TECHNIQUE: The patient was scanned from the apices of the lungs through the adrenals following administration of intravenous contrast.

FINDINGS: This examination is compared with a prior chest CT dated July 11. The patient is status post left mastectomy. Postsurgical changes are similar in appearance to the prior examination. Definite axillary adenopathy is not seen on this examination. Definite mediastinal adenopathy is not seen. No hilar adenopathy is identified. There are bilateral pleural effusions present on this examination. The right is larger than the left. The right effusion is larger than what was seen previously, and the left effusion is new. The liver appears heterogeneous, which presumably relates to the phase of enhancement at which it was scanned. Multiple hypodensities are associated with the liver. These were evaluated on a recent abdomen CT with follow-up suggested on that CT. Please refer to that report. The adrenal glands demonstrate the presence of scattered fibrotic change. Also, hazy opacity is present within the right lower lung zone. This may relate to atelectasis or infiltrate. I would recommend progress studies to document clearing of the opacities as well as the pleural effusions to exclude underlying lesions.

IMPRESSION:
1. Postsurgical changes of the left hemithorax.
2. Bilateral pleural effusions, worsened since the prior examination.
3. Hazy opacity seen within the right lower lung zone, which may relate to atelectasis or infiltrate.
4. Additional scattered fibrotic change noted within the lungs.

3-15A:

SERVICE CODE(S): ____________________

DX CODE(S): ____________________

CASE 3-16
3-16A CT Scan, Chest, Abdomen, and Pelvis

CASE 3-16

Report Dr. Monson's service.

ascites – cause of increasing girth

3-16A CT SCAN, CHEST, ABDOMEN, AND PELVIS

LOCATION: Outpatient, Hospital

PATIENT: Thelma Olson

PHYSICIAN: Gregory Dawson, M.D.

RADIOLOGIST: Morton Monson, M.D.

EXAMINATION OF: CT of chest, abdomen, and pelvis

CLINICAL SYMPTOMS: Right lower-lobe mass, abdominal aortic aneurysm, increasing girth, and fatigue.

CT OF CHEST, ABDOMEN, AND PELVIS: Technique: CT of the chest, abdomen, and pelvis was performed with oral and IV contrast material with delayed images through the kidneys. No previous CTs for comparison.

FINDINGS: Chest: Moderate-sized right pleural effusion with associated compressive atelectasis. Patchy, somewhat rounded infiltrate in the right mid and lower lung, which is nonspecific and could represent a neoplastic or infectious process. There is a 6.8-cm bleb or bulla in the right lower lobe. Emphysematous changes in both lungs. No mediastinal, hilar, or axillary adenopathy. Coronary artery calcification. No left pleural effusion. No focal adrenal masses. Atheromatous changes in the thoracic aorta. Slight fibrosis or linear atelectasis left lower lobe. Bullous formation in the posterior aspect of the right upper lobe.

ABDOMEN AND PELVIS: Moderate amount of ascites in the abdomen and pelvis, most marked in the right paracolic gutter. Normal-appearing small bowel and large bowel. No focal hepatic lesions. No focal adrenal masses. There is a prominent retrocrural node (images 40 and 41), which measures upper limits of normal. No abdominal or pelvic adenopathy. No free air. Tiny low-density lesion in the midportion of the left kidney is too small to characterize. Infrarenal abdominal aortic aneurysm, which measures 3.5 cm in maximum AP diameter and extends for a length of 3 to 4 cm and does not include the aortic bifurcation. Atheromatous changes in the abdominal aorta. No bony destructive lesions.

3-16A:

SERVICE CODE(S): ____________________

DX CODE(S): ____________________

CASE 3-16 DISCUSSION

This report is an excellent example of connecting the diagnoses to the service/procedure codes. A CT scan of the chest (thorax) was performed because of the right lower-lobe mass; the CT of the abdomen was done to assess the abdominal aortic aneurysm, and the pelvic scan was done to assess the bowels and kidneys. Since these services were provided and are now going to be reported, diagnoses to support the submission of each service must be provided.

The Findings section of the report indicates the following (Words from the report are underlined; comments follow in *italic* typeface.):

Pleural effusion, which is the presence of fluid in pleural space that can cause atelectasis *(incomplete expansion of the lung). Infiltrate into the right lung has occurred, but the physician indicates that this could be caused by a neoplastic (like a neoplasm) or infection process; and since outpatient coders do not report these types of probable diagnoses, these statements are not considered when reporting the diagnoses for this case.*

Presence of a bleb or bulla *(both words mean the same thing—a distended space in the lung associated with emphysema)* in right lower lobe, and emphysematous *(of the nature of emphysema)* changes in both lungs. *It would seem that the patient has emphysema, but the physician did not state this directly, and as such it is not coded.*

Coronary artery calcification. *This is not the reason the services were rendered, so this would be an incidental finding, which could or could not be reported.*

Atheromatous changes in the thoracic aorta. *Atheromatous describes the nature of atheroma, a gruel-type matter that fills a tumor. This is not a definitive diagnosis that can be reported.*

Slight fibrosis OR linear atelectasis left lower lobe. *Stated as a differential (one OR the other) diagnosis, which outpatient coders do not report.*

Bullous formation in the posterior aspect of the right upper lobe. *Bullous is derived from bulla, which means a distended space. This is not a diagnosis as much as it is a statement of what the lung area looks like (it is distended as in emphysema).*

None of these statements is a definitive diagnosis, so the reason for the x-ray of the thorax remains most definitively as "mass of right lower lobe."

Now for the abdomen and pelvis CT scan results in terms of diagnoses. Ascites *is an accumulation of fluid in the abdominal cavity and is the reason for the increased girth, as stated in the Clinical Symptoms section of the report.*

Tiny low-density lesion in the mid-portion of the kidney is too small to characterize. *This is an incidental finding and will not be coded.*

Infrarenal *(below or beneath the kidney)* **abdominal aortic aneurysm.** *This is the same as the entrance diagnosis and will be reported.*

Atheromatous changes in the thoracic aorta. *Atheromatous is the nature of atheroma, which is a gruel type matter that fills a tumor. This is not a definitive diagnosis that can be reported.*

In the end, after analysis of the report there is only one diagnosis that will be reported in addition to the entrance diagnoses of right lower lobe mass and abdominal aortic aneurysm—ascites. The right lower lobe mass (which is not a neoplasm, but a mass) is reported, the abdominal aortic aneurysm is reported, and the ascites is reported. The fatigue may be reported but does not support any of the services provided, so it is an incidental diagnosis.

CASE 3-17
3-17A CT Scan, Abdomen

CASE 3-17

This service is provided due to an abnormal radiological examination. You can begin your search for the correct diagnosis code in the Index of the ICD-9-CM under the term "Abnormal, radiological examination," subtermed by type of examination. Report Dr. Monson's service.

3-17A CT SCAN, ABDOMEN

LOCATION: Outpatient, Hospital

PATIENT: Jamal Johnson

PHYSICIAN: Ronald Green, M.D.

RADIOLOGIST: Morton Monson, M.D.

EXAMINATION OF: CT of abdomen

CLINICAL SYMPTOMS: Previous abdomen radiography indicated abnormality

CT OF ABDOMEN: This study is performed on July 5, and comparisons were made with the prior study of January 1.

Images were obtained from the hemidiaphragm through the inferior pubic rami. Seven-mm helical reconstructions through the abdomen were performed with 10-mm reconstructions through the pelvis. Nonionic intravenous contrast was used for the patient's safety and convenience. Oral contrast was also administered.

The cardiac silhouette is enlarged. There is evidence of bilateral pleural effusions, increased when compared with the previous study, particularly on the right. Atelectasis involving portions of the right lung base is seen. Midline sternotomy is noted. There is evidence of previous left mastectomy. On the initial study, the liver is extremely heterogeneous. I believe this is most likely due to an arterial phase resulting from poor cardiac output. Delayed images reveal the liver to be somewhat less inhomogeneous. At least three distinct cystic areas involving the liver are seen, one along the anterior right lobe, which on today's study measures 2 × 1.7 cm and has densities of approximately 8 Hounsfield units. The area within the left lobe measures 1.8 × 1.7 cm and has densities that are -5, which are most likely averaging. A smaller cystic area within the right lobe is seen on image 19. This is really too small to measure well or characterize. These are basically similar compared with the previous study insofar as I can determine. Evidence is also seen of abdominal and pelvic ascites at this time. This was also seen previously. The volume is small. Fluid is seen along the presacral region in the sigmoid colon. There is also what appears to be fluid surrounding portions of the lower bowel loops. A small midline uterus is noted. It is difficult to see clearly the tissue planes along the fluid and uterus. I cannot really rule out some soft-tissue density within this region, which may or may not be associated with the uterus. These findings are very similar, however, compared with the previous study. The pancreas is somewhat difficult to assess and appears to be small and atrophic. The adrenal glands are not enlarged. The spleen is not grossly enlarged. There is satisfactory excretory function within the kidneys, with partially opacified bladder being present. There is heavy aortoiliac ASVD without aneurysm. The remainder of the abdomen is basically stable and similar compared with the previous study.

CONCLUSION:

1. Status post midline sternotomy. There appears to be cardiac enlargement.
2. Bilateral pleural effusions, more prominent on the right, increased compared with the previous study. Atelectasis involving portions of the right lung base is also seen.
3. The initial study of the liver is quite inhomogeneous. I believe this is due to an arterial phase of the study resulting from the patient's apparent low cardiac output. The delayed images reveal the liver to be somewhat more homogeneous, although three apparent probable cystic areas are identified. These areas appear to be relatively stable and similar compared with the previous study. A small amount of abdominal ascites is also suggested. Fluid is seen within the pelvis, including the presacral region surrounding the sigmoid colon. These findings are relatively similar compared with the previous study. There are several low-lying bowel loops, which makes it difficult to assess whether there is fluid surrounding these bowel loops or some soft-tissue density. These findings, however, are basically unchanged compared with the previous study. The findings must be clinically correlated. An additional 6-month follow-up would be recommended to reassess again.
4. Aortoiliac ASVD without gross aneurysm. The remainder of the abdomen and pelvis is basically unchanged compared with the prior study.

3-17A:

SERVICE CODE(S): ______________________

DX CODE(S): ______________________

CASE 3-18
3-18A CT Scan, Abdomen and Pelvis

CASE 3-18

This service is provided due to an abnormal function study. You can begin your search for the correct diagnosis code in the Index of the ICD-9-CM under the term "Abnormal, function," subtermed by type of study. Report Dr. Monson's service.

3-18A CT SCAN, ABDOMEN AND PELVIS

LOCATION: Outpatient, Hospital

PATIENT: Amanda Longtree

PHYSICIAN: Larry Friendly, M.D.

RADIOLOGIST: Morton Monson, M.D.

EXAMINATION OF: CT of abdomen and pelvis

CLINICAL SYMPTOMS: Elevated liver function tests

CT OF ABDOMEN AND PELVIS: TECHNIQUE: 7-mm scans are obtained from the lung bases to the iliac crests and 10-mm scans from the iliac crests to the symphysis pubis. The study was done with oral and intravenous contrast. Limited comparison with CT scan of the chest from July 11.

Scattered fibrotic changes are seen in the lower lung zones. A 1.6-cm hypodense lesion is noted along the anterior aspect of the upper liver on image 10. Hounsfield units are upper limits of that expected for a cyst. Characterization, however, is limited because this is seen on one cut only. An additional hypodense lesion is seen in the left lobe of the liver anteriorly on image 12. This has Hounsfield units consistent with a cyst. These lesions appear unchanged since the previous study. Two additional small hypodensities are seen in the right lobe of the liver, but they are too small to characterize further. The evaluation of the liver overall is somewhat limited because of the phase of the bolus. This appears to be early regarding vascular enhancement. It is therefore difficult to assess the density of the liver compared with the spleen, and I am unable to assess for the presence or absence of fatty infiltration. The pancreas is grossly unremarkable. Adrenal glands and kidneys are grossly unremarkable. A small soft-tissue density is seen in the pelvis bilaterally, likely reflecting patient's ovaries. Vascular calcifications are seen. There is hazy density seen in the presacral space, and there appears to be a small amount of fluid. This includes adjacent to the rectum.

IMPRESSION:

1. Two hypodense lesions are noted along the anterior aspect of the liver. One of these appears to be a cyst. The other lesion is difficult to characterize because of its small size, but it may also be a cyst. These lesions do not appear significantly changed from July 11. Two additional tiny hypodensities are seen in the liver. Suggest additional short-term follow-up in 3 to 4 months to document stability.
2. Unable to assess for the presence or absence of fatty infiltration of the liver because of the phase of enhancement.

3-18A:

SERVICE CODE(S): ______________________

DX CODE(S): ______________________

CT Guidance

The CT scan is also used for guidance for procedures, such as needle placement for biopsies, tissue ablation (destruction), radiation therapy, and vertebroplasty. Guidance or marking is reported separately from the procedure. See the index of the CPT manual entries under CT Scan, Guidance, for the location of the codes to report these guidance or marking services.

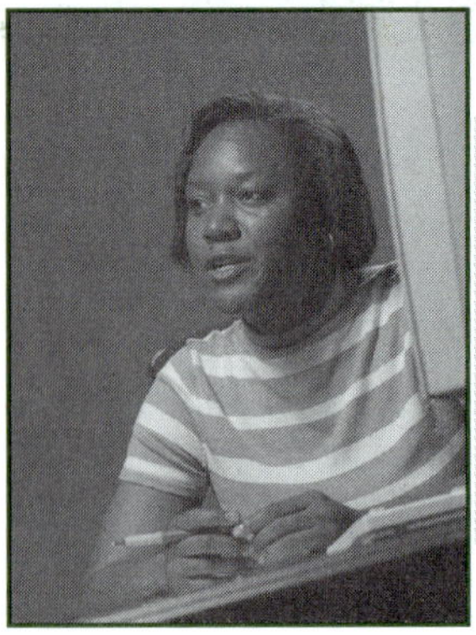

FROM THE TRENCHES

Letitia

"It's very important to be a multi-tasker in a work situation, especially when you don't have a lot of experience...familiarize yourself with the whole practice."

CASE 3-19
3-19A CT-Guided Kidney Biopsy

CASE 3-19

Dr. Riddle is an interventional radiologist who performed a CT-guided kidney biopsy. Report the biopsy service and the guidance services provided by Dr. Riddle.

3-19A CT-GUIDED KIDNEY BIOPSY

LOCATION: Outpatient, Hospital

PATIENT: Matt Barons

PHYSICIAN: Alma Naraquist, M.D.

RADIOLOGIST: Edward Riddle, M.D.

EXAMINATION OF: CT-guided kidney biopsy

CLINICAL SYMPTOMS: Severe chronic renal insufficiency and severe anemia

CT-GUIDED KIDNEY BIOPSY: HISTORY: This 70-year-old man presents with severe chronic renal insufficiency and severe anemia. The etiology of nephrotic syndrome and renal insufficiency is unknown.

FINDINGS: The procedure, risks, complications, and alternatives were explained to the patient and the patient's family. After questions and answers, they understand and agree to proceed.

The patient was prepped and draped in the standard fashion. With 1% Xylocaine with local anesthesia and conscious sedation with both Versed and fentanyl, the inferior third of the right lower pole kidney was selected with a van Sonnenberg needle. With a coaxial system, multiple 20-gauge core biopsies were obtained. Few glomeruli were evident. The tissue appeared very scarred and hyalinized. Then the middle third of the right kidney was selected, and similar results were obtained with the 20-gauge core biopsy. Then the inferior third of the left kidney was selected, this time with an 18-gauge ASAP needle. CT confirmed the position. Multiple core biopsies were obtained. Only one or two glomeruli were possibly evident but, similar to the other side of the tissue, appeared very scarred and hyalinized. At this point, we discussed the situation with the pathologist, and we agreed just to send the tissue out for further analysis.

Postprocedure CT scan through the retroperitoneal kidney region shows some mild bilateral retroperitoneal hemorrhage. The patient tolerated the procedure well, and we will follow-up with him this afternoon and make some decisions as to whether or not he can be discharged to home or needs to stay in the hospital overnight.

IMPRESSION: Successful CT-guided core biopsies of the right kidney and left kidney as described above.

3-19A:

SERVICE CODE(S): ______________________________

DX CODE(S): ______________________________

CASE 3-19A DISCUSSION

This service included CT scan guidance for biopsy needle placement, which is the first CPT code listed followed by the code for the bilateral (-50) kidney biopsy. Next, a follow-up (post-procedural) CT scan was performed, with -26 on this code to indicate that only the professional portion of the service is being reported.

The diagnoses stated in the Clinical Symptoms section of the report (renal insufficiency and anemia) and the nephrotic syndrome from within the body of the report are reported. Nephrotic syndrome is a name for a group of diseases involving defective renal glomeruli that result in proteinuria (excess protein in urine) and lipiduria (excess lipids in urine).

CASE 3-20
3-20A CT Scan, Brain

CASE 3-20

CT can provide excellent detail, as in the following case of brain hemorrhage and malignant neoplasm. Report Dr. Monson's service.

3-20A CT SCAN, BRAIN

LOCATION: Inpatient, Hospital

PATIENT: Daniel Quick

PHYSICIAN: Timothy Pleasant, M.D.

RADIOLOGIST: Morton Monson, M.D.

EXAMINATION OF: CT of brain

CLINICAL SYMPTOMS: Brain hemorrhage and primary malignant parietal lobe neoplasm

COMPUTED TOMOGRAPHIC EXAMINATION OF THE BRAIN was performed without contrast material and is compared with 2 days previously.

In the interim, the patient has had surgical procedure for parietal removal of neoplasm and hemorrhage in the right frontoparietal region. Anterior portions of the lateral ventricles again are noted to be expanded, and these now contain a considerable amount of gas from the operative procedure. There is also linear gas more posteriorly in the right hemisphere, surrounding a fluid-filled cavity that I believe represents the posterior portion of the lateral ventricle. The gas appears to be external or along the margin of the ventricle.

There is blood within the posterior portions of the lateral ventricles. I do not believe there is evidence of significant raised intracranial pressure. There is a small amount of gas in the scalp at the surgical site.

IMPRESSION: Partial removal of neoplasm and tumor from the right hemisphere. Findings as described above. I do not believe there is increased intracranial pressure. Small amount of gas in the scalp, which might represent postsurgical gas but might also represent a small dural leak if the dura was closed. It is recognized that this patient has had multiple surgical procedures, and there is most probably a significant amount of dural scarring.

3-20A:

SERVICE CODE(S): ______________________

DX CODE(S): ______________________

Ultrasound

Diagnostic ultrasound is the use of high-frequency sound waves to image anatomic structures and to detect the cause of illness and disease. The physician uses it in the diagnosis process. Ultrasound moves at different speeds through tissue, depending on the density of the tissue. Forms and outlines of organs can be identified by ultrasound as the sound waves bounce back from the tissue (echo).

Codes for ultrasound procedures are found in three locations:

- Radiology section, Diagnostic Ultrasound subsection, 76506-76886, divided on the basis of the anatomic location of the procedure (i.e, chest, pelvis)
- Medicine section, Non-Invasive Vascular Diagnostic Studies subsection, 93875-93990, divided on the basis of the anatomic location of the procedure (cerebrovascular, extremity)
- Medicine section, Echocardiography (ultrasound of the heart and great arteries), 93303-93350

The ultrasound codes for heart and vessels are in the Medicine section; all other ultrasound codes are in the Radiology section.

Modes and Scans

The four different types of ultrasound listed in the CPT manual are A-mode, M-mode, B-scan, and real-time scan.

- **A-mode:** one-dimensional display reflecting the time it takes the sound wave to reach a structure and reflect back. This process maps the structure's outline. *A* stands for amplitude of sound return (echo).
- **M-mode:** one-dimensional display of the movement of structures. *M* stands for motion.
- **B-scan:** two-dimensional display of the movement of tissues and organs. *B* stands for brightness. The sound waves bounce off tissue or organs and are projected onto a black-and-white television screen. Strong signals display as black, and weaker signals display as lighter shades of gray. B-scan is also called *gray-scale ultrasound.*

- **Real-time scan:** two-dimensional display of both the structure and the motion of tissues and organs. The display indicates the size, shape, and movement of the tissue or organ.

These modes and scans are used to describe the codes throughout the Diagnostic Ultrasound subsection. Codes are often divided on the basis of the scan or mode that was used. The medical record will indicate the scan or mode used.

Several codes within the subsection include the use of Doppler ultrasound. **Doppler ultrasound** is the use of sound that can be transmitted only through solids or liquids. It is a specific version of ultrasonography, or ultrasound. Doppler ultrasound can be standard black-and-white or color. Color Doppler translates the standard black-and-white into colored images, and the code descriptions will specifically state "color-flow Doppler."

There is component coding in the subheading of Ultrasonic Guidance Procedures. The parenthetic information will refer you to the surgical procedure code. For example, code 76946 is for the radiologic supervision and interpretation of ultrasonic guidance for amniocentesis. The radiologist guides (76946) the insertion (59000) of a needle by the surgeon to withdraw fluid from the uterus. If one physician, such as an interventional radiologist, performs both parts of the procedure, report both codes for the one physician.

CASE 3-21
3-21A Ultrasound, Right Lower Quadrant

CASE 3-21

Report Dr. Monson's service. This ultrasound is looking for an inflamed appendix because the patient presents with symptoms of appendicitis; however, no appendix is visualized.

3-21A ULTRASOUND, RIGHT LOWER QUADRANT

LOCATION: Outpatient, Hospital

PATIENT: Kathleen Lee

PHYSICIAN: Daniel G. Olanka, M.D.

RADIOLOGIST: Morton Monson, M.D.

RIGHT LOWER QUADRANT ULTRASOUND: Clinical information states right lower quadrant pain, chills, and fever. We are asked to look for an inflamed appendix. Right lower quadrant is imaged. There is bowel gas in that area. There is no fluid collection. There is no free fluid. There is no structure resembling the appendix.

IMPRESSION:
1. Normal ultrasound of right lower quadrant.
2. It must be remembered that failure to image an appendix does not exclude appendicitis.

3-21A:

SERVICE CODE(S): ______________________

DX CODE(S): ______________________

CASE 3-22
3-22A Ultrasound, Gallbladder

CASE 3-22

Report Dr. Monson's service.

3-22A ULTRASOUND, GALLBLADDER

LOCATION: Outpatient, Hospital

PATIENT: Mary Lou Moe

PHYSICIAN: Larry Friendly, M.D.

RADIOLOGIST: Morton Monson, M.D.

EXAMINATION OF: Gallbladder ultrasound

CLINICAL SYMPTOMS: Abdominal pain

GALLBLADDER ULTRASOUND: Findings: A right pleural effusion is present. Visualized portions of the liver have a normal sonographic appearance. A normal gallbladder is not identified. In the region of the gallbladder fossa, there is an echogenic structure that does produce prominent posterior shadowing. This is not peristalsis, and there is adjacent peristalsis of bowel. Common bile duct is 7 mm, which is upper normal.

IMPRESSION: Normal gallbladder is not identified. It is thought that there is a WES (wall echo shadow that occurs in patients with contracted gallbladders) sign consistent with a gallbladder packed with stones, but the differential diagnosis does include the absence of a gallbladder with echogenic bowel in the area. Clinical correlation is suggested.

3-22A:

SERVICE CODE(S): ______________________

DX CODE(S): ______________________

CASE 3-23
3-23A Ultrasound, Renal

CASE 3-23

Report Dr. Monson's service.

3-23A ULTRASOUND, RENAL

LOCATION: Outpatient, Hospital

PATIENT: Jerry Alcester

PHYSICIAN: Alma Naraquist, M.D.

RADIOLOGIST: Morton Monson, M.D.

CLINICAL SYMPTOMS: Nephrotic syndrome.

RENAL ULTRASOUND WITH ESTIMATION OF POSTVOID RESIDUAL URINARY BLADDER: No prior study. Right kidney is 11.6 × 6.6 × 5.3 cm. It shows some cortical thinning appropriate for age. No cystic or solid mass or hydronephrosis is noted. No echogenic density to suggest calculus. Left kidney is 11.8 × 5.8 × 4.8 cm. No cystic or solid mass or hydronephrosis noted. Prevoid estimated volume is 68.2 ml, postvoid urinary volume 7.94 ml. The prostate is enlarged, causing a bulge in the floor of the urinary bladder.

IMPRESSION:
1. Kidneys within normal limits.
2. Renal size normal bilaterally. No cystic or solid mass or hydronephrosis, right or left.
3. No significant urinary volume prevoid or postvoid.
4. Mild prostatic enlargement.

3-23A:

SERVICE CODE(S): ______________________

DX CODE(S): ______________________

CASE 3-24

Report Dr. Monson's service.

3-24A ULTRASOUND, GALLBLADDER

LOCATION: Outpatient, Hospital

PATIENT: Billy Zack

PHYSICIAN: Ronald Green, M.D.

RADIOLOGIST: Edward Riddle, M.D.

EXAMINATION OF: Gallbladder sonogram

CLINICAL SYMPTOMS: Abdominal pain in the right upper quadrant

GALLBLADDER SONOGRAM: This examination is difficult because of patient body habitus and position as well as the patient being on a ventilator. The liver is markedly enlarged and extends into the left abdomen. Longest measurement shown is greater than 21 cm. The gallbladder may demonstrate echogenic foci within it, which may be stones. No surrounding fluid is noted. No evidence of ductal dilatation is seen. The common hepatic duct and common bile duct measure 0.5 cm each.

3-24A:

SERVICE CODE(S): ______________________

DX CODE(S): ______________________

CASE 3-25
3-25A Ultrasound, Renal

CASE 3-25

Report Dr. Monson's service.

3-25A ULTRASOUND, RENAL

LOCATION: Outpatient, Hospital

PATIENT: Pat Highland

PHYSICIAN: George Orbitz, M.D.

RADIOLOGIST: Morton Monson, M.D.

EXAMINATION OF: Renal sonogram

CLINICAL SYMPTOMS: Chronic cholecystitis; chronic renal failure

RENAL SONOGRAM: FINDINGS: The right kidney measures 9.0 × 4.1 × 4.1 cm. The left kidney measures 9.8 × 4.4 × 4.6 cm. There is bilateral cortical thinning, consistent with the given history. Multiple cysts are seen bilaterally. On the right, the largest cyst measures 2.4 cm in maximum diameter. On the left, the largest cyst measures 1.4 cm in maximum diameter. The bladder volume after voiding is 16 cc. Incidental note of a large amount of ascites noted as well.

3-25A:

SERVICE CODE(S): ______________________

DX CODE(S): ______________________

A radiological procedure is often performed because of an abnormal test, such as an abnormal blood chemistry or abnormal function test. You can locate the diagnosis under the ICD-9-CM main term "Abnormal" and then subtermed by the test type. Take time now to review this important section of the ICD-9-CM index and become familiar with the subterms located there.

CASE 3-26

Increasing creatinine and BUN in the report represent a diagnosis of abnormal blood chemistry. Report Dr. Monson's service.

3-26A ULTRASOUND, RENAL

LOCATION: Outpatient, Hospital

PATIENT: Rosie O'Toole

PHYSICIAN: Ronald Green, M.D.

RADIOLOGIST: Morton Monson, M.D.

EXAMINATION OF: Renal ultrasound

CLINICAL SYMPTOMS: Increasing creatinine and BUN (blood urea nitrogen), low urine output (Oliguria)

RENAL ULTRASOUND: The right kidney measures 10.7 cm long and 5 cm wide; AP height is 6.8 cm. There appears to be a calculus involving the upper pole with shadowing. This measures approximately 6 mm. Gross hydronephrosis is not seen. The left kidney measures 11.8 × 5.9 × 5.6cm, respectively. No gross hydronephrosis or calculus is seen. Visualization of both kidneys is somewhat limited because of the patient's body habitus. A Foley catheter is in place. The urinary bladder cannot be assessed.

CONCLUSION: Somewhat limited visualization because of the patient's body habitus. I do not think there is gross hydronephrosis or solid mass involving either kidney, other than what may be a small stone involving the upper pole of the right kidney, which measures 6 mm.

3-26A:

SERVICE CODE(S): ______________________

DX CODE(S): ______________________

CASE 3-27
3-27A Ultrasound, Retroperitoneal

CASE 3-27

Report Dr. Monson's service.

3-27A ULTRASOUND, RETROPERITONEAL

LOCATION: Outpatient, Hospital

PATIENT: Shane Gustoworthy

PHYSICIAN: George Orbitz, M.D.

RADIOLOGIST: Morton Monson, M.D.

EXAMINATION OF: Renal ultrasound, limited

CLINICAL SYMPTOMS: Pyelonephritis

RETROPERITONEAL ULTRASOUND: FINDINGS: The right kidney measures approximately 10.8 cm in length and shows normal renal echotexture with no evidence of focal scarring, hydronephrosis, calculi, or mass. Suboptimal visualization of the right kidney is due to overlying bowel gas. The left kidney measures approximately 10.1 cm in length and shows normal renal echotexture with no focal scarring, mass, hydronephrosis, or calculi. Cholelithiasis is incidentally noted. Suprapubic catheter is in place.

3-27A:

SERVICE CODE(S): ______________________

DX CODE(S): ______________________

Ultrasound Guidance

Ultrasound is also used for guidance for such procedures as biopsy, aspiration, or injection. The radiologist determines the location where the needle is to be inserted and the best route to the site, including the exact measurements to the site. The term "marking" is sometimes used in the reports, but marking is reported with a guidance code since there is no separate code for marking. Ultrasound can also be used during the placement of the needle, catheter, or device. The radiology code does not include the actual procedure, only the marking; guidance for the procedure itself would be reported separately. For example, in the following thoracentesis, the surgeon would report thoracentesis, the radiology physician would report the professional component of the ultrasound guidance for marking, and the facility (hospital) would report the thoracentesis code (32000) along with the technical component of the ultrasound guidance.

CASE 3-28
3-28A Ultrasound, Right Lower Hemithorax—Marking

CASE 3-28

Report Dr. Monson's professional service. For the facility, report the thoracentesis and the facility portion of the ultrasound.

3-28A ULTRASOUND, RIGHT LOWER HEMITHORAX—MARKING

LOCATION: Outpatient, Hospital

PATIENT: Danny Hopmann

PHYSICIAN: Gregory Dawson, M.D.

RADIOLOGIST: Morton Monson, M.D.

ULTRASOUND OF THE RIGHT LOWER HEMITHORAX:

HISTORY: Right pleural effusion marking for thoracentesis.

FINDINGS: Limited ultrasound of the right lower hemithorax to mark for thoracentesis right-sided pleural effusion, which measures approximately 3.7 cm to the middle of the pocket of pleural fluid.

3-28A:

SERVICE CODE(S): ________________

DX CODE(S): ________________

Radiation Oncology

Radiation Oncology deals with both professional and technical treatments using radiation to destroy tumors. The codes are divided on the basis of treatment. Professional and technical components are used extensively. The codes within this subheading include codes for the initial consultation through management of the patient throughout the course of treatment. When the initial consultation occurs, the code for the service would be an E/M code.

Clinical Treatment Planning

Clinical Treatment Planning reflects professional services by the physician. It includes interpretation of special testing, tumor localization, treatment volume determination, treatment time/dosage determination, choice of treatment modality (method), determination of the number and size of treatment ports, selection of appropriate treatment devices, and any other procedures necessary to develop an adequate course of treatment. A treatment plan is set up for all patients who require radiation therapy.

The three types of clinical treatment plans are simple, intermediate, and complex.

- **Simple** planning requires that there be a single treatment area of interest that is encompassed by a single port or by simple parallel opposed ports with simple or no blocking (77261).
- **Intermediate** planning requires that there be three or more converging ports, two separate treatment areas, multiple blocks, or special time/dose constraints (77262).
- **Complex** planning requires that there be highly complex blocking, custom shielding blocks, tangential ports, special wedges or compensators, three or more separate treatment areas, rotational or special beam consideration, or a combination of therapeutic modalities (77263).

Simulation

Simulation aided field setting (77280-77299) is the service of determining treatment areas and placement of the ports for radiation treatment, but it does not include the administration of radiation. A simulation can be performed on a simulator designated for use only in simulations in a radiation therapy treatment unit or on a diagnostic x-ray machine. Codes are divided to indicate four levels of simulation-aided service:

- **Simple** simulation of a single treatment area, with either a single port or parallel opposed ports and simple or no blocking (77280).
- **Intermediate** simulation of three or more converging ports, with two separate treatment areas and multiple blocks (77285).
- **Complex** simulation of tangential ports, with three or more treatment areas, rotation or arc therapy, complex blocking, custom shielding blocks, brachytherapy source verification, hyperthermia probe verification, and any use of contrast material (77290).

- **Three-dimensional** computer-generated reconstruction of tumor volume and surrounding critical normal tissue structures based on direct CT scan and/or MRI data in preparation for noncoplanar or coplanar therapy; this is a simulation that utilizes documented three-dimensional beam's-eye view volume dose displays of multiple or moving beams. Documentation of three-dimensional volume reconstruction and dose distribution is required (77295).

Normal follow-up care is included for 3 months following completion of treatment that was reported using radiation oncology codes. You would not bill for the normal follow-up care that occurs within this 3-month period.

None of the codes in the subsection includes the radiopharmaceutical(s) used for diagnosis or therapy services. When radiopharmaceutical(s) are supplied for **diagnostic** purposes, use code 78990; when they are supplied for **therapeutic** purposes, use code 79900.

Medical Radiation Physics, Dosimetry, Treatment Devices, and Special Services codes (77300–77399) report the decision making of the physicians as to the type of treatment (modality), dose, and development of treatment devices (blocks, stents, bolus, etc.). It is common to have several dosimetry or device changes during a treatment course. **Dosimetry** is the calculation of the radiation dose and placement. It is reported on the basis of the level of treatment (simple, intermediate, complex).

Radiation Treatment Delivery (77401-77418) is the technical component of the service or the actual delivery of the radiation. Radiation treatment is delivered in units called *megaelectron* volts (MeV). A megaelectron volt is a unit of energy. The radiation energy delivered by the machine is measured in megaelectron volts; the energy that is deposited in the patient's tissue is measured in rads (radiation-absorbed dose). The therapy dose in a cancer treatment would typically be in the thousands of rads.

To code Radiation Treatment Delivery services, you need to know the amount of radiation delivered (6-10 MeV, 11-19 MeV) and the number of the following:

- Areas treated (single, two, three, or more)
- Ports involved (single, three or more, tangential)
- Blocks used (none, multiple, custom)

Radiation Treatment Management (77427-77499) reports the professional component. The codes are used to report weekly management of radiation therapy. The notes under the heading Radiation Treatment Management state that clinical management is based on five fractions or treatment sessions, regardless of the time interval separating the delivery of treatment. This means these codes can be used if the patient receives a treatment at least five times within a 7-day week; it also means that if the patient receives five treatments anytime during this week (i.e., skipping a day or two between treatments), these codes can still be used. If the patient receives five treatments and then receives an additional one or two fractions, you do not code for the additional fractions. Only if three or more fractions beyond the original five are delivered would you code using 77427 to indicate the additional treatment.

Bundled into the Radiation Treatment Management codes are the following physician services:

- Review of port films
- Review of dosimetry, dose delivery, and treatment parameters
- Review of patient treatment setup
- Examination of the patient for medical evaluation and management (e.g., assessment of the patient's response to treatment, coordination of care and treatment, review of imaging and/or lab test results)

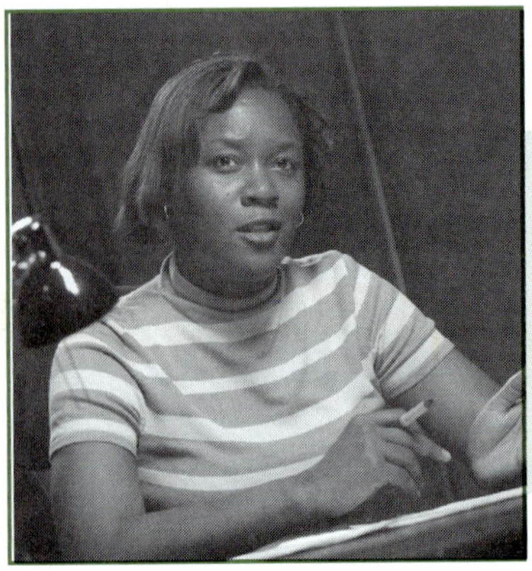

FROM THE TRENCHES

Letitia

"Employers want to make sure that whomever they hire actually has credentials to do the job...It gives more credibility. When you look at someone who is certified, you know they took the time to want to be an expert in a particular field."

Proton Beam Treatment Delivery

The delivery of radiation treatment using a proton beam utilizes particles that are positively charged with electricity. The use of the proton beam is an alternative delivery method for radiation in which photon (electromagnetic) radiation traditionally would be used. The Proton Beam subheading (77520-77525) was new in the 2000 edition of the CPT manual. The codes in the subheading are divided according to whether there was simple, intermediate, or complex delivery.

Hyperthermia

Hyperthermia is an increase in body temperature; it is used as a treatment for cancer. The heat source can be ultrasound, microwave, or another means of increasing the temperature in an area. When the temperature of an area is increased, metabolism increases, which boosts the ability of the body to eradicate cancer cells. The location of the heat source can be external (to a depth of 4 cm or less), interstitial (within the tissues), or intracavitary (inside the body). External treatment would be application to the skin of a heat source such as ultrasound. Interstitial treatment is insertion of a probe that delivers heat directly to the treatment area. Codes 77600-77615 are used to report external or interstitial treatment delivery.

Intracavitary treatment delivery requires insertion of a heat-producing probe into a body orifice, such as the rectum or vagina. Code 77620 is used to report intracavitary treatment and is the only code listed under Clinical Intracavitary Hyperthermia.

Clinical Brachytherapy

Clinical **brachytherapy** is the placement of radioactive material directly into or surrounding the site of the tumor. Placement may be **intracavitary** (within a body cavity) or **interstitial** (within the tissues), and material may be placed permanently or temporarily. The terms *source* and *ribbon* are used in the Clinical Brachytherapy codes (77750-77799). A **source** is a container holding a radioactive element that can be inserted directly into the body, where it delivers the radiation dose over time. Sources come in various forms, such as seeds or capsules, and are placed in a cavity (intracavitary) or permanently placed within the tissue (interstitial). **Ribbons** are seeds embedded on a tape. The ribbon is cut to the desired length to control the amount of radiation the patient receives. Ribbons are inserted temporarily into the tissue.

Codes are divided on the basis of the number of sources or ribbons used in an application:

- Simple 1-4
- Intermediate 5-10
- Complex 11+

The Clinical Brachytherapy codes include the physician's work related to the patient's admission to the hospital as well as the daily hospital visits.

CASE 3-29
3-29A Radiation Oncology Consultation Note
3-29B Radiation Oncology Treatment Planning Note
3-29C Radiation Oncology Simulation Note
3-29D Radiation Oncology Progress Note—Week 1, 5 Days
3-29E Radiation Oncology Progress Note—Week 2, 5 Days

CASE 3-29

3-29A RADIATION ONCOLOGY CONSULTATION NOTE

Dr. Eagle is a radiation oncologist who specializes in the treatment of cancer and is employed by the clinic. Dr. Eagle is requested by Dr. Avila to consult on Garrison O'Grady, a patient with long-standing prostate cancer.

LOCATION: Outpatient, Clinic

PATIENT: Garrison O'Grady

PHYSICIAN: Ira Avila, M.D.

RADIOLOGIST: James Eagle, M.D.

HISTORY: The patient is an 80-year-old male with a long-standing history of prostate cancer. He initially presented with right leg lymphedema and hematuria with an elevated PSA. Biopsies of the prostate were performed last year, demonstrating adenocarcinoma with a Gleason's score of 10. He was found to have a pelvic mass with bone metastases as well as a right hydronephrosis. Nephrostomy tubes were placed at that time. He received a course of palliative radiotherapy to 4620 cGy in 26 fractions to his pelvis, completed 9 months ago. Subsequently, he developed progressive right lower-extremity edema and initiation of left lower-extremity edema and scrotal edema. He received a second course of radiotherapy to the pelvis, receiving 4500 cGy in 25 fractions, completed 7 months ago. During the interim, the edema slowly increased involving both lower extremities and extending up to his waist. He has also developed a metastatic skin lesion involving the left flank. The patient has undergone several androgen blockade regimens consisting of Lupron, Casodex, and most recently ketoconazole and hydrocortisone. The patient reports that the metastatic skin lesion has increased in size and has become painful and associated with drainage. We have been asked to see the patient to discuss the role of palliative radiotherapy for the symptoms of skin metastasis.

ALLERGIES: Allergic to environmental bee stings; otherwise, no known drug allergies.

PAST MEDICAL HISTORY: Significant for:
1. Essential hypertension.
2. Hyperlipidemia.
3. Osteoarthritis.
4. Paget's disease.
5. Locally advanced prostate cancer with metastases as outlined.

PAST SURGICAL HISTORY: Placement of a right nephrostomy tube.

PRESENT MEDICATIONS:
1. Coumadin 5 mg q.d.
2. Dexamethasone 0.75 mg b.i.d.
3. Zaroxolyn 5 mg q.d.
4. Ketoconazole 200 mg t.i.d.
5. Hydrocortisone 20 mg q.a.m. and 10 mg q.p.m.

SOCIAL HISTORY: The patient lives with his younger brother in Marshville, 20 miles east. They have much difficulty with travel arrangements and have requested that he stay at the local elder care unit during his course of radiotherapy. He does have one sister, who accompanies him today. The patient reports that he is essentially unable to ambulate because of the lower-extremity peripheral edema.

FAMILY HISTORY: The patient had a brother who was diagnosed with prostate cancer.

REVIEW OF SYSTEMS: Significant for progressive pain and drainage associated with his skin metastases involving the left flank. It is also significant for progressive lymphedema involving both lower extremities, right greater than left, which has made ambulation essentially impossible. It is negative for fevers, chills, sweats, anorexia, weight loss, difficulty swallowing, cough, hemoptysis, shortness of breath, chest pain, chest tightness, chest pressure, nausea, vomiting, diarrhea, constipation, or musculoskeletal pain. EENT is within normal limits. Neurologic responses are normal. Review of systems is otherwise negative.

EXAMINATION: The patient is an 80-year-old man who appears to be in no apparent distress. Pulse is 90 and respiratory rate is 18. Head is normocephalic and atraumatic. The auricular canals and tympanic membranes are clear and intact bilaterally. Eyes have EOMI. PERRLA. Visual fields are full to confrontation. Sclerae are clear. Oral cavity is pink and moist without mucosal lesions. Dentition is in good repair. Lungs are clear to auscultation and percussion. Heart is regular without murmur. The left flank has a 13.5-cm wide lesion, which measures 5.5 cm in height and protrudes about 1.5 to 2 cm. The metastatic skin lesion is purplish and is mildly weeping throughout the consultation. A right nephrostomy tube is appreciated. There is pitting edema up through the ileal chest bilaterally and is significantly worse distally. Neurologically, he is oriented times three. Cranial nerves II through XII are intact. Gait is impossible, with the patient being wheelchair-bound.

IMPRESSION: Metastatic prostate cancer with symptomatic metastases to the left flank.

RECOMMENDATIONS: The patient is an 80-year-old man who presents with symptomatic skin metastases originating from his prostate cancer. I do believe he would benefit from palliative radiotherapy to the left flank for pain control as well as to decrease the drainage from the symptomatic skin metastases. The indications and goals of palliative radiotherapy have been discussed with the patient and his sister. Before initiating his palliative radiotherapy, the patient will require accommodations in the elder care unit. We contacted our social worker, who will facilitate living arrangements. Once the patient is able to become a resident within the elder care unit, he will then initiate his palliative radiotherapy. The patient and his family declined living arrangements in Marshville because of the difficulty with travel arrangements. All questions and concerns have been addressed.

We appreciate the opportunity to participate in the care of your patient.

3-29A:

SERVICE CODE(S): ______________________

DX CODE(S): ______________________

This patient is presenting for a consultation as stated in the last sentence of the History section of the report as: "We have been asked to see the patient to discuss the role of palliative radiotherapy for the symptoms of skin metastasis." The diagnosis for the secondary neoplasm of the skin (metastatic site) is listed first as per the directions in the Official Reporting and Coding Guidelines in C2. B. When the encounter is for the secondary site, the secondary site is listed first and the primary site (neoplasm of the prostate) is listed second.

3-29B RADIATION ONCOLOGY TREATMENT PLANNING NOTE

Mr. Garrison has been established at the elder care unit and is now ready to begin his palliative treatment. Palliative treatment is when the treatment is focused toward making the patient as comfortable as possible. The treatment is not intended to cure the condition but only to provide more comfort to a patient by relieving some of the pain. This is the clinical treatment planning of a complex level due to use of a custom-made Cerrobend block.

LOCATION: Outpatient, Clinic

PATIENT: Garrison O'Grady

PHYSICIAN: Ira Avila, M.D.

RADIOLOGIST: James Eagle, M.D.

DIAGNOSIS: Stage IV metastatic adenocarcinoma of the prostate with symptomatic metastasis to the skin involving the left flank.

CLINICAL CONSIDERATIONS: The patient is an 80-year-old man with symptomatic skin metastasis to the left flank from this prostate cancer. The indications, goals, and side effects of palliative radiotherapy for the symptomatic skin metastases have been discussed in detail. The patient and his family appear to understand and have verbalized a desire to proceed with this option. Arrangements have been made for the patient to proceed with his radiotherapy while a resident at the elder care unit.

TECHNICAL CONSIDERATIONS: The patient is an 80-year-old man with symptomatic skin metastasis from his metastatic prostate cancer. The target volume will include the skin of the left flank for a total of 15 fractions. Normal tissues, which need to be considered, include the surrounding normal skin, kidney, spine, and small bowel.

The fractionation is 3750 cGy in 15 fractions with an en face radiation treatment field at 100 SSD.

The palliative radiotherapy treatment field will be treated with 9 MEV electrons prescribed to the 90th percent isodose line. A custom-made **Cerrobend block** will be designed for the electron field. Bolus will also be used to enhance the skin dose. He will require a complex simulation, at which time dose calculations will be performed to ensure that the prescribed dose will be delivered to the target volume. The patient will initiate his radiotherapy thereafter. All questions and concerns have been addressed. We appreciate the opportunity to participate in the care of your patient.

3-29B:

SERVICE CODE(S): ______________________

DX CODE(S): ______________________

3-29C RADIATION ONCOLOGY SIMULATION NOTE

The simulation is now performed to calculate the amount of radiation that would be delivered during the treatment phase. The level of the simulation is indicated in the treatment- planning note in the previous report. The custom-made treatment block (treatment device) is reported with a separate CPT code. This is a complex simulation involving blocking.

LOCATION: Outpatient, Hospital

PATIENT: Garrison O'Grady

PHYSICIAN: Ira Avila, M.D.

RADIOLOGIST: James Eagle, M.D.

DIAGNOSIS: Stage IV symptomatic skin metastases involving the left flank originating from metastatic prostate cancer.

SIMULATION: After explaining to the patient the purpose of the simulation procedure, he was placed on the treatment table in the prone position. He was then placed in the treatment position.

THERAPEUTIC FIELD SETUP: An electron radiotherapy treatment field was clinically set at 100 SSD. A custom-made Cerrobend block (Note this is the treatment device) will be constructed for the radiotherapy treatment field. We anticipate using 9-MeV electrons prescribed to the 90th percent isodose line. Bolus will also be used to enhance the dose distribution to the skin. Dose calculations will be performed to ensure that the prescribed dose will be delivered to the target volume.

The entire simulation took approximately 40 minutes. The patient tolerated the procedure very well and was discharged in stable condition. We anticipate the patient initiating his radiotherapy later this week.

3-29C:

SERVICE CODE(S): ______________________________

DX CODE(S): ______________________________

Treatment Delivery

The physician writes one progress note for each week of treatment. Five fractions are delivered in a week, with one treatment a day for 5 days. The physician portion of the service is reported with 77427, once for each week with five fractions. The radiation oncology services are often provided in the hospital setting in an outpatient department, such as an oncology department. The hospital outpatient coder then reports the services for the facility on the UB92. The facility services are reported with different codes because the hospital is providing the physical location where the treatments are delivered and any additional service that may be required, such as in the following report, where port films are taken. The port films are x-rays that are taken to ensure the correct positioning of the treatment portals for the patient who is receiving external beam radiation therapy. Port films charges are for the technical component only, with no professional component provided or reported. The hospital would report the port films (77417), in addition to the radiation therapy treatment delivery (77413) on a per-session basis.

3-29D RADIATION ONCOLOGY PROGRESS NOTE—WEEK 1, 5 DAYS

This is the first week of treatment delivery.

LOCATION: Outpatient, Hospital

PATIENT: Garrison O'Grady

PHYSICIAN: Ira Avila, M.D.

RADIOLOGIST: James Eagle, M.D.

HISTORY: The patient is an 80-year-old man with stage IV prostate cancer with symptomatic skin metastases involving the left flank. He has received 1250 cGy in 5 fractions to his left flank. He has had a significant reduction in the metastatic lesion; however, he has also had a reaction from the tape required for his dressing. He denies any change in his energy level or changes in his bowel habits.

PHYSICAL EXAMINATION: Pulse is 84. Respiratory rate is 18. The neck is supple without adenopathy. Lungs are clear. Heart is regular without murmur. There is a palpable mass within the left flank that measures 12 × 5 cm, which protrudes less than at his consultation. There is a suggestion of necrosis with drainage from his tumor.

BEAM REVIEW: The patient's treatment position is as initially planned. The dose calculations have been reviewed and indicate the correct setting for all treatments.

PORT FILMS: The patient has been seen clinically with the setup being accepted.

DISPOSITION: The patient will continue with his radiation treatments as prescribed. He will continue with his dressings consisting of Telfa gauze and ABD dressing with the use of a tape. We will initiate the use of a tape prep to protect his skin during his treatment process. We will continue to monitor for further radiation side effects and treat as indicated.

3-29D:

SERVICE CODE(S): ______________________________

DX CODE(S): ______________________________

3-29E RADIATION ONCOLOGY PROGRESS NOTE—WEEK 2, 5 DAYS

This is the second week of treatment delivery.

LOCATION: Outpatient, Hospital

PATIENT: Garrison O'Grady

PHYSICIAN: Ira Avila, M.D.

RADIOLOGIST: James Eagle, M.D.

HISTORY: The patient is an 80-year-old man with a stage IV prostate cancer with symptomatic skin metastases involving the left flank. He has initiated a course of palliative radiotherapy and is receiving 25 Gy in 10 fractions. He continues to have drainage from tumor necrosis. He has also had a skin reaction from the tape required for his dressings. He denies any changes in his energy level or change in his bowel or bladder habits.

EXAM: Pulse 80. Respiratory rate is 18. The neck is supple without adenopathy. Lungs are clear to auscultation. Heart is regular without murmur. A palpable mass remains within the left flank, measuring 11 × 4.5, which protrudes much less than last week. There continues to be necrosis from the central portion of his tumor, which also has diminished from last week.

BEAM REVIEW: The patient's treatment position is as initially planned. The dose calculations have been reviewed and indicate the correct settings for all treatments.

PORT FILMS: The patient has been seen clinically with the setup being accepted.

DISPOSITION: The patient will continue with his radiation treatments as prescribed. He will continue with his dressings on a daily basis using Telfa gauze and an ABD dressing with the use of tape. The skin will be prepped before application of the gauze and tape. We will monitor for radiation side effects and treat as indicated.

3-29E:

SERVICE CODE(S): ______________________

DX CODE(S): ______________________

Nuclear Medicine

Nuclear medicine deals with the placement of radionuclides within the body and the monitoring of emissions from the radioactive elements.

There are two subsections in Nuclear Medicine: Diagnostic (78000-78999) and Therapeutic (79000-79999). The services listed do not include the radium or other radioelement, which are reported separately with 78990 (diagnostic radiopharmaceutical) or 79900 (therapeutic radiopharmaceutical). The Diagnostic Nuclear Medicine subsection is divided by body system organ system (i.e., Endocrine, Gastrointestinal, etc.). The codes report imaging, such as the organ system gastrointestinal subdivided into, for example, liver and salivary gland imaging. There are usually several imaging or studies that can be done; for example, there are three codes for salivary gland:

78230	Salivary gland imaging
78231	Salivary gland with serial imaging
78232	Salivary gland function study

For the imaging procedure, a radiotracer (radioactive isotope) is injected, and the salivary gland is imaged with a gamma camera (a special camera used to take images of the radiotracers). In the serial imaging procedure, several (a series of) images are taken, and then the patient is given a substance that stimulates the salivary gland (such as a lemon candy) and images are again taken. The function study includes a radioactive substance being placed under the tongue, which stimulates the salivary glands, and images then are taken of the salivary glands to assess the function.

The therapeutic services (79000-79999) contain codes for various thyroid treatments (79000-79035) in which radiopharmaceuticals are needed to treat lesions and thyroid malfunctions.

Intracavitary and interstitial radioactivity colloid therapies (79200-79300) are sources that are placed into the body at the site of the tumor, and over time the source emits radiation. An advantage of this method of treatment is that the source gives a high dose of radiation to the tumor and much lower dose to the surrounding areas.

Intravascular and intra-articular therapy involves the placement of radiopharmaceuticals directly into a vessel (intravascular) or a joint (intra-articular). After placement, the radiopharmaceutical destroys the lesion.

Nuclear medicine procedures are located in the index of the CPT manual under Nuclear Medicine.

CASE 3-30
3-30A Diagnostic Pulmonary Function Study

CASE 3-30

Dr. Monson provides the professional component of the study. To locate the correct CPT code, reference "Pulmonary, Diagnostic, Function Study."

3-30A DIAGNOSTIC PULMONARY FUNCTION STUDY

LOCATION: Outpatient, Hospital

PATIENT: Mary Blue

PHYSICIAN: Ronald Green, M.D.

RADIOLOGIST: Morton Monson, M.D.

EXAMINATION OF: Lungs

CLINICAL SYMPTOMS: Hypoxia, shortness of breath

VENTILATION-PERFUSION SCAN OF LUNGS: DOSE: The patient received 2.0 millicuries of technetium-99m DTPA by aerosol and 6.0 millicuries of technetium-99m labeled MAA intravenously.

FINDINGS: This examination is interpreted in conjunction with a chest radiograph dated last month. Overall perfusion appears better than ventilation. The ventilation is very patchy and inhomogeneous. Because of the inhomogeneity, this study is indeterminate for the possibility of pulmonary embolus. There is an apparent triple match present within the right lung base. This also makes the study indeterminate for the possibility of pulmonary embolus. A few scattered matched perfusion defects are seen. Definite unmatched perfusion defects are not seen on this examination.

IMPRESSION: Because of the inhomogeneous ventilation and the triple match within the right lung base, this study is indeterminate for the possibility of pulmonary embolus.

3-30A:

SERVICE CODE(S): ____________________

DX CODE(S): ____________________

CASE 3-31
3-31A Ventilation-Perfusion Lung Scan

CASE 3-31

Report Dr. Monson's service.

3-31A VENTILATION-PERFUSION LUNG SCAN

LOCATION: Outpatient, Hospital

PATIENT: Hilda Torgerson

PHYSICIAN: Marvin Elhard, M.D.

RADIOLOGIST: Morton Monson, M.D.

EXAMINATION OF: Ventilation-perfusion lung scan

CLINICAL SYMPTOMS: Right chest pain

VENTILATION-PERFUSION LUNG SCAN

DOSE: The patient received 2.0 millicuries of technetium-99m DTPA by aerosol and 6.0 millicuries of technetium-99m labeled MAA intravenously.

FINDINGS: This examination is interpreted in conjunction with a chest radiograph, which is dated last year. Evaluation of ventilation and perfusion images demonstrates the presence of small, scattered, matched ventilation and perfusion defects within both lungs. A moderately large perfusion defect is present within the right lung base. This matches on ventilation and perfusion images. A focal opacity is present within this area on the chest radiograph. The findings constitute a triple match, and the study is therefore indeterminate for pulmonary embolus. Definite perfusion mismatches are not seen on this examination.

IMPRESSION: Triple match identified within the right lower lung zone. The study is therefore indeterminate for the possibility of pulmonary embolus. Definite mismatch is not identified.

3-31A:

SERVICE CODE(S): ____________________

DX CODE(S): ____________________

Interventional Radiology

Component or combination coding means that a code from the Radiology section as well as a code from one of the other sections of the CPT manual must be used to fully describe the procedure. For example, an interventional radiologist may inject contrast material; place stents, catheters, or guide wires; or perform any number of procedures that could also be performed by two separate physicians—a radiologist and a surgeon. Interventional radiologists perform both the radiology and surgical portions of the procedure. Many times, before radiology procedures can be performed, a contrast material is used to make organs or vessels stand out more clearly on the radiographic image. When this contrast material is injected, a CPT code from the Surgery section must be used to indicate the injection service. For example, if the interventional radiologist performed a bronchoscopy in which a segment of the bronchi is injected with a contrast material (segmental bronchography) and x-rays taken of that area, the injection is reported with 31656 and the radiographic portion of the service is reported with 71040 (unilateral bronchography). If, however, the surgeon performed the injection procedure (31656) and the radiologist performed the bronchography (71040), each would report his or her portion of the service. Remember to use modifier -26 when reporting only the professional component of the radiology services.

Central Venous Access Procedures

Locate the Central Venous Access Procedures codes 36555-36565 in the CPT manual. Codes 36555 and 36556 are for **temporary** catheters (5-7 days). A tunneled catheter is one that is burrowed into the skin at a distance from the vascular access site. Codes 36557-36561 all are for tunneled catheters, but 36557 and 36558 are **level with the skin** with a button-type access. This access is like a PICC (peripherally inserted central catheter) that is used for direct access for long-term antibiotic IV therapy. Note that 36557 and 36558 are for "without subcutaneous port or pump" and 36560 and 36561 are for "with subcutaneous port." This means that the access on 36560 and 36561 is for those types of ports that would be accessed for therapies such as hemodialysis with a port that is placed **outside the skin.**

CASE 3-32
3-32A Radiology Report, Hemodialysis Catheter Placement

CASE 3-32

Code the professional interventional radiology services provided by Dr. Riddle.

3-32A RADIOLOGY REPORT, HEMODIALYSIS CATHETER PLACEMENT

LOCATION: Outpatient, Hospital

PATIENT: Harry Sportsmann

PERSONAL PHYSICIAN: George Orbitz, M.D.

RADIOLOGIST: Edward Riddle, M.D.

EXAMINATION OF: Placement of tunneled hemodialysis catheter

CLINICAL SYMPTOMS: Chronic renal failure.

PLACEMENT OF AN ANGIODYNAMICS MORE-FLOW HEMODIALYSIS CATHETER: The patient is a 54-year-old man with a history of renal failure. Placement of a tunneled hemodialysis catheter was requested by Dr. Orbitz.

Prior to the start of the study, the procedure was explained to the patient, including the risks, complications, and alternatives. The patient understood and consented to the exam.

The patient was prepped and draped in the usual sterile fashion. An Ioban II (antimicrobial film) was placed on the skin.

Using sterile technique under ultrasound guidance following administration of local anesthesia (1% lidocaine), a 21-gauge micropuncture needle was advanced into the right internal jugular vein in the lower neck region. Using a microvena kit, a 0.18 stainless steel wire was used to measure the distance from the junction of the right atrium/superior vena cava to the skin site, and the appropriate-sized catheter was obtained. A 5 French straight catheter was advanced into the internal jugular vein. The catheter was then placed to flush.

A small skin incision was placed in the upper chest region. Following administration of local anesthesia (1% lidocaine), a tunnel was obtained between the two skin incisions. A vascular sheath was then placed through the tunnel, and the More-Flow was then advanced through the peel-away sheath.

The 5 French straight catheter then was removed over an extra-stiff wire, and a peel-away sheath was placed into the right internal jugular vein. The dilator and wire were then removed, and the end of the peel-away sheath was crimped to avoid blood loss with the patient holding his or her breath. The tip of the catheter then was advanced through the peel-away sheath with the tip at the proximal right atrium. The peel-away sheath was removed, and the catheter was adjusted to obtain a smooth transition. The cuff of the catheter was approximately 1 to 2 cm from the incision site. A single 2-0 Prolene suture was then placed at the catheter insertion site, and two sutures were placed at the lower neck incision site. No obvious bleeding was seen. Contrast was infused through both ports, which revealed adequate placement.

The patient tolerated the procedure well. The patient denied pain and shortness of breath at termination of the study.

IMPRESSION: Placement of a 14.5-French AngioDynamics More-Flow hemodialysis catheter through the internal jugular vein as described above.

3-32A:

SERVICE CODE(S): ____________________

DX CODE(S): ____________________

CASE 3-33

Report Dr. Riddle's services. In this case a gastrojejunostomy catheter is placed (the service) for nutritional support of this atient who has nutritional deficiency (the diagnosis). This service requires a code from the Surgery section to report the percutaneous insertion of the gastrostomy tube and a radiology code to report the percutaneous placement of the tube.

3-33A GASTROJEJUNOSTOMY CATHETER PLACEMENT

LOCATION: Outpatient, Hospital

PATIENT: Brian Neilson

PERSONAL PHYSICIAN: Leslie Alanda, M.D.

RADIOLOGIST: Edward Riddle, M.D.

EXAMINATION OF: Placement of gastrojejunostomy catheter

CLINICAL SYMPTOMS: Nutritional support due to nutritional deficiency

PLACEMENT OF GASTROJEJUNOSTOMY CATHETER: The patient is a 63-year-old man with extensive medical history including intracranial hemorrhage. Placement of a percutaneous gastrojejunostomy catheter was requested by Dr. Alanda for nutritional support.

Before start of the study, the procedure was explained to the patient's wife, including the risks, complications, and alternatives. The patient's wife understood and consented to the exam.

The patient was prepped and draped in the usual sterile fashion. Using ultrasound guidance, the edge of the liver was localized. Through a previously placed nasogastric tube, the stomach was distended with air.

Using fluoroscopic guidance following administration of local anesthesia (1% lidocaine), gastropexy was performed using four Medi-Tech T-tacks at the mid to distal aspect of the stomach.

Using multiple wires and catheters, an extrastiff guide wire was ultimately placed with the tip in the proximal jejunum. Following multiple dilatations, a no. 14 French Shetty gastrojejunostomy was placed with the tip in the proximal jejunum. A small amount of contrast was administered, which revealed adequate placement. No evidence of extravasation or other significant abnormalities was seen.

The patient tolerated the procedure well. No evidence of bleeding was seen at the termination of the study.

IMPRESSION: Placement of a no. 14 French Shetty gastrojejunostomy catheter with the tip in the proximal jejunum as described above.

3-33A:

SERVICE CODE(S): ____________________

DX CODE(S): ____________________

CASE 3-34
3-34A Gastrojejunostomy Catheter Placement

CASE 3-34

There will be a code from the Surgery section to report the gastrostomy tube inserted percutaneously (with the addition of the modifier that indicates a discontinued procedure). The Impression section of the report indicates that the procedure was discontinued. Report Dr. Riddle's services.

3-34A GASTROJEJUNOSTOMY CATHETER PLACEMENT

LOCATION: Outpatient, Hospital

PATIENT: Malcolm Fox

PHYSICIAN: Ronald Green, M.D.

RADIOLOGIST: Edward Riddle, M.D.

EXAMINATION OF: Attempted placement of gastrojejunostomy catheter

CLINICAL SYMPTOMS: Abdominal pain and malnutrition

ATTEMPTED PLACEMENT OF GASTROJEJUNOSTOMY CATHETER: The patient is an 86-year-old man with an extensive medical history that includes abdominal pain and malnutrition. Placement of a gastrojejunostomy catheter was requested by Dr. Green.

Before start of the study, the procedure was explained to the patient's daughter, including the risks, complications, and alternatives. The patient's daughter understood and consented to the procedure.

The patient was prepped and draped in the usual sterile fashion. The patient was also sedated.

The gastrojejunostomy catheter could not be safely placed percutaneously because of the patient's anatomy. There is marked dilatation of what is thought to represent small bowel, which is displacing the stomach superiorly. If distension of the small bowel is relieved, percutaneous placement may be possible at a later date.

IMPRESSION: Percutaneous gastrojejunostomy catheter could not be placed because of the patient's anatomy, as described above.

3-34A:

SERVICE CODE(S): ____________________

DX CODE(S): ____________________

CASE 3-35
3-35A Gastrojejenostomy Catheter Placement

CASE 3-35

This service involves not only the percutaneous insertion of a gastrostomy tube by Dr. Riddle, but also x-ray guidance performed by Dr. Riddle. Because Dr. Riddle is an interventional radiologist, he has expertise in performing both the percutaneous insertion of the gastrostomy tube and the radiological guidance for the placement. Report Dr. Riddle's services.

3-35A GASTROJEJUNOSTOMY CATHETER PLACEMENT

LOCATION: Inpatient, Hospital

PATIENT: Jane Wellington

PERSONAL PHYSICIAN: Ronald Green, M.D.

RADIOLOGIST: Edward Riddle, M.D.

EXAMINATION OF: Placement of a gastrojejunostomy catheter

CLINICAL SYMPTOMS: CVA

PERCUTANEOUS GASTROJEJUNOSTOMY PLACEMENT: The patient is a 60-year-old woman with a history of a stroke and ARDS on a ventilator. Placement of a gastrojejunostomy catheter for nutritional support was requested by Dr. Green.

Before start of the study, the procedure was explained to the patient's husband on the phone, including the risks, complications, and alternatives. The patient's husband understood and consented to the procedure.

The patient was prepped and draped in the usual sterile fashion. Using ultrasound guidance, the edge of the liver was localized. Through a previously placed nasogastric tube, the stomach was distended with air.

Using fluoroscopic guidance following administration of local anesthesia (1% lidocaine), gastropexy was performed using four Medi-Tech T-tacks at the mid to distal aspect of the stomach.

Using multiple wires and catheters, an extrastiff guide wire was ultimately placed with the tip in the proximal jejunum. Following multiple dilatations, a 14 French Shetty gastrojejunostomy was placed with the tip in the proximal jejunum. A small amount of contrast was administered, which revealed adequate placement. There is no evidence of extravasation or other significant abnormalities.

The patient tolerated the procedure well. No evidence of bleeding was seen at termination of the study.

IMPRESSION: Placement of a 14 French Shetty gastrojejunostomy catheter with the tip in the proximal jejunum as described above.

3-35A:

SERVICE CODE(S): ______________________

DX CODE(S): ______________________

Glossary

A-mode one-dimensional ultrasonic display reflecting the time it takes a sound wave to reach a structure and reflect back; maps the structure's outline
anteroposterior from front to back
axial projection any projection that allows the x-ray beam to pass through the body part lengthwise

B-scan two-dimensional display of tissues and organs
brachytherapy therapy using radioactive sources that are placed inside the body

computed axial tomography (CAT or CT) procedure by which selected planes of tissue are pinpointed through computer enhancement, and images may be reconstructed by analysis of variance in absorption of the tissue

decubitus recumbent positions where the x-ray beam is placed horizontally
diagnostic ultrasound technique using high-frequency sound waves to determine the density of the outline of tissue to detect the cause of illness and disease
distal farther from the point of attachment or origin
Doppler ultrasound a diagnostic procedure using sound that can be standard black-and-white or color; can be transmitted only through solid or liquids
dosimetry scientific calculation of radiation emitted from various radioactive sources

interstitial within the body tissues
intracavitary within a body cavity

lateral away from the midline of the body (to the side)

M-mode one-dimensional display of movement of structures
magnetic resonance imaging (MRI) procedure that uses nonionizing radiation to view the body in a cross-sectional view

oblique view radiographic view in which the body or part is rotated so the projection is neither frontal nor lateral
odontoid position/view with the patient's mouth open

position placement of the patient during the x-ray examination
posteroanterior from back to front
projection the path of the x-ray beam
prone (ventral) lying on the stomach
proximal closer to the point of attachment or origin

radiologist physician who specializes in the use of radioactive materials in the diagnosis and treatment of disease and illnesses
radiology branch of medicine concerned with the use of radioactive substances for diagnosis and therapy
reconstruction the three-dimensional image created by putting together several cross-sectional views (CT scans, MRIs, etc.)
recumbent lying down
ribbons radioactive seeds embedded on a tape that is temporarily inserted into body tissues to deliver a radiation dose over time; can be cut to determine the amount of radiation the patient receives

source a container holding a radioactive element; can be inserted directly into the body to deliver a radiation dose over time
supine (dorsal) lying on the back
swimmers position/view in which the arms are over the head

tangential patient position that allows the beam to skim the body part; produces a profile of the structure of the body
tomography procedure that allows viewing of a single plane of the body by blurring out all but that particular level

Chapter 4

Pathology and Laboratory

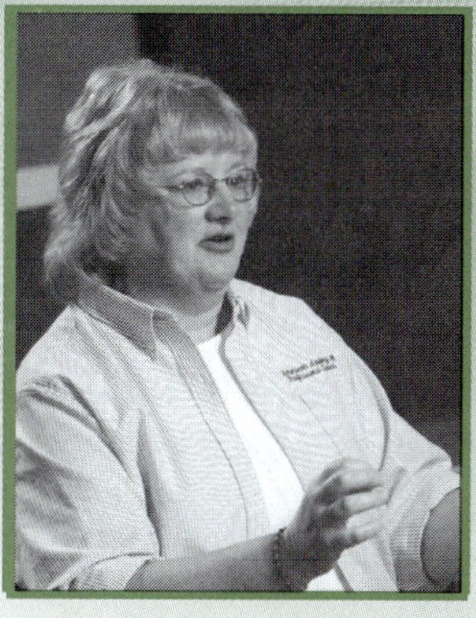

Patricia Feldner, MSW, CPC
Consultant
Madison, Wisconsin

ABBREVIATIONS

ABN	advanced beneficiary notice
ABO	three main blood types
ACTH	adrenocorticotropic hormone
Alb	albumin
Alkphos	alkaline phosphatase
ALT	alanine amino transferases
ANA	antinuclear antibodies
APTT	activated partial thromboplastin time
ASO	antistreptolysin O
AST	aspartate amino transferase
Bili tot	direct bilirubin, total and direct
BUN	blood urea nitrogen
Ca	calcium
CBC	complete blood count
CEA	carcinoembryonic antigen
Chol tot	total serum cholesterol
Cl	chloride
CK	creatine kinase
cm	centimeter
CO_2	carbon dioxide
CPK	creatine phosphokinase
Creat	creatinine
DAT	direct antiglobulin test
dL	deciliter
DM	diabetes mellitus
DNA	deoxyribonucleic acid
ds	double strand
ENA	extractable nuclear antigen
ESRD	end-stage renal disease
ESRF	end-stage renal failure
FSH	follicle stimulating hormone
g/dl	gram/deciliter
GERD	gastroesophageal reflux disease
GGT	gamma glutamyl transferase
Glu	glucose
HB_3Ag	lipoprotein
HCG	human chorionic gonadotropin
HCT	hematocrit
Hct	hematocrit
HDL	high-density lipoprotein
HGB	hemoglobin
Hgb	hemoglobin
HIV	human immunodeficiency virus
HTN	hypertension
IBC	iron-binding capacity
IgM	immunoglobulin M
K	potassium
LDH	lactate dehydrogenase
LDL	low-density lipoprotein
MCHC	mean corpuscular hemoglobin concentration
MCV	mean corpuscular volume
mg/dl	milligram/deciliter
ml	milliliter
ml/dl	milliliter/deciliter
mm/hr	millimeter/hour
N	negative
Na	sodium
NC	no charge
OB	obstetric
pH	potential of hydrogen
PLT	platelet
Prot tot	total protein
PSA	prostate-specific antigen
PT	prothrombin time
PTT	partial thromboplastin time
RBC	red blood cell
RDW	red cell distribution width
RF	rheumatoid factor
Rh	rhesus factor
Rh(D)	rhesus factor blood typing
RPR	rapid plasma reagin
stat.	*statim,* immediately
SGOT	serum glutamic oxaloacetic transaminase (AST)
SGPT	serum glutamic pyruvic transaminase (ALT)
TH	tumor 4 (thorium)
Trig	triglycerides
TSH	thyroid-stimulating hormone
UA	urine analysis
VCA	viral capsid antibody, viral capsid antigen
WBC	white blood cell
WNL	within normal limits

Types of Service

The codes in the Pathology and Laboratory section of the CPT manual cover a wide variety of services. The following are the types of services most commonly used:

Organ- or Disease-Oriented Panels (80048-80076)
Drug Testing (80100-80103)
Therapeutic Drug Assays (80150-80299)
Urinalysis (81000-81099)
Chemistry (82000-84999)
Hematology and Coagulation (85002-85999)
Immunology (86000-86849)

Superbill/Requisition Form

Tests are often requested by means of a form or **superbill** or requisition form as illustrated in **Figure 4-1**. Note on the superbill/requisition form that the area under the "Code" column would contain the CPT laboratory code, but for the purposes of this worktext, the codes have been deleted and you will be removing Figure 4-1 from the worktext and placing the codes on the form as you work through this chapter. When you are finished with the chapter, you will use the form to complete several coding cases using this form. In the office, the physician would place a check mark in the blank column to the left of the "Code" column as illustrated in **Figure 4-2** (see "Test ordered by physician"). The physician would complete the form, or the nursing staff would complete the form per the physician's direction. The form contains areas for the date and time the test was ordered, the priority of the test, whether the order is for a recurring test that will be conducted several times during the stated time, and any special instructions the physician wants to convey to the laboratory staff regarding the test(s). There is a space to indicate whether the collection of the specimen was conducted in the office or in the laboratory. An example of a physician collecting the specimen would be when the physician performed a spinal tap to aspirate spinal fluid for examination. The fluid then would be sent to the laboratory with a form indicating that the fluid was obtained by the physician in the office, along with directions from the physician for the specific laboratory test(s) requested. The aspiration service performed by the physician is reported separately. An example of the laboratory personnel collecting the specimen would be when the patient takes the General Laboratory Test Requisition to the laboratory where the technician performs the test(s) ordered by the physician. The requisition form is developed by the medical facility to reflect the organization's most commonly requested laboratory tests. There are also spaces on the form to request tests not listed on the form. The form also has a location for the written indication or diagnosis along with the ICD-9-CM code.

The services in the Pathology and Laboratory section of the CPT manual include **the laboratory test only. The collection of the specimen is coded separately.** For example, if a patient had a technician in a clinic laboratory withdraw blood by means of a venipuncture, and the blood sample was then analyzed in the laboratory, 36415 is coded for the venipuncture in addition to a code to report the test performed on the blood.

Indicators are written physician orders to the laboratory that set standards. When a test is found to be positive, the physician would want further information about the condition by means of additional laboratory tests. For example, if a routine urinalysis is performed, a culture is performed if a positive bacteria result is found. If a culture is performed to identify the organism, a sensitivity test is performed if the bacteria are of a certain type or count (as predetermined by the medical facility) to warrant the additional laboratory studies. Some indicators are also located on the form. For example, on Figure 4-1 under the Immunology (Blood) section, the ASO screen has an indicator specifying that another test is to be performed if the screening test is positive.

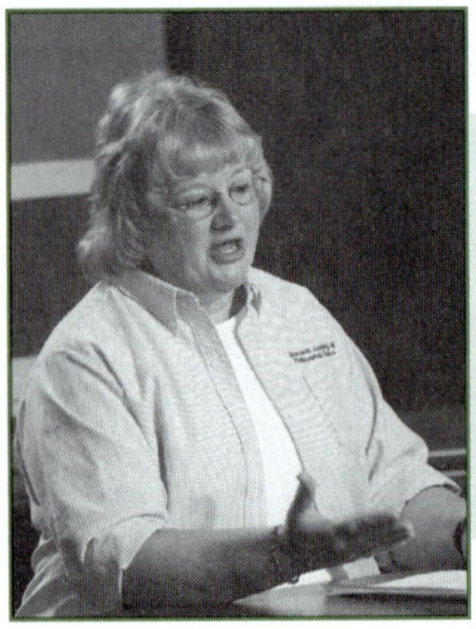

FROM THE TRENCHES

Pat

"Be as flexible as possible. You want to get into the job and learn the basics, but are able to move from specialty to specialty. By working in a multispecialty clinic, you are going to get a lot of background if you move from department to department."

General Laboratory Requisition

Order Date: ______________ Order Time: ______________

PRIORITY (Routine unless otherwise specified)
☐ ASAP ☐ STAT All tests: ☐ Yes ☐ No
If No, Specify Tests: ______________

☐ **RECURRING ORDER** (not to exceed 12 months)
Frequency: ________ Start Date: ________ End Date: ________

SPECIAL INSTRUCTIONS

FOR PHYSICIAN OFFICE COLLECTION ONLY:
Collected: Date: ________ Time: ________ By: ________

FOR LAB COLLECTION ONLY:
Collected: Date: ________ Time: ________ By: ________

Code	CHEMISTRY	DX
	Albumin/Serum	
	Alkaline phosphatase	
	ALT/SGPT	
	Amylase	
	Arterial Blood Gas	
	AST/SGOT	
	Bilirubin, direct	
	Bilirubin, total	
	BUN, Quant	
	Calcium, total	
	Carbon dioxide (CO_2)	
	CEA	
	Chloride, blood	
	Cholesterol, serum	
	CK (creatine kinase)	
	Creatinine, blood	
	FSH	
	Ferritin	
	Folic Acid (Folate), blood	
	GGT	
	Glucose, blood non-reag	
	Glycated Hgb (Hgb A1C)	
	HCG-Qualitative	
	HCG-Quantitative	
	HDL Cholesterol	
	-90 Immun. Electrophoresis	
	Iron	
	Iron Binding Capacity	
NC	% saturation requires iron & IBC to be ordered	
	LDH (lactate dehydrogenase)	
	LH (luteinizing hormone)	
	Magnesium	
	Phosphorus, blood	
	Potassium, blood	
	Prolactin, blood	
	Protein, total	
	-90 Protein Electrophoresis, serum	
	PSA, total	
	Sodium, serum	
	T4, free (thyroxine)	
	TSH	
	Triglycerides	
	Uric Acid, blood	
	Vitamin B12	
	CALCULATIONS	
NC	LDL requires Chol & HDL to be ordered	
NC	CHOL/HDL requires Chol & HDL to be ordered	

Code	TOXICOLOGY/ THERAPEUTIC DRUGS	DX
	Last Dose:	
	Carbamazepine	
	Digoxin	
	Lithium	
	Phenobarbital	
	Phenytoin (Dilantin)	
	Salicylate	
	Valproic Acid	
	Theophylline	

Code	IMMUNOLOGY (Blood)	DX
	ANA (FANA) Screen if ANA positive, 86039 titer performed, if titer >1:160 cascade performed (anti-ds DNA, ENA I & ENA II)	
	Anti-ds DNA	
	ENA I (Sm, RNP)	
	ENA II (SSA, SSB)	
	ASO screen (ASO titer if screen positive 86060)	
	Rheumatoid factor (qual)	
	RPR (Syphilis Serology), quant	
	Cold Agglutinin titer	
	Hep B surface antigen	
	-90 Hep B surface antigen OB (PHL)	
	-90 HIV	
	Mono test	
	Rubella Antibody	

Code	PANELS	DX
	Electrolytes CO_2, Cl, K, Na	
	Basic metabolic Ca, CO_2, Cl, Creat, Glu, K, Na, BUN	
	Comprehensive metabolic Alb, Bili tot, Ca, Cl, Creat, Glu, Alk phos, K, Prot tot, Na, AST, ALT, BUN, CO_2	
	Hepatic Function Alb, Bili tot and dir, Alk phos, AST, ALT, Prot tot	
	Lipid Chol tot, HDL, Trig., calc, LDL, Chol/HDL ratio	
	Gen health, Comp met, CBC, TSH	

Code	HEMATOLOGY	DX
	Hemogram WBC, auto WBC diff	
	Hemogram micro exam, WBC diff	
	Hemogram micro exam, w/o diff	
	Hemogram manual WBC diff, buffy	
	Hematocrit	
	Hemoglobin	
	Platelet count, auto	
	Reticulocyte count, manual	
	Sedimentation Rate, auto	
	WBC, automated	
	CBC, with diff Hgb, Hct, RBC, WBC, Platelet	
	CBC, w/o diff Hgb, Hct, RBC, WBC, Platelet	

Code	COAGULATION	DX
	☐ Coumadin ☐ Heparin	
	APTT	
	Prothrombin time	
	Bleeding time	

Code	OFFICE TESTING	DX
	UA, Dipstick in Office	

Code	URINE/STOOL	DX
	UA, Routine	
	UA SAVE (for possible urine culture if requested)	
	UA with microscopic	
	Urinalysis, Dipstick, Lab	
	Occult Blood	
	Urine HCG	
	Diabetic urine cascade	

Code	TIMED URINE	DX
	Hours:	
	Creatinine Clearance	
	Calcium, Urine, Quant.	
	Uric acid	

Code	BODY FLUID	DX
	Fluid Source:	
	Cell Count w/ Diff	
	Protein	
	Glucose	
	Semen Analysis	
	Semen Analysis, Comp	

Code	IMMUNOHEMATOLOGY	DX
	Blood type ABO, Rh(D) Weak D performed if Rh negative	
	Antibody Screen Identification, if positive, titer if indicated	
	Direct Coombs additional testing if positive	

WRITE-IN TESTS	DX	Lab Use

Medical Necessity Statement: Tests ordered on Medicare patients must follow CMS rules regarding medical necessity and FDA approval guidelines and must include diagnosis, symptoms, or reason for testing as indicated on the medical record. For any patient of any payor (including Medicare and Medicaid) that has a medical necessity requirement, order only those tests which are medically necessary for the diagnosis and treatment of the patient.

DX	ICD-9 CODE	WRITTEN INDICATION/DIAGNOSIS (Match Diagnosis # to Test)
1		
2		
3		
4		

LAB USE ONLY
Arterial Puncture
Venipuncture
Venipuncture MC/MA
Handling Fee
Urine Volume Measurement
-90 PKU

Chart #: ________ Date: ________
Name: ________ M/F
DOB: ________
Physician: ________

Medicare #: ________ Medicaid #: ________
☐ No ABN needed ☐ Patient refused to sign ABN
Nursing Home Part A Medicare: ☐ Yes ☐ No
Worker's Comp: ☐ Yes ☐ No
Company Account: ________

FIGURE 4-1 General Laboratory Requisition Form.

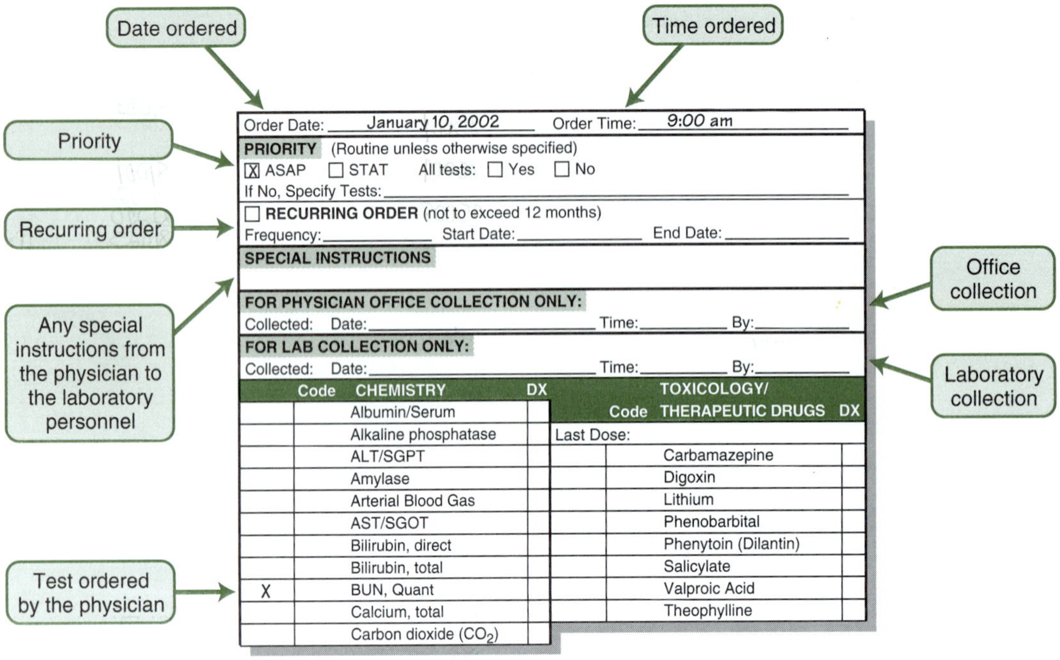

Order Date: January 10, 2002 Order Time: 9:00 am

PRIORITY (Routine unless otherwise specified)
☒ ASAP ☐ STAT All tests: ☐ Yes ☐ No
If No, Specify Tests:

☐ RECURRING ORDER (not to exceed 12 months)
Frequency: Start Date: End Date:

SPECIAL INSTRUCTIONS

FOR PHYSICIAN OFFICE COLLECTION ONLY:
Collected: Date: Time: By:

FOR LAB COLLECTION ONLY:
Collected: Date: Time: By:

Code	CHEMISTRY	DX
	Albumin/Serum	
	Alkaline phosphatase	
	ALT/SGPT	
	Amylase	
	Arterial Blood Gas	
	AST/SGOT	
	Bilirubin, direct	
	Bilirubin, total	
X	BUN, Quant	
	Calcium, total	
	Carbon dioxide (CO_2)	

Code	TOXICOLOGY/ THERAPEUTIC DRUGS	DX
Last Dose:		
	Carbamazepine	
	Digoxin	
	Lithium	
	Phenobarbital	
	Phenytoin (Dilantin)	
	Salicylate	
	Valproic Acid	
	Theophylline	

FIGURE 4-2 A physician would complete the form by placing a check mark in the blank column.

Organ- or Disease-Oriented Panels

The codes in the Organ- or Disease-Oriented Panels are grouped according to the usual laboratory work ordered by a physician for the diagnosis of, or screening for, various diseases or conditions. Groups of tests may be performed together, depending on the situation or disease. For example, during the first obstetric visit, the patient commonly has baseline laboratory tests performed to ensure that appropriate antepartum care can be given. CPT code 80055 describes an obstetric **panel** that would typically be used for the first obstetric visit. **To assign a panel code, each test listed in the panel description must be performed.** Additional tests are coded and billed separately. The development of panels saves the facility from having to bill for each test separately, and it is often more economical for the patient.

List each laboratory test separately unless the tests are part of a panel. You cannot use modifier -52 (reduced service) with a panel. For example, if all the tests in the obstetric panel were done except the syphilis test, you could not code 80055 (Obstetrical Panel) with modifier -52. You would instead list separately each of the tests that were performed with the corresponding CPT code.

Figure 4-3 illustrates the panel codes from the General Laboratory Test Requisition form. The types of codes on the form are based on the requirements of the medical facility. Not all panels are present on the form. Following each panel entry on the form is a list of abbreviations for the tests included in that panel.

Code	PANELS	DX
	Electrolytes CO_2, Cl, K Na	
	Basic metabolic Ca, CO_2, Cl, Creat, Glu, K, Na, BUN	
	Comprehensive metabolic Alb, Bili tot, Ca, Cl, Creat, Glu, Alk phos, K, Prot tot, Na, AST, ALT, BUN, CO_2	
	Hepatic Function Alb, Bili tot and dir, Alk phos, AST, ALT, Prot tot	
	Lipid Chol tot, HDL, Trig., calc, LDL, Chol/HDL ratio	
	Gen health, Comp met, CBC, TSH	

FIGURE 4-3 Panel codes.

CASE 4-1
4-1A Basic Metabolic Panel
4-1B Comprehensive Metabolic Panel
4-1C Hepatic Function Panel
4-1D Lipid Panel
4-1E General Health Panel

CASE 4-1

Identify the panel code and the meaning of the abbreviations by referring to the code description in the CPT manual. For example:

Code: 80051 Electrolyte

CO_2 carbon dioxide
Cl chloride
K potassium
Na sodium

4-1A BASIC METABOLIC PANEL

4-1A Code: ______________________

Ca ______________________
CO_2 ______________________
CI ______________________
Creat ______________________
Glu ______________________
K ______________________
Na ______________________
BUN ______________________

4-1B COMPREHENSIVE METABOLIC PANEL

4-1B Code: ______________________

Alb ______________________
Bili tot ______________________
Ca ______________________
CO_2 ______________________
CI ______________________
Creat ______________________
Glu ______________________
alk phos ______________________
K ______________________
Prot tot ______________________
Na ______________________
AST ______________________
ALT ______________________
BUN ______________________

4-1C HEPATIC FUNCTION PANEL

4-1C Code: ______________________

Prot tot______________________
Alb ______________________
Bili tot, dir (There are two separate tests represented here.)
____
alk phos ______________________
AST ______________________
ALT ______________________

4-1D LIPID PANEL

4-1D Code: ______________________

Chol tot ______________________
HDL ______________________
Trig ______________________

4-1E GENERAL HEALTH PANEL

4-1E Code: ____________________

Comp met ____________________

CBC ____________________

TSH ____________________

Now enter the panel codes onto the General Laboratory Test Requisition form in the blank to the left of the panel test name in the "Panels" section of the requisition form on Figure 4-1. When you have completed all the activities in this chapter, the superbill will have all the necessary codes and will be ready to use in several coding activities from that point on in your coding assignments.

Therapeutic Drug Assays

Figure 4-4 illustrates the Toxicology for Therapeutic Drugs section from the General Laboratory Test Requisition form. Note the location of the diagnosis number that is placed in the "DX" column. The DX is a number from 1 to 4 that identifies a specific ICD-9-CM code and a written diagnosis statement. For example, if a patient were prescribed phenobarbital for a clonic seizure disorder, the patient's blood ideally would contain a level of phenobarbital within the therapeutic drug range of 15 to 40 μg per milliliter (toxic range is about 40-100 μg per milliliter). Periodically, the physician would have the phenobarbital level of the patient's blood assessed to ensure that the level was within the therapeutic range. The physician or the assistant would complete the requisition form by placing the written diagnosis on the form, as illustrated in **Figure 4-5,** and placing number 1 after "Phenobarbital" in the "DX" column to indicate that the therapeutic drug assay was being performed because of the diagnosis of clonic epilepsy. Sometimes the physician or the assistant would also enter the diagnosis code, and in other instances the medical coder would assign the ICD-9-CM code based on the written description. The code is placed on the line that indicates the diagnosis. For example, if the physician indicated that diagnosis as clonic epilepsy (345.1), the medical coder would reference the patient's medical record to determine whether the fifth digit "0" (without mention of intractable epilepsy) or "1" (with intractable epilepsy) was documented in the medical record. *If it is not documented, the coder needs to query the physician as a fifth digit must be assigned to the code.*

It is important that the diagnosis and laboratory test correlate to ensure accurate reporting and reimbursement for services provided to the patient.

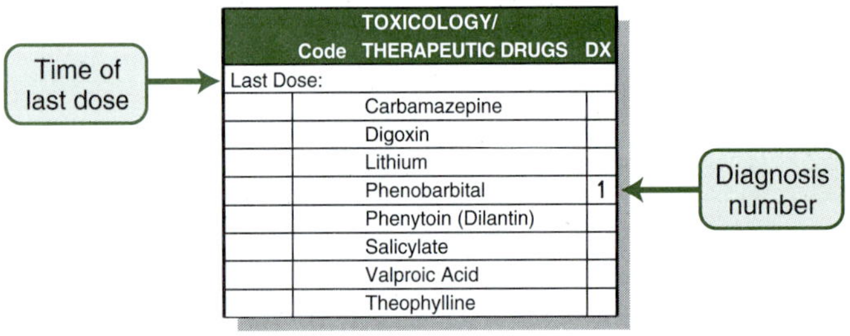

FIGURE 4-4 Toxicology for the Therapeutic Drugs section.

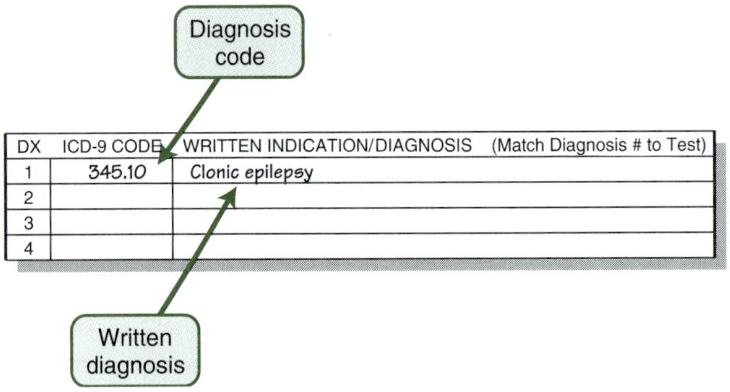

FIGURE 4-5 Diagnosis.

CASE 4-2
4-2A Therapeutic Drug Assays and Drug Monitoring
4-2B Drug Monitoring (Serum)

CASE 4-2

4-2A THERAPEUTIC DRUG ASSAYS AND DRUG MONITORING

Code the following drug assays that can be located in the Therapeutic Drug Assays subsection of the CPT manual (80150-80299):

CODE	DRUG	USED TO TREAT
1 _____	Carbamazepine, total	Seizures, neuralgia, depressive disorders, alcohol withdrawal, psychotic disorders
2 _____	Digoxin	Congestive heart failure, atrial fibrillation and flutter, tachycardia
3 _____	Lithium	Bipolar disorder, cluster headaches, premenstrual syndrome, alcoholism, dyskinesia, hyperthyroidism, mental disorders
4 _____	Phenobarbital	Seizures, hyperbilirubinemia
5 _____	Phenytoin, total (Dilantin)	Seizures, neuralgia, Bell's palsy, dysrhythmias, neuropathy pain
6 _____	Salicylate	Inflammation, pain (aspirin)
7 _____	Valproic acid	Seizures, migraines
8 _____	Theophylline	Bronchospasm

Enter the Therapeutic Drug Assay codes onto the form (Figure 4-1).

4-2B DRUG MONITORING (SERUM)

The following are drug-monitoring tests ordered on a variety of patients and the report generated in the laboratory and sent to the ordering physician. The > symbol means "greater than," and the < symbol means " less than." This patient's blood is 275, which the laboratory staff has flagged as abnormally high. The "Toxic" column indicates that for acetaminophen, any value greater than 250 (>250) is dangerous. This patient is 25 pg/ml (picogram/milliliter) higher than the top end of normal and would be contacted by the physician to adjust the amount of acetaminophen being taken. Code each of the following:

				NORMAL	TOXIC
9 _____	Acetaminophen* (UA)	275	H	10-20 pg/ml	>250
10 _____	Salicylate (serum)	50	L	100-250 pg/ml	>300
11 _____	Tobramycin (serum)	8		5-10 pg/ml	>10
12 _____	Phenobarbitol (serum)	60	H	15-40 pg/ml	>80
13 _____	Gentamicin (serum)	6		5-10 pg/ml	>10
14 _____	Aminophylline (serum) (another name for theophylline)	2	L	10-20 pg/ml	>20

*Some laboratory reports will draw the physician's attention to abnormal values with an asterisk.

The drugs are listed by their generic names, not their brand names. For example, 80162 is for the generic drug digoxin, sold under the brand names of Lanoxin, Purodigin, etc. A current copy of *Physician's Desk Reference* for drug reference will be helpful as you code drug assays.

Urinalysis and Chemistry

Many types of tests are located under the Urinalysis and Chemistry subsections of the CPT manual. **Urinalysis** codes are for nonspecific tests done on urine. Chemistry codes are used to report specific tests done on material from any source (e.g., urine, blood, breath, feces, sputum). For example, a urinalysis using a dipstick (81000-81003) would report the presence and quantity of the following constituents: **bilirubin, glucose, hemoglobin, ketones, leukocytes,** nitrite, pH **protein, specific gravity,** and **urobilinogen.** Any number of these constituents may be analyzed and reported using one code from the range 81000-81003. If the physician ordered an analysis of the urine specifically to determine the presence of urobilinogen (reduced bilirubin) and the exact amount of urobilinogen present (quantitative analysis), you would choose a code from the Chemistry subsection (84580). When coding from the Urinalysis or Chemistry subsection you need to know:

1. The identification of specific tests
2. Whether the test is automated (done by machine) or nonautomated (done manually)
3. The number of tests performed
4. The identification of combination codes for similar types of tests
5. Whether the results are qualitative (type) or quantitative (amount)
6. The methodology used for testing

Urine/Stool

Figure 4-6 illustrates the "Urine/Stool" analysis that the medical facility routinely performs. As you read the paragraphs below that refer to these analyses, place the code numbers on Figure 4-1 next to the correct test name.

A nonautomated urinalysis is performed when a dipstick or tablet **reagent** (a substance that changes color when exposed to another substance) is exposed to urine (81000-81003). The stick or reagent changes color, and that color is compared with a color chart that indicates the various levels of constitutes in the sample.

The sample may then be analyzed for any number of constituents in one reading (bilirubin, glucose, hemoglobin, ketones, leukocytes, nitrite, pH, protein, specific gravity, and/or urobilinogen). A manual (a comparison performed by a person without the aid of a machine—nonautomated) urinalysis is reported with 81000 (with microscopy) or 81002 (without microscopy). An automated urinalysis (using a machine) is reported with 81001 (with microscopy) or 81003 (without microscopy).

The "UA, Routine" on the General Laboratory Test Requisition form is an 81003 (automated without microscope) and would represent the most commonly ordered urinalysis. The "Diabetic urine cascade" under "Urine/Stool" on the form is also 81003 and is placed on the form developed by the medical facility because the physicians in the facility often refer to laboratory tests by that name. The "UA with microscopic" on the form is reported with 81001 (automated with microscope). The "Urinalysis, Dipstick, Lab" is 81002 (nonautomated without microscope). Be certain to read the full description of these codes in the CPT manual as you are placing the codes on the requisition form displayed in Figure 4-1.

The **Occult Blood** is an analysis of a stool sample to detect the presence of blood. Usually the patient takes a kit home and takes from one to three stool samples. The kit is then returned to a laboratory for analysis. Multiple samples improve the accuracy of the test. The test is reported with 82270 for consecutive collected specimens that are analyzed with a single determination. This test is sometimes called a *stool guaiac* ("gwi'ek"). Guaiac is the resin of a tree used as a reagent in tests for the presence of blood. 82270 reports only the presence or absence of blood in the stool sample (qualitative) and does not report the exact amount of blood present (quantitative).

The routine pregnancy test is reported with 81025 and is on the form as "Urine HCG" in the Urine/Stool section of the report. HCG stands for human chorionic gonadotropin and is the hormone that the reagent or strip reacts to and the presence of which indicates a positive pregnancy test.

You should now have all the code numbers for the Urine/Stool section entered onto Figure 4-1.

Code	URINE/STOOL	DX
	UA, Routine	
	UA SAVE (for possible urine culture if requested)	
	UA with microscopic	
	Urinalysis, Dipstick, Lab	
	Occult Blood	
	Urine HCG	
	Diabetic urine cascade	

FIGURE 4-6 Urine/Stool analysis.

Timed Urine

Timed urine tests are illustrated in **Figure 4-7**. The "Creatinine Clearance" is reported with 82575 and is a kidney function test. The assessment is conducted on a urine sample that is taken over a period of time—usually 24 hours—and calculates the creatinine expelled over that period. In a

Code	TIMED URINE	DX
Hours:		
	Creatinine Clearance	
	Calcium, Urine, Quant.	
	Uric acid	

FIGURE 4-7 Timed urine tests.

24-hour sample, the patient would discard the first urine passed in the day and then collect and refrigerate every void in the 24-hour period. The "Calcium, Urine, Quant" is reported with 82340 and is a 24-hour sample of urine that is analyzed to determine the amount of calcium expelled over the period. The "Uric acid" is reported with 84560 and is also a 24-hour urine sample that is analyzed for uric acid. Increased levels of uric acid are indicative of gout or increased risk for kidney stones.

Enter the codes above onto the form in Figure 4-1.

Chemistry

The Chemistry codes can appear to be the most challenging codes in all of the CPT because of the technical language used in the code descriptions. So let's start at the very beginning on this subsection so you can see that it is not really difficult if you adhere to a few simple steps. The tests in the Chemistry subsection can be from any source unless the code descriptions specifically indicate the source. Therefore, if no source is indicated in the code description, the code covers a sample from any source. An example of a code with a specified source in the code description is 82055 for alcohol by means of any specimen, except breath; 82075 is for a breath alcohol test. An example of a code without a specified source, 82003 is for acetaminophen (Tylenol), and the assessment could be used to report from any source (although the most common would be a dipstick urine test). Therefore, you should always note the source of the sample being tested before assigning a code.

The Chemistry codes are for **quantitative** assessment (exact amount present) unless otherwise stated. The alcohol tests measure not only the presence of (**qualitative**) but also the exact amount of alcohol present (quantitative)—whether the test was by blood or breath— because the code description does not state qualitative only.

The tests are listed in alphabetic order in the Chemistry subsection, and the tests are located in the CPT index by substance. For example, in the index of the CPT manual, "Acetone" is located in the "*As*" with the subterm "Blood or Urine" directing you to 82009-82010. The cross-referencing system in the CPT index is especially useful when locating chemistry tests, which are often stated in abbreviation form. For example, for BUN, you are directed by the notes in the CPT index under the entry (BUN) to *See* Blood Urea Nitrogen; Urea Nitrogen.

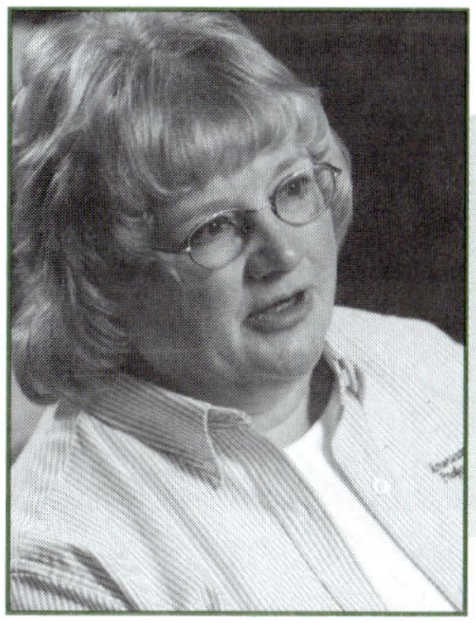

FROM THE TRENCHES

Pat

"You have to be very detail-oriented. You also have to have very strong character because you are subject to a lot of influence…there is a lot of pressure from different areas. You have to be able to take that and say, 'No, this is what we did and this is how we have to handle that.' You need to have a lot of integrity when you code."

CASE 4-3
4-3A Chemistry Tests

CASE 4-3

4-3A CHEMISTRY TESTS

Enter a code for each Chemistry test listed by first referencing the index of the CPT manual and then from the main portion of the CPT manual, choosing the correct code to place in the blank to the left of the chemistry test stated.

1 82040 Albumin, serum
2 ________ Alkaline phosphatase
3 ________ ALT/SGPT
4 ________ Amylase
5 ________ Arterial blood gas
6 ________ AST/SGOT
7 ________ Bilirubin, direct
8 ________ Bilirubin, total
9 ________ BUN, quant
10 ________ Calcium, total
11 ________ Carbon dioxide (CO_2)
12 ________ CEA
13 ________ Chloride, blood
14 ________ Cholesterol, serum
15 ________ CK (creatine kinase)
16 ________ Creatinine, blood
17 ________ FSH
18 ________ Ferritin
19 ________ Folic Acid (Folate), blood
20 ________ GGT
21 ________ Glucose, blood, non-reagent
22 ________ Glycated Hgb (Hgb A/C)
23 ________ hCG—Qualitative
24 ________ hCG—Quantitive
25 ________ HDL Cholesterol
26 ________ -90 Immunofixation Electrophoresis (*The medical facility sends the sample to an outside laboratory for analysis indicated by modifier -90.)*
27 ________ Iron
28 ________ Iron-Binding Capacity
NC % saturated requires iron and IBC to be ordered
29 ________ LDH (lactate dehydrogenase)
30 ________ LH (luteinizing hormone)
31 ________ Magnesium
32 ________ Phosphorus, blood
33 ________ Potassium, blood
34 ________ Prolactin, blood
35 ________ Protein, total, serum
36 ________ -90 Protein Electrophoresis, serum *(The medical facility sends the sample to an outside laboratory for analysis indicated by modifier -90.)*
37 ________ PSA, total
38 ________ Sodium, serum
39 ________ T_4, free (thyroxine)
40 ________ TSH
41 ________ Triglycerides
42 ________ Uric Acid, blood
43 ________ Vitamin B_{12}

Place the codes onto the form in Figure 4-1.

Code the following clinical chemistry (blood, serum, plasma) tests. Serum is the clear portion of any body fluid. For example, blood serum is the clear liquid that separates from the blood when blood is allowed to clot completely.

	06/06	**HIGH/LOW**	**NORMAL**
44 Insulin, fasting, plasma ________ (total)	2	L	5-25 μ/ml
45 Iron, serum ________	21	WNL	75-175 μ/dl
46 Iron-binding capacity ________	602	H	20-410 μ/dl
	02/27		**NORMAL**
47 Vitamin A, serum ________	10	L	20-80 μg/dl
48 Vitamin B_{12} ________	150	L	180-900 pg/ml
	04/30/XX		**NORMAL**
49 Creatinine ________ (CK) serum Male	0.6	H	0.2-0.5 mg/dl
50 Bilirubin, serum Direct ________	0.3	WNL	0.1-0.4 mg/dl
51 Bilirubin, serum Total ________	0.6	WNL	0.3-1.1 mg/dl

	12/24/XX		NORMAL
52 Thyroxine-binding globulin ________			
TBG	22	WNL	15.0-34.0 μg/ml
	07/02/XX		NORMAL
53 Prolactin, serum ________			
Male	18	H	1.0-15.0 mg/dl

Calculations

The "Calculations" section of the report located at the bottom of the Chemistry section (**Figure 4-8**) contains spaces for the physician to indicate that the technician is to calculate the LDL (low-density lipoprotein) and/or the HDL (high-density lipoprotein). This calculation does not have a separate code because it is not reported separately.

Chromatography

Chromatography is the measurement of a substance while the substance is moving (mobile phase) and while not moving (stationary phase or sorbent). Knowing about the mobile and stationary phase is important to the coder because each phase is reported separately. (For example, 82491 reports quantitative chromatography for a single analyte, with single mobile and stationary phase; however, if multiple analytes with a single stationary and mobile phase are performed, you would report with 82492.) The chemistry codes for chromatography are 82486-82492. The CPT index lists these specialized tests under "Chromatography."

Hematology and Coagulation

The Hematology and Coagulation subsection of the CPT manual contains codes based on the various blood-drawing methods and tests. The method used to do the test is often what determines code assignment. A common laboratory test is a **hemogram,** which is a graphic picture of the various blood constituencies. A **differential** is an actual count of the amount or number of the constituency. For example, a leukocyte (white blood cell [WBC]) differential would include the following constituencies:

Myelocytes
Band neutrophils
Segmented neutrophils
Lymphocytes
Monocytes
Eosinophils
Basophils

A physician would order a WBC, and the patient would arrive at the laboratory, where a technician will draw a specimen by venipuncture, finger stick, or heel stick for an infant. The blood would be analyzed and a report of the findings sent to the ordering physician. For example, a physician who ordered a WBC for a patient received the following laboratory information in the laboratory report:

WBC	01/03/02	NORMAL	
Myelocytes	2	H	0%
Band neutrophils	2	L	3-5%
Segmented neutrophils	50	L	54-62%
Lymphocytes	27	WNL	25-33%
Monocytes	5	WNL	3-7%
Eosinophils	4	H	1-3%
Basophils	2	H	0-1%

Note that the "Normal" ranges for each component of the WBC are displayed and represent the limits for a normal test result. Also, for each constituent above the "Normal" limit, an "H" is entered to indicate "high." For each constituent below "Normal," an "L" is entered to indicate "low" to enable the physician to locate quickly the constituents that vary from normal. WNL indicates "within normal limits." Although each medical facility has its own format for laboratory test results, the informational components displayed would be similar to these.

Laboratory Use Only

The codes in the Pathology and Laboratory section represent only the test performed, not the drawing of the sample. Note on **Figure 4-9** the section titled "Lab Use Only" in the lower-right corner of the form. The technician would place a check mark next to "Arterial Puncture" if the blood were drawn by means of an arterial puncture (36600); by "Venipuncture" if a venipuncture (36415) were performed and if the venipuncture was for a Medicare or Medicaid patient (Venipunctures MC/MA, G0001). Also note that there is a space to check off a handling fee if the sample is sent to an outside laboratory for analysis (99000). A urine volume measurement is reported with 81050. The PKU is a phenylketonuria, which is a urine and blood test performed in neonates to detect the presence of phenylketonuria, a genetic disease that if left untreated leads to brain damage (84030).

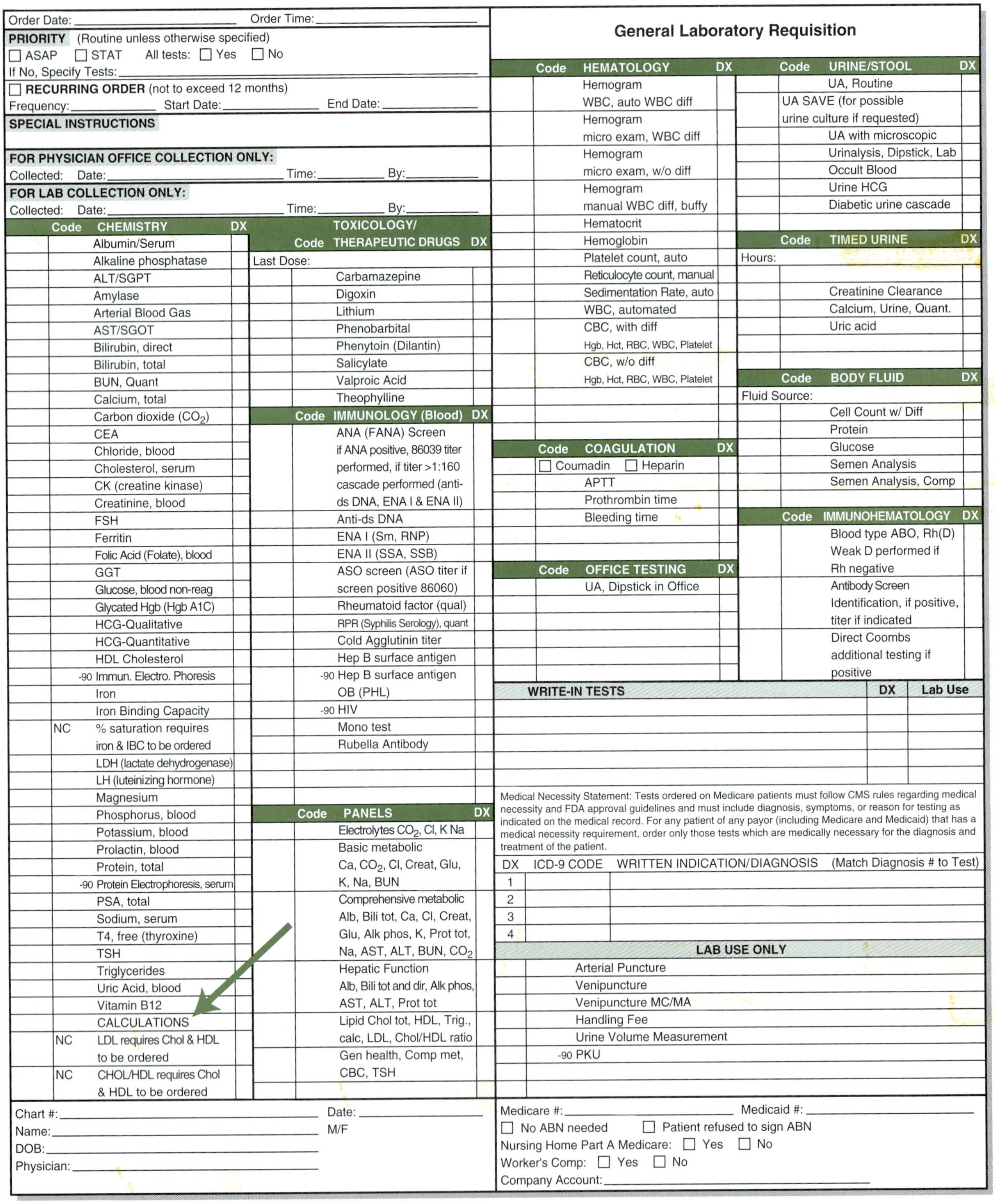

Order Date: ______ Order Time: ______
PRIORITY (Routine unless otherwise specified)
☐ ASAP ☐ STAT All tests: ☐ Yes ☐ No
If No, Specify Tests: ______
☐ RECURRING ORDER (not to exceed 12 months)
Frequency: ______ Start Date: ______ End Date: ______
SPECIAL INSTRUCTIONS
FOR PHYSICIAN OFFICE COLLECTION ONLY:
Collected: Date: ______ Time: ______ By: ______
FOR LAB COLLECTION ONLY:
Collected: Date: ______ Time: ______ By: ______

General Laboratory Requisition

Code	CHEMISTRY	DX
	Albumin/Serum	
	Alkaline phosphatase	
	ALT/SGPT	
	Amylase	
	Arterial Blood Gas	
	AST/SGOT	
	Bilirubin, direct	
	Bilirubin, total	
	BUN, Quant	
	Calcium, total	
	Carbon dioxide (CO_2)	
	CEA	
	Chloride, blood	
	Cholesterol, serum	
	CK (creatine kinase)	
	Creatinine, blood	
	FSH	
	Ferritin	
	Folic Acid (Folate), blood	
	GGT	
	Glucose, blood non-reag	
	Glycated Hgb (Hgb A1C)	
	HCG-Qualitative	
	HCG-Quantitative	
	HDL Cholesterol	
	-90 Immun. Electro. Phoresis	
	Iron	
	Iron Binding Capacity	
NC	% saturation requires iron & IBC to be ordered	
	LDH (lactate dehydrogenase)	
	LH (luteinizing hormone)	
	Magnesium	
	Phosphorus, blood	
	Potassium, blood	
	Prolactin, blood	
	Protein, total	
	-90 Protein Electrophoresis, serum	
	PSA, total	
	Sodium, serum	
	T4, free (thyroxine)	
	TSH	
	Triglycerides	
	Uric Acid, blood	
	Vitamin B12	
	CALCULATIONS	
NC	LDL requires Chol & HDL to be ordered	
NC	CHOL/HDL requires Chol & HDL to be ordered	

Code	TOXICOLOGY/ THERAPEUTIC DRUGS	DX
Last Dose:		
	Carbamazepine	
	Digoxin	
	Lithium	
	Phenobarbital	
	Phenytoin (Dilantin)	
	Salicylate	
	Valproic Acid	
	Theophylline	

Code	IMMUNOLOGY (Blood)	DX
	ANA (FANA) Screen if ANA positive, 86039 titer performed, if titer >1:160 cascade performed (anti-ds DNA, ENA I & ENA II)	
	Anti-ds DNA	
	ENA I (Sm, RNP)	
	ENA II (SSA, SSB)	
	ASO screen (ASO titer if screen positive 86060)	
	Rheumatoid factor (qual)	
	RPR (Syphilis Serology), quant	
	Cold Agglutinin titer	
	Hep B surface antigen	
	-90 Hep B surface antigen OB (PHL)	
	-90 HIV	
	Mono test	
	Rubella Antibody	

Code	PANELS	DX
	Electrolytes CO_2, Cl, K Na	
	Basic metabolic Ca, CO_2, Cl, Creat, Glu, K, Na, BUN	
	Comprehensive metabolic Alb, Bili tot, Ca, Cl, Creat, Glu, Alk phos, K, Prot tot, Na, AST, ALT, BUN, CO_2	
	Hepatic Function Alb, Bili tot and dir, Alk phos, AST, ALT, Prot tot	
	Lipid Chol tot, HDL, Trig., calc, LDL, Chol/HDL ratio	
	Gen health, Comp met, CBC, TSH	

Code	HEMATOLOGY	DX
	Hemogram WBC, auto WBC diff	
	Hemogram micro exam, WBC diff	
	Hemogram micro exam, w/o diff	
	Hemogram manual WBC diff, buffy	
	Hematocrit	
	Hemoglobin	
	Platelet count, auto	
	Reticulocyte count, manual	
	Sedimentation Rate, auto	
	WBC, automated	
	CBC, with diff Hgb, Hct, RBC, WBC, Platelet	
	CBC, w/o diff Hgb, Hct, RBC, WBC, Platelet	

Code	COAGULATION	DX
	☐ Coumadin ☐ Heparin	
	APTT	
	Prothrombin time	
	Bleeding time	

Code	OFFICE TESTING	DX
	UA, Dipstick in Office	

Code	URINE/STOOL	DX
	UA, Routine	
	UA SAVE (for possible urine culture if requested)	
	UA with microscopic	
	Urinalysis, Dipstick, Lab	
	Occult Blood	
	Urine HCG	
	Diabetic urine cascade	

Code	TIMED URINE	DX
Hours:		
	Creatinine Clearance	
	Calcium, Urine, Quant.	
	Uric acid	

Code	BODY FLUID	DX
Fluid Source:		
	Cell Count w/ Diff	
	Protein	
	Glucose	
	Semen Analysis	
	Semen Analysis, Comp	

Code	IMMUNOHEMATOLOGY	DX
	Blood type ABO, Rh(D) Weak D performed if Rh negative	
	Antibody Screen Identification, if positive, titer if indicated	
	Direct Coombs additional testing if positive	

WRITE-IN TESTS	DX	Lab Use

Medical Necessity Statement: Tests ordered on Medicare patients must follow CMS rules regarding medical necessity and FDA approval guidelines and must include diagnosis, symptoms, or reason for testing as indicated on the medical record. For any patient of any payor (including Medicare and Medicaid) that has a medical necessity requirement, order only those tests which are medically necessary for the diagnosis and treatment of the patient.

DX	ICD-9 CODE	WRITTEN INDICATION/DIAGNOSIS (Match Diagnosis # to Test)
1		
2		
3		
4		

LAB USE ONLY	
	Arterial Puncture
	Venipuncture
	Venipuncture MC/MA
	Handling Fee
	Urine Volume Measurement
	-90 PKU

Chart #: ______ Date: ______
Name: ______ M/F
DOB: ______
Physician: ______

Medicare #: ______ Medicaid #: ______
☐ No ABN needed ☐ Patient refused to sign ABN
Nursing Home Part A Medicare: ☐ Yes ☐ No
Worker's Comp: ☐ Yes ☐ No
Company Account: ______

FIGURE 4-8 Calculation section.

Order Date: ________ Order Time: ________

PRIORITY (Routine unless otherwise specified)

☐ ASAP ☐ STAT All tests: ☐ Yes ☐ No

If No, Specify Tests: ________

☐ **RECURRING ORDER** (not to exceed 12 months)

Frequency: ________ Start Date: ________ End Date: ________

SPECIAL INSTRUCTIONS

FOR PHYSICIAN OFFICE COLLECTION ONLY:

Collected: Date: ________ Time: ________ By: ________

FOR LAB COLLECTION ONLY:

Collected: Date: ________ Time: ________ By: ________

General Laboratory Requisition

Code	CHEMISTRY	DX
	Albumin/Serum	
	Alkaline phosphatase	
	ALT/SGPT	
	Amylase	
	Arterial Blood Gas	
	AST/SGOT	
	Bilirubin, direct	
	Bilirubin, total	
	BUN, Quant	
	Calcium, total	
	Carbon dioxide (CO_2)	
	CEA	
	Chloride, blood	
	Cholesterol, serum	
	CK (creatine kinase)	
	Creatinine, blood	
	FSH	
	Ferritin	
	Folic Acid (Folate), blood	
	GGT	
	Glucose, blood non-reag	
	Glycated Hgb (Hgb A1C)	
	HCG-Qualitative	
	HCG-Quantitative	
	HDL Cholesterol	
	-90 Immun. Electrophoresis	
	Iron	
	Iron Binding Capacity	
NC	% saturation requires iron & IBC to be ordered	
	LDH (lactate dehydrogenase)	
	LH (luteinizing hormone)	
	Magnesium	
	Phosphorus, blood	
	Potassium, blood	
	Prolactin, blood	
	Protein, total	
	-90 Protein Electrophoresis, serum	
	PSA, total	
	Sodium, serum	
	T4, free (thyroxine)	
	TSH	
	Triglycerides	
	Uric Acid, blood	
	Vitamin B12	
	CALCULATIONS	
NC	LDL requires Chol & HDL to be ordered	
NC	CHOL/HDL requires Chol & HDL to be ordered	

Code	TOXICOLOGY/ THERAPEUTIC DRUGS	DX
Last Dose:		
	Carbamazepine	
	Digoxin	
	Lithium	
	Phenobarbital	
	Phenytoin (Dilantin)	
	Salicylate	
	Valproic Acid	
	Theophylline	

Code	IMMUNOLOGY (Blood)	DX
	ANA (FANA) Screen if ANA positive, 86039 titer performed, if titer >1:160 cascade performed (anti-ds DNA, ENA I & ENA II)	
	Anti-ds DNA	
	ENA I (Sm, RNP)	
	ENA II (SSA, SSB)	
	ASO screen (ASO titer if screen positive 86060)	
	Rheumatoid factor (qual)	
	RPR (Syphilis Serology), quant	
	Cold Agglutinin titer	
	Hep B surface antigen	
-90	Hep B surface antigen OB (PHL)	
-90	HIV	
	Mono test	
	Rubella Antibody	

Code	PANELS	DX
	Electrolytes CO_2, Cl, K, Na	
	Basic metabolic Ca, CO_2, Cl, Creat, Glu, K, Na, BUN	
	Comprehensive metabolic Alb, Bili tot, Ca, Cl, Creat, Glu, Alk phos, K, Prot tot, Na, AST, ALT, BUN, CO_2	
	Hepatic Function Alb, Bili tot and dir, Alk phos, AST, ALT, Prot tot	
	Lipid Chol tot, HDL, Trig., calc, LDL, Chol/HDL ratio	
	Gen health, Comp met, CBC, TSH	

Code	HEMATOLOGY	DX
	Hemogram WBC, auto WBC diff	
	Hemogram micro exam, WBC diff	
	Hemogram micro exam, w/o diff	
	Hemogram manual WBC diff, buffy	
	Hematocrit	
	Hemoglobin	
	Platelet count, auto	
	Reticulocyte count, manual	
	Sedimentation Rate, auto	
	WBC, automated	
	CBC, with diff Hgb, Hct, RBC, WBC, Platelet	
	CBC, w/o diff Hgb, Hct, RBC, WBC, Platelet	

Code	COAGULATION	DX
☐ Coumadin ☐ Heparin		
	APTT	
	Prothrombin time	
	Bleeding time	

Code	OFFICE TESTING	DX
	UA, Dipstick in Office	

Code	URINE/STOOL	DX
	UA, Routine	
	UA SAVE (for possible urine culture if requested)	
	UA with microscopic	
	Urinalysis, Dipstick, Lab	
	Occult Blood	
	Urine HCG	
	Diabetic urine cascade	

Code	TIMED URINE	DX
Hours:		
	Creatinine Clearance	
	Calcium, Urine, Quant.	
	Uric acid	

Code	BODY FLUID	DX
Fluid Source:		
	Cell Count w/o Diff	
	Protein	
	Glucose	
	Semen Analysis	
	Semen Analysis, Comp	

Code	IMMUNOHEMATOLOGY	DX
	Blood type ABO, Rh(D) Weak D performed if Rh negative	
	Antibody Screen Identification, if positive, titer if indicated	
	Direct Coombs additional testing if positive	

WRITE-IN TESTS	DX	Lab Use

Medical Necessity Statement: Tests ordered on Medicare patients must follow CMS rules regarding medical necessity and FDA approval guidelines and must include diagnosis, symptoms, or reason for testing as indicated on the medical record. For any patient of any payor (including Medicare and Medicaid) that has a medical necessity requirement, order only those tests which are medically necessary for the diagnosis and treatment of the patient.

DX	ICD-9 CODE	WRITTEN INDICATION/DIAGNOSIS (Match Diagnosis # to Test)
1		
2		
3		
4		

	LAB USE ONLY
	Arterial Puncture
	Venipuncture
	Venipuncture MC/MA
	Handling Fee
	Urine Volume Measurement
	-90 PKU

Chart #: ________ Date: ________

Name: ________ M/F

DOB: ________

Physician: ________

Medicare #: ________ Medicaid #: ________

☐ No ABN needed ☐ Patient refused to sign ABN

Nursing Home Part A Medicare: ☐ Yes ☐ No

Worker's Comp: ☐ Yes ☐ No

Company Account: ________

FIGURE 4-9 Lab Use Only section.

Figure 4-10 illustrates the Hematology codes on the General Laboratory Test Requisition form representing commonly requested hematology procedures in a general outpatient setting. An automated hemogram with an automated WBC differential count is reported with 85004. When an automated blood count (hemogram) with an automated differential count of the leukocytes (WBC) is

Code	HEMATOLOGY	DX
	Hemogram WBC, auto WBC diff	
	Hemogram micro exam, WBC diff	
	Hemogram micro exam, w/o diff	
	Hemogram manual WBC diff, buffy	
	Hematocrit	
	Hemoglobin	
	Platelet count, auto	
	Reticulocyte count, manual	
	Sedimentation Rate, auto	
	WBC, automated	
	CBC, with diff Hgb, Hct, RBC, WBC, Platelet	
	CBC, w/o diff Hgb, Hct, RBC, WBC, Platelet	

FIGURE 4-10 Hematology codes.

not sufficient, the physician may order a manual microscopic review of the blood. Manual microscopic review of the blood is usually performed in one of three ways:

1. Manual differential WBC with a microscopy (85007)
2. Microscopic examination without manual differential (85008)
3. Manual differential WBC with buffy coat (a special study done when the leukocyte count is so low that the standard evaluation cannot be performed) (85009)

A complete CBC (complete blood count) is a hemogram that includes the RBC (red blood count), WBC (white blood count), HGB (hemoglobin), HCT (hematocrit), PLT (platelet or thrombocyte count), and indices (which includes MCHC, mean corpuscular hemoglobin; MCV, mean corpuscular volume; and RDW, red cell distribution width). There are two types of complete CBCs, 85025, which includes an automated differential WBC, and 85027, which does not include a differential.

Note that the hemogram codes in the 85032 to 85049 range are counts of certain constituents (i.e., red blood cells or reticulocyte) divided based on whether the test was manual or automated.

CASE 4-4

4-4A HEMATOLOGY

Fill in the hemogram code of each of the counts indicated on the Hematology section of the form as follows:

1 ________ Hemogram
blood count, auto WBC diff
2 ________ Hemogram
microexam, manual WBC diff
3 ________ Hemogram
smear, microexam, w/o diff
4 ________ Hemogram
manual WBC diff, buffy
5 ________ Hematocrit
6 ________ Hemoglobin
7 ________ Platelet count, auto
8 ________ Reticulocyte count, manual
9 ________ Sedimentation rate, auto
10 ________ WBC, automated
11 ________ CBC, with auto diff
Hgb, Hct, RBC, WBC, Platelet
12 ________ CBC, w/o diff
Hgb, Hct, RBC, WBC, Platelet

Enter the codes from the above activity onto the form in Figure 4-1.

The following laboratory tests were conducted on a variety of patients on January 21. The test performed appears in the left column, the results under the 01/21 column, an indication of an abnormal result in the "Rate" column, and the normal results for that test in the "Normal" column. Assign codes to the tests:

LABORATORY TEST	01/21	RATE	NORMAL
13 Coombs' test*			
Direct ________	N	N	Negative
14 Coombs' test			
Indirect, qual ________	P	P	Negative
15 Hematocrit (Hct)			
Male† ________	62	H	40-54 ml/dl
16 Hematocrit (Hct)			
Newborn† ________	30	L	49-54 ml/dl
17 Hemoglobin (Hgb)			
Female† ________	6	L	12.0-16.0 g/dl
18 Hemoglobin, fetal ________ chemical			
________ fetal qual	2	H	<1.0% of total
19 Hemoglobin A_2 quan ________	2	WNL	1.5-3.0% of total
20 Hemoglobin, plasma ________	4	WNL	0-5.0 mg/dl
21 Methemoglobin ________ qual			
________ quan	16	L	30-130 mg/dl
22 Sedimentation rate (ESR)			
Wintrobe test, Male ________ non-automated	4	WNL	0-5 mm/hr
________ automated			

*Coombs' test is also known as antierythrocyte antibodies (anti-RBC). **Direct Coombs'** measures the presence of the anti-RBC antibodies that are bound to the surface of circulating RBCs. **Indirect Coombs'** measures the "free" antibodies that are not bound to the surface of the circulating RBCs. The test is used to detect autoimmune anemia. As such, the negative test result (N) indicates the normal test result, and a positive test result (P) indicates an abnormal test result.

†Relates to laboratory value only and has nothing to do with code choice.

Code the following laboratory results:

LABORATORY TEST	01/21	RATE	NORMAL
23 Alkaline phosphates, leukocyte __________	58	WNL	14-100
24 Leukocytes, differential, manual __________			
Myelocytes	2	H	0%
Band neutrophils	4	WNL	3-5%
Segmented neutrophils	58	WNL	54-62%
Lymphocytes	27	WNL	25-33%
Monocytes	5	WNL	3-7%
Eosinophils	4	H	1-3%
Basophils	2	H	0-1%
25 Platelets, automated __________	150,000	WNL	150,000-350,000/mm^3
26 Reticulocytes, manual __________	33,000	WNL	25,000-75,000/mm^3 (0.5-15% of erythrocytes)

Coagulation

Many blood coagulation tests are located in the Hematology and Coagulation subsection. The codes are divided based on the particular factor being tested. Great care must be taken to ensure that the correct factor has been coded based on the information in the medical record.

The **Coagulation** codes represent frequent services to patients who take blood thinners. For example, Coumadin and heparin are prescribed to patients with conditions such as blood clots or heart attack. On the requisition form illustrated in **Figure 4-11,** the Coagulation section has a place for the physician to indicate whether the patient is currently taking Coumadin or heparin. The coagulation test is performed for that specific medication. The three assessments under the Coagulation section of the form are:

- APTT is an activated partial thromboplastin time, most often referred to as a PTT or partial thromboplastin time, and is used to assess coagulation. You can locate this test in the index of the CPT manual under the entry "Thromboplastin, Partial Time."
- A prothrombin time is a one-stage coagulation assessment using an automated device and is also used with patients who are on anticoagulation medications. You can locate the prothrombin time in the index of the CPT manual under the entry "Prothrombin Time."
- The bleeding time is measured by nicking the patient's vein and recording the amount of time it takes to stop the bleeding. This measures the platelet function or the coagulation of the blood. The physician then adjusts the patient's medication based on these bleeding times or coagulation assessments. You can locate the bleeding time assessments in the index of the CPT manual under the entry "Bleeding Time."

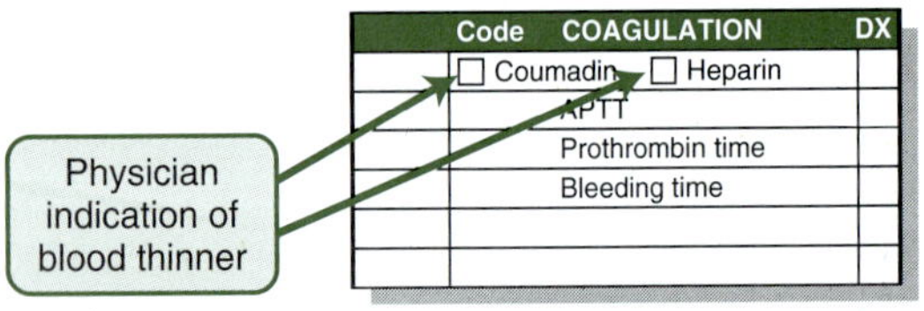

FIGURE 4-11 Coagulation section.

CASE 4-5

4-5A COAGULATION

Enter the codes for the following coagulation tests:

1 __________ PTT
2 __________ Prothrombin time
3 __________ Bleeding time

Record the codes for these coagulation tests on the form in Figure 4-1.

Code the following tests, some of which are not on the requisition form:

COAGULATION TESTS	02/09	RATE	NORMAL
4 Bleeding time (template) __________	2.32	L	2.75-8.0 min
5 Coagulation time (glass tube) __________	10	WNL	5-15 min
6 D-dimer, semiquant (Fibrin Degradation) __________	0.2	WNL	< 0.5 µg/ml
7 Factor VIII and other coagulation factors __________ (related antigen)	20	L	50-150% of normal
8 Fibrin split products (Thrombo-Welco test) __________ (paracoagulation)	8	L	>10 µg/dl
9 Fibrinogen, activity __________	300	WNL	200-400 mg/dl
10 Partial thromboplastin time (PTT) __________	29	H	20-15s
11 Prothrombin time (PT) __________	13	WNL	12.0-14.0s

Immunohematology

As illustrated in **Figure 4-12**, the Immunohematology section of the form indicates four tests that are commonly requested:

- Blood typing is identification of the patient's blood group as O, A, B, or AB. In addition, this test also indicates if there is an Rh factor present. You can locate this test in the index of the CPT manual under the entry "Blood Typing, ABO Only."
- Weak D is an Rh typing that determines whether the blood is positive or negative. You can locate this test in the index of the CPT manual under the entry "Blood Typing, Rh(D)."

Code	IMMUNOHEMATOLOGY	DX
	Blood type ABO, Rh(D) Weak D performed if Rh negative	
	Antibody Screen Identification, if positive, titer if indicated	
	Direct Coombs additional testing if positive	

FIGURE 4-12 Immunohematology section.

- Antibody screen is a test to detect a certain antibody that affects red blood cells, the presence of which may present difficulties during childbirth or blood transfusion. You can locate this test in the index of the CPT manual under the entry "Antibody, Red Blood Cell."
- Direct Coombs or a direct antiglobulin test (DAT) is used to identify the makeup of the surface of the red blood cell. The test is used to detect various types of anemia and other red blood cell conditions. You can locate the test in the CPT index under the entry "Coombs Test."

CASE 4-6
4-6A Immunohematology

CASE 4-6

Enter the codes for the following tests:

4-6A IMMUNOHEMATOLOGY

1 __________ Blood type ABO
2 __________ Rh(D) Weak D performed if Rh negative
3 __________ Antibody screen identification, if positive, titer if indicated
4 __________ Direct Coombs, additional testing if positive

Immunology

Figure 4-13 illustrates the **Immunology (Blood)** codes that deal with the identification of conditions of the immune system caused by the action of antibodies (e.g., hypersensitivity, allergic reactions, immunity, and alterations of body tissue). The tests on the form are as follows:

- ANA (FANA) screen, an antinuclear antibodies titer or a fluorescent antinuclear antibody, is a screen of the antibodies of the cell nucleus and is used as a diagnostic test for autoimmune disease, such as scleroderma or lupus. Note that an indicator is stated on the form that if the ANA screen is positive, an 86039 ANA titer should be done. If the titer is less than 1:160, another indicator, an anti-ds DNA, ENA I, and ENA II are to be performed, which are further analyses. You can locate these antibody tests in the index of the CPT manual under "Antinuclear Antibodies."
- Anti-ds DNA or deoxyribonucleic acid (DNA) antibody is a test that identifies the presence of certain antibodies that are not infectious, such as smooth-muscle antibody or mitochondrial antibody. The "*ds*" means double strand. This test is not a titer (a report on the level of the antibody) but rather a report of the presence or absence of the antibody. You can locate this antibody test in the index of the CPT manual under "DNA Antibody."
- ENA I, or extractable nuclear antigen, is an assessment of a number of antibodies that are listed in the parenthetical information of this code. The "Sm" and "RNP" are types of antibodies, but other types of antibodies may be reported with this code as listed in the code description. Each of the antibodies is indicative of certain conditions, for example, RNP is the ribonucleic protein, and the presence of this antibody is used in the diagnosis of lupus and scleroderma as well as other autoimmune diseases. This code has "×2" following it because each antibody assessment is reported separately. The physician orders the assessments (Sm and RNP) by placing a check next to ENA I. The next entry of ENA II is a second group of antigens—SSA, SSB; the physician places a check mark in the ENA II column to order assessment of these two antigens. You can locate this test in the index of the CPT manual under "Nuclear Antigen, Antibody."
- ASO stands for "antistreptolysin O" and is a laboratory test conducted to document a streptococcal infection. This test is routinely performed for patients with infectious mononucleosis or rheumatoid arthritis. There are two different ASO tests, one a screen (qualitative or presence of) and one a titer (quantitative or count). Also on the form is an indicator stating that if the screen is positive, the laboratory technician is to conduct a titer on the sample. You can locate this test in the index of the CPT manual under "Antistreptolysin O."
- Rheumatoid factor is often referred to as RF and is an immunoglobulin found in the blood of patients with rheumatoid arthritis. There is a screen code and a

	Code	IMMUNOLOGY (Blood)	DX
		ANA (FANA) Screen if ANA positive, 86039 titer performed, if titer >1:160 cascade performed (anti-ds DNA, ENA I & ENA II)	
		Anti-ds DNA	
		ENA I (Sm, RNP)	
		ENA II (SSA, SSB)	
		ASO screen (ASO titer if screen positive 86060)	
		Rheumatoid factor (qual)	
		RPR (Syphilis Serology), quant	
		Cold Agglutinin titer	
		Hep B surface antigen	
	-90	Hep B surface antigen OB (PHL) NC	
	-90	HIV NC	
		Mono test	
		Rubella Antibody	

FIGURE 4-13 Immunology (Blood) codes.

titer code. The RF test on the form is a qualitative test (presence of). You can locate this test in the index of the CPT manual under "Rheumatoid Factor."

- RPR is a rapid plasma reagin and is a syphilis test. There is a qualitative and a quantitative code. The test on the form is a qualitative test. You can locate this test in the index of the CPT under "Syphilis Test."
- Cold agglutinin is a test to assess for IgM (immunoglobulin M), which is the first immunoglobulin produced in an immune response. The presence of IgM may indicate *Mycoplasma pneumoniae*, anemia, or other conditions. There are codes for both a screen and titer. Screen is to separate from, and titer is an amount of one substance necessary to react with another substance. You can locate this test in the index of the CPT under "Cold Agglutinin."
- Hep B surface antigen identifies the presence of HBsAg, which is a lipoprotein that covers the surface of the virus that causes hepatitis B. There are two codes for hepatitis B surface antigen—one for the screening to identify the presence of HBsAg and a neutralization test, which is a further test performed when the hepatitis B surface antigen test is repeatedly positive; the neutralization test can rule out false-positives. You can locate this test in the index of the CPT under "Hepatitis Antigen, B surface."
- Hep B surface antigen OB is the same test as above, except that in the medical facility represented by the General Laboratory Test Requisition, the test for the pregnant patient is sent to an outside laboratory and, as such, modifier -90 is placed after the CPT code and NC (no charge) is indicated because the laboratory doing the analysis will submit the bill for the test directly to the third-party payer.
- HIV is a test for the human immunodeficiency virus. There are codes for HIV-1, HIV-2, or a combination code for HIV-1 and HIV-2 in one test. HIV-2 is a strain of HIV that originated in primates (monkeys). There is also a code for confirmation of HIV (86689). The code on the form is for HIV-1. You can locate this test in the index of the CPT under "HIV, Antibody."
- Mono test is a test for mononucleosis or heterophile antibody screen. There are many codes that can be used to report "mono tests." For example, 86663 reports an Epstein-Barr that tests for exposure to the virus and is called an early antigen test (EA). 86664 reports a test that is more extensive and assesses at the cellular level for the presence of the virus. 86665 reports a viral capsid antigen test (VCA) that is more efficient and is often used. 86308 is a screening test that is very inexpensive and efficient and is most often used for an Epstein-Barr virus screen. On the form in this text, the "mono test" is reported with 86308.
- Rubella Antibody is a titer for German measles, and it evaluates the level of antibodies in the patient's blood. You can locate this test in the index of the CPT under "Antibody, Rubella."

CASE 4-7
4-7A Immunology

CASE 4-7

Enter the codes for the following Immunology tests:

4-7A IMMUNOLOGY

1 __________ ANA (FANA) Screen
2 __________ Anti-ds DNA
3 __________ ENA I (Sm or RNP)
4 __________ ENA II (SS-A or SS-B)
5 __________ ASO screen
6 __________ Rheumatoid factor (qual)
7 __________ RPR (Syphilis Serology), quant
8 __________ Cold Agglutinin titer
9 __________ Hep B surface antigen
10 __________ -90 Hep B surface antigen OB, NC
11 __________ -90 HIV-1, NC
12 __________ Mono test*
13 __________ Rubella Antibody

*Mono = Epstein-Barr virus

Body Fluid

The Body Fluid section of the form illustrated in **Figure 4-14** has a selection of commonly performed laboratory tests that are done on a variety of body fluids.

- Cell count w/Diff is a cell count performed on miscellaneous body fluids, such as cerebrospinal fluid, pleural fluid, peritoneal fluid, or joint fluid. For example, cerebrospinal fluid can be analyzed for the presence of various bacteria (bacterial meningitis), such as *S. pneumoniae, E. coli,* or *N. meningitidis.*. The differential represented by the "w/Diff" is a study performed in addition to the basic cell count. The differential examination includes counting of types of cells present in the sample. You can locate this test in the index of the CPT under "Cell Count, Body Fluid."

Code	BODY FLUID	DX
Fluid Source:		
	Cell Count w/ Diff	
	Protein	
	Glucose	
	Semen Analysis	
	Semen Analysis, Comp	

FIGURE 4-14 Body Fluid section.

- The term "protein" represents a prostate specific antigen test (PSA) and is used to diagnose prostate cancer and to monitor recurrent prostate cancer. There are three different PSA tests, one for a complex PSA, one for total serum, and one for free PSA. The one on the form is for a free PSA. You can locate this test in the index of the CPT under "Prostate Specific Antigen."
- Glucose is found in many bodily fluids other than blood; for example, urine, and higher or lower levels than normal can indicate a disease condition. You can locate this test in the index of the CPT under "Glucose, Body Fluid."
- Semen Analysis is the analysis of the presence and/or motility of sperm that may include the Huhner test, which is an analysis of the sperm after intercourse. The sperm is removed from the vaginal area by means of a swab for analysis. You can locate this test in the index of the CPT under "Semen Analysis."
- Semen Analysis, Comp is a complete semen analysis that includes the volume, count, motility, and differential. This test can also be located in the index in the same location as the previous semen analysis.

CASE 4-8

4-8A BODY FLUID

Enter the codes for the following Body Fluid tests:

1 ____________ Cell Count w/Diff
2 ____________ Protein, total
3 ____________ Glucose (not blood)
4 ____________ Semen Analysis
5 ____________ Semen Analysis, Comp

Enter the CPT codes for the Body Fluid tests on the form in Figure 4-1.

Office Testing

Each medical facility will have tests that the physician does in the office rather than have the patient go to the laboratory for the test. In the medical facility represented on the General Laboratory Test Requisition, the physicians in the practice commonly have their nursing staff perform routine in-office urinalysis (UA) by means of a dipstick (nonautomated) as illustrated in **Figure 4-15**. Place the correct code for this service on the form.

Code	OFFICE TESTING	DX
	UA, Dipstick in Office	

FIGURE 4-15 Office testing.

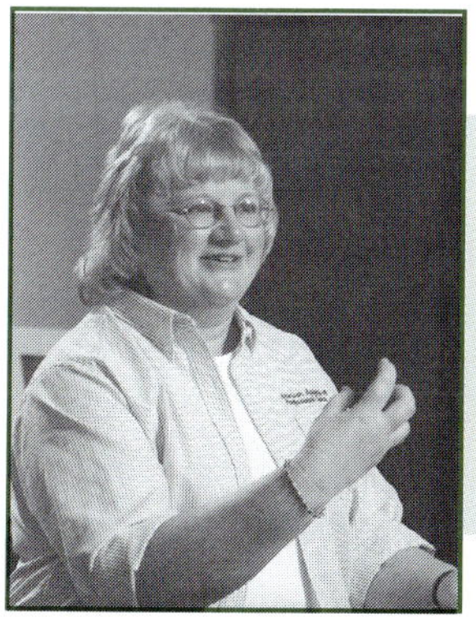

FROM THE TRENCHES

Pat

"Always have documentation, always be able to stand behind whatever you say. If you are saying something, as far as a coding rule, you better have the documentation to back yourself up."

CASE 4-9
4-9A Office Testing

CASE 4-9

Enter the code for the urinalysis.

4-9A OFFICE TESTING

1 ____________ UA, Dipstick in Office

There is no microscopic analysis with this office test. You can locate this test in the index of the CPT under "Urinalysis, Routine."
Enter the code on the form in Figure 4-1.

Other Laboratory and Pathology Services

In addition to the most commonly used laboratory codes, which are often placed on a superbill similar to the one you just coded, are the following:

- Drug testing (80100-80103)
- Evocative/Suppression Testing (80400-80440)
- Transfusion Medicine (86850-86999)
- Microbiology (87001-87999)
- Anatomic Pathology (88000-88099)
- Consultations (Clinical Pathology) (80500-80502)
- Cytopathology (88104-88199)
- Cytogenetic Studies (88230-88299)
- Surgical Pathology (88300-88399)
- Transcutaneous Procedures (88400)
- Other Procedures (89050-89356)

Drug Testing

Laboratory drug testing is done to identify the presence or absence of a drug. Testing that determines the presence or absence of a drug is **qualitative** (presence of). When the presence of a drug is detected in the qualitative test (80100 or 80101), a confirmation test is usually performed by using a second testing method; code 80102 is used to describe this test. Codes from the Therapeutic Drug Assay and Chemistry subsections are used to identify further the exact amount of drug that is present (quantitative).

The CPT manual lists the drugs most commonly tested for, although the use of the codes is not limited to the drugs listed. Modifier -51 is not used with pathology or laboratory codes; instead, each test is listed separately. For example, if confirmation tests were conducted for both alcohol and cocaine, code 80102 would be reported twice.

Diagnoses Coding in Drug Test and Drug Abuse

In the Index of the ICD-9-CM, locate the term "Test(s)." Note that the coder is directed to V codes for these tests except for the entry "Wassermann," which is a test for syphilis. The reason the coder is directed to 097.1 rather than a V code is that, as the Index entry states, this is a positive test. So, the patient presented for a blood test and the results are now known to be positive. Therefore, when reporting the services for the blood drawn and analysis of the blood, the coder would reference the Tabular for a full description of the code and then report 097.1 as the diagnosis for the test.

Now, locate the subterm "blood-alcohol" and "blood-drug," and note that you are referred to V70.4. When referencing the Tabular, the description of the code indicates "blood-alcohol tests" and "blood-drug tests." If the patient presents for a test to assess the presence or absence of drugs or alcohol, the service is reported with V70.4. Emergency departments often use this code.

Return to the term "Test(s)" in the Index. Review all of the subterms under this heading, and see that this is a good location for directions to many commonly reported diagnoses when coding laboratory services. For example, pregnancy tests, tuberculosis (Mantoux), paternity, and fertility tests.

If blood is drawn to assess the level of a therapeutic drug, such as when a patient takes Heparin (blood thinner), the diagnosis is reported V58.83.

If the laboratory test is performed as a confirmation, the patient is already known to have a more definitive diagnosis and it is that diagnosis that would be reported, not a V code for screening for the presence of a substance or condition. For example, if the patient had a drug screen to check for the presence of cocaine, the diagnosis code for the screening service would be V70.4. Upon return for a confirmation of the initial test, which is standard procedure, the diagnosis would be reported as 305.60, nondependent cocaine abuse. Turn to the term "Abuse" in the Index, and review the subterms listed there. You must *never* code directly from the Index of the ICD-9-CM and must *always* reference the Tabular before assigning a code. Using the Index is only half of the coding process, but it is the first step to locating the codes in the Tabular.

Many laboratory procedures are for conditions that are known or suspected. For example, if a patient presents to the laboratory for an insulin tolerance panel for suspected insulin deficiency, the diagnosis code would be 255.4 (Deficiency, corticoadrenal). This is another good example of how you must know your medical terminology (corticoadrenal), since there is no entry for insulin.

insulin

CASE 4-10
4-10A Drug Testing

CASE 4-10

4-10A DRUG TESTING

1. Martin Morison is a 17-year-old high school student sent to the laboratory for a routine drug screen conducted by chromatography that included multiple drugs (one phase).

SERVICE CODE(S): ____________________

DX CODE(S): ____________________

2. A confirmation of the drug screen is conducted when Martin's tests come back positive for cocaine.

SERVICE CODE(S): ____________________

DX CODE(S): ____________________

3. Alice Harnes, a nurse at the local hospital, is brought in to the laboratory for a drug screening that is to include amphetamine, cocaine, and barbiturates. Using a chromatograph, the technician conducts a test that includes one stationary phase and three mobile phases.

SERVICE CODE(S): ____________________

DX CODE(S): ____________________

Evocative/Suppression Testing

Evocative/Suppression testing is done to determine measurements of the effect of evocative or suppressive agents on chemical constituents. For example, code 80400 is reported when a patient undergoes testing to determine whether adrenocorticotropic hormone is being stimulated for production in the body. The physician may suspect that the patient suffers from adrenal gland insufficiency.

Note that following each of the code descriptions is a statement of the services that must have been provided for the code to be applicable. For example, the requirement to report 80400 ACTH stimulation panel is "Cortisol (82533 ×2)" or two cortisol tests as described in 82533. You will have to read the description for code 82533 to ensure that it is the correct test before you can report 80400.

CASE 4-11

4-11A EVOCATIVE/SUPPRESSION TESTING

1. Mary Hopewell is sent by her primary care physician to the laboratory in the clinic for an insulin tolerance panel that included five cortisol and five glucose assessments for what is suspected to be a deficiency in her adrenocorticotropic hormone (corticoadrenal deficiency).

SERVICE CODE(S): ______________________

DX CODE(S): ______________________

2. Joe Franklin is sent to the laboratory by his family physician to receive a complete pituitary panel (Evocative/Suppression test) for his suspected malignant tumor of the pituitary gland because of visual field impairment and headaches.

SERVICE CODE(S): ______________________

DX CODE(S): ______________________

Transfusion Medicine

The Transfusion Medicine subsection deals with tests performed on blood or blood products. Tests include screening for antibodies, Coombs testing, autologous blood collection and processing, blood typing, compatibility testing, and preparation of and treatments performed on blood and blood products.

CASE 4-12
4-12A Transfusion Medicine

CASE 4-12

4-12A TRANSFUSION MEDICINE

1. Jessi Welter presented to the laboratory for blood typing for a paternity test, which identified his ABO, Rh, and MN antigens.

SERVICE CODE(S): ______________________________

DX CODE(S): ______________________________

2. The blood bank technician prepares 6 units of blood for freezing.

SERVICE CODE(S): ______________________________

Microbiology

Microbiology deals with the study of microorganisms. Cultures for the identification of organisms as well as the identification of sensitivities of the organism to antibiotics (called *culture* and *sensitivity*) are found in this subsection. Culture codes must be read carefully because some codes are used to indicate screening only to detect the presence of an organism; some codes indicate the identification of specific organisms; and others indicate additional sensitivity testing to determine which antibiotic would be best for treatment of the specified bacteria. You should code all tests performed on the basis of whether they are quantitative or qualitative and/or a sensitivity study.

CASE 4-13
4-13A Microbiology

CASE 4-13

4-13A MICROBIOLOGY

1. Sally Jane Newman is brought to the laboratory by her father for a urinalysis for a bacterial culture that includes a quantitative colony count. Her pediatrician indicates a diagnosis of dysuria.

SERVICE CODE(S): ______________________

DX CODE(S): ______________________

2. Rachel Bose is sent to the laboratory by her obstetrician for a *Chlamydia* culture. According to physician documentation, the test was positive for *Chlamydia trachomatis.*

SERVICE CODE(S): ______________________

DX CODE(S): ______________________

Anatomic Pathology

Anatomic Pathology deals with examination of the body fluids or tissues in postmortem examination. Postmortem examination involves the completion of gross microscopic and limited autopsies. Codes are divided according to the extent of the examination. This subsection also contains codes for forensic examination and coroners' cases.

CASE 4-14
4-14A Anatomic Pathology

CASE 4-14

4-14A ANATOMIC PATHOLOGY

1. Grey Lonewolf performs an autopsy on a 13-year-old female who died in an automobile accident. The autopsy includes both gross and microscopic examinations and includes the brain and spinal cord.

SERVICE CODE(S): ______________________

2. The county coroner performs a forensic examination on an 18-year-old male who sustained fatal knife wounds to the chest during an altercation.

SERVICE CODE(S): ______________________

Consultations (Clinical Pathology)

A clinical pathologist, on request from a primary care physician, will perform a consultation to render additional medical interpretation regarding test results. For example, a primary care physician reviews laboratory test results and requests a clinical pathologist to review, interpret, and prepare a written report on the findings.

The two codes under the subsection Consultations (80500-80502) are reserved for clinical pathology consultations. These consultations are based on whether the consultation is limited or comprehensive. A **limited consultation** is one that is done without the pathologist's review of the medical record of the patient, and a **comprehensive consultation** is one in which the medical record is reviewed as a part of the consultative services. When either of these consultation codes is submitted to a third-party payer, it is accompanied by a written report.

These are not the only pathology consultation codes in the Pathology and Laboratory section of the CPT manual. There are also consultation codes toward the end of the section in the Surgical Pathology subsection, codes 88321-88332. These consultation codes are used to report the services of a pathologist who reviews and gives an opinion or advice concerning pathology slides, specimens, material, or records that were prepared elsewhere or for pathology consultation during surgery.

CASE 4-15
4-15A Consultations (Clinical Pathology)

CASE 4-15

4-15A CONSULTATIONS (CLINICAL PATHOLOGY)

1. Dr. Green's patient, Lonnie Glenn, was currently in the hospital when Dr. Green asked Dr. Lonewolf to consult with him on Lonnie's therapeutic drug levels. Dr. Lonewolf indicated that he provided a limited consultation.

SERVICE CODE(S): ______________________

DX CODE(S): ______________________

2. Dr. Alanda sent three slides to Dr. Lonewolf, asking him to review the slides that were prepared at the patient's hometown clinic's laboratory. Dr. Lonewolf reviews the slides and prepares a written report that is sent to Dr. Alanda. The patient has malignant primary prostate cancer.

SERVICE CODE(S): ______________________

DX CODE(S): ______________________

3. Dr. Green requests that Dr. Lonewolf provide a surgical pathology consultation during a surgical procedure for a patient with malignant primary breast cancer.

SERVICE CODE(S): ______________________

DX CODE(S): ______________________

Cytopathology and Cytogenetic Studies

The Cytopathology subsection deals with laboratory work done to determine whether cellular changes are present. For example, a common **cytopathology** procedure is the Papanicolaou smear (Pap smear). Cytopathology may also be performed on fluids that have been aspirated from a site to identify cellular changes. Cytogenetic studies include tests performed for genetic and chromosomal studies.

CASE 4-16
4-16A Cytopathology and Cytogenetic Studies

CASE 4-16

4-16A CYTOPATHOLOGY AND CYTOGENETIC STUDIES

1. A bone marrow sample is received in the laboratory with a request for a culture for a suspected generalized neoplastic disease.

SERVICE CODE(S): ____________________

DX Code:

2. A chromosome analysis for abnormalities of amniotic fluid, which included cell counts for 10 colonies and banding.

SERVICE CODE(S): ____________________

DX Code:

CMS1450 (a/k/a UB-92) used in hospitals

Surgical Pathology

A pathology department, usually located in a hospital, medical school, or outside medical laboratory facility, would analyze tissue removed from a patient during a surgical procedure, and that facility would report the analysis with codes from 88300-88309, Surgical Pathology. The clinic or other medical facility can send the tissue to an outside laboratory for analysis, reimburse the outside facility for the service, and then bill the third-party payer for reimbursement using modifier -90 to indicate that the service was actually provided by an outside laboratory. Pathology codes describe the evaluation of specimens to determine the pathology of disease processes. When choosing the correct code for pathology, you must identify the source of the specimen and the reason for the surgical procedure. The Surgical Pathology subsection contains codes that are divided into six levels (Levels I through VI) based on the specimen examined and the level of work required by the pathologist. Pathology testing is done on all tissue removed from the body. The surgical pathology classification level is determined by the complexity of the pathologic examination.

The 88300-88309 surgical pathology examination codes contain a technical and professional component. Let's look at three examples of settings and how the reporting of the examination would be handled:

1. The pathologist is an employee of the hospital, and the pathological examination of the surgical specimen was performed in the hospital's pathology laboratory. The hospital would report the professional employee (professional component) and the facility expenses of establishing and maintaining a laboratory (technical component). The professional component would be reported on the CMS1500 with modifier -26. The technical component would be reported on the CMS1450 with no modifier because the CMS1450 is only used to report the technical portion of services.
2. The pathologist is an employee of the clinic, and the pathologist went to the hospital and used the hospital facilities to perform the examination of the surgical specimen. The clinic would report the professional component on the CMS1500 with modifier -26 to indicate that only the physician portion of the service was being reported. The hospital would report the technical portion of the service on the CMS1450, again with no modifier.
3. The pathologist is an employee of the clinic and performed the surgical specimen examination at a clinic-based pathology laboratory. Using the CMS1500, the clinic would report the specimen examination code once, with no modifier to indicate that both the professional and technical portion of the service was provided.
4. The pathologist is an employee of the hospital and performed the surgical specimen examination at a clinic-based pathology laboratory. The hospital would report the professional component on the CMS1500, and the clinic would report the technical component on a CMS1500 with modifier -TC (technical component) to indicate that only the technical component of the service was provided.

As you can see from the above examples, who employs the professional and the location in which the services are provided are essential to correctly reporting the surgical pathology examination. For the purposes of this worktext, you will not be required to report the components of the surgical pathology examination codes (88300-88309). Usually the coder does not add modifier -26 because the clinic or hospital software systems automatically generate the necessary modifier to indicate where and by whom the service was provided. So, again, for this worktext and for the 88300-88309 codes only, you do not need to consider whether the service is technical, professional, or global (both technical and professional).

Level I pathology code 88300 identifies specimens that normally do not need to be viewed under a microscope for pathologic diagnosis (e.g., a tooth)—those for which the probability of disease or malignancy is minimal.

Level II pathology code 88302 deals with tissues that are usually considered normal tissue and have been removed, not because of the probability of the presence of disease or malignancy, but for some other reason (e.g., a fallopian tube for sterilization, foreskin of a newborn).

Level III pathology code 88304 is assigned for specimens with a low probability of disease or malignancy. For example, a gallbladder may be neoplastic (benign or malignant), but when the gallbladder is removed for cholecystitis (inflammation of the gallbladder), it is usually inflamed from chronic disease and not because of cancerous changes.

Level IV pathology code 88305 carries a higher probability of malignancy or decision making for disease pathology. For example, a uterus is removed because of a diagnosis of prolapse. There is a possibility that the uterus is malignant or there are other causes of disease pathology.

Level V pathology code 88307 classifies more complex pathology evaluations (e.g., examination of a uterus that was removed for reasons other than prolapse or neoplasm).

Level VI pathology code 88309 includes examination of neoplastic tissue or very involved specimens, such as a total resection of a colon.

The remaining codes at the end of the subsection classify specialized procedures, utilization of stains, consultations performed, preparations used, and/or instrumentation needed to complete testing.

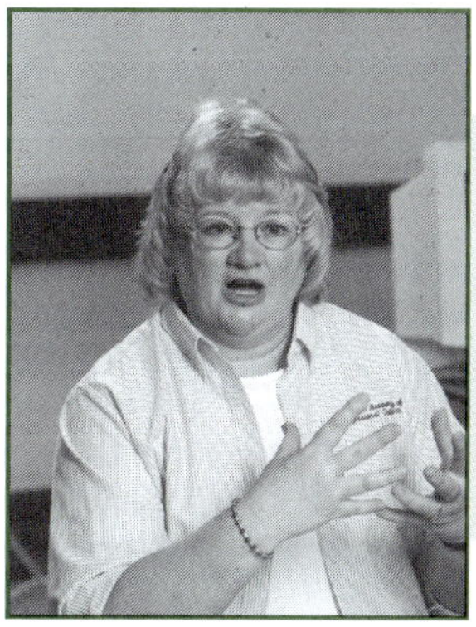

FROM THE TRENCHES

Pat

"I wish I had gotten into [coding] much earlier in my career. I think there is so much opportunity...I can't impress that enough on the people that I teach. They can go anywhere, they can do anything...It is not an 'end-all' type of thing."

CASE 4-17
4-17A Surgical Pathology Report

CASE 4-17

The following pathology report is a gastrointestinal pathology report from Chapter 7 of this worktext. Assign a CPT and ICD-9-CM code to the pathologist's service using the correct modifier to indicate that only that portion of the service is being reported:

4-17A SURGICAL PATHOLOGY REPORT

LOCATION: Outpatient Hospital

PATIENT: Jatin Al-Assad

SURGEON: Larry Friendly, M.D.

PATHOLOGIST: Morton Monson, M.D.

CLINICAL HISTORY: Polyp

TISSUE RECEIVED: Colon polyp

GROSS DESCRIPTION: The specimen is labeled with the patient's name and "colon polyps" and consists of five polypoid segments of colon mucosa up to 0.9 cm in greatest dimension. The two larger polyps are submitted in cassette 1, and the three smaller polyps in cassette 2. The specimen is submitted in toto in two cassettes.

MICROSCOPIC DESCRIPTION: Sections show five polyps showing surface epithelium and underlying glands lined by a serrated feathery surface epithelium.

DIAGNOSIS: Colon, polypectomy: Hyperplastic polyps (five).

4-17A:

SERVICE CODE(S): ______________________

DX CODE(S): ______________________

Throughout the remainder of this worktext, you will be presented with operative reports and the corresponding pathology reports to which you will assign the surgical pathology codes.

Other Procedures

Other Procedures include miscellaneous testing on body fluids, the use of special instrumentation, and testing performed on oocyte and sperm.

CASE 4-18

Report only the collection of the specimens, not the analysis.

(aspiration, duodenal) (Gastric, intubation)

4-18A OTHER PROCEDURES

1. Dr. Friendly performs a duodenal intubation and aspiration for duodenal cancer and obtains a single specimen for later analysis, which proved to be benign.

SERVICE CODE(S): ____________________

DX CODE(S): ____________________

2. Dr. Friendly performs a gastric secretory study that includes gastric stimulations lasting 2 hours for generalized abdominal pain.

SERVICE CODE(S): ____________________

DX CODE(S): ____________________

CASE 4-19

4-19A Pathology and Laboratory Section Review

CASE 4-19

Now that you have a reviewed the Pathology and Laboratory section of the CPT, it is time to combine the code laboratory tests from across the section. Code the following patient services and diagnoses.

4-19A PATHOLOGY AND LABORATORY SECTION REVIEW

Laboratory for a 60-year-old male patient with a chief complaint of heartburn with reflux (GERD):

SERVICE CODE(S)

1. *Helicobacter pylori* antibody ______________

DX CODE(S): ______________________________

Laboratory tests for a 50-year-old female patient with genital herpes simplex infection:

SERVICE CODE(S)

2. Tzanck smear with Wright stain (a special stain) ______________
3. Viral culture ______________
4. Herpes antibody testing ______________

DX CODE(S): ______________________________

Laboratory tests for a 24-year-old female with HIV screening due to high-risk lifestyle (Both the **screening** for a specified viral disease and the **problem** with lifestyle are reported with V codes):

SERVICE CODE(S)

5. Western blot ______________
6. Complete automated CBC ______________
7. ANA ______________

DX CODE(S): ______________________________

Laboratory tests for a 16-year-old diabetic male patient for confirmation of ketoacidosis:

SERVICE CODE(S)

8. Plasma glucose ______________
9. Serum ketones (ketone body, acetone) ______________
10. Electrolytes panel ______________
11. Arterial blood gases ______________

DX CODE(S): ______________________________

Laboratory tests for a 62-year-old female with hyperlipidemia:

SERVICE CODE(S)

12. Total cholesterol ______________
13. HDL cholesterol ______________

DX CODE(S): ______________________________

Laboratory tests for a 46-year-old man with impotence (organic):

SERVICE CODE(S)

14. CBC ______________
15. Thyroid (TSH) ______________
16. Prolactin ______________
17. Free testosterone ______________

DX CODE(S): ______________________________

Laboratory tests for a 26-year-old female with chronic myelocytic leukemia:

SERVICE CODE(S)

18. CBC ______________
19. Platelet count, including electrolytes ______________
20. Calcium ______________
21. Magnesium ______________
22. Uric acid/blood ______________
23. Prothrombin time ______________
24. Partial thromboplastin time ______________

DX CODE(S): ______________________________

Laboratory tests for a 6-year-old female with familial polycythemia:

SERVICE CODE(S)

25. BUN ______________
26. Creatinine ______________
27. CBC ______________
28. Blood smear ______________

DX CODE(S): ______________________________

Laboratory tests for a patient with suspected type I diabetes mellitus: Symptoms include weight loss and polydipsia. There is also a strong family history of type I diabetes. (There are three diagnoses to report here: weight loss, polydipsia, and family history of diabetes.)

SERVICE CODE(S)

29. Plasma glucose ______________

DX CODE(S): ______________________________

Laboratory tests for a morbidly obese 39-year-old female:

SERVICE CODE(S)

30. Blood glucose ______________
31. Lipid panel ______________

DX CODE(S): ______________________________

Laboratory tests for an 86-year-old male with endocarditis:

SERVICE CODE(S)

32. Sedimentation rate (automated) _______________
33. CBC _______________

DX CODE(S): _______________________________________

Laboratory tests for a 21-year-old female with endometriosis of uterus:

SERVICE CODE(S)

34. BUN _______________
35. Urinalysis (automated) _______________

DX CODE(S): _______________________________________

Laboratory tests for a 73-year-old male with Bell's palsy:

SERVICE CODE(S)

36. CBC _______________
37. Sedimentation rate _______________
38. Glucose _______________
39. Urea nitrogen, urine _______________
40. BUN _______________
41. Hepatic function enzymes panel _______________
42. Creatinine _______________

DX CODE(S): _______________________________________

43. BONE MARROW BIOPSY

PREOPERATIVE DIAGNOSIS: Amyloidosis.

POSTOPERATIVE DIAGNOSIS: Amyloidosis.

The patient was sterilized and anesthetized by standard procedure. One bone marrow core biopsy was obtained from the left posterior iliac crest with moderate to severe discomfort. At the end of the procedure, the patient did not have any discomfort. There were no obvious complications.

Pathology report on the specimen: _______________

Smear interpretation: _______________

DX CODE(S): _______________________________________

General Laboratory Requisition

Order Date: ______________ Order Time: ______________

PRIORITY (Routine unless otherwise specified)

[X] ASAP [ ] STAT All tests: [ ] Yes [ ] No

If No, Specify Tests: ______________

[ ] **RECURRING ORDER** (not to exceed 12 months)

Frequency: ________ Start Date: ________ End Date: ________

SPECIAL INSTRUCTIONS

FOR PHYSICIAN OFFICE COLLECTION ONLY:

Collected: Date: ________ Time: ________ By: ________

FOR LAB COLLECTION ONLY:

Collected: Date: ________ Time: ________ By: ________

Code	CHEMISTRY	DX
	Albumin/Serum	
	Alkaline phosphatase	
	ALT/SGPT	
	Amylase	
	Arterial Blood Gas	
	AST/SGOT	
	Bilirubin, direct	
X	Bilirubin, total	
	BUN, Quant	
	Calcium, total	
	Carbon dioxide (CO_2)	
	CEA	
	Chloride, blood	
	Cholesterol, serum	
	CK (creatine kinase)	
	Creatinine, blood	
	FSH	
	Ferritin	
	Folic Acid (Folate), blood	
	GGT	
	Glucose, blood non-reag	
	Glycated Hgb (Hgb A1C)	
	HCG-Qualitative	
	HCG-Quantitative	
	HDL Cholesterol	
	-90 Immun. Electrophoresis	
	Iron	
	Iron Binding Capacity	
	NC % saturation requires iron & IBC to be ordered	
	LDH (lactate dehydrogenase)	
	LH (luteinizing hormone)	
	Magnesium	
	Phosphorus, blood	
	Potassium, blood	
	Prolactin, blood	
	Protein, total	
	-90 Protein Electrophoresis, serum	
	PSA, total	
	Sodium, serum	
	T4, free (thyroxine)	
	TSH	
	Triglycerides	
	Uric Acid, blood	
	Vitamin B12	
	CALCULATIONS	
	NC LDL requires Chol & HDL to be ordered	
	NC CHOL/HDL requires Chol & HDL to be ordered	

Code	TOXICOLOGY/ THERAPEUTIC DRUGS	DX
Last Dose:		
	Carbamazepine	
	Digoxin	
	Lithium	
	Phenobarbital	
	Phenytoin (Dilantin)	
	Salicylate	
	Valproic Acid	
	Theophylline	

Code	IMMUNOLOGY (Blood)	DX
	ANA (FANA) Screen if ANA positive, 86039 titer performed, if titer >1:160 cascade performed (anti-ds DNA, ENA I & ENA II)	
	Anti-ds DNA	
	ENA I (Sm, RNP)	
	ENA II (SSA, SSB)	
	ASO screen (ASO titer if screen positive 86060)	
	Rheumatoid factor (qual)	
	RPR (Syphilis Serology), quant	
	Cold Agglutinin titer	
	Hep B surface antigen	
	-90 Hep B surface antigen OB (PHL)	
	-90 HIV	
	Mono test	
	Rubella Antibody	

Code	PANELS	DX
	Electrolytes CO_2, Cl, K, Na	
	Basic metabolic Ca, CO_2, Cl, Creat, Glu, K, Na, BUN	
X	Comprehensive metabolic Alb, Bili tot, Ca, Cl, Creat, Glu, Alk phos, K, Prot tot, Na, AST, ALT, BUN, CO_2	
	Hepatic Function Alb, Bili tot and dir, Alk phos, AST, ALT, Prot tot	
	Lipid Chol tot, HDL, Trig., calc, LDL, Chol/HDL ratio	
	Gen health, Comp met, CBC, TSH	

Code	HEMATOLOGY	DX
	Hemogram WBC, auto WBC diff	
	Hemogram micro exam, WBC diff	
	Hemogram micro exam, w/o diff	
	Hemogram manual WBC diff, buffy	
	Hematocrit	
	Hemoglobin	
	Platelet count, auto	
	Reticulocyte count, manual	
	Sedimentation Rate, auto	
	WBC, automated	
	CBC, with diff Hgb, Hct, RBC, WBC, Platelet	
	CBC, w/o diff Hgb, Hct, RBC, WBC, Platelet	

Code	COAGULATION	DX
	[ ] Coumadin [ ] Heparin	
	APTT	
	Prothrombin time	
	Bleeding time	

Code	OFFICE TESTING	DX
	UA, Dipstick in Office	

Code	URINE/STOOL	DX
	UA, Routine	
	UA SAVE (for possible urine culture if requested)	
	UA with microscopic	
	Urinalysis, Dipstick, Lab	
	Occult Blood	
	Urine HCG	
	Diabetic urine cascade	

Code	TIMED URINE	DX
Hours:		
	Creatinine Clearance	
	Calcium, Urine, Quant.	
	Uric acid	

Code	BODY FLUID	DX
Fluid Source:		
	Cell Count w/o Diff	
	Protein	
	Glucose	
	Semen Analysis	
	Semen Analysis, Comp	

Code	IMMUNOHEMATOLOGY	DX
	Blood type ABO, Rh(D) Weak D performed if Rh negative	
	Antibody Screen Identification, if positive, titer if indicated	
	Direct Coombs additional testing if positive	

WRITE-IN TESTS	DX	Lab Use

Medical Necessity Statement: Tests ordered on Medicare patients must follow CMS rules regarding medical necessity and FDA approval guidelines and must include diagnosis, symptoms, or reason for testing as indicated on the medical record. For any patient of any payor (including Medicare and Medicaid) that has a medical necessity requirement, order only those tests which are medically necessary for the diagnosis and treatment of the patient.

DX	ICD-9 CODE	WRITTEN INDICATION/DIAGNOSIS (Match Diagnosis # to Test)
1		Idiopathic renal stone recurrent
2		
3		
4		

LAB USE ONLY	
	Arterial Puncture
	Venipuncture
	Venipuncture MC/MA
	Handling Fee
	Urine Volume Measurement
	-90 PKU

Chart #: 1384 B Date: 01/10/0 2

Name: Mary Brown M (F)

DOB: 06/0 7/40

Physician: Ronald Green, MD

Medicare #: ________ Medicaid #: ________

[X] No ABN needed [ ] Patient refused to sign ABN

Nursing Home Part A Medicare: [ ] Yes [ ] No

Worker's Comp: [ ] Yes [ ] No

Company Account: ________

44.

SERVICE CODE(S): ______________________

DX CODE(S): ______________________

General Laboratory Requisition

Order Date: ______ Order Time: ______

PRIORITY (Routine unless otherwise specified)
[X] ASAP [ ] STAT All tests: [ ] Yes [ ] No
If No, Specify Tests: ______

[ ] **RECURRING ORDER** (not to exceed 12 months)
Frequency: ______ Start Date: ______ End Date: ______

SPECIAL INSTRUCTIONS

FOR PHYSICIAN OFFICE COLLECTION ONLY:
Collected: Date: ______ Time: ______ By: ______

FOR LAB COLLECTION ONLY:
Collected: Date: ______ Time: ______ By: ______

Code	CHEMISTRY	DX
	Albumin/Serum	
	Alkaline phosphatase	
	ALT/SGPT	
	Amylase	
	Arterial Blood Gas	
	AST/SGOT	
	Bilirubin, direct	
	Bilirubin, total	
	BUN, Quant	
	Calcium, total	
	Carbon dioxide (CO_2)	
	CEA	
	Chloride, blood	
	Cholesterol, serum	
	CK (creatine kinase)	
	Creatinine, blood	
	FSH	
	Ferritin	
	Folic Acid (Folate), blood	
	GGT	
	Glucose, blood non-reag	
	Glycated Hgb (Hgb A1C)	
	HCG-Qualitative	
	HCG-Quantitative	
	HDL Cholesterol	
	-90 Immun. Electrophoresis	
	Iron	
	Iron Binding Capacity	
NC	% saturation requires iron & IBC to be ordered	
	LDH (lactate dehydrogenase)	
	LH (luteinizing hormone)	
	Magnesium	
	Phosphorus, blood	
	Potassium, blood	
	Prolactin, blood	
	Protein, total	
	-90 Protein Electrophoresis, serum	
	PSA, total	
	Sodium, serum	
	T4, free (thyroxine)	
	TSH	
	Triglycerides	
	Uric Acid, blood	
	Vitamin B12	
	CALCULATIONS	
NC	LDL requires Chol & HDL to be ordered	
NC	CHOL/HDL requires Chol & HDL to be ordered	

Code	TOXICOLOGY/ THERAPEUTIC DRUGS	DX
Last Dose:		
	Carbamazepine	
	Digoxin	
	Lithium	
	Phenobarbital	
	Phenytoin (Dilantin)	
	Salicylate	
	Valproic Acid	
	Theophylline	

Code	IMMUNOLOGY (Blood)	DX
	ANA (FANA) Screen if ANA positive, 86039 titer performed, if titer >1:160 cascade performed (anti-ds DNA, ENA I & ENA II)	
	Anti-ds DNA	
	ENA I (Sm, RNP)	
	ENA II (SSA, SSB)	
	ASO screen (ASO titer if screen positive 86060)	
	Rheumatoid factor (qual)	
	RPR (Syphilis Serology), quant	
	Cold Agglutinin titer	
	Hep B surface antigen	
-90	Hep B surface antigen OB (PHL)	
-90	HIV	
	Mono test	
	Rubella Antibody	

Code	PANELS	DX
	Electrolytes CO_2, Cl, K, Na	
	Basic metabolic Ca, CO_2, Cl, Creat, Glu, K, Na, BUN	
	Comprehensive metabolic Alb, Bili tot, Ca, Cl, Creat, Glu, Alk phos, K, Prot tot, Na, AST, ALT, BUN, CO_2	
	Hepatic Function Alb, Bili tot and dir, Alk phos, AST, ALT, Prot tot	
	Lipid Chol tot, HDL, Trig., calc, LDL, Chol/HDL ratio	
	Gen health, Comp met, CBC, TSH	

Code	HEMATOLOGY	DX
	Hemogram	
	WBC, auto WBC diff	
	Hemogram micro exam, WBC diff	
	Hemogram micro exam, w/o diff	
	Hemogram manual WBC diff, buffy	
	Hematocrit	
	Hemoglobin	
X	Platelet count, auto	
	Reticulocyte count, manual	
	Sedimentation Rate, auto	
	WBC, automated	
	CBC, with diff Hgb, Hct, RBC, WBC, Platelet	
	CBC, w/o diff Hgb, Hct, RBC, WBC, Platelet	

Code	COAGULATION	DX
	[ ] Coumadin [ ] Heparin	
	APTT	
X	Prothrombin time	
X	Bleeding time	

Code	OFFICE TESTING	DX
	UA, Dipstick in Office	

Code	URINE/STOOL	DX
	UA, Routine	
	UA SAVE (for possible urine culture if requested)	
	UA with microscopic	
	Urinalysis, Dipstick, Lab	
	Occult Blood	
	Urine HCG	
	Diabetic urine cascade	

Code	TIMED URINE	DX
Hours:		
	Creatinine Clearance	
	Calcium, Urine, Quant.	
	Uric acid	

Code	BODY FLUID	DX
Fluid Source:		
	Cell Count w/o Diff	
	Protein	
	Glucose	
	Semen Analysis	
	Semen Analysis, Comp	

Code	IMMUNOHEMATOLOGY	DX
	Blood type ABO, Rh(D) Weak D performed if Rh negative	
	Antibody Screen Identification, if positive, titer if indicated	
	Direct Coombs additional testing if positive	

WRITE-IN TESTS	DX	Lab Use

Medical Necessity Statement: Tests ordered on Medicare patients must follow CMS rules regarding medical necessity and FDA approval guidelines and must include diagnosis, symptoms, or reason for testing as indicated on the medical record. For any patient of any payor (including Medicare and Medicaid) that has a medical necessity requirement, order only those tests which are medically necessary for the diagnosis and treatment of the patient.

DX	ICD-9 CODE	WRITTEN INDICATION/DIAGNOSIS (Match Diagnosis # to Test)
1		Thrombocytopenia
2		
3		
4		

	LAB USE ONLY
	Arterial Puncture
	Venipuncture
	Venipuncture MC/MA
	Handling Fee
	Urine Volume Measurement
	-90 PKU

Chart #: 8214J Date: 01/10/02
Name: Scott Jubelio (M) F
DOB: 08/01/64
Physician: Ronald Green, MD

Medicare #: ______ Medicaid #: ______
[X] No ABN needed [ ] Patient refused to sign ABN
Nursing Home Part A Medicare: [ ] Yes [ ] No
Worker's Comp: [ ] Yes [ ] No
Company Account: ______

45.

SERVICE CODE(S): ______

DX CODE(S): ______

General Laboratory Requisition

Order Date: ______________ Order Time: ______________

PRIORITY (Routine unless otherwise specified)

☒ ASAP ☐ STAT All tests: ☐ Yes ☐ No

If No, Specify Tests: ______________

☐ **RECURRING ORDER** (not to exceed 12 months)

Frequency: ________ Start Date: ________ End Date: ________

SPECIAL INSTRUCTIONS

FOR PHYSICIAN OFFICE COLLECTION ONLY:

Collected: Date: ________ Time: ________ By: ________

FOR LAB COLLECTION ONLY:

Collected: Date: ________ Time: ________ By: ________

Code	CHEMISTRY	DX
	Albumin/Serum	
	Alkaline phosphatase	
	ALT/SGPT	
	Amylase	
	Arterial Blood Gas	
	AST/SGOT	
	Bilirubin, direct	
	Bilirubin, total	
	BUN, Quant	
	Calcium, total	
	Carbon dioxide (CO_2)	
	CEA	
	Chloride, blood	
	Cholesterol, serum	
	CK (creatine kinase)	
	Creatinine, blood	
	FSH	
	Ferritin	
	Folic Acid (Folate), blood	
	GGT	
	Glucose, blood non-reag	
	Glycated Hgb (Hgb A1C)	
	HCG-Qualitative	
	HCG-Quantitative	
	HDL Cholesterol	
	-90 Immun. Electrophoresis	
	Iron	
	Iron Binding Capacity	
	NC % saturation requires iron & IBC to be ordered	
	LDH (lactate dehydrogenase)	
	LH (luteinizing hormone)	
	Magnesium	
	Phosphorus, blood	
	Potassium, blood	
	Prolactin, blood	
	Protein, total	
	-90 Protein Electrophoresis, serum	
	PSA, total	
	Sodium, serum	
X	T4, free (thyroxine)	
X	TSH	
	Triglycerides	
	Uric Acid, blood	
	Vitamin B12	
	CALCULATIONS	
	NC LDL requires Chol & HDL to be ordered	
	NC CHOL/HDL requires Chol & HDL to be ordered	

Code	TOXICOLOGY/ THERAPEUTIC DRUGS	DX
	Last Dose:	
	Carbamazepine	
	Digoxin	
	Lithium	
	Phenobarbital	
	Phenytoin (Dilantin)	
	Salicylate	
	Valproic Acid	
	Theophylline	

Code	IMMUNOLOGY (Blood)	DX
	ANA (FANA) Screen if ANA positive, 86039 titer performed, if titer >1:160 cascade performed (anti-ds DNA, ENA I & ENA II)	
	Anti-ds DNA	
	ENA I (Sm, RNP)	
	ENA II (SSA, SSB)	
	ASO screen (ASO titer if screen positive 86060)	
	Rheumatoid factor (qual)	
	RPR (Syphilis Serology), quant	
	Cold Agglutinin titer	
	Hep B surface antigen	
	-90 Hep B surface antigen OB (PHL)	
	-90 HIV	
	Mono test	
	Rubella Antibody	

Code	PANELS	DX
	Electrolytes CO_2, Cl, K, Na	
	Basic metabolic Ca, CO_2, Cl, Creat, Glu, K, Na, BUN	
	Comprehensive metabolic Alb, Bili tot, Ca, Cl, Creat, Glu, Alk phos, K, Prot tot, Na, AST, ALT, BUN, CO_2	
	Hepatic Function Alb, Bili tot and dir, Alk phos, AST, ALT, Prot tot	
	Lipid Chol tot, HDL, Trig., calc, LDL, Chol/HDL ratio	
	Gen health, Comp met, CBC, TSH	

Code	HEMATOLOGY	DX
	Hemogram WBC, auto WBC diff	
	Hemogram micro exam, WBC diff	
	Hemogram micro exam, w/o diff	
	Hemogram manual WBC diff, buffy	
	Hematocrit	
	Hemoglobin	
	Platelet count, auto	
	Reticulocyte count, manual	
X	Sedimentation Rate, auto	
	WBC, automated	
	CBC, with diff Hgb, Hct, RBC, WBC, Platelet	
	CBC, w/o diff Hgb, Hct, RBC, WBC, Platelet	

Code	COAGULATION	DX
	☐ Coumadin ☐ Heparin	
	APTT	
	Prothrombin time	
	Bleeding time	

Code	OFFICE TESTING	DX
	UA, Dipstick in Office	

Code	URINE/STOOL	DX
	UA, Routine	
	UA SAVE (for possible urine culture if requested)	
	UA with microscopic	
	Urinalysis, Dipstick, Lab	
	Occult Blood	
	Urine HCG	
	Diabetic urine cascade	

Code	TIMED URINE	DX
	Hours:	
	Creatinine Clearance	
	Calcium, Urine, Quant.	
	Uric acid	

Code	BODY FLUID	DX
	Fluid Source:	
	Cell Count w/o Diff	
	Protein	
	Glucose	
	Semen Analysis	
	Semen Analysis, Comp	

Code	IMMUNOHEMATOLOGY	DX
	Blood type ABO, Rh(D) Weak D performed if Rh negative	
	Antibody Screen Identification, if positive, titer if indicated	
	Direct Coombs additional testing if positive	

WRITE-IN TESTS	DX	Lab Use

Medical Necessity Statement: Tests ordered on Medicare patients must follow CMS rules regarding medical necessity and FDA approval guidelines and must include diagnosis, symptoms, or reason for testing as indicated on the medical record. For any patient of any payor (including Medicare and Medicaid) that has a medical necessity requirement, order only those tests which are medically necessary for the diagnosis and treatment of the patient.

DX	ICD-9 CODE	WRITTEN INDICATION/DIAGNOSIS (Match Diagnosis # to Test)
1		Hyperthyroidism
2		
3		
4		

LAB USE ONLY	
	Arterial Puncture
	Venipuncture
	Venipuncture MC/MA
	Handling Fee
	Urine Volume Measurement
	-90 PKU

Chart #: 1496B Date: 01/10/02

Name: Larry Blaine Ⓜ/F

DOB: 11/03/74

Physician: Alma Naraquist, MD

Medicare #: ________ Medicaid #: ________

☒ No ABN needed ☐ Patient refused to sign ABN

Nursing Home Part A Medicare: ☐ Yes ☐ No

Worker's Comp: ☐ Yes ☐ No

Company Account: ________

46.

SERVICE CODE(S): ______________

DX CODE(S): ______________

Order Date: ______________ Order Time: ______________

PRIORITY (Routine unless otherwise specified)

☒ ASAP ☐ STAT All tests: ☐ Yes ☐ No

If No, Specify Tests: ______________

☐ **RECURRING ORDER** (not to exceed 12 months)

Frequency: __________ Start Date: __________ End Date: __________

SPECIAL INSTRUCTIONS

FOR PHYSICIAN OFFICE COLLECTION ONLY:

Collected: Date: __________ Time: __________ By: __________

FOR LAB COLLECTION ONLY:

Collected: Date: __________ Time: __________ By: __________

General Laboratory Requisition

Code	CHEMISTRY	DX
	Albumin/Serum	
X	Alkaline phosphatase	
	ALT/SGPT	
	Amylase	
	Arterial Blood Gas	
	AST/SGOT	
	Bilirubin, direct	
	Bilirubin, total	
	BUN, Quant	
	Calcium, total	
	Carbon dioxide (CO_2)	
	CEA	
	Chloride, blood	
	Cholesterol, serum	
	CK (creatine kinase)	
	Creatinine, blood	
	FSH	
	Ferritin	
	Folic Acid (Folate), blood	
	GGT	
	Glucose, blood non-reag	
	Glycated Hgb (Hgb A1C)	
	HCG-Qualitative	
	HCG-Quantitative	
	HDL Cholesterol	
	-90 Immun. Electrophoresis	
	Iron	
	Iron Binding Capacity	
	NC % saturation requires iron & IBC to be ordered	
	LDH (lactate dehydrogenase)	
	LH (luteinizing hormone)	
	Magnesium	
X	Phosphorus, blood	
	Potassium, blood	
	Prolactin, blood	
	Protein, total	
	-90 Protein Electrophoresis, serum	
	PSA, total	
	Sodium, serum	
	T4, free (thyroxine)	
X	TSH	
	Triglycerides	
	Uric Acid, blood	
	Vitamin B12	
	CALCULATIONS	
	NC LDL requires Chol & HDL to be ordered	
	NC CHOL/HDL requires Chol & HDL to be ordered	

Code	TOXICOLOGY/ THERAPEUTIC DRUGS	DX
	Last Dose:	
	Carbamazepine	
	Digoxin	
	Lithium	
	Phenobarbital	
	Phenytoin (Dilantin)	
	Salicylate	
	Valproic Acid	
	Theophylline	

Code	IMMUNOLOGY (Blood)	DX
	ANA (FANA) Screen if ANA positive, 86039 titer performed, if titer >1:160 cascade performed (anti-ds DNA, ENA I & ENA II)	
	Anti-ds DNA	
	ENA I (Sm, RNP)	
	ENA II (SSA, SSB)	
	ASO screen (ASO titer if screen positive 86060)	
	Rheumatoid factor (qual)	
	RPR (Syphilis Serology), quant	
	Cold Agglutinin titer	
	Hep B surface antigen	
	-90 Hep B surface antigen OB (PHL)	
	-90 HIV	
	Mono test	
	Rubella Antibody	

Code	PANELS	DX
	Electrolytes CO_2, Cl, K, Na	
	Basic metabolic Ca, CO_2, Cl, Creat, Glu, K, Na, BUN	
	Comprehensive metabolic Alb, Bili tot, Ca, Cl, Creat, Glu, Alk phos, K, Prot tot, Na, AST, ALT, BUN, CO_2	
	Hepatic Function Alb, Bili tot and dir, Alk phos, AST, ALT, Prot tot	
	Lipid Chol tot, HDL, Trig., calc, LDL, Chol/HDL ratio	
	Gen health, Comp met, CBC, TSH	

Code	HEMATOLOGY	DX
	Hemogram WBC, auto WBC diff	
	Hemogram micro exam, WBC diff	
	Hemogram micro exam, w/o diff	
X	Hemogram manual WBC diff, buffy	
	Hematocrit	
	Hemoglobin	
	Platelet count, auto	
	Reticulocyte count, manual	
X	Sedimentation Rate, auto	
	WBC, automated	
	CBC, with diff Hgb, Hct, RBC, WBC, Platelet	
	CBC, w/o diff Hgb, Hct, RBC, WBC, Platelet	

Code	COAGULATION	DX
	☐ Coumadin ☐ Heparin	
	APTT	
	Prothrombin time	
	Bleeding time	

Code	OFFICE TESTING	DX
	UA, Dipstick in Office	

Code	URINE/STOOL	DX
X	UA, Routine	
	UA SAVE (for possible urine culture if requested)	
	UA with microscopic	
	Urinalysis, Dipstick, Lab	
	Occult Blood	
	Urine HCG	
	Diabetic urine cascade	

Code	TIMED URINE	DX
	Hours:	
	Creatinine Clearance	
	Calcium, Urine, Quant.	
	Uric acid	

Code	BODY FLUID	DX
	Fluid Source:	
	Cell Count w/o Diff	
	Protein	
	Glucose	
	Semen Analysis	
	Semen Analysis, Comp	

Code	IMMUNOHEMATOLOGY	DX
	Blood type ABO, Rh(D) Weak D performed if Rh negative	
	Antibody Screen Identification, if positive, titer if indicated	
	Direct Coombs additional testing if positive	

WRITE-IN TESTS	DX	Lab Use

Medical Necessity Statement: Tests ordered on Medicare patients must follow CMS rules regarding medical necessity and FDA approval guidelines and must include diagnosis, symptoms, or reason for testing as indicated on the medical record. For any patient of any payor (including Medicare and Medicaid) that has a medical necessity requirement, order only those tests which are medically necessary for the diagnosis and treatment of the patient.

DX	ICD-9 CODE	WRITTEN INDICATION/DIAGNOSIS (Match Diagnosis # to Test)
1		Osteoporosis
2		
3		
4		

	LAB USE ONLY
	Arterial Puncture
	Venipuncture
	Venipuncture MC/MA
	Handling Fee
	Urine Volume Measurement
	-90 PKU

Chart #: 4920C Date: 01/10/02

Name: Alma Covett M/F (F circled)

DOB: 06/09/40

Physician: Leslie Alanda, MD

Medicare #: __________ Medicaid #: __________

☒ No ABN needed ☐ Patient refused to sign ABN

Nursing Home Part A Medicare: ☐ Yes ☐ No

Worker's Comp: ☐ Yes ☐ No

Company Account: __________

47.

SERVICE CODE(S): ______________________

DX CODE(S): ______________________

General Laboratory Requisition

Order Date: ______________ Order Time: ______________

PRIORITY (Routine unless otherwise specified)

[X] ASAP [ ] STAT All tests: [ ] Yes [ ] No

If No, Specify Tests: ______________

[ ] **RECURRING ORDER** (not to exceed 12 months)

Frequency: ________ Start Date: ________ End Date: ________

SPECIAL INSTRUCTIONS

FOR PHYSICIAN OFFICE COLLECTION ONLY:

Collected: Date: ________ Time: ________ By: ________

FOR LAB COLLECTION ONLY:

Collected: Date: ________ Time: ________ By: ________

Code	CHEMISTRY	DX
	Albumin/Serum	
	Alkaline phosphatase	
	ALT/SGPT	
	Amylase	
	Arterial Blood Gas	
	AST/SGOT	
	Bilirubin, direct	
	Bilirubin, total	
	BUN, Quant	
	Calcium, total	
	Carbon dioxide (CO_2)	
	CEA	
	Chloride, blood	
	Cholesterol, serum	
	CK (creatine kinase)	
	Creatinine, blood	
	FSH	
	Ferritin	
	Folic Acid (Folate), blood	
	GGT	
	Glucose, blood non-reag	
	Glycated Hgb (Hgb A1C)	
	HCG-Qualitative	
	HCG-Quantitative	
	HDL Cholesterol	
	-90 Immun. Electrophoresis	
	Iron	
	Iron Binding Capacity	
NC	% saturation requires iron & IBC to be ordered	
	LDH (lactate dehydrogenase)	
	LH (luteinizing hormone)	
	Magnesium	
	Phosphorus, blood	
	Potassium, blood	
	Prolactin, blood	
	Protein, total	
	-90 Protein Electrophoresis, serum	
	PSA, total	
	Sodium, serum	
	T4, free (thyroxine)	
	TSH	
	Triglycerides	
	Uric Acid, blood	
	Vitamin B12	
	CALCULATIONS	
NC	LDL requires Chol & HDL to be ordered	
NC	CHOL/HDL requires Chol & HDL to be ordered	

TOXICOLOGY/ THERAPEUTIC DRUGS

Last Dose:

Code	TOXICOLOGY/ THERAPEUTIC DRUGS	DX
	Carbamazepine	
	Digoxin	
	Lithium	
	Phenobarbital	
	Phenytoin (Dilantin)	
	Salicylate	
	Valproic Acid	
	Theophylline	

Code	IMMUNOLOGY (Blood)	DX
	ANA (FANA) Screen if ANA positive, 86039 titer performed, if titer >1:160 cascade performed (anti-ds DNA, ENA I & ENA II)	
	Anti-ds DNA	
	ENA I (Sm, RNP)	
	ENA II (SSA, SSB)	
	ASO screen (ASO titer if screen positive 86060)	
	Rheumatoid factor (qual)	
X	RPR (Syphilis Serology), quant	
	Cold Agglutinin titer	
	Hep B surface antigen	
	-90 Hep B surface antigen OB (PHL)	
	-90 HIV	
	Mono test	
	Rubella Antibody	

Code	PANELS	DX
	Electrolytes CO_2, Cl, K, Na	
	Basic metabolic Ca, CO_2, Cl, Creat, Glu, K, Na, BUN	
	Comprehensive metabolic Alb, Bili tot, Ca, Cl, Creat, Glu, Alk phos, K, Prot tot, Na, AST, ALT, BUN, CO_2	
	Hepatic Function Alb, Bili tot and dir, Alk phos, AST, ALT, Prot tot	
X	Lipid Chol tot, HDL, Trig., calc, LDL, Chol/HDL ratio	
	Gen health, Comp met, CBC, TSH	

Code	HEMATOLOGY	DX
	Hemogram WBC, auto WBC diff	
	Hemogram micro exam, WBC diff	
	Hemogram micro exam, w/o diff	
	Hemogram manual WBC diff, buffy	
	Hematocrit	
	Hemoglobin	
	Platelet count, auto	
	Reticulocyte count, manual	
	Sedimentation Rate, auto	
	WBC, automated	
	CBC, with diff Hgb, Hct, RBC, WBC, Platelet	
	CBC, w/o diff Hgb, Hct, RBC, WBC, Platelet	

Code	COAGULATION	DX
	[ ] Coumadin [ ] Heparin	
	APTT	
	Prothrombin time	
	Bleeding time	

Code	OFFICE TESTING	DX
	UA, Dipstick in Office	

Code	URINE/STOOL	DX
	UA, Routine	
	UA SAVE (for possible urine culture if requested)	
	UA with microscopic	
	Urinalysis, Dipstick, Lab	
	Occult Blood	
	Urine HCG	
	Diabetic urine cascade	

TIMED URINE

Hours:

Code	TIMED URINE	DX
	Creatinine Clearance	
	Calcium, Urine, Quant.	
	Uric acid	

BODY FLUID

Fluid Source:

Code	BODY FLUID	DX
	Cell Count w/o Diff	
	Protein	
	Glucose	
	Semen Analysis	
	Semen Analysis, Comp	

Code	IMMUNOHEMATOLOGY	DX
	Blood type ABO, Rh(D) Weak D performed if Rh negative	
	Antibody Screen Identification, if positive, titer if indicated	
	Direct Coombs additional testing if positive	

WRITE-IN TESTS	DX	Lab Use

Medical Necessity Statement: Tests ordered on Medicare patients must follow CMS rules regarding medical necessity and FDA approval guidelines and must include diagnosis, symptoms, or reason for testing as indicated on the medical record. For any patient of any payor (including Medicare and Medicaid) that has a medical necessity requirement, order only those tests which are medically necessary for the diagnosis and treatment of the patient.

DX	ICD-9 CODE	WRITTEN INDICATION/DIAGNOSIS (Match Diagnosis # to Test)
1		Meniere's Disease
2		
3		
4		

	LAB USE ONLY
	Arterial Puncture
	Venipuncture
	Venipuncture MC/MA
	Handling Fee
	Urine Volume Measurement
	-90 PKU

Chart #: 2346B Date: 01/10/02

Name: Peter Bartlett (M) F

DOB: 04/04/47

Physician: Ronald Green, MD

Medicare #: ________ Medicaid #: ________

[X] No ABN needed [ ] Patient refused to sign ABN

Nursing Home Part A Medicare: [ ] Yes [ ] No

Worker's Comp: [ ] Yes [ ] No

Company Account: ________

48.

SERVICE CODE(S): ______________________

DX CODE(S): ______________________

General Laboratory Requisition

Order Date: ____ Order Time: ____

PRIORITY (Routine unless otherwise specified)
[X] ASAP [ ] STAT All tests: [ ] Yes [ ] No
If No, Specify Tests: ____

[ ] **RECURRING ORDER** (not to exceed 12 months)
Frequency: ____ Start Date: ____ End Date: ____

SPECIAL INSTRUCTIONS

FOR PHYSICIAN OFFICE COLLECTION ONLY:
Collected: Date: ____ Time: ____ By: ____

FOR LAB COLLECTION ONLY:
Collected: Date: ____ Time: ____ By: ____

Code	CHEMISTRY	DX
	Albumin/Serum	
	Alkaline phosphatase	
	ALT/SGPT	
	Amylase	
	Arterial Blood Gas	
	AST/SGOT	
	Bilirubin, direct	
	Bilirubin, total	
	BUN, Quant	
	Calcium, total	
	Carbon dioxide (CO_2)	
	CEA	
	Chloride, blood	
	Cholesterol, serum	
	CK (creatine kinase)	
	Creatinine, blood	
	FSH	
	Ferritin	
	Folic Acid (Folate), blood	
	GGT	
	Glucose, blood non-reag	
	Glycated Hgb (Hgb A1C)	
	HCG-Qualitative	
	HCG-Quantitative	
	HDL Cholesterol	
	-90 Immun. Electrophoresis	
	Iron	
	Iron Binding Capacity	
	NC % saturation requires iron & IBC to be ordered	
	LDH (lactate dehydrogenase)	
	LH (luteinizing hormone)	
	Magnesium	
	Phosphorus, blood	
	Potassium, blood	
	Prolactin, blood	
	Protein, total	
	-90 Protein Electrophoresis, serum	
X	PSA, total	
	Sodium, serum	
	T4, free (thyroxine)	
	TSH	
	Triglycerides	
	Uric Acid, blood	
	Vitamin B12	
	CALCULATIONS	
	NC LDL requires Chol & HDL to be ordered	
	NC CHOL/HDL requires Chol & HDL to be ordered	

Code	TOXICOLOGY/ THERAPEUTIC DRUGS	DX
	Last Dose:	
	Carbamazepine	
	Digoxin	
	Lithium	
	Phenobarbital	
	Phenytoin (Dilantin)	
	Salicylate	
	Valproic Acid	
	Theophylline	

Code	IMMUNOLOGY (Blood)	DX
	ANA (FANA) Screen if ANA positive, 86039 titer performed, if titer >1:160 cascade performed (anti-ds DNA, ENA I & ENA II)	
	Anti-ds DNA	
	ENA I (Sm, RNP)	
	ENA II (SSA, SSB)	
	ASO screen (ASO titer if screen positive 86060)	
	Rheumatoid factor (qual)	
	RPR (Syphilis Serology), quant	
	Cold Agglutinin titer	
	Hep B surface antigen	
	-90 Hep B surface antigen OB (PHL)	
	-90 HIV	
	Mono test	
	Rubella Antibody	

Code	PANELS	DX
	Electrolytes CO_2, Cl, K, Na	
	Basic metabolic Ca, CO_2, Cl, Creat, Glu, K, Na, BUN	
	Comprehensive metabolic Alb, Bili tot, Ca, Cl, Creat, Glu, Alk phos, K, Prot tot, Na, AST, ALT, BUN, CO_2	
	Hepatic Function Alb, Bili tot and dir, Alk phos, AST, ALT, Prot tot	
	Lipid Chol tot, HDL, Trig., calc, LDL, Chol/HDL ratio	
	Gen health, Comp met, CBC, TSH	

Code	HEMATOLOGY	DX
	Hemogram WBC, auto WBC diff	
	Hemogram micro exam, WBC diff	
X	Hemogram micro exam, w/o diff	
	Hemogram manual WBC diff, buffy	
	Hematocrit	
	Hemoglobin	
	Platelet count, auto	
	Reticulocyte count, manual	
	Sedimentation Rate, auto	
	WBC, automated	
	CBC, with diff Hgb, Hct, RBC, WBC, Platelet	
	CBC, w/o diff Hgb, Hct, RBC, WBC, Platelet	

Code	COAGULATION	DX
	[ ] Coumadin [ ] Heparin	
	APTT	
	Prothrombin time	
	Bleeding time	

Code	OFFICE TESTING	DX
	UA, Dipstick in Office	

Code	URINE/STOOL	DX
	UA, Routine	
	UA SAVE (for possible urine culture if requested)	
	UA with microscopic	
	Urinalysis, Dipstick, Lab	
	Occult Blood	
	Urine HCG	
	Diabetic urine cascade	

Code	TIMED URINE	DX
	Hours:	
	Creatinine Clearance	
	Calcium, Urine, Quant.	
	Uric acid	

Code	BODY FLUID	DX
	Fluid Source:	
	Cell Count w/o Diff	
	Protein	
	Glucose	
	Semen Analysis	
	Semen Analysis, Comp	

Code	IMMUNOHEMATOLOGY	DX
	Blood type ABO, Rh(D) Weak D performed if Rh negative	
	Antibody Screen Identification, if positive, titer if indicated	
	Direct Coombs additional testing if positive	

WRITE-IN TESTS	DX	Lab Use

Medical Necessity Statement: Tests ordered on Medicare patients must follow CMS rules regarding medical necessity and FDA approval guidelines and must include diagnosis, symptoms, or reason for testing as indicated on the medical record. For any patient of any payor (including Medicare and Medicaid) that has a medical necessity requirement, order only those tests which are medically necessary for the diagnosis and treatment of the patient.

DX	ICD-9 CODE	WRITTEN INDICATION/DIAGNOSIS (Match Diagnosis # to Test)
1		Prostatitis, acute
2		
3		
4		

	LAB USE ONLY
	Arterial Puncture
	Venipuncture
	Venipuncture MC/MA
	Handling Fee
	Urine Volume Measurement
	-90 PKU

Chart #: 6498 B Date: 01/10/0 2
Name: Loren Brown (M)/F
DOB: 01/30/56
Physician: Ronald Green, MD

Medicare #: ____ Medicaid #: ____
[X] No ABN needed [ ] Patient refused to sign ABN
Nursing Home Part A Medicare: [ ] Yes [ ] No
Worker's Comp: [ ] Yes [ ] No
Company Account: ____

49.

SERVICE CODE(S): ____________________

DX CODE(S): ____________________

Order Date: ______ Order Time: ______

PRIORITY (Routine unless otherwise specified)

☒ ASAP ☐ STAT All tests: ☐ Yes ☐ No

If No, Specify Tests: ______

☐ **RECURRING ORDER** (not to exceed 12 months)

Frequency: ______ Start Date: ______ End Date: ______

SPECIAL INSTRUCTIONS

FOR PHYSICIAN OFFICE COLLECTION ONLY:

Collected: Date: ______ Time: ______ By: ______

FOR LAB COLLECTION ONLY:

Collected: Date: ______ Time: ______ By: ______

General Laboratory Requisition

Code	CHEMISTRY	DX
	Albumin/Serum	
	Alkaline phosphatase	
	ALT/SGPT	
	Amylase	
	Arterial Blood Gas	
	AST/SGOT	
	Bilirubin, direct	
	Bilirubin, total	
	BUN, Quant	
	Calcium, total	
	Carbon dioxide (CO_2)	
	CEA	
	Chloride, blood	
	Cholesterol, serum	
	CK (creatine kinase)	
	Creatinine, blood	
X	FSH	
	Ferritin	
	Folic Acid (Folate), blood	
	GGT	
	Glucose, blood non-reag	
	Glycated Hgb (Hgb A1C)	
	HCG-Qualitative	
	HCG-Quantitative	
	HDL Cholesterol	
	-90 Immun. Electrophoresis	
	Iron	
	Iron Binding Capacity	
NC	% saturation requires iron & IBC to be ordered	
	LDH (lactate dehydrogenase)	
X	LH (luteinizing hormone)	
	Magnesium	
	Phosphorus, blood	
	Potassium, blood	
	Prolactin, blood	
	Protein, total	
	-90 Protein Electrophoresis, serum	
	PSA, total	
	Sodium, serum	
X	T4, free (thyroxine)	
X	TSH	
	Triglycerides	
	Uric Acid, blood	
	Vitamin B12	
	CALCULATIONS	
NC	LDL requires Chol & HDL to be ordered	
NC	CHOL/HDL requires Chol & HDL to be ordered	

Code	TOXICOLOGY/ THERAPEUTIC DRUGS	DX
	Last Dose:	
	Carbamazepine	
	Digoxin	
	Lithium	
	Phenobarbital	
	Phenytoin (Dilantin)	
	Salicylate	
	Valproic Acid	
	Theophylline	

Code	IMMUNOLOGY (Blood)	DX
	ANA (FANA) Screen if ANA positive, 86039 titer performed, if titer >1:160 cascade performed (anti-ds DNA, ENA I & ENA II)	
	Anti-ds DNA	
	ENA I (Sm, RNP)	
	ENA II (SSA, SSB)	
	ASO screen (ASO titer if screen positive 86060)	
	Rheumatoid factor (qual)	
	RPR (Syphilis Serology), quant	
	Cold Agglutinin titer	
	Hep B surface antigen	
	-90 Hep B surface antigen OB (PHL)	
	-90 HIV	
	Mono test	
	Rubella Antibody	

Code	PANELS	DX
	Electrolytes CO_2, Cl, K, Na	
	Basic metabolic Ca, CO_2, Cl, Creat, Glu, K, Na, BUN	
	Comprehensive metabolic Alb, Bili tot, Ca, Cl, Creat, Glu, Alk phos, K, Prot tot, Na, AST, ALT, BUN, CO_2	
	Hepatic Function Alb, Bili tot and dir, Alk phos, AST, ALT, Prot tot	
	Lipid Chol tot, HDL, Trig., calc, LDL, Chol/HDL ratio	
	Gen health, Comp met, CBC, TSH	

Code	HEMATOLOGY	DX
	Hemogram WBC, auto WBC diff	
	Hemogram micro exam, WBC diff	
	Hemogram micro exam, w/o diff	
	Hemogram manual WBC diff, buffy	
	Hematocrit	
	Hemoglobin	
	Platelet count, auto	
	Reticulocyte count, manual	
	Sedimentation Rate, auto	
	WBC, automated	
	CBC, with diff Hgb, Hct, RBC, WBC, Platelet	
	CBC, w/o diff Hgb, Hct, RBC, WBC, Platelet	

Code	COAGULATION	DX
	☐ Coumadin ☐ Heparin	
	APTT	
	Prothrombin time	
	Bleeding time	

Code	OFFICE TESTING	DX
	UA, Dipstick in Office	

Code	URINE/STOOL	DX
	UA, Routine	
	UA SAVE (for possible urine culture if requested)	
	UA with microscopic	
	Urinalysis, Dipstick, Lab	
	Occult Blood	
	Urine HCG	
	Diabetic urine cascade	

Code	TIMED URINE	DX
	Hours:	
	Creatinine Clearance	
	Calcium, Urine, Quant.	
	Uric acid	

Code	BODY FLUID	DX
	Fluid Source:	
	Cell Count w/o Diff	
	Protein	
	Glucose	
	Semen Analysis	
	Semen Analysis, Comp	

Code	IMMUNOHEMATOLOGY	DX
	Blood type ABO, Rh(D) Weak D performed if Rh negative	
	Antibody Screen Identification, if positive, titer if indicated	
	Direct Coombs additional testing if positive	

WRITE-IN TESTS	DX	Lab Use

Medical Necessity Statement: Tests ordered on Medicare patients must follow CMS rules regarding medical necessity and FDA approval guidelines and must include diagnosis, symptoms, or reason for testing as indicated on the medical record. For any patient of any payor (including Medicare and Medicaid) that has a medical necessity requirement, order only those tests which are medically necessary for the diagnosis and treatment of the patient.

DX	ICD-9 CODE	WRITTEN INDICATION/DIAGNOSIS (Match Diagnosis # to Test)
1		Hyperprolactinemia
2		
3		
4		

	LAB USE ONLY
	Arterial Puncture
	Venipuncture
	Venipuncture MC/MA
	Handling Fee
	Urine Volume Measurement
	-90 PKU

Chart #: 6241E Date: 01/10/02

Name: Manly Edwards Ⓜ/F

DOB: 07/04/33

Physician: Ronald Green, MD

Medicare #: ______ Medicaid #: ______

☒ No ABN needed ☐ Patient refused to sign ABN

Nursing Home Part A Medicare: ☐ Yes ☐ No

Worker's Comp: ☐ Yes ☐ No

Company Account: ______

50.

SERVICE CODE(S): ______

DX CODE(S): ______

Order Date: ____________ Order Time: ____________

PRIORITY (Routine unless otherwise specified)

☒ ASAP ☐ STAT All tests: ☐ Yes ☐ No

If No, Specify Tests: ____________

☐ **RECURRING ORDER** (not to exceed 12 months)

Frequency: ________ Start Date: ________ End Date: ________

SPECIAL INSTRUCTIONS

FOR PHYSICIAN OFFICE COLLECTION ONLY:

Collected: Date: ________ Time: ________ By: ________

FOR LAB COLLECTION ONLY:

Collected: Date: ________ Time: ________ By: ________

General Laboratory Requisition

Code	CHEMISTRY	DX
	Albumin/Serum	
	Alkaline phosphatase	
	ALT/SGPT	
	Amylase	
	Arterial Blood Gas	
	AST/SGOT	
	Bilirubin, direct	
	Bilirubin, total	
X	BUN, Quant	
	Calcium, total	
	Carbon dioxide (CO_2)	
	CEA	
	Chloride, blood	
	Cholesterol, serum	
	CK (creatine kinase)	
X	Creatinine, blood	
	FSH	
	Ferritin	
	Folic Acid (Folate), blood	
	GGT	
	Glucose, blood non-reag	
	Glycated Hgb (Hgb A1C)	
	HCG-Qualitative	
	HCG-Quantitative	
	HDL Cholesterol	
	-90 Immun. Electrophoresis	
	Iron	
	Iron Binding Capacity	
	NC % saturation requires iron & IBC to be ordered	
	LDH (lactate dehydrogenase)	
	LH (luteinizing hormone)	
	Magnesium	
	Phosphorus, blood	
	Potassium, blood	
	Prolactin, blood	
	Protein, total	
	-90 Protein Electrophoresis, serum	
	PSA, total	
	Sodium, serum	
	T4, free (thyroxine)	
	TSH	
	Triglycerides	
	Uric Acid, blood	
	Vitamin B12	
	CALCULATIONS	
	NC LDL requires Chol & HDL to be ordered	
	NC CHOL/HDL requires Chol & HDL to be ordered	

Code	TOXICOLOGY/ THERAPEUTIC DRUGS	DX
	Last Dose:	
	Carbamazepine	
	Digoxin	
	Lithium	
	Phenobarbital	
	Phenytoin (Dilantin)	
	Salicylate	
	Valproic Acid	
	Theophylline	

Code	IMMUNOLOGY (Blood)	DX
	ANA (FANA) Screen if ANA positive, 86039 titer performed, if titer >1:160 cascade performed (anti-ds DNA, ENA I & ENA II)	
	Anti-ds DNA	
	ENA I (Sm, RNP)	
	ENA II (SSA, SSB)	
	ASO screen (ASO titer if screen positive 86060)	
	Rheumatoid factor (qual)	
	RPR (Syphilis Serology), quant	
	Cold Agglutinin titer	
	Hep B surface antigen	
	-90 Hep B surface antigen OB (PHL)	
	-90 HIV	
	Mono test	
	Rubella Antibody	

Code	PANELS	DX
	Electrolytes CO_2, Cl, K, Na	
	Basic metabolic Ca, CO_2, Cl, Creat, Glu, K, Na, BUN	
	Comprehensive metabolic Alb, Bili tot, Ca, Cl, Creat, Glu, Alk phos, K, Prot tot, Na, AST, ALT, BUN, CO_2	
	Hepatic Function Alb, Bili tot and dir, Alk phos, AST, ALT, Prot tot	
	Lipid Chol tot, HDL, Trig., calc, LDL, Chol/HDL ratio	
	Gen health, Comp met, CBC, TSH	

Code	HEMATOLOGY	DX
	Hemogram WBC, auto WBC diff	
	Hemogram micro exam, WBC diff	
	Hemogram micro exam, w/o diff	
	Hemogram manual WBC diff, buffy	
	Hematocrit	
	Hemoglobin	
	Platelet count, auto	
	Reticulocyte count, manual	
	Sedimentation Rate, auto	
	WBC, automated	
	CBC, with diff Hgb, Hct, RBC, WBC, Platelet	
	CBC, w/o diff Hgb, Hct, RBC, WBC, Platelet	

Code	COAGULATION	DX
	☐ Coumadin ☐ Heparin	
	APTT	
	Prothrombin time	
	Bleeding time	

Code	OFFICE TESTING	DX
	UA, Dipstick in Office	

Code	URINE/STOOL	DX
	UA, Routine	
	UA SAVE (for possible urine culture if requested)	
	UA with microscopic	
	Urinalysis, Dipstick, Lab	
	Occult Blood	
	Urine HCG	
	Diabetic urine cascade	

Code	TIMED URINE	DX
	Hours:	
	Creatinine Clearance	
	Calcium, Urine, Quant.	
	Uric acid	

Code	BODY FLUID	DX
	Fluid Source:	
	Cell Count w/o Diff	
	Protein	
	Glucose	
	Semen Analysis	
	Semen Analysis, Comp	

Code	IMMUNOHEMATOLOGY	DX
	Blood type ABO, Rh(D) Weak D performed if Rh negative	
	Antibody Screen Identification, if positive, titer if indicated	
	Direct Coombs additional testing if positive	

WRITE-IN TESTS	DX	Lab Use

Medical Necessity Statement: Tests ordered on Medicare patients must follow CMS rules regarding medical necessity and FDA approval guidelines and must include diagnosis, symptoms, or reason for testing as indicated on the medical record. For any patient of any payor (including Medicare and Medicaid) that has a medical necessity requirement, order only those tests which are medically necessary for the diagnosis and treatment of the patient.

DX	ICD-9 CODE	WRITTEN INDICATION/DIAGNOSIS (Match Diagnosis # to Test)
1		Chronic renal failure
2		
3		
4		

	LAB USE ONLY
	Arterial Puncture
	Venipuncture
	Venipuncture MC/MA
	Handling Fee
	Urine Volume Measurement
	-90 PKU

Chart #: 5899 C Date: 01/10/0 2

Name: Randy Chalett e Ⓜ/F

DOB: 06/30/ 74

Physician: Leslie Alanda, MD

Medicare #: ________ Medicaid #: ________

☒ No ABN needed ☐ Patient refused to sign ABN

Nursing Home Part A Medicare: ☐ Yes ☐ No

Worker's Comp: ☐ Yes ☐ No

Company Account: ________

51.

SERVICE CODE(S): ____________

DX CODE(S): ____________

Glossary

bilirubin orange-colored pigment in bile; accumulation leads to jaundice

buffy coat a special study done when the leukocyte count is so low that the standard evaluation cannot be performed

cytopathology laboratory work done to determine whether any cellular changes are present

differential actual count of the amount or number of blood constituents

erythrocyte an element found in peripheral blood, also called red blood cell, corpuscle, and red cell

glucose blood sugar

gross postmortem examination a visual examination of a body after death to determine the cause of death and the presence of disease. The extent of the dissection and examination of the organs and tissues is variable. Performed by hospital pathologist, coroner, or medical examiner.

hemoglobin protein found in red blood cells that transport oxygen through the bloodstream

hemogram graphic picture (or written record) of a detailed blood assessment

indicators written physician orders to a laboratory that set standards for any tests performed

ketones carbon-based compounds that are a by-product of fatty acid metabolism; accumulation of ketone bodies in urine may indicate diabetes

leukocytes white blood cells

occult blood test to detect the presence of blood in stool samples

panel groups of laboratory tests that are performed together

postmortem examination see gross postmortem examination

qualitative only the presence of; not an exact amount

quantitative the exact amount present

reagent a substance that changes color when exposed to another substance

specific gravity weight of urine compared with an equal volume of water

superbill (encounter form) a form listing the most frequently used procedures and codes; the results of a patient's visit are checked off and used for billing purposes

thrombocyte a platelet (coagulates blood, also known as blood disk, blood platelet)

urinalysis the analysis of urine

urobilinogen a colorless compound formed in the intestines by the reduction of bilirubin

Chapter 5

Integumentary System

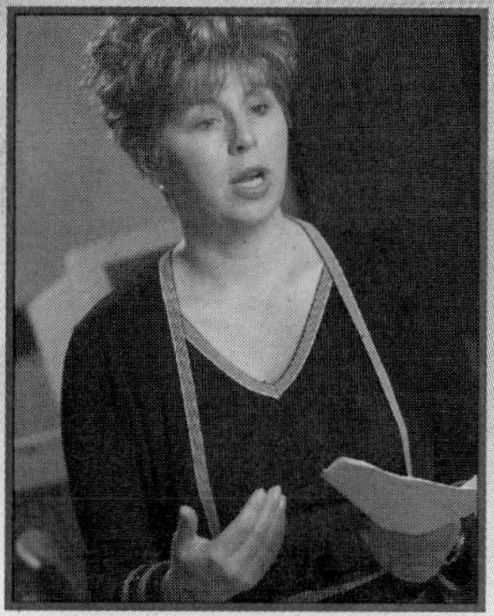

Christy A. Conway, CPC, CHCC, CMPE
Consultant
Past President, Greater Cincinnati Dayton AAPC
Troy, Ohio

ABBREVIATIONS

b.i.d.	twice a day
cc	cubic centimeter
cm	centimeter
DVT	deep vein thrombosis
FTSG	full-thickness skin graft
GI	gastrointestinal
lm	lumen
mg	milligram
mm	millimeters
NPO	*nucleus preopticus,* nothing by mouth
p.o.	by mouth
p.r.n.	as needed
q	each, every
STSG	split-thickness skin graft
t.i.d.	three times a day

Debridement

Debridement cleans surface areas and removes necrotic tissue. Codes in this category describe services of debridement based on depth, body surface, and condition. The first debridement codes (11000 and 11001) are used for eczematous debridement or infected skin. The dead tissue may have to be cut away with a scalpel or scissors or washed with saline solution. Code 11000 is used to report debridement of 10% of the body surface or less, and add-on code 11001 is used to report each additional 10%. Body surface percent is based on the rule of nines as illustrated in **Figure 5-1.** Codes 11010-11044 are used to report debridement based on the extent of the debridement of the skin/subcutaneous tissue or partial thickness.

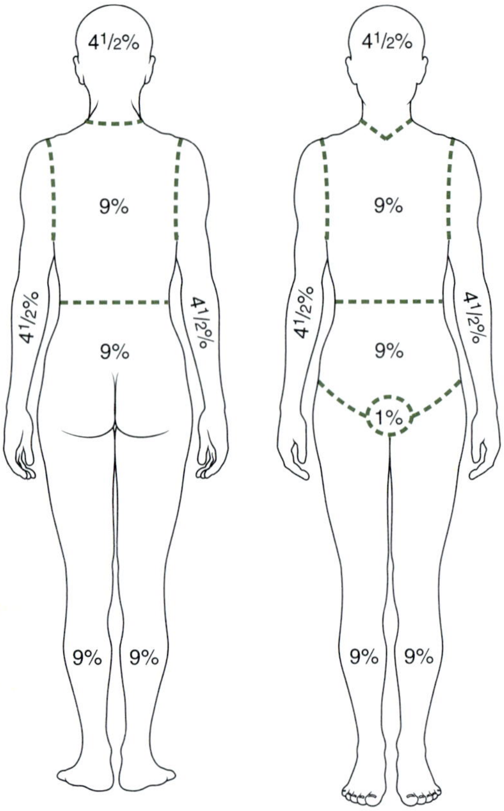

FIGURE 5-1 The rule of nines.

CASE 5-1
5-1A Operative Report, Excision Fat Necrosis

CASE 5-1

The postoperative period for this procedure is 30 days.

5-1A OPERATIVE REPORT, EXCISION FAT NECROSIS

LOCATION: Inpatient, Hospital

PATIENT: Terri Morgan

SURGEON: Gary Sanchez, M.D.

INDICATION FOR PROCEDURE: This patient has had extensive fat necrosis of the lower abdominal wound following a panniculectomy that I performed 24 days ago.

PREOPERATIVE DIAGNOSIS: Fat necrosis, lower abdominal wound

POSTOPERATIVE DIAGNOSIS: Fat necrosis, lower abdominal wound

SURGICAL FINDINGS: This is an area of about 10 × 6 cm diameter fat necrosis in the center of the wound and fat necrosis laterally in the wounds in a sulcus that was buried underneath the upper abdominal flap. The measurement of the wound from side to side was 50 cm in its total dimensions, and it was 6 cm proximally in its greatest width.

PROCEDURE PERFORMED: Excision of fat necrosis

ANESTHESIA: General endotracheal

ESTIMATED BLOOD LOSS: 25 cc

DESCRIPTION OF PROCEDURE: Under satisfactory general endotracheal anesthesia, the patient's abdomen was prepped with Betadine scrub and solution and draped in the routine sterile fashion. The dead fat was excised from the central portion of the wound, leaving the wound with about 6 mm width. We noted there was some dead fat in both lateral aspects of the wounds, which we excised, and there was an undermined area laterally in both aspects of the wound, which we opened up and curetted out at its base but remaining within the subcutaneous level. We also sharply removed the dead fat from these areas. We applied Silvadene cream and ABD pads for dressing. Estimated blood loss was 25 cc. The patient tolerated the procedure well and left the area in good condition.

5-1A:

SERVICE CODE(S): ____________________

DX CODE(S): ____________________

fat necrosis (abdominal wound) — degeneration, skin

CASE 5-1A DISCUSSION

A panniculectomy, which is a major surgical procedure in which excess skin and subcutaneous tissue is removed, is a major surgical procedure and would include at least a 30-day and probably a 90-day postoperative period within the global surgical package. The third-party payer would decide if this debridement would be paid separately or included within the initial surgical package. In many cases, the payer would include this complication within the global package and not pay separately for this complication, which included a return to the operating room. Since this patient was seen within the global period as stated in the directions for the case, you need to append modifier -78 to indicate a return to the operating room within the global period by the same physician that originally performed the surgical procedure.

As a result of the previous panniculectomy, the surgical incision developed "fat necrosis," a condition in which neutral fats in the cells of adipose (fatty) tissue are split and produce chalky white areas. In this surgical procedure, the physician removes the areas of necrosis by first using a scalpel or a dermatome (an instrument that slices layers of skin off) and removes the superficial necrotic areas. The epidermal layer is then excised to remove any areas of epidermal necrosis to the level of healthy tissue. This is a skin and subcutaneous tissue debridement.

The diagnosis is "fat necrosis," which is degeneration of the skin. This diagnosis is an excellent example of the directional feature of the Index of the ICD-9-CM. Let's follow the directions in the Index for this diagnosis. Look each entry up as we use this directional feature to help locate the correct code. When referencing the Index of the ICD-9-CM under the main term "Necrosis" and subterm "fat," the code is 272.8, but note that this is "generalized" fat necrosis and when the Tabular is referenced you will see that 272.8 is for disorders of the lipoid (fat) metabolism. The necrosis in this case was of a specific area (abdominal wound), so 272.8 is not the correct code. Returning to the Index under the terms "Necrosis, fat," the coder is directed to "*see also* degeneration, fatty." Upon referencing "Degeneration, fatty,

localized by site" the coder is directed to "*see* Degeneration, by site, fatty." Following this direction, the coder is directed to "Degeneration, skin, 709.3." When the Tabular is referenced, degeneration of the skin is listed in the code description, making this the correct code. One reference in the Index that initially looked promising was the "necrosis, fat, abdominal wall, 567.82"; however, the report indicates abdominal **wound** not abdominal **wall.**

CASE 5-2
5-2A Operative Report, Debridement
5-2B Radiology Report, Leg

CASE 5-2

The debridement in this case is performed to a deeper level than the debridement performed in 5-1A. In 5-1A, the depth was to the subcutaneous level; but in 5-2A the operative report indicates the debridement was to the level of bone, with cultures taken from the necrotic area.

5-2A OPERATIVE REPORT, DEBRIDEMENT

LOCATION: Inpatient, Hospital

PATIENT: Arnold Rolf

SURGEON: Gary Sanchez, M.D.

INDICATIONS FOR THIS PROCEDURE: This patient has had an apparent full-thickness loss of an area of previous surgery overlying the medial aspect of the left lower tibia. The patient sustained a compound tibial fracture 2 months previously, and this was immediately plated by Dr. Almaz. The patient subsequently developed a full-thickness loss in this area, and I saw him last week in an attempt to try to dry this area out and possibly salvage any tissue overlying the plate. When he was seen in the office, I felt he probably had a full-thickness loss and scheduled him for debridement. The patient was not set up at this time for soleus muscle flap, although that has been discussed as the possible definitive management, although it is slightly low for a soleus muscle flap. The only other alternative is a free flap.

PREOPERATIVE DIAGNOSIS: Full-thickness tissue loss, left lower extremity, medial aspect of lower third of leg. (This is an ulcer.)

POSTOPERATIVE DIAGNOSIS: Full-thickness tissue loss, left lower extremity, medial aspect of lower third of leg.

PROCEDURE PERFORMED: Debridement of soft tissue of left lower extremity, and culture and sensitivity of two deep soft-tissue sites and two bone sites, with the fourth bone site being from the medullary cavity.

ANESTHESIA: General endotracheal

SURGICAL FINDINGS: A 3-cm-diameter, full-thickness skin loss overlying a previously plated fracture. Lying on top of the plate and overlying two of the plate holes was a liquefactive *(conversion to liquid)* necrotic area. In one of the holes for the plate, there was some cloudy drainage of which we obtained a culture and sensitivity. We also obtained culture and sensitivity of another deep soft-tissue site and the other hole in the tibia in conjunction with the plate. There were actually loose bone particles in this area.

PROCEDURE: The patient's left leg was prepped with Betadine scrub and solution and draped in a routine sterile fashion. We lifted up the eschar (*slough produced by a heat burn*) with sharp dissection and noted there was liquefactive necrosis underneath the eschar and actually lying on top of the plate. We took some of the tissue from underneath the eschar on its deep surface and placed this for culture and sensitivity, labeling it "deep tissue with eschar, left lower extremity." Number two was also labeled "deep tissue over plate." Specimen number three was labeled "culture and sensitivity of bone and tissue." Number four was labeled "bone from medullary cavity, left tibia." After we obtained these cultures, we placed Xeroform on the wound and put a 4 × 4 over this. We wrapped it with a Kerlix roll and replaced the splint that the patient had arrived with. Estimated blood loss was zero. The patient seemed to tolerate the procedure well and left the operating room in good condition.

5-2A:

SERVICE CODE(S): ____________________

DX CODE(S): ____________________

5-2B RADIOLOGY REPORT, LEG

LOCATION: Inpatient, Hospital

PATIENT: Arnold Rolf

SURGEON: Gary Sanchez, M.D.

RADIOLOGIST: Morton Monson, M.D.

EXAMINATION OF: Left lower extremity ultrasound

CLINICAL SYMPTOMS: Extremity pain

LEFT LOWER EXTREMITY ULTRASOUND: HISTORY: History of fracture

FINDINGS: Ultrasound examination of the deep venous system of the left lower extremity is negative for DVT. The left popliteal, greater saphenous, and femoral veins are patent and negative for thrombus. Unable to evaluate the calf veins.

5-2B:

SERVICE CODE(S): ____________________

DX CODE(S): ____________________

CASE 5-2B DISCUSSION

This report is an excellent example of how the outpatient coder must only code the diagnostic statements made within the one report that is being coded. In this case, you know that the patient is in for debridement of an ulcer on his lower leg; however, the radiology report indicates the diagnosis under the Clinical Symptoms section of the report is "extremity pain." It is this pain in the leg that is reported as the reason for the radiology service by way of the diagnosis code.

Skin Tags

Skin tags are **benign lesions** that can appear anywhere but most often appear on the neck or trunk, especially in older people. Skin tags are removed by a variety of methods, such as scissors, blades, ligatures, electrosurgery, or chemicals, as illustrated in **Figure 5-2.** Whatever method of removal is used, simple closure is included in the skin tag codes, as is any local anesthesia used. Codes 11200 and 11201 are used to report skin tag removal and are based on the first 15 lesions and then on each additional 10 lesions after the first 15.

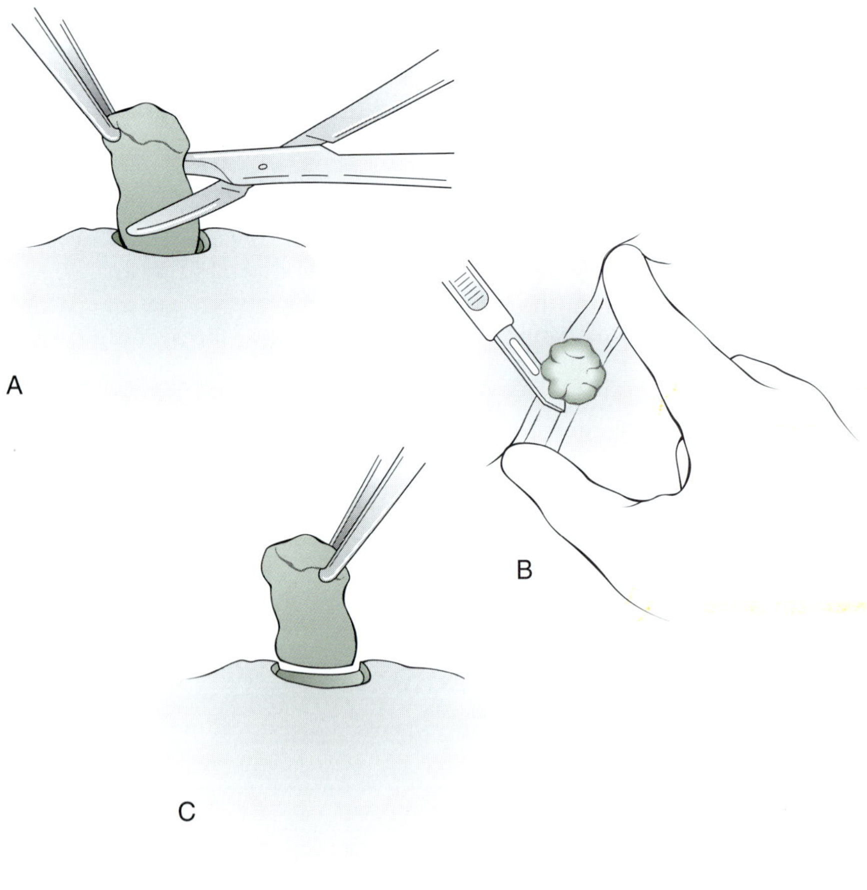

FIGURE 5-2 A, Scissors removal. **B,** Shaving of a lesion with a scalpel. **C,** Removal with tweezers.

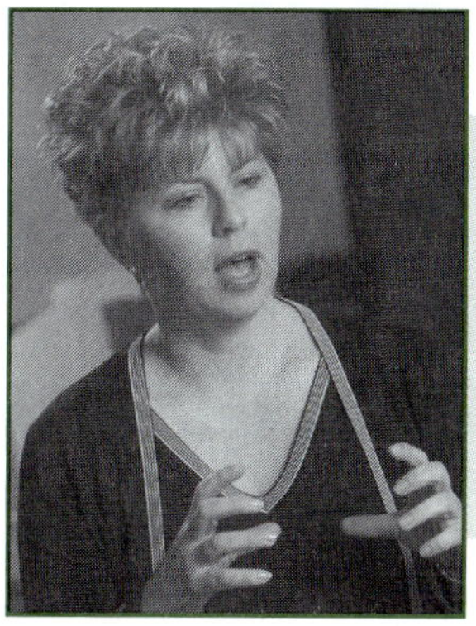

FROM THE TRENCHES

Christy

"Coding…it's like the center of a wheel…everything revolves around coding… You have to get reimbursed for the services that you provide. You have revenue, patient management, operations, HIPAA-and all of that ties into your monthly coding. It's the centerpiece."

CASE 5-3
5-3A Operative Report, Skin Tags

CASE 5-3

5-3A OPERATIVE REPORT, SKIN TAGS

LOCATION: Outpatient, Hospital

PATIENT: DiAnn Hopke

SURGEON: Gary Sanchez, M.D.

PREOPERATIVE DIAGNOSIS: Fibroepithelial skin tags of the neck

POSTOPERATIVE DIAGNOSIS: Fibroepithelial skin tags of the neck

PROCEDURE PERFORMED: Excision of multiple (ten) skin tags of neck

ANESTHESIA: General endotracheal, supplementing with 1% Xylocaine with 1:100,000 epinephrine, approximately 5 cc

SURGICAL FINDINGS: Fibroepithelial skin tags of the neck.

PROCEDURE: The neck was prepped with Betadine scrub and solution and draped in a routine sterile fashion. Skin tags were removed by electrocautery. The bases of the skin tag were cauterized where appropriate. Antibiotic ointment and Band-Aids were applied. The multiple skin tags were submitted for permanent sections (*biopsy section that takes several days to prepare, as compared to frozen section, which is immediately examined*). The patient tolerated the procedure well and left the area in good condition.

Pathology Report Later Indicated: Benign skin tags (10)

5-3A:

SERVICE CODE(S): ____________________

DX CODE(S): ____________________

CASE 5-3A DISCUSSION

The diagnosis is stated in the Postoperative Diagnosis section of the report as skin tags, and the ICD-9-CM index directs the coder to 701.9 under the entry "Tag, skin." The code description for 701.9 does not include the term "skin tag." This is an excellent example of how the coder must trust the Index of the ICD-9-CM to include terms that may not be in the Tabular.

Lesion Excision

Codes 11400-11646 are used to report the **excision** of **malignant** and benign lesions based on the **site, number,** and **size** and whether the lesion is **malignant or benign.** To calculate the sizes of the lesion, identify the lesion at the greatest dimension and the margin at the narrowest part as illustrated in **Figure 5-3** by the dotted line. The margin is the healthy skin that is taken from around the lesion to ensure that the entire lesion is removed. Take the measurements from the operative report because the preserving fluids in which the specimen is placed for processing when the specimen is sent to the laboratory for analysis may shrink the tissue sample. The pathology report should be used to identify the size of the lesion only if no other record of the size can be documented. For example, a benign lesion that measures 0.5 cm at the widest point that is removed with a 0.5-cm margin at the narrowest point is reported as a 1.0-cm lesion (11401).

The operative report must not be coded until the pathology report on the specimen has been prepared. The pathologist is a physician, and the diagnosis stated on the report prepared by the pathologist should be reported. For example, a surgeon removes a skin lesion and the operative report indicates a postoperative diagnosis of "skin lesion" but the pathology report indicates "malignant melanoma." The coder would report the diagnosis as malignant melanoma because it is the most definitive diagnosis.

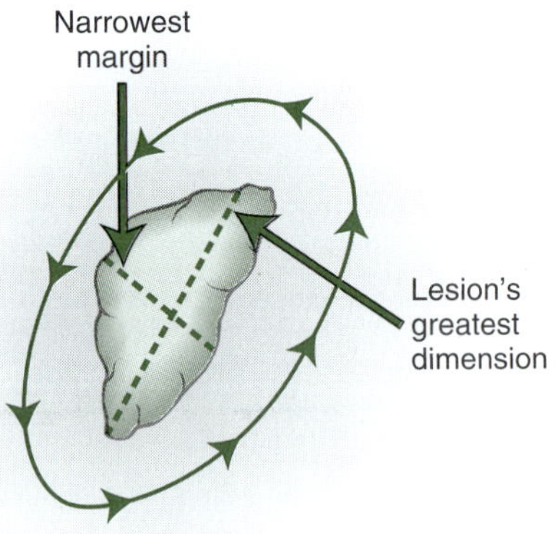

FIGURE 5-3 Calculating the size of a lesion.

If the specimen indicated "skin lesion" and the pathology report indicated "neoplasm of uncertain behavior," the neoplasm of uncertain behavior would be reported.

Do not code directly from the Neoplasm Table in the Index of the ICD-9-CM manual. Always locate the neoplasm morphology within the Index for instructions on how to use the Neoplasm Table, and then reference the Tabular of the ICD-9-CM.

The malignant lesion codes (11600-11646) are the same whether the lesion is malignant melanoma or basal cell carcinoma.

Read the notes that precede codes 11400 and 11600 before coding the reports that follow.

Keratosis

Keratosis is a callus or horny growth. For the purposes of reporting the CPT code, an excision of a keratosis is excision of a lesion.

CASE 5-4
5-4A Operative Report, Lesions
5-4B Pathology Report

CASE 5-4

5-4A OPERATIVE REPORT, LESIONS

LOCATION: Inpatient, Hospital

PATIENT: Tom Boll

SURGEON: Gary Sanchez, M.D.

PREOPERATIVE DIAGNOSIS: Lesions, left lower extremity

POSTOPERATIVE DIAGNOSIS: Undetermined lesion, right lower extremity, most likely benign with clear margins.

SURGICAL FINDINGS: There was a 2-cm diameter, raised erythematous lesion with a central pore of keratin. (This is keratosis.) Frozen section showed clear margins. Although it essentially looked benign, there is some question of well-differentiated squamous cell carcinoma, and this is reserved as a possible diagnosis.

SURGICAL PROCEDURE: Excision of lesion, left lower extremity

ANESTHESIA: Spinal

DESCRIPTION OF PROCEDURE: Under satisfactory spinal anesthesia, the patient's left leg was prepped with Betadine scrub and solution and draped in a routine sterile fashion. The lesion was excised with a 1-cm margin laterally and with a 2-cm margin proximally and distally tagging the superomedial aspect with a silk suture. Dissection was carried down to the deep layer of fascia, and bleeding was electrocoagulated. One 2-0 Monocryl suture was used subcuticularly to take tension off the wound, and then the skin was closed with interrupted vertical mattress sutures of 3-0 Prolene. We submitted the specimen for frozen section, and the frozen-section diagnosis was probably benign with the possibility of well-differentiated squamous cell carcinoma. The pathology report leaned in favor of this being a benign lesion; however, we went well around the lesion. I returned to the operating room, rescrubbed, and regloved and placed a Xeroform dressing, Kerlix fluffs over the wound, and Kerlix fluffs around the malleoli on the heels, wrapping the foot and leg from the foot to the knee with a Kerlix roll times two, Kling times two, and two Sof-Rol. The patient tolerated the procedure well and left the operating room in good condition.

Pathology Report Later Indicated: See report 5-4B.

5-4A:

SERVICE CODE(S): ____________________

DX CODE(S): ____________________

CASE 5-4A DISCUSSION

Note that in this case the pathologist had been in the operating room and taken a frozen section. The frozen section was examined by the pathologist immediately to determine if there was cancer in the specimen. The pathologist made the determination that the specimen was benign, and as such the surgeon returned to the operating room to close the wound. Although the frozen section is not as accurate as a permanent section, it provides a preliminary pathological diagnosis. The pathologist would also conduct a permanent section on the specimen, and the final pathological diagnosis would be made.

5-4B PATHOLOGY REPORT

Note that within this report the pathologist went to the operating room and provided an immediate consultation (frozen section). The heading "Intraoperative Frozen Section Diagnosis" is the indication for this service. Locate directions to this code in the Index of the CPT under "Pathology, Surgical, Consultation, Intraoperative." The frozen section is reported in addition to the pathological examination permanent section of the specimen.

LOCATION: Inpatient, Hospital

PATIENT: Tom Boll

SURGEON: Gary Sanchez, M.D.

PATHOLOGIST: Grey Lonewolf, M.D.

CLINICAL HISTORY: A 2-cm lesion, left leg

SPECIMEN RECEIVED: Lesion, left leg with FS

GROSS DESCRIPTION:

The specimen is labeled with the patient's name and "lesion left leg," which consists of a 4 × 2 × 0.8-cm skin ellipse with a central nodular area, 1.5 cm in diameter with scale crust. A suture identifies the superior medial ellipse, which is identified with black ink. The inferior/lateral ellipse is identified with green ink, the superior margin with red ink, and the inferior margin with blue ink. Representative sections are frozen and processed in cassettes.

Pathology Consultation

INTRAOPERATIVE FROZEN SECTION DIAGNOSES per Dr. Lonewolf. Lesion left leg, excision: Margins benign, defer to permanent sections.

Sections of skin show mild hyperkeratosis with pseudoepitheliomatous hyperplasia with central scale crust and underlying epidermal cysts. There are mild chronic inflammatory infiltrates. Margins are benign.

DIAGNOSIS: Skin lesion, left leg, excision: Skin showing mild hyperkeratosis with central scale crust, pseudoepitheliomatous hyperplasia, epidermal cysts, and mild chronic inflammation; margins are benign.

5-4B:

SERVICE CODE(S): ____________________

DX CODE(S): ____________________

CASE 5-4B DISCUSSION

Note that even tough the Diagnosis section of the report started off with "skin lesion," the diagnosis was hyperkeratosis later in the section, which is the highest level of specificity of the lesion and must be coded as such.

CASE 5-5
5-5A Operative Report, Lesions

CASE 5-5

5-5A OPERATIVE REPORT, LESIONS

This service is being provided to remove two chest lesions in a patient with a personal history of a malignant breast neoplasm. In addition to the code to report the current chest lesions, the history is reported with a V code. Locate directions to this code by referencing "History of, personal" in the Index of the ICD-9-CM, subtermed by type of history. Report only Dr. Sanchez's service, not the pathologist's service.

LOCATION: Outpatient, Hospital

PATIENT: Bernice Pries

SURGEON: Gary Sanchez, M.D.

PREOPERATIVE DIAGNOSIS: Lesions, chest, times two

POSTOPERATIVE DIAGNOSIS: Lesions, chest, times two

PROCEDURE PERFORMED: Removal of two lesions, chest, in previous total mastectomy site

HISTORY: This patient had a segmental mastectomy due to malignancy and then subsequently had radiotherapy in the past. She developed a recurrent breast cancer, and I did a total mastectomy. She now has two areas that are very hard; these are likely fat necrosis, but we are not sure. It is elected to remove them.

When I first saw her in the office, it was the most medial aspect of her incision that was hard, but I felt a new area right along the incision and a little more lateral toward the axilla, and she wanted that removed too. I marked both these areas in the same-day holding room with the patient's husband and the nurse present.

PROCEDURE: The patient was given an anesthetic. She was prepped and draped in a supine fashion. We started with the medial lesion. We made an incision and then developed superior flaps and inferior flaps. We removed this lesion going right down to the muscle. The first lesion measured approximately 1.7 cm, and the second lesion measured 2.0 cm. We obtained excellent hemostasis. I did the same with the smaller lesion that was on the lateral aspect. These both appeared to be fat necrosis. We did frozen sections, and they both appeared benign. We obtained excellent hemostasis and brought the subcutaneous tissues together with Vicryl. We closed the skin with subcuticular Vicryl also. We could not apply Steri-Strips because of her allergy to tape. That is why we used subcuticular Vicryl instead of my usual subcuticular Prolene with Steri-Strips. The patient tolerated this well and went the recovery room in good condition.
Pathology Report Later Indicated: Benign lesions

5-5A:

SERVICE CODE(S): ________________

DX CODE(S): ________________

CASE 5-6
5-6A Operative Report, Lipoma

CASE 5-6

5-6A OPERATIVE REPORT, LIPOMA

LOCATION: Outpatient, Hospital

PATIENT: Florence DeFrang

SURGEON: Gary Sanchez, M.D.

PREOPERATIVE DIAGNOSIS: Lesion, left lower neck anterior

POSTOPERATIVE DIAGNOSIS: Lesion, left lower neck anterior

PROCEDURE PERFORMED: Removal of lipoma

HISTORY: This patient has a small lipoma of her anterior lower neck. I tried removing it with EMLA cream (local anesthetic cream) in the ambulatory patient care center, but she completely lost it and it was impossible to do; so I elected to bring her to the operating room and do this with IV sedation.

DESCRIPTION OF PROCEDURE: The patient was prepped and draped in the supine position. We made a skin incision along Langer's lines. We removed the lesion in toto (*means in total*), and the lesion measured 0.8 cm, including margins. We obtained excellent hemostasis with cautery and then brought the subcutaneous tissue together with 3-0 Vicryl, and the skin was closed with a 5-0 Vicryl in a subcuticular fashion. Steri-Strips, gauze, and tape were applied. The patient tolerated the procedure well and went to the recovery room in excellent condition.

Pathology Report Later Indicated: Benign lipoma

5-6A:

SERVICE CODE(S): ____________________

DX CODE(S): ____________________

CASE 5-7
5-7A Operative Report, Nevus

CASE 5-7

5-7A OPERATIVE REPORT, NEVUS

LOCATION: Outpatient, Hospital

PATIENT: Beverly Weik

SURGEON: Gary Sanchez, M.D.

INDICATIONS FOR PROCEDURE: This patient has a giant congenital nevus of the anterior aspect of the midline of the neck, which has a 4% to 20% chance of development of malignant melanoma at some time in the patient's life.

PREOPERATIVE DIAGNOSIS: Giant congenital nevus (compound nevus), neck

POSTOPERATIVE DIAGNOSIS: Giant congenital nevus (compound nevus), neck

PROCEDURE PERFORMED: Excision of giant congenital nevus of the neck

SURGICAL FINDINGS: A 4 × 1.5-cm diameter irregular oval-shaped giant congenital nevus of the neck

ANESTHESIA: General endotracheal with 3 cc of 1% Xylocaine with 1:100,000 epinephrine

COMPLICATIONS: None

DRAINS: None

SPONGE AND NEEDLE COUNTS: Correct

PROCEDURE: The patient's neck was prepped with Betadine scrub and solution and draped in the routine sterile fashion. Anesthesia was administered in the concentration and amount mentioned above. The lesion was then excised elliptically with a margin of a few millimeters around it. Bleeding was electrocoagulated. The wound was closed with subcuticular 4-0 Monocryl, and $\frac{1}{2}$-inch Steri-Strips were applied. A soft cervical collar was not available, and we will attempt to use a firm cervical collar for the immobilization of the neck. Otherwise, the patient tolerated the procedure well and left the operating room in good condition.

Pathology Report Later Indicated: Benign giant nevus. (This is a benign skin lesion.)

5-7A:

SERVICE CODE(S): ______________________

DX CODE(S): ______________________

CASE 5-8

5-8A OPERATIVE REPORT, EPITHELIOMA

LOCATION: Outpatient, Hospital

PATIENT: Larry Harris

SURGEON: Gary Sanchez, M.D.

PREOPERATIVE DIAGNOSIS: Inclusion cyst, left eyebrow

POSTOPERATIVE DIAGNOSIS: Calcifying epithelioma (benign skin lesion) of Malherbe, left eyebrow, middle aspect

SURGICAL FINDINGS: A 0.7-cm-diameter ruptured calcifying epithelioma of Malherbe

SURGICAL PROCEDURE: Excision of calcifying epithelioma of Malherbe

ANESTHESIA: General endotracheal anesthesia plus 1 cc of 1% Xylocaine with 1:100,000 epinephrine

ESTIMATED BLOOD LOSS: Negligible

DESCRIPTION OF PROCEDURE: The patient's left eyebrow was prepped with Betadine scrub and solution and draped in a routine sterile fashion. We injected 1 cc of 1% Xylocaine with 1:100,000 epinephrine around it and waited about 5 minutes. We made an incision in the axis of the eyebrow and entered the capsule of the epithelioma. We were then able to dissect the capsule out completely along with the contents of the sac. There were no contents of the sac or sac left within the wound. We closed the wound with two plain sutures of 5-0 Prolene and a horizontal mattress suture of 5-0 Prolene. Surgical and an ophthalmic antibiotic ointment were applied. The patient tolerated the procedure well and left the operating room in good condition.

Pathology Report Later Indicated: Benign lesion (neoplasm)

5-8A:

SERVICE CODE(S): ______________________

DX CODE(S): ______________________

CASE 5-9
5-9A Operative Report, Keratosis Excision

CASE 5-9

5-9A OPERATIVE REPORT, KERATOSIS EXCISION

LOCATION: Outpatient, Hospital

PATIENT: Glen Croaker

SURGEON: Gary Sanchez, M.D.

PREOPERATIVE DIAGNOSIS: Bowen's disease, right cheek

POSTOPERATIVE DIAGNOSIS: Actinic keratosis, right cheek, by frozen section

PROCEDURE PERFORMED: Excision of keratosis, right cheek (1.5-cm diameter)

ANESTHESIA: Ten cc of 1% Xylocaine with 1:800,000 epinephrine with MAC anesthesia

ESTIMATED BLOOD LOSS: Negligible

COMPLICATIONS: None

SURGICAL FINDINGS: A 1.5-cm-diameter raised pink lesion with keratosis on surface, morphologically resembling Bowen's disease

DESCRIPTION OF PROCEDURE: The patient's face was prepped with Betadine scrub and solution and draped in a routine sterile fashion. A margin of about 0.5 cm was taken around the specimen, and we submitted this for frozen section, tagging the inferior aspect with a silk suture. It was the pathologist's opinion this was bowenoid keratosis, and the pathologist felt that we were sufficiently around this to forego any further surgery. The lesion had been closed with interrupted subcuticular 4-0 Vicryl and interrupted 5-0 Prolene. Xeroform and a 4 × 4 were applied for dressing. The patient tolerated the procedure well and left the area in good condition.

Pathology Report Later Indicated: Actinic keratosis, benign. (This is a benign skin lesion.)

5-9A:

SERVICE CODE(S): ______________________

DX CODE(S): ______________________

CASE 5-10

5-10A OPERATIVE REPORT, WIDE EXCISION, MELANOMA

LOCATION: Outpatient, Hospital

PATIENT: Roger Ulland

SURGEON: Gary Sanchez, M.D.

PREOPERATIVE DIAGNOSIS: Malignant melanoma, left shoulder (2 cm)

POSTOPERATIVE DIAGNOSIS: Malignant melanoma, left shoulder (2 cm)

PROCEDURE PERFORMED: Wide excision of malignant melanoma, posterior aspect of left shoulder

ANESTHESIA: General endotracheal with supplementary 1% Xylocaine with 1:100,000 epinephrine, approximately 10 cc

ESTIMATED BLOOD LOSS: Negligible

PROCEDURE: The shoulder was prepped with Betadine scrub and solution and draped in the routine sterile fashion. A margin of about 3 cm laterally and medially around the healed incision site was taken, tapering to a 4 to 5 cm proximally and distally. The incision was carried down to the muscle fascia, which was included with the specimen. Bleeding was electrocoagulated, and the wound was closed with subcuticular 2-0 Monocryl and some twists and pulley sutures of 2-0 Monocryl in the center of the wound, where the most tension was. Kerlix fluffs and a sling were applied followed by an external Ace bandage. The patient tolerated the procedure well and left the area in good condition.

Pathology Report Later Indicated: Malignant melanoma. (This is a primary, malignant neoplasm of the skin.)

5-10A:

SERVICE CODE(S): ____________________

DX CODE(S): ____________________

CASE 5-11
5-11A Operative Report, Squamous Cell Carcinoma

CASE 5-11

5-11A OPERATIVE REPORT, SQUAMOUS CELL CARCINOMA

LOCATION: Outpatient, Hospital

PATIENT: Kyle Pearce

SURGEON: Gary Sanchez, M.D.

PREOPERATIVE DIAGNOSIS: Nonhealing ulcer with eschar of the left temple

POSTOPERATIVE DIAGNOSIS: Squamous cell carcinoma of the left temple

SURGICAL FINDINGS: A 2-cm-diameter nonhealing ulcer of the left temporal region with an eschar overlying it

SURGICAL PROCEDURE: Excision of squamous cell carcinoma of the left temple

ANESTHESIA: Standby with 6.5 cc of 1% Xylocaine with 1:800,000 epinephrine

ESTIMATED BLOOD LOSS: Negligible

COMPLICATIONS: None

SPONGE AND NEEDLE COUNTS: Correct

DESCRIPTION OF PROCEDURE: The patient's face was prepped with Betadine scrub and solution and draped in a routine sterile fashion. A margin of 1 cm on each side of the lesion laterally and medially was outlined with 1-cm margins proximally and distally. We incised this elliptically down to the orbicularis oculi and the frontalis muscle. Bleeding was electrocoagulated. We tagged the medial end with a silk suture. This was submitted for frozen section, and there did not appear to be any residual squamous cell located within the lesion; the lesion was also widely clear on frozen section. We returned to the operating room, and after some undermining, we closed the wound with interrupted vertical mattress sutures of 3-0 Prolene. Xeroform and 4 × 4 dressing were applied. The patient tolerated the procedure well and left the operating room in good condition.

Pathology Report Later Indicated: Primary squamous cell carcinoma. (This is a primary, malignant neoplasm of the skin of temple.)

5-11A:

SERVICE CODE(S): ________________

DX CODE(S): ________________

CASE 5-12
5-12A Operative Report, Wide Excision, Malignant Melanoma

CASE 5-12

In this report there is a wide excision due to the location and extent of the lesion. In order to affect repair afterwards, the surgeon "undermined the skin after the manner of a subcutaneous facelift and brought the skin up…" However, note that the closure was only of the skin, there was no layered closure. If there had been a layered closure indicated in the report, an intermediate repair would also have been reported, but since there is only skin closure, there is no additional repair reported.

5-12A OPERATIVE REPORT, WIDE EXCISION, MALIGNANT MELANOMA

LOCATION: Outpatient, Hospital

PATIENT: Terry Uebe

SURGEON: Gary Sanchez, M.D.

PREOPERATIVE DIAGNOSIS: Malignant melanoma, left preauricular area. See clinic chart for depth of melanoma.

POSTOPERATIVE DIAGNOSIS: Malignant melanoma with clear margins on preauricular area

PROCEDURE PERFORMED: Wide excision of malignant melanoma, left preauricular area

ANESTHESIA: General endotracheal with supplementary 1% Xylocaine with 1:800,000 epinephrine

ESTIMATED BLOOD LOSS: Approximately 25 cc

PROCEDURE: The patient's left face and ear were prepped with Betadine scrub and solution and draped in a routine sterile fashion. The lesion was excised to include the crus of the left ear in the dissection because this was the only method to provide at least 2 cm of width around the excision site. We were able to get about 2.5 cm on the anterior excision site and at least 3 cm proximally and distally. We submitted the specimen, tagging the superior aspect with a silk suture, cauterized the bleeding, and then using separate instrument and gloves, we undermined the skin after the manner of a subcutaneous facelift and brought the skin up, suturing it to the more posterior edge with interrupted 3-0 Prolene. We dressed the wound with Xeroform, Kerlix fluffs, and a Kerlix roll plus Kling. The patient tolerated the procedure well and left the operating table in good condition.

Pathology Report Later Indicated: Malignant melanoma of ear.

5-12A:

SERVICE CODE(S): ____________________

DX CODE(S): ____________________

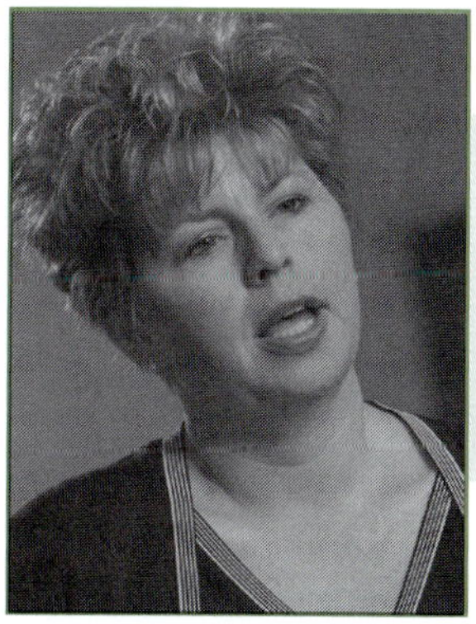

FROM THE TRENCHES

Christy

"Coding covers and encompasses every discipline and every specialty, but maybe there's something that you are particularly interested in. Just dive in! Find out all the information you can regarding that—coding newsletters, tools resources, books. Just read."

Nails

The codes in the category Nails (11719-11772) are for the trimming of fingernails and toenails, debridement of nails, removal of nails, drainage of hematomas, biopsies of nails, repair of nails, reconstruction of nails, and excision of cysts of the nails. Code 11719 is used to report trimming of nails that are not defective. This is a minimal service, and the code covers trimming one fingernail/toenail or many fingernails/toenails. Code 11720 is a more complex service that reports the manual cleaning of up to five nails and includes the use of tools to accomplish the service, cleaning materials/solutions, and files. Supplies used for nail services are included in the codes and not reported separately.

Codes 11730-11732 report avulsion of the nail, which is removal of the nail plate, leaving the root so the nail will grow back. After injection with local anesthetic, the nail is lifted away from the nail bed and all or a portion of the nail is removed.

The nail treatment codes do not require the use of modifier -51 because the codes indicate the number of nails included in the code. Units are used to report the service of multiple nails. For example, when reporting the removal of 3 nails, 11730 is used to report the first nail, and 11732 × 2 reports the second and third nails. Modifiers may be added, depending on the payer. Some payers will require the use of -RT and -LT to indicate right or left and others, such as Medicare, will require the use of the HCPCS modifiers F1-F9 and FA to report the fingers; T1-T9 and TA are used to report the toenails as illustrated in **Figure 5-4.**

A common condition that is treated by physicians and reported with the Nail subheading code is onychocryptosis (ingrown toenail). This is a painful condition in which the nail grows down and into the soft tissue of the nail fold and often leads to infection. Treatment for severe cases is a partial **onychectomy** (removal of the nail plate and root). The toe is anesthetized and a portion of the nail plate and root is removed (11750-11752). The nail will not grow back where the base has been removed. The local anesthetic and supplies necessary to remove the nail are included in the nail codes and are not reported separately.

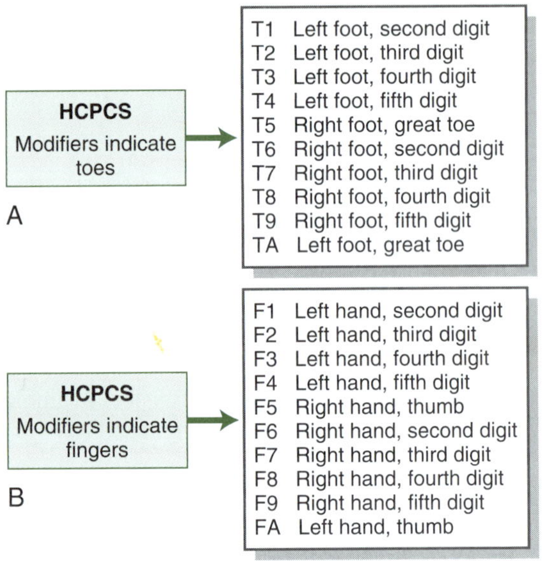

FIGURE 5-4 A, HCPCS modifiers for toes. **B,** HCPCS modifiers for fingers.

CASE 5-13

Violet Berg presents to Dr. Warner's office with a chronic ingrown toenail. Use HCPCS modifiers when reporting the service.

5-13A CLINIC PROGRESS NOTE

LOCATION: Outpatient, Clinic

PATIENT: Violet Berg

FAMILY PHYSICIAN: Leslie Alanda, M.D.

PODIATRIST: Samuel Warner, M.D.

This 14-year-old girl presents with her mom with a chronic ingrown lateral border, right great toenail. She has had the nail removed times two by Dr. Alanda, and it continues to come back. I would recommend that we do a more permanent-type procedure. She is not allergic to anything. She does get exercise-induced asthma. She is on Claritin and cold medications as needed. She has been dealing with this on and off for the last 3 years. She has actually had trouble with both great toenails. The only one sore today, though, is the right lateral border. She is quite nervous and anxious.

OBJECTIVE EVALUATION: Vascular status: Pulses are palpable, dorsalis pedis and posterior tibial. There is no ankle edema, swelling, or erythema. Feet are warm to touch. Dermatologic: She has paronychia, the lateral border of the right great toenail. Dr. Alanda mentioned in a note that it was the left great toenail, but the mother states that it was this toe times two. It is locally cellulitic. No signs of ascending cellulitis, paronychia, or pus formation. It is inflamed.

ASSESSMENT: Chronic ingrown lateral border, right great toenail with cellulitis (onychocryptosis)

PLAN:

1. I would recommend that we locally anesthetize the right great toe, prep and drape, and remove the lateral border in an attempt at permanent treatment to prevent regrowth. Consent was obtained.
2. We did locally anesthetize the right great toe. She was quite nervous during this but did tolerate it very well. We did prep and drape the right great toe in the standard sterile fashion. I did give her an additional 2 cc of 1% lidocaine and 0.5% Marcaine plain. Tourniquet was applied to the base of the right great toe. The lateral border of the right great toenail was avulsed. All nail spiculization and necrotic debris were removed as encountered. Phenol was applied to the nailbed and matrix tissues for the appropriate length of time and curetted aggressively between applications. Tourniquet was removed, and normal vascular status returned to the right great toe. Alcohol was used to wash the toe. Bacitracin ointment and a dry sterile dressing were applied. The patient tolerated the procedure and anesthesia well.

The patient was given written and verbal instructions on wound care regarding t.i.d. Epsom salt soaks for 5 to 10 minutes, two drops of Cortisporin otic solution, and cover with a dry sterile dressing or Band-Aid. I would recommend that she avoid tight-fitting shoes, take Tylenol as needed for pain, and we will see her back in 7 to 10 days for a postoperative check or sooner if any problems arise.

5-13A:

SERVICE CODE(S): ______________________

DX CODE(S): ______________________

Repair (Closure)

There are three types of wounds and three levels of repair or closure: simple, intermediate, and complex. A simple wound involves the **epidermis, dermis,** and/or **subcutaneous** tissue. A simple repair (one-layer) (12001-12021) is required to close a simple wound. Understanding what a simple repair is will provide useful knowledge because often you will have to report a closure that is more than a simple closure. A simple repair (closure) is bundled into excision codes, and if the wound required a closure that was more than a one-layer repair (simple), the closure may be reported separately. For example, if an excision of a lesion that would usually require a simple closure required an intermediate closure, you report the excision and the closure separately. An intermediate wound involves one or more layers of the subcutaneous tissue and superficial fascia. Fascia is the sheet of tissue that covers other tissue, such as the muscles. An **intermediate repair** (12031-12057) requires more than a single-layer closure in which the physician repairs deeper layers of tissue with dissolving stitches and then closes the epidermis, often with different type (number) of suture. If the documentation in the medical record indicates that a simple wound is extensively debrided (cleaned), an intermediate repair may be reported. A **complex repair** (13100-13160), such as revision, debridement, extensive undermining, stents or retention sutures, requires complicated wound closure, and more than layered closure.

After reading the medical documentation and making a decision about the **complexity** of the repair as simple, intermediate, or complex, the next step is to code correctly the repair and closure based on the location of the wound. The codes in the CPT manual are grouped together by complexity, which you already have learned about, and then by **location.** For example, 12001 reports superficial wounds of the scalp, neck, axillae, external genitalia, trunk, and/or extremities (including the hands and feet), and 12011 reports superficial repair of wounds of the face, ears, eyelids, nose, lips, and/or mucous membranes.

The codes are then further divided based on the **length** of the repair. The CPT measurements are in the metric system, so at first it is difficult to imagine the length of these measurements. An inch equals 2.54 cm. Physicians usually report the measurements using the metric system, but if they do not, you have to convert the measurements to metric to select the correct code. If the physician stated that the wound was 5 inches long, you would multiply 5 inches by 2.54 as a means of converting the measurement to 12.7 cm.

Repairs of the same complexity and location are added together and reported with one code. For example, two superficial (complexity) wounds are repaired. One 2.1 cm (length) wound is located on the arm (location), and another is 2.3 cm (length) and is on the neck (location). The wounds are of the same complexity, and grouped in the same locations as referred to in code description 12001 (neck and extremities). Add the two wounds together (4.4 cm) and report with 12002, which is assigned to repairs totaling 2.6 to 7.5 cm. If the wounds are of different complexity or location, you cannot add the lengths together but instead report them separately. When reporting multiple wounds, place the most complex repair first, and follow with the subsequent repair codes with modifier -51 added.

If the wound is grossly contaminated and requires extensive debridement, a separate debridement procedure may be coded. (11000-11044 for extensive debridement) A debridement code can also be used when the skin is broken and contaminated with an open fracture repair.

Do not report the following wound repair services separately:

- Simple **ligation** (tying) of vessels is considered part of the wound repair and is not listed separately.
- Simple **exploration** of surrounding tissue, nerves, vessels, and tendons is considered part of the wound repair process and is not listed separately.
- Normal **debridement** (cleaning and removing skin or tissue from the wound until normal, healthy tissue is exposed) is not listed separately.

There are substances, much like super strength household glue, that are used to glue the edges of wounds together. Dermabond is one of these special skin glues that the physician places in the wound, pulls the edges together, and then places a bandage over the area. HCPCS code G0168 is used to report skin closure for Medicare patients, and other third-party payers use the simple repair codes to report these skin closures using adhesives based on the location and length of the repair.

Read the notes preceding the Repair (Closure) codes to ensure that you understand wound repair before coding the cases that follow.

Section 3: Alphabetic Index to External Causes of Injuries and Poisonings (E Code). Section 3: Alphabetic Index to External Causes of Injuries and Poisonings is the index for the E codes. E codes have an index that is separate from the Section 1, Index of Diseases. It appears following the Table of Drugs and Chemicals and preceding the Tabular. The E codes index alphabetically lists environmental events (tornadoes, floods), circumstances, and other conditions as the cause of injury and other adverse effects. **E codes are never used as a principal diagnosis.** Rather, E codes are used to clarify the cause of an injury or adverse effect. E code terms describe the external circumstances under which an accident, injury, or act of violence occurred. The main terms in this section usually represent the type of accident or violence (e.g., assault, collision), with the specific agent or other circumstance listed below the main term. You must be sure to read all the information under a term in the E code index, then locate the code in the E code section of Volume 1, Tabular. V and E codes follow 999.9 in the Tabular. Be sure to check for fourth-digit specificity for railway accidents, motor vehicle traffic and nontraffic accidents, other road vehicle accidents, water transport accidents, and air and space transport accidents shown in the Index of the External Causes section. For an example, reference the fifth digits displayed above E810 in the ICD-9-CM Tabular.

In the outpatient setting, especially the emergency department, it is up to each facility to determine if they will record E codes, as recording E codes is not yet mandatory.

CASE 5-14
5-14A Operative Report, Laceration

CASE 5-14

While returning from a concert, Virgil Rhone fell asleep (there is a V code for this) at the wheel and lost control of his automobile. His car slid into a ditch and struck a tree. He sustained lacerations on both ears. Assign an E code to indicate how the accident happened.

5-14A OPERATIVE REPORT, LACERATION

LOCATION: Outpatient, Hospital Emergency Department

PATIENT: Virgil Rhone

SURGEON: Paul Sutton, M.D.

PREOPERATIVE DIAGNOSIS: Right and left ear lacerations

POSTOPERATIVE DIAGNOSIS: Right and left ear lacerations

PROCEDURE PERFORMED: Cleaning and suturing of right and left ear lacerations

ANESTHESIA: One-percent Xylocaine

INDICATIONS FOR PROCEDURE: The patient is a 45-year-old white male who was involved in a motor vehicle accident. The patient sustained bilateral ear lacerations, and he is now undergoing repair.

PROCEDURE: The patient was prepped and draped in the usual manner. Xylocaine was used as local anesthesia. The right ear was cleaned, and a 5.2-cm laceration was sutured with interrupted 5-0 nylon sutures. Next the left ear was cleaned and a 4.8-cm laceration was sutured with interrupted 5-0 nylon sutures. The patient tolerated the procedure well.

5-14A:

SERVICE CODE(S): ______________________

DX CODE(S): ______________________

CASE 5-15
5-15A Operative Report, Laceration

CASE 5-15

Don Ehlers was a passenger in Virgil Rhone's car and sustained a laceration of the lip. Report an E code in addition to the diagnosis code.

5-15A OPERATIVE REPORT, LACERATION

LOCATION: Outpatient, Hospital, Emergency Department

PATIENT: Don Ehlers

SURGEON: Paul Sutton, M.D.

PREOPERATIVE DIAGNOSIS: Laceration, left lip

POSTOPERATIVE DIAGNOSIS: Laceration, left lip

PROCEDURE PERFORMED: Complex repair of laceration

OPERATIVE NOTE: The 6-cm area of the laceration was inspected carefully and irrigated to remove all debris (pieces of glass and other debris). The laceration extends from the outside of the mouth, not through the lip itself, but below the lip into the mouth region. By turning the lip inside out, we were able to place some chromic sutures of 3-0 on the inside. The outside was then closed using 5-0 nylon in an interrupted fashion. The patient tolerated the procedure well and was discharged from the emergency room in stable condition.

(complicated due to debris)

5-15A:

SERVICE CODE(S): ____________________

DX CODE(S): ____________________

Modifier -59

Modifier -59 is used to indicate that services that are usually bundled into one Procedural Service payment were provided as separate services. The description of the modifier is as follows:

> Under certain circumstances, the physician may need to indicate that a procedure or service was distinct or independent from other services performed on the same day. Modifier -59 is used to identify procedures/services that are not normally reported together, but are appropriate under the circumstances. This may represent a different session or patient encounter, different procedure or surgery, different site or organ system, separate incision/excision, separate lesion, or separate injury (or area of injury in extensive injuries) not ordinarily encountered or performed on the same day by the same physician. However, when another already established modifier is appropriate, it should be used rather than modifier -59. Only if no more descriptive modifier is available, and the use of modifier -59 best explains the circumstances, should modifier -59 be used.

As the code description notes, modifier -59 is used to identify the following:

- Different session or patient encounter
- Different procedure or surgery
- Different site or organ system
- Separate incision/excision
- Separate lesion
- Separate injury or area of injury in extensive injuries

Modifier -59 is used with codes from all sections of the CPT manual except E/M and anesthesia codes. Medicare has lists of codes that cannot be reported together; they are called *edits*. These edits have been established to ensure that providers do not report services that are included in the bundle for a given code. For example, you would not report a standard preoperative visit related to a major surgical procedure and report separately the surgery and follow-up care. All three services-preoperative, intraoperative, and postoperative-are packaged together in one major surgical CPT code. The use of modifier -59 indicates that the service was not a part of another service but, indeed, was a distinct service.

Modifier -59 requests payment for a procedure performed on the same day as another procedure that normally would not be reported separately, e.g., a biopsy of one lesion on the right leg and an excision of another lesion on the same leg.

CASE 5-16
5-16A Operative Report, Excision Histiocytic Tumor

CASE 5-16

The following case involves the excision of a lesion that requires more than a simple closure. In addition, there are multiple procedures conducted during the same operative session.

5-16A OPERATIVE REPORT, EXCISION HISTIOCYTIC TUMOR

LOCATION: Hospital, Inpatient

PATIENT: Erik Moti

SURGEON: Gary Sanchez, M.D.

PREOPERATIVE DIAGNOSIS: Residual plexiform fibrous histiocytic tumor of the left costovertebral angle area

POSTOPERATIVE DIAGNOSIS: Residual plexiform fibrous histiocytic tumor of left costovertebral angle area

PROCEDURE PERFORMED: Excision of plexiform fibrous histiocytic tumor of left costovertebral angle and evacuation of hematoma, left costovertebral angle

ANESTHESIA: General endotracheal with approximately 20 cc of tumescent solution prepared by adding to 1 L of Ringer's lactate, 25 cc 2% Xylocaine, 1 cc of 1:100,000 epinephrine, and 3 cc of 8.4% sodium bicarbonate.

ESTIMATED BLOOD LOSS: Negligible

SURGICAL FINDINGS: There was a 50-cc hematoma beginning to organize in the area of the left costovertebral angle in the subcutaneous space on top of the latissimus dorsi muscle.

DESCRIPTION OF PROCEDURE: The patient was intubated and turned in the prone position. The area of the left costovertebral angle was prepped with Betadine scrub and solution and draped in a routine sterile fashion. An incision was made 2-cm and carried down to the fascia of the muscle where a hematoma was entered and drained. The skin portion of that lesion was removed, and the fascia and a portion of the muscle of the latissimus dorsi were removed secondarily. The lesion measured 2.9 cm at the widest point. Bleeding was electrocoagulated, and a no. 7 Jackson-Pratt drain was inserted in the depth of the wound. The wound was closed with interrupted 0 Monocryl for the deep fascia layer and subcuticular 4-0 Monocryl using a few vertical mattress sutures of 3-0 Monocryl. Steri-Strips and Kerlix fluffs plus Elastoplast were applied. The patient tolerated the procedure well and left the operating room in good condition.

Pathology Report Later Indicated: Benign lesion of clavicular area

5-16A:

SERVICE CODE(S): ____________________

DX CODE(S): ____________________

CASE 5-17
5-17A Operative Report, Umbilicoplasty

CASE 5-17

This case is of a complex repair in which the surgeon repaired an area of scarring by removal of the scarred area. The surgeon also removed a mass and then closed the area. The repair is the most resource- intensive procedure.

5-17A OPERATIVE REPORT, UMBILICOPLASTY

LOCATION: Outpatient, Hospital

PATIENT: Teresa Wiley

SURGEON: Gary Sanchez, M.D.

PREOPERATIVE DIAGNOSIS: Scarring and retraction of umbilicus, status post partial slough of umbilical skin

POSTOPERATIVE DIAGNOSIS: Scarring and retraction of umbilicus, status post partial slough of umbilical skin

SURGICAL FINDINGS:
1. There was a remnant of buried 1-cm diameter umbilical skin still attached to the umbilical stalk and some granulation tissue and scar tissue located within the depth of the umbilical wound.
2. Fat necrosis, left inguinal area.

SURGICAL PROCEDURES:
1. Excision of fat necrosis, left inguinal region
2. Umbilicoplasty utilizing a 3-cm diameter flap that was 5 mm wide

ANESTHESIA: General endotracheal. Supplementary local approximately 6 cc of 1% Xylocaine with 1:100,000 epinephrine.

DESCRIPTION OF PROCEDURE: The patient's abdomen was prepped with Betadine scrub and solution and draped in a routine sterile fashion. Several cc of 1% Xylocaine with 1:100,000 epinephrine was injected into the scar laterally, overlying the mass in the inguinal area. This mass measured about 1 cm in diameter. We excised the scar over the mass and came down on the mass, which had the appearance of fat necrosis and measured 2.9 cm at the greatest width. This was excised, and all the palpably firm tissue was removed. We cauterized the bleeding and closed the subcutaneous layer with 3-0 Vicryl and the subdermal layer with interrupted 3-0 Vicryl using 4-0 Prolene for the skin. A plain 4 × 4 was applied. The umbilicus was approached by excision of the scar for about 2 cm above the previous umbilical site beginning at the 12 o'clock position and also 2 cm below the 6 o'clock position. I incised the apparent scar tissue circumferentially and came down on a mass of apparent granulation tissue and fat necrosis, which I excised, trimming this off the umbilical stalk. Attached to the umbilical stalk was a nubbin of about 1 cm of umbilicus in a semicircular shape that was 5 mm wide and 3 cm from one side of the flap to the other. This flap was then sutured with half-mattress sutures to the 12 and 6 o'clock positions also, suturing it back to the original site with a subdermal half mattress suture of 3-0 Monocryl, following closure of the donor areas with interrupted 3-0 Prolene, and the completion of the closure of the outer ring of the bilateral flaps with interrupted 3-0 Prolene. Dressing consisted of a glycerin-soaked cotton ball and a 4 × 4. We did put some Nitro paste in the depth of the wound. The patient tolerated the procedure well and left the operating room in good condition.

Pathology Report Later Indicated: Necrotic, fatty mass; benign tissue

5-17A:

SERVICE CODE(S): ____________________

DX CODE(S): ____________________

CASE 5-17A DISCUSSION

The reason for this complex wound repair and excision of the benign lesion is because of the scar and the fat necrosis (709.x). The excision of the lesion would be the lesser of the two procedures, so the wound repair would be sequenced first followed by the lesion excision. Did you remember to use the multiple procedure modifier to indicate that both procedures took place during the same operative session?

CASE 5-18

5-18A Operative Report, Scar Revision, Dermabrasion

CASE 5-18

5-18A OPERATIVE REPORT, SCAR REVISION, DERMABRASION

LOCATION: Outpatient, Hospital

PATIENT: Daniel Vaa

SURGEON: Gary Sanchez, M.D.

PREOPERATIVE DIAGNOSIS: Unsightly widened scar of anterior chest wall

POSTOPERATIVE DIAGNOSIS: Unsightly widened scar of anterior chest wall

PROCEDURES PERFORMED:
1. Dermabrasion
2. Scar revision

ANESTHESIA: General endotracheal with approximately 7 cc of 1% Xylocaine and 1:100,000 epinephrine

ESTIMATED BLOOD LOSS: Less than 25 cc

COMPLICATIONS: None

SPONGE AND NEEDLE COUNTS: Correct

INDICATION: This patient has a widened scar with large suture marks as a result of resection of a dermatofibrosarcoma protuberans about 2 years ago.

SURGICAL FINDINGS: A 27-cm-long unsightly scar of left anterior chest wall with suture marks and widening of the scar. The scar is in the shape of a triangle with its base pointing medially and the apex pointing toward the coronoid process.

DESCRIPTION OF PROCEDURE: The patient's chest was prepped with Betadine scrub and solution and draped in a routine sterile fashion. The scar was injected with 7 cc of 1% Xylocaine and 1:100,000 epinephrine and dermabraded. It was excised to include parts of the suture marks. This was excised down to fat, but some residual scarring remained. This was left in to help provide support and blood supply. We closed the wound with subcuticular 3-0 Monocryl and interrupted twists of 5-0 Prolene. The dressing consisted of thymol iodide powder and 4 × 4s. The patient tolerated the procedure well and left the area in good condition.

5-18A:

SERVICE CODE(S): ______________________

DX CODE(S): ______________________

CASE 5-18A DISCUSSION

The complex repair codes 13100-13160 contain an interesting format that you need to understand to report the codes correctly. Turn to this code range in the CPT. With the text open to the code range, note that code 13100 is for a complex repair on the trunk that measures 1.1 cm to 2.5 cm and that 13101 is for a complex repair on the trunk that measures 2.6 cm to 7.5 cm. The add-on code 13102 is to be used for each additional 5 cm or less after the first 7.5 cm. In this case you had a 27 cm scar that was repaired. 13100 is only used for repairs between 1.1 cm and 2.5 cm, and per the note in the CPT the add-on code 13102 is *only used in conjunction with 13101*, not 13100. The first 7.5 is reported with 13101, because that is the maximum length you can report for the primary code. The remaining 19.5 cm are reported with the add-on code 13102, which is only used with 13101. Also note that the add-on code is for 5 cm **or less.** You would report the 27 cm scar repair with the following codes:

• 13101 for the first 7.5 cm	**7.5** cm (This is the primary code.)
• 13102 for the next additional 5 cm	**5** cm (This is an add-on code.)
• 13102 for the next additional 5 cm	**5** cm (This is an add-on code.)
• 13102 for the next additional 5 cm	**5** cm (This is an add-on code.)
• 13102 for the remaining 4.5 cm	**4.5** cm (This is an add-on code.)
	27 cm

CASE 5-19
5-19A Operative Report, Dermabrasion

CASE 5-19

5-19A OPERATIVE REPORT, DERMABRASION

LOCATION: Outpatient, Hospital

PATIENT: Florence DeFrang

SURGEON: Gary Sanchez, M.D.

PREOPERATIVE DIAGNOSIS: Scar of neck

POSTOPERATIVE DIAGNOSIS: Scar of neck

PROCEDURE PERFORMED: Dermabrasion of neck scar with revision of complex scar of neck (closure of complex wound)

ANESTHESIA: 7 cc of 1% Xylocaine with 1:100,000 epinephrine

ESTIMATED BLOOD LOSS: Negligible

DESCRIPTION OF PROCEDURE: The patient's neck was prepped with Betadine scrub and solution and draped in a routine sterile fashion. Dermabrasion was carried out with a hand engine, using one of the larger burs, and then we injected with 7 cc of 1% Xylocaine with 1:100,000 epinephrine. The scar measured 14 cm in length by about 1.5 cm in width with a 1.5-cm Y-extension. The scar was dermabraded, as noted, and then excised. Bleeding was electrocoagulated, and the wound was closed with subcuticular 3-0 and 4-0 Monocryl and interrupted twists of 5-0 Prolene using one horizontal mattress suture of 5-0 Prolene in the Y-portion of the scar. Thymol iodide powder was applied with Kerlix fluffs and a soft cervical collar was applied. The patient tolerated the procedure well and left the operating room in good condition.

5-19A:

SERVICE CODE(S): ______________________

DX CODE(S): ______________________

14 cm

CASE 5-20
5-20A Operative Report, Scar Revision

CASE 5-20

5-20A OPERATIVE REPORT, SCAR REVISION

LOCATION: Outpatient, Hospital

PATIENT: Kim Plante

SURGEON: Gary Sanchez, M.D.

PREOPERATIVE DIAGNOSIS: Foreign body granuloma of the nose and scar of dorsum of nose

POSTOPERATIVE DIAGNOSIS: Foreign body granuloma of the nose and scar of dorsum of nose

SURGICAL FINDINGS: There is about a 1.5-cm transverse scar located at about the level of the supratarsal fold, and beneath this there was extensive foreign body reaction extending beneath the procerus muscles over the nasal bone extending, in fact, down into the nasal bone in the nasal frontal angle area. There was extensive involvement of the subcutaneous tissue and the tissue extending all the way down to the nasal bone as mentioned.

PROCEDURE PERFORMED:
1. A 1.5-cm complex scar revision, dorsum of the nose
2. Excision of extensive (2.5 cm) foreign body granuloma of the nose involving the procerus and nasalis muscles

ANESTHESIA: General endotracheal with approximately 2 cc of 1% Xylocaine with 1:100,000 epinephrine

ESTIMATED BLOOD LOSS: Negligible

COMPLICATIONS: None

SPONGE AND NEEDLE COUNT: Correct

DESCRIPTION OF PROCEDURE: The patient's face was prepped with Betadine scrub and solution and draped in a routine sterile fashion. The scar was dermabraded and then we excised it. In the subcutaneous tissue, we came down on a foreign body granulomatous reaction that contained what appeared to be a mixture in the previous foreign body (glue). We excised this on top of the musculature, but some of the foreign body extended down below the musculature of the procerus muscles and obviously had separated the muscles at the midline. It (the glue) appeared that this had been injected underneath the muscles and went from the bridge of the nose at about the level of the canthi bilaterally up to the nasal frontal angle. This chronic inflammatory and granulomatous process was involved over about a 2.5 × 2.5-cm area of the nose. After removal of this, considerable dead space remained, and we cauterized the bleeding. I reapproximated the procerus muscles with 5-0 Monocryl, put subcuticular 5-0 Monocryl to close the dead space partially, but needed to use horizontal mattress sutures of 6-0 Prolene to complete closure of the dead space in the subcutaneous area. I did not think a subcuticular suture would be helpful in obtaining the type of closure that we wanted, and therefore the horizontal mattress sutures were used. We then better apposed the skin edges with interrupted 7-0 Prolene using a combination of twists and plain sutures. I applied Surgicel and antibiotic ointment. A portion of the specimen was submitted for frozen section and showed foreign body granulomatous reaction, which in fact had multiple sites of what appeared to be the previous injected glue surrounded by intense foreign body reaction. Interestingly, there were some muscle fibers present on the specimen. The patient tolerated the procedure well and left the operating room in good condition.

5-20A:

SERVICE CODE(S): ______________________

DX CODE(S): ______________________

Adjacent Tissue Transfers or Rearrangements

Adjacent **tissue transfers** are procedures in which a segment of skin is moved from one area to an adjacent area. One side of the moved skin (flap) is left attached to the blood supply to keep the area viable. The flap is then sutured into place. The procedures are often termed V-plasty, W-plasty, Z-plasty, rotation flaps, or advancement flaps.

Adjacent tissue transfers (14000-14350) are reported according to the size of the **recipient site** measured in square centimeters. Simple repair of the donor site is included in the tissue transfer code and is not coded separately. Complex closure or grafting of the donor site is reported separately. To code transfers, you need to know the location of the defect, the size of the defect, and any donor area.

Unlike the repair codes where lesion excision performed at the time of the repair was coded separately, when a lesion is excised at the site of the repair and then repaired by adjacent tissue transfer the lesion excision is included in the tissue transfer code and not reported separately.

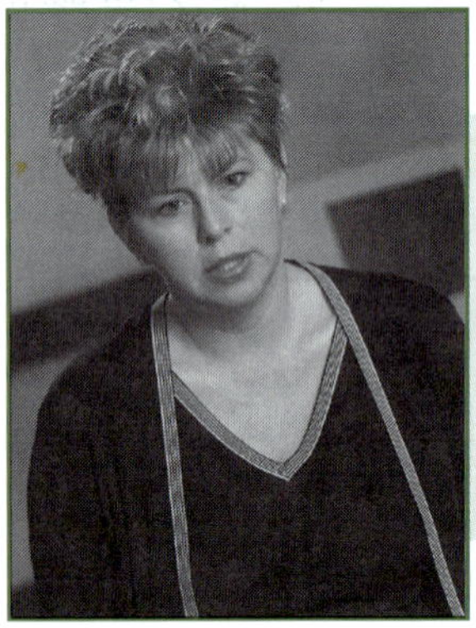

FROM THE TRENCHES

Christy

"I like to interact with people. One of the things that I find really rewarding is when I go in and I actually see the light turn on. When you're talking to somebody and it clicks. It's just there. That's a personal reward for me because it means that I've taught somebody something...and they've learned from their interaction with me."

CASE 5-21
5-21A Operative Report, Excision Ganglion Cyst

CASE 5-21

5-21A OPERATIVE REPORT, EXCISION GANGLION CYST

LOCATION: Outpatient, Hospital

PATIENT: Al Clark

SURGEON: Gary Sanchez, M.D.

INDICATIONS FOR PROCEDURE: This patient has had a ganglion of the second web space of the left hand just proximal to the web space but overlying the ulnar side of the A1 pulley. It has become annoying and occasionally painful.

PREOPERATIVE DIAGNOSIS: Ganglion cyst, left index finger (**location**), with protrusion into second web space on the ulnar side

POSTOPERATIVE DIAGNOSIS: Ganglion cyst, left index finger, with protrusion into second web space on the ulnar side

PROCEDURE PERFORMED: Excision of ganglion cyst, left index finger

SURGICAL FINDINGS: A 1-cm diameter, more or less dumbbell-shaped ganglion cyst of the left index finger arising from the ulnar side of the A1 pulley and extending into the base of the second web space.

ANESTHESIA: Intravenous block

ESTIMATED BLOOD LOSS: Zero

COMPLICATIONS: None

SPONGE AND NEEDLE COUNTS: Correct

PROCEDURE: Under satisfactory intravenous block anesthesia, the patient's left hand and arm were prepped with Betadine scrub and solution and draped in the routine sterile fashion. Using 2.5-power magnification, two 1-cm (**size**) long Z-plasty flaps (**repair type**) with a width of 2 cm each were marked out beginning at the central limb, which was situated over the site of the mass. After development of the flaps, dissection was carried down to the A1 pulley, which had a ganglion cyst arising from its surface more or less on the ulnar side and extending in an ulnar direction into the area of the base of the second web space. This cyst was dissected free intact. After completion of the ganglion removal and submission for permanent sections, we closed the wound with interrupted 6-0 Prolene sutures with Gillies sutures for the tips of the flaps. After cleaning Betadine off of the hand and the arm, dressing consisted of Xeroform, Kerlix, several Kerlix fluffs, Kerlix roll, Kling, Sof-Rol, and an Ace bandage from the fingers to the elbow. The patient tolerated the procedure well and left the operating room in good condition.

Pathology Report Later Indicated: Ganglion cyst

5-21A:

SERVICE CODE(S): ____________________

DX CODE(S): ____________________

CASE 5-22
5-22A Operative Report, Wide Excision, Basal Cell Carcinoma
5-22B Pathology Report

CASE 5-22

5-22A OPERATIVE REPORT, WIDE EXCISION, BASAL CELL CARCINOMA

LOCATION: Outpatient, Hospital

PATIENT: Irene Reep

SURGEON: Gary Sanchez, M.D.

PREOPERATIVE DIAGNOSIS: Basal cell carcinoma, left alar crease

POSTOPERATIVE DIAGNOSIS: Basal cell carcinoma, left alar crease

SURGICAL FINDINGS: A 7-mm-diameter raised lesion, morphologically resembling a cystic basal cell carcinoma, located in the left alar crease.

INTRAOPERATIVE FROZEN SECTION: Grey Lonewolf, M.D.

SURGICAL PROCEDURE: Wide excision of basal cell carcinoma, left alar crease with reconstruction of the defect by a 4 × 2.5-cm nasolabial flap.

ANESTHESIA: General endotracheal with 13 cc of 1% Xylocaine with 1:100,000 epinephrine.

ESTIMATED BLOOD LOSS: 25 cc

DESCRIPTION OF PROCEDURE: The patient's face was prepped with Betadine scrub and solution and draped in a routine sterile fashion. We initially outlined a margin of 5 mm around the lesion, excising it down to nasal musculature and the facial musculature lateral to the nasolabial (nose/lip) line. The margins were 1 cm on the proximal distal ends. The superior part was tagged with a silk suture. After excision of this lesion and once the inferior part was taken all the way down to the mucosa, we submitted it for frozen section, and there was involvement in both lateral and medial margins and some of the inferior margin. Also the deep margin was involved. I returned to the operating room and took another 5 mm of skin around this in continuity with the underlying musculature, going all the way down to the pyriform fossa and going all the way down to the mucosa of the nasal cavity. More laterally, we included some of the superficial musculature of the cheek and then obtained hemostasis. We cauterized the bleeding, following which a 4 × 2.5-cm nasolabial flap was developed from the cheek and rotated into the defect, insetting it with mostly interrupted horizontal mattress sutures of 4-0 Prolene. The wound was dressed with Surgicel and glycerin-soaked cotton with a few dry cotton balls on top and taped placed over this. The estimated blood loss was approximately 25 cc. As stated above, we did a second frozen section, which showed clear margins on all specimens. One margin was very close; however, I felt that grossly we had no tumor involvement in the margin in question.

Pathology Report Later Indicated: See 5-22B.

5-22A:

SERVICE CODE(S): ____________________

DX CODE(S): ____________________

CASE 5-22A DISCUSSION

You need to identify the location, size, and repair to correctly code this service. According to the Surgical Procedure section of the report and substantiated within the body of the report are these three items:

> SURGICAL PROCEDURE: Wide excision of basal cell carcinoma, left alar crease **(location is beside the ear)** with reconstruction of the defect by 4 × 2.5 cm **(size is 4 × 2.5 cm = 10 sq cm)** nasolabial flap **(repair type is a skin flap or an "adjacent tissue transfer")**.

In the index of the CPT you can locate the code for this transfer under "Skin Graft and Flap, Tissue Transfer." These codes are divided based on the location, such as trunk, arm, hands, etc., and total square centimeters.

5-22B PATHOLOGY REPORT

LOCATION: Outpatient, Hospital

PATIENT: Irene Reep

SURGEON: Gary Sanchez, M.D.

PATHOLOGIST: Grey Lonewolf, M.D.

CLINICAL HISTORY: A 7-mm lesion, left alar crease

SPECIMEN RECEIVED:
A. Lesion, left alar crease with FS
B. Re-excision of same lesion with FS

GROSS DESCRIPTION:
A. The specimen is labeled with the patient's name and "lesion, left alar crease," which consists of a 2 × 2 × 1.5-cm nodule. The superior aspect is tagged, which is also identified with black ink, the inferior aspect with green, the right (medial) aspect with red, and the left (lateral) aspect with blue ink. Frozen sections are processed in cassettes A1-4; the remaining tissue is in cassette A5.

INTRAOPERATIVE FROZEN-SECTION DIAGNOSIS per Dr. Lonewolf: Left alar crease skin lesion: Basal cell carcinoma involving margins.

B. The specimen is labeled with the patient's name and "re-excision left alar crease lesion, tagged superior," which consists of a 3.5 × 2.8 × 1.0-cm roughly spherical skin segment with a central biopsy cavity. The superior aspect is identified with black ink, inferior aspect with green ink, right (medial) aspect with red ink, and the left (lateral) aspect with blue ink. The specimen is serially sectioned and frozen. The frozen sections are processed in cassettes B1-9.

INTRAOPERATIVE FROZEN-SECTION DIAGNOSIS per Dr. Lonewolf: Re-excision left alar crease lesion: Focal residual basal carcinoma; margins benign.

MICROSCOPIC DESCRIPTION:
A. Permanent sections confirm the frozen-section diagnosis showing basal cell carcinoma involving the surgical margins. The tumor is characterized by downward growth of irregular nests of basaloid cells showing palisading of the peripheral cell layer. Tumor is associated with a reactive fibrous stoma.
B. Sections show skin with underlying subcutaneous adipose tissue with admixed skeletal muscle and focal hyaline cartilage. There is focal residual basal cell carcinoma similar in appearance to that described above in A. All margins are benign.

DIAGNOSIS:
A. Skin lesion, left alar crease excision: Basal cell carcinoma, involving margins.
B. Re-excision left alar crease excision: Focal residual basal cell carcinoma, margins benign.

5-22B:

SERVICE CODE(S): ______________________

DX CODE(S): ______________________

CASE 5-22A DISCUSSION

Based on the pathology report, the pathologist provided three services:

- First frozen section
- Second frozen section
- One microscopic examination.

An intraoperative consultation includes the pathologist's opinion provided during surgery. If the pathologist was present in the operating room and provided an opinion and only a gross examination (using the eyes only), the service is reported with 88239. If the pathologist was present at surgery, provided a gross examination, and took a frozen section (specimen that is immediately frozen in cold liquid or environment), the service is reported with 88331 for the first specimen and 88332 for each additional specimen. This report indicates that the pathologist was present in the operating room, provided a gross examination, and took two frozen sections.

In addition to the codes to report the intraoperative consultations, a microscopic examination (in the report labeled Microscopic Description) was conducted of one specimen. The microscopic description is reported with the correct level code from the 88300-88309 range. If there were two microscopic descriptions indicated in the report, then two codes from the 88300-88309 range would be reported.

Skin Grafts

A free **skin graft** is a piece of skin that is either of a split-thickness autograft (epidermis and part of the dermis) or a full-thickness autograft (epidermis and all the dermis). These grafts are completely freed from the donor site and are placed over the recipient site with a connection left between the graft and the donor site. As with adjacent tissue transfers, the free skin grafts are reported by the site, size, and type of repair to the **recipient** site.

The **recipient** site is specified within the code descriptions as the location, such as trunk, arms, or legs.

The **size** of the repair is reported in square centimeters for adults and in the Rule of Nines (see Figure 5-1) or the Lund-Browder for children **(Figure 5-5).** The Lund-Browder is similar to the Rule of Nines, with adjustments made in the percentages because the head of an infant is larger in proportion to the rest of his or her body.

The **types** of grafts are varied and specified within the codes as pinch, split, or full-thickness autograft. A *pinch graft* is a small, split-thickness repair; a *split graft* is a repair that involves the epidermis and some of the dermis; and a *full-thickness graft* is a repair that involves the epidermis and all of the dermis. Often a split-thickness skin graft is referred to in the patient record as STSG and a full-thickness skin graft as FTSG.

The **donor** site is the place from which the tissue for the graft is taken. If the donor site for the graft requires repair by grafting, an additional graft code is used. Simple repair (closure) of the donor site is included in the graft code and as such, simple repairs are not reported separately.

A temporary graft may be placed on the recipient site, such as a bilaminate (artificial skin). *Autografts* are grafts taken from the patient's body, *allografts* are taken from other persons (alive or cadaver), and *xenografts* are taken from other species (such as pigs).

Surgical preparation of the recipient site prepares the area to receive the graft and includes removal of scar tissue or lesions. If surgical preparation of a site is required, it is reported separately with codes 15000-15001.

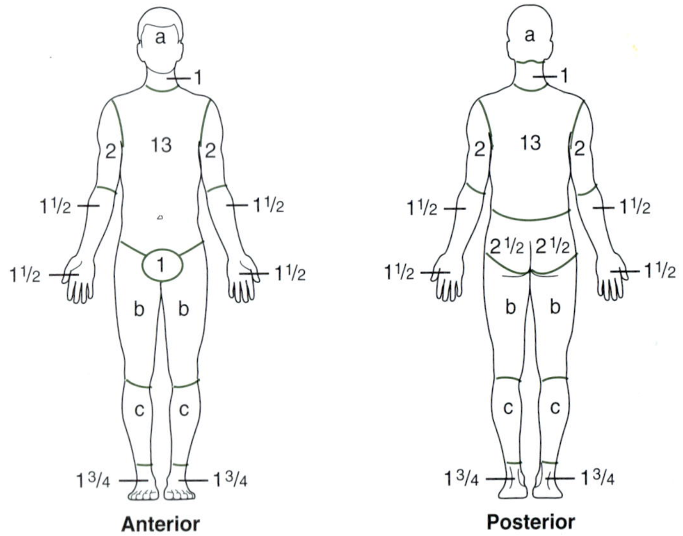

Relative percentage of body surface areas (% BSA) affected by growth

	0 yr	1 yr	5 yr	10 yr	15 yr
a – 1/2 of head	9 1/2	8 1/2	6 1/2	5 1/2	4 1/2
b – 1/2 of 1 thigh	2 3/4	3 1/4	4	4 1/4	4 1/2
c – 1/2 of lower leg	2 1/2	2 1/2	2 3/4	3	3 1/4

FIGURE 5-5 Lund-Browder chart for estimating the extent of burns in children.

CASE 5-23
5-23A Operative Report, Split-Thickness Autograft

CASE 5-23

The diagnosis on this report is that of a nonhealing wound, which can be located by first referencing the ICD-9-CM Index under the main term "Wound," followed by the subterms "open," "nonhealing surgical." The service is a split graft, which is a free skin graft.

5-23A OPERATIVE REPORT, SPLIT-THICKNESS AUTOGRAFT

LOCATION: Inpatient, Hospital

PATIENT: Roger Ulland

SURGEON: Gary Sanchez, M.D.

PREOPERATIVE DIAGNOSIS: Nonhealing wound of left lower quadrant of abdomen **(site)**

POSTOPERATIVE DIAGNOSIS: Nonhealing wound of left lower quadrant of abdomen

SURGICAL PROCEDURE: Split-thickness skin graft from the right thigh to the left lower quadrant of the abdomen measuring 2.5 × 2.5 cm

INDICATION: This patient has a nonhealing wound of a previous skin-grafted site of the lower abdomen.

SURGICAL FINDINGS: A 2.5 × 2.5-cm **(size)** nonhealing wound of the right lower abdomen with exuberant granulation tissue.

ANESTHESIA: Standby with about 6 cc of 1% Xylocaine with 1:800,000 epinephrine.

COMPLICATIONS: None

SPONGE AND NEEDLE COUNT: Correct

DESCRIPTION OF PROCEDURE: The patient's right thigh and abdomen were prepped with Betadine scrub and solution and draped in a routine sterile fashion. The right thigh was anesthetized with 1% Xylocaine with 1:800,000 epinephrine (6 cc), and Shur-Clens was applied. The skin graft was taken with a Goulian Weck blade with an 8-thousands-of-an-inch-thick shim on the blade. This was sewed to the defect with a running 5-0 Vicryl. A dressing of Xeroform glycerin-soaked cotton and a Kerlix fluff were then applied using Elastoplast to hold the dressing in place. The donor site was covered with scarlet red and an ABD pad. The patient tolerated the procedure well and left the area in good condition.

5-23A:

SERVICE CODE(S): ____________________

DX CODE(S): ____________________

right thigh (donor site)
left lower quadrant of abdomen (recipient site)
2.5 X 2.5 cm = 6.25 sq. cm.
split-thickness skin graft (STSG)

CASE 5-24
5-24A Operative Report, Muscle Flap
5-24B Radiology Report, Ultrasound, Lower Extremity

CASE 5-24

The procedure that Dr. Sanchez is performing involves deeper tissue than what is reported with the Free Skin Graft codes. In this case, the repair is of the muscle (muscle flap) and of the skin (skin graft), and both procedures are reported.

5-24A OPERATIVE REPORT, MUSCLE FLAP

LOCATION: Inpatient, Hospital

PATIENT: Josh Peterson

SURGEON: Gary Sanchez, M.D.

PREOPERATIVE DIAGNOSIS: Ulcer, left lower extremity, with exposed tibia and exposed plate

POSTOPERATIVE DIAGNOSIS: Ulcer, left lower extremity, with exposed tibia and exposed plate

PROCEDURES PERFORMED:

1. Soleus muscle flap
2. Split-thickness skin graft 2.5 × 2.5 cm from the left thigh to the left lower extremity

ANESTHESIA: General endotracheal

ESTIMATED BLOOD LOSS: 130 cc

DRAINS: One no. 10 Jackson-Pratt

SURGICAL FINDINGS: There was an open wound extending from the lower third of the tibia up into the middle third of the leg with an exposed plate, but tissue loss of the lower third of the leg was evident. Dr. Almaz, orthopedics, had previously inserted antibiotic beads.

PROCEDURE: An incision was made 2.5 cm medial to the tibial border. We developed a bilobed flap and identified the separation of the soleus muscle and the gastrocnemius medial head following incision of the deep fascia. I dissected the soleus muscle free distally as far as possible and then cut it distally at the Achilles tendon insertion, transposing it through a tunnel of the bilobed flap and covering the area of soft-tissue loss by using bolsters that were tied in place with 0 Prolene. This effectively covered the open area, and then we closed the remainder of the area with 0 Prolene, closing the donor area also with 0 Prolene. We put Nitro paste along the edges where there was some skin blanching and put a no. 10 Jackson-Pratt drain in the distal end of the wound, bringing it out through a separate stab wound incision. A split-thickness skin graft about 2.5 × 2.5 cm was taken from the left thigh, meshed with 1:1.5 mesher, and applied to the defect area measuring 2.5 × 2.5 cm with 2-0 Prolene sutures and staples. We dressed the wound with Xeroform, Kerlix fluffs, Kerlix roll, Kling, and Sof-Rol, and then a cast was applied by the orthopedic technician. The donor site was dressed with scarlet red and an ABD pad. The patient tolerated the procedure well and left the area in good condition.

5-24A:

SERVICE CODE(S): ____________________

DX CODE(S): ____________________

5-24B RADIOLOGY REPORT, ULTRASOUND, LOWER EXTREMITY

The diagnosis on this report is an ulcer of the skin of the lower leg, which requires a 707.xx code and aftercare for a fracture of the leg, which requires a V code. The service is the professional portion of a vascular study of the veins of the leg.

LOCATION: Inpatient, Hospital

PATIENT: Josh Peterson

SURGEON: Gary Sanchez, M.D.

RADIOLOGIST: Morton Monson, M.D.

EXAMINATION OF: Left lower extremity ultrasound

CLINICAL SYMPTOMS: Ulcer, lower extremity, calf

LEFT LOWER EXTREMITY ULTRASOUND: HISTORY: History of traumatic fracture

FINDINGS: Ultrasound examination of the deep venous system of the left lower extremity is negative for DVT. The left popliteal, greater saphenous, and femoral veins are patent and negative for thrombus. Unable to evaluate the calf veins due to existing cast.

5-24B:

SERVICE CODE(S): ____________________

DX CODE(S): ____________________

CASE 5-25
5-25A Operative Report, Full-Thickness Skin Graft

CASE 5-25

Avulsion is ripping or tearing apart. When referencing the Index of the ICD-9-CM under the term "Avulsion, skin and subcutaneous tissue," the coder is directed to "see Wound, open, finger*." Use an HCPCS modifier to indicate the location of the repair.*

5-25A OPERATIVE REPORT, FULL-THICKNESS SKIN GRAFT

LOCATION: Outpatient, Hospital

PATIENT: Brenda Payne

SURGEON: Gary Sanchez, M.D.

INDICATION: This patient had an avulsion injury of the dorsum of the left thumb.

PREOPERATIVE DIAGNOSIS: Partial-thickness avulsion, dorsum of left thumb **(location)**

POSTOPERATIVE DIAGNOSIS: Partial-thickness avulsion, dorsum of left thumb

SURGICAL FINDINGS: There is about a 4 × 2.5-cm **(size)** area of avulsion of the skin of the dorsum of left thumb extending from about the base of the nail to the metacarpophalangeal joint.

PROCEDURE PERFORMED: Full-thickness skin graft **(type of repair)**

ANESTHESIA: General

COMPLICATIONS: None

SPONGE AND NEEDLE COUNT: Correct

DESCRIPTION OF PROCEDURE: The arm and hand were prepped with Betadine scrub and solution and draped in a routine sterile fashion. The left groin was also prepped with Betadine scrub and solution and draped in a routine sterile fashion. The area of the left thumb was inspected, and a full-thickness graft was taken from the left groin and applied to the defect of the left thumb using a tie-over dressing of Xeroform and glycerin-soaked cotton balls. The donor site area was closed with subcuticular 3-0 Monocryl. The remainder of the hand dressing was Kerlix fluffs, Kerlix roll, Kling, Sof-Rol, and a short-arm fiberglass cast. The donor site was covered with Xeroform and 4 × 4. The patient tolerated the procedure well and left the area in good condition.

5-25A:

SERVICE CODE(S): ____________________

DX CODE(S): ____________________

5-24 A (1) Soleus muscle flap (bilobed)
(2) STSG 2.5 X 2.5 = 6.25 cm
donor – left thigh
recipient – left lower extremity

5-25 avulsion – left thumb
size = 4 X 2.5 cm = 10 cm
FTSG
(donor) left groin
(recipient) left thumb

CASE 5-26
5-26A Operative Report, Muscle Flap

CASE 5-26

5-26A OPERATIVE REPORT, MUSCLE FLAP

LOCATION: Outpatient, Hospital

PATIENT: Janet Larae

SURGEON: Gary Sanchez, M.D.

PREOPERATIVE DIAGNOSIS: Open wound, left lower extremity, with exposed tibia and exposed plate

POSTOPERATIVE DIAGNOSIS: Open wound, left lower extremity, with exposed tibia and exposed plate. (This is an ulcer.)

PROCEDURES PERFORMED:

1. Soleus muscle flap (muscle flap 15732-15738)
2. Split-thickness skin graft 5.0 × 5.0 cm from the left thigh to the left lower extremity (split autograft 15100-15121)

ANESTHESIA: General endotracheal

ESTIMATED BLOOD LOSS: 80 cc

DRAINS: One no. 1 Jackson-Pratt

SURGICAL FINDINGS: There was an open wound extending from the lower third of the tibia up into the middle third of the leg with an exposed plate, but tissue loss of the lower third of the leg was evident.

PROCEDURE: An incision was made 5.0 cm medial to the tibial border. We developed a bilobed flap and identified the separation of the soleus muscle and the gastrocnemius medial head following incision of the deep fascia. The soleus muscle was freed distally as far as possible and then cut distally at the Achilles tendon insertion. The bilobed flap was found covering the area of soft-tissue loss by using bolsters that were tied in place with 0 Prolene. The open area was covered, and then we closed the remainder of the area, closing the donor area also with 0 Prolene. We put Nitro paste along the edges where there was some skin blanching and put a no. 1 Jackson-Pratt drain in the distal end of the wound, bringing it out through a separate stab wound incision. A split-thickness skin graft about 5.0 × 5.0 cm was taken from the left thigh, meshed with a mesher, and applied to the defect with 2-0 Prolene, sutures, and staples. We dressed the wound with Xeroform, Kerlix fluffs, Kerlix roll, Kling, and a Sof-Rol, and then the orthopedic technician applied a cast. The donor site was dressed with scarlet red and an ABD pad. The patient tolerated the procedure well and left the area in good condition.

5-26A:

SERVICE CODE(S): ____________________

DX CODE(S): ____________________

Other Procedures

The next three reports will provide you with an opportunity to code a variety of services.

CASE 5-27

5-27A OPERATIVE REPORT, COMPOSITE GRAFT

(brown patch, generally on face)

LOCATION: Outpatient, Hospital

PATIENT: Doreen Anderson

SURGEON: Gary Sanchez, M.D.

PREOPERATIVE DIAGNOSIS: Lentigo maligna, right side of nose overlying alar cartilage

POSTOPERATIVE DIAGNOSIS: Lentigo maligna, right side of nose overlying alar cartilage

PROCEDURE PERFORMED: Excision, lentigo maligna ala of the right side of nose with repair by composite graft (**type**) from the right ear

SURGICAL FINDINGS: There is about a 5-mm raised scar along the nostril rim

ANESTHESIA: General endotracheal with 6 cc of 1% Xylocaine and 1:800,000 epinephrine

ESTIMATED BLOOD LOSS: Negligible

DESCRIPTION OF PROCEDURE: The patient's face and right ear were prepped with Betadine scrub and solution and draped in a routine sterile fashion. Both sites (i.e., the ear and nose) were injected with 1% Xylocaine and 1:800,000 epinephrine, and a through-and-through excision was accomplished of the right alar lesion with a margin of 1 cm from the farthest edge of the scar. This was excised in the form of a triangle and, after obtaining hemostasis, took a composite graft from the right ear with a no. 11 knife blade measuring about 2 cm in its maximal width. The cartilage was trimmed somewhat in this area. Then I sutured the vestibular lining in with interrupted 4-0 Monocryl using interrupted 5-0 Prolene for the external sutures. A dressing of Xeroform was rolled up and placed in the nose. It was placed in the right nostril and then a Xeroform and 4 × 4 were placed over it externally. The right ear had been repaired with interrupted 3-0 Prolene. Surgicel and a Band-Aid were applied to the right ear. The patient tolerated the procedure well and left the operating room in good condition.

Pathology Report Later Indicated: Carcinoma in situ.

5-27A:

SERVICE CODE(S): ____________

DX CODE(S): ____________

5-27 – Composite graft
(donor) – right ear
(recipient) – right side of nose

margin – 1 cm
lesion – 2 cm (?)
3 cm.

scar – 5 mm

CASE 5-28

5-28A Operative Report, Abdominoplasty

CASE 5-28

5-28A OPERATIVE REPORT, ABDOMINOPLASTY

LOCATION: Inpatient, Hospital

PATIENT: Harriet Bergh

SURGEON: Gary Sanchez, M.D.

INDICATIONS FOR PROCEDURE: This patient has a nonhealing vertical wound below the umbilicus for which we have attempted conservative management with failure of conservative management. This wound probably will not heal without removal of the large panniculus that the patient has. Complications were discussed with the patient, including hematoma, infection, pulmonary embolus, fat necrosis, skin necrosis, urinary tract infection, and atelectasis.

PREOPERATIVE DIAGNOSIS: Massive abdominal panniculus (localized fat)

POSTOPERATIVE DIAGNOSIS: Massive abdominal panniculus

SURGICAL FINDINGS: Massive abdominal panniculus weighing a total of 8.99 kg

SURGICAL PROCEDURE: Abdominoplasty (skin only) with relocation of the umbilicus

ANESTHESIA: General endotracheal

ESTIMATED BLOOD LOSS: 200 cc

FLUIDS: Three liters of Ringer's lactate

DRAINS: Four no. 10 Jackson-Pratt

DESCRIPTION OF PROCEDURE: A lower abdominal incision was marked out, and 400 cc of tumescent solution was infiltrated along the suture lines in the abdomen. Tumescent solution was prepared by adding 25 cc of 2% Xylocaine, 1 cc of 1:100,000 epinephrine, and 3 cc of sodium bicarbonate to 1L of Ringer's lactate. The umbilicus was circumscribed and cut down to the abdominal wall, undermining the skin at the supra-areolar fascial level on the abdominal wall, up to the costal margin. We then plexed the table, pulled the areas of resection down, and resected them by halving each side. We obtained a total of 8.99 kg from both sides, and after appropriate trimming, we closed the superficial layer with interrupted 0 Monocryl using subcuticular 0 Monocryl for the skin closure and staples. We then located the umbilicus by palpation underneath the abdominal wall. We had inserted four Jackson-Pratt drains and brought them out through separate stab wound incisions. After location of the abdominal wall, along the iliac crest, we made a 15-mm incision transversely over the proposed site of the umbilicus and brought it out in the skin, suturing to the skin with 3-0 Prolene. We did not suture it to the fascia because of the scarring around the umbilicus, and we inserted Xeroform in that using a dressing of ABD pads, Sof-Rol, and a plaster cast, on which we placed a 10-pound sandbag. Estimated blood loss was 200 cc. The patient tolerated the procedure well and left the operating room in good condition.

Pathology Report Later Indicated: Benign skin and fat.

5-28A:

SERVICE CODE(S): ____________________

DX CODE(S): ____________________

CASE 5-29
5-29A Operative Report, Post Skin Graft

CASE 5-29

This is a return to the operating room (during the postoperative period for the initial procedure) by the same surgeon who originally performed full-thickness graft 5 days before. This report describes the service of a dressing change and a diagnosis of admission for a change of surgical dressing.

5-29A OPERATIVE REPORT, POST SKIN GRAFT

LOCATION: Outpatient, Hospital

PATIENT: Helen Mittag

SURGEON: Gary Sanchez, M.D.

INDICATION: This patient had a thin, full-thickness graft from the groin applied to the dorsum of the right index finger 5 days ago after being burned by a bonfire. We are going to change her dressing under anesthesia to prevent any dislodgment of the graft secondary to movement.

PREOPERATIVE DIAGNOSIS: Status post full-thickness skin graft, right groin to dorsum of right index finger overlying the proximal phalanx.

POSTOPERATIVE DIAGNOSIS: Status post full-thickness skin graft, right groin to dorsum of right index finger overlying the proximal phalanx

SURGICAL FINDINGS:

1. A 2.5 × 1.5-cm intact full-thickness graft of the dorsum of the right index finger overlying the proximal phalanx.
2. Healed groin wound except for one 2-mm area of maceration of the skin in the center of the area. There was also a small amount of rash in the medial aspect of the groin.

PROCEDURE PERFORMED: Dressing change

ANESTHESIA: Local

COMPLICATIONS: None

SPONGE AND NEEDLE COUNT: Correct

DESCRIPTION OF PROCEDURE: Under satisfactory LMA anesthesia, the cast was removed and the dressing was removed. We removed the dressing down to the tie over portion of it and then draped it in a routine sterile fashion. The Monocryl sutures were cut near their origins, and the tie-over dressing was removed. The skin graft measuring about 2.5 × 1.5 cm was intact. There was a bit of serosanguineous drainage from one edge, and we took a culture and sensitivity of this. A dressing was reapplied using Xeroform immediately on top of the graft, followed by glycerin-soaked cotton ball, a 3-inch Kling, Kerlix roll, Kerlix fluffs at the base and the palm, and a 3-inch Kling for the outside of the dressing. For support and for immobilization, we taped the index and middle fingers to minimize motion in the fingers. A cast was not reapplied. The twists and single horizontal mattress suture in the groin were removed with a no. 11 knife blade, and a dry dressing was applied. There was one small 2-mm area of maceration of the center of the wound. The patient tolerated the procedure well and left the operating room in good condition.

5-29A:

SERVICE CODE(S): ____________________

DX CODE(S): ____________________

Pressure Ulcers

A pressure ulcer is a decubitus ulcer or a bedsore found on areas of the body that have bony projections, such as the hips, ankle projection, heel, and the area above the tailbone. Pressure on these areas causes decreased blood flow, and sores form. With continued pressure, the sores ulcerate, and deeper layers of tissue, such as fascia, muscle, and bone, may be affected. Ulcers are identified by stages—I, II, III, and IV.

Although a pressure ulcer can be seen, the depth to which the ulceration has penetrated cannot be seen. The ulcer may involve only superficial skin or may affect deeper layers. (Gangrene and/or osteomyelitis are possible complications.) The treatment for a pressure ulcer (15920-15999) is excision of the ulcerated area to the depth of unaffected tissue, fascia, or muscle. If a free skin graft is used to close the ulcer, that closure would be coded separately.

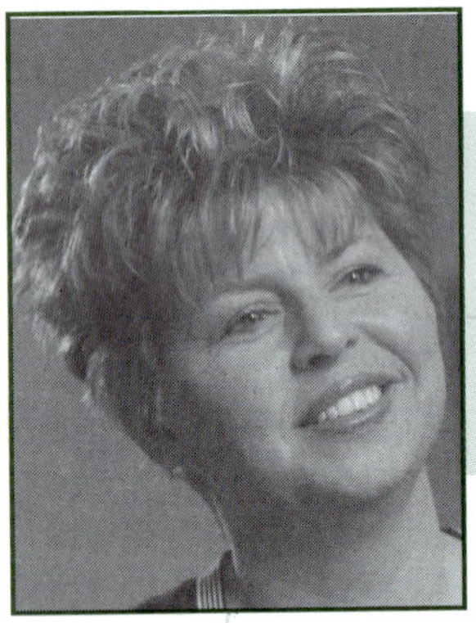

FROM THE TRENCHES

Christy

Coders have to be able to change and they have to be able to adapt. They have to be able to basically develop a method and some organization or some type of structuring… because everything changes from day to day, month to month, year to year."

CASE 5-30

5-30A OPERATIVE REPORT, DEBRIDEMENT

LOCATION: Inpatient, Hospital

PATIENT: Mabel Rud

SURGEON: Gary Sanchez, M.D.

PREOPERATIVE DIAGNOSIS:
1. Left ischial pressure ulcer
2. Osteomyelitis, left ischium

POSTOPERATIVE DIAGNOSIS:
1. Left ischial pressure ulcer
2. Osteomyelitis, left ischium

PROCEDURE PERFORMED: Debridement, left ischial ulcer, with ostectomy of the ischial tuberosity and primary closure

INDICATION: The patient had a recurrent left ischial ulcer secondary to osteomyelitis and shearing forces.

ESTIMATED BLOOD LOSS: 100 cc

DRAINS: One no. 10 Jackson-Pratt

DESCRIPTION OF PROCEDURE: Under satisfactory general endotracheal anesthesia, the patient was turned in the prone position and draped in a routine sterile fashion. She had been prepped with Betadine scrubbing solution. We excised the ulcer elliptically and dissected down to the ischial tuberosity, which was covered with granulation tissue, and we removed this as a unit with the osteotome. We took a piece of bone from deep in the ischial tuberosity and submitted it for culture and sensitivity. Bleeding was electrocoagulated, and we placed a no. 10 Jackson-Pratt in the wound, bringing it out through a separate stab wound incision laterally. I closed the wound by advancing the posterior thigh musculature to suture it to the gluteus maximus muscle with 0 Monocryl. The remainder of the wound was closed with no. 2 Prolene. We cauterized the granulation tissue on top of a 1.5-cm superficial sacral ulcer and then dressed the wound with Xeroform, Kerlix, and Elastoplast. The patient tolerated the procedure well and left the area in good condition.

5-30A:

SERVICE CODE(S): ____________________

DX CODE(S): ____________________

Breast Procedures

To report mastectomy procedures correctly, it is necessary to determine the extent of the procedure, that is, whether pectoral muscles, axillary lymph nodes, or internal mammary lymph nodes were also removed. The mastectomy codes are for unilateral procedures, and so bilateral procedures are reported with use of modifier -50 (bilateral procedures).

Breast biopsies can be performed by means of an incision made into the lesion, and a small portion of the lesion is taken out or by excisional biopsy in which the entire lesion is removed. The lesion may be marked preoperatively by placing a thin wire (radiologic marker) down to the lesion to identify its exact location. The placement of the wire is reported with 19290, and the excision of the lesions identified by the marker is coded separately with 19125 and 19126.

There are multiple codes for mastectomies (19140-19240). You should carefully review the operative report to confirm whether pectoral muscles, axillary lymph nodes, or internal mammary lymph nodes were also removed. This information will be necessary to determine the correct mastectomy code.

CASE 5-31
5-31A Operative Report, Breast Biopsy
5-31B Pathology Report
5-31C Progress Note

CASE 5-31

Use the HCPCS modifier that identifies the left side on the service code.

5-31A OPERATIVE REPORT, BREAST BIOPSY

LOCATION: Inpatient, Hospital

PATIENT: Marina Wild

SURGEON: Gary Sanchez, M.D.

PREOPERATIVE DIAGNOSIS: Left breast mass

POSTOPERATIVE DIAGNOSIS: Left breast mass

PROCEDURE PERFORMED: Biopsy, left breast mass

ANESTHESIA: General anesthesia

INDICATIONS: This is a 42-year-old female with a previous history of breast biopsy laterally in the left axillary tail (**previous location**) area. She has some scar tissue present in this area, and just lateral and superior to the tail of Spence in the axilla (**current location**), she has a firm area, which is worrisome to the patient. She has had a normal workup for breast mass.

DESCRIPTION OF PROCEDURE: She was taken to the operating room and laid supine on the operating room table, anesthetized, and put to sleep. The left axilla was prepped and draped in the usual fashion. We utilized a slightly oblique and transverse incision overlying the firm area and dissected down through the subcutaneous tissue with a combination of blunt and sharp dissection, tying off bleeding with silk suture material. The area represented breast tissue, and we grasped and elevated it with an Allis clamp and cored out a large area of tissue. The residual cavity had no palpable masses, and the area was closed. The dermal layer was closed with interrupted chromic, and skin edges were closed with interrupted nylon. Dressings were applied. She tolerated this well. Dr. Monson was present for the entire case.

Pathology Report Indicated: See 5-31B.

5-31A:

SERVICE CODE(S): ____________________

DX CODE(S): ____________________

5-31B PATHOLOGY REPORT

LOCATION: Inpatient, Hospital

PATIENT: Marina Wild

SURGEON: Gary Sanchez, M.D.

PATHOLOGIST: Morton Monson, M.D.

CLINICAL HISTORY: Breast lump

TISSUE RECEIVED: OR Consult

LEFT BREAST BIOPSY: Axillary tail area

GROSS DESCRIPTION: The specimen is labeled with the patient's name and "left breast lump," which consists of two yellow fatty tissues, one of which is 5 × 3.5 × 2.5 cm and the other 4 × 3 × 1.5 cm. Cut surfaces reveal largely yellow adipose tissue throughout. The specimen is serially sectioned and processed in toto in 25 cassettes with the smaller specimen in cassettes 1-9 and the larger specimen in cassettes 10-25.

INTRAOPERATIVE FROZEN SECTION DIAGNOSIS per Dr. Monson: Left breast biopsy, axillary tail area: Grossly benign, defer to permanent sections.

MICROSCOPIC DESCRIPTION: Sections show predominantly mature adipose tissue with intersecting bands of fibrous tissue. Sections from the smaller tissue segment show a focus of benign ducts. Sections of the large tissue section show a few benign lymph nodes with mild fatty change.

DIAGNOSIS: Left breast biopsy, axillary area: Adipose tissue with a single focus of benign ducts and nine benign axillary lymph nodes.

5-31B:

SERVICE CODE(S): ____________________

DX CODE(S): ____________________

5-31C PROGRESS NOTE

The diagnosis for this service is a V code to report after-care that involved the removal of dressing in a follow-up situation. The patient has no current symptoms or illness.

LOCATION: Outpatient, Clinic

PATIENT: Marina Wild

SURGEON: Gary Sanchez, M.D.

The patient comes in for a postoperative check after biopsy of a left breast mass. The biopsy specimen showed adipose tissue with a single focus of benign ducts and nine benign axillary lymph nodes. It was in the tail of Spence where the biopsy occurred. She has been doing well since her surgery. She complains of some pain and numbness, but this is improving. She takes Tylenol for the pain; no narcotics.

PHYSICAL EXAMINATION: The wound is clean and dry. No cellulitis. No evidence of a seroma. Stitches were removed. No Steri-Strips were applied.

IMPRESSION: Routine postoperative check

PLAN: Return to clinic p.r.n.

5-31C:

SERVICE CODE(S): ______________________

DX CODE(S): ______________________

CASE 5-32
5-32A Operative Report, Breast Mass
5-32B Pathology Report

CASE 5-32

5-32A OPERATIVE REPORT, BREAST MASS

LOCATION: Outpatient, Hospital

PATIENT: Donna Senne

SURGEON: Gary Sanchez, M.D.

PREOPERATIVE DIAGNOSIS: Right breast mass

POSTOPERATIVE DIAGNOSIS: Right breast mass

OPERATIVE NOTE: With the patient under general anesthesia, the right breast was prepped and draped in a sterile manner. A standard breast line incision was made over the palpated mass. Sharp dissection was carried down to the mass. The mass was grasped with an Allis clamp and then was excised from the surrounding breast tissue. Hemostasis was maintained with electrocautery, and then the breast tissue was reapproximated using 2 and 3-0 chromic. The skin was closed using 4-0 Vicryl in a subcuticular fashion. Steri-Strips were applied at the conclusion of the procedure. The patient tolerated the procedure well and was returned to the recovery area in stable condition. At the end of the procedure, all sponges and instruments were accounted for. Pathology Report Later Indicated: See report 5-32B.

5-32A:

SERVICE CODE(S): ______________________

DX CODE(S): ______________________

5-32B PATHOLOGY REPORT

LOCATION: Outpatient, Hospital

PATIENT: Donna Senne

SURGEON: Gary Sanchez, M.D.

PATHOLOGIST: Grey Lonewolf, M.D.

CLINICAL HISTORY: Right abnormal mammogram

SPECIMEN RECEIVED: Right breast biopsy

GROSS DESCRIPTION: The specimen is labeled with the patient's name and "right breast biopsy" and consists of a biopsy of white-tan lobulated tissue with adipose at the periphery, 4.7 × 3.5 × 2.0 cm. Surgical margins are inked black. Cut sections show a whit-tan, moderately firm, lobulated, somewhat glistening lesion, 3.5 × 2.8 × 1.6 cm. The lesion shows solid white-tan tissue throughout. Representative sections are submitted in six cassettes.

MICROSCOPIC DESCRIPTION: Sections show a well-circumscribed lesion showing a mildly cellular stroma consisting of spindled cells showing no cell atypia or mitotic activity. There is proliferation of variably sized glands with focal leaflike processes protruding into cystic spaces. Many of the ducts are collapsed into slitlike spaces. The epithelial elements consist of luminal epithelial cells and a myoepithelial layer.

DIAGNOSIS: Right breast biopsy: Benign fibroadenoma

5-32B:

SERVICE CODE(S): ______________________

DX CODE(S): ______________________

CASE 5-33
5-33A Operative Report, Breast Biopsy with Needle Localization
5-33B Pathology Report

CASE 5-33

5-33A OPERATIVE REPORT, BREAST BIOPSY WITH NEEDLE LOCALIZATION

This patient presents for the removal of a breast lesion that was previously marked prior to surgery with a radiological marker. Microcalcification of the breast is fibrosis of the breast.

LOCATION: Outpatient, Hospital

PATIENT: Marilyn Agnes

SURGEON: Gary Sanchez, M.D.

PREOPERATIVE DIAGNOSIS: Right breast microcalcification by mammogram

POSTOPERATIVE DIAGNOSIS: Right breast microcalcification by mammogram fibrosis of breast

PROCEDURE PERFORMED: Right breast biopsy with needle localization

ANESTHESIA: One percent Xylocaine local; 16 cc was used. The patient also received IV sedation.

INDICATIONS FOR SURGERY: The patient is a 77-year-old white female who had undergone mammography. The patient was found to have microcalcifications in her right breast. The patient was taken to the operating room for biopsy.

DESCRIPTION OF PROCEDURE: The patient had previously undergone needle localization on the right breast microcalcification. She was brought back to the operating room. The patient was then prepped and draped in the usual manner. One-percent Xylocaine was used as local anesthesia; a total of 16 cc was used. The patient also received IV sedation. An incision was made over the guidewire. The guidewire and surrounding breast tissue were incised and sent to radiology. Radiology confirmed that the microcalcifications had been removed. Hemostasis was obtained using Bovie cautery. The operative area was thoroughly irrigated. The incision was then closed with figure-of-eight 2-0 chromic sutures for the deep and superficial layers. The skin was closed with 4-0 Vicryl subcuticular stitch, and Steri-Strips were applied. The patient tolerated the operation and returned to recovery in stable condition.

Pathology Report Later Indicated: See Report 5-33B.

5-33A:

SERVICE CODE(S): ______________________

DX CODE(S): ______________________

5-33B PATHOLOGY REPORT

LOCATION: Outpatient, Hospital

PATIENT: Marilyn Agnes

SURGEON: Gary Sanchez, M.D.

PATHOLOGIST: Grey Lonewolf, M.D.

CLINICAL HISTORY: Right breast microcalcification

SPECIMEN RECEIVED: Right breast biopsy after wire localization

GROSS DESCRIPTION: Submitted in formalin and labeled with the patient's name and "right breast biopsy after wire localization" is a piece of lobulated yellow fatty tissue measuring 6.5 × 4 × 1.5 cm with an intact localizing wire. First, serial sections are submitted in cassettes 1-3, and sections from the region of the wire tip are submitted in cassettes 4-7. No gross lesion is identified. No gross lesions are identified in the remainder of the specimen, and representative sections are submitted in cassettes 8-12.

MICROSCOPIC DESCRIPTION: The slides show multiple sections of breast parenchyma featuring prominent adipose tissue replacement. A focus of mild fibrosis with coarse microcalcifications is present on slide 4, corresponding to the abnormality seen on accompanying specimen mammogram.

DIAGNOSIS: Breast, right, biopsy:

1. Focal fibrosis with coarse microcalcifications, corresponding to the abnormality seen on accompanying specimen mammogram.
2. Adipose tissue replacement of breast parenchyma.

DX: fibrosis of breast

5-33B:

SERVICE CODE(S): ______________________

DX CODE(S): ______________________

CASE 5-34
5-34A Operative Report, Segmental Mastectomy with Sentinel Node Injection

CASE 5-34

Glory Nisley had cancer of the right breast, and in this operative report, Dr. Sanchez performed a segmental mastectomy that removed a portion of her breast. Additionally, the surgeon injected dye into the patient, and when the dye reached the lymph nodes, the node appeared blue, which is "a hot node." The hot node was sampled and sent to the pathology lab for analysis. This injection procedure would be used when a lymphadenectomy (removal of the lymph node) is performed to ensure that all the nodes are removed. The sentinel node injection procedure is reported separately. Do not report the frozen sections, as this would be reported by the pathologist.

5-34A OPERATIVE REPORT, SEGMENTAL MASTECTOMY WITH SENTINEL NODE INJECTION

LOCATION: Outpatient, Hospital

PATIENT: Glory Nisley

SURGEON: Gary Sanchez, M.D.

PREOPERATIVE DIAGNOSIS: Cancer of right breast

POSTOPERATIVE DIAGNOSIS: Cancer of right breast

PROCEDURE PERFORMED: Segmental mastectomy with frozen-section margins, sentinel node biopsy times two, limited axillary dissection

ANESTHESIA: General

PROCEDURE: The patient was given a general anesthetic. I used 3 cc of isosulfan blue, and I injected just lateral to the cavity. I massaged for 5 minutes. Her right arm was free draped, and she was prepped and draped in this position. We marked 2 cm on every margin superior, inferior, medially, and laterally. We then developed our superior flap and went down to the chest wall. We developed the inferior flap and went down to chest wall. We then removed this segmental mastectomy going from medial to lateral. We oriented it with silk suture for pathological assessment. The frozen section margins came back negative. We then made an incision in the right axilla. We went down to the clavipectoral fascia and opened it up. We identified a very hot node that was blue. The counts are well documented in the chart. We sent another node, which was right against the first sentinel node. Both these nodes were blue. Once we got the second node out, our background was negligible. We sent both of these out for frozen section. We did a tissue to make sure that we did not have a false-negative result. After waiting, we found that the sentinel node biopsies times two were also benign. We then put a medium Hemovac drain in both sites and sutured the drains in place with silk sutures. We brought the subcutaneous tissue together with Vicryl. Staples were placed in the skin. Telfa, toppers, and gauze were applied. The patient tolerated the procedure well and went to the recovery room in good condition.

Pathology Report Later Indicated: Primary carcinoma of breast tissue

5-34A:

SERVICE CODE(S): ____________________

DX CODE(S): ____________________

CASE 5-35
5-35A Preoperative Consultation
5-35B Operative Report, Modified Radical Mastectomy
5-35C Pathology Report
5-35D Discharge Summary
5-35E Progress Note

CASE 5-35

5-35A PREOPERATIVE CONSULTATION

This is an E/M service at which a decision for surgery was made, which requires the use of modifier -57 on the E/M code. You report not only the diagnosis of breast mass but also the history of malignant breast neoplasm.

LOCATION: Outpatient, Clinic

PATIENT: Ann Rose

PHYSICIAN: Ronald Green, M.D.

CONSULTANT: Gary Sanchez

Mrs. Rose is a lady who in 1990 had a left modified radical mastectomy for breast cancer. She apparently had at least five lymph nodes positive at that time and underwent chemotherapy, and she has been symptom-free since then. She states that earlier in October, she noticed that there was a lump present in her right breast, which had not been there before. She only examines herself intermittently, and she says probably once about every 6 to 8 weeks. There has been no pain, no nipple discharge, and no history of trauma. She has had a partial evaluation by Dr. Green, including a bone scan and chest x-ray for the possibility of metastatic disease. The patient is otherwise doing well. She apparently lost her husband 8 years ago. He died of cancer, and she is concerned because her daughter's mother-in-law also has a cancer at the present time and apparently not doing well.

PHYSICAL EXAMINATION shows a lady who is very bright and oriented. Cervical and supraclavicular examination shows a soft lymph node in the posterior triangle of the left neck. There are no carotid bruits. The mastectomy site on the left has healed reasonably well. There is no evidence of any lymphadenopathy, and there is no evidence of recurrence. On the right side, in the 2 o'clock position, approximately 7 cm from the areola, there is a firm to hard mass that is approximately 2 cm in diameter. It is mobile within the breast tissue and not fixed to either the skin or the deeper structures. There is no evidence of any axillary node involvement. Periareolar area is normal.

Examination of the mammograms suggests a 2- to 2.5-cm lesion in the area of the palpable mass, and this is certainly suspicious for malignancy.

I went over in detail with the patient and her daughters the various options for her, but the patient basically wants to proceed with the biopsy of the area. Then, if it is malignant, she wants a mastectomy done at the same time. We did go through the risks of the procedure, and she is aware of these. I also reviewed in detail the other options, which would include lumpectomy with radiation therapy and chemotherapy, simple mastectomy with radiation, and axillary dissection, etc. After going through these, she says that she really is not inclined to proceed with anything other than the biopsy and breast resection, a modified radical, as indicated at the time of surgery, and she only wants to undergo one anesthetic. She apparently had significant problems with the biopsy the last time, and she does not want to proceed with this at this time. Consequently, we will be proceeding with the procedure. Because she is taking aspirin, even though it is only 80 mg a day, we will stop that today, and we will do the biopsy and probably mastectomy next week because I do feel this is most likely malignant.

5-35A:

SERVICE CODE(S): ______________________

DX CODE(S): ______________________

5-35B OPERATIVE REPORT, MODIFIED RADICAL MASTECTOMY

LOCATION: Inpatient, Hospital

PATIENT: Ann Rose

PHYSICIAN: Ronald Green, M.D.

SURGEON: Gary Sanchez, M.D.

PREOPERATIVE DIAGNOSIS: Lump in the right breast, upper, inner quadrant

POSTOPERATIVE DIAGNOSIS: Infiltrating intraductal carcinoma of the right breast

PROCEDURES PERFORMED: Right breast biopsy followed by a modified radical mastectomy with level II axillary dissection

This lady, in 1990, had a left mastectomy for breast cancer. This was done in Manytown, and she does not remember the surgeon's name. However, she presented with a mass in the right breast, and in further discussions had decided that, should this turn out to be a malignancy, then she wanted immediate mastectomy. She was not interested in breast reconstruction, nor was she interested in any other form of therapy such as lumpectomy. Risks have been explained in detail to her and her daughter.

Under general anesthesia, the right breast was prepped and draped, and then an incision was made parallel to a skin crease approximately 5 cm away from the areola at the 2 o'clock position. Because of the clinical characteristics, there was high probability of malignancy and the incision was placed in such a way that we could do the mastectomy as necessary with minimal risk. The skin incision was made, and then the lump itself was removed without difficulty. Electrocautery was not used because of the concern for interference with the histology. Once the lesion was removed, however, small bleeders were controlled with electrocautery. The skin was then closed with a subcuticular 4-0 Vicryl. At this time, the specimen was reviewed by pathology, and they confirmed the presence of probably a grade 2 infiltrating intraductal carcinoma.

The patient's drapes were removed, and then the right breast and axilla were prepped and draped secondarily. All surgeons also changed. Once this was completed, then a standard right modified radical mastectomy was completed to incorporate the incision from the biopsy site. The upper flap was able to be developed and not enter the biopsy site. The vessels were either suture ligated for the larger penetrating vessels or ligated and/or cauterized for the small flaps. Once the upper flap was developed, then the lower flap was developed in such a way that there would be an adequate amount of skin for closure. The axillary dissection was performed by initially dissecting along the pectoralis major and minor muscles, and the dissection stopped just at the pectoralis minor border. However, there was one lymph node that was more palpable up in probably a level III area, and because of this palpable nature, this was removed as an isolated node and marked for the pathologist. The majority of the dissection of the axilla was completed with blunt and then sharp dissection, but the larger lymphatics were ligated with 3-0 Vicryl. The arteries were ligated with 3-0 Vicryl as well. The intercostal brachial nerves were identified and preserved with the exception of one small branch, which went through a fairly dense area but was thought to be lymph nodes, and consequently this small branch was sacrificed. At completion of this procedure, the breast was then removed from the chest wall using electrocautery and, as noted above, the larger vessels being suture-ligated with 3-0 Vicryl. After the breast was removed, the entire area was irrigated. There were no further bleedings that required any intervention other than mild cautery. At this point, no. 10 Jackson-Pratts were placed, one into the axilla, and one into the subcuticular tissue through two separate stab wounds in the inferior flap. The skin was then approximated by using 2-0 Vicryl to approximate the deeper fatty tissue and then subcuticular 4-0 Vicryl for the skin. Half-inch Steri-Strips were then applied. The drains were sutured in place using 3-0 nylon, and then the dressing was applied around these. Total blood loss was less than 100 ml. The patient tolerated the procedure well. Further care will depend on the pathology in this area.

Pathology Report Later Indicated: See report 5-35C.

5-35B:

SERVICE CODE(S): ____________________

DX CODE(S): ____________________

5-35C PATHOLOGY REPORT

LOCATION: Inpatient, Hospital

PATIENT: Ann Rose

PHYSICIAN: Ronald Green, M.D.

SURGEON: Gary Sanchez, M.D.

PATHOGIST: Morton Monson, M.D.

CLINICAL HISTORY:
1. Lesion, right breast, upper inner quadrant
2. Suture at superior apical
3. Apical node (separate), just anterior axillary

TISSUE RECEIVED:
FA. RT breast BX (FS) FS = frozen section
A. RT breast BX (PS)
B. RT breast suture in apex
C. Apical node, right axilla

GROSS DESCRIPTION:
A. The specimen is labeled with the patient's name and "mass right breast" and consists of a piece of yellow and white fibrofatty tissue, 3.8 × 2.5 × 2 cm. Sectioning reveals a white solid mass measuring 2 × 1.8 × 1.4 cm with spiculated border.

INTRAOPERATIVE FROZEN SECTION DIAGNOSIS:
As per Dr. Monson: Infiltrating ductal carcinoma.

B. The specimen is labeled with the patient's name and "right breast" and consists of the product of a right modified radical mastectomy with skin ellipse measuring 23 × 12 cm with centrally placed everted nipple. Biopsy site is noted in the upper medical portion. Biopsy cavity reveals hemorrhagic tan tissue. No distinct evidence of residual neoplasm is seen. Representative section of nipple is placed in cassette labeled B1. Representative sections of biopsy site are placed in cassettes labeled B2 through B8. The remainder of the breast parenchyma is composed primarily of fat with occasional fibrous strands. Random representative sections of breast are placed in cassettes labeled B9 through B10. Sections of axillary tail reveal multiple lymph nodes ranging from 1 cm down to 0.3 cm.

C. The specimen is labeled with the patient's name and "apical node right axilla" and consists of a 0.5-cm diameter apparent lymph node.

MICROSCOPIC DESCRIPTION:

A. Sections of breast showing an infiltrating neoplasm consisting of sheets, cords, and nests of cells infiltrating the desmoplastic stroma. Cells are enlarged and have increased nuclear:cytoplasmic ratio.

B. Lymph nodes were negative for malignancy with normal cells throughout.

5-35C:

SERVICE CODE(S): ______________________

DX CODE(S): ______________________

5-35D DISCHARGE SUMMARY

LOCATION: Inpatient, Hospital

PATIENT: Ann Rose

PHYSICIAN: Ronald Green, M.D.

SURGEON: Gary Sanchez, M.D.

REASON FOR HOSPITALIZATION: Right breast mass

BRIEF HISTORY: This patient had left mastectomy for breast cancer in 1990. She was now found to have a right breast mass and decided that should this turn out to be a malignancy she wanted an immediate mastectomy.

HOSPITAL COURSE: The patient underwent a right breast biopsy with frozen section showing infiltrating ductal carcinoma. At that time, a right modified radical mastectomy was performed. The patient tolerated the procedure well and was transferred to the floor with two Jackson-Pratt drains in place. The patient's pain was controlled after surgery quite nicely. On postoperative day one, the patient was voiding without difficulty and tolerating her diet. She remained afebrile. Her wound did not show any signs of infection or drainage throughout her hospital course. The remainder of the patient's hospital course was uneventful, and she went home with her axillary Jackson-Pratt drain in place. Pathology on the specimen did reveal infiltrating ductal carcinoma grade 2 of 3 on her right breast. Six of six axillary nodes did not show any evidence of malignancy. One separate axillary node also did not show evidence of malignancy.

FOLLOW-UP: The patient was scheduled to return to the clinic in three to four days for follow-up and drain removal.

DISCHARGE INSTRUCTIONS:

1. Activity as tolerated
2. Diet as tolerated

DISCHARGE MEDICATIONS:

1. Lotensin 10 mg 1 p.o. q.d.
2. Metoprolol 25 mg 1 p.o. b.i.d.
3. Tylenol no. 3, 1-2 p.o. q. 4-6h. as needed for pain. The patient was sent home with 25.

PRINCIPAL DIAGNOSIS: Infiltrating ductal carcinoma grade 2 of 3, right breast, upper inner quadrant. Six of six axillary lymph nodes were negative. Now status post right modified radical mastectomy.

PRINCIPAL PROCEDURE: Right breast biopsy followed by a modified radical mastectomy with level II axillary dissection.

CONDITION ON DISCHARGE: Stable

5-35D:

SERVICE CODE(S): ______________________

DX CODE(S): ______________________

5-35E PROGRESS NOTE

This is a postoperative visit. The reason for the service is a follow up after surgery. A history of cancer code is not reported since the patient is still being followed for cancer, with her current referral to the oncologist.

LOCATION: Outpatient, Clinic

PATIENT: Ann Rose

PHYSICIAN: Ronald Green, M.D.

SURGEON: Gary Sanchez, M.D.

Mrs. Rose is now several weeks after her right modified mastectomy for invasive carcinoma of the breast. She had previous carcinoma of the breast and mastectomy in 1990. The patient states that she just had a fullness under her arms. She has noticed no problems with arm motion other than just a little bit of stiffening when she raises it above her head. She has no swelling of the arm.

PHYSICAL EXAMINATION: She is alert and oriented. Her chest is clear. The mastectomy site is healing well. There is a fold of fatty tissue in the posterior axillary area that is still a little edematous, and there is a mild amount of edema on the inferior flap on the medial aspect. Other than this, there is no sign of infection or fluid collections. The patient can move her arm relatively well. She is able to put the arm and hand up above her head.

The area is healing well. We did go over the issue regarding the swelling in these areas. She does not want anything done with respect to the fat fold in the area. I did caution her regarding the area of the swelling that if it gets worse or if there are any changes in the skin color, etc. Otherwise, I will see her in about a month's time for follow-up, and she is going to be seeing the surgical oncologist in the near future regarding any further therapy.

5-35E:

SERVICE CODE(S): ______________________

DX CODE(S): ______________________

CASE 5-36
5-36A Operative Report, Mammoplasty

CASE 5-36

Linda Halaas has been admitted to the hospital for a bilateral breast reduction (mammoplasty). The admission for breast reduction is the first listed code and is reported with a V code. The additional diagnoses are those conditions that support the reason the breast reduction is being performed. Report the services provided to her by Dr. Erickson, the clinic's plastic surgeon.

5-36A OPERATIVE REPORT, MAMMOPLASTY

LOCATION: Inpatient, Hospital

PATIENT: Linda Halaas

SURGEON: Mark Erickson, M.D.

PREOPERATIVE DIAGNOSIS:
1. Bilateral mammary hypertrophy and hyperplasia
2. Bilateral mammary ptosis

POSTOPERATIVE DIAGNOSIS:
1. Bilateral mammary hypertrophy and hyperplasia
2. Bilateral mammary ptosis

PROCEDURE PERFORMED: Bilateral reduction mammoplasty using inferior pedicle technique.
1. 615 g resected from the right side
2. 609 g from the left side

ANESTHESIA: General endotracheal with 225 cc of tumescent solution on the right side and 200 cc of tumescent solution on the left side. Tumescent solution was prepared by adding to 1 L of Ringer's lactate, 25 cc of 2% Xylocaine, 1 cc of 1:100,000 epinephrine, and 3 cc of 8.4% sodium bicarbonate.

ESTIMATED BLOOD LOSS: 75 cc

DRAINS: None

SPONGE AND NEEDLE COUNTS: Correct

COMPLICATIONS: None

SURGICAL FINDINGS: Predominantly fatty breasts with fibrocystic disease obvious throughout both breasts, particularly around the periareolar area

DESCRIPTION OF PROCEDURE: The patient's chest was prepped with Betadine scrub and solution and draped in a routine sterile fashion. In accordance with the preoperatively marked new nipple site at 22 cm from the sternal notch and 12.5 cm from the midsternal line, we marked out an inferior pedicle breast pattern using the 45-mm cookie cutter marker for the new areolar size and the new areolar window. We marked the 12, 6, 9, and 3 o'clock positions at these points, and then we resumed our marking of the inferior pedicle, making the vertical limb 5 cm long. After marking of the inferior pedicle pattern, de-epithelialization of the right side was carried out, leaving about a 1.5-cm cuff of the de-epithelialized tissue above the areola. Deep dissection started at the 12 o'clock position and came toward the 3 o'clock position between the upper end of the vertical limb and the lateral edge of the medial flap. We began to bevel away from the vertical limb, starting at the caudal edge of the medial flap and connecting with the inframammary incision. An incision was then made on the caudal edge of the medial flap to connect to the apex of the triangle with the inframammary incision, and we carried this down the pectoralis major fascia, resecting the medial triangle at that level. Bleeding was electrocoagulated using the insulated forceps for the cautery directly. At the edge of the pedicle, we used a no. 22 knife blade to incise down to pectoralis major fascia. Deep dissection was then started at the 12 o'clock position and came toward the 9 o'clock position coming between the upper and the vertical limb and the medial edge of the lateral flap. We began to bevel away from the vertical limb, starting at the caudal edge of the lateral flap, and we made our incision near the vertical limb with a no. 22 knife blade down to the pectoralis major fascia, connecting it at the inframammary level and the incision on the caudal edge of the lateral flap at the pectoralis major fascia. The incision on the caudal edge of the lateral flap was made in such a manner as to leave 1.5 mm of thickness on the flap and to include the tail of Spence in the resection. Hemostasis was achieved, and then we divided the lateral and medial flaps completely from the upper end of the vertical limb but did not extend this down to the pectoralis major fascia. The skin was dissected away from the superior triangular area, and then we resected the superior triangle by connecting our lateral and medial flap incisions between the respective vertical limbs with a periareolar window incision superiorly. After appropriate resection and trimming, we obtained a final weight of 615 g on the right side. The estimated amount was 750 g. I then separated the dermis from the skin inferiorly, and at the midpoint of the vertical limb, I inset the lateral and medial flaps with a horizontal half mattress suture of 0 Prolene. The points marked at the 3, 6, 9, and 12 o'clock positions were inset with subcuticular 3-0 Monocryl, and then the vertical limb was closed with an interrupted 3-0 Monocryl using subcuticular 3-0 Monocryl also for the inframammary limb. Where better apposition of the skin edges and eversion were needed, we used skin staples, particularly in the area of the areola. The circulation was excellent in the nipple areolar complex, and there was no apparent ischemia of either flap. The left breast was then approached in a similar manner, but we made the pedicle about 9 cm wide instead of 8 cm wide as on the right side. We had instilled 225 cc of tumescent solution in the right side, and we instilled 200 cc of tumescent solution in the left side through junctional incisions. I then de-epithelialized the vertical stalk and left a 1.5-cm cuff of de-epithelialized tissue above. Deep dissection was started at the 12 o'clock position and came, with the cautery, toward the 9 o'clock between the upper end of the vertical limb and the medial flap, beveling away from the vertical limb starting at the caudal edge of the medial flap and connecting with the inframammary incision, and an incision on the caudal edge of the medial flap was made in such a manner as to leave 1.5 cm of thickness on the flap. After resection of the medial triangle, a lateral triangle resection was started at the 12 o'clock position and came toward the 3 o'clock position, coming between the upper end of the vertical limb and the lateral flap. I then resected the lateral triangle by connecting with the lateral flap in such a manner as to leave 1.5 cm of thickness of the flap and to include the tail of Spence in the resection. The superior triangle was then resected, and hemostasis was obtained using the cautery. A no. 22 knife blade was used to make the incision near the vertical pedicle, and following separation of the dermis inferiorly of the vertical pedicle, I inset the lateral and medial flaps with a horizontal mattress suture of 0 Prolene. A running subcuticular suture was used for the inframammary area, and a few interrupted sutures of 3-0 Monocryl were used for the areolar inset and the vertical limb. Skin staples were used to appose the edges better, and the dressing consisted of Xeroform, Kerlix fluffs, a support bra, and an external Ace bandage. Estimated blood loss was 75 cc. The patient seemed to tolerate the procedure well and left the operating room in good condition.

Pathology Report Later Indicated: Benign breast tissue

5-36A:

SERVICE CODE(S): ______________________

DX CODE(S): ______________________

CASE 5-37

5-37A OPERATIVE REPORT, MAMMOPLASTY

The reason for this service is for admission for breast augmentation. Remember to use the bilateral modifier on this service as a mammoplasty code reports the procedure on only one breast.

LOCATION: Inpatient, Hospital

PATIENT: Sheila Lynch

SURGEON: Mark Erickson, M.D.

INDICATIONS FOR PROCEDURE: The patient has bilateral mammary hypoplasia following childbirth and wants to have an increase in breast volume just to fill out her clothes.

PREOPERATIVE DIAGNOSIS: Bilateral mammary hypoplasia

POSTOPERATIVE DIAGNOSIS: Bilateral mammary hypoplasia (only report if congenital)

PROCEDURE PERFORMED: Bilateral augmentation mammoplasty using McGhan style 468, 195-205 cc implant inflated to 205 cc. Lot number was 441693. The left side had a number designation of 4488. The right had 4489.

ANESTHESIA: General endotracheal plus 5 cc of 1% Xylocaine with 1:100,000 epinephrine and 250 cc total of tumescent solution prepared by adding 25 cc of 2% Xylocaine, 1 cc of 1:100,00 epinephrine, and 3 cc of 8.4% sodium bicarbonate to 1L of Ringer's lactate.

ESTIMATED BLOOD LOSS: Negligible

DESCRIPTION OF PROCEDURE: The patient's chest was prepped with Betadine scrub and solution and draped in a routine sterile fashion. Incision was made over the sixth rib and carried down through the subcutaneous tissue and fascia to the pectoralis muscle origin, which we incised along the rib, elevating it off of the rib and taking care not to dissect down on the rib or traumatize rib. We injected 150 cc of tumescent solution on the right side in the subpectoral space and used balloon dissection to further elevate the pectoralis muscle rapidly. Dissection was completed by sharp and blunt medially and inferiorly to detach the pectoralis insertion fibers. After detachment of those fibers, we inserted a balloon dissector and inflated to about 300 cc. We then went to the left side and made an incision over the sixth rib and dissected using the balloon dissector with some difficulty inserting 200-cc sizer. We left the balloon dissector in. We did insert the mammary sizer at this time. We left the balloon dissector in, went to the left side, made an incision over the sixth rib after injection of 1% Xylocaine and 1:100,000 epinephrine, carried down to the pectoralis fascia, incising the pectoralis major muscle, entering the subpectoral space where we injected 100 cc of tumescent solution, and then used the balloon dissector to elevate the pectoralis off the chest wall. We completed our pocket dissection, sharp and blunt dissection, and left the balloon dissector in place. We then went to the right side and removed the balloon dissector with some difficulty inserting a 200-cc sizer. The pocket was somewhat asymmetrical at this time, and we did further blunt dissection to enlarge the pocket. We went to the left side and removed our balloon dissector, completing the pocket dissection with very little bleeding. We inserted an inflatable saline implant, McGhan style 468, which we inflated to a total of 5 cc in the submuscular, subpectoral pocket. The muscle was closed with interrupted 3-0 Ethibond, the fascial layer was closed with interrupted 4-0 Vicryl, and a subcuticular Vicryl was used to complete the closure with a few twists of 6-0 Prolene. Steri-Strips were applied. On the right side, the pocket was clipped and completed to achieve symmetry, and after removal of the expander, we inserted the partially inflated McGhan style 468 with all the air removed, and after insertion of the pocket, we completed the filling to 205 cc. This brought the right breast implant into better asymmetry with the left side. Then we closed the muscle pocket with interrupted 3-0 Ethibond using interrupted 4-0 Vicryl for the fascial layer and subcuticular 4-0 Vicryl following by a few twists of 6-0 Prolene. Steri-Strips were applied. Dressing consisted of the Steri-Strips, Kerlix fluffs, Kerlix roll, Kling, and an Ace bandage. Estimated blood loss was negligible. The patient tolerated the procedure well and left the operating room in good condition.

5-37A:

SERVICE CODE(S): ____________________

DX CODE(S): ____________________

CASE 5-38
5-38A Operative Report, Removal of Tissue Expander

CASE 5-38

5-38A OPERATIVE REPORT, REMOVAL OF TISSUE EXPANDER

The reason for this service is a complication of a breast prosthetic, which was a tissue expander that was previously implanted and now is leaking. A tissue expander is placed to stretch the skin and can be a sac of fluid or air, or a plastic insert. The stretched skin can be harvested for skin grafting or as in this case, placed to expand the skin to allow for a breast implant at a later date. When the implant malfunctions, such as the one in this case that is leaking, it is considered a mechanical complication. Reference the Index of the ICD-9-CM under the main term "Complication" followed by subterms "mechanical, prosthetic, breast," which will direct you to the correct code. The service is removal of the malfunctioning tissue expander and the insertion of a prosthesis (breast).

LOCATION: Outpatient, Hospital

PATIENT: Donna Polanski

SURGEON: Gary Sanchez, M.D.

PREOPERATIVE DIAGNOSIS: Status post tissue expansion, left breast, with 500-cc tissue expander

POSTOPERATIVE DIAGNOSIS: Status post tissue expansion, left breast, with 500-cc tissue expander

SURGICAL FINDINGS: There was some exudate on the breast implant. There was a small amount of serosanguineous fluid within the pocket that appeared to be old. The capsule was very thin, and it was felt that it was indicated to leave this capsule intact.

SURGICAL PROCEDURE: Removal of tissue expander, left breast, with reinsertion of 440-cc inflatable McGhan implant. See details and appropriate labeling for model number.

ANESTHESIA: General endotracheal; approximately 3 cc of 1% Xylocaine with 1:100,000 epinephrine were used for the incision line.

ESTIMATED BLOOD LOSS: Negligible

DESCRIPTION OF PROCEDURE: The patient was prepped with Betadine scrub and solution and draped in a routine sterile fashion. The Betadine was removed from the incision site, and the scar was outlined with a fine marker. We injected 3 cc of 1% Xylocaine with 1:100,000 epinephrine along the suture line, excised the scar down to the capsule of the breast, which was opened with the cutting cautery set at 30. I noted that there was some exudate within the capsule, and culture and sensitivity of this were obtained. The cavity itself contained a small amount of serosanguineous fluid, perhaps 5 cc or so, and this was thought to be old and nonintroduced. We irrigated the pocket with about 250 cc of Ringer's lactate, and then I inspected the anterior aspect of the expander. There was some leakage upon rather extreme pressure from around the injection site, but this was minimal, and it was only produced with extreme pressure. The breast implant, which was a 440-460 McGhan inflatable textured anatomic-type implant, was inflated to 300 cc, and the air was removed from the implant. It was inserted in the pocket, and the complete inflation of the implant was then carried out, inflating it to 440 cc. The expander tube was then removed, and the capsule itself was closed with interrupted 2-0 Ethibond, following which the subcuticular layer was done with interrupted 4-0 Monocryl. One twist of 6-0 Prolene was placed in the lateral aspect of the incision, and Steri-Strips were applied. Kerlix fluffs and a support bra were applied. The patient tolerated the procedure well and left the area in good condition.

5-38A:

SERVICE CODE(S): ______________________

DX CODE(S): ______________________

Glossary

biopsy removal of a small piece of living tissue for diagnostic purposes

benign not progressive or recurrent

debridement cleansing of or removal of dead tissue from a wound

dermis second layer of skin, holding blood vessels, nerve endings, sweat glands, and hair follicles

donor site the site from which tissue is taken to repair another site

epidermis outer layer of skin

excision cutting or taking away (in reference to lesion removal, it is full-thickness removal of a lesion that may include simple closure)

excisional removal of an entire lesion for biopsy

frozen section a specimen of tissue that is obtained during an operative procedure for immediate analysis and preliminary diagnosis

global surgical procedure a set amount of preoperative, intraoperative, and postoperative services bundled into a service code

grafts *autograft* is taken from the patient's own body; *allograft* is taken from another person's body, either alive or cadaver; *xenograft* is one taken from another species; *bilaminate graft* is made of artificial skin; *pinch graft* is a small, split-thickness repair; *split graft* is a repair that involves the epidermis and some of the dermis; *full-thickness graft* is a repair that involves the epidermis and all of the dermis

lesion abnormal or altered tissue (e.g., wound, cyst, abscess, boil)

malignant used to describe a cancerous tumor that grows worse over time

mastectomy excision (removal) of the breast

onychectomy excision (removal) of a nail or nail bed

panniculectomy removal of abdominal fat and skin

parenchyma an essential element of an organ, functional elements, such as the renal parenchyma which is the tissue that contains the nephrons

permanent section a specimen of tissue obtained during an operative procedure that is mounted and analyzed by a pathologist for the most definitive diagnosis

recipient site the site that receives the tissue for repair

skin graft transplantation of tissue to repair a defect

subcutaneous tissue below the dermis, primarily fat cells that insulate the body

sulcus a groove, trench, or valley shape

tissue expander a sac of fluid or air or a plastic implant that is placed under the skin to stretch the skin; the stretched skin is used for grafting purposes or stretched to place an implant beneath the newly stretch skin

tissue transfer piece of skin for grafting that is still partially attached to the original blood supply and is used to cover an adjacent wound area

Chapter 6

Cardiovascular System

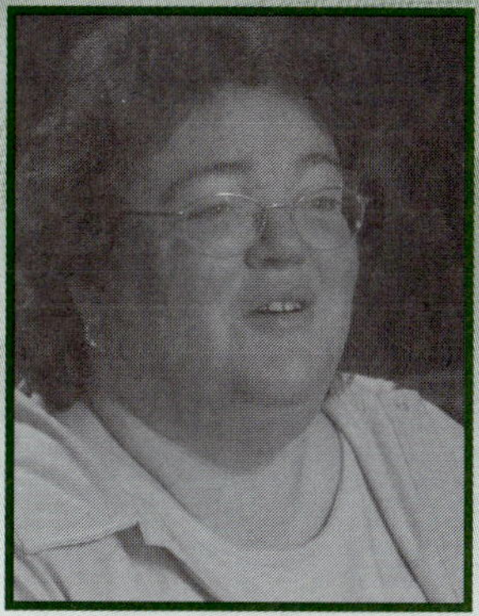

Lynn M. Anderson, CPC
Senior Coding Consultant
Healthcare Information Services, L.L.C.
Des Plaines, Illinois

ABBREVIATIONS

AAA	abdominal aortic aneurysm
AF or A Fib	atrial fibrillation
AM	acute marginal (branch of RCA)
AR	aortic regurgitation
AS	aortic stenosis
ASCVD	arteriosclerotic cardiovascular disease
AV	arteriovenous
BPG	bypass graft
CABG	coronary artery bypass graft
CAD	coronary artery disease
CCU	coronary care unit
CHD	congenital heart disease
CHF	congestive heart failure
CMP	cardiomyopathy
CPB	cardiopulmonary bypass
CPR	cardiopulmonary resuscitation
CVP	central venous pressure
CX	circumflex artery
D1 or D2	diagonal branch of the LAD artery
ECA	external carotid artery
ECC	extracorporeal circulation (or circuit) or external cardiac compression
ECG	electrocardiogram (see EKG)
ECHO	echocardiogram
EEG	electroencephalogram
EF	ejection fraction; the percent of the left ventricular volume ejected in a cardiac contraction
EKG	electrocardiogram (see ECG)
HR	heart rate
HTN	hypertension
IABP	intraaortic balloon pump
ICA	internal carotid artery
IVC	inferior vena cava
IVCD	intraventricular conduction defect
LAD	left anterior descending coronary artery
LBBB	left bundle branch block
LIMA	left internal mammary artery
LLL	left lower lobe
LMCA	left main coronary artery
LV	left ventricle
LVH	left ventricular hypertrophy
MI	mitral insufficiency or myocardial infarction
MR	mitral regurgitation
MS	mitral stenosis
MUGA	multiple gated acquisition scan; a radionuclide test of myocardial performance
MV	mitral valve
MVR	mitral valve repair
OM1 OM2	obtuse marginal
PAC	premature atrial contraction
PDA	posterior descending artery, part of the RCA
PND	paroxysmal nocturnal dyspnea
PSVT	paroxysmal supraventricular tachycardia
PTCA	percutaneous transluminal coronary angioplasty
PTT	partial thromboplastin time
PV	pulmonary valve
PVC	premature ventricular contraction
PVD	peripheral vascular disease
RBBB	right bundle branch block
RCA	right coronary artery
RIMA	right internal mammary artery
RV	right ventricle
RVH	right ventricular hypertrophy
S1 S2	sequential 1 and 2
SBP	systolic blood pressure
SIADH	syndrome of inappropriate secretion of anti-diuretic hormone
SPECT	single photon emission computed tomography
ST or S tach	sinus tachycardia
SVC	superior vena cava
SVG	saphenous vein graft
SVT or SV tach	supraventricular tachycardia
Tc-99M	technetium-99m
TEE	transesophageal echocardiography
TR	tricuspid regurgitation
TS	tricuspid stenosis
TV	tricuspid valve
VAD	ventricular assist device
VBR	ventricular branch
VF or V fib	ventricular fibrillation
VSD	ventricular septal defect
VT or V tach	ventricular tachycardia

The more common cardiovascular presenting problems are chest pain, hypertension, edema, murmur, mitral valve prolapse, palpitations, congestive heart failure, acute **ischemia,** abnormal **stress tests,** arrhythmias, congenital heart disease, syncope (fainting), hyperlipidemia, and claudication.

A cardiologist is a physician who specializes in diseases of the heart and vessels. A cardiothoracic surgeon is a physician who specializes in surgical procedures of the heart and chest. A variety of physicians frequently use the codes, as you will see as you code the services and procedures within this chapter. Examples of procedures include valve repair, beating heart surgery, aortic dissections, and excision of tumors of the chest wall.

When coding cardiovascular services, the coder will commonly use codes from the Evaluation/Management, Surgery, Medicine, and Radiology sections of the CPT manual.

Evaluation and Management Services

Often the E/M services provided to a patient with a cardiac condition are very complex and extensive. The history and physical examination of the patient with a suspected cardiovascular condition are of critical importance to proper medical management of the patient. The physician has training, skills, knowledge, and experience that cannot be replaced by a laboratory test; rather, the tests assist the physician in the diagnosis process. Through the history and physical examination, the physician gathers a wide range of information necessary to diagnose the patient. For example, the symptom of chest pain, which is a cardinal manifestation of cardiac disease, could be caused by conditions of the aorta, pulmonary **artery,** bronchopulmonary tree, pleura, mediastinum, esophagus, diaphragm, tissues of the neck or thoracic wall (including the skin, thoracic muscles, cervicodorsal spine, costochondral junctions, breasts, sensory nerves, or spinal cord), stomach, duodenum, pancreas, or gallbladder. There are many potential causes for just one of the symptoms of cardiac disease.

Consultations are a frequent cardiologist service. Cardiology consultations can be provided to the inpatient or outpatient, and the choice of the correct E/M for the consultation is based on documentation of key components and contributing factors. The cardiology consultation often produces lengthy, complex medical reports.

Arteriosclerosis

Arteriosclerosis is a chronic disease of the arterial system that results in thickened and hardened walls of the vessels resulting in loss of the artery elasticity. Gradually, the arterial lumen narrows. This results in increased blood pressure because the heart has to pump harder to force the blood through the artery, weakening of the arterial walls that then become more susceptible to rupture, and insufficient perfusion to the tissues of the body. **Atherosclerosis** is a form of arteriosclerosis in which deposits of fat and fibrin (insoluble protein) accumulate on the vessel walls. These accumulations are atheromas. When referencing atherosclerosis in the Index of the ICD-9-CM, the coder is directed to "*see* Arteriosclerosis." Under the main term "Arteriosclerosis, arteriosclerotic" the coder is directed to **440.9.** The code description indicates "Atherosclerosis." The subcategories are by the location of the disease, such as aorta (440.0), renal artery (440.1), extremities (440.2x), bypass graft of extremities (440.3x), of other specified arteries (440.8), or generalized or unspecified atherosclerosis (440.9).

When reporting atherosclerosis of the coronary artery, reference "Arteriosclerosis, coronary" in the Index of the ICD-9-CM. You are then directed to 414.00. The category **414** is for "Other forms of chronic ischemic heart disease," and 414.0 is for "Coronary atherosclerosis" and includes arteriosclerotic heart disease (ASHD), atherosclerotic heart disease, and coronary artery sclerosis. The fifth digit code classifications are based on the location of the atherosclerosis. For example, the following fifth digit classifications:

- "Of native coronary artery" indicates the atherosclerosis is within an original heart artery (414.01).
- "Of autologous biological bypass graft" indicates that the atherosclerosis is within a vein graft that was taken from within the patient (414.02).
- "Of nonautologous biological bypass graft" indicates the atherosclerosis is within a vessel grafted from other than the patient (414.03).
- "Of artery bypass graft" indicates the atherosclerosis is within an artery that was grafted from within the patient (414.04).
- "Of unspecified type of bypass graft" is for reporting atherosclerosis of a bypass graft, but the origin of the graft is unknown (414.05).

At this time, review the subterms listed under the main term "Arteriosclerosis, arteriosclerotic" in the Index of the ICD-9-CM to become familiar with the entries located there.

CASE 6-1

Time to put your cardiology coding knowledge to work by coding an E/M service provided by a cardiologist. A decision to perform surgery was made during this E/M visit, so remember to use the modifier that will indicate it.

6-1A CARDIOTHORACIC SURGERY CONSULTATION

LOCATION: Inpatient, Hospital

PATIENT: Manual Lopez

PHYSICIAN: David Barton, M.D.

REASON FOR CONSULTATION: Atherosclerotic heart disease

HISTORY OF PRESENT ILLNESS: This 62-year-old Hispanic male was being considered for knee replacement and in his preoperative workup underwent a stress test, which did not show any ischemia; however, because of angioplasty 6 months ago, the patient was considered a candidate for angiography.

CARDIAC RISK FACTORS: Risk factors include a remote history of cigarette smoking, hypertension, previous coronary stent, dyslipidemia, and adult-onset diabetes mellitus.

MEDICAL HISTORY: Previous operations include the following:

1. Rotator cuff surgery in December of last year
2. Right coronary artery stent 6 months ago after right coronary artery occlusion with myocardial infarction

CURRENT MEDICATIONS:

1. Lotrel, 5/20 mg, 1 p.o. daily
2. Atenolol, 50 mg p.o. daily
3. Protonix, 40 mg, 1 to 2 daily
4. Lipitor, 10 mg daily
5. Hydrocodone as needed for knee pain
6. Nitroglycerin sublingual, 4/10 of 1 mg as needed.
7. Zoloft, 150 mg daily
8. Celebrex, 200 mg p.o. b.i.d.
9. 1 adult aspirin daily
10. Isosorbide, 30 mg p.o. daily
11. Glucosamine and chondroitin sulfate, 1 tablet b.i.d.
12. Actos, 40 mg p.o. daily
13. Magnesium, 400 mg p.o. t.i.d.

FAMILY HISTORY: Positive for coronary disease

SOCIAL HISTORY: The patient is married and lives with his wife in Manytown. He drinks minimally and stopped smoking years ago.

REVIEW OF SYSTEMS: Review of systems is significant for bilateral knee osteoarthritis. Echocardiogram done last year showed normal ventricular size with concentric hypertrophy and apical area of aneurysm.

PHYSICAL EXAMINATION: On examination, the patient is a 272-pound, 6-foot Hispanic male in no apparent distress, supine after his cardiac catheterization. Jugular venous pressure is normal. Carotids were 2+, equal, and quiet. The CHEST is clear and equal. The HEART has a regular rhythm with a rate of 70 without murmur, gallop, or rubs. The ABDOMEN is soft and obese without organomegaly. The upper and lower EXTREMITIES show no cyanosis, clubbing, or edema. Pulses are intact peripherally. The patient is grossly and neurologically intact. The chest x-ray shows normal cardiothoracic ratio. LUNG fields are clear.

The ECG shows normal sinus rhythm with anterolateral ST segment and T-wave changes.

LABORATORY STUDIES: The laboratory shows sodium of 135, BUN of 24, glucose of 115. The lipids are within satisfactory limits. The protime is 12.7 and PTT is 31.6. White blood cell count is low at 3.5. Hemoglobin is 13.6, and platelets are 176,000.

Cardiac catheterization by Dr. Elhart 6 months ago showed good left ventricular contractility with, perhaps, some anterior early relaxation. The dominant right coronary artery had a 70% lesion at the posterior descending proximally. The left main was narrowed 40% distally. The left-to-left and right-to-left fill. The diagonal branch was diseased but small. The left circumflex was narrowed at two obtuse marginal branches at 70% to 90% proximally, respectively.

IMPRESSION: Three-vessel atherosclerotic heart disease in a 62-year-old Hispanic male with adult-onset diabetes mellitus, normal left ventricular function, and need for knee replacement.

DISPOSITION: The patient will be retained in the hospital and will undergo coronary vascularization on the 25th of the month. Operation, complications including blood transfusion, risks, and alternatives were discussed with the patient and his family.

6-1A:

SERVICE CODE(S): ______________________

DX CODE(S): ______________________

You will be coding other cardiovascular E/M services throughout this chapter.

Cardiac Artery Bypass Grafts

The Surgery section, Cardiovascular System subsection, codes are divided into Heart/Pericardium and Arteries/Veins. In the Arteries and Veins subheading, you will find many of the same types of procedures that are found in the Heart and Pericardium subheading, except the Arteries and Veins are for procedures on noncoronary vessels elsewhere in the body.

When coronary arteries clog with plaque (arteriosclerotic coronary artery disease [ASCAD]), the flow of blood is lessened. **Figure 6-1** is a drawing that was placed in the patient's medical record by the cardiologist to indicate the blockage of the patient's heart vessels. Note that the figure indicates the percentage of blockage of the involved vessels. For example, the right coronary artery (RCA) is 100% blocked by plaque. **Figure 6-2** illustrates an artery on fluoroscopy that is blocked with plaque. The heart muscle may begin to function below normal levels–*reversible ischemia*. If the heart muscle is denied adequate blood flow for an extended period, the muscle may die–*irreversible ischemia*. A coronary artery bypass graft (CABG) bypasses the clogged area(s) of the vessels to improve blood flow. There are three types of coronary artery bypass grafts:

1. CABG with venous graft only (33510-33516)
2. CABG with venous and arterial grafts (33517-33530)
3. CABG with arterial graft only (33533-33545)

The heart has two main coronary arteries-the left (left main) and right (right coronary artery). The left main (LM) artery divides into the left anterior descending (LAD) and left circumflex (LCA) arteries (**Figure 6-3**). The right coronary artery (RCA) supplies the right ventricle and continues down the back of the heart (posterior aspect), where it is called the posterior descending artery (PDA). The coronary artery can be bypassed with an artery using the internal mammary artery, gastroepiploic artery, epigastric artery, radial artery, and arterial grafts from other areas. Note in Figure 6-3 that the internal mammary artery (originates from the subclavian artery) is left attached to the subclavian artery on one end, and the distal end is detached from its origin and reattached to the coronary artery to bypass the area of damage. Other times, the surgeon removes a portion of a **vein** and uses it for a graft, such as a right or left saphenous vein that is removed and used for a bypass graft. The procurement of the artery or vein is included in the CABG code and would not be reported separately. If an upper-extremity **artery**,

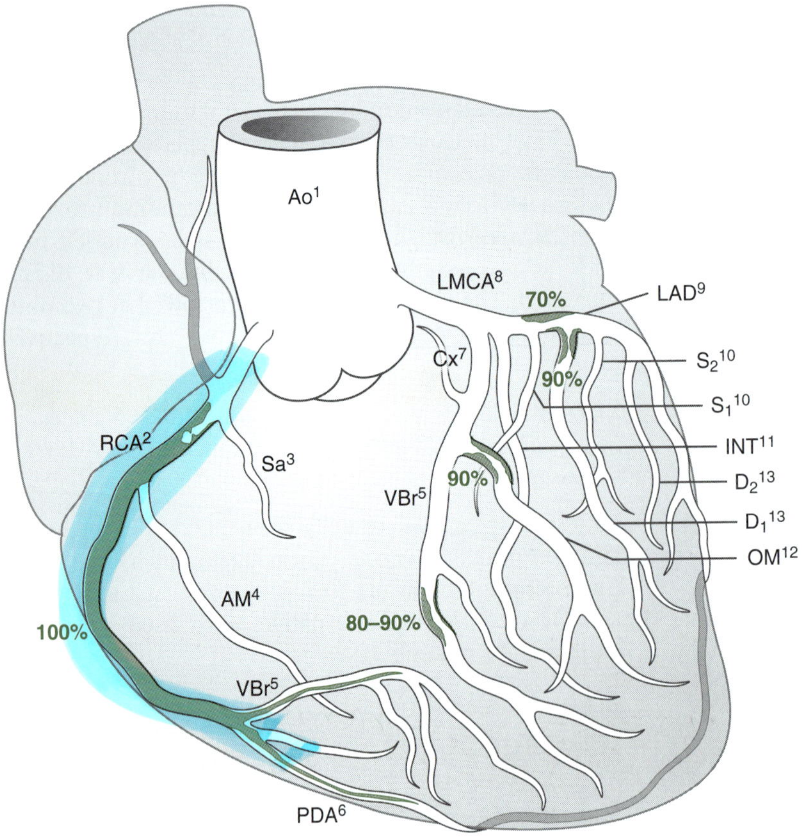

FIGURE 6-1 The percentages indicate the amount of blockage of the patient's heart vessels. The right coronary artery (RCA) is 100% blocked by plaque.

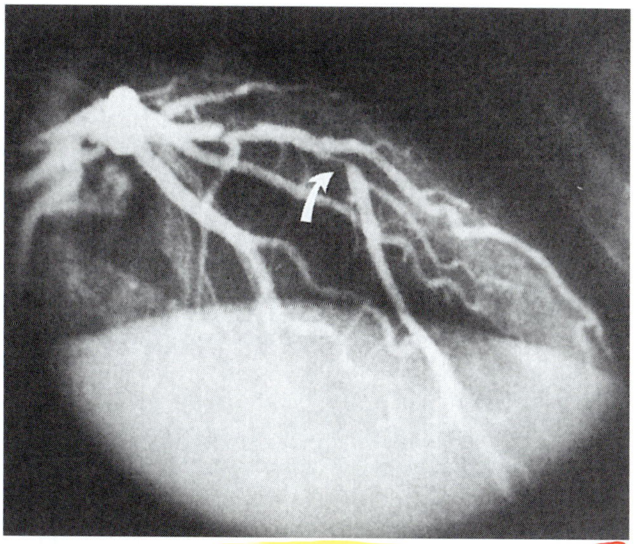

FIGURE 6-2 RAO cranial view showing the second LAD lesion *(arrow). (From Braunwald E:* Heart disease: a textbook of cardiovascular medicine, *vol 1, ed 3, Philadelphia, 1988, WB Saunders.)*

such as the radial artery, is harvested for grafting, however, the harvesting service can be reported separately with 35600 (Harvest of upper extremity artery, one segment for coronary artery bypass procedure) or harvesting of an upper-extremity **vein** can be reported separately with add-on code 35500 (Harvest of upper-extremity vein, one segment for lower extremity or coronary artery bypass procedure).

Codes are selected based on the type of graft (harvested) and the number of grafts placed on the coronary artery (recipient). For example, RCA and LAD receive two saphenous vein grafts. The type of graft is venous (harvested), and there were two grafts: one placed on the right coronary artery and one placed on the left anterior descending artery (recipients). The physician will often refer to the *harvested* and *recipient*, so you will need to know these terms to interpret the service provided correctly.

A CABG with venous and arterial grafts (33517-33530) is never used alone but only with the arterial codes (33533-33545). You can use the arterial codes alone (33533-33545) and the venous codes alone (33510-33516), but you can never report the Combined Arterial-Venous Grafting for Coronary Bypass codes alone. A helpful hint is to write "combination AV only" next to the codes 33517-33530 in your CPT as a reminder that these codes are used only when a combined arterial-venous graft is performed.

Cardiovascular surgeons often use artificial materials, such as Gore-Tex, to repair damaged areas of vessels. This artificial material is less susceptible to rejection and calcification than human tissue and can be readily available. The surgeon uses this material to repair a hole in a vessel as a seamstress would apply a patch to a hole in a pair of jeans. The material is cut to size and sewn over the hole. These artificial materials can also be formed into a tube and inserted into a vessel as a support for weakened or collapsed vessel walls.

FIGURE 6-3 Coronary artery bypass.

LAD = left anterior descending
RAD =

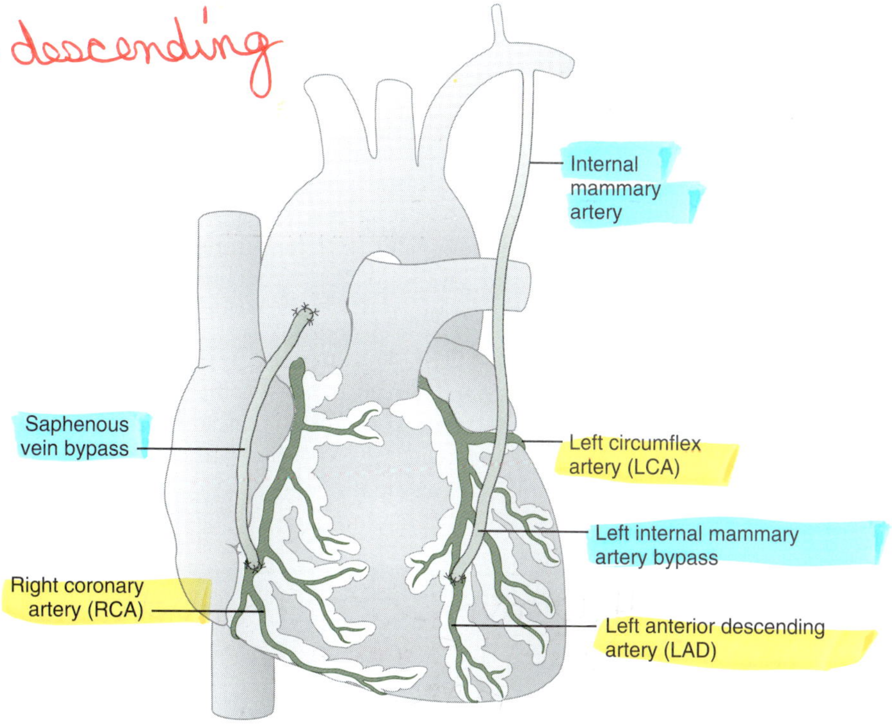

CASE 6-2
6-2A Coronary Artery Bypass

CASE 6-2

Code the following CABG. Be certain to identify the number, location, and type of grafts.

6-2A CORONARY ARTERY BYPASS

LOCATION: Inpatient, Hospital

PATIENT: Manual Lopez

SURGEON: David Barton, M.D.

PREOPERATIVE DIAGNOSIS: Atherosclerotic heart disease

POSTOPERATIVE DIAGNOSIS: Same

PROCEDURE PERFORMED: Coronary artery bypass grafts ×4 with left internal mammary artery to left anterior descending bypass and sequential saphenous vein bypass from the aorta to the first and second obtuse marginal branch of the left circumflex with an ongoing graft to the posterior descending coronary artery.

ANESTHESIA: General

INDICATIONS: This 62-year-old Hispanic male with a history of degenerative knee disease was considered a candidate for orthopedic surgical management; however, preoperatively he underwent stress testing, which was equivocal but prompted angiography, which showed severe three-vessel disease with normal ventricular function.

FINDINGS AT SURGERY: The vein was a 4-mm-diameter vessel of good quality and was used in reverse fashion. The left internal mammary artery was a 1.5-mm-diameter vessel of good quality. The left anterior descending was a 2-mm-diameter vessel of good quality. The first and second obtuse marginal branches were both 2 mm in diameter and of good quality. The posterior descending was, likewise, 2 mm in diameter and of good quality. All the grafts were appropriate prior to closure and were placed distal to palpable disease.

DESCRIPTION OF PROCEDURE: The patient was brought to the operating room and placed in the supine position. With the patient under general intubation anesthesia, the anterior chest, abdomen, and legs were prepped and draped in the usual manner. A segment of the greater saphenous vein was harvested from the left thigh using the endoscopic vein-harvesting technique and prepared for grafting. The pericardium was incised sharply and a pericardial well created. The patient was systemically heparinized and placed on single right atrial-to-aortic cardiopulmonary bypass with a stump in the main pulmonary artery for cardiac decompression. The patient was cooled to 26 degrees and, on fibrillation, aortic cross-clamp was applied and potassium-rich cold crystalline cardioplegic solution was administered through the aortic root with satisfactory cardiac arrest. Subsequent doses were given down the vein graft as the anastomosis was completed and also via the coronary sinus in a retrograde fashion. The end of the greater saphenous vein was then anastomosed to the proximal third of the posterior descending coronary artery using 7-0 Prolene. The graft was brought to the patient's left and then anastomosed side to side to the second obtuse marginal branch, followed by the first obtuse marginal branch, all with 7-0 continuous Prolene. The left internal mammary artery was then brought down to the midportion of the left anterior descending and anastomosed thereto with 8-0 continuous Prolene. The aortic cross-clamp was removed after 62 minutes with spontaneous cardioversion to a normal sinus rhythm. The patient was then warmed to 37 degrees esophageal temperature, during which time the vein graft was trimmed to size and anastomosed to the ascending aorta using 5-0 continuous Prolene technique. The patient was weaned from cardiopulmonary bypass without difficulty using no inotropes after 99 minutes. The patient was decannulated, protamine was given, and hemostasis was obtained. Temporary pacer wires were placed from the right atrium and right ventricles. The chest was drained with two Argyle chest tubes and closed in layers in the usual fashion. The leg was closed similarly. Sterile compression dressings were applied. The patient returned to the surgical intensive care unit in satisfactory condition. Sponge and needle counts were correct ×2.

6-2A:

SERVICE CODE(S): ____________________

DX CODE(S): ____________________

vein 4.0 mm
left IMA - 1.5 mm
LAD-2.0 mm
PDA = 2.0 mm
obtuse 2.0 mm

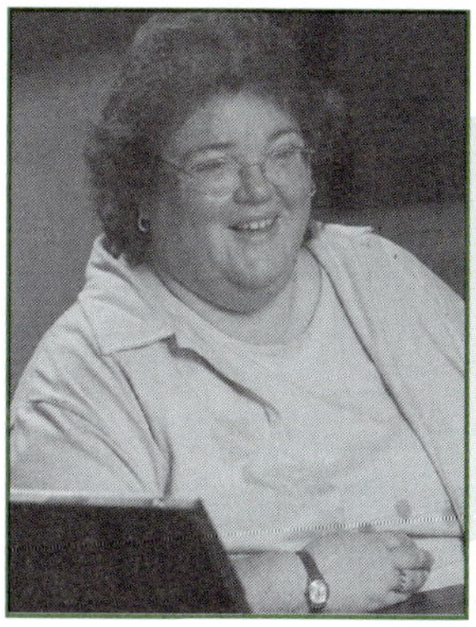

FROM THE TRENCHES

Lynn

What advice to do you give your coding students?

"To always have documentation. To always be able to stand behind whatever you say. If you are saying something, as far as a coding rule, you better have the documentation to back yourself up."

Pacemaker

A pacemaker is an electrical device that is inserted into the body to shock the heart electrically into regular rhythm. The two parts of a pacemaker are the battery and electrode. The electrode is the device that emits the electrical charge. The electrode is also called the *lead* and is a flexible, thin tube. The battery is also called a *pulse generator.* Some generators are programmable and have a wide range of programming options. The pulse generator is placed into a pocket either under the clavicle, as illustrated in **Figure 6-4,** or under the muscle of the abdomen below the rib cage.

Either an epicardial or transvenous approach can be used to implant the electrode portion of the pacemaker. The epicardial approach involves opening the chest to the view of the surgeon and the device being placed on the heart. The transvenous approach is most commonly used because it is the least traumatic to the patient and involves inserting a needle with a wire attached (guidewire) into a vein. The guidewire then directs the placement of the electrode into the heart while the surgeon views the progression using a fluoroscope. The electrode is then attached to the pulse generator.

The pacemaker can be a single- or dual-chamber unit. A single-chamber pacemaker uses one pulse generator and one electrode that is placed in either the atrium or the ventricle. A dual-chamber pacemaker uses a pulse generator and two electrodes-one placed in the atrium and the other placed in the ventricle.

Pacemakers can be permanent or temporary. A temporary pacemaker can be used when the heart needs only short-term pacing support. For example, when a patient is waiting for placement of a permanent pacemaker or postsurgical cardiac instability. After the pacemaker is placed, the physician will test the device to ensure that it is operating correctly. The pacemaker implantation report will indicate a statement such as "thresholds were obtained and were adequate."

FIGURE 6-4 Pacemaker insertion. The pulse generator is inserted into the upper chest area.

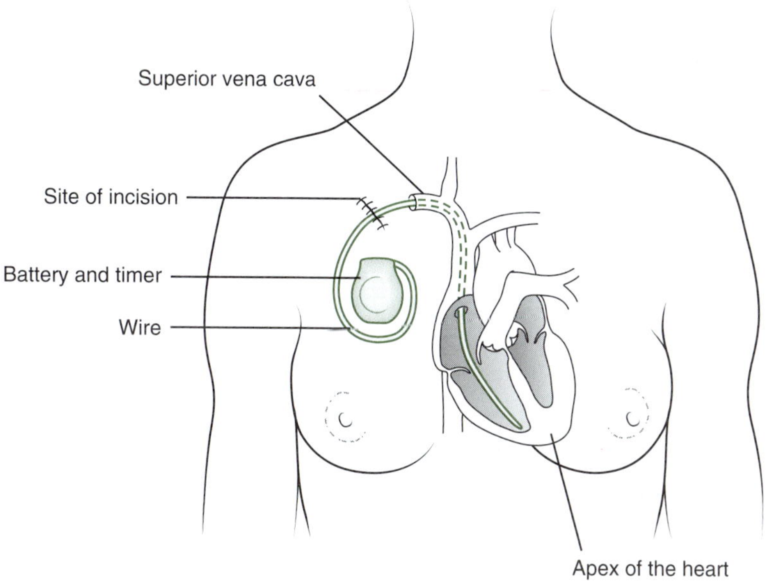

The testing and setting are included in the implantation service and are not reported separately. Special or extensive pacing, if noted in the report as those above the usual service, can be reported separately.

A **cardioverter-defibrillator** is an implantable electronic device that has both the pulse generator and the electrodes, but it is capable of more functions than the pacemaker. The device senses irregularities in the heart rhythm and emits electrical charges to regulate the heart rhythm and pace the heart to correct heart rhythm. The device can be programmed to sense a wide variety of heart irregularities and then further programmed to emit various electrical charges in response. The device is used for antitachycardia (stops rapid heartbeat) pacing, low-energy cardioversion (restoration of normal heartbeat), or defibrillating shocks to treat tachycardia or fibrillation (quivering).

A single-chamber cardioverter-defibrillator has a lead or leads inserted into a **single** chamber; a dual-chamber cardioverter-defibrillator has leads inserted into **both** the atrium and ventricle. The number of leads used does not indicate a single- or dual-chamber cardioverter-defibrillator because when a single chamber is being paced, multiple leads into that single chamber may be used. It is the number of **chambers** into which the leads are placed, *not* the number of leads used, which impacts code choice.

During insertion, electrophysiologic testing of a cardioverter-defibrillator and electrical analysis of a pacemaker would often be conducted as a part of the insertion or reinsertion procedure. This testing and analysis would be reported separately using Medicine section codes 93724-93744. Intraoperative testing is also reported separately with Medicine section codes 93640-93641. Remember to use modifier -26 if you are reporting only the professional component (physician) of the electrical analysis.

When a pacemaker or cardioverter-defibrillator battery is changed, it is actually the pulse generator that is replaced. As a part of the usual 90-day surgical package that accompanies the implantation service, follow-up visits would be considered part of the global service by the third-party payer and therefore not reimbursed.

If the pulse generator is replaced after the initial insertion, both the removal and the insertion of another pulse generator would be reported separately. Do not use modifiers -76 (Repeat procedure by same physician) or -77 (Repeat procedure by another physician) when reporting an implantation that occurs after the initial insertion because both the removal and insertion services would be considered a new service. This replacement of the pacemaker pulse generator in a single chamber is reported with 33212 and a dual chamber with 33213; cardioverter-defibrillator is reported with 33241, whether single or dual chamber.

Remember to use one code for an initial insertion and two codes for a removal and reinsertion of a subsequent pacemaker or cardioverter-defibrillator.

Sick Sinus Syndrome

Sick sinus syndrome is a group of abnormal heartbeats (arrhythmias). The exact cause of this syndrome is unknown, but it is thought to be caused by a malfunction of the sinus node, which is the heart's natural pacemaker. It can result in many arrhythmias, including tachycardia (fast heart rate), bradycardia (slow heart rate), sinus arrest, sinus node exit block, and sinus bradycardia. These arrhythmias are not reported separately because they are symptoms of the syndrome. Rather the syndrome is reported. You can locate direction to the code in the Index of the ICD-9-CM by referencing "Syndrome, sick, sinus."

CASE 6-3
6-3A Cardiology Follow-Up Note

CASE 6-3

With the information you just learned about pacemakers, code the following E/M services to a patient who, after several tests, will have a pacemaker implanted.

6-3A CARDIOLOGY FOLLOW-UP NOTE

LOCATION: Outpatient, Clinic

PATIENT: Herbert Gillford

PHYSICIAN: Marvin Elhart, M.D.

DIAGNOSES:
1. Symptomatic sick sinus syndrome
2. Dementia
3. Dilated cardiomyopathy with previous history of congestive heart failure

MEDICATIONS: Tylenol; Lasix 40 mg as needed; Vasotec 5 mg once daily; Colace; aspirin: Ambien; and Arthrotec.

I evaluated this patient approximately 2 years ago. He was seen by Dr. Pleasant again last year on referral from Dr. Green because of episodes of falling down. The episodes are significant to the point that he had a hip fracture. Apparently, he was transferred to a nursing home in his hometown.

The history from the patient is almost useless because he does not recollect any symptoms and he says he feels fine and has no shortness of breath or falling down. The patient has been diagnosed with dementia previously. We tried to contact his relative, but we got the answering machine.

We reviewed the previous notations from Dr. Green and Dr. Pleasant and myself. Predominantly the problem is that the patient has had repeated falls and has been diagnosed with sinus bradycardia with first-degree AV block and bundle-branch block; a Holter monitor read by myself recently revealed predominantly atrial block.

EXAMINATION today reveals an elderly man in a wheelchair in no acute distress. His blood pressure was 124/68 with a heart rate of 60. Lungs did not reveal any rales. Cardiovascular examination reveals distant heart tones with normal S1 and S2 with a holosystolic murmur, grade 1/6, over the mitral area. Abdomen was obese. Extremities: No edema.

ECG in the office reveals him to be in sinus bradycardia with a rate of 49 with first-degree AV block and left bundle-branch block. The Holter monitor revealed him to be predominantly in atrial fibrillation; his minimum rate was 49 and maximum 114 with an average of 74. At that time, the notation did show that he was taking Lanoxin, which apparently he is not taking at this time.

An echocardiogram also read by myself revealed the patient to have dilated cardiomyopathy with severe LV dysfunction with mild aortic insufficiency and significant mitral insufficiency.

IMPRESSION AND RECOMMENDATIONS: Symptomatic sick sinus syndrome with evidence of paroxysmal atrial fibrillation. It is very difficult to assess this patient symptom-wise because he does not have a lot of insight into his symptoms. He has been diagnosed with dementia. It seems to me that there is enough evidence that this patient's falling down episodes might be related to his rhythm because that is the most common finding. The only solution to this problem would be implantation of a dual-chamber pacemaker.

We attempted to contact his family to discuss this and to obtain a consent, but we did not find an answer. We will contact the family again and discuss with them the recommendations. If they consent to it and agree to proceed, we will bring him in for implantation of a dual-chamber pacemaker.

6-3A:

SERVICE CODE(S): ____________________

DX CODE(S): ____________________

In reports 6-5B and 6-5C, you will be coding the pacemaker implantation for the patient in report 6-3A, but you must learn a couple more things before you code the implantation service. Let us begin with **echocardiography** services.

Echocardiography

Cardiomyopathy (CMP) is a disease of the heart muscle. The exact cause(s) of cardiomyopathy are not known, and the symptoms of the disease are similar to those displayed in patients with myocarditis (infections caused by virus, bacteria, or parasites), toxic effects of various drugs, **myocardial** infarction, various cardiac disorders (pericarditis, congestive heart disease or stenosis), and various other conditions. As a part of the diagnostic process, the physician may order an electrocardiogram, chest x-rays, **Doppler** and echocardiography, radionuclide studies, cardiac catheterization, or blood tests.

Echocardiography obtains ultrasonic signals from the heart and coronary arteries with a two-dimensional image and/or Doppler ultrasound. Transthoracic echocardiography is a noninvasive procedure in which a transducer (transmitter) is placed on the skin and sound waves go through the structure of the body and bounce off the heart. From the frequency with which the waves return from the internal structures and bounce back to the transducer, the physician can determine the position and motion of the heart walls and internal structures of the heart and neighboring tissue.

Transesophageal echocardiography (TEE) is a procedure in which the transesophageal echography probe transducer is placed into the mouth and advanced into the esophagus, allowing a posterior view of the heart, as illustrated in **Figure 6-5.** Varieties of TEEs are reported with codes 93312-93318. The codes are divided into those done for congenital cardiac conditions (93315-93317) and those done for noncongenital cardiac conditions (93312-93314). The stand-alone codes 93312 and 93315 are for the full service, and the indented codes are for components of the service. For example, 93313 is used to report the service of the placement of the transesophageal probe. Code 93318 is used to report monitoring services using a previously implanted TEE. These monitoring functions are not limited to monitoring of the heart but also include monitoring of numerous organs, such as the lungs and mediastinum. These monitoring services are not the usual diagnostic service but instead are urgent services that are required for a critically ill or injured patient. (In Case 6-14A, you will be coding a TEE service prior to a cardioversion.)

Doppler echocardiography is a technique that records the flow of blood through the cardiovascular system by tracking the movement of the red blood cells by ultrasound. The pulsed-wave or continuous-wave Doppler produces

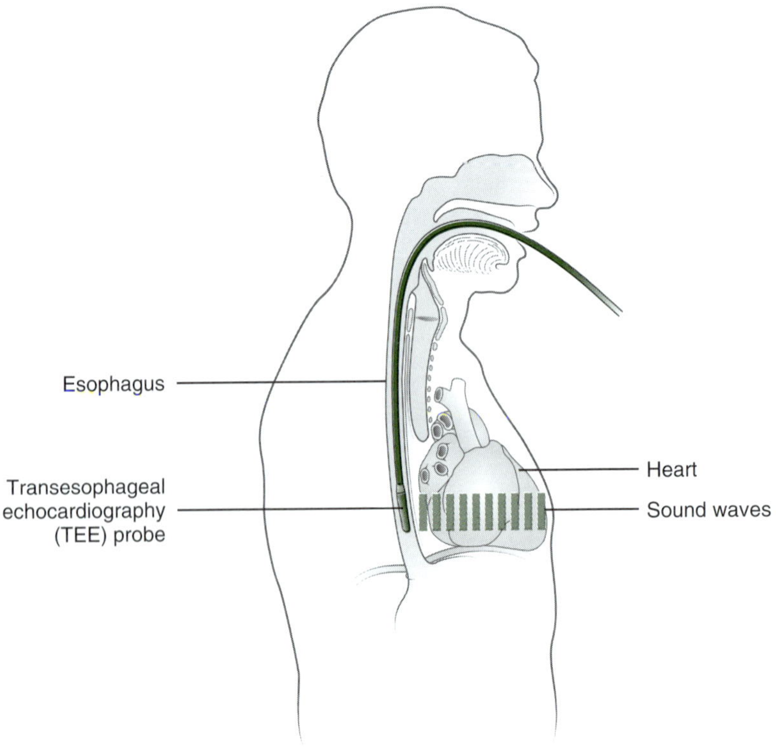

FIGURE 6-5 Transesophageal echocardiography (TEE).

a video recording or strip chart detailing the force with which the blood passes through the cardiovascular system and the direction of the blood. A **color-flow Doppler** is similar to the pulsed-wave or continuous Doppler but in addition to the color flow is a two-dimensional color display. The color makes identification of blood flow easier. A 2-D and color-flow Doppler echocardiography requires three codes to report the service: a code for the 2-D Doppler, a code for the pulse-wave Doppler, and a code for the color-flow Doppler. The Doppler codes are all add-on codes (93320-93325) and cannot be reported alone. For example, a patient has a transthoracic echocardiogram with pulsed-wave and color-flow Doppler. The service is coded 93307 for the echocardiogram, 93320 for the pulsed-wave Doppler, and 93325 for the color-flow Doppler. The echocardiogram service reported with 93307 results in only two-dimensional image, 93320 reports a fully dimensional image, and 93325 reports color enhancement of the image.

Valve Insufficiencies

Insufficiency of a heart valve means the valve does not close properly, which may lead to hypertrophy (enlargement) of the heart because blood will pool in the chambers. Rheumatic heart disease is a result of rheumatic fever, which is a febrile (fever) disease caused by a *streptococci* infection and results in valvular deformities. The ICD-9-CM separates codes for nonrheumatic valvular insufficiencies from valvular insufficiencies that are a result of (sequela) rheumatic heart disease. Code 424 is for **nonrheumatic** or **other specified** causes. This code is also assigned for **unspecified** causes when only **one valve** is involved. The documentation is often aortic stenosis (424.1) of unknown cause. When there are **multiple valves** involved in the diagnosis *or* the documentation specifies rheumatic, refer to 394-396. For example, a commonly documented diagnosis is aortic and mitral valve regurgitation (not specified as rheumatic), which is reported with 396.3. When both **mitral and aortic valves** are involved, the ICD-9-CM presumes an etiology (cause) of rheumatic heart disease and the physician does not need to document rheumatic heart disease. Also, when the diagnosis involves the **tricuspid valve,** the etiology also is presumed to be rheumatic heart disease.

CASE 6-4
6-4A Echocardiogram

CASE 6-4

The patient presented to Dr. Elhart with complaints of chest discomfort. A 2-D Doppler and color-flow Doppler was performed at the local hospital in the outpatient cardiology department, and Dr. Elhart monitored the echocardiography.

6-4A ECHOCARDIOGRAM

LOCATION: Hospital Outpatient

PATIENT: Herbert Gillford

PHYSICIAN: Marvin Elhart, M.D.

STUDY: The study is 2-D and a color-flow Doppler echocardiography.

INDICATION FOR STUDY: Sinus bradycardia.

Chamber dimension by M-mode:

1. The left atrial diameter is 62 mm, which is consistent with moderate atrial enlargement.
2. The aortic root is 39 mm.
3. Left ventricular diastolic diameter is 75 mm; systolic diameter is 65 mm.
4. Shortening fraction is 13%.
5. Ejection fraction is estimated at 26%.
6. Wall thickness is 7 mm.

DOPPLER:

1. Mild aortic insufficiency. The peak velocity across the aortic valve was estimated at 2 m/second. There is no evidence of significant aortic stenosis.
2. There is eccentric jet of mitral insufficiency. The E-velocity is estimated at 1.1 m/second, and that certainly corresponds with severe mitral insufficiency. There did not appear to be any significant mitral stenosis, even though the opening was decreased due to low cardiac output state.
3. There is moderate tricuspid insufficiency. The RV systolic pressure could not be estimated because of incomplete spectral envelopes.
4. Mild pulmonic insufficiency without stenosis.

2-D ECHO:

1. Mild to moderate left ventricular enlargement. The overall left ventricular systolic function is severely depressed, and ejection fraction is estimated at 15% to 20%.
2. There is severe global hypokinesia. The inferoposterior segment appears to be akinetic. The wall thickness is normal.
3. Right ventricle, right atrium, and aortic root are within the normal limits. The left atrium is moderately dilated.
4. The mitral valve is minimally thickened, and the excursion is decreased and most likely is due to low cardiac output state rather than mitral stenosis. The aortic valve is fibrocalcific without significant stenosis. The tricuspid valve is unremarkable.
5. There is no pericardial effusion.

CONCLUSION:

1. This is a markedly abnormal echocardiogram that reveals the presence of mild to moderate left ventricular enlargement with severe global left ventricular systolic dysfunction due to valvular insufficiency.
2. Mild aortic insufficiency.
3. Severe mitral insufficiency.

RECOMMENDATIONS:

1. I would suggest aggressive medical therapy with the use of ACE inhibitors, diuresis, and possible ACE inhibitors. SBE prophylaxis.

6-4A:

SERVICE CODE(S): ____________

DX CODE(S): ____________

CASE 6-4A DISCUSSION

This patient was referred for the symptom of sinus bradycardia (427.89); but there are more definitive diagnoses available based on the results of the test. Under the Conclusion section of the report, the physician indicates "left ventricular enlargement with severe global left ventricular systolic dysfunction due to valvular insufficiency." The ventricular enlargement and dysfunction are "due to" another more specific condition (valves are not functioning properly) and therefore are not reported separately. The physician also indicated both aortic and mitral insufficiency, but indicated no specific cause. There is a combination code available to report these two insufficiencies with one code. In the "Doppler" section of the report, the physician indicates that the patient also has tricuspid and pulmonary valve insufficiencies. There is no indication as to the cause of the insufficiency, and as such, the tricuspid is reported with the less specific 397.0 code; however, 397.1 is only for pulmonary valve insufficiency as a result of rheumatic disease. There is an Excludes note that indicates "excludes that not specified as rheumatic (424.3)," directing the coder to refer to 424.3 in the Tabular. When referencing 424.3, you will see an Includes note for "insufficiency NOS", which indicates that this is the correct code to assign to this pulmonary valve insufficiency.

Holter

Another commonly used cardiac diagnostic tool is the Holter monitor, which is a portable electrocardiography device that is worn by the patient, usually for 24 hours. The monitor records the electrical function of the heart and allows the physician to analyze the data to diagnose various cardiac conditions.

The sequence of events is important to know before you code the Holter monitor service. When the patient's physician evaluates the patient and determines that the patient requires the monitoring of cardiac function by means of a Holter monitor, the physician orders the monitoring, and at a later time the patient presents to the cardiology laboratory to be fitted with a monitor. The technician, under the supervision of the cardiologist, outfits the patient with the monitor and the patient leaves the department wearing the monitor for a specified period of time (24 hours), usually for a Holter. The patient returns to the cardiology department, and the technician removes the monitor. The cardiologist interprets tracing of the Holter and writes a report of findings that is sent to the physician who ordered the monitoring. In the meantime, after the monitoring has been performed, but before the results are returned and reviewed by the physician, the coder reports the services. This sequence is important in identifying the diagnosis for which the services were provided. The coder does not wait for the results of the various tests to be returned before reporting the services for reimbursement. The coder does, however, wait for the test to be conducted prior to submitting for reimbursement. The physician's diagnosis will be used to report the services for the Holter monitoring in the following report. After the physician reads the report, he or she may change the diagnosis of the patient to reflect the test results, but only the physician can make the determination of the diagnosis. Perhaps the physician ordered several tests and the interpretation as to the diagnosis varied. It is the ordering physician's responsibility to assess all test results and make the conclusion as to the final diagnosis. When coding the various reports in this worktext, you will be seeing the report results. However, you would usually only know that the test had been requested and performed, *not* the results.

CASE 6-5
6-5A Holter Report
6-5B Radiology Report, Preimplantation
6-5C Operative Report, Pacemaker Implantation
6-5D Radiology Report, Postimplantation

CASE 6-5

(also known as electrocardiographic monitoring, 24-hr.)

6-5A HOLTER REPORT

Code the following Holter service, assuming the test had been ordered and performed. For the diagnosis you would use the information presented in the "Indication" section of the report, because that would be the reason the physician ordered the test.

LOCATION: Outpatient, Clinic

PATIENT: Herbert Gillford

PHYSICIAN: Dr. Marvin Elhart

INDICATION: Patient with atrial fibrillation (1) on Lanoxin. Patient has known cardiomyopathy. (2)

BASELINE DATA: An 86-year-old man with congestive heart failure who is taking Elavil, Vasotec, Lanoxin, and Lasix.

The patient was monitored for 24 hours during which time the analysis was performed.

INTERPRETATION:

1. The predominant rhythm is atrial fibrillation. The average ventricular rate is 74 beats per minute, minimum 49 beats per minute, and maximum 114 beats per minute.
2. A total of 4948 ventricular ectopic beats were detected. There were four forms. There were 146 couplets with 1 triplet and 5 runs of bigeminy. There were two runs of ventricular tachycardia, the longest for 5 beats at a rate of 150 beats per minute. No ventricular fibrillation was noted.
3. There were no prolonged pauses.

CONCLUSION:

1. Predominant rhythm is atrial fibrillation with well-controlled ventricular rate.
2. There are no prolonged pauses.
3. Asymptomatic, nonsustained, ventricular tachycardia.

6-5A:

SERVICE CODE(S): ____________________

DX CODE(S): ____________________

Preimplantation, Implantation, and Postimplantation

A chest x-ray is performed prior to the pacemaker implantation. The pacemaker is implanted, and another chest x-ray is performed after the implantation to ensure proper pacemaker placement.

6-5B RADIOLOGY REPORT, PREIMPLANTATION

Code the preimplantation services.

LOCATION: Hospital Outpatient

PATIENT: Herbert Gillford

PHYSICIAN: Dr. Marvin Elhart

RADIOLOGIST: Dr. Morton Monson

EXAMINATION OF: Chest

CLINICAL SYMPTOMS: Sick sinus syndrome

CHEST, TWO VIEWS, FRONTAL AND LATERAL, 11:00 A.M.: Comparison is made to films taken 3 years ago. There is cardiomegaly. Overt failure is not identified. There is only a moderate degree of inspiration. Osseous structures show old compression deformity of the lower thoracic spine. Calcification is identified within a tortuous aorta. The portion of the abdomen that was seen is unremarkable.

IMPRESSION:
1. Sick sinus syndrome.
2. Cardiomegaly. There is a poor inspiration effort, but overt failure is not suggested grossly at this time.
3. Progress studies should be obtained as considered clinically warranted.

6-5B:

SERVICE CODE(S): ____________________

DX CODE(S): ____________________

6-5C OPERATIVE REPORT, PACEMAKER IMPLANTATION

LOCATION: Hospital Outpatient

PATIENT: Herbert Gillford

SURGEON: Dr. Marvin Elhart

PROCEDURE PERFORMED: Dual-chamber pacemaker implantation

INDICATION: Bradyarrhythmia

BRIEF HISTORY: This patient has been experiencing recurrent syncope. He was evaluated in the last year or so. Because of the presence of first-degree AV block, sinus bradycardia, and bundle-branch block, the cause for his syncope most likely is his bradyarrhythmia; for that reason, a dual-chamber pacemaker implantation was recommended after discussion with his cousin, who consented to the procedure. The cousin was informed of all potential complications, including infection, hematoma, pneumothorax, hemothorax, myocardial infarction, and even death. He agreed to proceed.

PROCEDURE: The patient was brought to the cardiac catheterization laboratory. He was placed on the catheterization table, where he was prepped and draped in the usual fashion. The procedure was extremely difficult to perform as a result of the patient's agitation despite adequate sedation. With reasonable hemostasis, the pacemaker pocket was performed in the left infraclavicular area after anesthetizing the area with 0.5 cc of Xylocaine. Hemostasis was secured with cautery. The patient had excessive venous oozing from Valsalva and straining, and that was controlled with pressure. A single stick was performed because of the patient's agitation. Using a 9 French peel-away sheath, we introduced an atrial and a ventricular lead and placed them in an excellent position. (dual pacer)

Thresholds were obtained adequately. The leads were sutured using 0 silk over their sleeves and secured. The pulse generator was connected. The pacemaker pocket was flushed with antibiotic solution. The pacemaker and leads were placed in the pocket and the pocket closed in two layers.

COMPLICATION: None

EQUIPMENT USED: Pulse generator was Medtronic model 60 Thera DRI, serial B28H. The ventricular lead was Medtronic serial L420V, model 4524 Link. The atrial lead was Medtronic 24-58, serial 326V.

The following parameters were obtained after implantation: Pacing threshold in the atrium was excellent at 0.5 msec and 0.5 V, and impedance was 445 ohms and sensing 2.1 mV. In the ventricle, 0.5 msec and 0.3 V with R wave of 19.9 mV and impedance 668.

The following parameters were left at implantation: DDDR with lower rate limit of 70 and an upper rate limit of 120. The amplitude was 3.5 V in the atrium at 0.4 msec with a sensitivity of 0.5 mV. The ventricle was 3.5 V and 0.4 msec at 2.8-mV sensitivity.

CONCLUSION: Successful implantation of dual-chamber pacemaker without immediate complications.

PLAN: Patient to return to recovery unit and to be discharged late this evening to the nursing home with routine postpacemaker care.

6-5C:

SERVICE CODE(S): ____________________

DX CODE(S): ____________________

6-5D RADIOLOGY REPORT, POSTIMPLANTATION

Two diagnoses are reported with this postimplantation service. The first listed diagnosis is a V code that indicates "Status, post, pacemaker, cardiac." The V code is listed first, as that is the reason for the service (checking on the placement of the pacemaker). The bradycardia is also reported, but sequenced after the V code.

LOCATION: Hospital Outpatient

PATIENT: Herbert Gillford

PHYSICIAN: Dr. Marvin Elhart

RADIOLOGIST: Dr. Morton Monson

EXAMINATION OF: Chest

CLINICAL SYMPTOMS: Status post pacemaker-placement, bradycardia

CHEST, SINGLE VIEW, FRONTAL: FINDINGS: This examination is compared with an examination performed earlier on the same day at 11:00 A.M. Since the previous examination, there has been interval placement of a pacemaker. One of the leads overlies the expected location of the right ventricle. The proximal lead overlies the expected location of the right atrium near the junction with the superior vena cava. Cardiomegaly is present on this examination. This is unchanged when compared with the previous examination. The pulmonary vascular markings appear within normal limits. The examination otherwise appears unchanged compared with the previous examination. Definite pneumothorax is not identified on this examination.

6-5D:

SERVICE CODE(S): ____________________

DX CODE(S): ____________________

Stress Tests

A cardiovascular **stress test** is a special type of echocardiogram that compares the electrical system of the heart at rest and under exertion. The test is used by the physician to diagnose various diseases, such as coronary artery disease (atherosclerosis), coronary ischemia (dead or dying heart muscle), and arrhythmias (irregular heartbeats). The technician administers the stress test under the direct supervision of the physician. Usually the test is conducted while the patient is exercised on a treadmill or bicycle and continuous recordings are made of the electrical activity of the heart. Electrodes are attached to the chest of the patient, as is a blood pressure monitor. The patient begins to exercise at a low speed. The speed is increased at set intervals until the patient's maximal or submaximal heart rate is reached and sustained. Three services are bundled into the complete stress test procedure as described in 93015:

- Physician supervision
- Tracing
- Interpretation with written report

Codes in the range 93016-93018 are used when only a component of the test is provided:

- Physician supervision (93016)
- Tracing only (93017)
- Interpretation and report (93018)

It would not be appropriate to report the entire service (93015) with the professional component modifier -26 or -TC because there are codes for each component of the complete service.

Sometimes, as the result of physical limitations, a patient is unable to exercise on a treadmill or bicycle. In these instances, the patient can be administered a drug to mimic the stress to the heart that would be brought about by exercise by dilating the vessels, such as Persantine, adenosine, Cardiolite, or dobutamine. These agents are administered in the outpatient setting at the hospital, and the hospital would report the cost of the pharmacologic agent, not the physician. *Where* tests are performed will have an effect on how the services are coded. If the test was administered at the local hospital, the physician would report the supervision and interpretation components of the service and the hospital would report the tracing portion of the service. If the outpatient facility employed a physician to do the supervision and interpretation and a technician to do the tracing, you would report the complete stress test service.

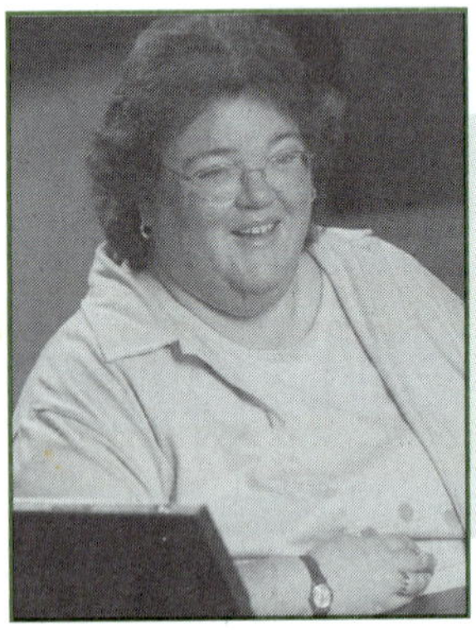

FROM THE TRENCHES

Lynn

What attracted you to coding, as a career?

"I liked the medical background—I was really interested in the medical part of it. Yet I really liked business and accounting, and I liked the patient contact. That worked out well for me... Coding gave me the best of both worlds!"

CASE 6-6
6-6A Adenosine Cardiolite Stress Test
6-6B Radiology Report, Perfusion Scan
6-6C Echo Doppler Report

CASE 6-6

6-6A ADENOSINE CARDIOLITE STRESS TEST

The stress test was conducted at the cardiology laboratory at the local hospital with the clinic physician supervising the test and interpreting the results.

LOCATION: Hospital Outpatient

PATIENT: Eleanor Montgomery

PHYSICIAN: Marvin Elhart, M.D.

INDICATIONS: Atherosclerotic heart disease with prior myocardial infarction, evaluate for potential ischemia

Electrocardiogram at rest in the exercise lead position reveals the presence of normal sinus rhythm with a somewhat atypical left bundle-branch block with related repolarization abnormalities. Subsequently the patient was injected with 140 µg per kilogram per minute of IV Adenoscan over a 6-minute period. At the 3-minute mark, Cardiolite was injected. At the 10-minute mark, the patient was brought for Cardiolite imaging. The patient had a little chest pain and chest tightness during this test that resolved by the end of the Adenoscan infusion. At no point did any diagnostic ST abnormalities develop beyond baseline.

No ectopy was seen other than one PVC.

The pulses ranged in the 60s to 70s during this test. Systolic blood pressures ranged in the 130s to 160s during this test.

CONCLUSION:
1. The patient did have some chest discomfort during this test, which could potentially represent an anginal equivalent.
2. By facility criteria, there was no evidence of any induction of ischemia.

6-6A:

SERVICE CODE(S): ____________________

DX CODE(S): ____________________

Myocardial Perfusion Scan

Depending on the results of the exercise stress test, the physician may recommend an additional test, such a **myocardial perfusion scan** or stress thallium scan. A **myocardial perfusion scan** or myocardial perfusion imaging is a radiology procedure performed to assess the amount of blood that is reaching the heart muscle, areas of blocked arteries, or the effectiveness of a coronary artery bypass or **angioplasty.** After an exercise stress test, the patient is injected with a radioactive tracer, such as adenosine or dipyridamole, and a specially equipped camera (gamma camera) is used to take a picture of the heart shortly after injection of the substance. The camera is attached to a computer, which displays the images. The tracer then circulates through the body and collects in the heart, at which time another image of the heart is taken that reveals areas where there are insufficient amounts of blood, which indicates dead or dying heart tissue. Myocardial perfusion scans are usually reported with codes from the Radiology section, Cardiovascular System subsection (78414-78499).

Ejection fraction (78480) is the percentage of blood pumped with each contraction of the heart and is related to the chamber volume. When the ejection fraction is low, the amount of blood pumped on each contraction is low. This test is done as a part of a myocardial perfusion scan (78460-78465).

6-6B RADIOLOGY REPORT, PERFUSION SCAN

LOCATION: Hospital Outpatient

PATIENT: Eleanor Montgomery

PHYSICIAN: Dr. Marvin Elhart

EXAMINATION OF: Stress and rest myocardial perfusion scan with ejection fraction quantifications

INDICATIONS: Arteriosclerosis, coronary vessel

CLINICAL SYMPTOMS: Postmyocardial infarction, 19xx, angiography, 19xx

STRESS AND REST MYOCARDIAL PERFUSION SCAN: TECHNIQUE: Yesterday 31.4 mCi of technetium 99 m sestamibi was administered following stress with adenosine. Today 24.4 mCi of technetium 99 m sestamibi was administered at rest. SPECT imaging was performed.

FINDINGS: There is minimal thinning of the cardiac apex on the stress images that shows some reversibility at rest. There is also a mild defect involving the inferolateral portion of the left ventricle extending from the periapical portion of the mid-left ventricle. This also shows reversibility in the inferior portion of the left ventricle.

IMPRESSION: Mild myocardial perfusion defects involving the apex and the periapical inferolateral portion of the left ventricle, which show reversibility on rest image. Diagnosis is coronary arteriosclerosis.

6-6B:

SERVICE CODE(S): ____________________

DX CODE(S): ____________________

In the information preceding case 6-4 of this chapter, you learned about coding a Doppler, and you once again have an opportunity to test your skills by coding the following report.

6-6C ECHO DOPPLER REPORT

The patient's chest pains may or may not be related to the aortic and mitral insufficiency, so the chest pain would be reported in addition to the insufficiencies.

LOCATION: Hospital Outpatient

PATIENT: Eleanor Montgomery

PHYSICIAN: Marvin Elhart, M.D.

INDICATION: Chest pain; evaluate heart function.

M-Mode, 2-D echo, and Doppler studies with color-flow analysis were performed. Findings are as follows:

1. CHAMBER SIZES: The left ventricle appears to be mildly enlarged on the 2-D images and mildly concentrically hypertrophied except for the septum, which is relatively thin compared with the rest of the left ventricle. The left atrium appears to be mildly enlarged and normal in thickness. The right ventricle and right atrium appear to be of normal size and thickness.
2. WALL MOTION (This is pulsed wave): All cardiac chambers contract normally except for the left ventricular interventricular septum; anterior wall appears to be hypokinetic with moderate impairment of LVEF, visually on the order of about 35% or so.
3. The AORTIC ROOT is normal in size.
4. There is no pericardial effusion.
5. VALVES: The aortic valve and mitral valve leaflets are nonspecifically fibrocalcific. The tricuspid valve and pulmonic valve appear normal. No cardiac valves appear to prolapse.
6. DOPPLER WITH COLOR-FLOW INTERROGATION reveals mild aortic insufficiency. There also appears to be moderate mitral insufficiency. No other valvular, stenotic, or regurgitation lesions are seen.

CONCLUSION: The present echo Doppler study reveals mild aortic insufficiency along with moderate mitral insufficiency. The left ventricle and left atrium appear to be moderately enlarged. (The hypertrophy is a result of the insufficiency.) There appears to be left ventricular septal and anterior-wall hypokinesis along with moderate impairment of LVEF in the order of about 35% or so. Please see above report for details.

6-6C:

SERVICE CODE(S): ____________________

DX CODE(S): ____________________

CASE 6-7
6-7A Cardiology Consultation
6-7B Hospital Service
7C Radiology Report, Chest
6-7D Cardiothoracic Surgical Consultation
6-7E Radiology Report, Chest

CASE 6-7

In Case 6-7, Eleanor Montgomery presents a year after the services you Coded in Case 6-6 with the chief complaint of chest tightness. She is initially seen by Dr. James Noonar, Cardiology, at the request of her internal medicine physician, Dr. Naraquist.

6-7A CARDIOLOGY CONSULTATION

LOCATION: Outpatient, Clinic

PATIENT: Eleanor Montgomery

CARDIOLOGIST: James Noonar, M.D.

DX

I have been asked by Dr. Naraquist to render an opinion regarding the patient's chest tightness. She has a history of chest discomfort that led to an angiogram that showed mild atherosclerotic heart disease, nothing critical enough to warrant any intervention, and thereafter she had a normal Cardiolite stress test. Over the years, she has had rare episodes of chest discomfort. Lately, however, she has had in the last several weeks three bouts of chest discomfort–all relieved with nitroglycerin sprays ×2 each time. She indicates that she is not doing anything in particular when the episodes occur. She became concerned about this. She had no associated diaphoresis, shortness of breath, or any lightheadedness, but these were retrosternal chest pressures radiating toward the back, all promptly relieved with the two nitroglycerin sprays done serially.

Her ECG in my office today shows normal sinus rhythm with left bundle-branch block with related repolarization abnormalities. This left bundle-branch block is a little more prominent in terms of the QRSs being slightly wider, but she did have a left bundle-branch block even back in December.

The patient has history of ALLERGY TO PENICILLIN AND SULFA DRUGS.

MEDICAL HISTORY includes the above as well as history of cancer of the uterus that has not recurred after having had TAH-BSO with incidental appendectomy. She has not had any other surgeries. There is also a history of right-wrist Colles fracture.

FAMILY HISTORY is negative for myocardial infarction and is otherwise noncontributory.

SOCIAL HISTORY: Nonsmoker. No history of alcohol abuse. No illegal drug use.

REVIEW OF SYSTEMS: Noncontributory except for above. General: No recent fevers, chills, or rigors. Weight has been stable. Neurologic: No strokelike or TIA-like symptoms. Endocrine: No diabetes mellitus or thyroid dysfunction noted. Hematologic: No anemia. Respiratory: No cough or hemoptysis. Cardiac: As per above with no PND, orthopnea, or pedal edema. No syncope or presyncope. No bright red blood per rectum, melena, hemoptysis, or hematemesis. Musculoskeletal: No arthritis complaints. Psychiatric: No depression. Integumentary: No rashes.

CARDIAC RISK FACTORS include the following:
1. Postmenopausal state
2. Age over 70 and otherwise negative

MEDICATIONS:
1. Detrol
2. Meclizine
3. Premarin
4. Vitamin B_{12}
5. Omega vitamins
6. Folic acid as per above

PHYSICAL EXAMINATION: Patient is a well-developed older female, age-appropriate for appearance, alert and oriented ×3. No apparent distress. Vital signs are stable. Afebrile. Blood pressure is 144/80. Pulse is 77 and regular. Weight is 152 pounds. Height is 5 feet 5 inches. HEENT examination is benign with head atraumatic and normocephalic. Oropharynx, teeth, and gums appear normal. Neck is supple without any significant jugular venous distention. No carotid bruits. No thyromegaly. Lungs are clear to auscultation. Cardiac examination: S1 and S2 are normal with a I-II/VI left sternal border soft systolic murmur. No other murmurs, gallops, clicks, or rubs are noted. The apical impulse is not palpable. No lifts, thrills, or heaves are noted. Abdominal examination: soft, nontender abdomen. Normoactive bowels sounds. No organomegaly or palpable masses. Back without CVAT and no spinal percussion tenderness. Extremities are without clubbing, cyanosis, or edema. Peripheral pulses are normal throughout.

No femoral bruits are present. Skin is without rashes. No xanthomas or xanthelasmas are seen. Neurologic exam is grossly normal.

Old clinic notes indicate that this patient has had a history of a remote MI; however, she did have a normal cardiac stress test 5 years ago.

IMPRESSION AND RECOMMENDATIONS: This elderly woman presents to me because of intermittent episodes of chest tightness. Of interest, she had an unremarkable angiogram back in 19xx or so. At this juncture, with her having this chest discomfort and having a possible heart murmur on exam, with a history of aortic insufficiency documented on echocardiogram a number or years ago, I will set her up for a Cardiolite stress test with an echocardiogram and return to clinic. If okay with her primary care physician, I will check screening lab results as ordered for further evaluation of this patient with a chest pain syndrome. I want to be sure that it is definitely not ischemia in someone who also has a history of atherosclerotic heart disease and a history of aortic insufficiency.

Thank you again for this consultation.

6-7A:

SERVICE CODE(S): ______________________

DX CODE(S): ______________________

Review of Previous History

If the physician reviews a recent history (ROS and PFSH) and then references this review in the current history, this reference qualifies the current history for the same level as the previously documented level if the date and location of the information are specified. For example, when the documentation from Case 6-7A, 10/14/xx is referenced, the ROS and PFSH are of a comprehensive level. This previous service qualifies the current service for a comprehensive level of ROS and PFSH. The physician must reference the specific date and service along with a statement of "changes included" or "no changes noted" for this review of documentation to qualify for the history portion of the current service.

6-7B HOSPITAL SERVICE

After Eleanor's cardiology consultation with Dr. Noonar, she was scheduled for a stress test. Dr. Noonar reviewed the results of the stress test and made arrangements to admit Eleanor to the hospital for further examination. Code the services provided to her.

LOCATION: Hospital Inpatient

PATIENT: Eleanor Montgomery

CARDIOLOGIST: James Noonar, M.D.

HISTORY: The patient is being admitted for an angiogram because of positive Cardiolite stress test for ischemia last week. At the present interview, she had no ongoing complaints. I did a full review at the clinic, and as part of the workup, because of her chest-tightness problems, a Cardiolite stress test was performed that unfortunately showed some evidence of ischemia. That is why she is being admitted. For full details of her medical history, social history, family history, review of systems, and so on, all of which have not changed since our last visit, please refer to the previous history dated August 10. Her cardiac risk factors and her medications are also summarized in that note.

PHYSICAL EXAMINATION: No changes since 10/14/xx with no stigmata of congestive heart failure. Normal heart tones except for a 1-2/6 left sternal border soft systolic murmur noted. She has no peripheral edema. LUNGS are clear. (*Note: Your review of the medical record of 10/14/xx [those in report 6-7A], indicates that a comprehensive level of history was done.*)

Recent echo Doppler study showed mild aortic insufficiency with moderate mitral insufficiency.

IMPRESSION/RECOMMENDATIONS: Patient is a woman with a history of intermittent chest tightness problems who recently had a Cardiolite stress test that was positive for ischemia. She also has a heart murmur on exam, and recent echocardiogram showed mild aortic insufficiency and moderate MR. Thus, at this point, I will set her up for a diagnostic cardiac cath and a view of her valvular heart disease when we do this cardiac cath. We will do this bilaterally. Further notes will follow pending the clinical course on this patient who has also had, on further review of systems, some fatigue problems. In view of her valvular disease, when we do the cardiac cath, we will do the cardiac cath bilaterally.

6-7B:

SERVICE CODE(S): ______________________

DX CODE(S): ______________________

6-7C RADIOLOGY REPORT, CHEST

LOCATION: Hospital Inpatient

PATIENT: Eleanor Montgomery

CARDIOLOGIST: James Noonar, M.D.

RADIOLOGIST: Morton Monson, M.D.

EXAMINATION OF: Chest, two views, frontal and lateral

CLINICAL SYMPTOMS: Positive cardiac stress test; chest pain

CHEST, TWO X-RAYS: Findings: No previous examination is available for comparison at this time. The heart size and pulmonary vascular markings appear within normal limits. There are atherosclerotic changes of the thoracic aorta. No focal infiltrates are seen within the lungs. No pleural effusions are seen. Hypertrophic changes are present within the thoracic spine.

IMPRESSION:
1. ASCVD
2. No evidence for congestive failure or infiltrate

6-7C:

SERVICE CODE(S): ____________________

DX CODE(S): ____________________

6-7D CARDIOTHORACIC SURGICAL CONSULTATION

LOCATION: Hospital Inpatient

PATIENT: Eleanor Montgomery

CARDIOTHORACIC SURGEON: David Barton, M.D.

CARDIOLOGIST: James Noonar, M.D.

PRIMARY CARE PHYSICIAN: Alana Naraquist, M.D.

REASON FOR CONSULTATION: Atherosclerotic heart disease and mitral insufficiency

HISTORY OF PRESENT ILLNESS: I have been asked by Dr. Barton to render an opinion regarding the patient's ASHD. Patient has a known history of atherosclerotic heart disease and has noted increasing symptoms of fatigability and intermittent chest pain over the past several months. She apparently did suffer a myocardial infarction in approximately 19xx. She remembers being given streptokinase at that time. She did have a coronary angiogram in 19xx that revealed mild atherosclerotic heart disease. A Cardiolite stress test in 19xx was normal by report. In the past several months, she has noted some increasing fatigability. She also has noticed some complaints of intermittent chest pain. She was given nitro spray to be used as needed and has used it approximately once per week for the past month or so according to her husband. The chest pain she has is retrosternal and occasionally radiates into the upper portion of the chest. She denies any accompanying shortness of breath, nausea, vomiting, or palpitations. The pain is relieved with nitroglycerin or rest. She also states that sometimes the pain is relieved with antacids. Today she underwent cardiac catheterization and coronary angiography revealing moderate atherosclerotic heart disease, preserved left ventricular systolic function, and moderate mitral insufficiency. Specifically, coronary angiography revealed a 50% stenosis of an obtuse marginal branch and a 70% stenosis of the left anterior descending artery. Distal to the stenosis, the LAD was quite small. There was also a 75% stenosis in the extreme apical portion of the left anterior descending artery. The distal right coronary artery has a 60% stenosis. There is 3+ mitral insufficiency. A recent Cardiolite stress test revealed mild perfusion defects involving the apex and the periapical inferolateral wall. Patient ejection fraction was calculated to be 41%. Cardiothoracic surgery was consulted to discuss the option of surgical revascularization and possibly mitral valve repair or replacement.

MEDICAL HISTORY:
1. Atherosclerotic heart disease as described above
2. History of uterine cancer
3. Arthritis

She specifically denies any known history of diabetes mellitus, cerebrovascular accident, hepatitis, tuberculosis, asthma, or seizures.

SURGICAL HISTORY:
1. Total abdominal hysterectomy with bilateral salpingo-oophorectomy
2. Appendectomy

MEDICATIONS ON ADMISSION:
1. Detrol 1.25 mg p.o. q.d.
2. Meclizine 12.5 mg p.o. q.d.
3. Premarin 1.25 mg p.o. q.d.
4. Aspirin 325 mg p.o. a.d.
5. Vitamin B_{12}
6. Omega-3
7. Folic acid
8. Nitro spray as described above

ALLERGIES: Penicillin and sulfa, which cause swelling and rashes. She also states that she is allergic to smoke, grapes, and oranges. The allergy to the grapes and oranges, however, appears to be a side effect (bloating and gas).

FAMILY HISTORY: Unremarkable for atherosclerotic heart disease according to the patient.

SOCIAL HISTORY: The patient is married and lives with her husband. He also has atherosclerotic heart disease and apparently had a stroke recently. She does not smoke cigarettes or drink alcohol.

REVIEW OF SYSTEMS: GENERAL: The patient denies any fever, chills, weight loss, or night sweats. CARDIAC:

Essentially as that described in the history of present illness. RESPIRATORY: Unremarkable for any hemoptysis, productive cough, or wheezing. GASTROINTESTINAL: Remarkable only for symptoms of GE reflux. She denies any jaundice, abdominal pain, or change in bowel habits. GENITOURINARY: Remarkable for intermittent incontinence. She denies any hematuria or dysuria. MUSCULOSKELETAL: Remarkable only for arthritic symptoms in her hands and fingers. She denies any muscle pain or joint swelling other than in her fingers. NEUROLOGIC: The patient denies any severe migraines or seizures of focal weakness. SKIN: Unremarkable for any new rashes or lesions. ENDOCRINE: Unremarkable for any polydipsia, polyuria, or temperature intolerance. HEMATOLOGIC: Unremarkable for any history of anemia or bleeding tendencies.

PHYSICAL EXAMINATION: The patient is a well-developed, well-nourished, thin, white female appearing her stated age in no acute distress. Blood pressure 140/80; pulse 74 and regular; respirations 14. HEENT: The patient is normocephalic. Pupils were equal, round, and reactive to light. Nose and throat exams were grossly unremarkable. The patient wears eyeglasses. The tympanic membranes were not examined. NECK: Supple without palpable adenopathy or thyromegaly. I could not detect any carotid bruits. There was no jugular venous distention with the patient sitting at 45 degrees. Auscultation of the CHEST reveals essentially clear breath sounds bilaterally. CARDIAC exam reveals a regular rhythm with a 1/6 systolic murmur heard best along the left sternal border. The murmur does not radiate. ABDOMEN: Soft abdominal organomegaly. GENITOURINARY/RECTAL: Deferred. The patient has a Foley catheter in place. Examination of the EXTREMITIES revealed palpable radial and femoral pulses. The left dorsalis pedis and posterior tibial pulse are faintly palpable. I could not detect any pedal pulses on the right foot. There is no significant peripheral cyanosis or edema. There are several superficial venous varicosities over both lower extremities. NEUROLOGIC: The patient is alert and oriented ×4. Gait was not tested. Strength was grossly normal in the upper extremities.

LABORATORY DATA: White blood cell count was 5600; hemoglobin 13.6; hematocrit 39.7; platelet count 244,000. Pro-time was 10.5; INR 0.8; PTT 25.2. Total cholesterol was 212 with an HDL fraction of 68 and an LDL fraction of 92. Sodium was 137, potassium 4.3, BUN 16, creatinine 1.3, and glucose 78.

A 12-lead ECG revealed a normal sinus rhythm with left bundle-branch block. Rate was 69.

IMPRESSION: The patient is a woman with a known history of atherosclerotic heart disease who has noticed increased fatigability and intermittent chest pain over the past several months. She has used nitroglycerin spray intermittently but only about once a week according to her and her husband. She is on no other cardiac medications. The results of the heart catheterization, Cardiolite stress test, and echocardiogram were reviewed with the physician. The prognosis as well as the risks and benefits of more aggressive medical therapy versus surgical revascularization and possible mitral valve surgery were discussed at length. Patient questions concerning her options for therapy were answered. I explained that because she had really been on minimal, if any, medical therapy that this certainly was an option. I explained that if she did not want to try a more aggressive medical therapy, surgery would be the next step. I also explained that if she wanted to try medical therapy and she experienced significant improvement in her symptoms, we could certainly try medical therapy for the time being. If, however, she did have breakthrough angina or developed symptoms of congestive heart failure, I think surgery would be her only other option. The patient appeared to understand the above findings and after a short discussion expressed the desire to proceed with a more aggressive medical therapy. I discussed the above findings with Dr. Noonar and Dr. Naraquist.

PLAN: The patient will be started on a more aggressive medical therapy. Dr. Naraquist will handle that. If she does not notice any improvement or experiences increasing symptoms, I think surgery should be strongly reconsidered.

6-7D:

SERVICE CODE(S): ____________________

DX CODE(S): ____________________

6-7E RADIOLOGY REPORT, CHEST

LOCATION: Hospital Inpatient

PATIENT: Eleanor Montgomery

CARDIOLOGIST: James Noonar, M.D.

RADIOLOGIST: Morton Monson, M.D.

EXAMINATION OF: Chest

CLINICAL SYMPTOMS: Rales, left lung, cough

PA & LATERAL CHEST, 11:05 A.M.: FINDINGS: Study is compared with the study of 11/01/xx at 8:40 A.M. Cardiac silhouette and pulmonary vasculature are within normal limits. No focal infiltrate or pleural effusion is identified. The aorta is tortuous with atherosclerotic change. Degenerative change involves the dorsal spine.

IMPRESSION: Stable chest

6-7E:

SERVICE CODE(S): ____________________

DX CODE(S): ____________________

CASE 6-8
6-8A Echo Doppler Report

CASE 6-8

In January, the patient returns to the hospital outpatient department for another echocardiography. Code the physician portion of the service that was provided in the cardiology laboratory of the hospital.

6-8A ECHO DOPPLER REPORT

LOCATION: Hospital Outpatient

PATIENT: Eleanor Montgomery

PRIMARY CARE PHYSICIAN: Alanda Naraquist, M.D.

CARDIOLOGIST: James Noonar, M.D.

INDICATIONS: Evaluation of mitral regurgitation

M-Mode, 2-D, and Doppler studies with color-flow analysis were performed, and the findings are as follows:

1. CHAMBER SIZES: The left ventricle on the 2-D image is mildly enlarged and mildly concentrically hypertrophied. The LA appears to be mildly enlarged and on the 2-D images is normal in thickness. The right ventricle and right atrium appear to be of normal size and thickness.
2. WALL MOTION: All cardiac chambers contract normally, except for the left ventricle, which displays interventricular septal and anterior lateral wall mild hypokinesis. There also appears to be a double kick on relaxation consistent with right bundle-branch block type of conduction. The overall LVEF by visual estimation is on the order of about 35% to 40% at best.
3. The aortic root is of normal size.
4. There is no pericardial effusion.
5. VALVES: The aortic valve and mitral valve leaflets are nonspecifically mildly fibrocalcific. The tricuspid valve and pulmonic valve appear to be grossly normal. No cardiac valves appear to prolapse.
6. Doppler with color-flow interrogation reveals mild mitral insufficiency, mild aortic insufficiency, and trace tricuspid insufficiency. No other valvular stenotic or regurgitant lesions are seen.

CONCLUSION: The present echo Doppler study reveals mild enlargement of the left ventricle and left atrium, along with some LVH. There also appears to be mild aortic insufficiency, mild mitral insufficiency, and trace tricuspid insufficiency. There appear to be regional wall motion abnormalities are discussed above, with an EF of around 35% to 40% at best. Please see above report for details.

ADDENDUM: Doppler interrogation of mitral valve inflow reveals a prominent A-wave suggestive of decreased left ventricular compliance for which I apologize for not mentioning above.

6-8A:

SERVICE CODE(S): abnormal echo

DX CODE(S): ______________

396.3 (insuff, mitral)
397.0 (insuff, tricuspid)
793.2 (abnormal, echo)
429.3 (hypertrophy, cardiac)

CASE 6-9
6-9A Cardiology Consultation

CASE 6-9

In February, the patient was again admitted through the emergency room for atrial fibrillation. Her primary care physician requested a cardiology consultation. Code the cardiology consultation services. The patient has atrial fibrillation, anemia, and a heart murmur; additionally a code to report that this anemia is a complication of a surgical procedure.

6-9A CARDIOLOGY CONSULTATION

LOCATION: Hospital ~~Outpatient~~ Inpatient

PATIENT: Eleanor Montgomery

CARDIOLOGIST: James Noonar, M.D.

REASON FOR ADMISSION: Rapid paroxysmal atrial fibrillation

HISTORY: I am being asked by Dr. Naraquist to render an opinion regarding this patient's paroxysmal atrial fibrillation. The patient was recently discharged after having bypass by Dr. Naraquist. During the admission she had some paroxysmal atrial fibrillation. She was discharged home yesterday and then, at about 3:00 in the morning today, she awakened with palpitations and a feeling of rapid heart rate. She saw her doctor, Dr. Naraquist, who found her to be in rapid atrial fibrillation. Apparently she was given verapamil and adenosine. I do not have those records at the time of this dictation, but by the time she arrived here she was in normal sinus rhythm with PACs occasionally, and that is what her rhythm is right now on telemetry (normal sinus rhythm with occasional PACs). She has not had any further atrial fibrillation. Lab results that have come back already include a digoxin level at 0.79 g/ml with TSH of 2.62, free T_4 1.0, BUN 14, sodium 135, potassium 4.3, chloride 102, glucose 140, creatinine 1.4, calcium 8.2, albumin 2.5, alkaline phosphatase 102, bilirubin total 0.3, SGOT 23, total protein 5.4, and CO_2 24.7.

On presentation showed a white blood cell count of 7170 with hemoglobin 8.6, hematocrit 26.2, and a normal platelet count and normal MCV. Recent hemoglobin around the time of her discharge earlier this week showed 8.6.

The patient at the present interview has no ongoing complaints.

Of interest, the patient had atrial fibrillation briefly during her hospitalization postbypass, which converted to sinus rhythm after getting some IV digitalis at that time.

MEDICAL HISTORY: Includes the above as well as prior myocardial infarction in 19xx; then in 19xx she had endometrial cancer treatment with TAH-BSO without any recurrence of that cancer and had apparently 29 or so radiation therapy treatments, after which there were no recurrences of that cancer. She is status post remote appendectomy.

ALLERGIES: Penicillin and sulfa

MEDICATIONS:
1. Detrol
2. Premarin
3. Vitamin B_{12}
4. Omega
5. Folic acid
6. Enteric-coated aspirin
7. Propranolol
8. Dyazide
9. Digoxin
10. KCl

The medications list said Lopressor 25 mg b.i.d., but I just started that here. She was on propranolol 10 mg b.i.d. prior to this admission at the time of her recent discharge.

SOCIAL HISTORY: Nonsmoker, nondrinker. No history of alcohol abuse. No illegal drug use. Married.

FAMILY HISTORY: Patient has two sisters and two brothers who have myocardial infarctions in their later years. The rest of the family history is noncontributory.

REVIEW OF SYSTEMS: Noncontributory except for above. GENERAL: Since her bypass, she has not had any reports of fever, chills, or rigors. Weight has been stable. NEUROLOGIC: No strokelike or TIA-like symptoms. ENDOCRINE: No diabetes mellitus or thyroid dysfunction noted. HEMATOLOGIC: Anemic since bypass, with hemoglobin as low as in the 7s postbypass that was 8.6 by the time of discharge without transfusion apparently given. RESPIRATORY: No cough or hemoptysis. CARDIAC: As per above with no PND, orthopnea, or pedal edema. No syncope or presyncope was noted. No angina that she recognized as similar to the angina that she used to have before her bypass. She has a little chest wall pain from her bypass. That is about it, and she feels that she is healing well. GI: No nausea, vomiting, bloody stools, or black stools were noted. GU: No reports of any dysuria or hematuria, but she has some occasional urinary frequency for which she takes the Detrol, and that is chronic for her. MUSCULOSKELETAL: No complaints of any arthritis other than her left wrist chronically bothering her where she has an old fracture site that did not heal well.

CARDIAC RISK FACTORS: Include her recent bypass and two prior myocardial infarctions and family history of myocardial infarction and history of hypercholesterolemia; otherwise, negative.

PHYSICAL EXAMINATION: Well-developed, older female, age-appropriate for appearance, alert and oriented ×3, in no apparent distress. VITAL SIGNS stable; afebrile; blood pressure, 138/70; pulse, 74, occasionally irregular consistent with PACs and otherwise regular; respirations 14 and normal. HEENT: Grossly benign with head atraumatic, normocephalic. Pharynx, teeth, and gums appear normal. NECK: Supple without any significant jugular venous distention. Carotids are normal in upstroke and volume. I do not appreciate any carotid bruits, but I can hear heart tones in her right neck. LUNGS: Clear to auscultation and percussion. CARDIAC: S1 and S2 normal with a 2/6 apical soft systolic murmur. Apical impulse is not palpable. No lifts, thrills, or heaves. ABDOMEN: Soft, nontender. Normoactive bowel sounds. No organomegaly, no palpable masses. BACK: Without CVA tenderness, no spinal percussion tenderness. EXTREMITIES: Without clubbing, cyanosis, or edema; both upper and lower extremities. Peripheral pulses are normal throughout, except for trace pedal pulses bilaterally. No femoral bruits. SKIN: Without rashes, no xanthomas, no xanthelasma. NEUROLOGIC: Grossly normal.

Chest-wall wound from recent bypass as well as epigastric drain site and saphenous vein strip site from her left thigh area all appear to be healing well without any stigmata of infection or dehiscence.

Admission ECG pending.

IMPRESSION/RECOMMENDATIONS: The patient is an older woman with a history of prior myocardial infarction in the early 19xxs, followed by the development of worsening angina recently that led to bypass recently. During that hospitalization, she had some brief paroxysmal atrial fibrillation after just being discharged home yesterday afternoon. At 3:00 in the morning today, she had rapid atrial fibrillation and was seen by her local physician; she apparently received some verapamil and adenosine, and by the time she arrived here, she was back in sinus rhythm with occasional PACs, which is her current status. She appears otherwise stable and looks well otherwise. I am not convinced there is anything active going on that we need to make any changes for except that she is on such a low dose of propranolol, which I will change to Lopressor 25 mg b.i.d., and that will be better for atrial fibrillation prophylaxis than the low-dose propranolol. I will keep her on telemetry, and as long as she remains otherwise stable I would recommend this patient up for discharge home tomorrow.

ADDENDUM: The patient is anemic. Her hemoglobin is only 8.6, and this is postsurgical because of blood loss with surgery as per prior records. I think ideally keeping her hemoglobin over 10 mg percent would help her and also help prophylaxis against recurrent atrial fibrillation. In this patient with recent bypass who now has a heart murmur on exam, that might be just a flow murmur due to her anemia. We will get her tanked up with some blood, get her hemoglobin over 10 mg percent, and if she continues to have a heart murmur, I recommend an echo. Thus, I will give her 2 units of packed cells.

Today the patient does have, in her right forearm area, a mildly cellulitic area that looks like it is an IV site infection from a prior IV placement in this patient with a history of penicillin and sulfa allergy. For this, I will empirically start her on Cipro 500 mg p.o. b.i.d. for 10 days.

6-9A:

SERVICE CODE(S): ______________________

DX CODE(S): ______________________

Cardiac Catheterization

Invasive cardiology is an area of medicine in which the physician not only diagnoses the cardiac condition but also performs the cardiac procedures that involve entry into the heart and circulatory system. For example, the cardiologist would perform cardiac catheterization, coronary angioplasty, and electrophysiologic studies of the heart.

Cardiac catheterization is an invasive procedure in which the physician percutaneously inserts a catheter into a vein and manipulates the catheter into the heart or coronary vessel. A fine-gauge needle is inserted into an artery, such as the right subclavian artery, internal jugular, femoral, external jugular, or brachial vessel. A guidewire, followed by a catheter, is then inserted into the artery. The surgeon manipulates the catheter into position by means of fluoroscopy (viewing on a monitor).

The three parts to a cardiac catheterization service are **placement** of the catheter, **injection** of dye into the vessel, and **imaging** of the vessel. Locate the Cardiac Catheterization subsection (93501-93572) of the CPT manual. Place a bracket beside the codes in the CPT manual in the range 93501-93533. Beside the bracket write "placement." Place a second bracket beside the codes in the range 93539-93545, and write "injection" next to the bracket. Place a third bracket beside the codes 93555-93556, and write "imaging" next to the bracket. During a cardiac catheterization service, these three services are provided, usually by the cardiologist.

Note that the placement, injection, and imaging codes are all modifier -51 exempt. This means that these three services, when performed together during the same operative session, are not subject to the usual reduction in reimbursement that would accompany the submission of the code if you added modifier -51 to the second and third services.

Once the catheter is positioned, for example, into the left coronary artery, and the catheter is repositioned into another vessel, for example, the left ventricle, the repositioning is included in the introduction. If, however, both the left coronary artery and left ventricle were injected and imaged, each injection (2) and each imaging service (2) would be reported separately.

The cardiac catheterization is often accompanied by placement of a **stent** or angioplasty. **Angioplasty** is repair of a vessel. Percutaneous transluminal coronary angioplasty (PTCA) is a procedure in which the physician makes an incision into a vessel and inserts a catheter. The catheter is manipulated into the vessel that is blocked with plaque. A second catheter with a balloon at the tip is threaded into the blocked area. The balloon is then inflated, pushing the plaque against the vessel wall (**Figure 6-6**). Angioplasty is done to improve the caliber of the vessel and thereby increases the blood flow. Angioplasty is reported with 92982 for the initial vessel and add-on code 92984 for each additional vessel.

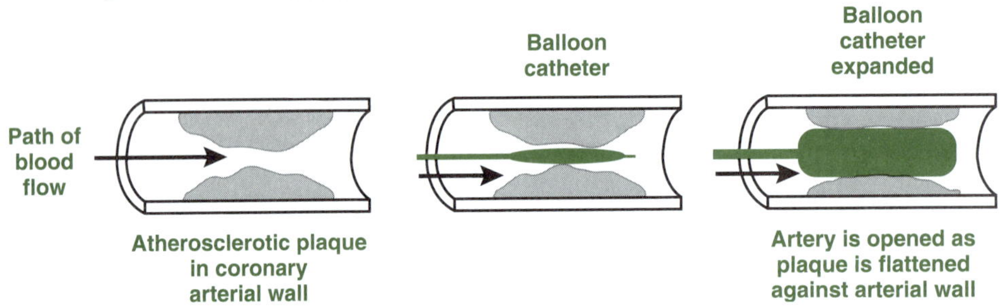

FIGURE 6-6 Balloon-tipped catheter with the balloon inflated is used to push back plaque against the wall of the vessel.

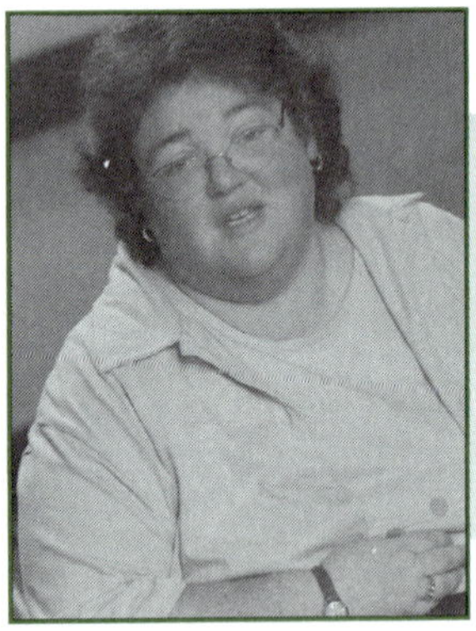

FROM THE TRENCHES

Lynn

"It is really hard to teach physicians to talk in CPT language...Some of them are really good at it, because they have taken the time to learn it... The new doctors that are coming out of medical school now are more in tune with coding. It is their bread and butter."

Stenting, illustrated in **Figure 6-7,** is reinforcing a weakened area in a vessel, in addition to forcing open and holding in place that area of a vessel that has weakened. For example, if it was discovered on cardiac catheterization that the patient's coronary vessel was obstructed with atherosclerosis, the physician could widen the area and place a stent into the vessel to maintain the vessel open, thereby increasing blood flow through the damaged area. The placement of the stent using the transcatheter approach (by means of the catheter) is reported with 92980 for the first vessel and 92981 for each additional vessel.

The terminology used in the cardiology services often refers not only to the location of the vessels but also the procedures, for example, the LAD (left anterior descending artery) and RCA (right coronary artery). A good medical dictionary and/or abbreviation text is a necessity as you begin to code from the various catheterization, angioplasty, and stenting records.

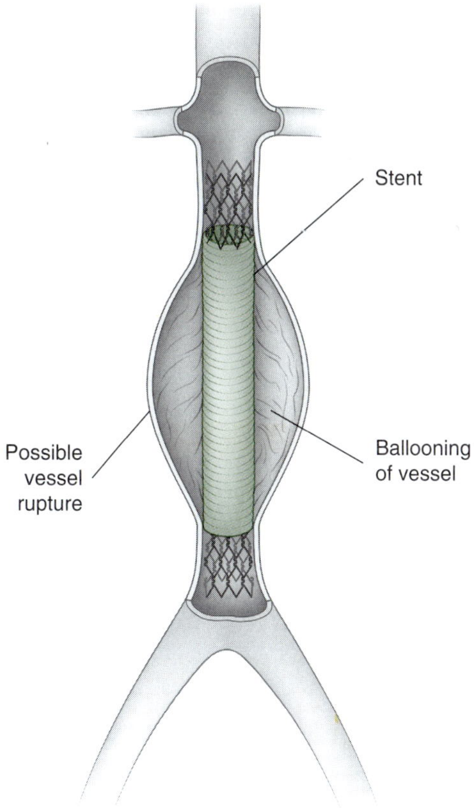

FIGURE 6-7 Stenting.

CASE 6-10
6-10A Emergency and Outpatient Record
6-10B Radiology Report, Chest
6-10C Hospital Admission
6-10D Cardiac Catheterization Report
6-10E PTCA/Stenting Report

CASE 6-10

The following reports are for a 50-year-old white male who is seen in the emergency department of the local hospital. The patient was first seen in the emergency department by the physician on staff. The emergency department physician then turned the case over to Dr. Elhart, the cardiologist from the local clinic who was on call. Dr. Elhart admitted the patient to the hospital. Code the emergency outpatient services provided to the patient by Dr. Sutton.

6-10A EMERGENCY AND OUTPATIENT RECORD

LOCATION: Hospital Outpatient

PATIENT: Kenneth Peters

PHYSICIAN: Paul Sutton, M.D.

SUBJECTIVE: This is a 50-year-old white male who has a history of hypertension. He has no other significant ongoing medical problems and takes no other medications. He is on aspirin and nifedipine. He has no known allergies. He presents acutely to the emergency room today with a history of suddenly developing substernal chest pressure radiating to his jaw that started about 1 hour prior to his arrival. He had diaphoresis and some nausea associated with this. He had no significant dyspnea, however. Other than his history of hypertension and remote smoking history when he quit smoking about 23 years ago, he has no significant risk factors for coronary artery disease.

REVIEW OF SYSTEMS: CONSTITUTIONAL: No fevers, sweats, or chills. GASTROINTESTINAL: No vomiting or diarrhea. GU: No urgency, frequency, or dysuria. RESPIRATORY: No cough or significant shortness of breath. CARDIOVASCULAR: Chest pain as outlined above. No history of peripheral edema.

OBJECTIVE: He is afebrile (99) and stable. VITAL SIGNS: There is no evidence of diaphoresis or dyspnea at this time. His HEENT exam is grossly unremarkable. NECK: Supple. There is no thyromegaly or adenopathy. HEART: S1 and S2, no S3 or S4. The rhythm is regular. No murmur. LUNG sounds are clear. ABDOMEN: Bowel sounds are present and active. No organomegaly, masses, or hernias are noted. Generally, soft and nontender. There is no evidence of a pulsatile mass, and his femoral pulses are equal bilaterally. EXTREMITIES: Negative for cyanosis or edema.

His ECG revealed a sinus rhythm with obvious inferior ST elevation changes. He had taken aspirin at home prior to his arrival here. He was started on IV nitroglycerin at 5 μg/min. He was started on nasal-prong oxygen and given two sublingual nitroglycerin sprays, all of which did afford some improvement. He was given a bolus with 5000 units of IV heparin and started on 1000 units per hour heparin drip. The remainder of a cardiac panel was ordered and is pending at this time.

ASSESSMENT: Acute myocardial ischemic event

PLAN: The case was discussed with Dr. Elhart, who was on call for Cardiology. He arrived to evaluate further and assume care, and the patient was admitted and transferred to the cath lab.

6-10A:

SERVICE CODE(S): ____________________

DX CODE(S): ____________________

6-10B RADIOLOGY REPORT, CHEST

Even though you know from the previous report that this patient had an acute myocardial ischemic event, you can only code the diagnostic statement made on this one report, which is chest pain.

LOCATION: Hospital Outpatient

PATIENT: Kenneth Peters

PHYSICIAN: Paul Sutton, M.D.

RADIOLOGIST: Morton Monson, M.D.

EXAMINATION OF: Chest

CLINICAL SYMPTOMS: Chest pain

ONE-VIEW CHEST, 9/22/xx, 4:15 P.M.: A portable AP supine view was obtained of the chest. No previous examinations were available for comparison. Cardiac size is within normal limits. Pulmonary vascularity is grossly unremarkable. No focal pulmonary infiltrates are seen. There is no evidence of pulmonary edema.

IMPRESSION:
1. Portable AP view of the chest shows no evidence of pulmonary edema or focal pulmonary infiltrates.
2. Scattered degenerative/hypertrophic changes are noted in the dorsal spine.

6-10B:

SERVICE CODE(S): ______________________

DX CODE(S): ______________________

6-10C HOSPITAL ADMISSION

The angina is a symptom of myocardial infarction and is not reported separately.

LOCATION: Hospital Inpatient

PATIENT: Kenneth Peters

PHYSICIAN: Marvin Elhart, M.D.

REASON FOR ADMISSION: Acute inferior-wall MI and unstable angina (not reported separately)

HISTORY: This 50-year-old man came to the emergency room with acute inferior-wall MI with ongoing unstable angina. He has ST elevation in the inferior leads, reciprocal lateral changes in leads 1 and L. He has never had any prior MI. His chest pain began about 1 hour ago when he was sitting around at his home without any activities going on, and this suddenly developed retrosternally associated with some diaphoresis, but nothing else was going on otherwise. He came to the emergency room, where oxygen and sublingual nitroglycerin were administered. Right now, his chest discomfort is down to about 2/10 in intensity. He has no other ongoing complaints.

MEDICAL HISTORY: Notable for recurrent diagnosis of hypertension made by Dr. Naraquist. He was started on some medication, but I do not have the name of the medication this admission. Otherwise, he has not been on any medications. No known drug allergies; no prior operations.

His medical history is notable for the above problem and is otherwise totally unremarkable except for the fact that he was born with retinitis pigmentosa and is on social security disability for that because of tunnel vision that is related to his retinitis pigmentosa and his recent documentation of hypertension. That is about it in his health history; this man has otherwise been healthy.

SOCIAL HISTORY: Former five- to six-pack-year smoker. He quit smoking more than 23 years ago. No history of alcohol abuse. No illegal drug use is noted.

FAMILY HISTORY: Negative for MI and otherwise noncontributory

REVIEW OF SYSTEMS: Noncontributory except for above. In general, no recent fevers, chills, or rigors. Weight has been stable. NEUROLOGIC: No history of any strokelike or TIA-like symptoms. ENDOCRINOLOGIC: No diabetes mellitus or thyroid dysfunction is noted. HEMATOLOGIC: No anemia. PSYCHIATRIC: No depression. RESPIRATORY: No cough or hemoptysis. CARDIAC: As per above with no PND, orthopnea, or pedal edema. No syncope or presyncope. No palpitations. GI: No nausea, vomiting, bloody stools, or black stools. GU: No dysuria or hematuria. MUSCULOSKELETAL: No arthritis.

CARDIAC RISK FACTORS: Scant remote cigarette use and recent documentation of hypertension. Otherwise negative.

PHYSICAL EXAMINATION: Man with no known drug allergies. Well-developed, middle-aged man who is age-appropriate for appearance, alert, and oriented ×3. complaining of mild chest discomfort. Age is appropriate for appearance. Medium build. VITAL SIGNS: Stable. He is afebrile. Blood pressure is 130/74. Pulse is 63 and regular. Respirations are 20. HEENT EXAMINATION: Benign with head atraumatic and normocephalic. Pharynx, teeth, and gums appear normal. NECK: Supple without any significant jugular venous distention. Carotids are normal in upstroke and volume. No carotid bruits. No thyromegaly. LUNGS: Clear to auscultation and percussion. CARDIAC EXAMINATION: S1 and S2 normal. No audible murmurs, gallops, clicks, or rubs. Apical impulse is not palpable. No lifts, thrills, or heaves. ABDOMINAL EXAM: Soft, nontender abdomen. Normoactive bowel sounds. No organomegaly, no palpable masses. No abdominal bruits. BACK: Without CVA tenderness, no spinal percussion tenderness. EXTREMITIES: Without clubbing, cyanosis, or edema. Peripheral pulses are normal throughout. No femoral bruits. SKIN: Without rashes, no xanthomas, no xanthelasmas. NEUROLOGIC EXAM: Grossly normal.

In discussion with the patient, I advised him about the risks and benefits of cardiac catheterization with potential acute intervention with angioplasty and stenting versus thrombolytic therapy. He and I both agree that there is an edge to going right to the cath lab as we can get our cath mobilized right away. We will bring him stat to the cath lab and do an emergency angiogram and, if need be, go ahead and do angioplasty and stenting, all depending, of course, on the results of our cardiac cath. Further notes will follow pending upcoming clinical course in the cath lab.

6-10C:

SERVICE CODE(S): ______________________

DX CODE(S): ______________________

6-10D CARDIAC CATHETERIZATION REPORT

LOCATION: Hospital Inpatient

PATIENT: Kenneth Peters

SURGEON: Marvin Elhart, M.D.

PROCEDURES PERFORMED: Left-sided heart catheterization, selective coronary arteriography, left ventriculography

INDICATION: Ongoing unstable angina with acute inferior-wall MI. See the present records for further details.

PROCEDURE NOTE: Please refer to the procedure note in the enclosed cardiac catheterization log sheet. This procedure is done through the modified Seldinger technique via the right femoral approach without any complications. At the end of the case, the right femoral arterial sheath was left in place and the decision was made to intervene with angioplasty and stenting. See the upcoming angioplasty and stenting reports for details. The patient suffered no complications from the angiogram.

RESULTS: Results are as follows.

I. HEMODYNAMICS: Hemodynamics are listed fully on separate sheets within this report. Please refer to those separate sheets for details.

II. FLUOROSCOPY: Fluoroscopy reveals no valvular calcifications. No coronary artery calcifications are noted.

III. ANGIOGRAPHY:

A. LEFT MAIN CORONARY ARTERY: The left main coronary artery is normal.

B. LEFT ANTERIOR DESCENDING CORONARY ARTERY: The anterior descending coronary artery at its midportion has a 75% focal stenosis followed by a 50% focal stenosis in its midportion. The remainder of the LAD system is normal.

C. LEFT CIRCUMFLEX ARTERY: The left circumflex artery is an anatomically dominant vessel. The left circumflex artery is stump-occluded at its midportion. Just before this midportion stump occlusion, the left circumflex artery gives rise to its major marginal branch. This major marginal branch has a 95% focal stenosis proximally. The rest of the left circumflex system appears normal.

D. RIGHT CORONARY ARTERY: The right coronary artery is an anatomically nondominant, small 2-mm-caliber vessel. The right coronary artery is diffusely diseased at its proximal through early midsection over about a 20-mm length with up to 95% luminal compromise. The rest of this RCA system is normal.

IV. VENTRICULOGRAPHY:

A. QUALITATIVE: The left ventricle displays normal contractility except there is slight localized inferior hypokinesis near the apex. No mitral valve prolapse or mitral regurgitation is seen on normal sinus rhythm beats.

B. QUANTITATIVE: The calculated left ventricular ejection fraction is 65%.

Note that the coronary artery lesions described above are atherosclerotic in nature.

CONCLUSION:

1. Severe three-vessel atherosclerotic heart disease with the culprit for his MI being a stump-occluded dominant circumflex.
2. Well-preserved left ventricular function with only slight inferior-wall localized hypokinesis.
3. Angiographically normal cardiac output.
4. See report above for details.

RECOMMENDATIONS: Angioplasty and stenting of the patient's culprit for the MI being his stump-occluded circumflex. While we are at this procedure, if this goes smoothly, I will go ahead and angioplasty and consider stenting his circumflex marginal and also angioplasty his RCA system and LAD system.

6-10D:

SERVICE CODE(S): ____________________

DX CODE(S): ____________________

CASE 6-10D DISCUSSION

There are three parts to this service:

1. Placement: 93501-93572 (reporting physician portion only, add -26)
2. Injection: 93539-93545 (no modifier, as the physician performs the injection)
3. Imaging: 93555-93556 (reporting physician portion only, add -26)

In this report the catheter was placed, then two injections and two images were performed in different vessels. Point III indicates an angiography; this requires an injection code and an imagining code. Point IV indicates a ventriculography; this requires an injection code and an imagining code. The initial introduction of the catheter includes repositioning–in this case from the left coronary artery to the left ventricle (separate vessels).

6-10E PTCA/STENTING REPORT

Use appropriate HCPCS modifiers to indicate stenting locations.

LOCATION: Hospital Inpatient

PATIENT: Kenneth Peters

SURGEON: Marvin Elhart, M.D.

PROCEDURE PERFORMED: Percutaneous transluminal coronary angioplasty/stenting of the left circumflex, left circumflex marginal, and LAD, with angioplasty of the RCA.

INDICATION: Culprit circumflex occlusion with this patient having severe disease in these other vessels as mentioned. See the present records for further details on this patient with an acute inferior-wall MI and arteriosclerosis of the coronary artery.

PROCEDURE NOTE: Please refer to the procedure log in the enclosed cardiac catheterization log sheet. This procedure is done through the modified Seldinger technique via the right femoral approach without any complications. At the end of the procedure, the right femoral arterial sheath was left in place and the patient was brought to the ICU for monitoring purposes. He suffered no complications from this procedure. Note that ReoPro was given during this procedure per the ReoPro protocol. Results are as follows.

A. PREANGIOPLASTY ANGIOGRAPHY of the right and left coronary systems is well-described in the earlier cath report. See that earlier cath report for details.

B. POSTANGIOPLASTY AND STENTING ANGIOGRAPHY of the left coronary system shows the former 75% mid-LAD lesion has been reduced to 9% luminal residual post-PTCA/stenting. The circumflex marginal has been reduced from 95% to 0% luminal residual post PTCA/stenting. The former 100% stump-occluded circumflex itself has been reduced to 0% luminal residual post PTCA/stenting. The remainder of the left coronary system is otherwise unchanged compared with prior to angioplasty and stenting. The LAD still has a residual midportion 50% lesion that I left alone at this time.

The RCA system, which was nondominant and small in caliber, had the former 95% diffuse proximal and midportion disease angioplastied successfully to 20% to 30% smooth luminal residual post PTCA.

Note that there was good TIMI grade 3 filling seen into the entire right and left coronary systems postprocedure. The patient was free of chest pain after the procedure.

CONCLUSION: Successful multivessel angioplasty and stenting, with angioplasty and stenting done of an occluded circumflex as well as angioplasty and stenting done of the diseased LAD and circumflex marginal and angioplasty of the RCA. This multivessel angioplasty and stenting procedure was highly successful. The patient was brought to the ICU for monitoring purposes, chest pain free, after the procedure.

6-10E:

SERVICE CODE(S): ______________________

DX CODE(S): ______________________

CASE 6-11
6-11A Hospital Admission
6-11B General Chemistry
6-11C Hematology
6-11D Electrocardiography
6-11E Radiology Report, Chest

CASE 6-11

This 63-year-old male presents to the ED with the chief complaint of palpitations and is seen by his cardiologist, Dr. Elhart. He had been discharged from the same hospital the day before this visit. He is again admitted into the hospital by Dr. Elhart where a history and physical, blood workup, electrocardiography, and chest x-ray are done. Code the services provided to this patient.

6-11A HOSPITAL ADMISSION

LOCATION: Hospital Inpatient

PATIENT: Randall Meyers

PHYSICIAN: Marvin Elhart, M.D.

HISTORY: The patient is 63 years old and complaining of palpitations. Although initially he mentioned that he has had these symptoms for the last week or two, with the help of his brother, he clarified that he has been having this for 1 or 2 years, although infrequent. It has occurred more often in the last week or two. Last Saturday he was hospitalized for palpitations. He felt his heart beating fast and hard and also had some shooting pains in the left arm and a burning sensation in the left chest. He states that x-rays and ECGs were done. He apparently had low sodium, potassium, and magnesium levels that were replaced. He was told that he had an "irregular heartbeat." He also has a history of irregular heartbeat according to his records.

He was discharged on Wednesday. Wednesday night, however, he returned to the hospital because he again experienced fast heartbeats. He was just discharged yesterday. He comes in today because this morning he had another episode when he felt his heart was beating fast. He states that it was about 100 beats per minute. He tells me that when he was in the hospital during the second hospitalization, he was found to have a heart rate of 120. This was during the night. He also had what sounds like a 2-second pause within that time. He also had a CT scan done of his head and an EEG. He is uncertain exactly why this was done. He did not state that he had any strokelike problems. He is scheduled to have an echocardiogram Tuesday in the hospital. At this time he does not complain of palpitations and has no shortness of breath or chest pains.

MEDICAL HISTORY: History of palpitations for 1 to 2 years. There has been some question in his old medical records about whether he has had atrial fibrillation in the past. History of open-heart surgery at age 16 for what sounds like aortic coarctation. (His brother knows that since then he has been able "always to feel his heart beating.") History of TURP and bladder spasms, appendectomy, and hypertension.

SOCIAL HISTORY: He is married. He does not smoke; he quit 7 years ago. Prior to that, he smoked one-half pack per day since his teenage years. Alcohol: He drinks about three whiskies a day. He states that he waters these down; however, he initially stated he did not drink, and his brother helped to clarify this history.

REVIEW OF SYSTEMS: Patient denies any history of migraines or seizures. EENT: Negative. CARDIAC: Per HPI. No PND or orthopnea. RESPIRATORY: No chronic cough or hemoptysis. GI: No melena or hematochezia. No vomiting or diarrhea. GU: History of TURP. He has no problems with his stream now. EXTREMITIES: Negative. No clubbing NEUROLOGIC: Normal.

MEDICATIONS: Cardura, K-Dur, Prinivil, amitriptyline, phenazopyridine, over-the-counter Pepcid, Cipro, and magnesium tablets.

ALLERGIES: None to drugs known.

PHYSICAL EXAMINATION: Sixty-three-year-old in no acute distress. VITAL SIGNS: Blood pressure, 167/80. Pulse 88. Respirations 20. Temperature 36.5°C. HEENT: Head, normocephalic. Eyes are clear. TMs are normal. PERL. EOMs intact. Nose without congestions or discharge. Oral pharynx without inflammation or exudate. NECK: Supple, no lymphadenopathy or thyromegaly. No JVD. HEART: Tones regular. S1, S2, no murmur appreciated. LUNGS: Clear bilaterally with good air entry. ABDOMEN: Soft, nontender. No guarding or rebound. No hepatosplenomegaly. GU: Negative. EXTREMITIES: Without cyanosis or edema.

CHEST X-RAY: PA and lateral show no acute pulmonary disease. Radiology report pending. ECG showed sinus tachycardia, poor R-wave progression V1 through V4. Appreciate no ischemic changes.

CBC was unremarkable. Electrolytes, BUN, and creatinine within normal limits. Glucose 114.

ASSESSMENT: Palpitations

PLAN: An echo will be performed and also a Holter monitor will be set up. Patient is comfortable with these recommendations.

6-11A:

SERVICE CODE(S): ______

DX CODE(S): ______

6-11B GENERAL CHEMISTRY

The services in Cases 6-11B, 6-11C, 6-11D, and 6-11E were performed as part of the ER services. The diagnosis for 6-11B, 6-11C, and 6-11D is palpitations.

LOCATION: Inpatient, Hospital

PATIENT: Randall Meyers

PHYSICIAN: Marvin Elhart, M.D.

TIME:	REF RANGE	UNITS	+0905
BUN	7-22	mg/dl	12
Sodium	135-145	mmol/L	135
Potassium	3.6-5.5	mmol/L	5.2
Chloride	98-109	mmol/L	100
Carbon dioxide	23-33	mmol/L	29.3
Timed glucose	70-110	mg/dl	H 114
Creatinine	0.5-1.2	mg/dl	0.9
Calcium	8.4-10.6	mg/dl	9.1

6-11B:

SERVICE CODE(S): ______

DX CODE(S): ______

6-11C HEMATOLOGY

There are two services to be coded in 6-11C–an automated blood cell count with manual differential and an automated differential.

LOCATION: Inpatient, Hospital

PATIENT: Randall Meyers

PHYSICIAN: Marvin Elhart, M.D.

AUTOMATED BLOOD COUNT WITH MANUAL DIFFERENTIAL

DATE:		02/10/XX	
TIME:	REF RANGE	UNITS	+0905
WBC	3.6-11.0	K/UL	6.23
RBC	4.40-5.90	M/UL	4.82
HGB	13.0-18.0	g/dl	14.5
HCT	40-52	%	42.2
MCV	80-100	FL	87.6
MCH	26-34	PG	30.1
MCHC	32-36	g/dl	34.4
RDW	37-50	FL	42.3
PLT	150-440	K/UL	296
MPV	8.0-13.0	FL	9.8

AUTO WBC DIFFERENTIAL

DATE:		02/10/XX	
	REF RANGE	UNITS	+0905
Neutrophil	54-74	%	70.5
Lymphocyte	22-42	%	L 18.6
Monocyte	2-8	%	H 9.3
Eosinophil	0-6	%	1.1
Basophil	0-2	%	0.5
Neutrophil	1.5-8.5	K/UL	4.39
Lymphocyte	1.1-3.5	K/UL	1.16
Monocyte	0.2-0.8	K/UL	0.58
Eosinophil	0.0-0.6	K/UL	0.07
Basophil	0.0-0.2	K/UL	0.03

6-11C:

SERVICE CODE(S): ______

DX CODE(S): ______

6-11D ELECTROCARDIOGRAPHY

The physician you are coding for, Dr. Naraquist, did the tracing and the interpretation with a report for the following electrocardiography. Note that there is a code for the tracing only and a code for the interpretation with report only as well as a code for the complete service, which includes the tracing and the interpretation with the report.

LOCATION: Inpatient, Hospital

PATIENT: Randall Meyers

PHYSICIAN: Marvin Elhart, M.D.

Age: 63-year-old male

Clinical Presentation: Palpitation
Time: 7:42:02
Previous ECG: 23 December, 12:20:04 (8 years ago)

133	Sinus tachycardia, rate 104	Normal P axis, rate >=100
99	Late translation	QRS negative in V5 and V6
195	Borderline low voltage in	6 frontal leads <0.6mV
	QMART Artifact in leads (s_ II, III, aVF)	

6-11D:

SERVICE CODE(S): ______________________

DX CODE(S): ______________________

6-11E RADIOLOGY REPORT, CHEST

LOCATION: Inpatient, Hospital

PATIENT: Randall Meyers

PHYSICIAN: Marvin Elhart, M.D.

RADIOLOGIST: Morton Monson, M.D.

EXAMINATION OF: Chest, two views

CLINICAL SYMPTOMS: Palpitations

CHEST, TWO VIEWS: Comparison is made to a previous examination dated 12-24.

FINDINGS: The heart size and pulmonary vascular markings appear within normal limits. There is new focal density present within the right lung base, which may reflect either atelectasis or infiltrate. Please correlate this clinically. There is radiographic evidence of COPD. Rib changes are seen on the left, suggesting previous thoracotomy.

IMPRESSION:
1. Chronic obstructive pulmonary disease
2. Focal density is present within the right lung base, which may represent either atelectasis or infiltrate.

6-11E:

SERVICE CODE(S): ______________________

DX CODE(S): ______________________

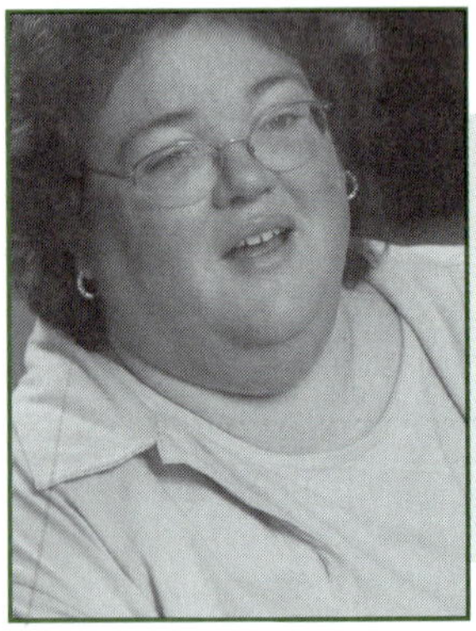

FROM THE TRENCHES

Lynn

What is the most important quality for a coder?

"I think a really important quality is motivation. Be aggressive. Continue the education. ...You still have to have motivation to get where you want to be in coding. You have to work with your employers a lot of time. You have to prove to them that it's worth it. You have to be somewhat on your own, to accomplish [your goals.]"

CASE 6-12
6-12A Hospital Admission
6-12B Cardiology Consultation
6-12C Radiology Report, Chest
6-12D Cardiac Catheterization Report
6-12E Radiology Report, GI

CASE 6-12

6-12A HOSPITAL ADMISSION

The patient in Case 6-11 was subsequently discharged to home. Twenty-three days after the discharge, the 63-year-old male patient was again admitted to the hospital by Dr. Elhart with a chief complaint of chest pain.

LOCATION: Outpatient, Hospital

PATIENT: Randall Meyers

PHYSICIAN: Marvin Elhart, M.D.

REASON FOR ADMISSION: Chest pain

HISTORY IS AS FOLLOWS: This 63-year-old man came to my service for admission and a Cardiolite stress test. Even before we started, he started having chest pain and became bradycardic after a sublingual nitroglycerin spray and he had to be given atropine. His heart rate was down to about 40. After the atropine, the heart rate returned to normal. Blood pressure was briefly down to the 90s and high 80s systolic, but then after a fluid bolus, it returned to normal. The chest pain, which was retrosternal chest pressure, slowly ameliorated, although it is still about 1 to 2/10, and I decided to cancel the Cardiolite stress test and admit him to the ICU.

He has had a history the last several months of exertional and resting chest pains, which he describes as burning in intensity and also has had pounding in his chest occasionally. This man had an echocardiogram showing borderline concentric LVH with mild aortic insufficiency and mild aortic stenosis with a negative non-Cardiolite stress test about 1 year ago. At the present interview, when I had him admitted, he was still having mild chest pain. He was admitted to ICU at the time that I initially had him admitted and was started on IV nitroglycerin.

His MEDICAL HISTORY is notable for multiple cystoscopies for urethral stricture, prostatitis, aortic coarctation that was repaired as a child, what sounds like paroxysmal atrial fibrillation, history of hypertension and history of SIADH in the past, and gastroesophageal reflux disease.

SOCIAL HISTORY reveals him to be married with no children. He was a former smoker, about 50 to 60 pack years. He quit smoking about 6 to 7 years ago. No history of alcohol abuse. No illegal drug use.

FAMILY HISTORY: Negative for a mycocardial infarction otherwise, noncontributory.

REVIEW OF SYSTEMS: Noncontributory except for above with no PND, orthopnea, pedal edema, and no syncope or presyncope. No bright red blood per rectum, melena, hemoptysis, or hematemesis.

CARDIAC RISK FACTORS: History of essential hypertension and tobacco use, and all other systems are otherwise negative.

ALLERGIES: None known, although on Floxin he gets nausea and vomiting.

CHRONIC MEDICATIONS FOR THIS MAN HAVE INCLUDED AS PER NURSING ADMISSION NOTES:

1. Cardura
2. Hydrochlorothiazide
3. Atenolol
4. Magnesium
5. KCl
6. Amitriptyline

EXAMINATION AT PRESENT: Well-developed, elderly man, age-appropriate for appearance, fully oriented, comfortable and in apparent distress, somewhat vague historian, but fully oriented ×3 and alert. Vital signs are stable. Afebrile. Blood pressure at present now is 120/70; pulse 70 and regular; respirations 22 and normal; weight 172 pounds; height 5 feet 10 inches. HEENT: Grossly benign. Fundi not examined. NECK: Supple without any significant jugular venous distention. Carotids are normal in upstroke and volume. No carotid bruits. No thyromegaly. LUNGS: clear. CARDIAC: S1 and S2 normal with 1/6 apical to left sternal border soft systolic murmur. No other murmurs heard. No gallops, clicks, or rubs. Apical pulse is not palpable. No lifts, thrills, or heaves. ABDOMEN: Soft, nontender abdomen. Normoactive bowels sounds. No organomegaly; no palpable masses. BACK: Without CVA clubbing, cyanosis, or edema. Peripheral pulses are normal throughout. No femoral bruits. SKIN: Without rashes; no xanthomas; no xanthelasmas. NEUROLOGIC: Grossly normal.

ADMISSION LABORATORY AND ECG: Pending, except an ECG done at the time we were going to do the Cardiolite stress test showed no evidence of any ischemia or infarction and was otherwise unremarkable. Palpation of the chest wall shows no evidence of any tenderness, and the abdominal examination is totally benign with no evidence of abdominal tenderness.

OVERALL IMPRESSIONS AND RECOMMENDATIONS are that this man with recent chest pains, which is difficult to sort out, was scheduled for Cardiolite stress today. Before we even hooked him up, he was having burning chest pain. He had no significant ECG changes, but because of that and the fact that he became hypotensive after sublingual nitroglycerin for which we had to start IV fluids and IV atropine, my feeling is that the best decision is to place him in the ICU, cancel his Cardiolite stress test, and schedule him for a cardiac catheterization. The patient agrees with this strategy. By the way, he had chest pain, which I did not mention off and on all last night as well. With this story, we really must consider that he has unstable angina and rule out myocardial infarction. He is scheduled for a cardiac catheterization today. I think there is no reason now to do a Cardiolite stress test because we are going to do a cardiac catheterization. The cardiac catheterization will be scheduled later today. Further notes to follow pending his clinical course.

ADDENDUM: Please note that the H and P was dictated somewhat late as I already had an admission thereafter and could not dictate this until now; but after I did this dictation, we subsequently brought him down to the cardiac catheterization laboratory and found normal coronary arteries! Therefore, I will undertake a noncardiac workup for chest pain and do an upper GI in the morning. I am going to ask Dr. Noonar to consult on this patient.

6-12A:

SERVICE CODE(S): ____________________

DX CODE(S): ____________________

6-12B CARDIOLOGY CONSULTATION

The patient was discharged and now presents for a consultation.

LOCATION: Outpatient, Clinic

PATIENT: Randall Meyers

ATTENDING PHYSICIAN: Marvin Elhart, M.D.

CONSULTANT: James Noonar, M.D.

REASON FOR CONSULTATION: The patient has been referred for an opinion on the problem of chest pain.

HISTORY IS AS FOLLOWS: He is a somewhat vague historian, a nice man who is 63 years of age and has noticed in the last several months intermittent exertional and resting chest pains during which he feels his chest burning. He also has had palpitations. A recent 24-hour Holter monitor showed some nonsustained PSVT for which he tried to increase his atenolol to 100 mg a day, but that slowed his pulse down to the 40s and he went back to his usual 50 mg of atenolol per day and still is having palpitation problems. On the Holter monitor, there is also a suggestion of some ischemia on the monitored ECGs. Echocardiogram was done in May that also showed borderline concentric left ventricular hypertrophy with mild aortic insufficiency and aortic stenosis. He had a negative non-Cardiolite stress test about one year ago. Back then he was not having any chest pain per se he tells me. Note that the patient has never had a myocardial infarction. He is presently on Cardura 2 mg daily; hydrochlorothiazide a half tablet daily; atenolol 50 mg daily; magnesium 64 mg, two tablets b.i.d.; KCl 20 mEq b.i.d.; amitriptyline 10 mg q.h.s. He has no known true drug allergies, although when he is taking Floxin he has nausea and vomiting.

MEDICAL HISTORY is notable for the above. Additionally:
1. He has had multiple cystoscopes for urethral stricture.
2. Prostatitis.
3. Repair of aortic coarctation as a child.
4. History in the past of what sounds like paroxysmal atrial fibrillation.
5. History of hypertension.
6. History of hyponatremia believed in the past to be due to SIADH.
7. He also has had a history suggestive of gastroesophageal reflux disease.

SOCIAL HISTORY: He is married with no children, a former smoker, about 50 to 60 packs per year. He quit smoking 6 to 7 years ago. No history of alcohol use or abuse. No illegal drug use.

FAMILY HISTORY: Negative for myocardial infarction and otherwise noncontributory.

REVIEW OF SYSTEMS: Noncontributory except for above with no PND, orthopnea, or pedal edema; no syncope or presyncope, no bright red blood per rectum, melena, hemoptysis, or hematemesis.

CARDIAC RISK FACTORS: History of essential hypertension and tobacco use; all organ systems are otherwise negative.

ALLERGIES: He has no known true drug allergies, although when taking Floxin he gets nausea and vomiting.

PRESENT MEDICATIONS include:
1. Cardura 2 mg daily
2. Hydrochlorothiazide, ½ tablet daily
3. Atenolol 50 mg daily
4. Magnesium 64 mg, 2 tablets t.i.d.
5. KCl 20 mEq b.i.d.
6. Amitriptyline 10 mg q.h.s.

PHYSICAL EXAMINATION: Well-developed older man, age-appropriate for appearance. Fully oriented, comfortable, and in no apparent distress. Vital signs are stable. Afebrile. Blood pressure is 130/74. Pulse is 72 and regular. Respirations are 20 and normal. Weight is 172 pounds. Height: 5 feet 10 inches. HEENT examination is grossly benign. Fundi are not examined. Neck is supple without any significant jugular venous distention. Carotids are normal in upstroke and volume; no carotid bruits; no thyromegaly. Lungs are clear. Cardiac examination: S1 and 2 are normal with a I/VI apical to left sternal border soft systolic murmur. No other murmurs are heard; no gallops, clicks, or rubs. Apical impulse is not palpable. No lifts, thrills, or heaves. Abdominal examination reveals a soft, nontender abdomen with normoactive bowel sounds. There is no organomegaly. There are no palpable masses. Back reveals no CVAT and no spinal percussion tenderness. Extremities are without clubbing, cyanosis, or edema. Peripheral pulses are normal throughout. No femoral bruits. Skin without rashes. No xanthomas. No xanthelasmas. Neurologic examination is grossly normal.

ECG today: Normal sinus rhythm with right bundle-branch block with diffuse ST-T abnormalities.

My IMPRESSION/RECOMMENDATIONS for this patient with a history of some recent chest pain problems are somewhat difficult to sort out given that he has a history suggestive of gastroesophageal reflux disease. It sounds to me that, with his cardiac risk factors, he is developing angina, and at this point what I would suggest the following:

1. An ECG.
2. Set up a Cardiolite stress test in the morning.
3. Given his slight heart murmur and mild aortic insufficiency, he is given SBE prophylaxis card.

ADDENDUM: The patient has a history of a coarctation in the aorta repaired many years ago. When I check his radial pulses both in the left and right arm and check that against his femoral pulses in the right and left legs, I see no timing delay in his femorals. Because there is no timing delay between radial and femoral pulses, there is no clinical evidence of any significant recurrent coarctation.

Thank you for the consultation. I will make further comments about what to do next for this man who also has had some nonsustained PSVTs seen on a recent 24-hour Holter monitor that did not tolerate higher doses of a beta-blocker. Right now, though, I want to see how he does on a stress test and then make a decision about whether he needs to have an angiogram. I suspect his Cardiolite stress test will be positive. His clinical story and recent 24-hour Holter monitor did suggest some ischemic problems potentially. Further notes will follow pending the clinical course. Thank you for the consultation.

6-12B:

SERVICE CODE(S): ____________________

DX CODE(S): ____________________

6-12C RADIOLOGY REPORT, CHEST

LOCATION: Outpatient, Hospital

PATIENT: Randall Meyers

ATTENDING PHYSICIAN: Marvin Elhart, M.D.

RADIOLOGIST: Morton Monson, M.D.

EXAMINATION OF: Chest

CLINICAL SYMPTOMS: Chest pain, precatheterization

CHEST, SINGLE VIEW: COMPARISON: Comparison is made to a previous examination dated 1 year ago.

FINDINGS: The heart size appears at the upper limits of normal. The pulmonary vascular markings appear within normal limits. This examination is somewhat rotated. This accentuates the right paratracheal markings. Definite focal infiltrates are not seen within the lungs. No pleural effusions are seen.

IMPRESSION: No evidence for infiltrate or congestive failure.

6-12C:

SERVICE CODE(S): ____________________

DX CODE(S): ____________________

6-12D CARDIAC CATHETERIZATION REPORT

LOCATION: Outpatient, Hospital

PATIENT: Randall Meyers

ATTENDING PHYSICIAN: Marvin Elhart, M.D.

SURGEON: Marvin Elhart, M.D.

PROCEDURES PERFORMED: Left-sided heart catheterization, selective coronary angiography, left ventriculography

INDICATION: Clinical unstable angina. See the present hospital records for further details.

PROCEDURE NOTE: Refer to the procedure log in the enclosed cardiac catheterization log sheet. Note that this procedure was done via the modified Seldinger technique via the right femoral approach without any complications. At the end of the case, sheaths were removed and good hemostasis was achieved. The patient suffered no complications from this procedure.

RESULTS:

I. HEMODYNAMICS: Hemodynamics are listed fully on separate sheets within this report and are normal.

II. FLUOROSCOPY: Fluoroscopy reveals no valvular calcifications. No coronary artery calcifications are noted.

III. ANGIOGRAPHY (This is the injection and interpretation of the arteries):

A. LEFT MAIN CORONARY ARTERY: Normal

B. LEFT ANTERIOR DESCENDING CORONARY ARTERY and its branches are normal.

C. LEFT CIRCUMFLEX ARTERY: Normal.

D. There is a ramus intermedius branch. This ramus intermedius branch is normal.

E. RIGHT CORONARY ARTERY: The right coronary artery is an anatomically dominant vessel. The right coronary artery and its branches are normal.

IV. VENTRICULOGRAPHY (This is the injection and interpretation of the ventricle, a different [separate] vessel):

A. QUALIFICATIONS: The left ventricle displays normal contractility. No regional wall motion abnormalities are identified. No mitral valve prolapse or mitral regurgitation is seen.

B. QUANTITATIVE: The calculated left ventricular ejection fraction is pending at the time of this dictation but by visual estimation is normal.

CONCLUSION:

1. Normal coronary arteries
2. Normal left ventricular systolic function
3. Angiographically normal cardiac output
4. See report above for details

RECOMMENDATIONS: Noncardiac workup of chest pain. The patient has no underlying coronary artery disease seen at this time, and even though he clinically had unstable angina in retrospect with his normal angiogram study, one must consider pursuing a noncardiac workup of chest pain.

6-12D:

SERVICE CODE(S): ______________________

DX CODE(S): ______________________

6-12E RADIOLOGY REPORT, GI

Immediately after the cardiac catheterization, the following x-ray was taken.

LOCATION: Outpatient, Hospital

PATIENT: Randall Meyers

ATTENDING PHYSICIAN: Marvin Elhart, M.D.

RADIOLOGIST: Morton Monson, M.D.

EXAMINATION OF: Upper GI

CLINICAL SYMPTOMS: Chest pain

UPPER GI: CLINICAL HISTORY: Chest pain

FINDINGS: A biphasic examination of the upper gastrointestinal tract was performed. The esophagus, stomach, and duodenum appear morphologically normal. There is no evidence of ulceration. During the course of the examination, multiple episodes of gastroesophageal reflux were noted. This reflux is considered of mild to moderate degree. Definite hiatal hernia was not seen.

IMPRESSION: DX's

1. Mild to moderate gastroesophageal reflux
2. No evidence of ulceration

6-12E:

SERVICE CODE(S): ______________________

DX CODE(S): ______________________

Miscellaneous Reports

Cardioversion

Cardioversion is electrical stimulation of the heart to achieve normal heart rhythm. The procedure can be performed on as an emergency procedure or a planned procedure to correct an abnormal heart rhythm. There are two approaches used for cardioversion–an internal procedure (92961, the heart is exposed and paddles are placed directly on the heart) and an external procedure (92960, the paddles are placed directly on the chest).

CASE 6-13

The patient had a diagnosis of atrial fibrillation and atrial flutter, and Dr. Noonar has recommended cardioversion to correct the abnormal rhythm.

6-13A CARDIOVERSION

LOCATION: Outpatient, Hospital

PATIENT: Karen Blackwell

PHYSICIAN: James Noonar, M.D.

PROCEDURE PERFORMED: Cardioversion

INDICATIONS: Atrial fibrillation and atrial flutter

DESCRIPTION OF PROCEDURE: Informed consent was obtained. After adequate sedation and while the patient's heart rate, blood pressure, and O_2 saturation were being monitored, cardioversion was done successfully using 300 synchronized joules with which the patient converted to sinus bradycardia; however, she had frequent PACs.

RECOMMENDATIONS: We will lead the patient up with 1 g of procainamide in an attempt to maintain her sinus mechanism.

6-13A:

SERVICE CODE(S): ____________________

DX CODE(S): ____________________

CASE 6-14
6-14A Transesophageal Echocardiogram Report

CASE 6-14

6-14A TRANSESOPHAGEAL ECHOCARDIOGRAM REPORT

LOCATION: Outpatient, Hospital

PATIENT: Mary South

PHYSICIAN: David Barton, M.D.

RADIOLOGY: Morton Monson, M.D.

PROCEDURE: Transesophageal echocardiogram

INDICATION: To evaluate the patient for the presence of atrial thrombi prior to cardioversion

DESCRIPTION OF PROCEDURE: Informed consent was obtained. The patient was premedicated with intravenous Versed and fentanyl. (Note: These drugs indicate conscious sedation.) The throat was anesthetized with Hurricaine spray. After adequate sedation and local anesthesia were obtained, the transesophageal echocardiogram was performed in the usual manner.

FINDINGS:

CARDIAC CHAMBER: The left atrium was dilated. The left atrial appendage was dilated. There was no evidence of atrial thrombi. The left ventricle was normal sized. There was moderate diffuse hypokinesis. The overall left ventricular systolic function was moderately reduced with an ejection fraction of about 30%, markedly better than her echocardiogram from a couple of days ago. The right atrium and right ventricle were markedly dilated. The aortic root was normal sized.

VALVES: The mitral valve was mildly thickened but opened normally. There was mild aortic sclerosis without stenosis. The tricuspid valve was grossly normal. The pulmonic valve was also normal.

DOPPLER AND COLOR DOPPLER INTERROGATION revealed the presence of moderate mitral insufficiency and what appeared to be also moderate tricuspid insufficiency.

CONCLUSION:
1. No evidence of atrial thrombi
2. Dilated left atrium
3. Dilated right atrium and right ventricle
4. Moderate mitral and what appears to be (?)moderate tricuspid insufficiency

DX

6-14A:

SERVICE CODE(S): ____________________

DX CODE(S): ____________________

CASE 6-15
6-15A Operative Report, Thromboendarterectomy

CASE 6-15

6-15A OPERATIVE REPORT, THROMBOENDARTERECTOMY

LOCATION: Outpatient, Hospital

PATIENT: Mary Heidorn

SURGEON: Gary Sanchez, M.D.

PREOPERATIVE DIAGNOSIS: Right carotid stenosis

POSTOPERATIVE DIAGNOSIS: Right carotid stenosis

PROCEDURE PERFORMED: Right carotid thromboendarterectomy

This patient was monitored with EEG. There were some depressions when we clamped, but this returned to normal after re-establishing circulation.

ANESTHESIA: General

DESCRIPTION OF PROCEDURE: Under general anesthesia, the patient's right side of the neck was prepped and draped in the usual manner. An incision was made across the medial border of the sternocleidomastoid. The platysma was divided. The common carotid artery was localized. We then put a LigaLoop around it, and then we isolated the external and internal carotid arteries and placed LigaLoops around them. We saw the hypoglossal nerve. We put the retractors in and retracted on the upper end of the wound, and then we gave the patient heparin and proceeded with the arteriotomy.

After placing clamps on the internal, common, and external carotid arteries, the arteriotomy was done. This was a severe stenosing atherosclerotic plaque. This was removed. We then sutured the artery up with a 5-0 Prolene at the distal and then at the proximal and meeting in the middle, producing back bleeding, and then we closed the artery. The wound was then closed in layers after placing a Hemovac in the wound. The wound was approximated with 2-0 chromic, 2-0 plain, and surgical staples on skin. A dressing was applied. The patient was discharged to recovery.

6-15A:

SERVICE CODE(S): ________________

DX CODE(S): ________________

CASE 6-16
6-16A Radiology Report, Venogram
6-16B Operative Report, Arteriovenous Fistula

CASE 6-16

6-16A RADIOLOGY REPORT, VENOGRAM

This patient has chronic renal failure, and the nephrologist is going to create a fistula (channel between two structures) between a vein and an artery to be used for hemodialysis. Prior to the surgery, a venogram is performed to ensure the vessels are adequate for the fistula creation. The hospital provides the technician and equipment and Dr. Monson provides the supervision, interpretation, and report of the radiology service.

LOCATION: Outpatient, Hospital

PATIENT: Maggie Sodium

PHYSICIAN: George Orbitz, M.D.

RADIOLOGIST: Morton Monson, M.D.

EXAMINATION OF: Limited venogram of left upper extremity

CLINICAL SYMPTOMS: CRF, intraoperative evaluation of veins of the left forearm

LIMITED VENOGRAM OF LEFT UPPER EXTREMITY

Injection of a vein in the region of the wrist was performed, and there was visualization of the veins predominantly at and above the antecubital region. There is no evidence of thrombus within the veins, and there is no evidence of extravasation. This examination was performed for a roadmap for planned surgery due to CRF.

6-16A:

SERVICE CODE(S): ____________________

DX CODE(S): ____________________

6-16B OPERATIVE REPORT, ARTERIOVENOUS FISTULA

LOCATION: Outpatient, Hospital

PATIENT: Maggie Sodium

SURGEON: George Orbitz, M.D.

PREOPERATIVE DIAGNOSIS: Chronic renal failure

POSTOPERATIVE DIAGNOSIS: Chronic renal failure

PROCEDURE PERFORMED: Placement of primary arteriovenous fistula, left wrist

ANESTHESIA: General

PROCEDURE: With the patient under general anesthesia, the arm was marked for the vein. There was a fairly large cephalic vein at the wrist on the left, but we are not certain as to whether there was a continuous vein going up the arm. We then prepped and draped the arm. We first made a small incision about midway up the forearm over an area where we could no longer palpate the vein. After marking this incision and freeing up the vein in this location, we could see that there was an adequate vein going up to just below the elbow. With this in mind, we then made an extended incision at the wrist and were able to mobilize the cephalic vein toward the radial artery. We were also able to free the radial artery. We took down some tributaries of the vein with 4-0 silk ligatures and then in a similar fashion took down tributaries of the artery. Once we had both vessels well immobilized, we brought them together with vascular loops, gave the patient 5000 units of heparin, and then performed a primary anastomosis between the artery and vein using 6-0 Prolene. With completion of the anastomosis, there was excellent flow with a palpable thrill. We ligated three tributary branches of vein to increase the flow up the arm. We passed a Fogarty catheter all the way up the arm and then gently pulled it back with the balloon partially inflated to dilate the vein. This showed that we had a patent vein all the way up the arm and that we were able to dilate the vein back down to the anastomosis. This Fogarty catheter was introduced through the distal venous segment, which was then ligated using 2-0 silk. On completion of the procedure, the patient had an intact vascular anastomosis with good flow documented to the hand in both the radial and ulnar arteries. The patient had a palpable thrill going up the lower portion of the arm. The incisions were then closed using an inner layer of 3-0 chromic and a skin layer of 4-0 nylon. Sterile dressings were applied. The patient tolerated the procedure well and was discharged from the operating room in stable condition.

6-16B:

SERVICE CODE(S): ____________________

DX CODE(S): ____________________

CASE 6-17

6-17A OPERATIVE REPORT, ARTERIOVENOUS FISTULA

LOCATION: Hospital Inpatient

PATIENT: Samuel Mortonson

SURGEON: Gary Sanchez, M.D.

PREOPERATIVE DIAGNOSIS: End-stage renal disease

POSTOPERATIVE DIAGNOSIS: End-stage renal disease

OPERATIVE PROCEDURE: Primary arteriovenous fistula, right radiocephalic.

INDICATION: This 48-year-old man has end-stage renal disease and is on hemodialysis. He has fair-sized cephalic vein clinically. I discussed the primary AV fistula between the radial artery and cephalic vein. I had previously discussed this procedure with him. I said that we should try to get this to work first. Sometimes, though, veins do not dilate up nicely, depending on how many times they have been "poked" for IV access and blood draws. He has been in the hospital a number of times, and so they have had some access to this but overall clinically it looks pretty good.

PROCEDURE: The patient was brought to the operating theater and placed in a supine position on the operating room table. After receiving some IV sedation, he was prepped and draped in a sterile fashion. His cephalic vein was marked out as was as his radial artery. An incision line was marked halfway between these two. This was longitudinal. It was infiltrated with 0.5% Marcaine with epinephrine, which was left to set for a couple of minutes. An incision was then made. We dissected out the cephalic vein first. This was done sharply. We were able to get around the circumferential. A couple of small side branches were ligated with 4-0 silks and transected. We were able to dissect up a good segment of the cephalic vein and then dissected out the radial artery. This was also done sharply. We were able to dissect down to it and dissect it sharply in a circumferential manner. This had a fair amount of calcifications within it. Two tiny side branches were taken down with 4-0 silks and transected. We then put a right-angle clamp on the distal aspect of the cephalic vein. It was transected. We ligated this with 2-0 Vicryl and attached a Titus needle onto the end of the cephalic vein. This dilated nicely and flushed out easily. We then occluded the radial artery proximally and distally with mini vessel loops in a Potts loop fashion. Arteriotomy was made. Bleeding was still coming distally. This was controlled then with a small profunda clamp. This worked well. We then irrigated it out with a heparinized saline both proximally and distally for heparinization and spatulated the end of the vein and cut it to length. We then performed an end-to-side anastomosis using Gore-Tex CV-7 suture. Prior to placing the last couple of bites, we back-bled and forward-bled and flushed everything out with heparinized saline. We then placed the last couple of suture bites and secured the suture line. We opened up the vein and then the proximal radial artery. We let the flow initially go through this and into the vein. We then opened up the distal radial artery. A light thrill was present. Pulses were heard with the Doppler of the radial artery on the wrist distally to our anastomosis as well as on the ulnar artery. The palmar arch also had good flow both proximally and distally. There was distal artery flow and good capsular refill in all fingers. There was good long diastolic flow through the cephalic vein up the forearm. A light thrill was present over the area. A good bruit was also audible with a sterile stethoscope. Hemostasis was present. We closed the subcutaneous tissue with 3-0 Vicryl in interrupted fashion. The skin was closed with 4-0 Vicryl in a running subcuticular fashion. Sterile dressings of Telfa and Tegaderm were applied. The patient tolerated the procedure well and went to the recovery room in stable condition.

graft

6-17A:

SERVICE CODE(S): ______________________

DX CODE(S): ______________________

CASE 6-18
6-18A Operative Report, Abdominal Aortic Aneurysm
6-18B Pathology Report

CASE 6-18

6-18A OPERATIVE REPORT, ABDOMINAL AORTIC ANEURYSM

LOCATION: Hospital Inpatient

PATIENT: Tom Hoff

SURGEON: Gary Sanchez, M.D.

PREOPERATIVE DIAGNOSIS: Ruptured abdominal aortic aneurysm

POSTOPERATIVE DIAGNOSIS: Ruptured abdominal aortic aneurysm. Anemia due to acute blood loss

OPERATIVE PROCEDURE: Repair of ruptured abdominal aortic aneurysm with a 20 × 10 bifurcated aortobifemoral graft

ANESTHESIA: General

INDICATIONS FOR SURGERY: The patient is a 36-year-old male who came to the emergency room with severe back and abdominal pain. The patient was found to have a ruptured abdominal aortic aneurysm, and he was taken immediately to the operating room for surgery.

DESCRIPTION OF OPERATION: The patient was taken to the operating room with a ruptured abdominal aortic aneurysm. A midline abdominal incision was made. The abdomen was entered. The patient's entire right side and middle part of his abdomen were full of blood. Attempts were made, and finally control was obtained by clamping the aorta at the level of the diaphragm. The aneurysm was then opened, and there was aneurysmal wall on the anterior surface. It had completely blown out. After searching, we were able to find the neck of the aneurysm and the aorta. A clamp was placed on this level, and the clamp at the hilum was released. The distal iliac arteries were also aneurysmal, and these were located with some difficulty. After these were packed off, the proximal aneurysmal aorta was partially transected, leaving the posterior wall intact. A 20 × 10-mm bifurcated Dacron graft was then sewn end to end to the aorta using a running 3-0 Prolene suture. The vascular clamp then was placed on the graft, and the clamp on the aorta was then released. There was some bleeding on the left lateral aspect of the anastomosis, and this was controlled with 3-0 Prolene sutures. After this, the anastomosis was tight. The distal iliac artery openings were then oversewn. It was difficult to ascertain the openings in the distal iliac arteries because of the aneurysmal dilatation. Before this was done, the bleeding from the iliac arteries was controlled by dissecting both femoral arteries and clamping the femoral arteries to decrease the backflow. The iliac arteries were oversewn from the inside; at least this attempt was made. The right and left limbs were then tunneled into each groin area. An end-to-side anastomosis was then done on each femoral artery. Just prior to completion of the left femoral anastomosis, the clamp on the aortic graft was released to allow flow to go through the left limb of the graft. When this occurred, there was extreme backflow of blood into the abdomen through the iliac arteries. We did not sew the opening closed. After multiple attempts to try to control this, we were unable to do so and again a large amount of blood loss was obtained because of this bleeding. Therefore, we packed the artery off and opened up the abdomen initially from the left groin into the abdomen lying out the iliac artery. When this was done, we then ligated the iliac artery with 0 silk sutures. After we completed this, the anastomosis was completed on the left side and blood was allowed to flow in the left femoral artery. The right anastomosis was completed and then blood was allowed to flow into this artery. The patient's blood pressure was initially below 50, but blood pressure was finally over 100. The estimated blood loss was unable to be obtained because of the huge amount of blood loss sustained during the operation. The patient received 5351 cc of Cellsaver, 24,000 cc of crystalloid, 500 cc of albumin, 6978 cc of RBCs, 245 cc of platelets, 1051 cc of fresh frozen plasma, and 6000 cc of lactated Ringer's. The patient's incisions were partially closed, and the abdominal wound was left open. Steri-Drapes were placed within the abdominal wall, and then towels were placed over the Steri-Drapes, followed by Jackson-Pratt drains, and then followed by adhesive Ioban drapes. This would allow for expansion of the abdomen because of the edema that occurred during surgery. Also, the right colon appeared to have a large amount of ecchymosis in this area, and there is some question as to whether or not this will be survivable. The patient put out less than 100 cc of urine during the entire operation, which lasted over 5 hours. The patient was taken back to the intensive care unit in critical condition.

6-18A:

SERVICE CODE(S): ____________________

DX CODE(S): ____________________

6-18B PATHOLOGY REPORT

LOCATION: Hospital Inpatient

PATIENT: Tom Hoff

SURGEON: Gary Sanchez, M.D.

PATHOLOGIST: Grey Lonewolf, M.D.

CLINICAL HISTORY: Leaking abdominal aortic aneurysm, ruptured

SPECIMEN RECEIVED: Abdominal aortic plaque and clot

GROSS DESCRIPTION: The specimen is labeled with the patient's name and "abdominal aortic plaque and clot," which consists of multiple pink-tan laminated fibrin thrombus fragments up to 6 cm in greatest dimension. Admixed are numerous fragments of dark red blood clots up to 7 cm in greatest dimension. A few tan-yellow atherosclerotic plaque segments up to 2.5 cm in greatest dimension were seen, with representative sections in five cassettes.

MICROSCOPIC DIAGNOSIS: Fibrohyalinzed tissue with severe atherosclerosis and plaque hemorrhage with laminated fibrin thrombus and blood clot consistent with abdominal aortic aneurysm.

6-18B:

SERVICE CODE(S): ______________________

DX CODE(S): ______________________

CASE 6-19

6-19A OPERATIVE REPORT, FEMORAL ARTERY LACERATION

You will be coding the services of both the surgeon and the assistant surgeon in the following case. The diagnosis code for this service will be the complication, which was an accidental puncture or laceration that occurred during the initial stenting procedure.

LOCATION: Hospital Inpatient

PATIENT: Nora Hycliff

ATTENDING PHYSCIAN: Ronald Green, M.D.

SURGEON: Gary Sanchez, M.D.

ASSISTANT SURGEON: Terry Moltz, M.D.

PREOPERATIVE DIAGNOSIS:
1. Retroperitoneal bleed
2. Right femoral artery laceration

POSTOPERATIVE DIAGNOSIS:
1. Retroperitoneal bleed
2. Right femoral artery laceration

PROCEDURE PERFORMED: Repair of femoral artery laceration

INDICATIONS: This is a 57-year-old female who underwent a heart catheterization/stenting today. This actually had been performed through a left femoral artery; however, the procedure started with an attempt on the right. They had to take a few sticks apparently to get into the right femoral artery. They were able to cannulate it, though, and were able to pass a guidewire a short distance. They were unable to pass it any farther. This was removed. They subsequently then went over to the left groin and performed their procedure. Actually, I had been called to see her regarding a stenosis of the left common femoral artery. She had a pulseless left foot; however, decreasing to a 4 French catheter, there was no flow by the catheter noted on angiography. The catheter was then subsequently removed and was closed with a VasoSeal. She had a pulse in the anterior tibial artery on the left and seemed to have at times weak pulse in the posterior tibial on the right. She was subsequently transferred up to the medical ICU. I checked on her shortly thereafter. She was awake, alert, and doing okay. We could not identify any pulses in the left foot but could on the right foot. Arterial Doppler study also could not find any pulses in the foot. I therefore contacted interventional radiology about performing a left leg angiogram. They were going to do this within the hour. Subsequently, she apparently became hypotensive, and she was managed for this by Dr. Noonar and then by Dr. Green.

When she came down to interventional radiology, she was rather hypotensive. She then had a CT ordered by Dr. Green and was brought there. I was notified that she was going to the scanner. I went to see her. She was noted to have a large retroperitoneal bleed on the right side. I thought this was most likely coming from her right femoral stick.

I met with the patient's husband. I discussed the patient's diagnosis and my recommendations of a right femoral artery exploration and possibly a left femoral artery exploration to re-establish flow in the left foot as necessary.

PROCEDURE: The patient was brought to the operating room as a class 1. She went right back to room 9 and had a cardiac arrest at this point. She became pulseless. We started chest compressions. She had, of course, already been intubated. Code was managed by anesthesia. We kept giving her IV boluses of fluids. We were able to get her pressure back. We then quickly prepped and draped her. Even while I was scrubbing in, she had another episode of pulseless electrical activity. They were able to get her pulse back again. We then prepped and draped in a sterile fashion. A vertical incision was made in the right groin. Dissection was carried down through the subcutaneous tissues. I tried to come in high on this to be sure that we could get in proximally to the lesion. We came down on the external oblique and cleaned this all off down to the artery. It was at this point that some bleeding occurred. We could see that there was a laceration in the anterior wall of the common femoral artery; however, we did not really have the artery very cleaned out at this point, nor could I get proximal control. We tried to get proximal control above this, but with the bleeding and the patient being obese, we just could not get control. We then extended the incision in hockey-stick fashion up the right side. We carried this down to the fascia. We divided this and entered the retroperitoneal space. There was a huge amount of sanguineous fluid but no clot in this. Again, because of the body habitus, we still could not get down to really good control in the external iliac. I was able, though, to control it somewhat with a finger. Dr. Moltz then came in to provide surgical assistance. I was then able to take 5-0 Prolene stitch to oversew the laceration. This was on the anterior wall of the common femoral artery. We were able to fix this with a figure-of-eight ligature. This had been bleeding rather profusely. I am not sure whether the wire had caught on something as it came out or if it had been kind of tangentially lacerated with the needle, but there was a hole of approximately 3 to maybe even 4 mm. With this controlled, visualization was much better in the groin. She had a couple of other bleeding points from our dissection that were controlled with either Prolene ligatures or through Vicryl ligatures. A small branch had been avulsed off the common femoral vein. Again, this was a small branch. The soft tissue site was ligated with 3-0 Vicryl. A small hole in the vein was ligated with and repaired with a 6-0 Prolene suture. We packed Gelfoam and thrombin in these areas. We then reinspected the wound after a little while. Again, we continued to achieve hemostasis in the soft tissues with either 3-0 Vicryl ligatures or cautery. She had a lot of soft-tissue areas that were just oozing. The patient had received multiple units of blood and had also received FFP as well as platelets. She was going into DIC. With packing of the wound, though, things actually seemed to settle down and seemed to be rather hemostatic overall. We placed a no. 10 flat Jackson-Pratt drain and brought this out through a separate stab wound. This was attached to the skin with 2-0 silk. We closed the retroperitoneal exposure site and the fascia overlying it with 2-0 Vicryl suture. The ilioinguinal ligament also had been partially divided in a vertical fashion prior to this. This was also repaired with interrupted sutures of 2-0 Vicryl in a figure-of-eight fashion. We then closed the subcutaneous tissues in three layers of interrupted 2-0 Vicryl. The skin was closed with staples. Sterile dressings were applied. We had checked for pulses in the feet during the procedure. Pulses were present, but she had excellent capillary refill. She had good flow through her femorals on both sides. Distally to our anastomotic repair, she had a good pulse and also good flow through Doppler with good diastolic waves. I could even feel a thrill in the artery. On the left side, she had a good Doppler flow again with long diastolic waves. Her feet and toes showed very good capillary refill and were pink. The patient was in no condition at this time to undergo an exploration of her left femoral artery to see what we could do to improve the flow in her left foot. She may develop an occlusion here, but again she is going into DIC. She has had multiple units of blood. She has had two codes of pulseless electrical activity (PEA). I have been trying to keep her pressure just up to diastolic of 90. The amount of fluid was huge. We are taking the risk of potentially having a limb loss, but I think at this time we are going to have to do everything we can just to get her to survive all of this. She was then transferred to the surgical ICU in critical and unstable condition.

6-19A:

SERVICE CODE(S): ______________________

DX CODE(S): ______________________

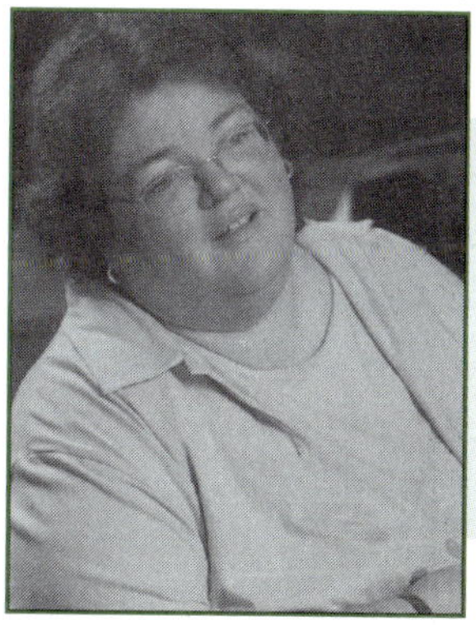

FROM THE TRENCHES

Lynn

What makes you take the most pride in your career?

Helping others with their careers. That's probably my greatest joy—that I can help others. People can trust that I know my job and know what I do. And I can help them…and I can teach them. I think that's probably the best reward."

Glossary

angioplasty surgical or percutaneous procedure in a vessel to dilate the vessel opening; used in the treatment of atherosclerotic disease.
artery vessel that carries oxygenated blood from the heart to body tissue.

cardioverter-defibrillator surgically placed device that directs an electric current shock to the heart to restore rhythm.

Doppler ultrasonic measure of blood movement.

echocardiography radiographic recording of the heart or heart walls or surrounding tissues.
ejection fraction the percentage of blood pumped with each contraction of the heart.

ischemia deficiency of blood in a body part, usually due to constriction or obstruction of a blood vessel.

myocardial pertaining to the heart muscle.
myocardial perfusion scan a radiologic procedure performed to assess the amount of blood reaching a given area.

stent mold that holds a surgically placed graft in place.
stress test test that assesses cardiovascular health and function (by echocardiogram) after application of stress to the heart, usually in the form of exercise, but sometimes with atrial pacing, a cold pressor test, or specific drugs.

transesophageal echocardiography (TEE) echocardiogram performed by placing a probe down the esophagus and sending out sound waves to obtain images of the heart and its movement.

vein vessel that carries unoxygenated blood to the heart from body tissues.

Chapter 7

Digestive System, Hemic/Lymphatic System, and Mediastinum/ Diaphragm

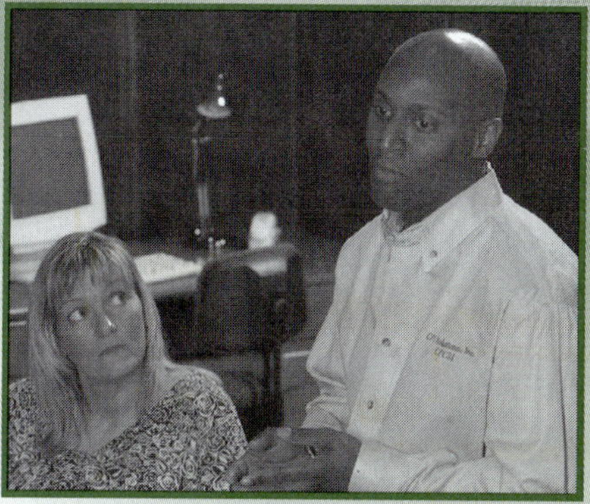

Betty Johnson, CPC, CCP
President/CEO
Terence Johnson, JD, CPC, CCP
Vice-President/CFO
CPC Solutions, Inc.
Country Club Hills, Illinois

HEMIC/LYMPHATIC SYSTEM

ABBREVIATIONS

ABD Adriamycin, bleomycin, dacarbazine
AST aspartate aminotransferase (SGOT)
AV arteriovenous
C. difficile *Clostridium difficile*
CEA carcinoembryonic antigen
CMV cytomegalovirus
EGD esophagogastroduodenoscopy
GERD gastroesophageal reflux disease
GI gastrointestinal
HIDA hydroxy iminodiacetic acid (imaging test)
I&D incision and drainage
IVP intravenous pyelogram
KUB kidney, ureter, bladder
NG nasogastric
NSAID nonsteroidal anti-inflammatory drug
PTH plasma thromboplastin antecedent
TPN total parenteral nutrition
ZE Zollinger-Ellison syndrome

Digestive System

Digestive system complaints are common and are treated by a wide variety of physicians. The **gastrointestinal** tract includes the items indicated in **Figure 7-1.** Common gastrointestinal symptoms are abdominal pain, nausea, vomiting, difficulty swallowing, heartburn, indigestion, bleeding, diarrhea, and constipation. Common conditions are stomatitis, peptic ulcer, gastroesophageal reflux, hemorrhoids, diverticulitis, bowel obstruction, gastritis, appendicitis, and colorectal cancer.

Conditions of the liver, gallbladder, and bile ducts are part of the gastrointestinal system; common signs or symptoms include jaundice, ascites (fluid in the abdominal cavity), and abnormal liver function tests. Common conditions of the liver are cirrhosis, hepatitis, and hyperbilirubinemia; of the gallbladder, gallstones and cholecystitis; of the pancreas, pancreatitis and carcinomas.

A physician who specializes in the diagnoses and treatment of the digestive system is a **gastroenterologist.** These specialists provide operative services using various approaches, such as rectal, endoscopic, laparoscopic, and open surgical procedures. The approach will be a determining factor in the code you choose.

General surgeons often use digestive system codes because they perform many of the abdominal procedures. For example, a gastroenterologist would diagnose a patient with appendicitis, and the general surgeon would remove the appendix. The gastroenterologist usually does the endoscopic procedures (through the mouth or the anus) and diagnoses gastrointestinal system conditions; if the conditions require surgery, the general surgeon would do the laparoscopic (through the abdomen) and open (incisional) procedures.

Not all the codes in the Digestive System subsection are for procedures that you think of as being in the gastrointestinal system, for example, the Abdomen, Peritoneum, and Omentum (49000-49999), in which you will find codes such as those for laparotomy (49000-49010), subdiaphragmatic and retroperitoneal abscess drainage (49020-49062), **laparoscopy** (49320-49329), and abdominal insertion procedures, just to name a few. When an abdominal laparoscopic procedure is performed for diagnostic purposes and no procedure is conducted, you would report the diagnostic procedure with a Digestive section code. For example, the surgeon performs a diagnostic laparoscopy (49320) for the purpose of examining the adrenal gland. The surgeon takes a biopsy of a suspicious lesion on the adrenal gland, and the procedure becomes a surgical laparoscopy (60650). Read the notes above 60650, and you will find that the note refers you to 49320, depending on whether the laparoscopy was diagnostic or surgical.

The Introduction, Revision, and/or Removal (49400-49429) contains codes for insertion, revision, or removal of air, contrast, **catheter,** or shunt into the abdomen (peritoneal/intraperitoneal cavity). For example, placement (insertion) of a dialysis catheter for peritoneal **hemodialysis.**

E/M Services

Report 7-1A is a surgical consultation for a patient with a bowel obstruction. A bowel obstruction is a blockage of the small or large intestine. Postoperative adhesions are the most common cause of bowel obstruction of the small intestine, with hernias and neoplasms also being common. Cancer is the most common cause of large intestine obstruction; volvulus (twisting of intestine) and diverticulitis

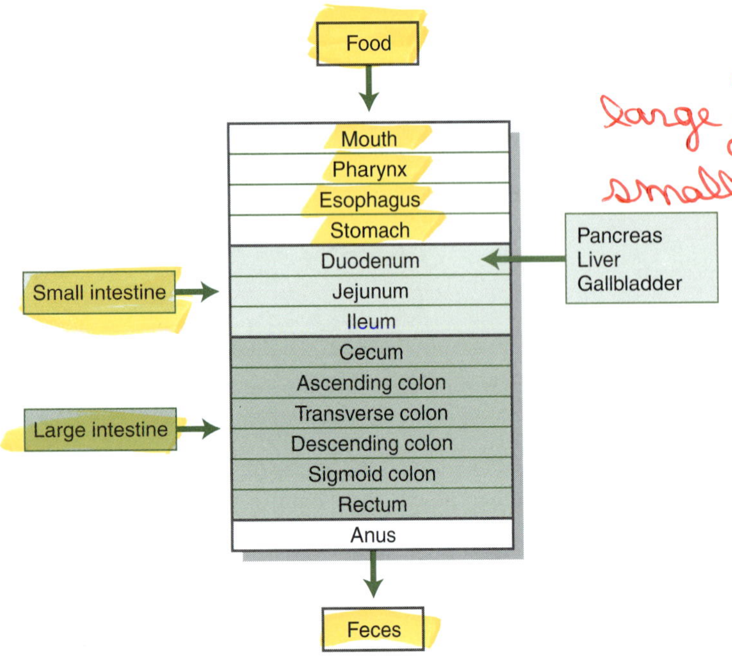

FIGURE 7-1 Gastrointestinal tract.

are also common. Clinical presentations would often be abdominal pain, nausea, vomiting, or bloating. Clinical findings include blood in the stool, fever (especially if the bowel is perforated), absence of bowel sounds or a tinkling sound, and abdominal tenderness. No laboratory tests are available that can be used to indicate bowel obstruction. X-ray, contrast studies, and CT scan are the main tests that the physician would use to assist in the diagnostic process.

If the diagnosis is obstructed bowel, a general surgeon would usually perform an open surgical procedure and nearly all complete obstructions require surgery. After an abdominal surgery, although uncommon, the anastomosis can leak and allow air and bowel contents into the abdominal cavity and could place the patient in an emergency situation requiring immediate attention.

Intestinal Obstruction

Obstruction of the intestinal tract can occur in a variety of ways. **Intussusception** (560.0) is the prolapse of part of the intestine into another adjacent part of the intestine. Intussusception may be enteric (ileoileal, jejunoileal, jejunojejunal), colic (colocolic), or intracolic (ileocecal, ileocolic). See Figure 7-2. Usually this causes strangulation of the blood supply (causing ischemic colon, gangrene) and is most common in infants. **Paralytic ileus** (560.1) is the loss of the peristaltic action of the intestine. Usually this occurs after intestinal trauma or a gastrointestinal surgical procedure (complication code 997.4) and can occur in the large and small intestines. **Volvulus** (560.2) is the twisting of a segment of the intestine (also known as torsion), and is most common in the large intestine of the elderly. **Impaction** of the intestine (560.3x) can occur through fecal material impacted in the colon (560.30), gallstone obstruction of the intestine (560.31), or other types of obstruction (560.39) such as calculus. Other specified types of intestinal obstructions, such as intestinal or peritoneal adhesions, occur after an operation or an infection (560.81). **Unspecified intestinal obstruction** (560.9) is assigned to those obstructions where there is no clear indication of the type of obstruction.

FIGURE 7-2 Types of intussusception.

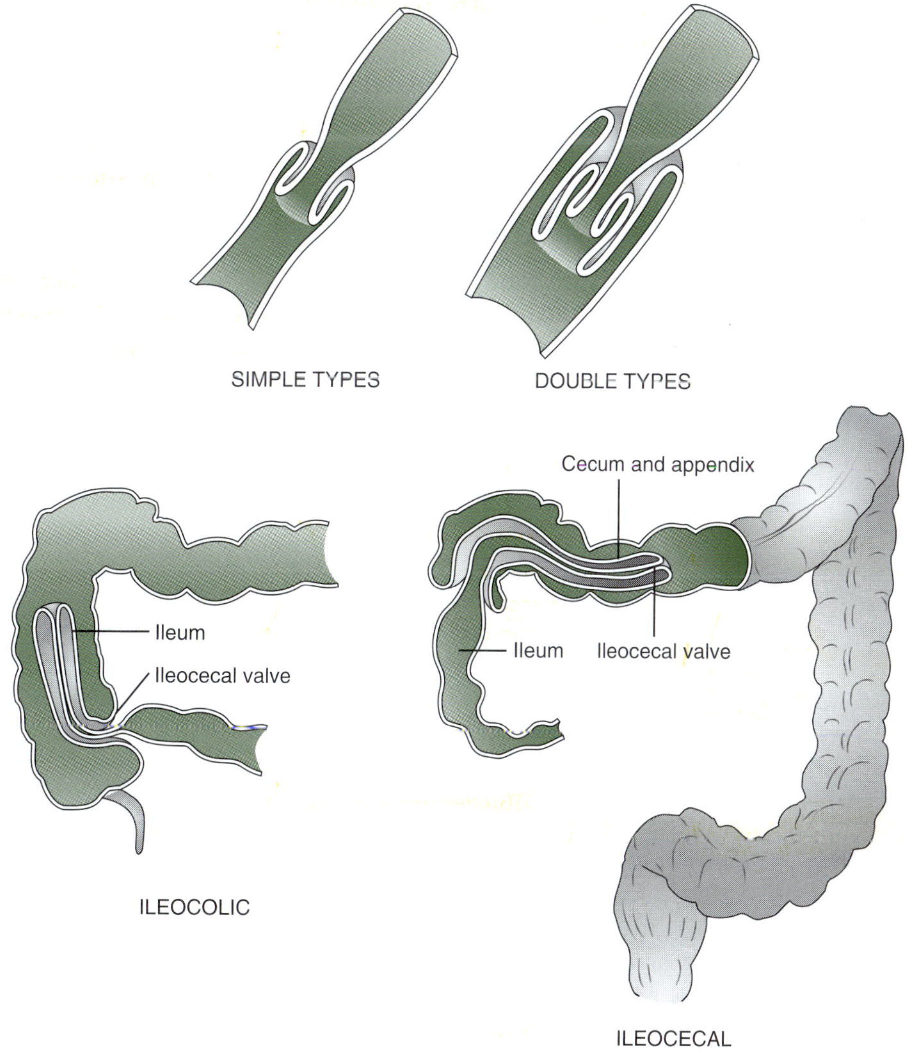

CASE 7-1
7-1A Surgical Consultation

CASE 7-1

7-1A SURGICAL CONSULTATION

The patient had a gastrointestinal operation four weeks ago, but the report does not clearly indicate that the current obstruction is due to the surgical procedure, therefore, a "complication of surgery" code would not be appropriate in this case.

LOCATION: Inpatient Hospital

PATIENT: Martin Newwell

PHYSICIAN: Alma Naraquist, M.D.

CONSULTANT: Daniel Olanka, M.D.

HISTORY OF PRESENT ILLNESS: This patient was operated on by Dr. Sanchez approximately 4 weeks ago for a misdiagnosis of appendicitis. He underwent ileocecal resection. He has had a variety of problems in the postoperative period, including renal failure, respiratory failure, tracheostomy, etc. He is currently under the care of Dr. Naraquist and is off the ventilator and breathing through the tracheostomy. He has been intermittently fed through small bowel Cor-Flo tube, but this has the appearance of a bowel obstruction. Dr. Naraquist has asked me to evaluate the patient, and the family has requested that another surgeon get involved in his care, and so I have been tagged to review his case.

PHYSICAL EXAMINATION: On examination, the patient is resting comfortably in bed. He does have a tracheostomy in place. He is alert and does respond. The chest is clear to auscultation. There is a catheter in place for dialysis, although the patient is not currently on dialysis. The abdomen is markedly distended. It is tympanitic. Tinkling bowel sounds are heard. There are no rushes. The midline scar is well healed. There is no particular focal tenderness, and no hernias are appreciated.

Review of the patient's films shows marked dilatation of the small bowel. Review of the CT scan shows marked dilatation of the small bowel with what appears to be a transition zone in the distal ileum. The colon is deflated.

DISCUSSION: By physical examination, this patient has chronic bowel obstruction, at least partial in nature. Certainly his x-rays support that there is a major problem intra-abdominally. My recommendation would be that the patient should be considered for re-exploration for bowel obstruction. I do not know whether the problem is at the anastomosis or near the anastomosis. I think patient would benefit from some total parenteral nutrition (TPN) and aggressive hydration over the next few days, and then we will plan to take him to the operating room next week.

7-1A:

SERVICE CODE(S): ____________________

DX CODE(S): ____________________

External Procedures

External procedures are those that can be performed in the area of the rectum, such as drainage of rectal abscess or hemorrhoidectomy. These external procedures performed with an **anoscope,** as illustrated in **Figure 7-3,** are coded with **endoscopy** codes. The anoscope codes are located in the Endoscopy subcategory (46600-46615) of the Anus category. The stand-alone code 46600 states "Anoscopy; . . . " and is then followed by the indented codes based on the procedure performed, such as **biopsy,** foreign body removal, or control of bleeding. Note that there is a distinction made for the method of removal of tumors (46610-46611); 46612 is for removal of multiple tumors, polyps, or lesions using hot biopsy forceps, cautery, or snare. This means that if one tumor was removed with cautery, you would code

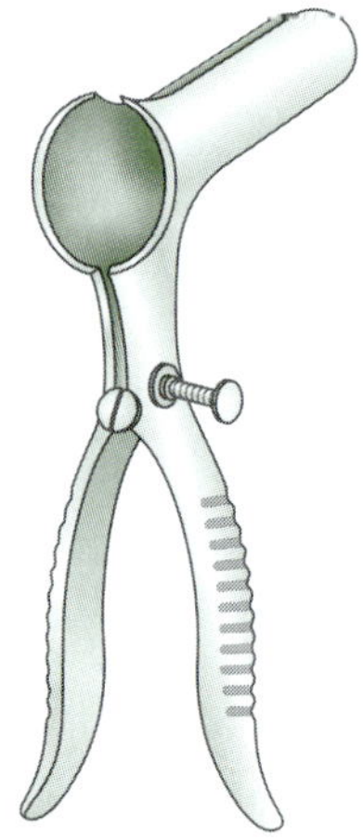

FIGURE 7-3 Anoscope.

46610, and if multiple tumors were removed, you would code with 46612. It would *not* be appropriate to list the single tumor removal code with modifier -51 on the second code (i.e., 46610 and 46610-51); rather, you must list only 46612 to report the multiple removal.

A **fistula** (565.1) is an abnormal channel that connects two places that would ordinarily not be connected, for example, an anal fistula in which a channel leads from the anal canal into the tissue surrounding the channel. The channel then becomes clogged with fecal material, and often an abscess (566) will form at the end of the channel. The channel can be closed with sutures or excised. Codes to report the excision of anal fistula are in the Excision subcategory (46200-46320). If a diagnostic anoscopy were performed (46600) as well as the surgical excision of a fistula, each is coded separately with modifier -51 added to the exploration anoscope. If both a fistula and an abscess are present, each is reported separately. Packing placed into an abscessed area is not reported separately.

Some gastroenterologists perform these anal procedures, or a general surgeon may be called in to perform the procedure at the request of the gastroenterologist or other physician who diagnosed the condition. Most gastroenterologists perform the procedures that use a endoscope and refer the open abdominal procedures to a general surgeon. Smaller facilities have no gastrointestinal specialists, and these procedures are performed by general surgeons.

CASE 7-2
7-2A Operative Report, Anal Fistula

CASE 7-2

7-2A OPERATIVE REPORT, ANAL FISTULA

LOCATION: Inpatient Hospital

PATIENT: Russell Cornwall

SURGEON: Larry P. Friendly, M.D.

PREOPERATIVE DIAGNOSIS: Anal fistula

POSTOPERATIVE DIAGNOSIS: Anal fistula

TITLE OF PROCEDURE:
1. Fistulotomy.
2. Anoscopy.

ANESTHESIA: General

INDICATIONS: The patient is a 46-year-old male with fever of unknown origin whom I had seen several months ago with perianal fistula. Since that time, he has had decreased drainage but still has pain and fevers. He presents today for elective fistulotomy, and he understands the risk of bleeding and infection and the possible risk of damage to the sphincter muscle, and he wishes to proceed with procedure.

The patient was brought to the operating room, placed under spinal anesthesia, placed in the jackknife position, and prepped and draped sterilely. Digital rectal examination was first performed, and there were no masses. Anoscopy was then performed, and there was no internal anal fistulous opening. At the 4 o'clock position, we could feel this hard, indurated mass that drained purulent material. We then opened this with a no. 15 blade and debrided a necrotic capsule from this area. We then cauterized the base, injected it with 30 cc of 0.5% Sensorcaine with epinephrine solution, and packed it with 4 × 4 gauze. The patient tolerated this well and was taken to the postanesthesia recovery room in stable condition.

7-2A:

SERVICE CODE(S): ____________________

DX CODE(S): ____________________

If an abscess is simply lanced and drained, report the services with an incision code (46020-46083).

CASE 7-3
7-3A Operative Report, Intersphincteric Abscess

CASE 7-3

7-3A OPERATIVE REPORT, INTERSPHINCTERIC ABSCESS

LOCATION: Inpatient Hospital

PATIENT: Mortica Kellogg

PHYSICIAN: Ronald Green, M.D.

SURGEON: Larry P. Friendly, M.D.

PREOPERATIVE DIAGNOSIS: Rectal pain

POSTOPERATIVE DIAGNOSIS: Intersphincteric abscess

OPERATIVE PROCEDURE: Examination under anesthesia and drainage of perirectal abscess

OPERATIVE NOTE: The patient was placed under general anesthesia and was placed in the lithotomy position. The rectal area was prepped and draped in a sterile manner. Examination of the external anus showed no evidence of a fissure or obvious perirectal abscess. I palpated around the anus carefully and could not really appreciate any pathology. We then proceeded to dilate the anus to three fingers and introduced the bivalve speculum. While carefully inspecting the inner lining of the anus in the lithotomy position proximally at the 6 or 7 o'clock location, we encountered a fluctuant feeling area, which with mild pressure from the finger ruptured and drained purulent material. This was cultured. We were then in a small abscess cavity, which appeared to be in an intersphincteric location in between the subcutaneous and the deep sphincters. This was completely drained and then irrigated with some saline. We then packed the area with gauze. The patient tolerated the procedure well and was discharged to the recovery room in stable condition.

7-3A:

SERVICE CODE(S): ____________________

DX CODE(S): ____________________

CASE 7-4
7-4A Operative Report, Perirectal Fistulectomies

CASE 7-4

7-4A OPERATIVE REPORT, PERIRECTAL FISTULECTOMIES

In this case a fistula is removed with no mention of an abscess.

LOCATION: Inpatient, Hospital

PATIENT: George Papenfuss

SURGEON: Larry Friendly, M.D.

PREOPERATIVE DIAGNOSIS: Perirectal fistulas

POSTOPERATIVE DIAGNOSIS: Perirectal fistulas

PROCEDURE PERFORMED: Perirectal fistulectomies

ANESTHESIA: General anesthetic.

INDICATIONS FOR SURGERY: The patient is a 61-year-old white male who had draining perirectal fistulas, which had been incised and drained in the past. The patient is now being admitted for incision of these fistulas.

DESCRIPTION OF PROCEDURE: The patient was placed in a jackknife position. He was prepped and draped in the usual manner. The patient was given a general anesthetic. The fistulous tracts were in the 2 and 11 o'clock positions. The fistulous tracts were excised; one had an abscessed pocket, which was excised in its entirety. The tracts continued over the 12 o'clock midline position over into about the 2 o'clock position. All these tracts were combined into one large incision, and all the inflammatory tissue was excised sharply. The rectum was also dilated up and examined. No evidence of any tract could be seen draining directly into the rectum at this time, and no induration was seen. The inflammatory tissue present on the outer skin area was completely excised. The operative area was thoroughly irrigated. Hemostasis was obtained using Bovie cautery. The wounds were left open, and dressings were applied. The patient tolerated the operation and returned to recovery in stable condition.

7-4A:

SERVICE CODE(S): ______________________________

DX CODE(S): ______________________________

Hemorrhoids

Hemorrhoids (piles) are caused by increased pressure on the hemorrhoid veins, such as constipation, straining during heavy lifting, lesions, or pregnancy. This pressure causes the hemorrhoid vein to bulge (*like a varicose vein*), causing anal bleeding, itching, and/or pain. Hemorrhoids are graded, similar to how ulcers are graded.

- Grade I hemorrhoids project into the anal canal but do not protrude outside of the anus.
- Grade II hemorrhoids protrude (*external*) from the anus on straining, but return upon cessation of straining.
- Grade III hemorrhoids protrude upon straining and only return if manually reducted (returned to normal position).
- Grade IV hemorrhoids permanently protrude.

The complexity of the procedure depends on the type of hemorrhoid and the complexity of repair.

A common term when speaking of hemorrhoids is *thrombosed,* which means one containing clotted blood.

The diagnosis code for hemorrhoids is (455.x) with fourth digit subcategories for internal, external, unspecified, and those with or without mention of complication or thrombosed. If the hemorrhoid occurs during pregnancy, 671.8, Other venous complications, is used to report the diagnosis.

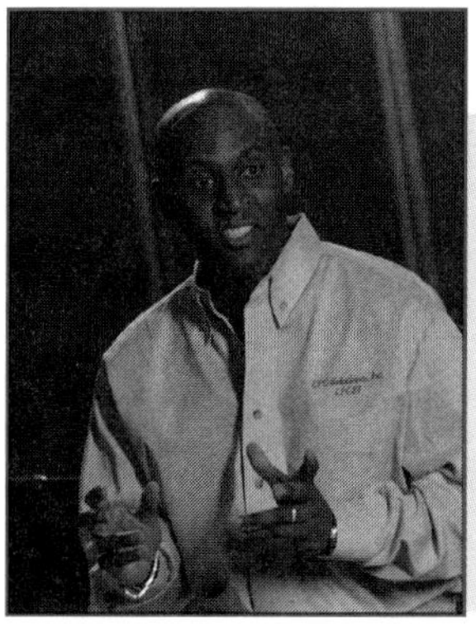

FROM THE TRENCHES

Terry

"The training you get in certification classes—that training is invaluable. If you're a new coder, there's no way you can learn the ins and outs of coding without preparing for certification... That's what people are looking for now. What facilities want is to know that you are going to be accountable. They know what you're putting down is going to be accurate... It gives them security."

CASE 7-5
7-5A Operative Report, Hemorrhoidectomy

CASE 7-5

7-5A OPERATIVE REPORT, HEMORRHOIDECTOMY

LOCATION: Outpatient, Hospital

PATIENT: Pricilla Stephanopolis

PHYSICIAN: Gary Sanchez, M.D.

SURGEON: Ronald Ripple, M.D.

PREOPERATIVE DIAGNOSIS: Symptomatic internal hemorrhoid, grade II

POSTOPERATIVE DIAGNOSIS: Symptomatic internal hemorrhoid, grade II

PROCEDURE PERFORMED: Hemorrhoidectomy (excision of single internal hemorrhoid). This is the largest and the only bleeding hemorrhoid.

ANESTHESIA: General endotracheal anesthesia plus 30 cc of 0.5% Marcaine with epinephrine

The patient, on examination under anesthesia, had other smaller, Grade I hemorrhoids that were higher up in the anal canal, but the decision was made not to excise these because they were not bleeding.

PROCEDURE IN DETAIL: After good general endotracheal anesthesia, the patient was carefully placed in the prone position. After this, a total of 30 cc of Marcaine was infiltrated into the area around the hemorrhoid. The hemorrhoid was grasped with an Allis clamp, and a straight clamp was placed across the base. A running stitch was then placed below the clamp for hemostasis. Next the hemorrhoid was excised above the clamp, and a running stitch going in the opposite direction was then looped over the straight clamp. The straight clamp was removed, and the looped stitch was then tightened up. Another layer of suture was then run down the length of the excised hemorrhoid. Hemostasis was obtained with this maneuver. No other large thrombosed or extruding hemorrhoids were noted. After this, Vaseline gauze was placed over the wound. ABD dressing and knit mesh pants were placed on the patient to hold the dressing in place. She was returned to the recovery room in good condition.

7-5A:

SERVICE CODE(S): ____________________

DX CODE(S): ____________________

Catheters

Intraperitoneal catheters are inserted into the abdomen (peritoneal cavity) for the purposes of drainage. The choice of catheter depends on the purpose for which the catheter is being placed and the physician's preference. Reports often refer to the catheters by brand name, such as Tenkhoff, oley, and Swan neck. Catheters are inserted on either a permanent or a temporary basis. The approach for placement can be closed (percutaneous) or open. The closed placement requires a puncture wound made on the abdomen with the catheter threaded through the incision and into the abdominal cavity. During an open procedure, the surgeon may place a drain, securing the catheter in place outside of the abdomen. The drain placement is bundled into the procedure and not reported separately.

CASE 7-6
7-6A Operative Report, Dialysis Catheter

CASE 7-6

7-6A OPERATIVE REPORT, DIALYSIS CATHETER

LOCATION: Inpatient, Hospital

PATIENT: Gladys Hanson

SURGEON: Gary Sanchez, M.D.

PREOPERATIVE DIAGNOSIS: End-stage renal disease

POSTOPERATIVE DIAGNOSIS: End-stage renal disease

PROCEDURE PERFORMED: Placement of a peritoneal dialysis catheter

INDICATION: This 23-year-old female has end-stage renal disease and is going to need permanent dialysis. She elected peritoneal dialysis. Please see clinic consultation for further details of the discussion of procedure and risks involved.

PROCEDURE: The patient was brought to the operating theater and placed in the supine position on the operating room table. After receiving a general anesthetic, she was prepped and draped in a sterile fashion. An incision line that was infraumbilical and vertical was infiltrated with 0.5% Marcaine. An incision was then made and carried down through the subcutaneous tissues down to the anterior fascia. The anterior fascia was grasped and divided sharply. The peritoneum was also divided sharply. The peritoneal cavity was entered. A peritoneal dialysis catheter was then inserted using a Bozeman catheter into the pelvis. The patient had been placed in a Trendelenburg position. We then were able to place the catheter with ease. We placed a 2-0 Vicryl in a pursestring fashion through the peritoneum. This was also attached to the cuff in adjacent spots. This was then secured. Interrupted sutures of 2-0 Vicryl were then used to close the fascia. The sutures in the cuff were also placed through the cuff to help secure this in place. It was then tunneled out to the left side. The cuff was buried in the subcutaneous tissues. The subcutaneous tissues and vertical midline incision were closed with interrupted sutures of 3-0 Vicryl around and over the catheter. The skin was closed with 4-0 Vicryl in a running subcuticular fashion. Steri-Strips and a sterile dressing were applied. The catheter-retaining device was used at the exit site to help secure it in place. We had also flushed this intermittently with heparinized saline during the procedure at various steps and then let the drain back out at all times as well as at the end of the procedure. This flushed well and irrigated well. The patient tolerated the procedure well and went to the recovery room in stable condition. No family was present to meet with postoperatively to discuss the results.

7-6A:

SERVICE CODE(S): ____________________

DX CODE(S): ____________________

Endoscopy Procedures

Procedures are often performed by means of an endoscope and laparoscopy. The surgical approach determines the code. For example, if the patient has a lesion on the outside of the intestine, the physician would open the abdomen (open procedure) or use a laparoscopy (tube inserted through the abdominal wall) to excise the lesion. Codes for the open procedure are located in the Intestine, Excision category (44100-44160). Codes for the laparoscopic approach are located in the Intestine, Laparoscopy category. If the lesion was inside the intestine and the surgeon used an endoscope inserted through the anus to remove the lesion, you would report the service with a code from Intestine, Endoscopy (44360-44397). There are endoscopic, laparoscopic, and open approaches in many of the subheadings of the Digestive System subsection.

> The **endoscopic** procedure uses an existing orifice (opening), a **laparoscopic** procedure uses a small incision, and an **open** procedure uses a larger incision.

There are endoscopic and laparoscopic codes for the gastrointestinal tract, such as the esophagus, stomach, intestines, and anus as well as abdomen, peritoneum, and omentum.

Remember to code to the full extent of the procedure, which is the point at which the procedure terminates. For example, if the procedure begins by an endoscope being placed into the mouth, through the esophagus, and terminating in the stomach, the full extent is the stomach. Although the operative report will state the procedure performed in the identifiers of the report, such as "Procedure Performed," you must always read the full operative report to ensure the full extent is reported. For example, the Procedure Performed identifier may state esophagogastroscopy (full extent is the stomach), but upon reading the report, you find that the duodenum was referenced, making the procedure an esophagogastroduodenoscopy (full extent is the duodenum).

Use the correct approach and code to the fullest extent of the procedure.

Gastritis and Duodenitis

Gastritis is a severe inflammation of the stomach. **Acute gastritis** (535.0) is usually superficial erosions of the surface epithelium brought about by drugs, chemicals, or *Helicobacter pylori* bacteria. **Atrophic gastritis** (535.1x) is a chronic inflammation of the stomach that results in destruction of the cells of the mucous lining of the stomach. **Duodenitis** (535.6x) is a severe inflammation of the duodenum. There is a fifth digit subclassification used with the category code 535. These fifth digits indicate without mention of hemorrhage (0) and with hemorrhage (1).

Ulcer

Ulcer is an erosive area or a break. The term peptic pertains to pepsin or to digestion. A peptic ulcer occurs on the mucosal lining of the stomach (531) or duodenum (532) and results in the submucosal areas being exposed to the gastric secretions. The site may be unspecified (533) in the medical record. All three categories also have fourth digit subcategories for acute or chronic with or without hemorrhage, and/or perforation. These categories of codes have a fifth digit available to indicate those diagnoses without mention of obstruction (0) and with mention of obstruction (1).

Hiatal Hernia

Hernias of the groin are the most common type of hernia, accounting for 80 percent of all hernias. There are two major types of inguinal hernias (550.xx): indirect (oblique) and direct. **Indirect inguinal hernias** result when the intestines emerge through the abdominal wall in an indirect fashion through the inguinal canal. **Direct inguinal hernias** penetrate through the abdominal wall in a direct fashion. **Femoral hernias** occur at the femoral ring where the femoral vessels enter the thigh. In both inguinal and femoral hernia classifications, there is a fifth digit to indicate unilateral (0, 1) or bilateral (2, 3). Classification of hernias is based on the location of the hernia and whether there is obstruction and/or gangrene present. If the documentation indicates incarcerated or strangulated, the hernia is classified as obstructed. A common type of hernia is a hiatal or esophageal hernia, also referred to as a sliding hernia or diaphragmatic hernia. When the diaphragmatic hernia is mentioned with obstruction, report the diagnosis with 552.3; when it is without obstruction report the diagnosis with 553.3.

CASE 7-7
7-7A Operative Report, Esophagogastroduodenoscopy

CASE 7-7

7-7A OPERATIVE REPORT, ESOPHAGOGASTRODUODENOSCOPY

LOCATION: Outpatient, Hospital

PATIENT: David Amron

PHYSICIAN: Larry Friendly, M.D.

PREOPERATIVE DIAGNOSIS: Upper gastrointestinal bleeding

POSTOPERATIVE DIAGNOSIS: Mild gastritis, mild duodenitis, a 5-mm gastric ulcer, not actively bleeding; biopsies obtained for *Helicobacter pylori;* also hiatal hernia

INDICATION: A 70-year-old white man who has chronic renal failure secondary to amyloidosis presents with 1 week of coffee-ground emesis. He smokes two to three packs per day and has two to three melenic stools per day. We do not have any results of laboratory tests. He was just admitted. We suspect upper gastrointestinal bleeding. He has not been on any NSAIDs. He has never had an ulcer. He has no other gastrointestinal symptoms.

PROCEDURE PERFORMED: Esophagogastroduodenoscopy

PREOPERATIVE MEDICATION: Demerol 50 mg IV; Versed 4 mg IV

FINDINGS: The Pentax video pediatric endoscope was passed without difficulty into the oropharynx. The gastroesophageal junction was seen at 40 cm. Inspection of the esophagus revealed no erythema, ulceration, exudate, friability, or other mucosal abnormalities. From 40 to 43 cm, there was a 3-cm hiatal hernia. Along the lower border of the hernia sac, there was a 5 × 2-mm ulceration. It was not actively bleeding. Photograph was obtained. The stomach proper was entered. Coffee-ground material was present, but no fresh blood. Endoscope was advanced to the second duodenum. Inspection of the second duodenum revealed no abnormalities. The first duodenum and duodenal bulb revealed some mild patchy erythema and no ulceration. The antrum revealed patchy erythema but no ulceration. Retroflexion revealed the previously described minimal ulcer and hiatal hernia. Nothing was seen in the fundus or cardia. Biopsies were obtained of the antrum to rule out *H. pylori.* The patient tolerated the procedure well.

IMPRESSION: Some old blood present, no active bleeding. A 5-mm gastric ulcer along the inferior border of the 3-mm hiatal hernia, not bleeding. Mild gastritis and mild duodenitis are present. Biopsies obtained for *Helicobacter pylori.*

PLAN: Will observe patient for 24 hours and possibly discharge, follow hemoglobins. At this point, it does not appear that the patient has amyloid of the gastrointestinal tract.

7-7A:

SERVICE CODE(S): ____________________

DX CODE(S): ____________________

Rectal Procedures

Rectal endoscopic procedures are:

- Proctosigmoidoscopy: Endoscopic examination of the rectum (proct/o = rectum) and the sigmoid colon (45300-45327)
- Sigmoidoscopy: Endoscopic examination of the sigmoid colon and may include the descending colon (45330-45345)
- Colonoscopy: Endoscopic examination of the colon (from rectum to cecum, which is the uppermost portion of the large intestine and may include the lower portion of the small intestine, ileum) (45378-45387)

The codes are divided based on the extent and the purpose of the procedure. Note that the stand-alone codes 45300, 45330, and 45378 each have a list of indented codes based on the purpose (such as biopsy, foreign body removal, ablation, control of bleeding, etc.).

If the patient is fully prepared for the endoscopic procedure, and the procedure has begun but is not completed due to extenuating circumstances, use modifier -53, Discontinued Procedure, with the endoscopic code. Some payers, such as Medicare, require the coder to report -53 (Discontinued Procedure) to report a procedure that could not be completed. These extenuating circumstances could be that the patient has become unstable, the bowel preparation for the surgery was not sufficient to continue the procedure, or an equipment failure has occurred.

Polyps

A polyp is a growth on a pedicle (stem) that bleeds easily and may become malignant. In the ICD-9-CM, the codes for a diagnosis of polyp(s) is located under the main term "Polyp, polypus" subtermed by location, such as nose (471.9), labia (624.6), and gum (523.8). These codes are then referenced in the Tabular for further information regarding code assignment. A polyp is not a neoplasm, rather it is an abnormal growth of normal cells. Sometimes the term *hyperplastic* is used in the pathology report of a polyp specimen. The term means that there is an increase in the number of normal cells.

CASE 7-8
7-8A Operative Report, Colon Polypectomy
7-8B Pathology Report

CASE 7-8

CASE 7-8A OPERATIVE REPORT, COLON POLYPECTOMY

Report the services for the following case. When reporting the diagnosis for the operative procedure, reference the pathology report located in 7.8B.

LOCATION: Outpatient Hospital

PATIENT: Jatin Al-Assad

SURGEON: Larry Friendly, M.D.

SCOPE USED: Pentax video colonoscope

MEDICATIONS GIVEN: Fentanyl 75 µg and Versed 3 mg IV prior to the procedure

PREOPERATIVE DIAGNOSIS: Polyp on sigmoidoscopy

POSTOPERATIVE DIAGNOSIS: Colon polyps

INDICATION: The patient is a 48-year-old male who presented for screening sigmoidoscopy on January 15. He was found to have several adenomatous polyps in the sigmoid colon and rectum. This procedure is being done to remove those polyps and any other polyps in the more proximal colon.

FINDINGS: About five polyps were seen, three pedunculated and two sessile. These were snared. The remainder of the colon and rectum were normal.

DESCRIPTION OF TECHNIQUE: After informed consent was obtained, the patient was prepared for colonoscopy. He was placed in the left lateral decubitus position. A digital rectal examination was performed and was unremarkable. The lubricated Pentax video colonoscope was then guided digitally into the rectum and advanced to the cecum. The scope was withdrawn and the mucosa inspected. The cecum, ascending colon, transverse colon, and descending colon were normal. Through the sigmoid colon and rectum, five polyps were seen. The largest measured about 1 cm in diameter. These were pedunculated. These were snared. Two others were smaller. The distal rectum was normal. The scope was withdrawn. The patient tolerated the procedure well and was discharged ambulatory with a driver.

RECOMMENDATIONS: Follow-up colonoscopy in 2 years due to the relatively large number of polyps seen on this examination in a relatively young man.

7-8A:

SERVICE CODE(S): ____________________

DX CODE(S): ____________________

7-8B PATHOLOGY REPORT

LOCATION: Outpatient Hospital

PATIENT: Jatin Al-Assad

SURGEON: Larry Friendly, M.D.

PATHOLOGIST: Morton Monson, M.D.

CLINICAL HISTORY: Polyp

TISSUE RECEIVED: Colon polyp

GROSS DESCRIPTION: The specimen is labeled with the patient's name and "colon polyps" and consists of four polypoid segments of colon mucosa up to 0.9 cm in greatest dimension. The two larger polyps are submitted in cassette 1 and the three smaller polyps in cassette 2. The specimen is submitted in toto in two cassettes.

MICROSCOPIC DESCRIPTION: Sections reveal five polyps showing surface epithelium and underlying glands lined by a serrated feathery surface epithelium.

DIAGNOSIS: Colon, polypectomy: hyperplastic polyps (five)

7-8B:

SERVICE CODE(S): ____________________

DX CODE(S): ____________________

Abnormal Findings

When a patient has an abnormal finding as the preoperative diagnosis, reference "Abnormal" in the ICD-9-CM Index. In the following case, the patient presents for a sigmoidoscopy because of abnormal findings on x-ray. This would be a common reason for the patient to have an endoscopic procedure of the lower gastrointestinal tract. Also, if the patient has a family history or personal history of gastrointestinal lesions, the physician will recommend a screening endoscopic procedure.

As you read the reports, if there are terms you do not understand, you should take the time now to look them up in a medical dictionary. Your medical terminology skills will increase quickly and greatly if you make a practice of doing this.

Coder's Rule: Never pass by a medical term that you do not understand.

CASE 7-9

7-9A OPERATIVE REPORT, SIGMOIDOSCOPY

LOCATION: Outpatient, Hospital

PATIENT: James Acheson

SURGEON: Larry Friendly, M.D.

PREOPERATIVE DIAGNOSIS: Abnormal findings on x-ray; GI tract

POSTOPERATIVE DIAGNOSIS: Normal flexible sigmoidoscopy; no volvulus. Normal mucosa, just a few diverticula in the descending sigmoid colon

PROCEDURE PERFORMED: Flexible sigmoidoscopy

INDICATION: The patient is a 19-year-old white male who apparently had a perforated appendix with abscess. He had a cecectomy and has had a complicated hospital course with renal failure and sepsis. He has been getting tube feedings, which have been poorly tolerated. His CT scan showed dilated bowel in the midabdomen and pelvis and also a loop in the sigmoid colon, which is abnormal, thought to be possibly a volvulus or inflammatory infectious process in that area. The procedure is indicated to determine whether obstruction is present.

PREOPERATIVE MEDICATION: None

FINDINGS: The Pentax video sigmoidoscope was inserted without difficulty to 60 cm. Careful inspection in the mid-descending (*this is the colon*), distal descending, sigmoid, and rectum revealed no erythema, ulceration, exudate, friability, or other mucosal abnormalities. There were a few diverticula present. The mucosa was normal. No volvulus were noted. No diverticulitis and no obstructing lesion were seen. The patient tolerated the procedure well.

IMPRESSION: Normal flexible sigmoidoscopy to 60 cm. No obstruction or volvulus was noted. The mucosa was normal.

DISCUSSION/PLAN: The patient needs to have a small bowel obstruction ruled out. We have recommended small bowel series.

7-9A:

SERVICE CODE(S): ____________________

DX CODE(S): ____________________

CASE 7-10
7-10A Operative Report, Sigmoidoscopy
7-10B Pathology Report

CASE 7-10

7-10A OPERATIVE REPORT, SIGMOIDOSCOPY

LOCATION: Outpatient, Hospital

PATIENT: Jason Bell

SURGEON: Larry Friendly, M.D.

SCOPE USED: Pentax video sigmoidoscope

MEDICATIONS GIVEN: None

PREOPERATIVE DIAGNOSIS: Screen

POSTOPERATIVE DIAGNOSIS: Sigmoid and rectal polyps

INDICATION: The patient is a 51-year-old man who presents for screening sigmoidoscopy. He is asymptomatic. There is no family history of colon cancer or polyps.

FINDINGS: Four polyps were seen on this examination scattered between the rectum and proximal sigmoid colon. The largest measured about 1 cm in diameter. The others were diminutive, about 4 or 5 mm in diameter. Biopsies were taken of two of these polyps.

DESCRIPTION OF TECHNIQUE: After informed consent was obtained, the patient was prepared for a sigmoidoscopy. He was placed in the left lateral decubitus position and given no medication. A digital rectal examination was performed and was unremarkable. The lubricated Pentax video sigmoidoscope was guided digitally into the rectum and advanced to 60 cm. Four polyps were seen to range from 4 to 10 mm in diameter between the sigmoid colon and the proximal rectum. Biopsies were taken of two of these. They appeared to be adenomas. There were no diverticula. The distal rectum was normal. The scope was withdrawn. The patient tolerated the procedure well and was discharged ambulatory.

RECOMMENDATIONS: Review polyp biopsies. These appear to be adenomas, and the patient will be scheduled for colonoscopy for polypectomy.

Pathology Report Later Indicated: See Report 7-10B.

7-10A:

SERVICE CODE(S): ____________________

DX CODE(S): ____________________

7-10B PATHOLOGY REPORT

LOCATION: Outpatient, Hospital

PATIENT: Jason Bell

SURGEON: Larry Friendly, M.D.

PATHOLOGIST: Morton Monson, M.D.

CLINICAL HISTORY: Screening for colon polyps

SPECIMEN RECEIVED: Colon polyps biopsy

GROSS DESCRIPTION: Received in a container labeled "colon polyps biopsy" are two frozen fragments of tan tissue measuring 0.1 to 0.4 cm in greatest dimension. The specimen is totally submitted.

MICROSCOPIC DESCRIPTION: The colon biopsy demonstrates a polyp showing adenomatous and villous epithelial features within the glandular and surface epithelium. The glands vary in size and configuration and are separated by an intact lamina propria. The cells are enlarged with elongated hyperchromatic nuclei. Pseudostratification and crowding are evident.

DIAGNOSIS: Colon and rectum biopsy, mucosal: tubulovillous adenoma (*this is a benign neoplasm*).

7-10B:

SERVICE CODE(S): ____________________

DX CODE(S): ____________________

Abdominal Pain

Abdominal pain is a common complaint with many possible problems. The physician must rely on his or her expert clinical skills in obtaining a thorough history and examination that will lead to the correct diagnosis and correct treatment. The history would include assessment of the onset (chronic or acute), progression, location, type, and associated signs and symptoms, such as vomiting or change in bowel habits.

CASE 7-11
7-11A Operative Report, Colonoscopy
7-11B Surgical Consultation
7-11C Operative Report, Hemicolectomy
7-11D Pathology Report

CASE 7-11

7-11A OPERATIVE REPORT, COLONOSCOPY

Dr. Friendly performs a colonoscopy on a patient with a history of diarrhea for the past month.

LOCATION: Inpatient, Hospital

PATIENT: Gloria Hathorne

PRIMARY PHYSICIAN: Ronald Green, M.D.

SURGEON: Larry Friendly, M.D.

PROCEDURE PERFORMED: Colonoscopy with biopsies

PREPROCEDURE DIAGNOSIS: Abdominal pain, anemia

POSTPROCEDURE DIAGNOSIS: Ulcerative circumferential mass in the ascending colon consistent with either adenocarcinoma or lymphoma

PREOPERATIVE MEDICATION: Demerol 50 mg IV; Versed 2 mg IV

INDICATION: This is a very pleasant 40-year-old white female who I referred for evaluation of anemia and lower abdominal pain. The patient has had bilateral lower abdominal pain for 4 weeks. She has also developed diarrhea in the last few months. She had a gastric lymphoma 1 year ago that was treated with chemotherapy, and I believe also radiation. Her pain has disappeared, but her hemoglobin is 8.7. The patient had a CT scan that showed thickening in the ascending colon and cecum.

PROCEDURE: The Pentax video colonoscope was inserted without difficulty to the cecum. The ileocecal valve was identified. The appendiceal orifice was seen. The cecum was normal; however, just above the cecum in the proximal ascending colon was a large circumferential mass with ulceration and friability. Biopsies were obtained and a photograph obtained. Inspection in the remainder of the ascending colon, hepatic flexure, transverse colon, splenic flexure, descending colon, sigmoid colon, and rectum revealed no erythema, ulceration, exudate, friability, or other mucosal abnormalities. The patient tolerated the procedure well.

IMPRESSION: Large circumferential mass in the proximal ascending colon consistent with adenocarcinoma of the colon versus lymphoma

PLAN: Will await biopsy results, test accordingly, and do esophagogastroduodenoscopy.

Pathology Report Later Indicated: Adenocarcinoma, ascending colon

7-11A:

SERVICE CODE(S): ____________________

DX CODE(S): ____________________

7-11B SURGICAL CONSULTATION

Dr. Sanchez serves as a consultant to assess the feasibility of undergoing resection of the colon the following Monday.

LOCATION: Inpatient, Hospital

PATIENT: Gloria Hathorne

PRIMARY PHYSICIAN: Ronald Green, M.D.

CONSULTANT: Gary Sanchez, M.D.

HISTORY OF PRESENT ILLNESS: The patient is a 40-year-old white female who has been having difficulty with diarrhea for the past month. The patient was recently admitted to the hospital because of abdominal pain and this diarrhea problem. The patient has a history of gastric lymphoma 2 years ago that was treated with chemotherapy and radiation therapy. The patient underwent evaluation for abdominal pain. Dr. Friendly did an upper endoscopy that showed radiation gastritis in the stomach area, and colonoscopy revealed an ascending colon lesion. Biopsies taken by Dr. Friendly showed an adenocarcinoma. The patient is now being seen for consideration of resection of her right colon for adenocarcinoma of the ascending colon.

PAST MEDICAL HISTORY:

OPERATIONS:
1. Open cholecystectomy
2. Total abdominal hysterectomy
3. Coronary artery bypass graft

ILLNESSES:
1. Diabetes mellitus
2. Hypertension
3. History of lymphoma

MEDICATIONS:
1. Advil
2. Compazine
3. Furosemide
4. Insulin
5. Lorazepam
6. Paxil
7. Remeron
8. Ultram
9. Zestril
10. Aciphex
11. Iron

ALLERGIES: None known.

REVIEW OF SYSTEMS: The patient does not smoke or drink. Neuro: The patient denies any history of seizure disorder, headaches, or dizziness. Cardiac: No history of myocardial infarction or congenital heart disease. The patient has hypertension and had heart bypass surgery in 1998. Pulmonary: No history of asthma, hay fever, or pneumonia. No history of hemoptysis. GI: See history of present illness. GU: The patient denies any urgency, frequency, or dysuria. GYN: Gravida 1, para 1, AB 0. Status TAH-BSO. Hematologic: The patient has received blood transfusions recently during this hospitalization. She has not noted any rectal bleeding. However, the patient does have bleeding from her colon cancer.

EXAMINATION: Mrs. Hathorne is a 40-year-old white female who is oriented to time, place, and person. Chest: Lungs are clear. No rales or rhonchi are heard. Heart: Regular rhythm. No murmur. Abdomen: Normal bowel sounds. No masses or hepatosplenomegaly. The patient's abdomen is nontender at this time. She has a right subcostal incision scar and lower abdominal incision scar from her previous surgeries.

IMPRESSION:
1. Ascending colon adenocarcinoma
2. Status post lymphoma treatment 2 years ago
3. Hypertension
4. Diabetes mellitus
5. Pacemaker

PLAN: The patient has been counseled for resection of her colon cancer. She has agreed to the operation. All her questions about the surgery were answered. The patient will undergo a bowel prep tomorrow and surgery on Monday.

Thank you for the consultation.

7-11B:

SERVICE CODE(S): ______________________

DX CODE(S): ______________________

A **hemicolectomy** is resection of about half the colon. The designations of right and left indicate the location of the resection as either the left or right half of the colon from the middle of the transverse segment to the rectum. This procedure is performed for a variety of reasons, such as cancer or Crohn's disease (inflamed, ulcerated, thickened, and sometimes obstructed intestine). The colon is then joined with the ileum. Great care is taken to ensure that the anastomosis (joining of the two ends of the intestine) is secure so that it does not leak into the abdominal cavity. A hemicolectomy is a partial excision of the colon.

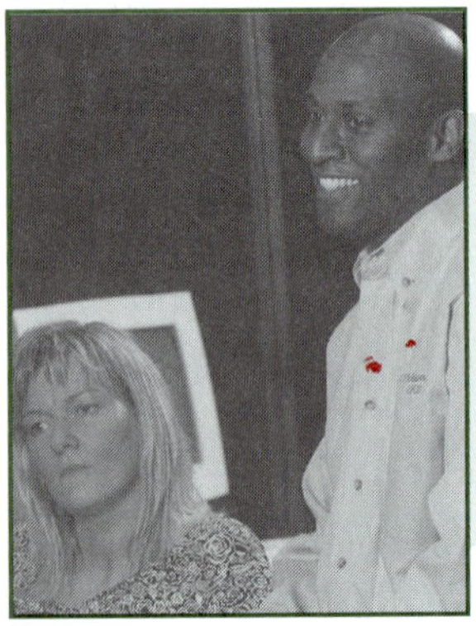

FROM THE TRENCHES

Betty

"[In] our profession, you never stop learning. I've been [in coding] for over 15 years, and I'm always learning something new, whether it be from one of my students or from going to seminars. These change every year with us, so we always have to be updated."

7-11C OPERATIVE REPORT, HEMICOLECTOMY

Some time later, the patient is taken to the operating room for a hemicolectomy by Dr. Sanchez. When assigning the diagnoses codes to this report, be certain to use the pathology report for the most definitive diagnosis. This report is an example how if you use only the surgical report, you would report only the ascending colon adenocarcinoma; but upon referencing the pathology report you will see that there is metastasis from the primary site to the mesentery, the secondary site.

PATIENT: Gloria Hathorne

PRIMARY PHYSICIAN: Ronald Green, M.D.

SURGEON: Gary Sanchez, M.D.

PREOPERATIVE DIAGNOSIS: Adenocarcinoma of the ascending colon

POSTOPERATIVE DIAGNOSIS: Perforated adenocarcinoma of the ascending colon with attachment to the lateral abdominal wall

PROCEDURE PERFORMED: Right hemicolectomy with anastomosis

ANESTHESIA: General

INDICATIONS FOR SURGERY: Mrs. Hathorne is a 40-year-old white female who is having difficulties with her bowels. The patient was found to have an adenocarcinoma of the ascending colon that was proven by biopsy. The patient is taken to the operating room after a bowel prep yesterday for surgery.

PROCEDURE: The patient was prepped and draped in the usual manner. A midline abdominal incision was made. The patient has had previous surgeries, which included an appendectomy, hysterectomy, cholecystectomy, and radiation treatment to her abdomen for lymphoma. The patient had adhesions from her multiple previous surgeries and radiation therapy. These adhesions were taken down sharply using the Bovie cautery and Metzenbaum scissors. After this was done, the right colon was elevated using the Bovie cautery to divide the peritoneum on the right lateral gutter. The colon was then brought up into the operative area. The small bowel ileum was adherent down into the pelvis from her previous surgeries. These were taken down using Metzenbaum scissors and then allowed the small bowel to be freed up into the incision area. The dissection was carried to the transverse colon in about the midpoint of the transverse colon. A Penrose drain was then placed around the transverse colon and also one around the ileum. During the dissection of the cancer from the lateral abdominal wall, the cancer was firmly adherent to the abdominal wall. When this was finally freed up, there was an opening in the colon, which appeared to be a perforation of the area of cancer, which had been sealed by the lateral abdominal wall. No gross evidence of any tumor on the abdominal wall was seen. The opening in the colon was closed with a 2-0 silk suture. Next the mesentery was scored using the Bovie cautery. The mesentery was clamped and divided using Kelly clamps and tied with interrupted 2-0 silk sutures. After this was completed, the bowel clamp was placed on the proximal ileum and also on the distal colon. Kocher clamps were placed on the specimen side of the ileum and the colon. The colon and ileum were then transected, and the specimen was sent to pathology. An end-to-end anastomosis was then done. A two-layer closure was done. Interrupted 3-0 silk sutures were placed on either end of the anastomosis, and the posterior layer was then placed. All sutures were placed before they were tied. After this was completed, the inner layer was then run using a running 3-0 Vicryl suture using a locking stitch for the posterior layer and a running stitch on the anterior layer. After this was completed, the bowel clamps were removed. The anterior outer layer was then placed using interrupted 3-0 silk sutures. There was an excellent anastomosis following this procedure. The opening in the mesentery was closed with a running 2-0 Vicryl suture. The operative area was thoroughly irrigated. There were a few small bleeders that were found after the irrigation, and these were controlled by 2-0 silk ties or Bovie cautery. An additional adhesion was taken down of the omentum attached to the pelvis down into the pelvic gutter, and this was freed. After all the adhesions were taken down, *(Don't be tempted to code the adhesions separately)* the operative area again was thoroughly irrigated. The bowel was returned to the abdomen. The anastomosis was again checked and was excellent. The abdominal incision was then closed with a running no. 1 looped PDS suture for the fascia and the peritoneum in a single-layer closure. The subcutaneous tissues were then thoroughly irrigated, and the skin was closed with skin clips. The patient tolerated the operation and returned to recovery in stable condition.

Pathology Report Later Indicated: See Report 7-10D.

7-11C: ileum removed

SERVICE CODE(S): 44160

DX CODE(S): ______________________

7-11D PATHOLOGY REPORT

PATIENT: Gloria Hathorne

PRIMARY PHYSICIAN: Ronald Green, M.D.

SURGEON: Gary Sanchez, M.D.

PATHOLOGIST: Morton Monson, M.D.

CLINICAL HISTORY: Ascending colon adenocarcinoma

SPECIMEN RECEIVED: Right colon

GROSS DESCRIPTION:

The specimen is labeled with the patient's name and "right ascending colon" and consists of a right hemicolectomy specimen including 4 cm of distal ileum including ileocecal valve with attached cecum and approximately 10 cm of colon. Also attached is mesentery. The appendix is absent. Approximately 5 cm from the ileocecal valve, a constricting lesion is noted grossly, which puckers the serosal surface. Cut section reveals a somewhat excavating circumferential mass measuring approximately 3 cm in length that consists of gritty tan tissue. On cut section, it appears that the above-described lesion penetrates the full thickness of the bowel wall on the mesenteric side. Multiple small lymph nodes are found in the mesenteric fat and are placed in cassettes labeled 8-15.

MICROSCOPIC DESCRIPTION:

Sections of proximal and distal resection margins show no evidence of neoplasm. Sections of the previously described neoplasm consist of an excavating tumor consisting of small glandular strictures with abundant mucin production. The tumor infiltrates to the full thickness of the wall to the mesenteric fat. Several small foci of tumor are noted in the mesenteric fat. Sections of 11 lymph nodes show no evidence of neoplasm.

DIAGNOSIS:

Right hemicolectomy:

1. Moderately differentiated infiltrating adenocarcinoma with full-thickness penetration and multiple small discrete mesenteric metastatic nodules.
2. Twelve mesenteric lymph nodes showing no evidence of neoplasm.
3. Proximal and distal resection margins negative for tumor.

COMMENT: Although no tumor is seen in microscopically recognizable lymph nodes, several small tumor nodules are present in the mesenteric fat.

7-11D:

SERVICE CODE(S): ____________________

DX CODE(S): ____________________

CASE 7-12
7-12A Hospital Inpatient Service
7-12B Infectious Disease Consultation
7-12C Operative Report, Colonoscopy
7-12D Operative Report, Esophagogastroduodenoscopy
7-12E KUB
7-12F KUB
7-12G KUB
7-12H Discharge Summary

CASE 7-12

7-12A HOSPITAL INPATIENT SERVICE

In this next case, you will have the opportunity to code an extensive case (7-12A to 7-12H) for a patient initially admitted for nausea, vomiting, and diarrhea. The patient was in the hospital for 6 days and had multiple and varied services.

LOCATION: Hospital Inpatient

PATIENT: Maynard Peters

ATTENDING PHYSICIAN: George Orbitz, M.D.

Patient is being admitted primarily because of intractable nausea, vomiting, and diarrhea.

The patient is a 32-year-old white gentleman who was diagnosed as having type 1 diabetes mellitus at 12 years of age. His diabetes has been complicated by diabetic retinopathy/blindness with multiple eye laser treatments; diabetic vascular neuropathy/autonomic neuropathy manifested by significant gastroparesis and erectile dysfunction; and diabetic nephropathy. He has had a kidney and pancreas transplant performed in May 2001 and January 2002, respectively. According to the patient, he has not had any episodes of rejection of either organ per repeated biopsies.

History started around 1 to 2 weeks prior to admission, when the patient started to have intermittent episodes of diarrhea, which have been attributed to some irritable bowel syndrome component. During the course of his evaluation in the clinic and in the hospital, the patient was noted to have a significant cytomegalovirus infection, for which he was placed on ganciclovir intravenous treatment.

In the ensuing days, the patient continued to have persistent nausea, vomiting, and diarrhea. He has been coordinating his care with Dr. Jayco as well as with the transplant center in Denver. It is believed his diarrhea and other gastrointestinal symptoms stem primarily from either the cytomegalovirus infection and/or the intravenous ganciclovir treatment per se, thereby necessitating that his dose of ganciclovir be reduced to every 24 hours instead of every 12 hours as he had been taking. This dosage adjustment was done fairly recently, within the past 2 days.

The patient was seen by Dr. Jayco in the clinic on Monday and was advised to go to the emergency room, where he was given 2 L of intravenous fluids. After coming home, the patient relates that he continued to have persistent diarrhea, and this time he has had vague epigastric abdominal discomfort, nonradiating, not related to meals or change in position or bowel movements. On examination, he did not really have a surgical abdomen, as there is no evidence of rebound or guarding. Furthermore, his bowel sounds seem to be normal. A KUB was performed, however, which did show evidence of air fluid levels, which would be suggestive of small bowel obstruction. Please note that the serum potassium is 5.4.

At this time, the plan is to admit the patient to the medical floor. We will check his daily weights and his inputs and outputs, and we will give him IV fluids, mainly 0.9% normal saline infusing at a rate of 150 to 200 ml per hour. I will continue the same medications, including rapamycin, Prograf, and ganciclovir every 24 hours as he has been taking. We will ask Dr. Olanka from gastroenterology to evaluate the patient in the morning to see if he has any recommendations. With absence of significant distention of the abdomen, I do not feel compelled to place a nasogastric tube at this time. Again, it is possible that these gastrointestinal symptoms may stem primarily from a long-standing history of diabetic autonomic neuropathy/gastroparesis plus/minus ganciclovir treatment per se plus/minus cytomegalovirus infection. In the morning, Dr. Jayco will assume care from the nephrology standpoint, and he will be coordinating with the Denver transplant coordinators.

PAST MEDICAL/SURGICAL HISTORY:

1. Type 1 insulin-dependent diabetes mellitus
   - A. Diabetic retinopathy with multiple laser surgeries; status post vitrectomy right eye ×2, left eye ×1.
   - B. Diabetic vascular neuropathy, erectile dysfunction
   - C. Diabetic autonomic neuropathy, gastroparesis, gastroesophageal reflux disease, chronic nausea, and vomiting (?)
   - D. Diabetic nephropathy, history of hemodialysis requirement

2. Status post toenail surgery, right and left
3. Status post angiography, February 2001, showing minimal atherosclerotic disease with normal LV function and some LV dilatation
4. Hyperlipidemia
5. Chronic mild metabolic acidosis most likely relating to chronic renal insufficiency/pancreas transplant draining into the bladder
6. Depression
7. Asthma
8. Hypertension secondary to diabetic nephropathy/chronic renal insufficiency/renal failure

SOCIAL HISTORY: He is married and has two children. He is on disability, I believe. He denies any current or previous history of alcohol, tobacco, or intravenous or recreational drugs.

FAMILY HISTORY: Positive for heart disease. Negative for hypertension, diabetes, stroke, cancer, kidney disease, bleeding disorder, or dyscrasia. A cousin has had spina bifida, heart disease, and seizures. Mother was diagnosed as having Crohn's disease.

CURRENT MEDICATIONS:
1. Rapamycin 2 mg q.d.
2. Prograf 2 mg b.i.d.
3. Lipitor 10 mg q.h.s.
4. Aspirin 81 mg q.d.
5. Sodium bicarbonate 650 per tab, 2 tabs q.i.d.
6. Zoloft 100 mg q.d.
7. Ganciclovir IV q.24h (recently adjusted from 12h dosing; see note above).

ALLERGIES: ACE inhibitors apparently cause some swelling. Penicillin and sulfa medications cause rash.

LABORATORY TESTS: Sodium 135, potassium 5.4, chloride 98, CO_2 21, BUN and creatinine are 28/3.1, glucose 135, calcium 8.8. Hemogram shows an H&H of 12.5/37, WBC 8.6, and platelets 319. There is a slight left shift as neutrophils are 89.8%.

REVIEW OF SYSTEMS: CONSTITUTIONAL: No fever or chills. Positive weight loss. He appears to be fairly nourished. No night sweats. SKIN: No skin lesions. No active dermatosis. EYES: No eye discharge. No eye itching. Positive diabetic retinopathy/legally blind. ENT: No ear discharge. No hearing difficulty. No pharyngeal hyperemia, congestion, or exudate. LYMPH NODES: No lymphadenopathy in the neck, axillae, or groin. NEUROLOGIC: No headaches. No gait instability. No falls. No seizures. PSYCHIATRIC: No behavioral changes. NECK: No thyromegaly. RESPIRATORY: No cough. No colds. No hemoptysis. No shortness of breath. CARDIOVASCULAR: No chest pain. No palpitations. No orthopnea. No paroxysmal nocturnal dyspnea. GASTROINTESTINAL: Positive anorexia. Positive nausea. Positive vomiting. No dysphagia. No odynophagia. No constipation. Positive diarrhea. Positive abdominal pain. No fecal incontinence. Positive history of irritable bowel syndrome is questionable. No hematemesis. No hematochezia. No melena. GENITOURINARY: No urgency. No frequency. No dysuria. No hematuria. No urinary incontinence. No nocturia. No penile discharge. No penile lesion. Positive history of erectile dysfunction related to diabetic vascular neuropathy. MUSCULOSKELETAL: No joint pains. No muscle pain/weaknesses. HEMATOLOGIC: No bleeding tendencies. No purpura. No petechia. No ecchymosis. ENDOCRINOLOGIC: No heat/cold intolerance.

PHYSICAL EXAMINATION: Vital signs are stable. Blood pressure 120s/80s. Heart rate in the 80s to 90s. Respirations 20. He is afebrile. Normocephalic and atraumatic. Pink palpebral conjunctivae, anicteric sclerae. No nasal or aural discharge. Moist tongue and buccal mucosa. No pharyngeal hyperemia, congestion, or exudates. Supple neck. No lymphadenopathy. Symmetric chest expansion. No retractions. Positive rhonchi. No crackles or wheezes. S1 and S2 are distinct. No S3 or S4. Regular rate and rhythm. Abdomen: Positive bowel sounds, soft. No rebound. No guarding. Positive direct tenderness over the epigastrium only on deep palpation but not on light palpation. No abdominal bruits appreciated during this examination. Renal allograft appears to be nontender without any bruits appreciated. No edema. No arthritic changes noted on both upper and lower extremities. Pulses are fair.

ASSESSMENT/PLAN: Impression for this patient is as follows:
1. Nausea, vomiting, and diarrhea, questionable etiology.
   A. Gastroenteritis unlikely because of the chronic nature of his symptomatology.
   B. Medications, namely ganciclovir. Questionable Prograf. Will need to discuss with transplant coordinators. Will check Prograf levels. Agree with decreasing ganciclovir to every 24-hour dosing.
   C. Diabetic autonomic neuropathy/gastroparesis/irritable bowel syndrome, questionable.
   D. Cytomegalovirus infection per se.

At this time, plan is to hydrate the patient with IV fluids, namely, 0.9% normal saline. We will continue to monitor his chemistries, labs, etc.

Because of the air fluid levels on the KUB, which suggest a small bowel obstruction, I am going to ask Dr. Olanka from gastroenterology to give us his opinion regarding this patient. Please note this patient does not have any evidence of ileus or hypokalemia.

2. Chronic renal failure, hypertensive, (latest creatinine clearance is 43 ml/min with a creatinine of 1.8, total volume of 2000 ml, and 1.36 g proteinuria performed last month), status post kidney, pancreas transplant with no previous episodes of rejection. Will check urinary amylase because this patient's pancreas is allegedly draining into the urinary bladder. If urinary amylase is slow, this may suggest rejection. Please note that this patient's creatinine has been in the 2.8 to 3.1 range over the past several weeks to months. His baseline creatinine is in the 1.4 to 1.6 range.

Aggressive IV fluid hydration as noted above.

3. Hyperlipidemia. Continue Lipitor 10 mg at q.h.s.
   A. Questionable mild atherosclerotic heart disease (see past medical/surgical history). Continue aspirin 81 mg q.d.
   B. Mild chronic metabolic acidosis related to pancreatic drainage into the urinary bladder. Continue bicarbonate supplements.
   C. Depression. Continue Zoloft 100 mg q.d.

PLAN: As dictated above. Dr. Jayco will take over in the morning and will reassume care. Dr. Olanka of gastroenterology will evaluate the patient in the morning.

I have spent a total of 90 minutes evaluating and reviewing this patient's medical records and formulating a treatment strategy. An additional 20 minutes was spent discussing the case in great detail with the patient and his family.

7-12A:

SERVICE CODE(S): ______________________

DX CODE(S): ______________________

CASE 7-12A DISCUSSION

There are so many diagnoses to consider in this report. When deciding which diagnosis to report, consider why the patient initially presented for care. In an inpatient setting, all of the diagnoses would be reported, but in the outpatient setting, those conditions that prompted the encounter and demonstrate medical necessity are reported. Under the Assessment/Plan section of the report, the first-listed statement is the nausea, vomiting, and diarrhea, which must be reported as it was the primary reason for the patient presenting for care. There is a combination code for the nausea with vomiting and another code for the diarrhea. The hypertensive renal failure could be reported, as indicated in point 2 of the Assessment/Plan section of the report, and most coders would definitely report that. The diabetes with the diabetic retinopathy and neuropathy could be reported. The history of transplants (kidney, V42.0 and pancreas, V42.83) also has major impact on the care of this patient, so that also could be reported.

7-12B INFECTIOUS DISEASE CONSULTATION

On this report, the order of the diagnoses has changed. The physician lists as the first point under the Impression section the diarrhea and vomiting. There is no mention of the nausea on this report. In points 2 and 3, the kidney and pancreas transplants are noted with indication that the patient's immune system is depressed due to the transplants. When people undergo organ transplants, the patient is given immunosuppressants to decrease the likelihood of rejection of the transplanted organ.
The transplant status should be reported using V codes. You can find direction to the correct V codes by locating "Transplant" in the Index of the ICD-9-CM.

LOCATION: Hospital Inpatient

PATIENT: Maynard Peters

PHYSICIAN: Gordon Jayco, M.D.

CONSULTANT: Lou Lin, M.D.

REASON FOR REFERRAL: Diarrhea in an immunocompromised host.

IMPRESSION:

1. Two-week duration of diarrhea, vomiting, night sweats, and chills, progressing on ganciclovir.
2. Immune compromise secondary to transplantation.
3. Renal transplant with apparently a living related donor in May 2001 with a pancreatic cadaver transplant in December 2002 with drainage to the bladder in a patient who apparently is CMV positive and has not had any opportunistic infections or complications. Now on an immunosuppressive regimen of sirolimus and FK-506. For approximately 2 months after each transplant, the patient received a course of ganciclovir and a month or two ago completed 2 to 3 months of oral acyclovir for apparent herpes of the eye.
4. Hyperlipidemia
5. Diabetes mellitus type 1 with complications of retinopathy, vasculopathy, autonomic neuropathy, gastroparesis, and neuropathy
6. Chronic renal failure with a creatinine clearance of 43 in December 2002, status posttransplant as above
7. Hematuria, etiology unclear
8. Depression
9. Asthma
10. Hypertension
11. Coronary artery disease with an angiogram done in January 2001 when he had minimal coronary disease

RECOMMENDATIONS:

1. I think it is important that we try to make a diagnosis to see whether this is an infectious etiology versus a partial small bowel obstruction. He will need a colonoscopy and upper endoscopy. Certainly, if lesions are found, biopsy should be obtained for specific viral studies.
2. *C. difficile* toxin should be obtained.
3. Stool cultures and white blood cell stains should be obtained.
4. CMV titer of either a CMV P-65 or a quantitative CMV titer should be obtained.
5. CT scan
6. Consideration of surgical consultation as well

HISTORY OF PRESENT ILLNESS: This 32-year-old gentleman is status post renal transplant and pancreatic transplant in May 2001 and January 2002 for underlying diabetic nephropathy. His transplant has been uneventful. He has been on sirolimus and FK-506. First, he has had a chronic history of constipation followed by diarrhea for years, which he usually takes Imodium, which stops his diarrhea. About 2 weeks ago, he developed increasing diarrhea that was not responsive to Imodium with vomiting, night sweats, and chills. He was treated with acyclovir for a week and it had no effect. Apparently, he had a CMV titer that was positive at the transplant center in Denver and then was started on IV ganciclovir. Despite that, he continues to get worse with worsening diarrhea and cramps.

When seen in the emergency room, he was hydrated. He continues to have relapses with dehydration. Subsequently, he was admitted to the hospital for hydration as well as diagnosis. Because of this, an infectious disease consultation was obtained.

FAMILY HISTORY: Father died at age 39 of cardiac problems. Mother died at 76 and had recently been diagnosed with Crohn's disease. A cousin has spina bifida, heart disease, and seizures of unknown origin.

PAST MEDICAL HISTORY: He has had diabetes mellitus now for 19 years, on insulin. It has been complicated by retinopathy requiring multiple laser treatments. He is essentially blind. He had vasculopathy, autonomic neuropathy, gastroparesis, neuropathy, and nephropathy that eventually required the transplant. He also had a long history of irritable bowel syndrome, hyperlipidemia, depression, asthma, and hypertension. He has coronary artery disease. He had an angiogram in January 2001 that showed minimal disease. He had his transplant in May 2001, which was apparently a living related donor from his wife and a pancreatic cadaver transplant in January 2002 with drainage to the bladder. Apparently, he has not had any opportunistic infections. He was treated with prophylactic ganciclovir for 2 months, approximately after the kidney transplant and then again for about 2 months after the pancreatic transplant. About 2 months ago, he completed 2 to 3 months of acyclovir for what sounds like herpes of the eye.

MEDICATIONS: Besides the antirejection medications sirolimus and FK-506, he is on atorvastatin, an aspirin a day, Prevacid, and Zoloft.

ALLERGIES: ACE inhibitors cause swelling. Penicillin and sulfa cause manifestation of rash.

REVIEW OF SYSTEMS: Complete, negative except he has had a little bit of dyspnea related to this illness. He had some dysuria yesterday. Although he had some chronic low back pain and some chronic arthralgias, predominantly hip and shoulders, it seems to have become worse in the last week or two. OPHTHALMOLOGIC: Negative. OTOLARYNGOLOGIC: Negative. CARDIOVASCULAR: Negative. RESPIRATORY: Negative. GU: Negative. MUSCULOSKELETAL INTEGUMENTARY: Negative. NEUROLOGIC: Negative. PSYCHIATRIC: Negative. ENDOCRINE: Negative. HEMATOLOGIC: Negative. LYMPHATIC: Negative.

TRAVEL: No recent travel, hunting, or fishing.

ANIMAL EXPOSURE: He does have animal exposure to cats, dogs, and horses. He does not have any direct care of these.

SOCIAL HISTORY: He is married and has three children. No tobacco use. No alcohol use.

PHYSICAL EXAMINATION: He is alert. His T-max is 37.2. Pulse is 110. Respiratory rate is 22. Blood pressure is 126/75. HEENT: Head, nontraumatic. The tympanic membranes are clear bilaterally. The conjunctivae are clear. Red reflex is seen. Pupils are irregular, probably related to prior surgery. He has evidence of the fundus with multiple laser treatments. The nasal membranes are clear. The pharynx is clear. Moist mucous membranes. I do not hear a carotid bruit. NECK is supple. There is no cervical adenopathy. No thyroid tenderness. There is no supraclavicular adenopathy. Chest is symmetrical. PULMONARY exam is clear. There are no secondary muscles of respiration and no axillary or epitrochlear adenopathy. ABDOMEN: He is distended. I can hear tinkling bowel sounds. There is no tenderness with deep palpation. No rebound. There is no groin adenopathy. INTEGUMENTARY: No other rashes or eruptions.

LABORATORY DATA: He has a white count of 8.6, hemoglobin of 21.5, and platelet count of 319. Urinalysis showed 10-15 RBCs. Sodium was 135, potassium 5.4. BUN was 38. Creatinine was 3.1. His glucose was 135. Blood cultures: He had urine cultures, stool, and cultures done 2 months ago. Apparently, no pathogen has been identified.

I have discussed the case with Dr. Jayco, and we will implement the interventions.

7-12B:

SERVICE CODE(S): ____________________

DX CODE(S): ____________________

Cytomegalovirus

Cytomegalovirus (CMV) is a herpes virus that infects humans, monkeys, and rodents. CMV is also known as salivary gland virus. The virus produces unique large cells. Transmission is associated with close contact, not only sexual contact. It does not produce genital symptoms, but rather produces nonspecific and often mild clinical symptoms, such as colitis.

Infectious versus Noninfectious Colitis

When reporting infectious colitis, turn in the Index of the ICD-9-CM to the main term "Colitis," subterm "infectious," where you are directed to "009.0 *see also* Enteritis, due to, specific organism." When the "Enteritis, due to" is referenced, you are presented subterms that represent the various infectious agents that cause enteritis. These subterms will refer the coder to 001-009, Intestinal Infectious Diseases. **Infectious** colitis (009.0) includes the terms colitis, dysentery, enteritis, and gastroenteritis. 009.1 reports colitis of a **presumed** infectious origin. Codes 555-558, **Noninfectious** Enteritis and Colitis, is used to report intestinal conditions that are not due to an infectious agent. In the Index of the ICD-9-CM, under the main term "Colitis," note that the term "(noninfectious)" is in the list of terms that follow that main term entry. From this main term "Colitis," the coder is directed to the Tabular to reference 558.9. Also, under the main term "Enteritis," note that included in the list of terms is "(noninfectious)" with a direction to reference 558.9 in the Tabular.

7-12C OPERATIVE REPORT, COLONOSCOPY

LOCATION: Hospital Inpatient

PATIENT: Maynard Peters

ATTENDING PHYSICIAN: Gordon Jayco, M.D.

SURGEON: Daniel Olanka, M.D.

PROCEDURE: Colonoscopy with multiple biopsies

PREOPERATIVE DIAGNOSIS: Rule out cytomegalovirus colitis

POSTOPERATIVE DIAGNOSIS: Mild patchy erythema in the descending, sigmoid, and rectum, nonspecific, not characteristic of colitis

INDICATION: This is a 32-year-old white man with pancreatic and kidney transplant secondary to diabetes who presents with 1 week of diarrhea, abdominal cramping, and nausea and vomiting. He was treated with ganciclovir at the transplant center in Denver for presumed CMV enteritis based on rising CMV serology. He was not seen, however, by anyone. He presents now dehydrated and with creatinine of 3.1. The procedure is indicated to rule out CMV colitis.

PREOPERATIVE MEDICATION: Demerol 50 mg IV; Versed 4 mg IV

FINDINGS: The Pentax video colonoscope was inserted easily into the cecum. Ileocecal valve was identified. The appendiceal orifice was seen. The terminal ileum was entered a distance of 5 cm. No lesions were seen. Inspection of the cecum, ascending colon, hepatic flexure, transverse colon, and splenic flexure revealed no erythema, ulceration, exudate, or friability in the mucosa. Biopsies were obtained in the right colon of normal mucosa. The distal distending, sigmoid, and rectum revealed patchy erythema without ulceration, no friability, and really no loss of vascular pattern. There was erythematous area, nonspecific. Biopsies were obtained of these areas also. The patient tolerated the procedure well.

IMPRESSION: Nonspecific mild erythema in the distal descending, sigmoid, and rectum, not characteristic of CMV colitis. Biopsies of terminal ileum were benign as per pathology. Normal colon otherwise.

PLAN: Esophagogastroduodenoscopy.

7-12C:

SERVICE CODE(S): ______________________

DX CODE(S): ______________________

7-12D OPERATIVE REPORT, ESOPHAGOGASTRODUODENOSCOPY

In this report, the diagnosis changed to gastritis.

LOCATION: Hospital Inpatient

PATIENT: Maynard Peters

ATTENDING PHYSICIAN: Gordon Jayco, M.D.

SURGEON: Daniel Olanka, M.D.

OPERATIVE PROCEDURE: Esophagogastroduodenoscopy

PREOPERATIVE DIAGNOSIS: Rule out cytomegalovirus gastritis

POSTOPERATIVE DIAGNOSIS: Mild gastritis, nonspecific; biopsied

INDICATION: A 32-year-old white male with diabetes who had kidney and pancreatic transplant, presents with 1 week of nausea, vomiting, and diarrhea. He was treated for a presumptive CMV enteritis elsewhere with ganciclovir, and he continues to be ill. We just performed colonoscopy, which showed nonspecific erythema in the distal descending sigmoid and rectum.

PREOPERATIVE MEDICATION: As per colonoscopy.

FINDINGS: The Pentax video pediatric endoscope was passed without difficulty into the oropharynx. The gastroesophageal junction was seen at 42 cm. Inspection of the esophagus revealed no erythema, ulceration, exudate, friability, varices, or other mucosal abnormalities. The stomach proper was entered, and the endoscope advanced to the second duodenum. Inspection of the second duodenum, first duodenum, duodenal bulb, and pylorus revealed no abnormalities. Retroflexion revealed no lesions of the cardia or fundus. Inspection of the body revealed no abnormalities. The antrum revealed some patchy and linear erythema; no friability. There were some coffee-ground specks present. Biopsies were obtained, and photograph was obtained. The patient tolerated the procedure well.

IMPRESSION: Mild gastritis, biopsied.

PLAN: We placed a nasogastric tube for this patient because he is having severe vomiting of large amounts of liquids. Will treat the patient conservatively and hydrate him and see how he does, and then we will review the biopsy.

Pathology Report Later Indicated: Gastritis.

7-12D:

SERVICE CODE(S): ____________________

DX CODE(S): ____________________

7-12E KUB

A barium study is a contrast barium enema, also known as air-contrast barium enema, air-contrast study, or barium-contrast study of the colon.

LOCATION: Inpatient Hospital

PATIENT: Maynard Peters

PRIMARY PHYSICIAN: Gordon Jayco, M.D.

RADIOLOGIST: Morton Monson, M.D.

EXAMINATION OF: KUB

CLINICAL SYMPTOMS: Nausea, vomiting, and diarrhea in a patient with kidney and pancreas transplants.

KUB DONE PRIOR TO BARIUM STUDY: There is no prior study for comparison. No bony lesion is appreciated. There are surgical clips over the right side of vertebral body L5 and the right side of the sacrum. That is presumably either transplanted kidney or transplanted pancreas site. There are vascular or surgical clips over the left sacroiliac joint, midportion, and that is again either the site of the transplanted kidney or site of the pancreas transplant presumably. Bowel gas pattern is nonspecific. No distended bowel loops are seen. There is bowel gas from stomach to rectum. No enlargement of liver or spleen. No significant calcification seen. Entirety of pelvis not imaged on film.

IMPRESSION:
1. History of kidney and pancreas transplants
2. Nonspecific bowel gas pattern
3. Surgical clips, low abdomen/upper pelvis
4. No bony lesion seen

7-12E:

SERVICE CODE(S): ____________________

DX CODE(S): ____________________

7-12F KUB

Two days after the initial KUB, the patient was returned to the radiology department for a recheck.

LOCATION: Inpatient Hospital

PATIENT: Maynard Peters

ATTENDING PHYSICIAN: Gordon Jayco, M.D.

RADIOLOGIST: Morton Monson, M.D.

EXAMINATION OF: KUB

CLINICAL SYMPTOMS: Barium recheck in patient with diarrhea, vomiting in a patient with a history of kidney and pancreas transplant.

KUB, 8 A.M.: FINDINGS: There is barium throughout the decompressed colon to the level of the rectum. Gaseous distention of a few loops of small bowel that are of normal caliber in the midabdomen. NG tube with tip in the distal stomach. Surgical clips projected over the left aspect of the pelvis.

7-12F:

SERVICE CODE(S): ____________________

DX CODE(S): ____________________

7-12G KUB

The next day, the patient was returned to the radiology department for "barium in the belly," which refers to the previous day's results that indicated there was heavy barium residue in the colon. This residue would prevent clarity on visualization. Dr. Jayco wants the patient to have a CT scan.

LOCATION: Inpatient Hospital

PATIENT: Maynard Peters

ATTENDING PHYSICIAN: Gordon Jayco, M.D.

RADIOLOGIST: Morton Monson, M.D.

EXAMINATION OF: KUB

CLINICAL SYMPTOMS: Barium in belly in patient with diarrhea, vomiting in a patient with a history of kidney and pancreas transplant.

KUB: This is performed pre-CT to determine whether barium has cleared adequately to obtain a CT. This is 8:45 A.M. Comparison is made with previous study performed yesterday. Heavy barium is again seen within portions of the descending and sigmoid colon. This is decreased compared with the previous study; however, the heavy barium still would create a significant artifact. I would recommend that CT be rescheduled for perhaps tomorrow or Monday to ensure that this heavy barium is no longer present. The gastrointestinal air pattern is relatively nonspecific.

CONCLUSION: Residual heavy barium seen within portions of the transverse, descending, and sigmoid colon. It is decreased compared with the previous study, and yet still a significant amount is present, which I believe would create significant artifact on the CT scan that is planned. I would recommend delaying it until this barium has cleared.

7-12G:

SERVICE CODE(S): ____________________

DX CODE(S): ____________________

7-12H DISCHARGE SUMMARY

LOCATION: Inpatient Hospital

PATIENT: Maynard Peters

ATTENDING PHYSICIAN: Gordon Jayco, M.D.

FINAL DIAGNOSES:

1. Small-bowel obstruction, etiology to be determined
2. Dehydration, secondary to no. 1
3. Acute renal failure, secondary to no. 1, recovering
4. Status post kidney transplant
5. Status post pancreas transplant
6. Diabetes mellitus type 1
7. Immunocompromised state, secondary to transplantation, hyperlipidemia
8. History of asthma
9. Minimal history of coronary artery disease
10. Metabolic acidosis and electrolyte imbalance, secondary to acute renal failure

HOSPITAL COURSE: This patient was admitted for dehydration, electrolyte imbalance, and acute renal failure superimposed on his living unrelated donor kidney transplant and pancreas transplant. The kidney was significantly involved, and the pancreas was not affected. They were on the mend during his hospital course. He received electrolyte repletion. He had both ends scoped and was believed not to have CMV colitis, for which he was being empirically treated. *C. difficile* was negative, and there was no other obvious explanation for his problem except that we suspected a partial small-bowel obstruction on admission. This did not resolve. It actually got worse, and the situation was severe enough for us to proceed with our evacuation plan, which was devised on Friday; that is, if he did not continue to get better, we would transfer him to the primary transplant center for further evaluation. There was an area in the middle of the small bowel that was abnormal and that we could not visualize well, and we were trying to get a CT scan done, but his barium was not cleaning out properly. In any case, that will be resolved at the transplant center.

Time spent preparing and reviewing his chart was 30 minutes.

7-12H:

SERVICE CODE(S): ____________________

DX CODE(S): ____________________

Laparoscopic Procedures

Laparoscopic procedures are those in which a scope is inserted into the abdomen by way of small incisions as illustrated in **Figure 7-4.** Trocar ports are introduced. The port is a sharp-ended hollow tube that is inserted into the abdomen and serves as an entry point for the scope. The surgeon will place additional trocar ports as needed to view the internal structures from the correct angle and to insert instruments as needed. The number of ports has no influence on the code choice. The physician then performs the procedure by means of manipulation of the instruments inserted through the ports. Many abdominal procedures can be accomplished using this less invasive method that reduces the recovery time for the patient and is less painful because the incision size is reduced. These procedures are often done in an ambulatory surgery center, that is, at the hospital, clinic, or free-standing surgical center. The patients seen in these centers are outpatients, even if the center is part of a hospital. The physician reports his or her services, and the hospital reports the facility service.

Closed Procedures Converted to Open Procedures

V code V64.41 reports operative procedures that began as a closed procedure (a procedure being performed by means of scope) that was converted to an open procedure (operation completed through an incision). Also note that V64.1 is available for assignment for surgical or other procedures not carried out because of contraindications. Contraindication means literally "against indication" that would be recommended by the physician. V64.2 is a surgical procedure not carried out because of the patient's decision. V64.3 is assigned for procedures not carried out for other reasons. The V code is sequenced last.

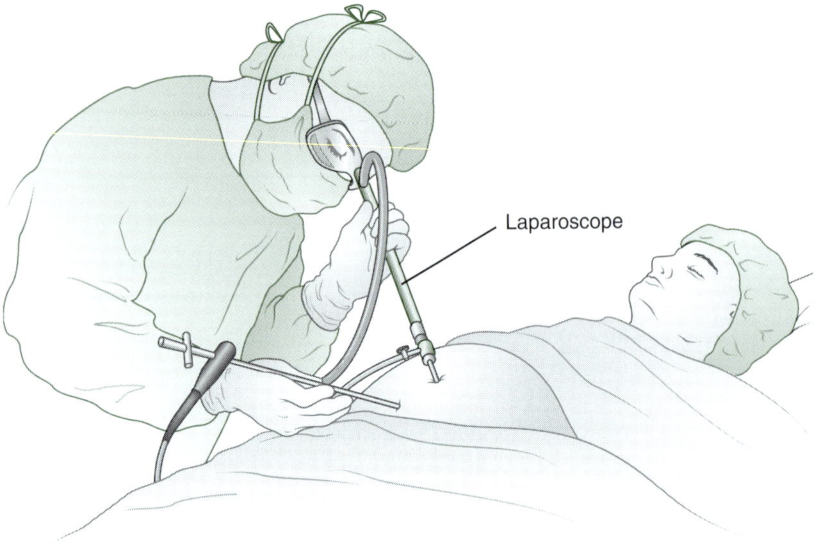

FIGURE 7-4 Laparoscopic procedure.

CASE 7-13
7-13A Operative Report, Appendectomy

CASE 7-13

7-13A OPERATIVE REPORT, APPENDECTOMY

°In this report, note that there was a complication (see highlighted area on the report) in which a small serosal tear was created by one of the surgical instruments (Kitner). This is reported with two codes, one for the complication (998.x) and one for the location of the complication (the tear). Begin the code assignment process for the location of the complication in the Index of the ICD-9-CM under the main term "Injury" and subterm by location of the injury. You will be directed to the Tabular to assign the code. Never code directly from the Index.

LOCATION: Outpatient Hospital

PATIENT: Samantha Young

PHYSICIAN: Larry Friendly, M.D.

PREOPERATIVE DIAGNOSIS: Colitis, terminal ileitis, and possible appendicitis.

POSTOPERATIVE DIAGNOSIS: Acute appendicitis. No evidence of abscess or peritonitis. No pus in the abdomen.

PROCEDURE PERFORMED: Laparoscopic abdominal exploration, laparoscopic mobilization of the cecum converted to open appendectomy.

SPECIMEN: Appendix

COMPLICATIONS: A small serosal tear in the terminal ileum was a retraction injury. This was repaired during the open part of the case with 3-0 silk.

ESTIMATED BLOOD LOSS: Less than 100 cc

ANESTHESIA: General endotracheal with 30 cc of Marcaine local augmentation.

PROCEDURE IN DETAIL: After good general endotracheal anesthesia, the patient was prepped and draped in the usual sterile fashion. A Foley and OT tube were both placed to decompress the stomach and also the bladder. A small infraumbilical incision was made, and under direct vision the fascia was nicked. The Veress needle was placed in the fascia, and the abdomen was insufflated to 16 Torr. After this, the fascial incision was lengthened, and a no. 10 trocar was placed. The camera was placed through this, and the abdomen was inspected. The cecum was quite inflamed. The base of the appendix was noted. The appendix itself was stuck down to the cecum. The area of terminal ileum just adjacent to the cecum was inflamed. The cecum was mobilized, and the peritoneal reflection was taken down. This was done with hot scissors. Care was taken not to injure bowel. The ovary was inspected and was normal. The appendix was felt to be quite friable, and there was a small serosal tear created in the ileum with the Kitner while mobilizing the cecum (*this represents a complication during surgery*). We were unable to determine laparoscopically whether this is just a serosal tear, and additionally the tissue was so friable that we were not confident that we would be able to close the stump of the appendix with an endoscopic stapler. Therefore, the decision was made to open the abdomen. This was done with appendiceal incision. A Rocky-Davis incision was made after anesthetizing the area with Marcaine. The external oblique and transversus abdominis fascia was incised, and a muscle-sparing technique was applied. The peritoneum was entered, and the cecum was brought up into the wound. The base of the appendix was identified, and it was so friable that we could not simply tie off the base of the appendix and amputate the appendix distally. It was necessary to close the cecum where the appendix was attached and to divide the appendix off the cecum. This was done with running 3-0 Vicryl. After this, some imbricating 3-0 silk stitches were placed. Attention was then turned to the serosal injury. This indeed turned out to be just serosa. This was on the terminal ileum. The serosal injury was repaired with interrupted 3-0 silk. Next the abdomen was irrigated and pneumoperitoneum was sucked out. The pneumoperitoneum was released. The two ports, the no. 10 port and the no. 5 subport, were removed. The camera port was also removed. This was done prior to opening the abdomen. All the fascial stitches were used to close the umbilical port and also the left no. 10 port sites. The appendiceal wound was closed in layers with the peritoneum, and two layers of fascia were closed separately. The skin was closed with 4-0 Vicryl. Steri-Strips and sterile dressings were applied. The patient tolerated the procedure well, and sponge and needle counts were correct. She was extubated in the operating room and returned to the recovery room in good condition.

7-13A:

SERVICE CODE(S): ______________________

DX CODE(S): ______________________

Cholecystectomy

Removal of the gallbladder, **cholecystectomy**, is a procedure performed for diseased or malfunctioning gallbladder conditions. The procedure can be performed either open (47600-47620) or laparoscopic (47562-47570, **Figure 7-5**). The CPT codes are divided based on the method (open/laparoscopic) and the extent of the procedure (with or without exploration of the common bile duct, repairs, removal of portion of bile duct or intestine). The preferred method continues to be the open cholecystectomy due to a higher complication rate from hemorrhage or bile leakage following laparoscopic procedures. One benefit of the laparoscopic procedure is that the hospital stay is an average of 4 days compared with the more invasive open procedure with a hospital stay of 7 days.

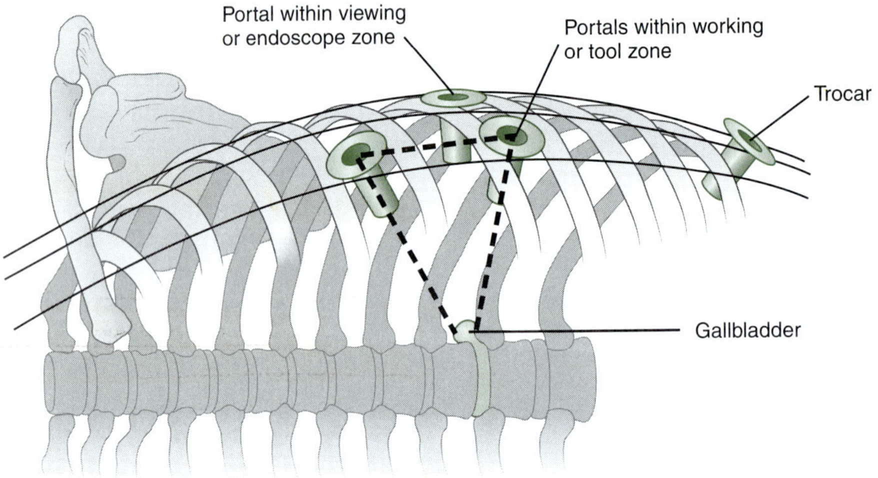

FIGURE 7-5 Laparoscopic cholecystectomy.

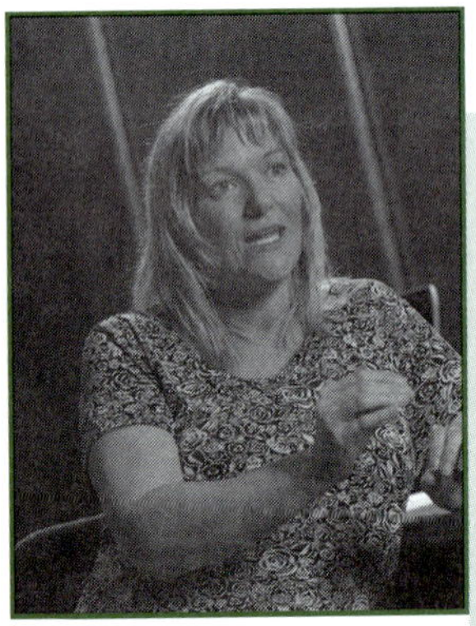

FROM THE TRENCHES

Betty

What advice would you give an entry-level coder?

"Ask questions. There's no such thing as a stupid question ... Ask your physician. Ask the nurses. Ask the insurance companies. Ask anybody that you can talk to if you don't understand something. Ask or you're never going to understand."

Terry

"Don't be afraid to use your resources. You're not on your own as an entry-level coder. There are a lot of people that have walked before you that are willing to help ... the path to finding the answer might not be in the book. You need to use your resources."

CASE 7-14
7-14A Operative Report, Cholecystectomy

CASE 7-14

7-14A OPERATIVE REPORT, CHOLECYSTECTOMY

The patient in this case presents with biliary dyskinesia (gallbladder dysfunction). The gallbladder of a patient with biliary dyskinesia appears normal on ultrasound scan, but when the gallbladder is stimulated to contract with food or with the stimulating hormone CCK, the gallbladder does not contract properly. Another diagnostic tool often used is the HIDA scan, which is a special type of isotope scan used to visualize the gallbladder empty (ejection fraction). The patient in the following case has an abnormal CCK and HIDA and is having the gallbladder removed.

LOCATION: Outpatient Hospital

PATIENT: Karen Daniels

PHYSICIAN: Larry Friendly, M.D.

PREOPERATIVE DIAGNOSIS: Biliary dyskinesia

POSTOPERATIVE DIAGNOSIS: Biliary dyskinesia

PROCEDURE PERFORMED: Laparoscopic cholecystectomy

ANESTHESIA: General

INDICATION: The patient is a 39-year-old female who presents with an abnormal CCK HIDA scan. She presents today for elective laparoscopic cholecystectomy. She understands the risks of bleeding, infection, possible damage to the biliary system, and possible conversion to open procedure, and she wishes to proceed.

PROCEDURE: The patient was brought to the operating table and placed under general anesthesia. Foley catheter and orogastric tubes were inserted, and she was prepped and draped sterilely. A supraumbilical skin incision was made with a no. 11 blade, and dissection was carried down through subcutaneous tissues. Bluntly, midline fascia was grasped with a Kocher clamp, and 0 Vicryl sutures were placed on either side of the midline fascia. The Veress needle was then inserted into the abdominal cavity; drop test confirmed placement within the peritoneal space. The abdomen was insufflated with carbon dioxide, and a 10-mm trocar port and laparoscope were introduced, showing no damage to the underlying viscera. Under direct vision, three additional trocar ports were placed, one upper midline 10 mm, two right upper quadrant 5 mm. The gallbladder was grasped and elevated from its fossa. The cystic duct and artery were dissected and doubly clipped proximally and distally, dividing them with the scissors. The gallbladder was then shelled from its fossa using electrocautery and brought up and out of the upper midline incision. The abdomen was irrigated with saline until returns were clear. There was no bleeding from the liver bed. Clips were in with no evidence of bleeding. When we were removing the final port, we could see down in the right groin, and she had small, indirect inguinal hernia, which was about 3 mm in size. We removed the remaining trocar port with no evidence of bleeding, closed the supraumbilical and upper midline ports and fascial defects with interrupted 0 Vicryl sutures, and closed the skin at all port sites with subcuticular 4-0 undyed Vicryl. Steri-Strips and sterile bandages were applied.

Pathology Report Later Indicated: Benign tissue

7-14A:

SERVICE CODE(S): ____________________

DX CODE(S): ____________________

could report w/550.90

CASE 7-15
7-15A Surgical Consultation
7-15B Emergency and Outpatient Record
7-15C Critical Care
7-15D Operative Report, Ulcer and Cholecystitis
7-15E Intraoperative Cholangiogram
7-15F Pathology Report
7-15G Discharge Summary

CASE 7-15

7-15A SURGICAL CONSULTATION

In Case 7-12, you coded a case with extensive inpatient services for Maynard Peters. In this case, you will code these same types of services, except these services are on an outpatient and inpatient basis.

LOCATION: Outpatient Clinic

PATIENT: Alma Kincaid

PHYSICIAN: Larry Friendly, M.D.

REASON FOR CONSULTATION: Alma is in the clinic today after being referred to us from Dr. Alanda for a nonhealing gastric ulcer.

HISTORY OF PRESENT ILLNESS: She is a 60-year-old white female who states that she has had an ulcer since March 2000. She has failed medical treatment with both Zantac and Prilosec. She has had several upper endoscopies, which revealed a large ulcer at the greater curvature of the antrum. A biopsy was taken, which was benign. She has also tested negative for *Helicobacter pylori.* There has been no healing of this ulcer since it was discovered. On January 30, she underwent an exploratory laparoscopy. This all turned out to be normal also. She denies any hematemesis. She denies any nausea; however, she is unable to eat secondary to the pain. She states she has been basically living off of Ensure for the past few months and has lost quite a bit of weight. She denies any blood in her stool. She denies any fever or chills.

CURRENT MEDICATIONS:
1. Prilosec, 1 b.i.d.
2. Zantac, 1 b.i.d.
3. Tylenol as needed
4. Tylox as needed for pain

ALLERGIES:
1. Penicillin
2. Toradol

PHYSICAL EXAMINATION: Neck is supple and without lymphadenopathy. There is no supraclavicular or infraclavicular and lymphadenopathy. Lungs are distant breath sounds but clear. Heart: S1 and S2 heard. No apparent murmurs are noted. Regular rate and rhythm. Abdomen is soft and moderately tender in the epigastric area with palpation. Bowel sounds are positive. Two well-healing port sites from her laparoscopy are noted, with no signs of infection. Extremities: No edema is noted. Dorsalis pedis and posterior tibial pulses are palpable and symmetric.

IMPRESSION: Nonhealing gastric ulcer, failure of medical treatment.

PLAN: At this time, we would like to obtain an upper gastrointestinal series on this patient. This still could be cancer until proven otherwise. Once we have this and re-evaluate, the patient will probably have to undergo a partial gastrectomy. The patient is willing to proceed with this, and she understands the risks and benefits of the procedure. We will discuss this with her after we get the upper gastrointestinal results. We will also have her seen by internal medicine for clearance for surgery.

7-15A:
SERVICE CODE(S): ____________________

DX CODE(S): ____________________

7-15B EMERGENCY AND OUTPATIENT RECORD

LOCATION: Outpatient Hospital

PATIENT: Alma Kincaid

PRIMARY CARE PHYSICIAN: Leslie Alanda, M.D.

EMERGENCY DEPARTMENT PHYSICIAN: Paul Sutton, M.D.

SUBJECTIVE: This 60-year-old white female is currently diagnosed with gastric ulcer and is having workup for potential surgical treatment. She also has gastroesophageal reflux disease.

MEDICATIONS: She is taking Prilosec, Zantac, amitriptyline, and p.r.n. GI cocktails.

ALLERGIES: She has allergies to penicillin and Toradol.

She presents acutely in the Emergency Room stating that she is scheduled in the morning for some x-ray procedures for which she has to be NPO. She is having significant abdominal discomfort and is wondering whether she can get something for pain until she has the procedures done in the morning. She is scheduled for 8 o'clock; apparently, upper GI. She is also scheduled for a preoperative evaluation by Dr. Green and is going to be seeing Dr. Sanchez. She is a chronic smoker who has chronic obstructive pulmonary disease, being evaluated regarding that prior to surgery.

OBJECTIVE: She is afebrile. Blood pressure is elevated at 159/78. She is obviously uncomfortable. She has tenderness in the abdominal area. There is slight guarding but no rebound tenderness. The ABDOMINAL EXAM is otherwise grossly unremarkable.

ASSESSMENT:
1. Abdominal pain
2. Gastric ulcer

PLAN: We gave her 100 mg of Demerol and 100 mg of Vistaril IM, which did afford some improvement. She was discharged with a recommendation to return here if she has increasing problems. Otherwise, plan on following up for evaluation in the morning.

7-15B:

SERVICE CODE(S): ____________________

DX CODE(S): ____________________

7-15C CRITICAL CARE

Dr. Alanda, Alma Kincaid's primary care physician, requested a consultation from Dr. Green, whose caseload includes many of the critical care patients for the clinic, regarding the pending gastric resection.

LOCATION: Outpatient Clinic

PATIENT: Alma Kincaid

PRIMARY CARE PHYSICIAN: Leslie Alanda, M.D.

CONSULTANT: Ronald Green, M.D.

Dr. Alanda asked me to evaluate the patient for preparation for pending gastric resection. The patient was examined and the chart reviewed.

HISTORY OF PRESENT ILLNESS: She has been having problems with recurrent peptic ulcer disease in spite of therapy with Zantac and Prilosec. She had several endoscopies, which revealed a large ulcer, which was reported to be benign. The patient was also noted to have a slightly elevated CEA of 11. Two months ago, the patient underwent laparoscopy, which turned out to be normal as well. There were no signs of any lymphadenopathy.

PAST SURGICAL HISTORY:
1. Hysterectomy
2. Tubal ligation

The patient never has problems with surgery or anesthesia.

SOCIAL HISTORY: Positive for smoking. The patient denies alcohol abuse. She smokes about a pack per day, with a total of a 40-pack-year history.

FAMILY HISTORY: Negative for colonic carcinoma, premature coronary artery disease, but positive for severe peptic ulcer disease in her sister.

ALLERGIES: Penicillin and Toradol

REVIEW OF SYSTEMS: Negative for melena, hematochezia, and hematemesis

PHYSICAL EXAMINATION: demonstrates a slender white female in no acute distress. She is uncomfortable, however, because of epigastric discomfort. Her neck is supple. There is no thyromegaly or regional lymphadenopathy. No subclavicular or supraclavicular lymph nodes. ENT is within normal limits. Eyes: Sclerae anicteric. Conjunctivae are pale. Funduscopic exam shows no AV nicking, hemorrhages, exudates, or papilledema. Chest is barrel-shaped without dullness to percussion but with rhonchi scattered throughout the lung fields. Prolonged expiratory phase was noted. Cardiac exam: Regular rhythm. Distant heart sounds, 1/6 systolic ejection murmur at the base. Abdomen is soft and tender to palpation. Epigastric area without rebound, tenderness, or guarding. Liver span is 7 cm; edge at right costal margin. Aorta diameter is normal. Extremities: No edema, cyanosis, or clubbing. Neurologic exam is nonfocal.

REVIEW OF LABORATORY ANALYSIS revealed hypercalcemia of 10.3, which is probably exaggerated by a low albumin and is likely to be more significant than that. Creatinine is 0.5. AST is 15. Carcinoembryonic antigen is 11.5. *H. pylori* is 4.8 three months ago.

IMPRESSION/PLAN: Nonhealing peptic ulcer disease. Patient's doctor increased her Prilosec to twice daily and is continuing Zantac at the present dose. In fact, one might increase it to 300 mg b.i.d. if necessary. There is certainly need to rule out ZE and hyperparathyroidism in the source of the patient's nonhealing ulcer. C-terminal PTH will be checked along with ionized calcium. One might plan a parahyperthyroidectomy simultaneous with gastrectomy should patient have high PTH, which I suspect will be the case, although in the case of treatment with H_2 blockers and Prilosec, a gastrin level might be elevated. Anyhow, we will check it and make sure that it is not extreme. If the gastrin level is very high, one might consider complete gastrectomy rather than a partial one on the presumption of

Zollinger-Ellison syndrome. The patient will be reevaluated after results of the aforementioned tests are available and scheduled for surgery. Elevated CEA is bothersome. She has had no colonoscopy for some time; if it is again elevated, one might consider colonoscopy simultaneously during the same admission. I am concerned with her pulmonary status. She is advised to curtail her cigarette consumption as low as possible and to switch to low-tar nicotine cigarettes in the interim. Once she is admitted, therapy with beta-agonists and Atrovent will be immediately initiated, and the patient will be started on incentive spirometry.

Thank you for letting me see this interesting patient. We discussed the aforementioned problem with Dr. Sanchez, who will hold surgery for one week until all laboratory analyses are completed. A total of 135 minutes was spent with patient, and going over data; 55 of those minutes was spent consulting the patient.

7-15C:

SERVICE CODE(S): ____________________

DX CODE(S): ____________________

7-15D OPERATIVE REPORT, ULCER AND CHOLECYSTITIS

The patient is admitted by Dr. Alanda for an operative procedure for the duodenal ulcer. Dr. Sanchez is the general surgeon who will perform the procedures. You will be reporting a partial gastrectomy with gastrojejunostomy, vagotomy, and cholecystectomy with cholangiogram, with the diagnoses of duodenal ulcer and cholecystis to support the medical necessity for the three procedures.

LOCATION: Inpatient Hospital

PATIENT: Alma Kincaid

ATTENDING PHYSICIAN: Leslie Alanda, M.D.

SURGEON: Gary Sanchez, M.D. ①

② PREOPERATIVE DIAGNOSIS: Nonhealing duodenal ulcer. Chronic cholecystitis.

POSTOPERATIVE DIAGNOSIS: Nonhealing duodenal ulcer. Chronic cholecystitis.

PROCEDURES PERFORMED:

1. Exploratory laparotomy
2. Partial gastrectomy (antrectomy) w/#4
3. Truncal vagotomy
4. Gastrojejunostomy
5. Cholecystectomy with intraoperative cholangiogram

INDICATION: The patient is a 60-year-old female who presented with a nonhealing gastric ulcer. She has had symptoms for about a year. She complains of epigastric pain. She failed medical therapy with Prilosec and therapy for *H. pylori.* Biopsy of the ulcer showed it to be benign. The patient had a negative workup for gastrinoma. Calcium level was also normal. The patient now presents for exploratory laparotomy and partial gastrectomy. The risks and benefits were discussed with the patient in detail. She understood and agreed to proceed.

PROCEDURE: The patient was brought to the operating room. Her abdomen was prepped and draped in a sterile fashion. A midline umbilical incision was made. The peritoneal cavity was entered. Initial inspection of the peritoneal cavity showed normal liver, spleen, colon, and small bowel. There was an ulcer along the first portion of the duodenum just beyond the pylorus with some scarring. There was also an ulcer in the posterior part of the duodenal bulb, which was penetrating to the pancreas. We started dissection along the greater curvature of the stomach. Vessels were ligated with 2-0 silk ties. There was an enlarged lymph node along the greater curvature of the stomach, which was sent for frozen section. It proved to be a benign lymph node. This was the only enlarged node found during dissection. We then proceeded with truncal vagotomy. The anterior vagus and posterior vagus were identified. They were clipped proximally and distally, and a segment of each nerve was excised and sent for frozen section. A segment of both vagus nerves was excised and confirmed by frozen section. An incision was made around the gastrohepatic ligament. The mesentery along the lesser curvature of the stomach was dissected. The vessels were ligated with 2-0 silk ties along the lesser curvature of the stomach. A Kocher maneuver was performed to aid mobilization. The pancreas was completely normal. No masses were seen in the pancreas. There was penetration of the ulcer in the superior part of the head of the pancreas. Dissection was continued posterior to the stomach. The adhesions posterior to the stomach were taken down. The ulcer was in the posterior segment of the duodenal bulb just beyond the pylorus and it had penetrated the pancreas. All the posterior layer of the ulcer that was left adherent to the pancreas was shaved off. The stomach was divided with the GIA stapler so that the complete antrum would be in the specimen. The duodenum was divided between clamps. The stomach pylorus and first part of the duodenum were sent to pathology for examination. Then the duodenal stump was closed with running suture. Using 3-0 Lembert sutures, the posterior wall of the ulcer was incorporated for duodenal closure. The base of the duodenum was rolled over the ulcer, and it was all-incorporating to the duodenal closure. Our next step was to proceed with cholecystectomy. The gallbladder was separated from the liver, reflected, and taken down, and the gallbladder was divided from the liver with blunt dissection and cautery. The cystic artery was doubly ligated with silk. The cystic duct was identified. The cystic duct and gallbladder junction and gallbladder ducts were identified. Intraoperative cholangiogram was performed showing free flow of bile into the intrahepatic duct and into the duodenum. No leaks were seen. The cystic duct was doubly ligated, and the gallbladder was sent to pathology. The staple line in the proximal stomach was oversewn with 3-0 silk Lembert sutures. A retrocolic isoperistaltic Hofmeister-type gastrojejunostomy was performed on the remaining stomach and loop of jejunum. This was an isoperistaltic end-to-side two-layer anastomosis with 3-0 chromic and 3-0 silk. The stomach was secured to the transverse mesocolon with several interrupted silk sutures to prevent any herniation along the retrocolic space. The anastomosis had a good lumen and good blood supply. There was no twist along the anastomosis. Prior to finishing the anastomosis, a nasogastric tube was placed along the afferent limb of the jejunum to decompress the duodenum and prevent blowout of the duodenal stump. Extra holes were made in the NG tube to provide adequate drainage. The anastomosis was marked with two clips on each side, and a Jackson-Pratt drain was placed over the duodenal stump. The peritoneal cavity was irrigated until clear. Hemostasis was adequate. The fascia was then closed with interrupted 0 Ethibond sutures. Skin edges were approximated with staples. Subcutaneous tissues were irrigated before closure. Estimated blood loss throughout the procedure was 200 ml. IV fluids: 3400 ml. Urine output: 840 ml.

FINDINGS:
1. Nonhealing benign ulcer in the posterior duodenal bulb penetrating into the head of the pancreas.
2. Partial gastrectomy (antrectomy performed) and excision of the pylorus, first portion of the duodenum along with ulcer.
3. Hofmeister-type retrocolic isoperistaltic gastrojejunostomy.
4. Posterior wall of the ulcer that was penetrating into the pancreas incorporated into closure of the duodenal stump.
5. Truncal vagotomy performed with intraoperative frozen section confirming both vagus nerves.
6. Cholecystectomy performed with normal intraoperative cholangiogram.
7. Jackson-Pratt drain placed over the duodenal stump.

Pathology Report Later Indicated: See Report 7-15F.

7-15D:

SERVICE CODE(S): ____________________

DX CODE(S): ____________________

7-15E INTRAOPERATIVE CHOLANGIOGRAM

LOCATION: Inpatient Hospital

PATIENT: Alma Kincaid

ATTENDING PHYSICIAN: Leslie Alanda, M.D.

SURGEON: Gary Sanchez, M.D.

RADIOLOGIST: Morton Monson, M.D.

DIAGNOSIS: Chronic cholecystitis

INTRAOPERATIVE CHOLANGIOGRAM: Two views were obtained portably in the Operating Room during the intraoperative cholangiogram. Catheter is in the cystic duct remnant. No definitive filling defects are seen in the common duct. There is incomplete visualization of the intrahepatic ducts. There is contrast seen within the proximal duodenum without evidence of obstruction.

7-15E:

SERVICE CODE(S): ____________________

DX CODE(S): ____________________

Gastric ulcers (531) are lesions of the stomach that result in the death of the tissue and a defect of the surface as illustrated in **Figure 7-6**. **Perforated ulcers** are those in which the lesion penetrates the gastric wall, leaving a hole, as illustrated in **Figure 7-7**. Peptic refers to the gastric juice, pepsin. **Duodenal ulcers** (532) are lesions of the duodenum. **Peptic ulcers** are lesions of the stomach or the duodenum, which do not necessarily cause necrosis or perforation. The site may be unspecified (533). All three categories also have fourth digit subcategories for acute or chronic with or without hemorrhage and/or perforation. These categories of codes have a fifth digit available to indicate those without mention of obstruction (0) and with mention of obstruction (1).

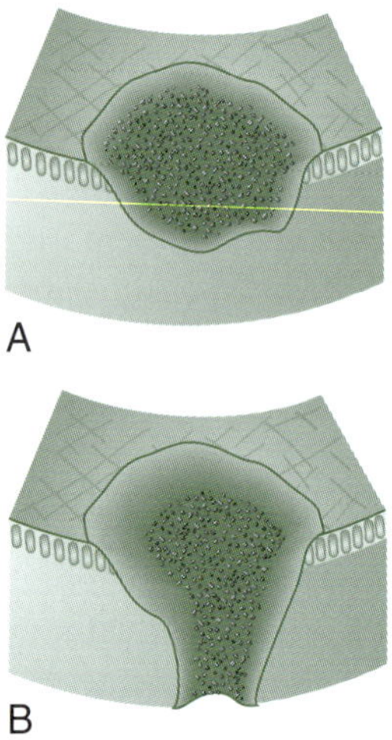

FIGURE 7-6 **A.** Ulcer. **B.** Perforated ulcer.

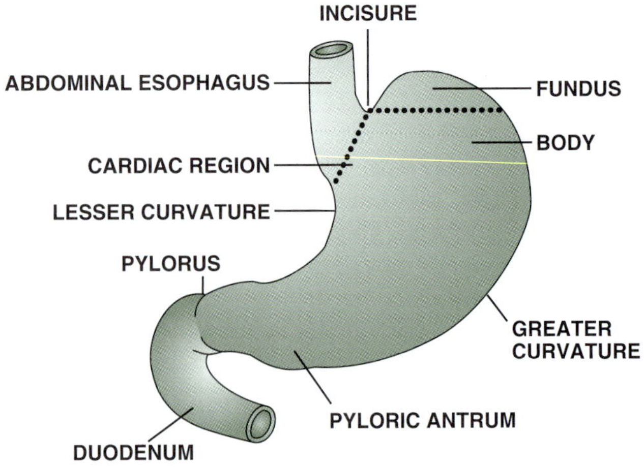

FIGURE 7-7 Parts of the stomach.

7-15F PATHOLOGY REPORT

During and following the operative procedure, the surgeon sends specimens of the tissue removed to the pathologist for examination and a written report of documents. The report has been highlighted to assist in coding.

LOCATION: Inpatient Hospital

PATIENT: Alma Kincaid

ATTENDING PHYSICIAN: Leslie Alanda, M.D.

SURGEON: Gary Sanchez, M.D.

PATHOLOGIST: Grey Lonewolf, M.D.

CLINICAL HISTORY: Nonhealing ulcer gastric ulcer, failure of medical treatment.

A. Gastroepifleur lymph node
B. Anterior vagus nerves
C. Posterior vagus nerves
D. Ulcer bed
E. Gallbladder

TISSUE RECEIVED:

FA. Gastroepifleur lymph node (FS) *(2 cassettes, 1 specimen)*
A. Gastroepifleur lymph node (FS) *(2 cassettes, 1 specimen)*
FB. Anterior vagus (FS)
B. Anterior vagus (FS)
FC. Posterior vagus (FS)
C. Posterior vagus (FS)
FD. Ulcer bed (FS)
D. Ulcer bed (FS)
E. Gallbladder

GROSS DESCRIPTION:

A. The specimen is labeled with the patient's name and "gastroepifleur lymph node," which consists of a 1.0 × 0.6 × 0.5-cm pink-tan lymph node. The specimen is bisected and processed in toto in two cassettes *(1 lymph node)*.

INTRAOPERATIVE FROZEN SECTION DIAGNOSIS: *(1, FS)*
Gastriepifleur lymph node: Benign lymph node.

B. The specimen is labeled with the patient's name and "anterior vagus," which consists of two linear pink-tan tissues, up to 6.0 cm in length and 0.1 cm in width. The specimen is process in toto in two cassettes.

INTRAOPERATIVE FROZEN SECTION DIAGNOSIS: *(2, FS)*
Peripheral nerve identified.

C. The specimen is labeled with the patient's name and "posterior vagus," which consists of a 0.6-cm pink-tan soft tissue. The specimen is processed in toto in one cassette.

INTRAOPERATIVE FROZEN-SECTION DIAGNOSIS: *(3, FS)*
Posterior vagus: Peripheral nerve identified.

D. The specimen is labeled with patient's name and "ulcer bed," which consists of a 14 × 8cm-segment of pink-tan stomach with attached fatty tissue along with the lesser and greater curvatures. Multiple lymph nodes are identified on the greater curvature, and these range in size from 0.3 to 1.5 cm in size and are pink-tan. Approximately 2 mm from the distal resection margin, there is a 3 × 2-cm ulcer. Approximately 1.5 cm proximal to this ulcer, there is another 2 × 0.5 cm linear ulcer. The stomach mucosa is pink-tan with no other obvious gross lesions. Representative sections are processed in 19 cassettes.

INTRAOPERATIVE FROZEN-SECTION DIAGNOSIS: (*4, FS*)
Ulcer bed: Benign ulcer.

E. The specimen is labeled with the patient's name and "gallbladder," which consists of a previously opened collapsed gallbladder 7 × 2.5 × 1 cm. The serosal surface is stained bile green. The wall is 1 to 2 mm thick, and the mucosa is dark green and velvety. No stones accompany the specimen. Representative sections are processed in two cassettes.

MICROSCOPIC DESCRIPTION:

A. Permanent sections confirm the frozen-section diagnosis showing a benign lymph node (*micro 1*) with mild follicular hyperplasia.
B. Permanent sections confirm the frozen-section diagnosis showing fibrofatty tissue with peripheral nerve segments (*micro 2*).
C. Permanent sections confirm the frozen-section diagnosis showing fibrofatty tissue with peripheral nerve segments (*micro 3*).
D. Permanent sections confirm the frozen-section diagnosis showing a benign antral ulcer (*stomach ulcer*) (*micro 4*) characterized by fibrinous neutrophilic exudate with underlying granulation tissue and fibrosis with acute inflammatory infiltrates. The region of the ulcer wall is markedly thinned with fibrosis extending in the adjacent perigastric fatty tissue. The adjacent mucosa shows an intact glandular architecture with reactive and regenerative glands. The lamina propria is mildly edematous with mild lymphocytic, plasma cell, and eosinophilic infiltrates. The muscular wall adjacent to the ulcer site shows hypertrophy with scattered lymphoid aggregates and lymphoid follicles. Sections of the linear ulcer show gastric body mucosa with benign ulceration. The adjacent gastric body mucosa shows intact glandular architecture with reactive and regenerative glands showing increased cytoplasmic basophilia with slightly enlarged hyperchromatic nuclei and occasional mitoses. The lamina propria is mildly edematous with mildly increased lymphocytic, plasma cell, and eosinophilic infiltrates. A rare gland shows intraluminal neutrophils. There is submucosal edema with lymphoid aggregates and lymphoid follicles. Random sections of the stomach show intact gastric body-type mucosa. The superficial lamina propria shows mildly increased lymphocytic, plasma cell, and eosinophilic infiltrates. Multiple lymph nodes show mild reactive follicular hyperplasia.
E. Sections of the gallbladder (*micro 5*) show mild mucosal atrophy and intermuscular fibrosis. There is mild smooth-muscle hypertrophy with an occasional Rokitansky-Aschoff sinus.

DIAGNOSIS:

A. Gastric epifleur lymph node: Mild follicular hyperplasia, benign
B. Peripheral nerve segment, consistent with anterior vagus nerve
C. Peripheral nerve segment, consistent with posterior vagus nerve
D. Partial gastrectomy:
   1. Benign antral ulcer with acute inflammation (*DX 1*).
   2. Benign gastric body ulcer with acute inflammation (*DX 2*).
   3. Multiple lymph nodes: mild follicular hyperplasia (*DX 3*), benign.
E. Gallbladder, excision: chronic cholecystitis (*DX 4*)

7-15F:

SERVICE CODE(S): ______________________

DX CODE(S): ______________________

7-15G DISCHARGE SUMMARY

LOCATION: Inpatient Hospital

PATIENT: Alma Kincaid

ATTENDING PHYSICIAN: Leslie Alanda, M.D.

REASON FOR ADMISSION: Nonhealing gastric ulcer.

SUMMARY OF HOSPITAL COURSE: The patient is a 60-year-old female with a history of ulcer disease, which failed medical management. She was subsequently referred to Dr. Sanchez for partial gastrectomy. The patient was admitted and taken to the operating room, where she underwent exploratory laparotomy with partial gastrectomy, truncal vagotomy, gastrojejunostomy, and a cholecystectomy with intraoperative cholangiogram. All pathology reports were benign. The patient tolerated the procedure well. She had an epidural in place following this, and she was transferred to the ICU for observation postoperatively. The patient did well in the ICU, and by the following Monday, she was ready for transfer to the floor. By Wednesday, her ileus was resolving, her NG discontinued, and she was started on a diet. By Friday, the patient was tolerating a regular diet. Her Jackson-Pratts were removed. She was afebrile with stable vital signs and was ready for discharge to home.

DISCHARGE INSTRUCTIONS: Activity as tolerated. Diet as tolerated.

DISCHARGE MEDICATIONS: Tylenol no. 3, 1-2 tablets p.o. q.4 h. p.r.n. pain.

FOLLOW-UP: The patient is to call for an appointment.

CONDITION ON DISCHARGE: Improved

DISCHARGE DIAGNOSES:

1. Nonhealing duodenal ulcer, chronic
2. Chronic cholecystitis

PROCEDURE PERFORMED: Exploratory laparotomy with partial gastrectomy, truncal vagotomy, gastrojejunostomy, and a cholecystectomy with intraoperative cholangiogram.

7-15G:

SERVICE CODE(S): ______________________

DX CODE(S): ______________________

Incisional (Open) Surgical Procedures

Unlike laparoscopic (closed) procedures, which must be viewed through an endoscope during an open procedure, the surgical site is opened to the view of the surgeon. The following are a variety of open surgical procedures for you to code.

CASE 7-16
7-16A Operative Report, Cystectomy

CASE 7-16

7-16A OPERATIVE REPORT, CYSTECTOMY

LOCATION: Inpatient Hospital

PATIENT: Tiffany Blue

ATTENDING PHYSICIAN: Ronald Green, M.D.

SURGEON: Gary Sanchez, M.D.

PREOPERATIVE DIAGNOSIS: Right intra-abdominal cyst on CT scan

POSTOPERATIVE DIAGNOSIS: Right descending sigmoid colon area mesenteric cyst (of colon)

PROCEDURE PERFORMED: Exploratory laparotomy, excision of descending sigmoid colon area mesenteric cyst

ANESTHESIA: General

INDICATIONS FOR PROCEDURE: The patient is a 27-year-old white female who was found to have an abdominal mass in the left lower abdominal area. The patient underwent a CT scan, and Dr. Monson found a cyst in what appeared to be the mesentery of the colon. The patient was taken to the operating room for exploratory laparotomy and excision.

DESCRIPTION OF PROCEDURE: The patient had previously undergone a bowel prep the day before. She was then prepped and draped in the usual manner. She received Mefoxin 2 g intravenously preoperatively. The lower midline abdominal incision was made. The abdomen was entered, and a large cyst was found in the lateral wall along the colon mesentery in the area about the junction of the descending and sigmoid colon. This cyst was then sharply and bluntly dissected free from the surrounding tissues and excised and sent to pathology. Hemostasis was obtained using pressure and Bovie cautery.

Thorough examination of the abdomen was then done. The liver, spleen, stomach, duodenum, and gallbladder all felt within normal limits. The colon and small bowel also appeared within normal limits. The uterus, both ovaries, and tubes were in place and also appeared within normal limits. There was what may be a small fibroid on the right apex of the uterus. No abnormalities were found. The cyst was sent to pathology.

After thorough examination of the abdomen and no other abnormalities were noted, the appendix also appeared normal and was left in place. The abdominal incision was then closed using a running no. 1 double-stranded suture. The subcutaneous tissues were irrigated and closed with a running 3-0 Vicryl suture. The skin was closed with skin clips. The patient tolerated the operation and returned to recovery in stable condition.

Pathology Report Later Indicated: Benign neoplasm

7-16A:

SERVICE CODE(S): ______________________

DX CODE(S): ______________________

CASE 7-17
7-17A Operative Report, Hemicolectomy

CASE 7-17

44160 – ileum removed

7-17A OPERATIVE REPORT, HEMICOLECTOMY

LOCATION: Inpatient Hospital

PATIENT: Sally Ortez

ATTENDING PHYSICIAN: Leslie Alanda, M.D.

SURGEON: Gary Sanchez, M.D.

PREOPERATIVE DIAGNOSIS: Adenocarcinoma of the ascending colon

POSTOPERATIVE DIAGNOSIS: Perforated adenocarcinoma of the ascending colon with attachment to the lateral abdominal wall.

ANESTHESIA: General

INDICATIONS FOR SURGERY: The patient is a 56-year-old white female who is having difficulties with her bowels. The patient was found to have adenocarcinoma of the ascending colon that was proven by biopsy. The patient is taken to the operating room after a bowel prep yesterday for surgery.

PROCEDURE: The patient was prepped and draped in the usual manner. A midline abdominal incision was made. The patient has had previous surgeries, which included an appendectomy, hysterectomy, cholecystectomy, and radiation therapy to her abdomen for a lymphoma. The patient had adhesions from her multiple previous surgeries and radiation therapy. These adhesions were taken down sharply using the Bovie cautery and Metzenbaum scissors. After this was done, the right colon was elevated using the Bovie cautery to divide the peritoneum on the right lateral gutter. The colon was then brought up into the operative area. The small bowel ileum was adherent down into the pelvis from her previous surgeries. These were taken down using the Metzenbaum scissors; then the small bowel was freed up into the incision area. The dissection was carried out to the transverse colon in about the midpoint of the transverse colon. A Penrose drain was then placed around the transverse colon and also one around the ileum. During dissection of the cancer from the lateral abdominal wall, the cancer was firmly adherent to the abdominal wall. When this was finally freed up, there was an opening in the colon that appeared to be a perforation of the area of cancer, which had been sealed by the lateral abdominal wall. There was no gross evidence of any tumor on the abdominal wall. The opening in the colon was closed with a 2-0 silk suture. Next the mesentery was scored using the Bovie cautery. The mesentery was clamped and divided using Kelly clamps and tied with interrupted 2-0 silk sutures. After this was completed, the bowel clamp was placed on the proximal ileum and also on the distal colon. Kocher clamps were placed on the specimen side of the ileum and colon. The colon and ileum were then transected and the specimen was sent to pathology. An end-to-end anastomosis was then done. A two-layer closure was done. Interrupted 3-0 silk sutures were placed on either end of the anastomosis and then the posterior layer was then placed. All sutures were placed before they were tied. After this was completed, the inner layer was then run using a running 3-0 Vicryl suture using a locking stitch for the posterior layer and a running stitch on the anterior layer. After this was completed, the bowel clamps were removed. The anterior outer layer was then placed using interrupted 3-0 silk sutures. There was an excellent anastomosis following this procedure. The opening in the mesentery was closed with a running 2-0 Vicryl suture. The operative area was thoroughly irrigated. A few small bleeders were found after the irrigation, and these were controlled by 2-0 silk ties or Bovie cautery. An additional adhesion was taken down from the omentum attached to the pelvis down into the pelvic gutter, and this was freed. After all the adhesions were taken down, the operative area was again thoroughly irrigated. The bowel was returned to the abdomen. The anastomosis was again checked and was excellent. The abdominal incision was then closed with a running no. 1 looped PDS suture for the fascia and the peritoneum in a single-layer closure. The subcutaneous tissues were then thoroughly irrigated, and the skin was closed with skin clips. The patient tolerated the operation and returned to recovery in stable condition.

Pathology Report Later Indicated: Adenocarcinoma of both the colon (primary) and abdominal wall neoplasm (secondary)

7-17A:

SERVICE CODE(S): ____________________

DX CODE(S): ____________________

CASE 7-18
7-18A Initial Hospital Services
7-18B Operative Report, Laparotomy
7-18C Discharge Summary

CASE 7-18

7-18A INITIAL HOSPITAL SERVICES

The patient, Mary Black, was brought to the hospital emergency room by ambulance from Manytown. Mary recently moved to Manytown to be located closer to her son. Her primary care physician in Manytown is Dr. Gregory Whipple. Dr. Paul Sutton treated the patient in the emergency department and then contacted Dr. Larry Friendly, who admitted the patient to the hospital.

LOCATION: Inpatient Hospital

PATIENT: Mary Black

ATTENDING PHYSICIAN: Larry Friendly, M.D.

Please see Dr. Sutton's note. His history was reviewed, the patient was interviewed, and then Dr. Whipple was contacted at Manytown; finally, the patient was examined.

Briefly, I was called about this lady earlier this morning. There was a history of questionable diverticulitis and pneumonia. She was brought in, and the pneumonia seemed to be well treated; however, she developed distention when they tried to feed her. They then did a barium enema, which did not show any diverticulitis. There was diverticulosis but definitely no active diverticulitis. There was question of a lesion at the splenic flexure, and there was no dye going into the small bowel. A CT scan was done 2 days ago, which showed very distended small bowel and completely collapsed small bowel, and, again, no signs of diverticulitis.

When we went in to do a history and examine the patient, she was very confused. She has a Duragesic patch, which was started, according to Dr. Whipple, because of her abdominal pain. He did not want to stop it during transfer because he wanted the patient to be free of pain during transfer. That was a good decision because the medication worked very well for her pain. According to Dr. Whipple, she was really quite with it prior to having the patch put on.

She cannot tell what surgery she has had done. When I talked to Dr. Sutton, he suggested that she had a hysterectomy, some stomach surgery, a right hemicolectomy, and an aortic aneurysm repair; however, the CT that was done on the outside shows no evidence that aortic surgery ever was done because she has a 4-cm aneurysm that goes down to her iliacs. I am also not clear about the right colon resection because the staples are in the left upper quadrant.

According to the chart, she had *Klebsiella* pneumonia, some hypertension, and underlying renal insufficiency.

PHYSICAL EXAMINATION: She is really quite distended with a silent abdomen. When I push, she does show signs that she is in pain. I reviewed her x-rays with Dr. Monson. There indeed is a questionable lesion at the splenic flexure, but this is where the staples are. It could easily be that what the barium enema is showing is old changes from previous surgery, but obviously there could be another lesion there. I am not even sure whether this was a cancer operation or a benign etiology, and nor was Dr. Sutton. Her CT showed massively distended small bowel and completely collapsed small bowel; so she has an obvious complete obstruction. According to the patient, she has not passed any gas for the last 2 days.

ASSESSMENT: She has a severe problem, and the treatment is extremely high risk. If I operate, there is a reasonable chance that she is not going to make it through the perioperative and postoperative periods. I told her this, and she made it very clear that she wanted to go ahead with surgery. It is impossible, however, to get an informed consent from this patient. Apparently, the family is on their way, and I will talk to them when they arrive. According to Dr. Sutton, the patient and her family had understood that they were coming to town likely for an operation, and they had consented to that, but I do want to hear it from them.

I was worried enough about this patient that I will get Dr. Green involved from critical care preoperatively. He will help us also with her postoperative care.

7-18A:

SERVICE CODE(S): ____________________

DX CODE(S): ____________________

7-18B OPERATIVE REPORT, LAPAROTOMY

LOCATION: Inpatient Hospital

PATIENT: Mary Black

ATTENDING PHYSICIAN: Larry Friendly, M.D.

SURGEON: Gary Sanchez, M.D.

PREOPERATIVE DIAGNOSIS: Complete small bowel obstruction

POSTOPERATIVE DIAGNOSIS:
1. Ischiorectal hernia with obstruction
2. Enterocolic fistula
3. Intestinal adhesions

PROCEDURE PERFORMED:

1. Exploratory laparotomy and lysis of adhesions
2. Release of small bowel obstruction
3. Takedown of enterocolonic fistula

ANESTHESIA: General anesthesia

IV FLUIDS: 3800 Crystalloid; 500 albumin

URINE OUTPUT: 40 cc

NG TUBE OUTPUT: 1100 cc

COMPLICATIONS: None

INDICATIONS: The patient was referred from her local care facility after having been admitted there for 3 to 4 days with the presence of a nonresolving small bowel obstruction. The patient had multiple intra-abdominal surgeries, including two gastric surgeries for peptic ulcer disease, a right hemicolectomy for benign polyps, and a total abdominal hysterectomy for benign disease. The patient had been having signs of complete bowel obstruction for at least 4 days that did not respond to medical therapy. The patient was transferred to our institution, and after confirming the diagnosis, she was taken to the operating room for exploration.

DESCRIPTION OF PROCEDURE: The patient was informed about indications and alternatives of the procedure. Her family members were informed as well, and she was made a code I. After discussing the situation with the family, we took her to the operating room. An informed written consent was obtained. The patient was placed in the supine position and given general anesthesia. Her abdomen was prepped and draped in the usual sterile fashion. The patient had several surgical scars from previous procedures. A midline supra and infraumbilical incision was performed. We gained access to the abdominal cavity from the most superior aspect of the incision. At this area we found heavy adhesions from the small bowel and transverse colon to the anterior abdominal wall. Through a meticulous dissection, we took down the adhesions and were able then to divide the fascia at the midline. In the lower-most aspect, there were many adhesions, and we were actually able to release all the small bowel from this area. The patient had a mild amount of straw-colored free fluid inside the abdomen. We subsequently proceeded to perform adhesiolysis, releasing all the small intestine and adhesed to the anterior wall to both sides. The transverse colon was also released from the anterior abdominal wall, which gave us exposure of the whole intra-abdominal contents. At this point, we proceeded to perform a formal exploratory laparotomy. The most superior organs of the abdomen were not evaluated because our incision did not extend to this area, and the patient had dense adhesions all over. We did not get to the area of the stomach or the liver. The patient does have evidence of a previous right hemicolectomy with an ileocolonic anastomosis that was localized in the right upper quadrant. We checked the transverse colon, the splenic flexure, and the descending colon including the sigmoid and the rectum, which showed normal characteristics. No evidence of obstruction in the sigmoid area was seen as previously suggested on CT scan. The colon itself looked normal in all its extent.

We proceeded then to inspect the small bowel, starting at the ligament of Treitz. There was dilated small bowel proximally. Approximately at the level of the transition between the jejunum and ileum, there was an area of transition caused by an internal hernia that was created by an enterocolonic fistula from the distal ileum to the colon almost at the area of the anastomosis from the previous right hemicolectomy. To be able to reduce the hernia and decompress the small bowel, we had to take down the fistula itself. Initially we dissected all the inflammatory tissue around this with Metzenbaum scissors. Once we got down to the fistula itself, we fired a GIA 75 across. Both ends of the fistula were completely sealed with no evidence of leak. At this point, we were able to run the small bowel completely. As already mentioned, the fistula was localized in the distal ileum approximately 30 cm away from the ileocecal valve. The area of transition was in the distal jejunum and proximal ileum. The hernia was completely reduced without any difficulty. A 1-cm segment in this area looked somewhat dusky but was definitely viable. This did not prompt us to perform any small bowel resection because once the pressure of the hernia was released, it looked completely viable. The pelvis itself looked normal with an absent uterus. The rest of the exploratory laparotomy was essentially normal. We then irrigated the abdominal cavity copiously until clear returns were obtained. Once this was achieved, we proceeded to close the wound at the level of the fascia with a running stitch of 2-0 nylon, and the skin was closed with staples. The patient tolerated the procedure well without any difficulty. Note – hernia was reducible small bowel resection not done

7-18B:

SERVICE CODE(S): 44650 (colon, suture fistula)

DX CODE(S): ____________________

7-18C DISCHARGE SUMMARY

LOCATION: Inpatient Hospital

PATIENT: Mary Black

ATTENDING PHYSICIAN: Larry Friendly, M.D.

DIAGNOSES:

1. Small bowel obstruction diagnosed at the time of transfer. Ischiorectal hernia with obstruction.
2. Enterocolonic fistula.
3. Acute respiratory distress syndrome.
4. Failure to extubate—challenge to extubate, challenge to wean.
5. Atherosclerotic heart disease.

SUMMARY: The patient was admitted for adhesiolysis because of bowel obstruction and underwent surgery. Unfortunately, in the postoperative period, she developed increasing respiratory problems, most likely *Klebsiella pneumoniae* complicated by acute respiratory distress syndrome. She was on prolonged mechanical ventilation but continued to be fairly difficult to wean because of respiratory and muscle fatigue and also problems with a pulmonary toilet. At one time the patient was on pressure support alone, but intermittently she had episodes of heart failure, undoubtedly as a result of high demand of breathing on patients with marginal coronary status and poor left ventricular systolic function. She continues to be a challenge to wean and is being transferred to Manytown Critical Care Unit for chronic acute care, to be followed by Dr. Green.

7-18C:

SERVICE CODE(S): ____________________

DX CODE(S): ____________________

Crohn's Disease

Crohn's disease is an inflammatory bowel disease (IBD) that is a group of conditions that can affect any portion of the gastrointestinal tract. The disease produces inflammatory lesions, and the type of Crohn's is named for the location of the inflammation, for example, colonic, ileocolonic, small bowel, or upper gastrointestinal Crohn's disease. The inflammation causes pain and diarrhea. The cause of Crohn's disease is unknown, but suspected causes are bacterial, genetics, suppressed immune system, or environmental factors.

The treatment for Crohn's disease is medications, such as the antiinflammatory drug prednisone, but surgical management of complications may be necessary for complications such as abscess, fistula, obstruction, or hemorrhage. Surgery is not a cure but is only used to manage complications that arise as a part of the disease process.

Crohn's Disease Diagnosis

Crohn's disease (555.x), also known as regional enteritis, is a chronic inflammatory disease of the intestines. Classification is based on the location in the small (duodenum, ileum, jejunum) or large (cecum, colon, rectum, anal canal) intestine.

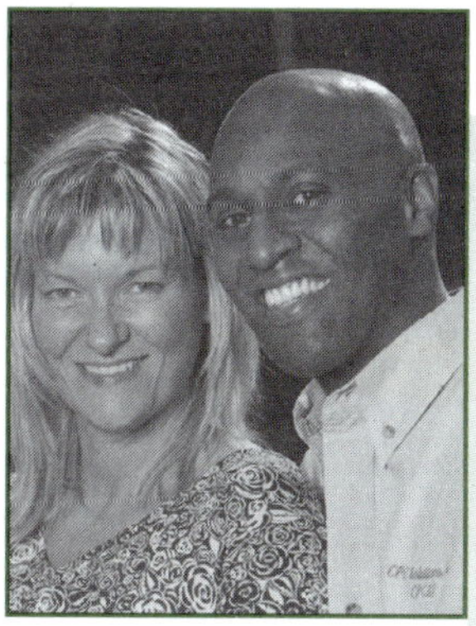

FROM THE TRENCHES

Terry

What is the most interesting part of your job?

"The different people that we meet. With our job we have the benefit of being able to go to a lot of different locations because we're our own company… and we get *the chance to meet the people that are 'in the trenches!'"*

Betty

"I think the most interesting part is teaching someone… to take people and walk them through coding…You see they're getting it, you see that they're progressing. To me that's not only the most interesting but the most enriching part of what we do."

CASE 7-19
7-19A Operative Report, Gastrojejunostomy/Tracheostomy

CASE 7-19

7-19A OPERATIVE REPORT, GASTROJEJUNOSTOMY/TRACHEOSTOMY

Bill Stillman is admitted by Dr. Naraquist, his PCP, for placement of a tracheostomy tube and a feeding tube. Dr. Riddle, Interventional Radiologist, attempted to place a gastrointestinal tube, but the colon was punctured during the procedure. The patient is now scheduled for an open procedure by Dr. Sanchez.

LOCATION: Inpatient Hospital

PATIENT: Bill Stillman

ATTENDING PHYSICIAN: Leslie Naraquist, M.D.

SURGEON: Gary Sanchez, M.D.

PREOPERATIVE DIAGNOSIS: Crohn's disease

POSTOPERATIVE DIAGNOSIS: Crohn's disease

PROCEDURE PERFORMED:
1. Repair of intestinal wound
2. Gastrojejunostomy with no. 18 French Moss tube
3. Tracheostomy with no. 8 Shiley tube

ANESTHESIA: General.

INDICATIONS: The patient is a 61-year-old male with Crohn's disease. He is now on the ventilator, ventilatory dependent, in need of feeding tube placement, and in need of tracheostomy to further assist in weaning the patient from the ventilator. Interventional radiology had attempted to place a feeding tube, but their needle had entered the colon; so he presents today for elective exploration, placement of feeding tube, possible repair of colon, and then tracheostomy. I discussed with the brother the surgery and its risks. He understands and wishes to proceed.

PROCEDURE: The patient was brought to the operating room, placed under general anesthesia, and prepped and draped with Betadine solution. A midline incision with a no. 10 blade and dissection was carried down through subcutaneous tissues using electrocautery. We entered the abdominal cavity sharply and encountered the transverse colon, which was dilated, and we could see a puncture site within the transverse colon. There was a leak of some air from the puncture site but no purulence in the peritoneal cavity. We oversewed the colon with 3-0 silk Lembert sutures. We then evaluated our small bowel anastomoses, and these appeared normal. There was also clear fluid within the peritoneal cavity. We irrigated and removed the clear fluid. We then placed two concentric pursestring sutures on the stomach, made our gastric opening, and then placed a no. 18 French Moss gastrojejunostomy tube through a left upper quadrant stab incision, passed it into the stomach, inflated the balloon, and passed the distal tip around the duodenum to the third portion of the duodenum. We secured our two pursestring sutures and then anchored it to the anterior abdominal wall with 3-0 silk sutures. We then once again closed the midline fascia with a combination of interrupted 0 Vicryl and running 0 PDS. The skin was left open and packed with Kerlix. The patient was then placed in the reverse Trendelenburg position with his neck slightly extended. We made a collar-type incision about two fingerbreadths above the manubrium. We carried our dissection through platysma using electrocautery and then divided the strap muscles along the midline. We encountered the thyroid cartilage and then the first tracheal ring. We placed a tracheal retractor, divided the second and third tracheal rings sharply with a no. 11 blade, withdrew the endotracheal tube above our opening into the trachea, placed a 3-0 Prolene suture on either side of the trachea, and then passed a no. 8 Shiley tracheostomy tube. We insufflated the balloon and had good returns. We then placed trach ties on and sterile dressing. All sponge and needle counts were correct. He tolerated this well and was taken to recovery in stable condition.

7-19A:

SERVICE CODE(S): ______________________

DX CODE(S): ______________________

CASE 7-20
7-20A Operative Report, Appendectomy
7-20B Pathology Report

CASE 7-20

7-20A OPERATIVE REPORT, APPENDECTOMY

LOCATION: Inpatient Hospital

PATIENT: Sally Jacobson

ATTENDING PHYSICIAN: Leslie Alanda, M.D.

PREOPERATIVE DIAGNOSIS: Acute appendicitis

POSTOPERATIVE DIAGNOSIS: Acute appendicitis

ANESTHESIA: General anesthesia

INDICATION: The patient is a 17-year-old female with insulin-dependent diabetes mellitus who presents with crampy, colicky right lower quadrant abdominal pain and an ultrasound showing a question of appendicitis. Her white count is within normal limits. She continues to have pain in the right lower quadrant. She presents today for elective open appendectomy.

We discussed the risks of bleeding, infection, and possible abscess formation with the patient's mother, and they wish to proceed.

PROCEDURE: The patient was brought to the operating room and prepped and draped sterilely. A right lower quadrant skin incision was made with a no. 10 blade and carried down through subcutaneous tissues using electrocautery. The anterior sheath of the rectus was scored. The rectus retracted medially, and the posterior sheath and peritoneum were grasped with curved clamps and sharply incised, thus allowing entry into the peritoneal cavity. Some serous fluid was found in the right lower quadrant, and this was aspirated. The cecum was grasped, and the appendix was delivered up and into the wound. The mesoappendix was taken down between the right angle clamps. The base of the appendix was transected sharply and sent to pathology for permanent. The tip was cauterized and inverted into the cecum with a 3-0 silk pursestring suture. Two to three feet of the terminal ileum were explored, with no evidence of Meckel's diverticula. The remainder of the abdominal cavity was within normal limits.

The abdomen was irrigated with saline solution, and then the posterior sheath and peritoneum were closed with running 3-0 Vicryl. The anterior sheath was closed with interrupted 3-0 Vicryl. The skin was closed with subcuticular 4-0 undyed Vicryl. Steri-Strips and sterile bandage were applied.

SPONGE AND NEEDLE COUNT: All sponge and needle counts were correct.

The patient tolerated the procedure well and was taken to recovery in stable condition.

Pathology Report Later Indicated: See Report 7-20B.

7-20A:

SERVICE CODE(S): ____________________

DX CODE(S): ____________________

7-20B PATHOLOGY REPORT

LOCATION: Inpatient Hospital

PATIENT: Sally Jacobson

ATTENDING PHYSICIAN: Leslie Alanda, M.D.

PATHOLOGIST: Grey Lonewolf, M.D.

CLINICAL HISTORY: Rule out acute appendicitis

TISSUE RECEIVED: Appendix

GROSS DESCRIPTION:
The specimen is labeled with the patient's name and "appendix" and consists of 7.3-cm veriform appendix with attached mesoappendix. The serosal surface is smooth pink-tan. Cut sections show a white-tan wall with a pinpoint lumen. Representative sections are submitted in two cassettes.

MICROSCOPIC DESCRIPTION:
Cross-sections of appendix show intact mucosal epithelium. No evidence of acute inflammation is seen. There is fibrofatty obliteration of the distal tip.

DIAGNOSIS:
Appendix, excision. Fibrofatty obliteration of the distal tip; no acute inflammation identified.

7-20B:

SERVICE CODE(S): ____________________

DX CODE(S): ____________________

CASE 7-21
7-21A Hospital Inpatient Service
7-21B Operative Report, Cecectomy
7-21C Discharge Summary

CASE 7-21

7-21A HOSPITAL INPATIENT SERVICE

In the Impression section of the report, the physician indicates this patient has an abdominal mass with rule out diagnosis. Rule out diagnoses are not reported by outpatient coders, so the abdominal mass would be reported. Also the urinary tract infection requires two codes, one for the "infection" and one for the causative agent "E. coli." Begin your search for both codes under the main term "Infection" in the Index of the ICD-9-CM. Always list the "infection" first followed by the infectious agent, which in this case is the E. coli.

LOCATION: Inpatient Hospital

PATIENT: Dominick Miller

PHYSICIAN: Larry Friendly, M.D.

The patient is a 69-year-old white male who was admitted to the hospital approximately 5 days ago because of faintness and slight neurologic difficulties. This patient has a history of having multiple strokes in the past. The etiology of the strokes has never been determined. The patient had a CT scan at the other facility, which showed evidence of old strokes but nothing new at this time. The patient was initially rehydrated because he was dehydrated, and his condition remained stable. He was also found to have urinary tract infection, greater than 100,000 colonies of *E. coli.* He has been on Unasyn for this problem. The patient improved. On Friday, he stated that he began having abdominal pain and pain in the right lower quadrant area. Because of this continued abdominal pain, the patient was transferred today for further evaluation and treatment of this problem. The patient also has a history of having blood in his stool, and he is also anemic. Because of these findings, the patient needs further evaluation. He is also presently taking Coumadin for his strokes, and this complicates any surgical intervention at this time. The patient is stable. He states that he is hungry and wants to eat and otherwise complains of pain in the right lower quadrant area. The patient has a history of having some type of an endoscopic procedure done about a year and a half ago at the Manytown Hospital. He is not sure whether it was a colonoscopy or a flexible sigmoidoscopy; therefore, we do not know if his right colon was fully evaluated. The patient is again stable at this time.

PAST MEDICAL HISTORY:

OPERATIONS:
1. Bilateral herniorrhaphies
2. TURP
3. Laparoscopic cholecystectomy

ILLNESSES:
1. Multiple strokes
2. Hypertension
3. Arthritis

MEDICATIONS:
1. Labetolol 200 mg t.i.d.
2. Sulindac 200 mg b.i.d.
3. Coumadin 5 mg half a tablet on Mondays, Wednesdays, and Fridays and 1 tablet on the other days
4. Detrol LA 4 mg q.d. or b.i.d. as needed.
5. Colace b.i.d.
6. Multiple vitamins
7. Calcium 600 mg b.i.d.

ALLERGIES: IVP dye and sulfa

REVIEW OF SYSTEMS: The patient states that he does not smoke and does not drink. Neuro: The patient denies any history of seizure disorder or headaches. He does have trouble with dizziness and has had multiple strokes in the past. Cardiac: No history of myocardial infarction or congenital heart disease. The patient does have hypertension. Pulmonary: No history of asthma, hay fever, or pneumonia. No hemoptysis. GI: The patient denies any nausea, vomiting, diarrhea, or constipation. He has a history of rectal bleeding. The patient has complaints of pain in the right lower quadrant; see present illness. GU: The patient has a urinary tract infection of *E. coli,* which is being treated presently. Hematologic: The patient has received blood transfusions in the past but otherwise presently has not had any recently, even though he is anemic, and he also has rectal bleeding.

EXAMINATION: The patient is a 69-year-old white male. Eyes: Pupils are equal, round, and react to light and accommodation. Ears: TMs are normal. Nose within normal limits. Throat within normal limits. The patient has his own teeth. Neck is supple. No carotid bruits are heard.

Lungs: The patient has bilateral basilar rales. Heart: Regular rhythm, grade 2/6 systolic murmur. Abdomen: Normal bowel sounds. The patient has tenderness in the right lower quadrant area and questionable palpable mass in this area.

IMPRESSION:

1. Right lower quadrant mass, rule out ruptured appendicitis, rule out tumor
2. Urinary tract infection of *E. Coli*
3. Hypertension

PLAN: The patient will be admitted to the hospital. He will be kept on IV antibiotics. His Coumadin will be stopped. He will undergo a CT scan of his abdomen for evaluation of this mass. The patient is not critical to the point where he requires emergency surgery at this time. We will rehydrate the patient and continue him on IV antibiotics and see whether we can treat this medically and, possibly, if there is an abscess pocket, drain it percutaneously. If this is possible, we will continue on this plan, but if it is not, then the patient may require surgery.

7-21A:

SERVICE CODE(S): ____________________

DX CODE(S): ____________________

7-21B OPERATIVE REPORT, CECECTOMY

LOCATION: Inpatient Hospital

PATIENT: Dominick Miller

PHYSICIAN: Larry Friendly, M.D.

SURGEON: Gary Sanchez, M.D.

PREOPERATIVE DIAGNOSIS: Right lower quadrant mass.

POSTOPERATIVE DIAGNOSIS: Inflamed ruptured appendix with mass palpable in the cecum, possibly inflammatory, possibly cancer.

OPERATION PERFORMED: Right cecectomy with anastomosis. Appendectomy.

ANESTHESIA: General

INDICATIONS FOR SURGERY: The patient is a 69-year-old white male who was recently admitted to the hospital with a right lower quadrant mass and tenderness, possible appendicitis. The patient has also been anemic for quite some time, and no etiology could be found for the anemia. The patient was taken to the operating room after bowel prep for surgery.

DESCRIPTION OF PROCEDURE: The patient was prepped and draped in the usual manner. A midline abdominal incision was made. The patient was also receiving Zosyn 4.5 g, and he was given a dose prior to surgery. Examination of the right lower quadrant revealed an inflamed appendix, which appeared to be ruptured, but the cecum was also quite inflamed, and there is a solid mass in this area. An appendectomy was then performed. It was difficult to ascertain whether or not this mass was inflammatory only or possible cancer. Because of this, a cecectomy was performed. The ascending colon was transected using a GIA stapler followed by the ileum resection. The mesentery was then clamped and divided using Pean clamps and tied with interrupted 2-0 silk sutures. The specimen was sent to pathology, and then a stapled anastomosis was done using the GIA stapler and the TA-60 stapler to close the opening that remained after the stapling procedure. There was excellent anastomosis following this procedure. The staple line was reinforced with several interrupted 3-0 silk sutures. The operative area was thoroughly irrigated. The opening in the mesentery was closed with a running 3-0 Vicryl suture. The bowel was returned to the abdomen, and the fascia was then closed with running no. 1, double-stranded PDS suture. The subcutaneous tissues were thoroughly irrigated. The skin was left open, and a dressing was applied. The patient tolerated the operation and returned to recovery in stable condition.

7-21B:

SERVICE CODE(S): ____________________

DX CODE(S): ____________________

7-21C DISCHARGE SUMMARY

You will note that this is a very long discharge summary that details a complex case in which the patient died. Report all of the diagnoses indicated in the Principal Diagnosis and Secondary Diagnosis sections of the report.

LOCATION: Inpatient Hospital

PATIENT: Dominick Miller

PHYSICIAN: Larry Friendly, M.D.

SURGEON: Gary Sanchez, M.D.

INDICATIONS FOR ADMISSION: Abdominal pain with pain mainly in the right lower quadrant.

This 69-year-old gentleman was transferred from another hospital. He was admitted to the other hospital with history of neurological difficulties and feeling faint. Subsequent CT showed multiple old strokes but no new infarcts. The patient had a UTI with more than 100,000 colonies of *E. coli* and was subsequently treated with Unasyn at the other hospital. He was also hydrated. At the other hospital, he started having right lower quadrant abdominal pain, for which the patient was transferred to this facility for evaluation and treatment. The patient also had history of having blood in the stool and was taking Coumadin for strokes.

PAST MEDICAL HISTORY on this gentleman is significant for multiple strokes, hypertension, and arthritis.

PAST SURGICAL HISTORY: He underwent laparoscopic cholecystectomy, transrectal resection of prostate, and bilateral inguinal herniorrhaphies in the past.

PHYSICAL EXAMINATION revealed a grade 2.6 systolic murmur and tenderness in the right lower quadrant of the abdomen. Questionable palpable mass was seen in the area. The patient underwent an ultrasound examination of the right lower quadrant, which showed complex structure in the right lower quadrant measuring about 4.3 × 4.1 × 2 cm, which does not compress during the ultrasound examination and demonstrates bowel nature. On a few of the views, there is a tubular structure, which may be separate from the more complex-looking area. The complex structure may represent a cecum according to the radiologist's report on the ultrasound examination. These findings could be compatible with a contained perforation. The patient also underwent a CT scan examination of the abdomen and pelvis on 05/03/xx. Findings at this examination include a phlegmonous-type mass density noted in the right lower quadrant adjacent to and cannot be separated from the cecum. This was at least 3 cm in diameter. The differential considerations include inflammation/infection and also a mass arising from the cecum. There is inflammatory change in the inferior aspect of the right lower abdominal musculature. Nonspecific hypodensity is noted in the anterior aspect of the left lobe. Small bilateral pleural effusions with patchy opacity were seen in the lung bases and were compatible with volume loss. The right kidney appears slightly larger than the left, with some stranding noted in the perirenal fat on the right side. The patient also underwent cardiac evaluation prior to surgery. As part of this workup, the patient underwent an echocardiogram, which showed a normal left ventricular size with left ventricular systolic function, mild left ventricular hypertrophy, mild mitral insufficiency without stenosis, and trace tricuspid insufficiency without stenosis. The left ventricular inflow pattern was suggestive of early diastolic dysfunction not borderline. The patient was recommended for acute bacterial endocarditis prophylaxis, which was given prior to surgery.

The patient underwent right cecectomy with primary stapled anastomosis between ileum and ascending colon on Monday. Findings at surgery included an inflamed, ruptured appendix with mass palpable in the cecum, most probably inflammatory, but neoplastic could not be ruled out. Pathologic examination of this resected cecal specimen showed acute inflammation of the appendix, which was severe and extensive, with perforation and excision of inflammation into the mesoappendix and mesocolon with abscess formation. The cecum showed that the acute inflammation was terminal ileum. No evidence of neoplasm in the cecum or in the appendix or ileum was seen. The patient developed spiking temperature immediately after the surgery. The patient was cared for in the major postoperative period in the medical ICU, where he was given nitroprusside drip and was on arterial monitoring. The patient was transferred back to the floor, where he developed some confusion. His medications were stopped, especially the narcotic analgesics, to help with his confusion. The patient developed chest infection with sputum Gram stain showing gram-positive bacteria and yeast. He was started on IV antibiotics and IV fungal agents on Monday. The patient desatted again on Tuesday. There was evidence of aspiration into the bronchial tree. We found large amounts of gastric contents as part of the suction. The patient had to be intubated and ventilated and was transferred to the surgical care unit on Wednesday as treatment for this aspiration pneumonitis. The patient was started on TPN in the meantime. Critical care service was involved in the management of this patient in view of the aspiration pneumonitis and associated problems. The patient continued to be managed on ventilator for his respiratory failure secondary to *Pseudomonas* pneumonia. The sputum culture showed presumptive *Pseudomonas* species, which were rare. There was some yeast, but it was not *Candida albicans.* The patient was started on tube feeds. Subsequently, the patient developed symptoms suggestive of respiratory distress syndrome secondary to the pulmonary insult he had sustained. The patient was managed in the surgical critical care unit all the time and had central venous access for TPN and also resuscitative efforts. The patient had problems with continued pyrexia. The exact source of the pyrexia was not easily ascertained after multiple investigations, and the lines were changed. The patient had a CT scan of the abdomen on Thursday as part of workup for pyrexia. The CT scan showed at that time that he had pleural effusions that were present even previously. He had scattered fluid throughout the abdomen and pelvis which was new. There could be some postoperative changes. There was no definite fluid collection noted to suggest an abscess. There were distended bowel loops of both large and small bowel consistent with generalized ileus. There was atelectasis and/or infiltrates at both lung bases, part of which was new. The patient also underwent a CT scan examination of the paranasal sinuses, which showed some mucosal thickening in most of the ethmoidal sinuses. The bilateral sphenoid sinuses showed considerable mucosal thickening with the possibility of fluid level in either of the sphenoid sinuses. The maxillary sinus showed mucosal thickening, particularly posteriorly. The patient had deteriorating renal function and was started on renal dialysis on Friday. The patient had tunneled hemodialysis catheter placed on the Thursday prior to the start of dialysis. The patient underwent tracheostomy tube placement on Friday without complications. The patient had some altered neurologic status and subsequently underwent CT scan of the brain on Saturday. This showed questionable low density of the superior margin of the left temporal lobe, which might represent a recent ischemic change.

There were no hemorrhages in the brain noted on that study. The patient continued to have hemodialysis performed in the surgical critical care unit. The patient developed failure of the lateral aspect of the left lower extremity for which he underwent a skin biopsy, and the pathology of the lesion showed minimal chronic dermatitis and dermal edema, which was nonspecific and without evidence of cellulitis. The patient continued to spike temperature. The patient continued to have problems with multiple organ systems and was acutely ill and was treated in the surgical critical care unit.

The patient continued to have some intermittent problems with the GI function with KUB showing persistent small bowel distention consistent with possible obstruction of the persistent ileum. The patient was weaned off the ventilator and was put on trach mask on Tuesday. The patient tolerated this transition. The patient's urine output started to pick up, and the patient was continued on dialysis to augment his renal function. Repeated sputum culture showed *Pseudomonas* with yeast. The patient underwent CT scan of the abdomen on Wednesday, which showed dilated bowel in the mid-abdomen and pelvis. A portion of this dilated bowel was found to be sigmoid colon. The rectum was also of abnormal appearance, and the wall appears to be thickened. There was stranding about both the kidneys noted. There was abnormal appearance of a loop of bowel in the inferior pelvis, which was most likely sigmoid colon and could be from continued inflammatory or infected change. The patient had a flexible sigmoidoscopy subsequent to this on Friday. The patient had an attempted placement of a GJ catheter by interventional radiology but was not successful due to overlying bowel, and this was tried on Friday. The patient's care transferred to Dr. Alanda on Friday at request of the patient's family. The patient underwent a repeat CT scan of the abdomen, which showed prominently dilated loops of small bowel, the findings of which were worrisome for small bowel obstruction. This obstruction could be traced to the level of the operative site in the right lower quadrant. Free fluid was noted in the pelvis, and infiltrate/volume loss in the lung bases has improved compared with the previous surgery. The patient underwent exploratory laparotomy, adhesiolysis, and closure of enterotomies and multiple serosal tears along the insertion of Moss tube. Findings at surgery included internal hernia with a small bowel loop stuck to the anterior abdominal wall with proximal dilated and distal collapsed small bowel. Multiple small bowel adhesions were noted. Anastomosis was intact. The patient needed increased amount of fluid secondary to the third spacing from the surgery. The patient needed repeat dialysis in view of the significant third spacing. Prior to this surgery, he had a dialysis-free period of about 10 days. The repeat dialysis was initiated after the surgery to clear his fluids secondary to third spacing. The patient was taken off the ventilator. The patient had significant amount of serious fluid draining from this main abdominal wound initially after the surgery, but it reduced over a period of time. The patient was transferred to the floor. The patient was restarted on tube feedings and tolerated them reasonably well. He developed attacks of fast atrial fibrillation and was started on digoxin for it. The patient was restarted on Coumadin for this as part of treatment for atrial fibrillation. The patient's renal function again deteriorated, with urine output falling and patient developing acidosis. The patient became hypotensive with mottling and tachypnea. The impression was that he might have started developing sepsis and also possible dehydration secondary to dialysis. The patient was given extra fluids; despite these measures, the patient died on Saturday.

PRINCIPAL DIAGNOSIS: Acute appendicitis with perforation and abscess formation

SECONDARY DIAGNOSES:

1. Anemia
2. Hypertension
3. Respiratory failure
4. Renal failure, acute and chronic
5. Postoperative small bowel obstruction due to internal hernia
6. Urinary tract infection secondary to *E. coli*

PROCEDURES PERFORMED:

1. Right colectomy with primary anastomosis
2. Intubation and mechanical ventilation
3. Insertion of central venous catheter
4. Placement of right femoral central line
5. Placement of tunneled triple lumen catheter
6. Placement of hemodialysis catheter
7. Tracheostomy placement
8. Skin biopsy of the cellulitic area over the right hip
9. Flexible sigmoidoscopy
10. Attempt at placement of gastrojejunostomy catheter
11. Exploratory laparotomy and reduction of internal small bowel hernia, lysis of adhesions, repair of multiple enterotomies, and serosal tears with placement of Moss gastrojejunostomy tube
12. Multiple sittings of hemodialysis

7-21C:

SERVICE CODE(S): ____________________

DX CODE(S): ____________________

CASE 7-22
7-22A Operative Report, Placement of Gastrostomy Tube

CASE 7-22

7-22A OPERATIVE REPORT, PLACEMENT OF GASTROSTOMY TUBE

This patient, George Powers, returned to the hospital for a procedure to treat a bowel obstruction. The procedure in Case 7-22A is performed during the postoperative period of the previous surgery.

LOCATION: Inpatient

PATIENT: George Powers

SURGEON: Gary Sanchez, M.D.

PREOPERATIVE DIAGNOSIS: Bowel obstruction

POSTOPERATIVE DIAGNOSIS: Bowel obstruction

PROCEDURES PERFORMED:
1. Adhesiolysis and repair of bowel enterotomy
2. Placement of Moss gastrostomy tube

OPERATIVE NOTE: With the patient under general anesthesia, the abdomen was opened, extending the midline incision from below the xiphoid to below the umbilicus. Most of the old incision was open. We were able to get into the abdominal cavity without too much difficulty. There were minimal adhesions to the anterior abdominal wall. There was marked dilatation of the small bowel, and we began by taking down multiple adhesions. There were multiple incidents of serosal tear due to the marked dilatation of the small bowel. Once we got started, we could identify a loop of small bowel that was approximately 6 or 12 inches from the ileocecal valve, which was stuck into the pelvis. The rest of the small bowel was volvulized around this as an internal hernia and was creating the bowel obstruction. There was a clear transition zone from the dilated bowel and to the nondilated bowel. As we worked to take down all these adhesions doing extensive adhesiolysis, we entered the bowel at one point with an enterotomy. Very tough, tenacious, almost stool-like material was within the small bowel, suggesting that this has been obstructed for quite some time. We attempted to keep all of this out of the abdominal cavity, and we were successful, but we did have some spillage of this tenacious small bowel material. It was so thick that we really could not suction it out of the bowel with the sucker. We had to allow it to run out of the opening in the bowel into a basin as we squeezed; it was too thick to come through a sucker. In any event, we finally got all the bowel lysed such that we could run from the bowel from the ligament of Treitz to the ileum. We could see that the point of obstruction was not at the anastomotic site, and the anastomosis appeared widely patent. Multiple serosal tears were repaired with interrupted silk sutures. The enterotomy into the bowel was repaired in two layers using an inner layer of Vicryl and an outer layer of interrupted silk. With this accomplished, we copiously irrigated the abdominal cavity and then proceeded to return to the bowel to the abdominal cavity. We then placed a Moss gastrostomy tube into the stomach. This was brought through the anterior abdominal wall through a stab incision, and then a double pursestring was placed into the stomach and the tube introduced. The balloon was inflated, and the distal portion of the tube was threaded through the pylorus into the duodenum. The stomach was tacked up to the anterior abdominal wall. The abdominal cavity was again copiously irrigated with saline, and then the abdomen was closed using running 0 loop nylon. We did tack the sutures around the umbilicus and then left the wound packed with some wet saline gauze. A sterile dressing was applied. The patient tolerated the procedure well and was discharged from the operating room on the ventilator but in stable condition. He went directly to the surgical intensive care unit. At the end of the procedure, all sponges and instruments were accounted for.

7-22A: consider coding 44050

SERVICE CODE(S): ____________________

DX CODE(S): ____________________

Hernia

A hernia is a protrusion of tissue or an organ through an abdominal opening. Hernias are named for the type and location of the hernia. Reference a medical dictionary under the main term *hernia* for the various types of hernias, for example, an inguinal hernia (into the inguinal canal) or a sliding hernia (cecum and sigmoid colon that involves the viscera).

Hernias can be strangulated (cut off from the blood supply) or incarcerated (cannot be returned to original location). In a surgical reduction of a hernia, the surgeon returns the hernia to the original location. Sutures and/or mesh may be used to repair the area and provide support. The strangulated hernia may involve an organ, such as the large or small intestine, and that organ may also require repair. Additional organ repair would be reported in addition to the hernia repair.

Hernia codes in the CPT are divided based on whether the repair is initial/recurrent, incarcerated/strangulated, patient age, and type (i.e., femoral, inguinal), etc. Add-on code 49568 is used to report the implantation of mesh or other supports for incisional or ventral hernia repairs.

Diagnosis coding of hernias was discussed prior to Case 7-7.

CASE 7-23
7-23A Hospital Inpatient Service
7-23B Operative Report, Right Inguinal Hernia Repair
7-23C Pathology Report

CASE 7-23

7-23A HOSPITAL INPATIENT SERVICE

LOCATION: Inpatient, Hospital

PATIENT: Doris Craven

ATTENDING PHYSICIAN: Gary Sanchez, M.D.

CHIEF COMPLAINT: Right inguinal hernia.

HISTORY OF PRESENT ILLNESS: The patient is a 39-year-old female who reports a 1-year history of an intermittent painful lump in the right groin area. She states that it will come out every so often, more frequently toward the end of the day or with exertion. It is painful while it is out; however, she has always been able to reduce it. She did have one episode approximately a week ago when she could not reduce it at first and had to leave work to go home and lie down before it reduced. She saw Dr. Friendly for this problem, and he referred her to us. She has been seen several times in the clinic. She denies any GI symptoms, specifically no nausea, vomiting, or change in bowel habits.

PAST MEDICAL HISTORY: She is essentially healthy. She takes no medications.

ALLERGIES: No known drug allergies.

FAMILY HISTORY: Her father had a cerebral aneurysm; otherwise, family history is unremarkable.

SOCIAL HISTORY: She smokes one pack of cigarettes per day. Rarely uses alcohol.

REVIEW OF SYSTEMS: Negative. Specifically, she denies any syncope, shortness of breath, hemoptysis, chest pain, GI, or GU symptoms. She denies any muscle or joint pain.

PHYSICAL EXAMINATION: This slender white female is appropriate for stated age. She is afebrile. Stable vital signs. Blood pressure is 112/72. Her weight is 116 pounds. HEENT is unremarkable. Neck is supple with no masses. Chest: The lungs are clear to auscultation bilaterally. Heart is regular rate and rhythm without murmur. Abdomen has positive bowel sounds, soft without masses. GU: There is no reducible hernia in the right inguinal region. No hernias noted on the left. Extremities: Appropriate pulses, reflexes, and muscle strength. Neurologic: She is grossly intact.

ASSESSMENT: Right inguinal hernia.

PLAN: I discussed the nature of the disease and the treatment options with the patient. The patient understood and wished to proceed with surgical repair.

7-23A:
SERVICE CODE(S): Decision for surgery

DX CODE(S): ______________________

7-23B OPERATIVE REPORT, RIGHT INGUINAL HERNIA REPAIR

LOCATION: Inpatient, Hospital

PATIENT: Doris Craven

SURGEON: Gary Sanchez, M.D.

PREOPERATIVE DIAGNOSIS: Right inguinal hernia

POSTOPERATIVE DIAGNOSIS: Right direct and right indirect inguinal hernias

PROCEDURE PERFORMED: Right inguinal hernia repair

PROCEDURE: The patient was brought to the operating room and placed in the supine position on the operating table. After satisfactory general anesthesia had been induced, the patient's abdomen and groins were prepped and draped in a sterile manner. A short transverse incision was made over the right inguinal area. Subcutaneous tissue was divided sharply. Ties and cautery were used for hemostasis. The external oblique aponeurosis was identified and opened from above downward. The ilioinguinal nerve was identified and protected. The patient had a direct inguinal hernia about 1 cm superior and medial to the internal ring. It was properitoneal fat pushed through a very small opening about 0.5 cm in size. We reduced this and closed this hole with interrupted Ethibond, which gave a solid closure without tension. We then dissected up the round ligament and ligated it distally. Proximally we then separated the round ligament from a small internal sac. We ligated the round ligament and the sac separately and then closed the internal ring with Ethibond suture in a Bassini repair. This gave us a solid repair with fixed hernias. We then irrigated the wound with Neomycin. Final sponge and needle counts were taken; they were correct. We then closed the external oblique aponeurosis with Vicryl; subcutaneous tissue was closed with chromic and skin with nylon. Blood loss during the procedure was minimal. Sponge and needle counts were correct. The patient tolerated the procedure well and left for the recovery room in stable condition.

Pathology Report Later Indicated: See Report 7-23C.

7-23B:

SERVICE CODE(S): ______________________

DX CODE(S): ______________________

7-23C PATHOLOGY REPORT

LOCATION: Inpatient, Hospital

PATIENT: Doris Craven

PHYSICIAN: Gary Sanchez, M.D.

PATHOLOGIST: Grey Lonewolf, M.D.

CLINICAL HISTORY: Right inguinal hernia

TISSUE RECEIVED: Round ligament

GROSS DESCRIPTION:

The specimen was labeled with the patient's name and "round ligament" and consists of two membranous pink-tan tissues, 2.0 and 2.5 cm in greatest dimension. Submitted in one cassette.

MICROSCOPIC DIAGNOSIS:

Mesothelial-lined fibrovascular tissue with skeletal muscle, consistent with right inguinal hernia.

7-23C:

SERVICE CODE(S): ______________________

DX CODE(S): ______________________

CASE 7-24
7-24A Surgical Consultation
7-24B Operative Report, Umbilical Herniorrhaphy

CASE 7-24

7-24A SURGICAL CONSULTATION

LOCATION: Outpatient, Clinic

PATIENT: Rose Scheibler

PRIMARY CARE PHYSICIAN: Gary Sanchez, M.D.

CONSULTANT: Ronald Green, M.D.

CHIEF COMPLAINT: Umbilical hernia

HISTORY OF PRESENT ILLNESS: The patient is an otherwise healthy 35-year-old female who presents with a symptomatic umbilical hernia that has been present for some time. She thinks it may have occurred during work and now is tender when she exercises. It is occasionally tender when she moves patients. She is a nurse. She denies any symptoms of obstruction or incarceration and denies any chronic cough, chronic constipation, or difficulty with urination.

PAST MEDICAL HISTORY:
1. Normal spontaneous vaginal delivery ×3
2. History of hypothyroidism

MEDICATIONS: Synthroid

ALLERGIES: None

REVIEW OF SYSTEMS: Otherwise healthy

PHYSICAL EXAM: Chest is clear. Cardiovascular: Regular rate and rhythm. Abdomen: Soft and nontender. There are no masses. She has an easily reducible umbilical hernia. She has no inguinal hernias. Musculoskeletal: Negative. Extremities: Negative. EENT: Negative. Lymph nodes: Negative.

IMPRESSION: Umbilical hernia

RECOMMENDATIONS/PLAN: I have discussed umbilical hernia repair along with the risks of bleeding, infection, and possible recurrence. She appears to understand and wishes to proceed. Will plan to proceed at her earliest convenience. She states that due to work she wishes to have this repaired on Monday. I will make arrangements. Letter to Dr. Sanchez.

7-24A CODES:

SERVICE CODE(S): ______________________________

DX CODE(S): ______________________________

7-24B OPERATIVE REPORT, UMBILICAL HERNIORRHAPHY

LOCATION: Inpatient, Hospital

PATIENT: Rose Scheibler

SURGEON: Gary Sanchez, M.D.

PREOPERATIVE DIAGNOSIS: Umbilical hernia

POSTOPERATIVE DIAGNOSIS: Umbilical hernia

PROCEDURE: Umbilical herniorrhaphy

DATE OF OPERATION:

ANESTHESIA: General

INDICATIONS: The patient, a 35-year-old female, noticed increasing periumbilical pain. She has a noticeable bulge that has increased in size over the past several weeks. She denies any symptoms of obstruction or incarceration. She presents today for elective repair. She understands the risks of bleeding, infection, or possible recurrence and wishes to proceed.

PROCEDURE: The patient was brought to the operating room and placed under general anesthesia, prepped, and draped sterilely. An infraumbilical skin incision was made with a no. 15 blade and carried down through the subcutaneous tissues using sharp dissection. We carried the dissection down to the fascia and then dissected the umbilicus free from its fascial attachment. We opened the hernia sac, reduced the hernia contents, and then repaired the fascial defect with interrupted 0 Vicryl sutures. The umbilicus was packed back down to the fascia with a single interrupted 4-0 undyed Vicryl. Steri-Strips and sterile Band-Aids were applied. Sponge and needle counts were correct prior to leaving the operating room. The wound was anesthetized with 30 cc of 0.5% Sensorcaine with epinephrine solution.

7-24B:

SERVICE CODE(S): ______________________________

DX CODE(S): ______________________________

Hemic/Lymphatic System

The hemic system is the blood-forming system of the body and includes blood cells and bone marrow. The lymphatic system is the drainage system of the body and is closely related to the blood system. The lymph carries waste from the body to the bloodstream. The system is part of the immune system that protects the body, and as such, the physician assesses the status of the lymphatic system by palpating (feeling) the various lymph nodes that are located throughout the body. Enlarged lymph nodes are a sign of infection.

The lymphatic channels are the vessels throughout which the lymph circulates. The lymph nodes are lymph tissue located along the channel. The lymph nodes can be the site of tumor, such as in Hodgkin's disease, which is a malignant tumor of the lymph tissue and spleen. There are several types of non-Hodgkin's lymphoma, such as lymphocytic lymphoma and histiocytic lymphoma. Radiation and/or chemotherapy are used to halt the progress of the disease.

The CPT codes for the lymph nodes and lymphatic channels are 38300-38999. Biopsy of nodes is reported based on the method used to obtain the sample (open or percutaneous) and the nodes sampled (cervical, axillary, internal mammary). Biopsy and excision are usually in a separate section, such as Excision and Biopsy, but for these lymph node codes, both an excision and/or a biopsy can be reported with the same code, for example, 38510 Biopsy or excision of lymph node(s); open, deep cervical node(s). Note that the description indicates both biopsy and excision. Also note that the method (open) and node (cervical) are specified in the code.

Laparoscopy can be used to repair retroperitoneal lymph nodes (38570-38572). Resection of the lymph node differs from the excision of a lymph node. Resection is when the nodes as well as the surrounding tissue are removed and excision is only the lymph node(s).

The **spleen** is composed of lymph tissue located in the left upper quadrant (LUQ). The surgical removal of the spleen is a splenectomy, which can be either total or partial. The spleen is sometimes removed due to extensive disease and is reported with 38100-38101. The spleen can be ruptured as in motor vehicle accidents and requires a splenorrhaphy (38115).

Bone marrow and stem cells (38204-38242) are part of the Hemic and Lymphatic Systems subsection in the CPT and include service codes for bone marrow aspirations and transplantation. Most of these codes are for preparation and preservation of marrow and stem cell transplantation.

Diagnosis Coding of Hematopoietic and Lymphatic Neoplasms

Hematopoietic and lymphatic neoplasms do not spread to secondary sites; rather the cells travel through the hemic and lymphatic systems and then occur in multiple sites within the system. All of these sites are considered primary sites. For example, if the diagnosis is lymphosarcoma of the face, axilla, and intra-abdominal lymph nodes, you would report 200.18 with the fifth digit 8 indicating multiple lymph node sites. (Note the fifth digits available for use with categories 200-202 that appears in the ICD-9-CM before code 200.) Only assign the 200-202 codes when the neoplasm originates in the lymphatic or hematopoietic systems. If a neoplasm spreads from another location in the body to the lymph node, a 196 code is assigned to indicate the lymph node is a secondary site.

Leukemia is a progressive, malignant disease of the blood-forming organs. Leukemias are reported with codes from 204-208 with a fourth digit to indicate the condition as subacute, acute, or chronic. Lymphoid leukemia (204) is a proliferation of the lymphoblasts (immature lymphocytes) referred to as lymphocytic, lymphoblastic, lymphatic, and lymphogenous leukemia. Myeloid leukemia (205) is a proliferation of the myeloblasts (immature myelocytes) referred to as granulocytic, myeloblastic, myelocytic, myelogenous, myelomonocytic, myelosclerotic, and myelosis. Codes in the 204-208 categories have a fifth digit to indicate without mention of remission (0) and in remission (1). Monocytic leukemia (206) is a myelogenous leukemia with a blastic phase. The diagnosis of the blastic phase requires greater than 30% myeloblasts in marrow or blood. Patients in blastic phase live an average of 3 to 6 months.

CASE 7-25
CASE 7-25A Operative Report, Axillary Node Dissection
7-25B Pathology Report

CASE 7-25

CASE 7-25A OPERATIVE REPORT, AXILLARY NODE DISSECTION

LOCATION: Inpatient, Hospital

PATIENT: Gloria Polenske

SURGEON: Gary Sanchez, M.D.

PREOPERATIVE DIAGNOSIS: Left axillary nodes

POSTOPERATIVE DIAGNOSIS: Left axillary nodes, possible malignancy

PROCEDURE PERFORMED: Left axillary node dissection

ANESTHESIA: General

INDICATIONS FOR SURGERY: The patient is a 37-year-old white female who was noted to have left axillary nodes on a physical examination and scan. The patient has a history of having a right breast cancer removed many years ago. The patient is now undergoing left axillary node dissection for diagnosis.

DESCRIPTION OF PROCEDURE: The patient was prepped and draped in the usual manner. She was given a general anesthetic. An incision was made on the lateral border of the pectoralis major muscle. The dissection was carried down into the axilla. Multiple enlarged lymph nodes were identified and excised. All lymph nodes that could be found were removed and sent to pathology. Pathology stated that the lymph nodes were not breast cancer; however, they were highly suspicious for some type of malignancy. Hemostasis was obtained using Bovie cautery and also 3-0 silk ties. The operative area was thoroughly irrigated. The deep layer was closed with a running 3-0 Vicryl suture. The subcutaneous tissue was closed with a running 3-0 Vicryl suture. The skin was closed with 4-0 Vicryl subcuticular stitch. Steri-Strips were applied. The drain was sutured in place using a 3-0 nylon suture. The patient tolerated the operation and returned to recovery in stable condition.

Pathology Report Later Indicated: See Report 7-25B.

7-25A:

SERVICE CODE(S): ______________________

DX CODE(S): ______________________

7-25B PATHOLOGY REPORT

LOCATION: Inpatient, Hospital

PATIENT: Gloria Polenske

SURGEON: Gary Sanchez, M.D.

PATHOLOGIST: Morton Monson, M.D.

CLINICAL HISTORY: History of breast cancer, left axillary nodes

SPECIMEN RECEIVED: A: Left axillary nodes with frozen section. B: Additional axillary nodes, left.

GROSS DESCRIPTION:
A. The specimen is labeled with the patient's name and "left axillary lymph nodes" and consists of a 4 × 2 × 1 cm ovoid fatty lymphoid tissue.

INTRAOPERATIVE FROZEN-SECTION DIAGNOSIS: No evidence of breast carcinoma; rule out lymphoma on permanent sections

B. The specimen is labeled with the patient's name and "additional axillary nodes, left" and consists of three, up to 2-cm, pieces of tan lymphoid-appearing tissue.

MICROSCOPIC DESCRIPTION:
A. and B. Sections show lymph nodes showing a diffuse proliferation, lymphocytes, which are uniform in size and shape and replace the normal lymphoid architecture. Occasional histiocytic-type cells are scattered throughout the proliferation, and prominent vasculature is noted in the interstitium. Immunohistochemical stain for CD20 shows positive diffusion.

DIAGNOSIS:
A. and B. Small lymphocytic lymphoma, left axillary nodes.

COMMENT: The case was reviewed with Dr. Sanchez.

7-25B:

SERVICE CODE(S): ______________________

DX CODE(S): ______________________

CASE 7-26
7-26A Operative Report, Splenectomy
7-26B Pathology Report

CASE 7-26

7-26A OPERATIVE REPORT, SPLENECTOMY

LOCATION: Inpatient, Hospital

PATIENT: Morgan Hillard

SURGEON: Gary Sanchez, M.D.

PREOPERATIVE DIAGNOSIS: Idiopathic thrombocytopenic purpura refractory to medical therapy

POSTOPERATIVE DIAGNOSIS: Same

PROCEDURE PERFORMED: Splenectomy, total

HISTORY: This gentleman has ITP refractory to medical therapy. It was elected to do an open splenectomy. It was difficult to consider a laparoscopic splenectomy in a person who has had such severe vascular disease, but more importantly he had perforated diverticulitis with a colon resection and then had an incisional hernia repair with mesh. I felt that the wiser approach would be to do a left-sided Kocher incision and try to stay away from the mesh and away, hopefully, from the adhesions.

PROCEDURE: The patient was given a general anesthetic. He had a Foley catheter inserted. He was prepped and draped while in a supine fashion. We made a left-sided Kocher incision. We looked way into the abdomen. He had a lot of adhesions, but they were below our lower-most incision so that turned out great. We used the Omni retractor and got everything set up. We then identified a very large spleen. It was about 60% the size of the liver. We lifted up the spleen and brought it through the wound. We identified the major vessels, which we controlled with right angles, and then we divided them. There were short gastric vessels that we dealt with the same way. We then removed the spleen and made sure that there was no tear of the spleen and no chance of splenosis. We then doubly tied all areas and made sure we suture ligated the major vessels in addition to tying them. We then looked along the greater curve. There were two small short gastric vessels that were not bleeding that had been dealt with during the dissection, but we elected to lift these up and clip them. We had excellent hemostasis at the end. The pancreas looked normal. We looked around and made sure that there were no signs of any accessory spleens. We then irrigated and suctioned out copiously and closed the wound with no. 2 Vicryl stitches in a two-layer fashion. We then irrigated out the wound and put in some staples. We put some 0.25% plain Marcaine into the wound. Telfa, Toppers, and gauze were applied. The patient tolerated this well and went to the recovery room in good condition.

7-26A:

SERVICE CODE(S): ____________________

DX CODE(S): ____________________

7-26B PATHOLOGY REPORT

LOCATION: Inpatient, Hospital

PATIENT: Morgan Hillard

SURGEON: Gary Sanchez, M.D.

PATHOLOGIST: Morton Monson, M.D.

CLINICAL HISTORY: Idiopathic thrombocytopenia, purpura

SPECIMEN RECEIVED: Spleen

GROSS DESCRIPTION:

Received in a container labeled "spleen" is a spleen measuring 18 × 9.5 × 6 cm in greatest dimension and weighing 620 g. The surface contains a capsule that is mildly wrinkled and has a gray-purple appearance. The hilum demonstrates small superficial lacerations. The specimen is step-sectioned and demonstrates a uniform red-purple color. A faintly distinct nodular appearance is present. Representative portions are submitted.

The spleen demonstrates a prominent red pulp with congestion of the sinusoids. Scattered follicles showing normal morphology are widely separated by the expanded red pulp. The sinusoids exhibit megakaryocytic and erythroid metaplasia.

DIAGNOSIS:
Spleen, excision: Splenomegaly, marked, with severe congestion. Extramedullary hematopoiesis with megakaryocytic and erythroid hyperplasia.

COMMENT: The above-described findings have been noted in idiopathic thrombocytopenic purpura.

Case reviewed by Dr. Melon from the university.

7-26B:

SERVICE CODE(S): ____________________

DX CODE(S): ____________________

CASE 7-27
7-27A Bone Marrow Biopsy

CASE 7-27

7-27A BONE MARROW BIOPSY

In the following report, there were two procedures performed during one operative session. The aspiration procedure is the least intensive procedure.

LOCATION: Inpatient, Hospital

PATIENT: Sammy Schultz

SURGEON: Gary Sanchez, M.D.

PREOPERATIVE DIAGNOSIS: Anemia, acute renal failure, diffuse skeletal pain — bone pain

POSTOPERATIVE DIAGNOSIS: Same

PROCEDURE PERFORMED: Bone marrow aspiration and biopsy

DESCRIPTION OF PROCEDURE: The patient was sterilized and anesthetized by standard procedure. One bone marrow core biopsy was obtained from the right posterior iliac crest with moderate to severe discomfort. At the end of the procedure, the patient had no obvious discomfort and no obvious complications. On three different occasions, I attempted to obtain bone marrow aspiration from the right posterior iliac crest and was unsuccessful. It seemed to be a dry tap. I went over to the left posterior iliac crest and was able to obtain some bone marrow aspirate with some minimal to moderate discomfort. Most of the patient's discomfort was from having to lie on his right shoulder because he has been having discomfort there.

At the end of the procedure, the patient had no discomfort, and there was no obvious complication.

7-27A:

SERVICE CODE(S): ____________________

DX CODE(S): ____________________

CASE 7-28

7-28A BONE MARROW BIOPSY

LOCATION: Inpatient, Hospital

PATIENT: George Orwell

SURGEON: Gary Sanchez, M.D.

PREOPERATIVE DIAGNOSIS: Acute myelogenous leukemia

POSTOPERATIVE DIAGNOSIS: Acute myelogenous leukemia

PROCEDURE PERFORMED: Bone marrow biopsy

PROCEDURE: The patient was sterilized and anesthetized by standard procedure. One bone marrow core biopsy was obtained from the left posterior iliac crest with minimal discomfort. At the end of the procedure, the patient denied discomfort, and there were no obvious complications. I did obtain one bone marrow aspirate from the left posterior iliac crest with minimal to moderate discomfort. At the end of the procedure, the patient denied discomfort, and there were no obvious complications.

7-28A:

SERVICE CODE(S): ____________________

DX CODE(S): ____________________

Glossary

anoscope instrument used in an examination of the anus

biopsy removal of a small piece of living tissue for diagnostic purposes

catheter tube placed into the body to put fluid in or take fluid out

cholecystectomy removal of the gallbladder

endoscopy inspection of body organs or cavities using a lighted scope that may be inserted through an existing opening or through a small incision

fistula abnormal opening from one area to another area or to the outside of the body

gastroenterologist a physician who specializes in the diagnosis and treatment of the digestive system

gastrointestinal pertaining to the stomach and intestine

hemodialysis cleansing of the blood outside of the body

laparoscopy exploration of the abdomen and pelvic cavities using a scope placed through a small incision in the abdominal wall

Chapter 8

Musculoskeletal System

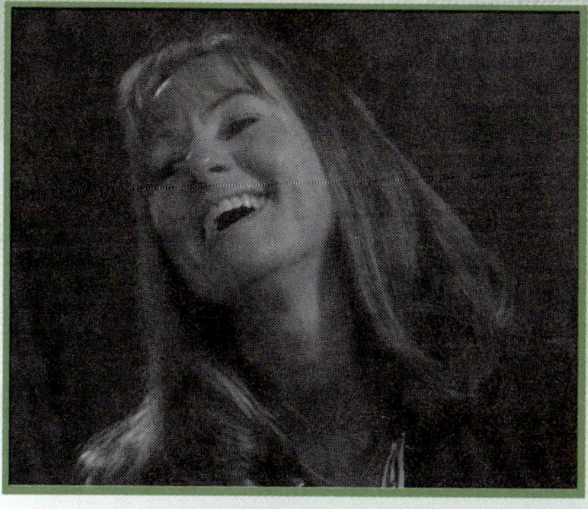

Sharon Parr, CPC
Patient Accounts Supervisor
Cardiology Specialists, Inc.
St. Louis, Missouri

ABBREVIATIONS

A1 pulley	tendon on anterior surface of finger
ACL	anterior cruciate ligament
AKA	above-knee amputation
AP	anteroposterior
BKA	below-knee amputation
C1-C7	cervical vertebrae
CTS	carpal tunnel syndrome
CVA	cerebrovascular accident (stroke)
fx	fracture
I&D	incision and drainage
L1-5	lumbar vertebrae
M-1 tibia	tibial insert
MAC	monitored anesthesia care
MRI	magnetic resonance imaging
OA	osteoarthritis
ORIF	open reduction, internal fixation
PCL	posterior cruciate ligament
RA	rheumatoid arthritis
T1-12	thoracic vertebrae
TMJ	temporomandibular joint

Common musculoskeletal complaints are pain of the neck, knee, shoulder, elbow, wrist, hand, back, hip, ankle, and foot. Conditions commonly related to the musculoskeletal system are sprains, bursitis, tendonitis, dislocations, fractures, nerve entrapments (such as carpal tunnel syndrome), and gout. A physician who specializes in the diagnosis and treatment of musculoskeletal disorders is an **orthopedist.** An **orthopedic surgeon** is one who not only diagnoses and treats musculoskeletal disorders but also performs musculoskeletal surgical procedures, for example, repairs involving the placement of pins, wires, screws, cranial halos, spinal instrumentation, and other fixation devices. Reconstruction surgeries such as hip replacements and other joint replacements are now performed frequently. Endoscopic procedures are often used in the orthopedic specialty. Most major clinics would have orthopedic physician(s)/surgeon(s) on staff, and in other settings the orthopedic services would be provided by an orthopedist in independent practice. Orthopedic physicians frequently receive referrals from other physicians to consult on musculoskeletal conditions.

Arthrocentesis

Arthrocentesis is injection and/or aspiration of a joint and is a commonly used treatment for joint conditions. A needle is inserted into the joint to anesthetize it. Drugs such as Depo-Medrol (synthetic glucocorticoid) or cortisone can then be injected into the joint, or fluid can be withdrawn. Bundled into the arthrocentesis are the dual services of injection and aspiration. For example, 20610 is reported when a physician withdraws fluid from the knee joint and then injects Depo-Medrol into the knee joint. The drug injected would be reported separately with a HCPCS code. HCPCS J code (drug code) descriptions identify the drug by the generic name, not the brand name. When reporting the drug with a HCPCS code, it is necessary to translate the brand name into the generic name; this is when the cross-reference feature of the Table of Drugs will be useful. For example, if the medical record indicates a Depo-Medrol injection, the Table of Drugs entry for Depo-Medrol (brand name) refers you to the generic name of the drug, methylprednisolone acetate (J1020-J1040). A current medical drug reference is also often necessary to translate brand names into the generic names to locate the drug in the HCPCS manual.

If image guidance was used during an arthrocentesis reported with 20600-20610, report the radiographic service separately with 76003, 76360, 76393, or 76942.

Injections into the tendon sheath, origin, or muscle are reported with 20550-20553 and are reported one time per service visit when the same tendon sheath, tendon origin/insertion, or muscle is injected, no matter how many injections were placed in that specific sheath, origin/insertion, or muscle. If, however, a tendon sheath and a tendon insertion were injected, both injections are reported.

- One sheath, origin/insert, or muscle injected, report one injection code.
- Multiple sheaths, origins/insertions, or muscle sites injected, report multiple injection codes.

Use modifier -59 (distinct service) when reporting multiple injections during the same service visit to make it clear that documentation indicates that separate services were provided. The drug injected would be reported separately with a CPT or HCPCS code. If image guidance was used during an injection reported with 20550-20553, report the radiographic service separately with 76003, 76393, or 76942.

Fractures

The categories used to report fractures are 800-829 as follows:

Skull (800-804)
Neck and Trunk (805-809)
Upper Limb (810-819)
Lower Limb (820-829)

The codes within these categories are usually divided based on the exact location of the fracture and/or open/closed type. For example:

802	Fractures of face bones		
	802.2	Mandible, closed	
		802.25	Angle of the jaw
		802.29	Multiple sites
	802.3	Mandible, open	
		802.35	Angle of the jaw
		802. 39	Multiple sites

There are many other 802.2x and 802.3x five-digit codes to choose from; these are displayed as an example of the closed/open codes. **Closed fractures** are those in which the bone does not protrude outside the skin and usually include terms such as compound, infected, missile, puncture, or with foreign body. **Open fractures** are those in which the bone does protrude outside the skin and include terms such as comminuted, compound, depressed, elevated, fissured greenstick, impacted, linear, simple, or spiral. If the documentation indicates both open and closed fracture terminology, assign an open fracture code. The type of treatment does not necessarily correlate to type of fracture; for example, an open reduction of a closed fracture.

Vertebral column fractures are reported with 805, without mention of spinal cord injury, and 806, with mention of spinal cord injury. If the injury was only of the spinal cord, report with a 952 category code, spinal cord injury without evidence of spinal bone injury. Cervical injuries (805.0, closed, and 806.1, open) are reported with a fifth digit (0-8) to indicate the level as C1-C7, unspecified, or multiple cervical vertebrae.

Fractures of the rib(s), sternum, larynx, and trachea are assigned to 807 based on the status of open/closed and specific location. There are fifth digits available (0-9) to indicate the number of ribs involved.

Fractures of the upper limbs (810-819) are divided by the specific location as are the fractures of the lower limbs (820-829). There are fifth digits available for many of the codes.

E codes are only reported at the time of initial episode of care and only if the facility policy indicates that E codes will be assigned. If, as per facility policy, E codes are assigned, and since fractures usually are a result of an accident of some type an E code would be assigned to indicate the way in which the accident happened (circumstances of the accident).

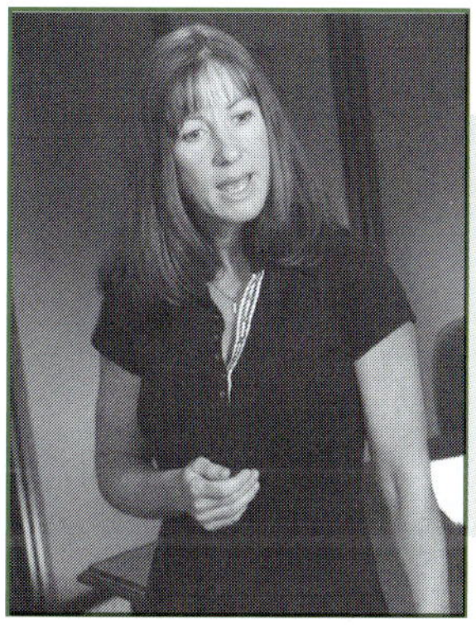

FROM THE TRENCHES

Sharon

What's the most interesting part of your job?

"There's so much to learn and I just think that's the great part…I like [coding] and you have to like doing it, or you're not going to do it right. You have to enjoy it. You have to like to study, and you have to do a lot of self-study…It's difficult, but it's a lot of fun."

CASE 8-1
8-1A Orthopedic Consultation

CASE 8-1

Dr. Green referred Janelle Masche to Dr. Almaz, an orthopedic physician/surgeon, for an opinion about her right tennis elbow (epicondylitis), which is an overuse syndrome. The lateral epicondyle is the outside bony portion of the elbow where the tendons attach from the muscle to the elbow. Repetitive motion can injure the tendon, causing pain. X-rays are usually normal. Local cortisone may be injected.

8-1A ORTHOPEDIC CONSULTATION

LOCATION: Outpatient, Clinic

PATIENT: Janelle Masche

PRIMARY CARE PHYSICIAN: Ronald Green, M.D.

CONSULTANT: Mohomad Almaz, M.D.

HISTORY OF PRESENT ILLNESS: The patient is a 52-year-old woman who works in coding at the local hospital. Dr. Green referred her for right tennis elbow.

She explained that her right wrist started hurting about 6 months ago when she was pulling some charts. Then, about 4 months ago, she developed some pain along the lateral aspect of her right elbow. She saw Dr. Green and states that he treated her with an injection. I am unable to find evidence of this injection in the chart, but she explained that it was done probably in 1989. She has also been treated with a tennis elbow strap.

PHYSICAL EXAMINATION: The physical examination today finds that she localizes her pain to the lateral aspect of the right elbow near the lateral humeral epicondyle. She has pain in the area with dorsiflexion of her wrist against resistance. She has a full range of motion of her right elbow, including supination and pronation. No areas of erythema are noted.

X-rays of her right elbow found the bony architecture to appear essentially within normal limits.

IMPRESSION: Right lateral humeral epicondylitis

RECOMMENDATION: I have elected to inject the tender area over the right lateral humeral epicondyle with 80 mg of Depo-Medrol and 1 cc of 1% Xylocaine following Betadine prep. I have asked that she let me know if she has further problems. She understands that a tennis elbow release may be necessary if the pain returns following these injections.

8-1A:

SERVICE CODE(S): ______________________

HCPCS DRUG CODE: ______________________

DX CODE(S): ______________________

Fixation

Fixation can be internal or external and is used to hold a bone in place. **Internal fixation** is the placement of wires, pins, screws, plates, or rods onto or into the bone to repair bones. The fixations can also be inserted into the bone **percutaneously** (skeletal fixation) to serve as attachments for traction devices. **External fixation** is the application of a device that holds the bone in place from the outside. Fasteners are driven into the bone percutaneously, and the external fixation device is attached to the fasteners.

Both application and removal of the device are reported with one code. If a physician other than the physician who applied the device removes the device, the removal is reported separately. When reporting a fracture repair with the application of a fixation device, the device is usually reported separately; however, use caution when reporting the repair and application, because some fracture codes include application of devices in the code description (so then you would not report the services separately). Routine adjustment of the device is included in the application code unless the adjustment requires anesthesia.

CASE 8-2
8-2A Operative Report, Application of Halo

CASE 8-2

Dr. Almaz applies a cranial halo to stabilize a C1-2 fracture, as illustrated in Figure 8-1. This is the initial treatment of the injury. Assign an E code to indicate how the accident happened.

8-2A OPERATIVE REPORT, APPLICATION OF HALO

LOCATION: Outpatient, Hospital

PATIENT: Ella German

SURGEON: Mohomad Almaz, M.D.

PREOPERATIVE DIAGNOSIS: Fracture of C1 and C2

POSTOPERATIVE DIAGNOSIS: Fracture of C1 and C2

PROCEDURE PERFORMED: Application of halo

PROCEDURE: The patient's head was prepped and draped. The halo was applied to the head. Lidocaine was used in the area where the pins enter. We then placed the pins and fitted the patient with the rest of the vest. The patient is comfortable. She can get mobilized with the halo. She is 89 years old. You wonder whether she will ever heal after this fall. We will keep her in the halo for 3 to 4 months and see if she heals properly.

8-2A:

SERVICE CODE(S): ____________________

DX CODE(S): ____________________

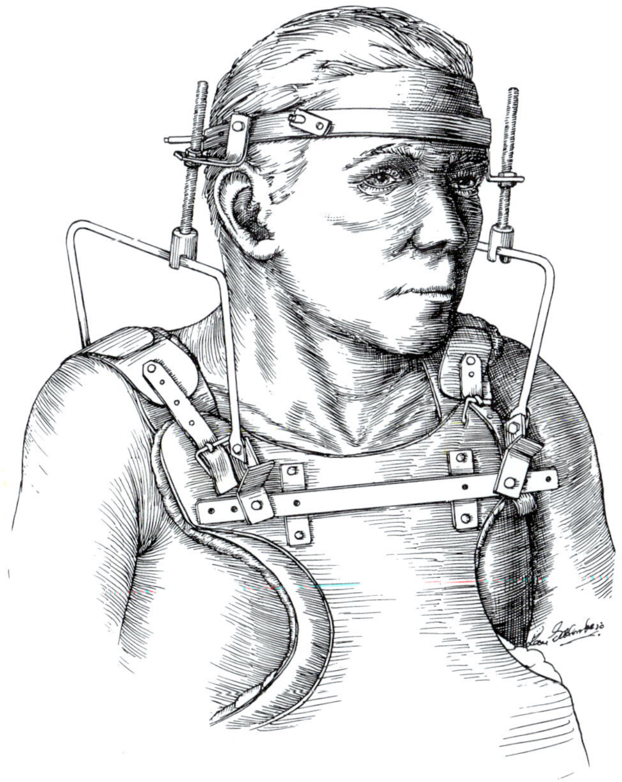

FIGURE 8-1 A cranial halo device. *(From Johnson RM, et al: Surgical approaches to the spine. In Herkowitz HN, et al., eds: Rothman-Simeone the spine, ed 4, vol II. Philadelphia, 1999, WB Saunders.)*

CASE 8-3
8-3A Operative Report, Hardware Removal

CASE 8-3

Removal of hardware is not included in the insertion procedures when the procedure is done outside the global period, as in this case in which the hardware was placed last year and is being removed now and reported separately. Code the removal service in the following case (Remember to report the diagnosis as a fracture **aftercare** *with a V code.):*

8-3A OPERATIVE REPORT, HARDWARE REMOVAL

LOCATION: Outpatient, Hospital

PATIENT: Gary Leiser

SURGEON: Mohomad Almaz, M.D.

PREOPERATIVE DIAGNOSIS: Healed comminuted fracture, right distal radius

POSTOPERATIVE DIAGNOSIS: Healed comminuted fracture, right distal radius

NAME OF OPERATION: Removal of hardware, right distal radius

INDICATIONS FOR SURGERY: This patient had a traumatic distal radius fracture treated last year with a Synthes dorsal distal radius plate. Because of the risk of atraumatic rupture of the extensor tendons running over the plate, it was elected to remove the plate at this time.

OPERATIVE PROCEDURE: After a suitable general anesthesia was achieved, the patient's right wrist, hand, and forearm were prepped and draped. Before prepping, an arm tourniquet was applied and after draping inflated to 250 mmHg. Scar on the dorsal aspect of the wrist was used as the site of the incision. The extensor pollicis longus tendon was incised in line with the tendon. The tendon was then retracted. The extensor retinaculum was elevated off at the plate bone level. The plate was then easily exposed. Screws were removed, and the plate was easily elevated. The wound was then irrigated. Skin edges were infiltrated with 0.5% Marcaine with adrenaline. The retinaculum was closed with 2-0 Tycron, subcutaneous tissue with 3-0 Vicryl, and the skin with interrupted 4-0 nylon horizontal mattress sutures (*this indicates the plate removal was from "deep" layers*). The patient tolerated the procedure well and returned to the recovery room in stable condition.

8-3A:

SERVICE CODE(S): ______________________

DX CODE(S): ______________________

Excision

Throughout the Musculoskeletal System subsection, there are excision codes. These codes are used to report excisions from the deeper levels. Recall that excision codes are also located in the Integumentary System subsection. It is the depth of the excision that differentiates the codes. For example if a superficial benign lesion was removed from the skin of the leg, the service is reported with a code from 11400-11406 (Integumentary System). If the excision was of a lesion located on the muscle of the leg, the service is reported with 27619 (Musculoskeletal System). Watch for terms that indicate the extent or depth of the excision, such as resection, deeper layers, extensive undermining, muscles, bones, and other terms that indicate those deeper structures.

CASE 8-4

8-4A OPERATIVE REPORT, PREAURICULAR AREA EXCISION

LOCATION: Outpatient, Hospital

PATIENT: Doris Fisher

SURGEON: Mohomad Almaz, M.D.

PREOPERATIVE DIAGNOSIS: Malignant melanoma, skin of left preauricular area

POSTOPERATIVE DIAGNOSIS: Malignant melanomas with clear margins on the skin of the left preauricular area

PROCEDURE PERFORMED: Wide excision (*this indicates radical excision*) of malignant melanoma, skin of left preauricular area

ANESTHESIA: General endotracheal with supplementary 1% Xylocaine with 1:800,000 epinephrine

ESTIMATED BLOOD LOSS: Approximately 25 cc

PROCEDURE: The patient's left face and ear were prepped with Betadine scrub and solution and draped in a routine sterile fashion. The lesion was excised to include the crus of the left ear in the dissection, because this was the only method to provide at least 2 cm of width around the excision site. We were able to get about 2.5 cm on the anterior excision site and at least 3 cm proximally and distally. We submitted the specimen, tagging the superior aspect with a silk suture, and cauterized the bleeding. A small section of the fascia and muscle was repaired and then, using separate instrument and gloves, we undermined the skin after the manner of a subcutaneous facelift and brought the skin up, suturing it to the more posterior edge with interrupted 3-0 Prolene. We dressed the wound with Xeroform, Kerlix fluffs, and a Kerlix roll plus Kling. The patient tolerated the procedure well and left the operating table in good condition.

Pathology Report Later Indicated: Malignant melanoma

8-4A:

SERVICE CODE(S): ____________________

DX CODE(S): ____________________

CASE 8-5
8-5A Operative Report, Carbuncle Removal

CASE 8-5

Not all deep tissue excisions are reported with Musculoskeletal System codes. For example, the services in the next two cases are reported with Hemic and Lymphatic Systems codes. Note the two diagnoses bolded in this report. This is another good example of why a coder ***must*** *read the report and not code from the Postoperative Diagnosis section of the report.*

8-5A OPERATIVE REPORT, CARBUNCLE REMOVAL

LOCATION: Outpatient, Hospital

PATIENT: Jennifer Carlin

PRIMARY CARE PHYSICIAN: Ronald Green, M.D.

SURGEON: Gary Sanchez, M.D.

PREOPERATIVE DIAGNOSIS: Two separate **carbuncles,** left axilla

POSTOPERATIVE DIAGNOSIS: Two separate carbuncles, left axilla

PROCEDURE PERFORMED: Removal of two separate carbuncles, left axilla. Tissue was submitted for aerobic and anaerobic cultures as well as permanent section.

INDICATION: This patient for the last 6 months has had a couple of carbuncles in her left axilla. They have been observed, and she has been placed on antibiotics. Attempts at drainage have been made, however, without results. Finally, the patient wants to have these tumors removed.

PROCEDURE IN DETAIL: After good MAC, the patient was prepped and draped in the usual sterile fashion. The left arm was adducted to expose the axilla. The two areas were infiltrated separately with 1% lidocaine after the incisions were made over both affected areas, and dissection was carried down to encompass subdural and deeper tissue. An **inflamed lymph node** was also identified, and this was taken with the more superficial tissue. After this, the wounds were irrigated and closed with 4-0 subcuticular stitch. Steri-Strips and sterile dressings were applied. The patient tolerated the procedure well and was returned to the recovery room in good condition.

Pathology Report Later Indicated: Lymph node was negative for neoplastic behavior.

8-5A:

SERVICE CODE(S): ______________________

DX CODE(S): ______________________

CASE 8-6

8-6A OPERATIVE REPORT, DISSECTION AND EXCISION

LOCATION: Outpatient, Hospital

PATIENT: Sara Henre

PRIMARY CARE PHYSICIAN: Ronald Green, M.D.

SURGEON: Gary Sanchez, M.D.

PREOPERATIVE DIAGNOSIS: History of palpable right axillary mass

POSTOPERATIVE DIAGNOSIS: History of palpable right axillary mass

OPERATIVE PROCEDURE: Superficial right axillary dissection and excision of lymphatic tissue

COMPLICATIONS: None

ESTIMATED BLOOD LOSS: 50 cc

ANESTHESIA: General endotracheal with 30 cc of 0.5% Marcaine augmentation

SPECIMEN: Superficial axillary contents. No large mass was identified.

PROCEDURE: After good general endotracheal anesthesia, the patient was prepped and draped in the usual sterile fashion. The arm and axilla were prepped, and the hand and forearm were covered with a stockinette to allow mobilizing. The patient was previously interviewed in the preoperative area, and the palpable little mass had been marked with ink. An incision was made over this area, which was in the axillary skin fold just above the axillary hairline, and this was after anesthetizing the skin. Dissection was carried down right under the skin in search of this nodule. We did find some fatty tissue, which could have represented a small lipoma in this area. This was resected. The axillary fascia was identified and incised, and similar fatty tissue was excised upward at the border of the latissimus and then down toward the posterior border of the axilla. An exploring finger was placed up in the axilla up toward the axillary vein, and no palpable adenopathy was noted, nor was there any adenopathy noted when the rest of the axilla was explored with a finger. We did continue to take away small pieces of lymphatic tissue in the entire area where the patient felt the lump and submitted this as axillary fatty and lymphatic contents. The wound was thoroughly irrigated. Bleeding was controlled using electrocautery. The wound was then closed in layers with 3-0 Vicryl and 4-0 Vicryl subcuticular. The patient tolerated the procedure well and was returned to the recovery room in good condition.

Pathology Report Later Indicated: Benign encapsulated lipoma (*of skin of breast*) ① axilla

8-6A:

SERVICE CODE(S): ______________________

DX CODE(S): ______________________

Rationale was unclear { 38525-RT or 38740

CASE 8-7
8-7A Operative Report, Nevus Removal

CASE 8-7

A congenital nevus is a mole that is present at birth. There is a difference between a small and a giant nevus. Usually a giant congenital nevus is larger than 20 cm, and the small nevus is usually about 1.5 cm. In the CPT, the excision codes for nevus are based on the depth of subcutaneous or intramuscular excision.

8-7A OPERATIVE REPORT, NEVUS REMOVAL

LOCATION: Outpatient, Hospital

PATIENT: Earl Oukek

PRIMARY CARE PHYSICIAN: Ronald Green, M.D.

SURGEON: Mohomad Almaz, M.D.

PREOPERATIVE DIAGNOSIS: Giant congenital nevus, left pectoral region involving the left areola

POSTOPERATIVE DIAGNOSIS: Giant congenital nevus, left pectoral region involving the left areola

PROCEDURE PERFORMED: Excision of giant congenital nevus and portion of areola of the left chest

SURGICAL FINDINGS: A 7 × 4-cm giant congenital nevus (common nevus) involving about 50% of the areola on the left side

ANESTHESIA: General endotracheal plus 4 cc of 0.5% Xylocaine and 1:100,000 epinephrine

COMPLICATIONS: None

SPONGE AND NEEDLE COUNTS: Correct

DESCRIPTION OF THE PROCEDURE: The patient's chest wall was prepped with Betadine scrub and solution and draped in a routine sterile fashion. I injected 4 cc of 0.5% Xylocaine with 1:100,000 epinephrine along the suture line and excised the lesion down to carpus fascia being sure to include the complete dermis and a little subcutaneous fat. We cauterized the bleeders and tagged the superior aspect of the specimen with a silk suture. We closed the wound with subcuticular 3-0 Monocryl and three twists of 6-0 Prolene. One-half-inch Steri-Strips were applied, plus a clavicle strap for immobilization. Estimated blood loss was less than 5 cc. The patient tolerated the procedure well and left the operating room in good condition.

Pathology Report Later Indicated: Benign tissue (*chest skin*)

8-7A:

SERVICE CODE(S): ______________________

DX CODE(S): ______________________

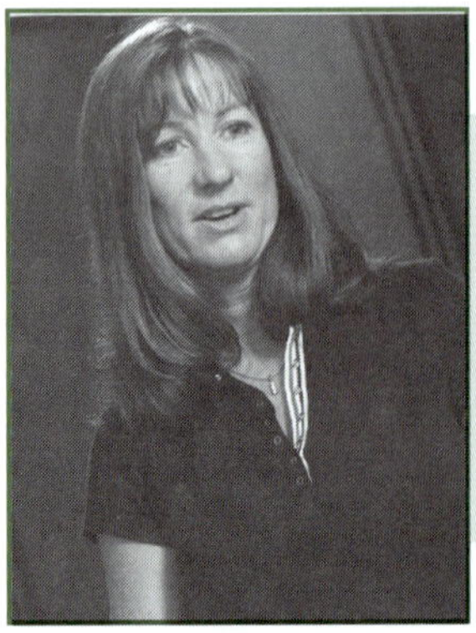

FROM THE TRENCHES

Sharon

"I think, unfortunately, there are people out there that don't do things fairly... You need to be steadfast to know and tell them 'I'm not doing that. That is not the right thing, and if that is what you want me to do, then I can't work here anymore.' That's the stand that you have to take as a coder. That's your profession, so stand behind it."

CASE 8-8
8-8A Operative Report, Costovertebral Tumor

CASE 8-8

8-8A OPERATIVE REPORT, COSTOVERTEBRAL TUMOR

LOCATION: Outpatient, Hospital

PATIENT: Leif Hanson

PRIMARY CARE PHYSICIAN: Leslie Alanda, M.D.

SURGEON: Mohomad Almaz, M.D.

PREOPERATIVE DIAGNOSIS: Residual plexiform fibrous histiocytic tumor of left costovertebral angle area (back)

POSTOPERATIVE DIAGNOSIS: Residual plexiform fibrous histiocytic tumor of left costovertebral angle area

PROCEDURE PERFORMED: Excision of plexiform fibrous histiocytic tumor (*this is a mast cell tumor*) of left costovertebral angle (*this is connective tissue of the back*) and evacuation of hematoma (*this is a postoperative hematoma*), left costovertebral angle

ANESTHESIA: General endotracheal was with approximately 20 cc of tumescent solution prepared by adding to 1L of Ringer's lactate, 25 cc 2% Xylocaine, 1 cc of 1:100,000 epinephrine, and 3 cc of 8.4% sodium bicarbonate.

ESTIMATED BLOOD LOSS: Negligible

SURGICAL FINDINGS: There was a healing 2.5-cm incision of the left costovertebral angle, and in the subcutaneous space on top of the latissimus dorsi muscle, there was about a 50-cc hematoma that was beginning to organize.

DESCRIPTION OF PROCEDURE: The patient was intubated and turned in the prone position. The area of the left costovertebral angle was prepped with Betadine scrub and solution and draped in a routine sterile fashion. An incision was made 2 cm around in the previous incision site and carried down to the fascia of the muscle, where a hematoma was entered. The skin portion of that lesion was removed, and the fascia and a portion of the muscle of the latissimus dorsi were removed secondarily. Bleeding was electrocoagulated, and a no. 7 Jackson-Pratt drain was inserted in the depth of the wound. The wound was closed with interrupted 0 Monocryl for the deep fascia layer and subcuticular 4-0 Monocryl using a few vertical mattress sutures of 3-0 Monocryl. Steri-Strips and Kerlix fluffs plus Elastoplast were applied. The patient tolerated the procedure well and left the operating room in good condition.

Pathology Report Later Indicated: Mast cell tumor

8-8A:

SERVICE CODE(S): ____________________

DX CODE(S): ____________________

CASE 8-9
8-9A Operative Report, Shoulder Mass Excision
8-9B Pathology Report

CASE 8-9

8-9A OPERATIVE REPORT, SHOULDER MASS EXCISION

LOCATION: Outpatient, Hospital

PATIENT: Verner Fox

SURGEON: Mohomad Almaz, M.D.

PREOPERATIVE DIAGNOSIS: Giant mass of right shoulder

POSTOPERATIVE DIAGNOSIS: Giant mass of right shoulder, probable lipoma

PROCEDURE PERFORMED: Excision of a giant shoulder mass. The mass was excised and measured 14 × 14 inches × 6 inches deep. This was found to be superficial to the trapezius fascia.

DRAIN: One Jackson-Pratt

PROCEDURE IN DETAIL: After good sedation, the area around the giant mass was anesthetized with a total of 60 cc of 0.5% Marcaine with epinephrine. An incision was along Langer's line over the apex of the mass. Dissection was carried down through the skin down to the mass itself. Very large skin flaps were created in both directions measuring 6 inches and 6 inches. The mass was quite adherent, and any fibrous septa were dissected free to mobilize it. Eventually we were able to mobilize the bottom of the mass, and we were able to reflect it back from the fascia. We then dissected it free of its fascial attachments going medially to laterally. We then removed it from the lateral attachments that were very close to the skin. After the mass was excised, the wound was thoroughly irrigated. Meticulous hemostasis was obtained with electrocautery. A no. 10 flat Jackson-Pratt was placed and brought out inferior to the wound. The wound was then closed in two layers with 3-0 Vicryl subdermal and 2-0 nylon mattress sutures. The drain was secured with 0 Prolene and placed to bulb suction. The patient tolerated the procedure well and was returned to the recovery room in good condition.

Pathology Report Later Indicated: See 8-9B.

8-9A:

SERVICE CODE(S): ______________________

DX CODE(S): ______________________

8-9B PATHOLOGY REPORT

LOCATION: Outpatient, Hospital

PATIENT: Verner Fox

SURGEON: Mohomad Almaz, M.D.

PATHOLOGIST: Morton Monson, M.D.

CLINICAL HISTORY: Right shoulder mass

SPECIMEN RECEIVED: Right shoulder mass

GROSS DESCRIPTION: The specimen is labeled with the patient's name and "right shoulder mass" and consists of a 635-globulated mass of adipose-like tissue. The exterior surgical margins are inked in black. The mass is approximately 16 × 15 × 5 cm in thickness. Cut sections show adipose tissue throughout. Representative sections are submitted in 13 cassettes.

MICROSCOPIC DESCRIPTION: Sections show adipose throughout intersected by fine strands of fibrous tissue.

DIAGNOSIS: Right shoulder mass: benign lipoma

8-9B:

SERVICE CODE(S): ______________________

DX CODE(S): ______________________

CASE 8-10

8-10A OPERATIVE REPORT, TUMOR EXCISION

LOCATION: Outpatient, Hospital

PATIENT: Ervin Gulman

SURGEON: Mohomad Almaz, M.D.

PREOPERATIVE DIAGNOSIS: Malignant melanoma, left shoulder (6/10 mm thick)

POSTOPERATIVE DIAGNOSIS: Malignant melanoma, left shoulder (6/10 mm thick)

PROCEDURE PERFORMED: Radical excision of malignant melanoma, posterior aspect of skin of left shoulder

ANESTHESIA: General endotracheal with supplementary 1% Xylocaine with 1:100,000 epinephrine, approximately 10 cc

ESTIMATED BLOOD LOSS: Negligible

PROCEDURE: The shoulder was prepped with Betadine scrub and solution and draped in the routine sterile fashion. A margin of about 3 cm laterally and medially around the healed incision site was taken, tapering to a 4 to 5 cm proximally and distally. The incision was carried down to the muscle fascia, which was included with the specimen. Bleeding was electrocoagulated, and the wound was closed with subcuticular 2-0 Monocryl and some twists and pulley sutures of 2-0 Monocryl in the center of the wound, where the most tension was. Kerlix fluffs and a sling were applied followed by an external Ace bandage. The patient tolerated the procedure well and left the area in good condition.

Pathology Report Later Indicated: Malignant melanoma of shoulder (*this is an upper limb.*)

8-10A:

SERVICE CODE(S): ____________________

DX CODE(S): ____________________

CASE 8-11
8-11A Operative Report, Ganglion Cyst

CASE 8-11

The service code in this case requires a HCPCS modifier.

8-11A OPERATIVE REPORT, GANGLION CYST

LOCATION: Outpatient, Hospital

PATIENT: Lilah Coan

SURGEON: Mohomad Almaz, M.D.

INDICATIONS FOR PROCEDURE: This patient has had a ganglion cyst of the second web space of the left hand just proximal to the web space but overlying the ulnar side of the A1 pulley. It has become annoying and occasionally painful.

PREOPERATIVE DIAGNOSIS: Ganglion cyst, left index finger, with protrusion into second web space on the ulnar side

POSTOPERATIVE DIAGNOSIS: Ganglion cyst, left index finger, with protrusion into second web space on the ulnar side

PROCEDURE PERFORMED: Excision of ganglion cyst, left index finger

SURGICAL FINDINGS: A 1-cm diameter more or less dumbbell-shaped ganglion cyst of the left index finger arises from the ulnar side of the A1 pulley and extending into the base of the second web space.

ANESTHESIA: Intravenous block

ESTIMATED BLOOD LOSS: Zero

COMPLICATIONS: None

SPONGE AND NEEDLE COUNTS: Correct

PROCEDURE: Under satisfactory intravenous block anesthesia, the patient's left hand and arm were prepped with Betadine scrub and solution and draped in the routine sterile fashion. Using 2.5-power magnification, two 1-cm-long Z-plasty flaps were marked out beginning at the central limb, which was situated over the site of the mass. After development of the flaps, dissection was carried down to the A1 pulley, which had a ganglion cyst arising from its surface more or less on the ulnar side and extending in an ulnar direction into the area of the base of the second web space. This cyst was dissected free intact. After completion of the ganglion removal and submission for permanent sections, we closed the wound with interrupted 6-0 Prolene sutures with Gillies sutures for the tips of the flaps. After cleaning Betadine off the hand and the arm, dressing consisted of Xeroform, Kerlix, several Kerlix fluffs, Kerlix roll, Kling, Sof-Rol, and an Ace bandage from the fingers to the elbow. The patient tolerated the procedure well and left the operating room in good condition.

Pathology Report Later Indicated: Ganglion cyst, benign

8-11A:

SERVICE CODE(S): ____________________

DX CODE(S): ____________________

Repair, Revision, and Reconstruction

Most of the anatomic subheadings (e.g., Shoulder or Humerus [Upper Arm] Elbow) in the Musculoskeletal System subsection include a Repair, Revision, and Reconstruction category. The procedures are osteoplasty, osteotomies, arthroplasty, tendon transplants or transfers, and various other repairs, revisions, and reconstructive procedures with numerous grafting procedures for bones, tendons, and muscles. Be certain to identify the correct location and extent of the procedure before assigning a code. A good medical dictionary is an important tool as you report muscle repairs, as only by understanding all of the medical terminology in each report can you be certain to report the service accurately.

CASE 8-12
8-12A Operative Report, Rotator Cuff Repair

CASE 8-12

This report states that the reconstruction procedure was a repair with acromioplasty. An acromioplasty is the surgical removal of a portion of the acromion (the highest point on the shoulder) to relieve compression of the rotator cuff when the joint moves. The acromioplasty is bundled into the repair procedure and is not reported separately.

8-12A OPERATIVE REPORT, ROTATOR CUFF REPAIR

LOCATION: Outpatient, Hospital

PATIENT: Casey Chaput

SURGEON: Mohomad Almaz, M.D.

PREOPERATIVE DIAGNOSIS: Left, nontraumatic, rotator cuff tear

POSTOPERATIVE DIAGNOSIS: Left, nontraumatic, rotator cuff tear

PROCEDURE PERFORMED: Repair of left rotator cuff repair with Neer acromioplasty

ANESTHESIA: General with endotracheal intubation

FINDINGS: The patient was found to have a complete tear of the rotator cuff. This extended from approximately the level of the long head of the biceps around posteriorly about 2 cm.

We created an incision over the left acromion in a shoulder-strap fashion and dissected down through the subcutaneous tissue until we identified the acromion. We reflected the deltoid sharply off the anterior and anterolateral aspect of the acromion. We were then able to view the subacromial space, and we immediately noted a large tear in the rotator cuff. We were careful not to split the deltoid more than about 1 cm.

We then thought there was a rather prominent inferior corner to the anterolateral edge of the acromion. We elected to proceed with a Neer acromioplasty. We then removed the inferior corner of the anterolateral aspect of the acromion using an oscillating saw. We smoothed the undersurface of the acromion with a rasp. After thoroughly irrigating the area with saline, we were able to achieve a very nice view of the rotator cuff tear. We found that the rotator cuff had essentially split into two layers, and they were both avulsed from the humeral head from the long head of the biceps around the articular surface about 2 cm. We freshened the edges of the rotator cuff and then created a bony trough along the margin of the articular surface, starting from the long head of the biceps posteriorly about 2 cm. We then used two sutures of no. 1 Nurolon. We passed each suture through the proximal humerus and out through the bony trough. We then entered the rotator cuff and then again through the bony trough such that when we tied the sutures, the rotator cuff was pulled nicely into the bony trough. We thoroughly irrigated this area before we tied the sutures and then abducted the shoulder as the sutures were tied. Again, the rotator cuff was pulled nicely into the trough without undue tension. We then freshened the margins of the acromion and repaired the deltoid back to the acromion with no. 1 Panacryl suture. We closed the subcutaneous tissue using 2-0 Vicryl, and the skin was closed using 4-0 nylon suture. A sterile Xeroform dressing was applied. Then we placed the patient's left arm into a sling with an abduction pillow to keep the arm abducted slightly. She was then taken from the operating room in good condition and breathing spontaneously. The final sponge and needle counts were correct. She was given 1g of Kefzol intravenously preoperatively and will be continued on 1g of Kefzol q.8h. for 2 days.

Pathology Report Later Indicated: Benign tissue and bone morsels

8-12A:

SERVICE CODE(S): ____________________

DX CODE(S): ____________________

Sprains and Strains

Although sprain and strain do not mean the same thing (a sprain is a ligament injury and strain is a muscle/tendon injury), in the ICD the codes for Sprains and Strains of Joints and Adjacent Muscles (840-848) are used to report both. Read the Includes notes that precede 840-848, and you will note that the following conditions of the joint capsule, ligament, muscle and tendon are included in these codes:

Avulsion (ripping or tearing)
Hemarthrosis (blood in joint)
Laceration (torn, ragged, mangled)
Rupture (forcible tearing or disruption)
Sprain (ligament injury)
Strain (muscle/tendon injury)
Tear (pulling apart)

CASE 8-13
8-13A Consultation, Tendon Rupture
8-13B Radiology Report, Shoulder
8-13C Operative Report, Open Tendon Repair
8-13D Discharge Summary

CASE 8-13

Since this is the initial episode of treatment of the injury, assign an E code to indicate how the injury occurred.

8-13A CONSULTATION, TENDON RUPTURE

LOCATION: Outpatient, Clinic

PATIENT: Lyle Conard

ATTENDING PHYSICIAN: Ronald Green, M.D.

CONSULTANT: Mohomad Almaz, M.D.

CHIEF COMPLAINT: Right pectoralis major tendon rupture

HISTORY OF PRESENT ILLNESS: This 22-year-old right-hand-dominant student at the University of Manytown presents with an injury of his right pectoralis major that occurred approximately 2 weeks ago. He was doing a bench press at the time and had sudden loss of shape and function of the right pectoralis major. Follow-up examinations confirmed evidence of damage to that tendon.

PAST MEDICAL HISTORY: He had nasal reconstruction done four years ago. He has had no other operations. He has had no other ongoing medical concerns.

MEDICATIONS: He takes no medications.

ALLERGIES: He has no allergies.

FAMILY HISTORY: His mother is diabetic, but there have been no other problems within the family for medical concerns.

SOCIAL HISTORY: He is a student living here in Manytown. He is a nonsmoker.

REVIEW OF SYSTEMS: Systems inquiry shows he is otherwise healthy. No weight loss. There is no history of asthma, diabetes, high blood pressure, or cancer. He has no cardiac or pulmonary concerns. There is no hepatic or renal dysfunction. He has no other joint problems related to tendon problems. There are no neurologic, vascular, or skin-related concerns.

PHYSICAL EXAMINATION shows him to have a height of 5 feet 11 inches. Weight of 250 pounds. Blood pressure is 108/80. Head and neck examinations are normal. The chest is symmetrical and clear. The first and second heart sounds are normal; there are no extra heart sounds or murmurs. Abdominal, soft; examination shows no tenderness. Musculoskeletal examination is normal with the exception of the right pectoralis major, which shows obvious evidence of disruption. The neurologic and vascular examinations are normal.

SURGICAL PLAN: The patient will be admitted overnight for repair of the right pectoralis major.

8-13A:

SERVICE CODE(S): ____________________

DX CODE(S): ____________________

8-13B RADIOLOGY REPORT, SHOULDER

Assign an E code to indicate how the injury occurred.

LOCATION: Outpatient, Clinic

PATIENT: Lyle Conard

PRIMARY CARE PHYSICIAN: Ronald Green, M.D.

SURGEON: Mohomad Almaz, M.D.

RADIOLOGIST: Morton Monson, M.D.

DIAGNOSIS: Sprain right pectoralis major

RIGHT SHOULDER, ONE VIEW:

FINDINGS: There is no definite evidence for acute fracture or dislocation of the visualized bony structures identified on this examination. The bone mineral density appears to be within normal limits. Please correlate clinically the need for additional more advanced imaging or other evaluation.

8-13B:

SERVICE CODE(S): ____________________

DX CODE(S): ____________________

8-13C OPERATIVE REPORT, OPEN TENDON REPAIR

Since this is the initial treatment episode of the injury, assign an E code to indicate how the injury occurred. Remember, E codes are only assigned on the initial episode of care in both the outpatient and inpatient settings.

LOCATION: Outpatient, Clinic

PATIENT: Lyle Conard

PRIMARY CARE PHYSICIAN: Ronald Green, M.D.

SURGEON: Mohomad Almaz, M.D.

PREOPERATIVE DIAGNOSIS: Right shoulder pectoralis major tendon rupture

POSTOPERATIVE DIAGNOSIS: Complete right pectoralis major tendon rupture

PROCEDURE PERFORMED: Open repair, right pectoralis major

CLINICAL HISTORY: This 22-year-old gentleman injured his right pectoralis major while weight lifting approximately 14 days ago. He presented to orthopedics yesterday. It was determined that he had a complete rupture of his right pectoralis major and that surgery was necessary. He was advised that because of the delay there was some further risk if we went any further before having this repaired, and we recommended that surgery be done as soon as possible. After the risks and benefits of anesthesia and surgery were explained to both the patient and his parents, the decision was made to undertake the procedure.

OPERATIVE REPORT: Under general anesthetic, the patient was laid in a beach-chair position on the operating table. He was given 1g of cefazolin intravenously before the onset of surgery. The right shoulder was prepped and draped in the usual fashion. A deltopectoral incision approximately 10 cm long was made and was deepened through subcutaneous tissue to expose the deltoid fascia. Immediately apparent was that there was complete avulsion of the pectoralis major with retraction of the muscle medially. The tendinous portion of the muscle was quite inflamed and macerated. It was typical of the type of softened tendon we would expect 14 days post injury. The area on the humerus where the tendon had been avulsed was exposed. Just lateral to the biceps tendon, three Mitek super anchors were then placed down into the bone with no. 2 Ethibond sutures coming from them. A series of no. 5 Ethibond sutures were then woven through the tendon medially to act as stay sutures. These allowed us to place traction on the muscle and bring it toward the arm attachment. The no. 2 Ethibond sutures were then placed through tendinous structures from the top to bottom and sewn down into position. The tendon was then further anchored using the no. 5 Ethibond sutures to the surrounding structures laterally. When this was done, there was quite a firm repair. Because of the length of time in contracture, however, the muscle itself was not flexible enough to allow substantial external rotation. The wound was then thoroughly irrigated with normal saline and closed in layers with absorbable suture and Steri-Strips. The wound was then infiltrated with Marcaine and dressed with Vaseline gauze, 4 × 4s, and HypaFix. The arm was then placed in a CryoCuff sling. The patient awakened, was placed on his hospital bed, and was taken to the recovery room in good condition. Estimated blood loss for the procedure was less than 100 cc. The sponge and needle counts were correct.

8-13C:

SERVICE CODE(S): ____________________

DX CODE(S): ____________________

8-13D DISCHARGE SUMMARY

Since this is the initial treatment episode of the injury, assign an E code to indicate how the injury occurred. Remember, E codes are only assigned on the initial episode of care in both the outpatient and inpatient settings.

LOCATION: Outpatient, Clinic

PATIENT: Lyle Conard

PRIMARY CARE PHYSICIAN: Ronald Green, M.D.

SURGEON: Mohomad Almaz, M.D.

FINAL DIAGNOSIS: Right pectoralis major tendon rupture

CLINICAL HISTORY: This 22-year-old gentleman injured his right pectoralis major 2 weeks ago. He was doing a bench press at that time. He had a sudden pain in the right pectoral area.

Surgical examination confirmed that he has complete rupture of the right pectoralis major.

The patient was taken to surgery yesterday for repair of the tendon of the right pectoralis major. No perioperative complications occurred. The patient's pain was controlled with the usual analgesics postoperatively. He was discharged home in the care of his parents today. Arrangements were made for him to be seen by myself in follow-up in 7 to 8 days. He will be sent home with Lorcet for analgesic in the interval.

8-13D:

SERVICE CODE(S): ____________________

DX CODE(S): ____________________

CASE 8-14
8-14A Operative Report, Tendon Repair

CASE 8-14

Since this is the initial treatment of the injury, assign an E code to indicate how the injury occurred. In this report, there is no indication of how the injury occurred, so you assign an unspecified accident E code.

8-14A OPERATIVE REPORT, TENDON REPAIR

LOCATION: Outpatient, Hospital

PATIENT: Melvin Brodern

ATTENDING PHYSICIAN: Mohamad Almaz, M.D.

SURGEON: Mohomad Almaz, M.D.

sprain/strain

PREOPERATIVE PROCEDURE: Quadriceps tendon rupture, right knee

POSTOPERATIVE PROCEDURE: Quadriceps tendon rupture, right knee

OPERATIVE PROCEDURE: Repair of quadriceps tendon, right knee

OPERATIVE PROCEDURE: After suitable spinal anesthesia had been achieved, the patient's right knee was prepped and draped in the usual manner. Prior to prepping, a thigh tourniquet was applied. A midline skin incision was made from the inferior pole of the patella to one handbreadth above the superior pole of the patella. The patient had a thickened prepatellar bursa and chronic bursitis. This was partially excised. The quadriceps tendon was exposed. The patient had complete rupture of the quadriceps tendon extending to the medial and lateral retinacula. The interposed clot was removed. Four blocking stitches of no. 5 Ethibond were then placed into the central aspect of the quadriceps tendon. These were passed through drill holes, going from the superior pole of the patella to the inferior pole of the patella. The sutures were then tied over a bone bridge at the inferior pole of the patella securing the main portion of the quadriceps tendon back to the patella. The medial and lateral retinacula tears were then repaired with interrupted no. 1 Panacryl. Before wound closure, a Hemovac drain was inserted into the knee joint. Subcutaneous tissue was then closed with 2-0 Vicryl, and the skin was closed with staples. A fiberglass cylinder cast was then applied. The tourniquet was released before cast application. After tourniquet release, good circulation was noted to return to the foot. The patient tolerated the procedure well and returned to the recovery room in stable condition.

8-14A:

SERVICE CODE(S): ______________________

DX CODE(S): ______________________

CASE 8-15
8-15A Operative Report, Arthroplasty

CASE 8-15

8-15A OPERATIVE REPORT, ARTHROPLASTY

LOCATION: Inpatient, Hospital

PATIENT: Jack Baglien

SURGEON: Mohomad Almaz, M.D.

PREOPERATIVE DIAGNOSIS: Osteoarthritis, right knee

POSTOPERATIVE DIAGNOSIS: Osteoarthritis, right knee

PROCEDURE PERFORMED: Right cemented posterior stabilized total knee arthroplasty

COMPONENTS USED: Duracon size extra-large femur, size large 2 tibia, 9-mm posterior stabilized tibial insert, and 33-mm symmetric patella

OPERATIVE PROCEDURE: After suitable epidural anesthesia had been achieved, the patient's right knee was prepped and draped in the usual manner. Before prepping, the thigh tourniquet was applied, but initially it was not inflated. A long anterior midline skin incision and a long anteromedial arthrotomy were performed. The patient was noted to have marked synovitis in his knee. Once the synovial bleeders, capsular bleeders, and skin bleeders were cauterized, the leg was stripped with an Esmarch, and the tourniquet inflated to 275 mmHg.

A partial fat pad excision was performed. The patella was dislocated laterally. An entry hole was made in the distal femur for the intramedullary alignment rod. Rotation was selected off the interepicondylar axis. Anterior referencing instruments were used. Using the intramedullary alignment, the anterior shim cut and then the distal femoral cuts were performed. The tibia was then subluxed forward. The proximal tibial cut was performed. Nine millimeters of bone was excised, referencing off the intact lateral femur. The extension gap was then measured. The flexion gap was assessed, and a mark was placed on the distal femur to reproduce the identical flexion gap. This indicated the femoral component should be extra-large sized. An extra-large 4-in-1 jig was then applied. Anterior and posterior chamfer cuts were then performed. A trial femur was then placed to fit very well. A trial tibia with a 9-mm insert was placed, and there was excellent alignment and good stability. The patella was then everted and prepared for resurfacing technique using free-hand cuts with a saw. A symmetrical 3-mm trial component was placed and fit quite well. The box was then cut for the posterior stabilized femoral component, and the slot in the tibia was cut for the keel of the tibial component. The wounds were then thoroughly irrigated and dried. Bone graft was placed into the lug holes in the distal femur and the entry hole in the distal femur. The large 2-tibial component was then cemented into place. The extra large femoral component was cemented into place. A trial tibial insert was in place, and the leg was placed into full extension. The patellar component was then cemented into place. Once the cement was hard, stability was reassessed and found to be very good. A trial component was removed. The knee was carefully examined for any cement debris, which was carefully removed. The actual 9-mm posterior stabilized insert was then placed, and a locking screw was placed. The knee was then thoroughly irrigated. Autotransfusion Hemovac drain was placed. The wound was closed in layers. The capsule was closed with no. 1 Panacryl, the subcutaneous tissue with 2-0 Vicryl, and the skin with staples. A Robert Jones dressing and anterior splint were then applied. Before wound closure, an autotransfusion Hemovac drain was placed. The patient tolerated the procedure well and returned to the recovery room in stable condition.

Pathology Report Later Indicated: Benign bone.

8-15A:

SERVICE CODE(S): ______________________

DX CODE(S): ______________________

Late Effects

Sometimes an acute illness or injury leaves a patient with a residual health problem that remains after the illness or injury has resolved. The residual effect or manifestation is coded first, and then the late effects code is assigned to indicate the cause of the residual. An example would be scars (residual) that remain after a severe burn (cause). The late effects code is accessed in the Index under the main term "Late."

In most instances, two codes will be assigned—one code for the **residual** that is being treated (chief complaint) and one code that indicates the **late effect** (cause). There is no time limit for the development of a residual. It may be evident at the time of the acute illness, or it may occur months after an injury. It is also possible that a patient may develop more than one residual. For example, a patient who has had a stroke may develop right-sided hemiparesis (paralysis of one side) and aphasia (loss of ability to communicate). A person cannot have a current hip fracture (820.8) and a late effect of hip fracture (905.3). The code is either a current injury or a condition caused by a prior injury. It cannot be both at the same time. (The only exception to this rule is in category 438, Late effects of cerebrovascular disease.)

CASE 8-16

8-16A OPERATIVE REPORT, FUSION WITH AUTOGRAFT

Assign a diagnosis code for the osteoarthritis of the foot and a late effects code for the bone fracture of the extremity. Note the "due to old calcaneal fracture," which is the indication for the late effects code.

LOCATION: Outpatient, Hospital

PATIENT: Rose Stich

SURGEON: Mohomad Almaz, M.D.

PREOPERATIVE DIAGNOSIS: Posttraumatic subtalar osteoarthritis, left hindfoot, due to old calcaneal fracture

POSTOPERATIVE DIAGNOSIS: Posttraumatic subtalar osteoarthritis, left hindfoot, due to old calcaneal fracture

PROCEDURE PERFORMED: Left subtalar fusion using moldable autograft obtained from the left iliac crest

OPERATIVE PROCEDURE: After suitable general anesthesia had been achieved, the patient's left iliac crest and left foot and ankle were prepped and draped in the usual manner. Before prepping, a thigh tourniquet was applied but initially not inflated. Bone graft was harvested from the left iliac crest. A 10-cm incision was made and carried down through the subcutaneous fat. The fascia was incised in line, with the crest starting about 2 cm back from the anterior-superior iliac spine. Cortical cancellous bone graft was then harvested from the inner table. Defect was packed with Gelfoam. The wound was closed in layers. The skin was closed with staples.

The leg was then elevated. The tourniquet was inflated. The incision was made from the tip of the fibula to the base of the fourth metatarsal. The distally based flap of the extensor digitorum brevis was elevated off the lateral aspect of the calcaneus. Fat pad and the sinus tarsi were split in line with the skin incision. Anterior process of the calcaneus was excised. The capsule was incised. A lot of thickened synovial tissue was removed. The joint surfaces were noted to be substantially damaged from the old calcaneal fracture. The remaining articular cartilage and scar tissue were removed with a curet and rongeur. The subchondral bone was then carefully burred down to a bleeding surface. Autograft from the iliac crest was then packed in between the bone surfaces. Using an image intensifier, a large-fragment cannulated screw was then placed starting at the talar neck across the posterior face of the subtalar joint into the central aspect of the calcaneal body. Further gap in the fusion at the sinus tarsi area was filled with autograft and allograft. The wound was then closed. Skin was closed with 4-0 nylon. Dressing and a Robert Jones dressing with a posterior fiberglass splint were then applied. The tourniquet was released. Following tourniquet release, good circulation was noted to return to the foot. The patient tolerated the procedure well and returned to the recovery room in stable condition.

8-16A:

SERVICE CODE(S): ______________________

DX CODE(S): ______________________

Fusion (arthrodesis) — 28725 - LT
Graft — 20902 - LT

Fractures

Several methods are employed to repair fractures. **Open treatment** of a fracture is when a surgeon opens the tissue and the fracture is exposed; the fractured bone can then be visualized by the physician. **Closed treatment** is when the fracture is repaired without the physician directly visualizing the fracture. Fractures are reported by the specific anatomic site and the reason for the repair. **Manipulation** is manually returning the bone (pushing or pulling) to proper alignment without an incision. The codes are often divided based on whether or not manipulation was performed in closed treatment of a fracture.

The CPT defines the key fracture repair terms as follows:

- **Closed Treatment:** This terminology is used to describe procedures that treat fractures by one of three methods: (1) without manipulation, (2) with manipulation, or (3) with or without traction.
- **Manipulation** is a reduction, which is an attempt to maneuver the bone back into proper alignment. The physician may bend, rotate, pull, or guide the bone back into position.
- **Closed treatment without manipulation** is a procedure in which the physician immobilizes the bone with a splint, cast, or other device but without having to manipulate the fracture into alignment first.
- **Closed treatment with manipulation** is a procedure in which the physician has to reduce (put back in place) the fracture.
- **Open treatment** is used when the fracture is surgically opened (exposed to the external environment). In this instance, the fracture (bone) is open to view and internal fixation (pins, screws, etc.) may be used. Open treatment can also mean that a remote site (not directly over the fracture) is opened to place a nail (intramedullary) across the fracture site.
- **Percutaneous skeletal fixation** describes fracture treatment that is neither open nor closed. In this procedure, the fracture is not open to view, but fixation (e.g., pins) is placed across the fracture site, usually under x-ray imaging.

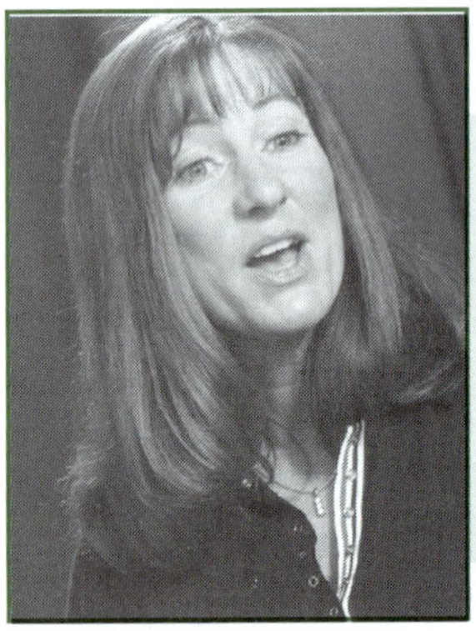

FROM THE TRENCHES

Sharon

"I think everyone needs to read the [coding reference] books. It's a great practice tool for everybody—even if you're not coding—to know what you're doing in the office...that all comes back to the coding portion at the end of the day. You still have to figure out what [the physicians] did...I don't think a lot of people understand that, but physicians are starting to."

CASE 8-17
8-17A Operative Report, Open Reduction
8-17B Radiology Report, Wrist

CASE 8-17

Fracture not specified as open or closed is reported as closed.

8-17A OPERATIVE REPORT, OPEN REDUCTION

Since this is the initial treatment of the injury, assign an E code to indicate how the injury occurred.

LOCATION: Outpatient, Hospital

PATIENT: Doyle Dryhdahl

SURGEON: Mohomad Almaz, M.D.

PREOPERATIVE DIAGNOSIS: Displaced fracture, right scaphoid

POSTOPERATIVE DIAGNOSIS: Displaced fracture, right scaphoid

OPERATIVE PROCEDURE: Right scaphoid open reduction internal fixation with bone grafting

CLINICAL HISTORY: This gentleman presents with a history of having injured his right scaphoid in 2001 and had an open reduction internal fixation at that time. He had been managing quite well until a week ago, when his arm was hit by a sledgehammer. Follow-up x-rays showed displacement of the scaphoid area. It was unclear whether this was a new fracture or displacement of a nonunion. After the risks and benefits of anesthesia and surgery were explained to the patient, a decision was made to undertake the procedure.

PROCEDURE: Under a general anesthetic, the patient was laid supine on the operating table. The right hand was prepped and draped in the usual fashion. He was given 1g of cefazolin intravenously before the onset of surgery. A tourniquet was then inflated around the right upper arm to 250 mmHg. We used the same volar incision for access that had been used previously. It was deepened through subcutaneous tissue and down through the scar to expose the volar carpal ligaments, which were then incised longitudinally to allow access to the scaphoid tubercle and the wrist joint. With this done, we were then able to expose the scaphoid fully. We could see that there was some scar tissue present in the area of the fracture. This was all excised to get us down to hard bone. Distally, there was reasonable blood supply. Proximally, it was not clear that there was any evidence of blood supply to the proximal pole. A curet was then used to remove the sclerotic bone along the margins of the area. When this was done, a single K-wire was then introduced across the fracture on the ulnar side to stabilize it. We had to open the bone because there was a tendency toward a humpback deformity. With the gap created, we then removed the Herbert screw that had been placed previously. We then switched to the AcroMed screw system. A single guide pin was then placed down the central axis of the scaphoid, and we then viewed this with anteroposterior and lateral fluoroscopic imaging. Satisfied that the position of the guide pin was accurate, we then drilled the hole for the AcroMed screw. We measured it and decided that a 20-mm screw would be sufficiently long to stabilize the fracture. A 20-mm AcroMed was then introduced and then held firmly. It gave good support, and the temporary K-wire was then removed and the guide pin removed.

We now had a gap of approximately 1 cm on the volar cortex. We elected to treat this with local graft from the distal radius.

Accordingly, at the proximal end of our incision, the distal radius was exposed through the pronator quadratus. An osteotome was then used to remove a triangular shape bone cortical graft. The cancellous graft was then harvested with a curet.

The cancellous graft was then packed firmly into the cavity of the scaphoid. When this was completed, we had filled the cavity. The cortical graft was then wedged into the defect on the volar cortex of the scaphoid and tamped into place with a bone tamp. When this was completed, we had a very secure solid construct of the volar cortex and the scaphoid was filled with cancellous bone.

The wound was then thoroughly irrigated with normal saline. The volar carpal ligaments were then repaired with 2-0 Vicryl suture. Fascial layers were then closed with absorbable sutures, and the skin was closed with Monocryl. The wound edges were also opposed with Steri-Strips and then infiltrated with Marcaine. The wound was then dressed with Vaseline gauze, 4 × 4s, and sterile Sof-Rol, and a thumb spica splint was then placed on and held in position with Kerlix and an Ace wrap. The patient's arm was then placed in a sling. The tourniquet was deflated after a total of 80 minutes. The patient was then awakened, placed on his hospital bed, and taken to the recovery room in good condition. Estimated blood loss for the procedure was less than 20 cc. The sponge and needle counts were correct.

8-17A:

SERVICE CODE(S): ______________________

DX CODE(S): ______________________

8-17B RADIOLOGY REPORT, WRIST

Since this is the initial treatment of the injury, assign an E code to indicate how the injury occurred.

LOCATION: Outpatient, Hospital

PATIENT: Doyle Dryhdahl

SURGEON: Mohomad Almaz, M.D.

RADIOLOGIST: Morton Monson, M.D.

CLINICAL FINDINGS: Displaced fracture, right scaphoid

AP AND LATERAL VIEWS OF THE RIGHT WRIST PERFORMED INTEROPERATIVELY:

FINDINGS: Screw fixation across a fracture of the right scaphoid

8-17B:

SERVICE CODE(S): ____________________

DX CODE(S): ____________________

CASE 8-18
8-18A Operative Report, Closed Reduction

CASE 8-18

Do not report the x-ray service provided; only report the surgeon's service and diagnoses code(s).

8-18A OPERATIVE REPORT, CLOSED REDUCTION

LOCATION: Outpatient, Hospital

PATIENT: Scott Laranzo

SURGEON: Mohomad Almaz, M.D.

DIAGNOSIS: Right hand fourth metacarpal fracture, transverse and displaced. Patient was injured in a fight.

PROCEDURE PERFORMED: Closed reduction, percutaneous pin fixation of right fourth metacarpal fracture

PROCEDURE: Under a satisfactory level of sedation and regional block, the extremity was prepped and draped. At this time, the fracture was reducible with distraction and manipulation. This was then further augmented with intramedullary retrograde pinning.

This was demonstrated in AP lateral and oblique views to maintain virtually anatomic position. I elected, at this time, to leave the pin proud and dress the pin, and then applied an ulnar gutter spica cast, fiberglass, about the extremity, keeping free and mobile the thumb and the index finger. There were no other complicating events. Fluoroscopy photos were obtained. The patient tolerated the procedure well.

8-18A:

SERVICE CODE(S): ______________________

DX CODE(S): ______________________

percutaneous skeletal fixation

CASE 8-19
8-19A Radiology Report, Right Femur
8-19B Orthopedic Consultation, Thigh Pain
8-19C Operative Report, Femur Repair, Intramedullary Nailing
8-19D Discharge Summary

CASE 8-19

8-19A RADIOLOGY REPORT, RIGHT FEMUR

Becky Bradley fell while walking to her car today and was seen in the emergency department by Dr. Sutton, who called Becky's primary care physician, Dr. Green. Dr. Sutton had ordered an x-ray, and when Dr. Green arrived at the emergency department he reviewed the x-ray. Report Dr. Monson's radiology service. Assume from this point on in this chapter that the health care facility requires E codes to be assigned for all initial treatments of injuries. This is a case for good medical terminology because the word "shaft" does not appear in the report. The coder needs to know epiphysis from diaphysis and distal from proximal. Other femur codes mention epiphysis, but none mention diaphysis.

LOCATION: Outpatient, Hospital

PATIENT: Becky Bradley

PRIMARY CARE PHYSICIAN: Ronald Green, M.D.

EMERGENCY DEPARTMENT PHYSICIAN: Paul Sutton, M.D.

RADIOLOGIST: Morton Monson, M.D.

EXAMINATION OF: Right femur

CLINICAL SYMPTOMS: Right leg pain, status post fall while walking to car today

RIGHT FEMUR, TWO VIEWS: No prior studies are available for comparison. There is evidence of an acute fracture involving the proximal diaphysis of the femur. This is severely angulated laterally and anteriorly. It is slightly impacted. Additional acute fractures are not seen, although views of the femur are somewhat limited. The femoral head appears to be seated within the acetabulum. There is some cortical thickening involving the slightly more distal femoral diaphysis. I do not know whether this is from a previous injury or some sort of a benign cortical thickening. I do not see gross destructive change. This should be clinically correlated, however.

CONCLUSION: Acute displaced fracture involving the proximal diaphysis of the right femur. Additional fractures are not seen, although views are somewhat limited. There is also an incidental finding of cortical thickening involving the slightly more distal femoral diaphysis. I believe this is most likely a benign cortical thickening because I do not see obvious destructive change involving the cortex. This could even be sequelae from perhaps a previous injury. This, of course, must be clinically correlated.

8-19A:

SERVICE CODE(S): ____________________

DX CODE(S): ____________________

8-19B ORTHOPEDIC CONSULTATION, THIGH PAIN

Based on the x-ray and Dr. Sutton's notes (which are not available to you here), Dr. Green decided to admit Becky to the hospital immediately. Dr. Green also contacted Dr. Almaz, an orthopedist, to provide a consultation regarding Becky's care.

LOCATION: Inpatient, Hospital

PATIENT: Becky Bradley

ATTENDING PHYSICIAN: Ronald Green, M.D.

CONSULTANT: Mohomad Almaz, M.D.

CHIEF COMPLAINT: Pain, right thigh

HISTORY OF PRESENT ILLNESS: This patient was walking to her car this afternoon and twisted and then developed acute pain in the right thigh. She fell. She had marked deformity of the thigh. X-rays revealed a midshaft fracture of the femur. The patient states that she has had right thigh pain for several months. She has been evaluated by Dr. Sutton. Bone scan was performed last month, and it suggested a stress fracture of both femurs. Right side has been much more symptomatic than the left. She has been prescribed Fosamax and Evista.

PAST MEDICAL HISTORY: History of hypothyroidism. She is taking Synthroid. She has a history of osteoporosis and is taking Fosamax and Evista. Patient denies any history of diabetes, coronary artery disease, or lung problems.

ALLERGIES: PENICILLIN, which results in a rash.

The patient is using a cane because of her thigh pain.

PHYSICAL EXAMINATION: On examination, she is in moderate distress. Blood pressure was initially 200/104. Pulse is 80 and regular. There is no neck tenderness. She has a contusion on the left frontal area. There was no loss of consciousness with this fall. She has no chest wall tenderness.

Upper extremities are nontender. Left lower extremity is nontender. Right lower extremity has marked shortening and marked deformity of the midthigh. She has good pedal pulses and normal sensation in the foot.

X-rays reveal a transverse fracture of the midshaft of the femur on the right side.

It sounds like she has had some ongoing problems with thigh pain from a stress fracture, and I think she completed the stress fracture this evening. I do not see any evidence on the plane x-ray to suggest anything else going on other than osteoporosis. Certainly she could also have osteomalacia. I see no evidence of any metastatic disease for the femurs.

I recommended to the family that we stabilize this evening with an intramedullary nail. In addition to taking Fosamax and Evista, because of her problems with the left femur, I recommend we add calcitonin, and we should also add a high dose of vitamin D for osteomalacia. If the left side becomes more symptomatic, we may want to consider prophylactic intramedullary nailing.

Operative procedure was discussed with the patient and family. Risks and benefits were discussed and typical post-operative course discussed. I advised that the patient has already lost blood into the femur fracture and may lose further blood with the surgery and may require transfusion. Risks and benefits of transfusion were discussed with the family. All questions were answered.

8-19B:

SERVICE CODE(S): ______________________

DX CODE(S): ______________________

8-19C OPERATIVE REPORT, FEMUR REPAIR, INTRAMEDULLARY NAILING

Becky has been scheduled for repair of her fractured right femur. Report Dr. Almaz's surgical services.

LOCATION: Inpatient, Hospital

PATIENT: Becky Bradley

ATTENDING PHYSICIAN: Ronald Green, M.D.

SURGEON: Mohomad Almaz, M.D.

PREOPERATIVE DIAGNOSIS: Transverse midshaft fracture, right femur

POSTOPERATIVE DIAGNOSIS: Transverse midshaft fracture, right femur

PROCEDURE PERFORMED: Intramedullary nailing, right femur (open reduction, internal fixation)

OPERATIVE PROCEDURE: After suitable general anesthesia had been achieved, the patient was positioned on the fracture table for right femoral nailing. The patient's right buttock, thigh, and knee were prepped and draped. A 7-cm incision (open) was made on the lateral aspect of the buttock. The incision was carried down to fascia. The fascia was split just above the greater trochanter. A guide pin was inserted into the piriformis fossa. A 13-mm reamer was used over the guide pin to establish the entry hole. A guide wire was then easily passed across the fracture site and impacted into the distal femoral metaphysis. Reaming was then done to 14 mm. A 13-mm × 360 mm Synthes titanium-cannulated nail was then inserted. (internal fixation) Proximal and distal locking was performed. The incisions were then irrigated. The wounds were closed in layers, and the skin was closed with staples. Estimated blood loss for the procedure was 100 ml. The patient tolerated the procedure well and returned to the recovery room in stable condition.

8-19C:

SERVICE CODE(S): ______________________

DX CODE(S): ______________________

8-19D DISCHARGE SUMMARY

LOCATION: Inpatient, Hospital

PATIENT: Becky Bradley

PRIMARY CARE PHYSICIAN: Ronald Green, M.D.

PRINCIPAL DIAGNOSIS: Transverse midshaft fracture, right femur, secondary to osteoporosis/osteomalacia.

PRINCIPAL PROCEDURE: Yesterday the patient underwent an intramedullary nailing, right femur.

HISTORY OF PRESENT ILLNESS: The patient had thigh pain for several months. X-rays suggested possible stress fracture, as did bone scan. She was placed on Fosamax and Evista. On the day of admission, she was turning to get into the car and her right femur snapped.

COURSE IN HOSPITAL: She was seen by Dr. Elhart from cardiology for preoperative evaluation regarding her hypertension. He thought her hypertension was up a little bit secondary to pain, but otherwise she was stable for surgery. On the day of admission, she was taken to the operating room and an open intramedullary nailing of the right femur was performed. There were no intraoperative or postoperative complications. She will be seen at the rehabilitation center for continued therapy.

DISCHARGE RECOMMENDATIONS: Remove staples 2 weeks postoperatively. Follow-up is with me in 3 to 4 weeks postoperatively.

8-19D:

SERVICE CODE(S): ______________________

DX CODE(S): ______________________

CASE 8-20
8-20A Orthopedic Consultation, Supracondylar Fracture
8-20B Operative Report, Supracondylar Fracture

CASE 8-20

8-20A ORTHOPEDIC CONSULTATION, SUPRACONDYLAR FRACTURE

LOCATION: Outpatient, Clinic

PATIENT: Lourene Bohn

PRIMARY CARE PHYSICIAN: Maxamillian Conclave, M.D.

CONSULTATION: Mohomad Almaz, M.D.

CHIEF COMPLAINT: Left thigh pain

HISTORY OF PRESENT ILLNESS: The patient is a 54-year-old woman accompanied today by her son. They were referred by Dr. Conclave from Anytown. She explained that she was walking in the hallway in her house when she just fell, injuring her left femur. She was brought by ambulance to see Dr. Conclave, who obtained an x-ray that revealed a comminuted displaced supracondylar fracture of her left femur. She was transported here. She is complaining of pain only in her left thigh and denies pain elsewhere. She denies any loss of sensation. She did tell me she had had a stroke, I believe, in 1999, resulting in left-sided weakness. She has regained much of the function of her left arm but still has a weak left leg. She walks with a walker outside but can sometimes get along without the walker at home. She also is a diabetic and recently developed bronchitis. I am told that the ambulance crew had a hard time keeping her stats above 90% on her way here today. This was with the use of oxygen. She lives at home with her husband and one son.

PAST MEDICAL HISTORY reveals that she has no known allergies to medications. She has a history of hypertension along with marked obesity. She had a CVA in 1999. She told me that she has had cellulitis of her legs in the past but not currently.

PHYSICAL EXAMINATION today finds that she is an alert and cooperative, obese woman lying in the supine position. She appears to be fairly comfortable. All extremities are symmetrical. She is able to move her upper extremities and her right leg. She is unable to move her left leg because of pain in her left thigh. She can dorsiflex and plantarflex her toes slightly, although she does not have a full range of motion. She does not have a full range of motion of her ankle. She explains that she has not been able to move her left leg well since she had her stroke in 1999. She does have rather leathery skin involving the distal two thirds of her leg between her knee and her ankle. There are no lacerations or abrasions. I am unable to palpate the dorsalis pedis or the posterior tibialis pulse in her left foot, but the foot is warm and sensation is intact to light touch. She is unable to move her left leg without pain.

X-rays of her left distal femur found that she does have a comminuted supracondylar fracture, which is displaced. It appears that she may have some early osteophytes forming about her left knee. No other fractures are noted.

IMPRESSION:
1. Comminuted displaced supracondylar fracture, left distal femur
2. History of diabetes mellitus
3. History of recent onset bronchitis
4. Obesity
5. History of hypertension
6. Status post cellulitis, lower extremities

RECOMMENDATIONS: I have thoroughly discussed this fracture with her and her son, who accompanied her today. I have recommended that we proceed with an open reduction internal fixation of this supracondylar fracture. I have discussed the procedure along with the risks involved and specifically mentioned the possibility of an infection or the possibility of loss of fixation, malunion, or nonunion. We have also discussed the possibility of a stroke or a heart attack, especially because she has had a previous stroke. Certainly there are very significant risks involved here. They understand this and would like to proceed. We have mentioned other forms of treatment including the possibility of traction; however, due to her size and the length of traction required, I do not think this is a good option. I have asked Dr. Green to see her preoperatively. If he believes that she is an acceptable candidate for surgery, we will plan this for tomorrow. Their questions have been answered.

8-20A:

SERVICE CODE(S): ____________________

DX CODE(S): ____________________

8-20B OPERATIVE REPORT, SUPRACONDYLAR FRACTURE

LOCATION: Inpatient, Hospital

PATIENT: Lourene Bohn

PRIMARY CARE PHYSICIAN: Maxamillian Conclave, M.D.

CONSULTATION: Mohomad Almaz, M.D.

PREOPERATIVE DIAGNOSIS: Supracondylar fracture, left distal femur

POSTOPERATIVE DIAGNOSIS: Supracondylar fracture, left distal femur

ANESTHESIA: General

FINDINGS: The patient was found to have a markedly comminuted supracondylar fracture. This fracture extended down to the condyles but not between them. We were able to achieve a near anatomic output, but we bone grafted this fracture as well.

PROCEDURE: The patient was brought from the intensive care unit, where she had already been intubated for several days. She was placed under a general anesthetic and then transported carefully to the operating room table. She is a very heavy woman, weighing nearly 300 pounds, and we had to be very careful with her. We padded all bony prominences.

We then prepped the patient's left leg by applying traction to the leg and supporting it during the prep. We prepped with Betadine and then draped it in a sterile fashion.

We then created a longitudinal incision over the anterolateral aspect of her left knee and leg. We carried the dissection down through the subcutaneous tissue and identified the fascia longitudinally. We reflected the vastus lateralis off the lateral intermuscular septum, and we were able to identify the femur and the fracture. We cauterized the perforators as we approached them. We then exposed the lateral femoral condyle, and we could identify the patellofemoral joint. We found that the supracondylar fracture was a markedly comminuted fracture with multiple fragments. We elected first of all to apply a cerclage wire (*an encircling loop*) around the distal fragment to more or less hold this in position as there were some longitudinal cracks, especially over the anterior surface of the distal femur. This seemed to help hold things in position as we manipulated the fracture into a more anatomic position. After having done this, we used the guide for the 95 supracondylar C-arm image intensifier to identify the location of this wire because we certainly could not palpate the distal end of the wire due to her obesity.

We eventually passed a reamer over this guide wire and reamed to a depth of about 65 mm. We then placed a 70-mm lag screw across the condyles and eventually attached a 16-hole 95 supracondylar plate. We were able to position this adjacent to the femur quite nicely and hold the fracture in a near anatomic position. We eventually used a second cerclage wire around the femur and removed the first. We used a cable lock to enhance our fixation on the distal fragment. We were able to get two good cancellous screws and this cable lock around the distal fragment. This seemed to provide excellent fixation, together with the lag screw. We placed cortical screws in the remainder of the plate, and this provided again excellent fixation of the proximal fragment as well. These screws were somewhat difficult to insert, and we did end up twisting the heads off two of the screws in midportion of the plate. In the end, however, we obtained excellent fixation of the proximal fragment, and we felt that we had good fixation of the distal fragment as well. There was no motion of the fracture site with range of motion of the knee. The bone at the fracture site, however, appeared to be quite thin, and we will need to be very careful in moving her leg in the future until this fracture heals. We felt that bone grafting this area would be a good idea. We then used cancellous bone chips from the Red Cross and scattered these about the fracture site. There were several of her bone fragments, which we had removed. We were able to place these into the femur as in completing a jigsaw puzzle.

We thoroughly irrigated the area frequently with saline throughout this procedure. We finally tightened the cable lock on the distal fragment at the end of the procedure so that we could be certain that it would be tight after we had inserted all those screws. We crimped the cable and cut off the excess cable.

We then repaired the fascia using 0 Vicryl and the subcutaneous tissue with 2-0 Vicryl. We closed the skin with skin staples. A sterile Xeroform dressing was applied, and we very carefully lifted the leg by lifting behind the distal femur and knee as well as the foot as we applied a knee immobilizer. With the knee immobilizer in place, we were able to transport her back to her hospital bed. She was left intubated and transported to the ICU. She was given IV antibiotics ahead of time and will be continued on IV antibiotics for several days postoperatively. She tolerated the procedure well.

8-20B:

SERVICE CODE(S): ______________________

DX CODE(S): ______________________

Amputation

An **amputation** is the removal of a limb or an appendage that has been so damaged or diseased that the amputation is the procedure of last resort. Persons with diabetes or vascular disease often have great difficulties with their legs and feet because the blood flow can be so decreased as to cause death to the tissues. In colder climates, frostbite, a condition in which the tissue is frozen and dies, is often a reason for amputation because the necrotic tissue will lead to gangrene and blood poisoning.

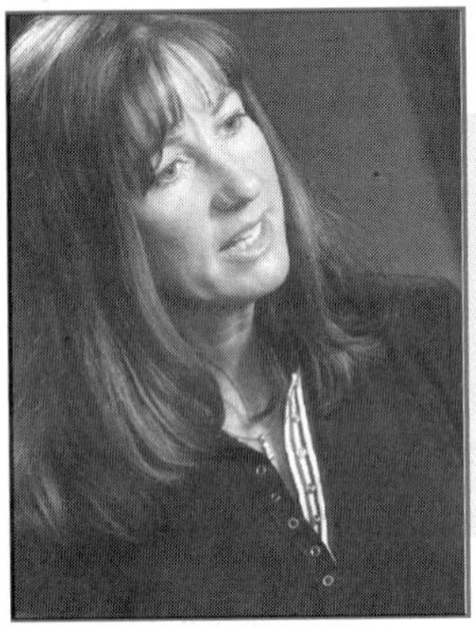

FROM THE TRENCHES

Sharon

"This is how I make my living, and I care about the people I work for and the physicians I work for...for me it is very personal. It's not just a job. Those people make a living partially because of me. They are doing a job, but if I don't code it correctly, they're not going to get paid for the job. It is important to me."

CASE 8-21
8-21A Operative Report, Amputation

CASE 8-21

8-21A OPERATIVE REPORT, AMPUTATION

LOCATION: Inpatient, Hospital

PATIENT: Edwin Burslie

SURGEON: Loren White, M.D.

PREOPERATIVE DIAGNOSIS: Gangrene and severe peripheral vascular disease, left leg due to diabetes

POSTOPERATIVE DIAGNOSIS: Gangrene and severe peripheral vascular disease, left leg due to diabetes

PROCEDURE PERFORMED: Left below-knee amputation

ANESTHESIA: Spinal with sedation

INDICATIONS: The patient is a 51-year-old male with diabetes and severe peripheral vascular disease who is post left-foot toe amputation by Dr. Sanchez. He has ischemia and gangrene of the foot and had seen Dr. Green, and they talked about a left below-knee amputation. Dr. Sanchez is out of town and asked me to perform the procedure. I discussed this with the patient. Also discussed the possibility of above-knee amputation, postoperative wound infections, and bleeding. He understands all this and wishes to proceed.

DESCRIPTION OF PROCEDURE: The patient was brought to the operating room, given spinal sedation and given sedation, and then prepped and draped with Betadine solution. An incision was made approximately 8 cm below the tibial tuberosity on the left leg. With a no. 10 blade, we carried our dissection down through subcutaneous tissues sharply. We raised a posterior flap using popliteal muscles, and our dissection through subcutaneous tissues found multiple enlarged venous bleeders and venous hypertension. We had to tie off nearly all the vessels, and we did this with 3-0 silk and 3-0 Vicryl free-ties. We used a periosteal elevator to elevate the tibial periosteum and divided this with the Gigli saw. We used the bone cutter to divide the fibula and then used sharp dissection to go through the popliteal muscles. We irrigated with saline until returns were clear and then rasped the bone edges so that there was no sharpness, and we assured that the vessels were tied as well as the nerves up above the bone edges themselves. After we had irrigated, we closed the popliteal flap over the top of the tibia and the fibula and did a deep layer of 3-0 Vicryl sutures. The skin was then closed with vertical mattress 3-0 Ethilon. The leg was then packed with fluffs and then wrapped with Ace wrap. All sponge and needle counts were correct. He tolerated this well and was taken to recovery in stable condition.

8-21A:

SERVICE CODE(S): ______________________________

DX CODE(S): ______________________________

Arthroscopy

Arthroscopy is fast becoming the treatment of choice for many surgical procedures. The incisions are smaller, which decreases the risk of infection and speeds recovery time. Several small incisions are made through which lights, mirrors, and instruments are inserted. The arthroscopy codes are located separately at the end of the Musculoskeletal subsection. If multiple procedures are performed through a scope, they are reported with modifier -51. Bundled into all surgical arthroscopic procedure codes is the diagnostic arthroscopy, so do not unbundle and code a diagnostic arthroscopy and a surgical arthroscopy if both were performed during the same encounter. Do not report separately things done during a procedure that are considered a part of the procedure, such as shaving, removing, evacuating, casting, splinting, or strapping.

A note preceding the Endoscopy/Arthroscopy codes states, "When arthroscopy is performed in conjunction with arthrotomy, add modifier -51." This note indicates that if a surgeon performs an arthroscopy and during the procedure also does an arthrotomy, you can report both services. For example, a physician performs an arthroscopic shaving of the articular cartilage and also does an open capsulotomy (posterior capsular release) of the knee. Both the arthroscopic shaving (29877) and the capsulotomy (27435) would be reported, and to the least expensive procedure you would add modifier -51 (multiple procedures).

The codes in this subheading are divided according to body area—elbow, shoulder, knee—and then according to the type and extent of procedure performed. An example of type of service is as follows: code 29805 is for an arthroscopy of the shoulder for diagnostic purposes, whereas code 29819 is an arthroscopy of the shoulder for a surgical procedure. Not only are there two different codes for surgical and diagnostic arthroscopy procedures, but also the surgical procedure is significantly more expensive than the diagnostic procedure. Great care must be taken to select the code that correctly describes the services supported in the medical record.

Note the description for code 29805: "Arthroscopy, shoulder, diagnostic, with or without synovial biopsy (separate procedure)." You will find the term "separate procedure" several times in the Endoscopy/Arthroscopy subheading because often an arthroscopic procedure is part of a larger procedure. You cannot report the service of the arthroscopy unless it has been performed as an independent, separate procedure. Also note that the parenthetical information following the codes indicates the codes to use if the procedure was done as an open (incisional) procedure rather than as an endoscopic (*closed*) procedure.

CASE 8-22

This is not the first treatment of the injury.

8-22A OPERATIVE REPORT, SHOULDER

LOCATION: Outpatient, Hospital

PATIENT: Deb Slover

SURGEON: Mohomad Almaz, M.D.

PREOPERATIVE DIAGNOSIS: Right shoulder pain

POSTOPERATIVE DIAGNOSIS: Normal right shoulder

PROCEDURE PERFORMED: Diagnostic arthroscopy, right shoulder

CLINICAL HISTORY: This 67-year-old woman presents with a history of having fallen on her right side and injuring her right shoulder. She is experiencing severe pain in the shoulder area. X-rays were normal. Preoperative MRI showed no evidence of skeletal or soft-tissue damage. The patient continued to have pain and discomfort. After the risks and benefits of anesthesia and surgery were explained to the patient, the decision was made to undertake the procedure.

OPERATIVE REPORT: Under general anesthetic, the patient was laid in the beach-chair position on the operating table. The right shoulder was examined and found to be stable with full range of motion. The shoulder was then prepped and draped in the usual fashion. A standard posterior arthroscopic portal was created and the camera was introduced into the back of the joint. Inspection of the articular surfaces showed no evidence of damage of the glenoids or the humerus. The anterior ligamentous structures were normal. The biceps attachment and its transit through the joint were normal. Subscapularis was intact with no abnormality. The undersurface of the rotator cuff showed no fraying or inflammation. It was well attached laterally with no evidence of damage. The inferior recess showed no abnormalities.

The camera was then taken out of the glenohumeral joint and placed in the subacromial space. We had excellent visualization of this region. The rotator cuff surface showed absolutely no evidence of fraying or disruption. We had good visualization right out the lateral-most recess. No abnormalities could be identified, and there was no evidence of impingement taking place. The camera was then removed from the subacromial space, and the area was infiltrated with Marcaine. The posterior portal was then closed with absorbable sutures and Steri-Strips, and a Mepore dressing was placed on it. The arm was then placed in a sling; the patient awakened and was placed on her hospital bed and taken to the recovery room in good condition.

8-22A:

SERVICE CODE(S): ____________________

DX CODE(S): ____________________

CASE 8-23
8-23A Operative Report, Debridement

CASE 8-23

8-23A OPERATIVE REPORT, DEBRIDEMENT

LOCATION: Outpatient, Hospital

PATIENT: Viola Reynolds

SURGEON: Mohomad Almaz, M.D.

PREOPERATIVE DIAGNOSIS: Left frozen shoulder

POSTOPERATIVE DIAGNOSIS: Left frozen shoulder adhesive pericapsulitis

PROCEDURE PERFORMED: Arthroscopic debridement, left shoulder.
Joint manipulation, left shoulder.

CLINICAL HISTORY: This 73-year-old woman presents with a history of progressive pain and discomfort of her left shoulder. Evaluation confirmed evidence of a left frozen shoulder. After the risks and benefits of anesthesia and surgery were explained to the patient, the decision was made to undertake the procedure.

PROCEDURE: Under general anesthetic, the patient was laid in the beach-chair position on the operating room table. The left shoulder was prepped and draped in the usual fashion. A standard posterior arthroscopic portal was created, and the camera was introduced into the back of the joint. We had excellent visualization. It was immediately apparent that there was substantial inflammation and adhesions throughout the entirety of the joint. Using a switch-stick technique, an anterior portal was created and the 7-mm cannula was then brought in from the front. Using a 4.0 double-biter resector, the synovium was then debrided throughout the entirety of the rotator cuff over the surface of the biceps and the anterior ligamentous structures as well as inferior ligamentous structures. With this completed, the joint was then thoroughly irrigated to remove any blood. The articular surfaces were inspected and were found to be normal. The attachment of the biceps was normal, although it had been covered with synovium. Anterior ligamentum structures were free from the subscapularis. The joint was then infiltrated with 80 mg of Depo-Medrol and 12 cc of Marcaine. The instruments were removed. The arthroscopic portal was closed with absorbable sutures and Steri-Strips. The joint was then manipulated. Before the manipulation, we had about 90 degrees of elevation passively. After manipulation, evaluation was free up to 180 degrees, and external rotation in an abducted position was possible to 90 degrees, as was internal rotation. Extension was possible to 40 degrees, and adduction was possible to 50 degrees. The wounds were then dressed with Myopore dressing. The patient was then placed in a CryoCuff sling, awakened, placed on her hospital bed, and taken to the recovery room in good condition.

8-23A:

SERVICE CODE(S): ____________________

DX CODE(S): ____________________

resection of adhesions

CASE 8-24
8-24A Operative Report, Knee Repair

CASE 8-24

Before you code this case, let's take a moment to review some of the terms that you will find in this report. The medial meniscus is C-shaped and is wider on the posterior horn (point) than on the anterior horn. The term medial means the middle of, and lateral is the farthest point from the middle or midline. A bucket handle tear is a vertical tear in the meniscus, which can be either the medial meniscus or the lateral meniscus. A plica is a fold in the lining of the knee joint, and chondromalacia is softening of the kneecap. Understanding of these terms will be necessary to correctly code this case.

8-24A OPERATIVE REPORT, KNEE REPAIR

LOCATION: Outpatient, Hospital

PATIENT: Glenn Arch

SURGEON: Mohomad Almaz, M.D.

PREOPERATIVE DIAGNOSIS: Medial meniscus tear

POSTOPERATIVE DIAGNOSES:
1. Right knee medial meniscus tear (*this is a derangement*)
2. Right knee plica
3. Right knee diffuse chondromalacia, grade 2-3

PROCEDURE PERFORMED: Right knee arthroscopy with partial medial meniscectomy and removal of plica

ANESTHESIA: General

ESTIMATED BLOOD LOSS: Minimal

No drains.

A 36-year-old male suffered with chronic right knee pain. MRI demonstrated a medial menicus tear. The patient was taken to surgery today. After an appropriate level of anesthesia was achieved, the right knee was appropriately prepped and draped in an orthopedic manner. We made two portal sites in the knee, one medial and the other lateral to the patellar tendon at the joint line. On examination of the joint, we appreciated that the patient had grade 1-2 chondromalacia involving the patella. On the articulating surface on the femur anteriorly, the patient had grade 2-3, a rather large area about 2 cm in diameter. He had a large plica medially, and this was debrided with a shaver. The medial lateral gutters and patella fascia were cleared of some loose bodies. At the joint space level, I appreciated some cartilage floating around, coming off these various sites of chondromalacia. In the medial compartment, he had a complex posterior horn medial meniscus tear, which was debrided back to the stable tissue. I appreciated that the patient had significant grade 2-3 chondromalacia and a 2-3 × 5-cm area on the weight-bearing surface of the knee, starting with the knee flexed to about 10 degrees. Laterally, the patient had a 1 × 2-cm area of chondromalacia on the weight-bearing surface. The lateral meniscus was probed and considered intact. The anterior cruciate ligament was noted to be intact, as was the remainder of the medial meniscus. We irrigated the knee copiously and injected 20 cc of 0.5% Marcaine to the portal spaces in the joint. We reapproximated the portal sites with interrupted nylon sutures, dressed the knee sterilely, and placed the patient in the knee immobilizer. The patient appeared to tolerate the procedure well and left the operating room in good condition.

8-24A:

SERVICE CODE(S): ____________

DX CODE(S): ____________

CASE 8-25

8-25A Operative Report, Acromioplasty
8-25B Operative Report, Debridement and Irrigation

CASE 8-25

8-25A OPERATIVE REPORT, ACROMIOPLASTY

LOCATION: Inpatient, Hospital

PATIENT: Else Wavia

SURGEON: Mohomad Almaz, M.D.

PREOPERATIVE DIAGNOSIS: Right shoulder rotator cuff tear

POSTOPERATIVE DIAGNOSES:
1. Loose body, right shoulder joint
2. A 4-cm rotator cuff tear (*rupture*)
3. Grade 3 osteoarthritis, right shoulder

OPERATIONS PERFORMED:
1. Removal of loose body, right shoulder joint
2. Right shoulder arthroscopic acromioplasty
3. Mini-open right rotator cuff repair

CLINICAL HISTORY: This 81-year-old woman presents with a history of pain and discomfort of her right shoulder. She had undergone an MRI done preoperatively with confirmed evidence of a full-thickness rotator cuff tear. After the risks and benefits of anesthesia and surgery were explained to the patient, the decision was made to undertake this procedure.

PROCEDURE: Under general anesthetic, the patient was laid in a beach-chair position on the operating table. The right shoulder was prepped and draped in the usual fashion. A standard posterior arthroscopic portal was created, and the camera was introduced into the back of the joint. Visualization was good. The undersurface of the rotator cuff was substantially inflamed. The articular surface of the glenoid and humerus showed several areas of substantial degenerative change. There was a full-thickness articular cartilage loss through some smaller segments. There were broader areas of grade 3 articular cartilage change. The biceps tendon was well attached. The anterior labrum was normal.

Using a switching stick technique, an anterior portal was created, and a 7-mm cannula was brought in from the front. Using a 4.0 double-biter resector, the undersurface of the rotator cuff was then debrided. The damaged edges of the glenoid and humeral articular surfaces were then debrided back to a smooth surface. We then found an 8 × 12-mm loose body in the inferior recess. This was then removed without difficulty. (*Procedure 1: removed loose body through scope*) The remainder of the inspection of the joint showed no other abnormalities. The camera was then taken out of the glenohumeral joint and placed into the subacromial space. We had good visualization once again. There was fraying on the undersurface of the acromion. A lateral portal was then created, and a 5.5 resector blade was brought in. The undersurface of the acromion was then denuded of soft tissue. A very large anterior bone spur was curving inferiorly. This was then removed, and the undersurface of the acromion was thinned through a depth of approximately 4 mm extending from the acromioclavicular joint over to the lateral margin and from the anterior margin posteriorly for 2.5 cm. When this was completed, the camera was then placed into the lateral portal and the shaver placed posteriorly. Using a "butcher-block technique," the undersurface of the acromion was then smoothed to a flat surface. When this was completed, the camera was then placed so that we could see the rotator cuff more fully. We could see evidence of substantial damage through the central portion of the cuff, although no full-thickness injury could be identified. (*Procedure 2: acromioplasty through scope*)

Instruments were removed from the subacromial space. The lateral portal was then extended to a 4-cm incision (*Procedure is converted to open*), and the deltoid split to expose the rotator cuff. We could now see more fully that there was an area about the size of a silver dollar where the cuff had been substantially thinned and was atrophic. This was then sharply excised. Side-to-side repair was done with a series of no. 2 Panacryl sutures. (*Procedure 3: mini-open rotator cuff repair.*) When this was completed, the arm was then placed through a range of motion. No further stress appeared on the repair.

The deltoid was then repaired with no. 1 Vicryl suture. The skin was closed in layers with Monocryl suture and Steri-Strips. The wound was then infiltrated with Marcaine and dressed with Mepore dressing. The arm was then placed in a CryoCuff sling. The patient was awakened and placed on her hospital bed and taken to the recovery room in good condition. Estimated blood loss for the procedure was less than 50 cc. The sponge and needle counts were correct.

8-25A:

SERVICE CODE(S): ____________________

DX CODE(S): ____________________

8-25B OPERATIVE REPORT, DEBRIDEMENT AND IRRIGATION

Else had surgery 2 months ago to repair her torn rotator cuff. The surgeon who performed the cuff repair is now returning her to the operating room for an incision and drainage of the infected wound (previous incision) on her right shoulder within the postoperative period. This wound is a complication of her original surgical procedure and occurs within the postoperative period.

LOCATION: Outpatient, Hospital

PATIENT: Else Wavia

SURGEON: Mohomad Almaz, M.D.

PREOPERATIVE DIAGNOSIS: Infected wound, right shoulder

POSTOPERATIVE DIAGNOSIS: Infected wound, right shoulder

PROCEDURE PERFORMED: Debridement and irrigation of infected wound, right shoulder

CLINICAL HISTORY: This 81-year-old woman had previously undergone an arthroscopic mini-open repair of a right rotator cuff tear, which I performed. At about the 4-week stage postoperatively, she developed drainage from the wound. This was culture positive for *Staphylococcus aureus.* She was then placed on oral antibiotics and did show some improvement, but there has been persistent drainage for the last 2 weeks without evidence of resolution. Because of the continuation of this problem, the decision was made to undertake the procedure.

ANESTHESIA: General

PROCEDURE: Under general anesthetic, the patient was laid in the beach-chair position on the operating table. The right shoulder was prepped and draped in the usual fashion. The anterior 3 cm of the surgical wound was excised. There was fluid drainage from this area. A sinus tract was identified that went down to the area of the anterior acromial area. We followed the tract down. No further purulence could be identified. The rotator cuff was exposed, and the repair was holding well with no evidence of disruption. The edges of the sinus tract area were then fully debrided and then irrigated using a power lavage system and 4 L of normal saline. Once the irrigation was completed, we repaired the soft tissues around the sinus tract with interrupted no. 1 Vicryl suture and then closed the skin with Monocryl suture. The wound was then dressed with Vaseline gauze, 4× 4s, and Hypafix. The arm was placed in a sling. The patient was then awakened and placed on her hospital bed and taken to the recovery room in good condition. Estimated blood loss for the procedure was negligible. Sponge and needle counts were correct.

8-25B:

SERVICE CODE(S): ____________________

DX CODE(S): ____________________

sinus tract – reported as the complication of a "fistula"

CASE 8-26
8-26A Operative Report, Debridement

CASE 8-26

This is the initial treatment for the injury. The neoplasm is listed first followed by the sprain code and E code.

8-26A OPERATIVE REPORT, DEBRIDEMENT

LOCATION: Outpatient, Hospital

PATIENT: Anita Aune

SURGEON: Mohomad Almaz, M.D.

PREOPERATIVE DIAGNOSIS: Right wrist pain

POSTOPERATIVE DIAGNOSES:
1. Partial-thickness chondral lesion, right distal radial articular surface
2. Partial thickness tear, right scapholunate ligament

PROCEDURE PERFORMED: Right wrist arthroscopy and debridement

CLINICAL HISTORY: This 35-year-old woman was involved in a motor vehicle accident. She sustained injuries to both wrists. She has had continuing pain on the right side, and after the risks and benefits of anesthesia and surgery were explained to the patient, the decision was made to undertake this procedure.

PROCEDURE: Under a general anesthetic, the patient was laid supine on the operating table. The right hand was prepped and draped in the usual fashion and placed in the fingertip traction with 10 pounds of weight around the upper arm. A tourniquet was inflated around the right upper arm after prepping. The joint was infiltrated with saline. Only 3 cc of saline could enter into the joint. The standard 3-4 arthroscopic portal was created, and the camera was introduced into the joint. We had excellent visualization. The undersurface of the carpus showed a small flap tear in the scapholunate junction. The same corresponding region on the distal radial articular surface showed a ridge of heaped up scar tissue. More ulnarly, the triangular fibrocartilage was inspected and was found to be intact with no evidence of damage through it.

The 6-R portal was created, and a 2.5 full radius resector was then brought in. The surface of the radius was then smoothed to a flat surface, and the flap tear in the scapholunate ligament was debrided. No further abnormalities could be identified. The instruments were then removed, and then the two arthroscopic portals closed with absorbable suture. Wound edges were also closed with Steri-Strips, and then the wound was dressed with Vaseline gauze, 4 × 4s, Kerlix, and an Ace wrap. The tourniquet was deflated, and the patient awoken, placed on her hospital bed, and taken to the recovery room in good condition. Sponge and needle counts were correct.

Pathology Report Later Indicated: Benign lesion of radius.

8-26A:

SERVICE CODE(S): ____________________

DX CODE(S): ____________________

Chondral means "cartilage" (articular surface)

(Tear, ligament by site) - coder is directed to sprain, by site, eg "Sprain, wrist"

CASE 8-27
8-27A Operative Report, Knee

CASE 8-27

overexertion

This is the initial care for the injury. Darrell was working out in the gymnasium when he attempted to lift a 150-pound weight. Dr. Almaz diagnoses the condition as a dislocation of the patella with fracture of the right knee, and he is performing a repair procedure today. Any dislocation at the same site as a fracture is included in the fracture diagnosis code and not reported separately.

8-27A OPERATIVE REPORT, KNEE

LOCATION: Outpatient, Hospital

PATIENT: Darrell Backer

SURGEON: Mohomad Almaz, M.D.

PREOPERATIVE DIAGNOSIS: Prepatellar dislocation with osteochondral fracture, inferior pole of patella, right knee

POSTOPERATIVE DIAGNOSIS: Acute patellar dislocation with osteochondral fracture, inferior pole of patella, right knee; an old posterior horn tear, medial meniscus, posterior horn of right knee

PROCEDURE PERFORMED:
1. Right knee arthroscopy and partial arthroscopic lateral meniscectomy 29881
2. Arthrotomy and attempted open reduction and internal fixation of osteochondral fracture, inferior pole of patella, right knee
3. Removal of osteochondral body, right knee

OPERATIVE PROCEDURE: After suitable general anesthesia had been achieved, the patient's right knee was prepped and draped in the usual manner. Before prepping, the thigh tourniquet was applied after draping, inflated to 300 mmHg. Inflow cannula was inserted in the suprapatellar pouch on the medial side. Hemarthrosis was evacuated from the knee. Arthroscopic anteromedial and anterolateral portals were established. Thickened inferior plica was noted and excised for visualization of the ACL. The ACL was intact and stable to probing. The medial compartment was intact. The articular surfaces were stable with intact medial meniscus. Examination of the lateral compartment revealed a tear on the medial aspect of the posterior horn. Using combination punch and shaver, the torn area was excised. The articular surfaces laterally looked in good shape. Examination of the patellofemoral joint revealed some evidence of tearing of the medial retinacular structures. There was an osteochondral fragment off the inferior pole. This was stuck to the synovium. The shaver was placed. Clot around the fragment was evacuated. The fragment was then mobilized. It looked like there was a reasonable area of osseous tissue on the undersurface of the fragment. The fragment was too large to be manipulated arthroscopically, and it was elected to do an arthrotomy of the knee and possible repair, possible excision.

Arthroscope was removed. Incision was made from the tibial tubercle to about two fingerbreadths above the patella over the midline. A medial arthrotomy was made from the superior pole of the patella to the joint line. The patella was everted. A defect off the inferior aspect of the patella on the inferior tongue of the patella was noted. The osteochondral fragment was retrieved from the knee. The osseous surface covered about 40% of the fragment. Attempts to try to reduce the fragment revealed some plastic deformation of the fragment, but I could not get this to align appropriately. With the deformation of that fragment and the very thin area of osseous component affecting about 40% of the fragment, it was felt that repair would not be something that would have a high likelihood of success. For this reason, the fragment was excised.

Hemovac drain was then inserted. Synovium and the medial patellofemoral ligament were repaired. Medial capsule was repaired and bursa repaired. Skin was closed with 3-0 Vicryl subcuticular sutures and staples. Hemovac drain was inserted through the superolateral portal prior to wound closure. A dressing and a hinged-knee immobilizer with a hinge lock in full extension were then applied. The patient tolerated the procedure well and returned to the recovery room in stable condition.

8-27A:

SERVICE CODE(S): ____________________

DX CODE(S): ____________________

CASE 8-28
8-28A Operative Report, Meniscectomy and Chondroplasty

CASE 8-28

8-28A OPERATIVE REPORT, MENISCECTOMY AND CHONDROPLASTY

LOCATION: Outpatient, Hospital

PATIENT: Doyle Dryhdahl

SURGEON: Mohomad Almaz, M.D.

PREOPERATIVE DIAGNOSIS: Chondromalacia patella, left knee

POSTOPERATIVE DIAGNOSIS: Chondromalacia patella, left knee; anterior horn tear, lateral meniscus, left knee; focal grade 2 chondromalacia, medial femoral condyle (10 cm in diameter).

PROCEDURE PERFORMED: Left knee arthroscopy, partial arthroscopic lateral meniscectomy, and chondroplasty patella and medial femoral condyle.

PROCEDURE: After suitable general anesthesia had been achieved, the patient's left knee was prepped and draped in the usual manner. Before prepping, a thigh tourniquet was applied; after draping, it was inflated to 300 mmHg. The arthroscope was inserted through an anteromedial portal. Operative anterolateral portal was established. The lateral compartment was examined; it had intact articular surfaces, stable intact meniscus. Examination of the notch revealed some hypertrophic synovium, which was cauterized with the radiofrequency probe. ACL and PCL were intact. Examination of the medial compartment revealed about a 10-mm diameter area of grade 2 chondromalacia with loose articular cartilage flap and about 20 degrees of flexion. The loose articular cartilage flap was divided with the shaver and further smoothing down with the radiofrequency probe at a very low setting. The patient was noted to have a marked multiple fraying of the anterior horn with multiple tears. Using a combination of punch and shaver, the unstable meniscus was excised and contoured. The meniscus was intact medially. Examination of the patellofemoral joint revealed diffuse grade 3 changes of the lateral facet of the patella but minimal articular cartilage flaps where there was loose collapse at the inferior pole, and these smoothed with the shaver. The knee joint was then thoroughly irrigated and the arthroscope removed. The tourniquet was released. Following the tourniquet release, good circulation was noted to return to the foot. The patient tolerated the procedure well and returned to recovery room in stable condition.

8-28A:

SERVICE CODE(S): ____________________

DX CODE(S): ____________________

Glossary

amputation the removal of a limb or appendage that has been too damaged or diseased for treatment.
arthrocentesis puncture and aspiration of a joint.
arthroscopy examination of the interior of joint with an arthroscope (specialized endoscope).

closed treatment procedure in which a fracture is repaired without exposure direct fascia: fibrous tissue that lies creates an investment for muscles and organs.

external fixation application of a device that holds bones in place from the outside.

internal fixation placement of hardware (rods, pins, etc.) onto or into the bone to hold it in place for repair.

manipulation an attempt to maneuver a bone back into proper alignment.

open treatment a procedure in which a fracture site is surgically exposed and visualized.
orthopedist a physician who specializes in the diagnosis and treatment of musculoskeletal disorders.

percutaneous through the skin.

Chapter 9

Respiratory System

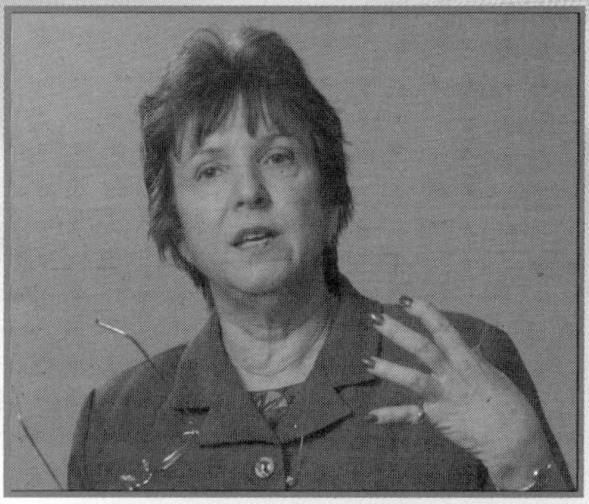

Maryann Ward, CPC
Billing Production
Unit Manager
Baltimore, Maryland

ABBREVIATIONS

ABG	arterial blood gas
AFB	acid-fast bacillus
ARDS	acute respiratory distress syndrome
AU	both ears (aures unitas) or each ear (aures uterque)
BAL	broncho alveolar lavage
BiPAP	bilevel positive airway pressure
COPD	chronic obstructive pulmonary disease
CPAP	continuous positive airway pressure
DLCO	diffuse capacity of lungs
EIA	exercise-induced asthma
FEF	forced expiratory flow
FEV1	forced expiratory volume in one second
FEV1:FVC ratio	forced expiratory volume in one second to forced vital capacity ratio
FRC	functional residual capacity
FVC	forced vital capacity
HHN	handheld nebulizer
IPAP	inspiratory positive airway pressure
MDI	metered dose inhaler
MVV	maximum voluntary ventilation
PAWP	pulmonary artery wedge pressure
PCWP	pulmonary capillary wedge pressure
PEAP	positive end-airway pressure
PEEP	positive end-expiratory pressure
PFT	pulmonary function test
PND	paroxysmal nocturnal dyspnea
PPH	primary pulmonary hypertension
RDS	respiratory distress syndrome
RSV	respiratory syncytial virus
RV	respiratory volume, residual volume
RV:TLC	respiratory volume to total lung capacity ratio
SOB	shortness of breath
TLC	total lung capacity
TLV	total lung volume
UPPP	uvulo-palato-pharyngoplasty
V/Q scan	ventilation/perfusion scan

The respiratory system often reflects diseases in other organ systems of the body. The process of respiration includes not only the lungs but also the diaphragm, the brain (regulates respiration through cerebral regulatory centers), and the cardiovascular system. The physician treating the patient with pulmonary disease must take into consideration a wide variety of pathological considerations. For example, areas of density on a chest x-ray may be caused by pulmonary infection or tumor. Dysfunction of the lungs could represent a systemic disease, such as an embolism or a cardiac disturbance. The physician will begin the diagnostic process with a complete history and physical.

E/M Services

During the history portion of the service, the physician will be seeking information about factors that would have an effect on the patient's lungs, such as exposure to tobacco smoke, pollution, asbestos, coal, and other irritating respiratory factors. A family history of lung disease, such as asthma, allergies, lung cancer, or chronic obstructive lung disease, is significant for making a diagnosis. The personal history includes eliciting information about previous lung infections, such as tuberculosis or pneumonia, and other factors that have an effect on the respiratory system, such as drug abuse or human immunodeficiency (HIV). The patient's history of medications is important, as some drugs can affect long-term lung function.

The physical examination will reveal much to the skilled clinician. For example, if there is an absence of breath sounds during inspiration over a certain area of the lung, the absence may indicate **atelectasis** (incomplete expansion of the lung) or a pleural **effusion** (liquid in the pleural space). Tenderness over the sinus area may indicate a sinus infection, or clubbed fingers may indicate lung cancer or cystic fibrosis. Each element in the physical examination is important in the diagnostic process and is noted in the medical documentation.

Common respiratory symptoms are chronic cough, sore throat, and **hemoptysis** (blood in sputum). Conditions of the respiratory system frequently include upper respiratory infection, laryngitis, croup, bronchiolitis, asthma, bronchitis, chronic obstructive pulmonary disease, pneumonia, atelectasis, and pulmonary embolus. Common procedures include endotracheal intubation, tracheostomy, **thoracentesis,** biopsies, and various endoscopic procedures, such as sinus endoscopy or bronchoscopy. Pulmonary specialty studies include pulmonary function, oxygen saturation, polysomnogram, and sleep studies. X-rays and computed tomography (CT) scans are often part of the medical documentation for patients with respiratory conditions.

Physicians who specialize in treatment of the nose and throat are otolaryngologists, and physicians who specialize in treatment of the respiratory system are **pulmonologists.**

Enzyme Immunoassay

An EIA (enzyme immunoassay) is screening for strep. *Streptococcus* organisms are classified by means of the Lancefield classification into Groups A through O. The CPT manual divides *Streptococcus* into Groups A and B. Group A is *Streptococcus pyogenes,* which can be a cause of sore throat **(pharyngitis).** A culture allows identification of the cause of the pharyngitis. The patient presents to the laboratory, and laboratory personnel will swab the pharyngeal wall and tonsillar area. The material on the swab is placed into a medium (culture medium) that allows for the growth of the microorganism over a period of time. Newer methods allow results to be known more quickly, termed *rapid detection methods,* which are not cultured (noncultured). Noncultured is also known as primary source, which means that instead of waiting for the overnight incubation, as is required in the cultured method, the swabbed material is incubated with an acid solution or an enzyme that extracts the Group A antigen. EIA that utilizes this fast test method is manufactured in a kit, much like the commercially available pregnancy test kits that are now readily available. A plus sign appears to

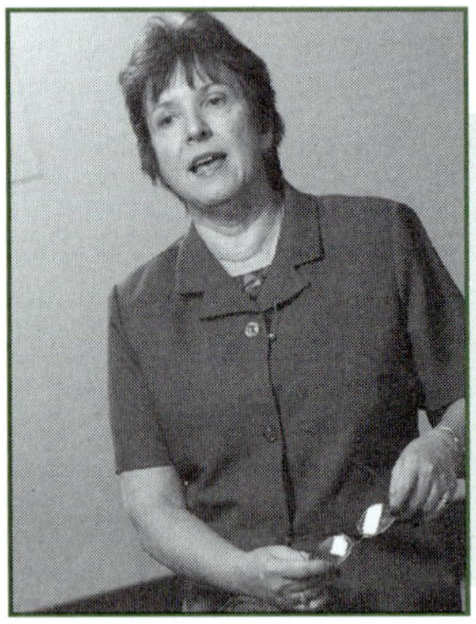

FROM THE TRENCHES

Maryann

"Physicians are very involved with performing the surgery and the clinical aspects [and] are a little less apt to be involved in the actual coding process. I realized early on that in order to be able to accurately bill for them I would have to A) become educated on the procedures that they were doing and B) be able to find the appropriate codes in order to bill for them and be reimbursed fairly for what they are actually doing."

indicate that *Streptococcus* was detected, and a minus sign appears to indicate that no *Streptococcus* was found in the sample. These results are stated on a laboratory report that is sent to the physician for review.

The diagnosis for the laboratory tests is not stated in the laboratory report; rather, when the service is submitted for reimbursement, the reason for the service is stated as the diagnosis assigned by the physician. Laboratory results are not used for diagnosis unless a physician has interpreted the results.

You can locate the various enzyme immunoassays in the index of the CPT manual under Antigen Detection.

CASE 9-1
9-1A Evening Clinic, Sore Throat
9-1B Laboratory, Respiratory Cultures

CASE 9-1

9-1A EVENING CLINIC, SORE THROAT

LOCATION: Outpatient, Clinic

PATIENT: Cindy Byer

PHYSICIAN: Ronald Green, M.D.

This established patient presents to the evening clinic on May 9. She relates that she has had a sore throat for one day. No fever. No nausea, vomiting, or diarrhea. No significant runny nose or congestion. She has had occasional nonproductive cough, which she attributes to smoking.

EXAMINATION: The patient is an alert, cooperative 36-year-old white female with a temperature of 99.6. AU TMs are clear. The nose is inflamed but patent. Sinuses are nontender. The oropharynx is hyperemic. The are no exudates. There is a bit of food debris in the right tonsillar crypt. Neck is supple without significant nodes. Lungs are clear to auscultation. A 4-hour EIA strep screen is pending.

ASSESSMENT:
1. Food debris in right tonsil (*not significant*)
2. Rhinopharyngitis

PLAN: An EIA strep screen is pending. We will call her back with the results but will have her call back if she has not heard from us by 11 o'clock tomorrow morning. Hygiene precautions are discussed, and over-the-counter medication is also discussed. Further treatment pending the results of the strep screen.

9-1A:

SERVICE CODE(S): ____________________

DX CODE(S): ____________________

9-1B LABORATORY, RESPIRATORY CULTURES

Dr. Green sends Cindy to the laboratory for an EIA.

LOCATION: Outpatient, Clinic

PATIENT: Cindy Byer

PHYSICIAN: Ronald Green, M.D.

INDICATION: Rhinopharyngitis

STREP SCREEN EIA

SPECIMEN SOURCE: Throat

SPECIAL REQUESTS: None

STREP FA: Negative for group A beta strep by EIA

9-1B:

SERVICE CODE(S): ____________________

DX CODE(S): ____________________

Residents

As a part of the medical resident's education, each resident is required to serve a rotation in a variety of health care settings under the direct supervision of a qualified physician who serves as the resident's supervisor and teacher. When the health care services provided by the resident are not directly reported to all the third-party payers (e.g., Medicare), the HCPCS modifier -GC (performed in part by a resident) or-GE (performed completely by a resident) is sometimes used on the code submitted for the teaching physician to indicate that the resident, under supervision of the teaching physician, performed a portion of the service and that the resident's notes have been considered when reporting the teaching physician's service. For example, in the following case, the teaching physician dictated a history and physical on admitting a patient to the hospital. The resident alsodictated a history and physical. The coder uses both the teaching physician's notes and the resident's notes to report the teaching physician's services of a hospital admission.

Most third-party payers will not reimburse a facility for services performed completely by a resident.

CASE 9-2
9-2A Admission History and Physical (Physician's and Resident's Notes)
9-2B Radiology Report, Chest
9-2C Radiology Report, Chest
9-2D Thoracic Medicine/Critical Care Progress Report
9-2E Thoracic Medicine/Critical Care Progress Report
9-2F Thoracic Medicine/Critical Care Progress Note
9-2G Discharge Summary

CASE 9-2

Dr. Dawson admitted Mr. Gulman to the hospital and prepared an admission history and physical. Dr. Grovedahl is a resident being supervised by Dr. Dawson. When completing the audit form for the admission service, place a "✓" on the form to indicate elements Dr. Dawson provided and a "×" to indicate elements Dr. Grovedahl provided. Dr. Grovedahl performed only part of the service because Dr. Dawson also contributed to the service. Assume that the third-party payer requires the use of the HCPCS modifiers for those services provided in part by a resident.

9-2A ADMISSION HISTORY AND PHYSICAL (PHYSICIAN'S AND RESIDENT'S NOTES)

LOCATION: Inpatient, Hospital

PATIENT: Ervin Gulman

PRIMARY CARE PHYSICIAN: Ronald Green, M.D.

ATTENDING PHYSICIAN: Gregory Dawson, M.D.

PHYSICIAN ADMISSION NOTES:
The emergency room notified that the patient presented himself there with increasing shortness of breath, and of course he had an abnormal chest x-ray. This is the same patient I tried to talk into coming into the emergency room earlier, and Dr. Green also tried even a week before that, and he has now agreed that perhaps he is sick enough to come in.

He is a patient who is well known to me, so a lot of history is already in the clinic chart. His past medical history, social history, family history, and review of systems are outlined in detail by my resident. Please see the resident's note for complete details of the entrance history and physical.

The patient has significant chronic obstructive pulmonary disease (COPD) with hypoxic, hypercarbic respiratory failure on today's blood gases. He has had diminished appetite for a couple of weeks and dry mouth, and he is too short of breath really to eat well. He is on home O_2 (*report dependence on supplemental oxygen with a V code*), and he has been on Avalax since the 10th. Before that he had a week's worth of antibiotics as well, but I do not know what they were. No fevers, sweats, or chills were present. He had increasing malaise, and he had some fever, with a temperature of 101° F to 102° F before admission.

The time I saw the patient revealed a very ill-appearing white male. HEENT is benign. No blood in the nose or posterior pharynx. The neck is supple without adenopathy. No JVD. Thyroid is not palpably enlarged. Lungs have diminished air movement everywhere, with rales in the right. No wheezes, rhonchi, or rubs. Heart shows a heart rate of about 110. I thought it was regular, without an S3 or S4. No diastolic sounds, clicks, or rubs; maybe a grade 1 murmur over the fourth intercostal, but his heart is so fast I am not sure what exactly I am hearing at this point. Abdomen is benign without hepatosplenomegaly. Normal bowel sounds are present. No bruits are heard in either flank. No masses are palpable, nontender, somewhat distended and tympanitis but within the range of normal. Neurologically he is awake and alert. Extremities show no edema, rashes, clubbing, cyanosis, or tremor except some ecchymosis in his upper arms, probably from steroid use. Neurologic: Cranial nerves II-XII are intact, and there is symmetrical strength in all four extremities. A detailed exam is not done because of his respiratory distress. Lymphatics: There are no nodes in the neck, clavicular, or axillary area.

IMPRESSION:
1. Acute *pneumonia,* organism unknown with secondary acute bronchospasm superimposed in a patient with significant COPD and respiratory failure.
   He will be admitted for antibiotic use and bronchodilator therapy, and we will have to look more into this hypercarbia. If the problem gets too great, we might have difficulty because this patient did not tolerate the BiPAP mask because of claustrophobia.
2. Chronic anxiety: In fact, that is why he is on BuSpar. We will try to get into him as soon as we can, but I do not really want to do it right today because of the elevated pCO_2 (*not reported*).

Resident's Admission Notes

LOCATION: Inpatient, Hospital

PATIENT: Ervin Gulman

PRIMARY CARE PHYSICIAN: Ronald Green, M.D.

ATTENDING PHYSICIAN: Gregory Dawson, M.D.

RESIDENT: Mandy Grovedahl, M.D.

CHIEF COMPLAINT: Increasing shortness of breath and malaise

HISTORY OF PRESENT ILLNESS: This 73-year-old male was seen in Dr. Green's office 1 week ago to follow up on pneumonia. The patient had been taking quinolone for a week for a pneumonia that had been diagnosed approximately 2 weeks previously when he had presented with cough, fever, chills, and shortness of breath. Since then, those symptoms have resolved. The patient complained of a decreased appetite at home and complaining of a dry mouth. He is on home O_2 and has been on Avelox since the 10th when he went to the office to see Dr. Green. Over the past 2 days he has complained of increasing shortness of breath, increasing malaise, temperature 101° F to 102° F yesterday. He denies any nausea, vomiting, or diarrhea.

PAST MEDICAL HISTORY:
1. Severe chronic obstructive pulmonary disease
2. Congestive heart failure
3. Elevated PSA in the past

MEDICATIONS:
1. BuSpar 10 mg b.i.d.
2. Lasix 40 mg q.d.
3. Ibuprofen 1 tab p.r.n.
4. Albuterol 0.5% nebulizer q.6h.
5. Aerobid inhalers 4 puffs b.i.d.
6. Albuterol sulfate 0.5 mg with each nebulizer treatment.
7. Serevent 2 puffs q.12h
8. Atrovent 2 puffs q.i.d.

ALLERGIES: Aspirin

PAST SURGICAL HISTORY: Right jaw repair following a broken jaw. No other surgeries.

FAMILY HISTORY: Father passed away at age 86 of congestive heart failure. Mother passed away at age 78 of colon cancer. The patient has three brothers and one sister alive. Two brothers have pacemakers. One sister has COPD.

SOCIAL HISTORY: Patient one pack daily × 45-year smoker. He quit approximately 15 years ago. He does have a history of heavy drinking in the past but denies any current use. He currently lives in Manytown with his wife.

REVIEW OF SYSTEMS: Constitutional: The patient indicates that there was an 18-pound weight loss approximately 2 months ago secondary to some fluid overload. He denies any headaches. He has had a decreased appetite in the past week or so, and he sleeps well with no problems. Eyes: Denies any history of glaucoma and has no eye pain or blurry or double vision. Ears, nose, mouth, and throat: No hearing problems reported. No bleeding from the nose or mouth. Cardiovascular: Denies palpitations. Denies any pressure or racing heartbeat. He does complain of some substernal chest pain off and on with exertion, last experienced approximately 1 week ago. Respiratory: Chronic cough, which is productive of white sputum. Dyspnea on exertion. GI: No history of ulcers. No digestive problems. He has had some positive stools recently. GU: History of prostate problems. Positive burning with urination recently. Skin: Complaint of dryness around the nares. No rashes. No nonhealing lesions. Musculoskeletal: No arthritis. No complaints of joint pain. No loss of muscle strength. Psych: Patient does have a history of anxiety secondary to shortness of breath. Neuro: No epilepsy or history of seizures. Hematology: Patient states he bruises easily. He does not have a bleeding problem. Endocrine: No kidney problems. No thyroid problems.

PHYSICAL EXAMINATION: Vitals: Pulse 105. Blood pressure 132/157. O_2 saturation on 3L nasal cannula is 82% to 89%. Respirations are mid 20s to 30s. Temperature 36.8° C. HEENT: Normocephalic and atraumatic. Extraocular movements are intact. Neck is soft. No cervical adenopathy. Pharynx is without erythema. There are no oral lesions. Cardiovascular: Tachycardia. No murmurs, rubs, or gallops heard. Respiratory: Diminished air movement in bilateral bases. Minimal respiratory wheeze heard. No rhonchi or rales appreciated. Abdomen: Soft, positive bowel sounds, nondistended. The patient complains of positive tenderness to palpation over the right upper quadrant. Musculoskeletal: Strength is 5/5 and equal bilaterally upper and lower extremities. Extremities: No clubbing, cyanosis, or edema. Full range of motion times four. Neuro: Cranial nerves II-XII grossly intact. Sensation is intact.

LABORATORY: Sodium 142, potassium 4.4, chloride 96, CO_2 greater than or equal to 41.8, BUN 17, creatinine 0.7, and glucose 129. Calcium 8.9. White blood cells 9.7, hemoglobin 15.6, and platelets 202. ABGs from this morning: pH 7.439, pCO_2 52.9, pO_2 55.2, bicarbonate 35.1, O_2 saturation 94% on 3L nasal cannula from 9:30 this morning, when he came in through the emergency department. Chest x-ray from 2 weeks ago revealed extensive opacities on the right side, awaiting results of x-ray from the emergency room this morning. I will review those this afternoon with Dr. Dawson.

ASSESSMENT/PLAN: Pneumonia right-sided in someone with COPD. Patient is oxygen dependent due to chronic respiratory failure. He has been placed on Claforan, Zithromax, and Solu-Medrol as well as a variety of breathing treatments. We will monitor labs, ABGs, and x-ray. See orders for remainder.

9-2A:

SERVICE CODE(S): ____________________

DX CODE(S): ____________________

9-2B RADIOLOGY REPORT, CHEST

This radiology report indicates that there were two parts to the chest (upper and lower); however, this is a single view (anteroposterior, front to back). It is the number of views that is reported.

LOCATION: Inpatient, Hospital

PATIENT: Ervin Gulman

PRIMARY CARE PHYSICIAN: Ronald Green, M.D.

ATTENDING PHYSICIAN: Gregory Dawson, M.D.

RADIOLOGIST: Morton Monson, M.D.

EXAMINATION OF: Chest

CLINICAL SYMPTOMS: Pneumonia, COPD, and chronic respiratory failure

PORTABLE CHEST: SINGLE VIEW: FINDINGS: Study is compared today with the study dated 2 weeks ago. Cardiac monitor leads overlie the patient. This chest film is obtained in two parts—one contains the upper portion of the chest, the second the lower portion of the chest. Cardiac silhouette is prominent but stable. Pulmonary vasculature also mildly prominent but stable. The left lung appears relatively clear. There is some linear opacity, left infrahilar area, consistent with segmental volume loss. Opacity is seen in the right lung with some mild sparing of the right apex. This is a mixed interstitial and alveolar pattern with a more focal area of opacity in the right mid-lung extending to the lateral chest wall. Pleural density is seen along the right lateral chest wall, and there is an unusual lucency over the right heart border. Osseous structures are stable.

IMPRESSION:

1. Increasing consolidation in the right mid-lung and infiltrate in the right lung base. Clinical correlation is suggested.
2. Pleural density is new since previous exam on the right, likely related to a pleural effusion. Again, clinical correlation is suggested. These findings may represent an acute infiltrate likely secondary to infectious process, but it can also be seen with other etiologies, such as pulmonary embolism.
3. There is an unusual lucency over the right lung base adjacent to the heart border. This may represent aerated lung against consolidation, but other etiologies, including pneumatocele, could have this appearance, and clinical correlation suggests the need for further imaging.

9-2B:

SERVICE CODE(S): ____________________

DX CODE(S): ____________________

9-2C RADIOLOGY REPORT, CHEST

Dr. Monson suggested further imaging, and based on that recommendation, Dr. Dawson ordered a posteroanterior (PA) and lateral chest x-ray.

LOCATION: Inpatient, Hospital

PATIENT: Ervin Gulman

PRIMARY CARE PHYSICIAN: Ronald Green, M.D.

ATTENDING PHYSICIAN: Gregory Dawson, M.D.

EXAMINATION OF: Chest

CLINICAL SYMPTOMS: Pneumonia, COPD, and chronic respiratory failure

PA AND LATERAL CHEST X-RAY, 9:15 A.M.: Previous portable upright only yesterday

CLINICAL INFORMATION: There is cardiomegaly, as there has been on previous x-rays for this patient. The vascular markings on the left are within normal limits. On the left, there is what appears to be interstitial fibrosis, mid-lung and base. No left effusion suggested. On the right, there is abnormal density throughout the right lung that is interstitial in nature and could be unilateral failure pattern. That is less confluent than it was in the right upper lobe compared with the previous report. The remainder of the right lung (mid-lung and base) shows no change from previous report. There is blunting of the right costophrenic angle and the right posterior sulcus suggesting a small effusion that is stable. There is some pleural density along the right lateral chest wall and over the apex that is assumed to be scarring. There is degenerative change of the thoracic spine, mild. No destructive lesion or fracture is seen.

IMPRESSION:

1. Cardiomegaly stable
2. No vascular congestion on the left. The left lung shows scar but no active parenchymal disease and no left effusion.
3. On the right, there is a pleural scar along the right lateral chest wall and over the apex.
4. There is abnormal interstitial finding throughout the entire right lung except for the apex. That is abnormal and is new compared with the previous film, indicating that it is an acute finding. It could be a unilateral failure pattern. It could be interstitial pneumonia. There is slightly improved aeration in the periphery of the right upper lobe compared with the film taken 2 days ago. The remainder of the chest is stable.
5. Suggestion of small effusion on the right.

9-2C:

SERVICE CODE(S): ____________________

DX CODE(S): ____________________

9-2D THORACIC MEDICINE/CRITICAL CARE PROGRESS REPORT

Note that the physician changed the diagnosis from "pneumonia" to "pneumonia, interstitial-type," which is in the inner spaces of the lung linings. Since the outpatient coder reports only those diagnosis(es) stated on that current report being coded, the diagnoses for this patient will need to reflect this more current diagnosis.

LOCATION: Inpatient, Hospital

PATIENT: Ervin Gulman

PRIMARY CARE PHYSICIAN: Ronald Green, M.D.

ATTENDING PHYSICIAN: Gregory Dawson, M.D.

The patient has a right-lung pneumonia, interstitial-type; COPD and chronic respiratory failure. Yesterday's x-ray showed maybe some clearing. The sputum culture so far is not very helpful. The Gram stain does show evidence of gram-positive disease with moderate gram-positive cocci and moderate gram-positive cocci in clusters. He is taking Claforan and Zithromax, which should cover that. He seems to be responding and is a little more energetic.

OBJECTIVE: He has been afebrile since he has been here. HEENT: Benign. Neck: Supple without JVD. Chest: Symmetrical. Rales on the right. Very distant breath sounds. Left sounds pretty good. I do not hear any rales, anyway, but again, distant breath sounds. Heart: S1 and S2 are regular with a grade 1/6 murmur at the fourth interspace near the sternum that really does not radiate much. Abdomen: soft. Benign without hepatosplenomegaly. Extremities: No clubbing. No edema.

The patient is a significant CO_2 retainer but does not really tolerate BiPAP much at all, and he tried that in the past. He seems to be quite claustrophobic and just cannot do it. I will put him back on his BuSpar, put him back on his Lasix today 40 mg a day, and we will continue the rest of the drugs. We will start physical therapy with him a little bit to see if we cannot get him moving. His Solu-Medrol is every 6; go down to every 8 today. I would like to discharge him after a good 5 days of antibiotics, as I am sure the x-ray is better.

9-2D:

SERVICE CODE(S): ______________________

DX CODE(S): ______________________

9-2E THORACIC MEDICINE/CRITICAL CARE PROGRESS REPORT

LOCATION: Inpatient, Hospital

PATIENT: Ervin Gulman

PRIMARY CARE PHYSICIAN: Ronald Green, M.D.

ATTENDING PHYSICIAN: Gregory Dawson, M.D.

The patient has significant COPD, is oxygen dependent, and has chronic respiratory failure. He had an extensive right-lung pneumonia, interstitial type, basically sparing the apex. Gram stain showing gram-positive *cocci* in the chains and clusters. No pathogen was grown. He is actually doing better. He was able to walk in the hallway a little bit.

EXAMINATION: He has fewer rales. He still has a little bit of wheeze. His weight, however, has gone up. He has some edema in his legs. We will have to give him some Lasix today. I am sure this is fluid retention from steroids. He weighs about 3 pounds more now than he did on the 27th (186 pounds).

The plan is to finish out this week with steroids. I will taper him off so he will be done on the 2nd. With any luck, he can be discharged on the 3rd. Recheck a chest x-ray tomorrow. Recheck his oxygen level. He gets a little dizzy when he stands up, and that may be from hypercarbia, which he is prone to have. Hopefully things are improving enough that we can get him home on Friday.

9-2E:

SERVICE CODE(S): ______________________

DX CODE(S): ______________________

9-2F THORACIC MEDICINE/CRITICAL CARE PROGRESS NOTE

On this report the physician indicates that the interstitial is now clear, and so the diagnosis for the pneumonia is no longer the interstitial type.

LOCATION: Inpatient, Hospital

PATIENT: Ervin Gulman

PRIMARY CARE PHYSICIAN: Ronald Green, M.D.

ATTENDING PHYSICIAN: Gregory Dawson, M.D.

The patient is here for pneumonia that is clearing on x-ray. Interstitially clear. On exam, it is clearing. He is symptomatically better and is afebrile. On exam, he still has a few rales at the base. Very distant breath sounds, but he has extremely severe COPD. His O_2 requirement is back down to his usual 2L. His pO_2 60, pCO_2 77, pH 7.38, and that is his usual set of blood gases. He still has a little edema on exam. Heart shows a regular flow as well as a regular rhythm.

DISPOSITION: We will switch from IV antibiotics to oral antibiotics. If he is doing this well tomorrow, I can discharge him at that time, and with any luck we can get him discharged tomorrow and home.

9-2F:

SERVICE CODE(S): ____________________

DX CODE(S): ____________________

9-2G DISCHARGE SUMMARY

LOCATION: Inpatient, Hospital

PATIENT: Ervin Gulman

PRIMARY CARE PHYSICIAN: Ronald Green, M.D.

ATTENDING PHYSICIAN: Gregory Dawson, M.D.
The patient was admitted with pneumonia, increasing shortness of breath, and failure to thrive. He had been treated as an outpatient for similar things but has gradually declined and become quite fatigued and increasingly short of breath. He had acute pneumonia, unknown organism, and at the time of admission. I do not think our cultures helped much in identifying a causative organism. His case was gradual slow improvement. He was able to take care of himself a little bit, and he was able to be discharged.

The Gram stain suggested a streptococcal or even a streptococcal organism with moderate gram-positive *cocci* in pairs and gram-negative *cocci* in clusters, but no cultures actually revealed pathogenic diagnosis.

We finally were able to discharge him today to his home under the care of his family.

MEDICATIONS: he was discharged with were:

1. Albuterol nebulizer four times a day and then q.3h. p.r.n.
2. BuSpar 10 mg q.d.
3. Vantin 200 mg b.i.d.
4. Atrovent four times a day with the albuterol
5. TheoDur 200 mg q.d.
6. Oxygen

The Vantin will be discontinued on the 5th after his dose on that day. Follow-up will be in a week in the office to repeat his chest x-ray. His O_2 was set at 4 L with 2 L continuously.

DISCHARGE DIAGNOSES:

1. Pneumonia
2. Chronic respiratory failure
3. Chronic obstructive pulmonary disease, O_2 dependent

9-2G:

SERVICE CODE(S): ____________________

DX CODE(S): ____________________

CASE 9-3
9-3A Thoracic Medicine/Critical Care Consultation
9-3B Thoracic Medicine/Critical Care Progress Note
9-3C Radiology Report, Chest
9-3D Thoracic Medicine/Critical Care Progress Note
9-3E Thoracic Medicine/Critical Care Progress Note
9-3F Radiology Report, Chest
9-3G Discharge Summary

CASE 9-3

Dr. Dawson was called to the emergency department for a consultation regarding Kurt Troy who presented with pulmonary edema and respiratory failure. During the consultation, Dr. Dawson decided to admit Mr. Troy to the hospital. The consultation then becomes a hospital admission and is reported as an admission, not as a consultation, even though you will note that the report is titled a consultation. Dr. Dawson admitted the patient, and is the attending physician. There is a ventilation service to be coded in this case. Ventilation service is reported based on if it is an initial or subsequent service (94656 and 94657). The physician must document the ventilator settings to report the service. Usually ventilator service is reported in addition to an E/M service. Append modifier -25 to the E/M code to indicate that the E/M service was separate from the ventilator service. This patient has a myriad of problems; when reporting the diagnoses, report the chief reason(s) the patient reported for this service. In Case 9-3, you will find the diagnoses highlighted for you, to illustrate how the diagnosis changes slightly from report to report.

9-3A THORACIC MEDICINE/CRITICAL CARE CONSULTATION

LOCATION: Inpatient, Hospital

PATIENT: Kurt Troy

ATTENDING PHYSICIAN: Gregory Dawson, M.D.

CHIEF COMPLAINT: Pulmonary edema with respiratory failure

HISTORY OF PRESENT ILLNESS: This is a 57-year-old male admitted through the emergency department at 6:04 A.M. in respiratory distress leading to intubation. The patient did vomit in the emergency department and was suctioned with possible aspiration. The patient has no significant cardiac arrhythmia since intubation, and no CPR was performed in the emergency room. The patient is currently on a vent with settings of tidal volume 650, rate 21, PEEP 7, FIO_2 50%, SIMV mode PSV of 15. Family reports that the patient had complained of chest pain and pressure and severe back pain in the previous 2 days since falling a week ago. He was seen in the emergency room on that date. CT and x-ray were done and indicated that there were some lumbar spine transverse process fractures. The patient also hit his head in the fall, but there was no loss of consciousness.

PAST MEDICAL HISTORY:
1. COPD
2. Atherosclerotic heart disease with CABG performed 10 years ago
3. History of silent MI 10 years ago
4. Chronic congestive cardiomyopathy
5. Congestive heart failure
6. Questionable hypertension
7. Increased cholesterol
8. Diabetes diagnosed in February of last year

CURRENT MEDICATIONS IN HOSPITAL:
1. Cozaar 10 mg b.i.d.
2. Nitroglycerin IV titration
3. Midazolam IV titration
4. Bumex 1 mg q.6h.
5. Morphine IV 2-4 mg p.r.n

ALLERGIES: No known drug allergies

PAST SURGICAL HISTORY:
1. Coronary artery bypass graft 10 years ago
2. Hemorrhoid surgery sometime in the past

SOCIAL HISTORY: The patient lives at home with wife and daughter. He smoked one pack per day ×41 years, quit 1 year ago. No alcohol.

FAMILY HISTORY: Father with history of multiple MIs after the age of 55, congestive heart failure, and pacemaker. Mother passed away when patient was fifteen.

REVIEW OF SYSTEMS: Not obtainable at this time other than above from family as patient is sedated.

EXAMINATION: VITAL SIGNS: Afebrile (98), pulse 72, blood pressure 127/69, O_2 saturation 98% on 50% FIO_2, and rate 21. GENERAL: The patient is a 57-year-old white male who appears his stated age; he is well nourished and well hydrated. CARDIOVASCULAR: S1 and S2; no murmur appreciated. ECG indicates a rate of 85 and left bundle-branch block. Cardiac enzymes × 1 indicate CK of 378, MB of 4, and troponin I of 0.3. Cardiac enzymes will be repeated in triplicate. PULMONARY: Diminished breath sounds at bilateral bases. ABGs were drawn at 10:30 A.M. indicating a pH of 7.409, pCO_2 of 35.0, O_2 saturation 99.6%, pO_2 is 213.3, and bicarb is 21.7. FIO_2 was set at 50% with PEEP of 7, pressure support of 15, and rate of 21 during this draw. (*The preceding are the ventilator settings.*) Chest x-ray done in the emergency department indicated congestive heart failure and infiltrate. Antibiotics have been started secondary to the likely aspiration. GI and GU: Soft, positive bowel sounds, nontender, and nondistended. Foley catheter and NB tube in place. ELECTROLYTES: Sodium 133, potassium 5.1, chloride 94, creatinine 1.1, BUN 30, magnesium 2.2. ENDOCRINE: Blood glucose 233 this A.M.; insulin sliding scale has been implemented, and Accu-Chek will be done every 4 hours. INFECTIOUS DISEASE: We have ordered cultures for blood, urine, and sputum. Antibiotics have been started. NEUROLOGICAL: The patient is sedated at this time.

DISPOSITION: Likely aspiration, questionable angina of 5 days' duration, leading to flash pulmonary edema. Cardiology has been consulted. Echo for left ventricular function. Added a third set of cardiac enzymes to be drawn. Aspirin now 325 mg. Blood, urine, sputum, cultures, and sensitivities ordered. Morphine drip at 1 mg continuous with 0.5-mg bolus q. 10 minutes p.r.n. Begin Unasyn. Change vent settings to PEEP of 5, drop tidal volume to 600; recheck ABGs in 30 minutes.

9-3A:

SERVICE CODE(S): ______________________

DX CODE(S): ______________________

9-3B THORACIC MEDICINE/CRITICAL CARE PROGRESS NOTE

LOCATION: Inpatient, Hospital

PATIENT: Kurt Troy

ATTENDING PHYSICIAN: Gregory Dawson, M.D.

The patient is on ventilator with aspiration and acute pulmonary edema and respiratory failure. His chest x-ray is now clearing up. He still has some clutter, but it is much better than it was. He still has residual changes of pulmonary edema pattern, right greater than left, but much better and his oxygenation is better.

REVIEW OF SYSTEMS/PHYSICAL EXAM:

CARDIOLOGY REVIEW OF SYSTEMS: Fairly stable. Blood pressures are holding their own, with systolic in the 110 range and diastolic in the 50 range with sinus rhythm of about 80. Troponins have not really risen very much. I think the highest we had was 0.8 and is now down to 0.6, so I do not think we had an acute MI, just a troponin leak. No S3 or S4. I do not appreciate any murmurs. Echocardiogram, however, shows a really depressed left ventricular function down to 10% to 15%. Right ventricular pressure is 45, which is mild pulmonary hypertension. He shows marked hypokinesis of the septum. He has some calcification of the aortic leaflets and mitral leaflets, and apical and periapical segments are also severely hypokinetic and probably akinetic. We have a really bad pump.

PULMONARY SYSTEM REVIEW was just excellent. The pH is 7.53, pCO_2 29, pO_2 152. On exam, he has a few scattered rales, much improved over his initial exam.

GASTROINTESTINAL SYSTEM REVIEW: He has really low residuals. Abdomen is soft and nontender. No ascites.

GENITOURINARY SYSTEM REVIEW: He had 1.7 L more out than in with a creatinine clearance exceeding 100. He has no edema on exam.

ENDOCRINOLOGY: Blood sugars are holding their own at 152.

ELECTROLYTES: Potassium is a little low; we will have to replace that. Sodium 135, potassium 3.2, chloride 102, CO_2 21.8, calcium 7.2, magnesium 1.6, phosphorus 2.4; we will have to replace that as well.

HEMATOLOGIC: White count is coming down, but it is still high at 15,530. Hemoglobin is 15.8 with normal platelets of 178,000.

INFECTIOUS DISEASE: White count is coming down. Cultures so far have not grown much. There is a gram-negative *Diplococcus*, but it is rarely seen on Gram stain and may be causative organism, and he is on Unasyn anyway, and he has been afebrile.

NEUROLOGIC: He is too sedated right now.

DISPOSITION: We will not start any tube feedings because I think we will be extubating him this afternoon. Will try to wean him off the ventilator. Will replace his potassium. Dr. Elhart will be by later to see him and adjust his medications. At this point, I think the reason for the flash pulmonary edema was really poor cardiac function.

We spent a total of 45 minutes discussing the case with Dr. Elhart and discussing with the family, examining the patient, reviewing his labs, especially digging up the microbiology, reviewing his x-rays, writing the orders, and dictating the note. This is a pivotal day for this patient. He seems to be getting better but has such precarious cardiac function that it still makes him a critical care patient, and it is somewhat tedious to make decisions. Mostly, we will spend in and out all day today watching how he responds to the ventilator changes because his cardiac function is so precarious that just the extra work of breathing might be enough to cause more trouble with pulmonary edema. So we may have to go slower than I expect.

9-3B:

SERVICE CODE(S): ______________________

DX CODE(S): ______________________

9-3C RADIOLOGY REPORT, CHEST

LOCATION: Inpatient, Hospital

PATIENT: Kurt Troy

ATTENDING PHYSICIAN: Gregory Dawson, M.D.

EXAMINATION OF: Chest

CLINICAL SYMPTOMS: Follow-up congestive heart failure

REFERRING DR: None stated

PORTABLE CHEST: ONE VIEW: 5:00 A.M. Comparisons are made with the previous study taken on admission at 5:00 A.M. The heart is enlarged. Central vascularity is mildly prominent. Endotracheal tube lies at the level of the aortic arch. Nasogastric tube transverses the esophagus and lies beyond our field of view within the region of the stomach. Effusions are not seen.

CONCLUSION:

1. There is persistent cardiomegaly, perhaps slightly worsened compared with the previous study. Central vessels are also mildly prominent.
2. Multiple support apparatuses as discussed above.

9-3C:

SERVICE CODE(S): ____________________

DX CODE(S): ____________________

9-3D THORACIC MEDICINE/CRITICAL CARE PROGRESS NOTE

LOCATION: Inpatient, Hospital

PATIENT: Kurt Troy

ATTENDING PHYSICIAN: Gregory Dawson, M.D.

The patient was seen and examined at 8:30 A.M. He remains unresponsive secondary to sedation. The acute pulmonary edema is improved on x-ray following diuresis.

Vitals: Pulse 95. Blood pressure 111/53. O_2 saturation 97% on 35% FIO_2; rate is 15. Patient is afebrile (98.6° F). Cardiovascular: Regular rate and rhythm. No edema is noted. Ejection fraction is 15% per echo done by cardiology in April. Cardiac enzymes are negative ×3. Pulmonary: Decreased breath sounds, scattered rales. Improved chest x-ray this morning with decreased infiltrate. ABG at 8 A.M. shows a pH of 7.465, pCO_2 of 35.6, pO_2 of 125.1, bicarbonate of 25.1, FIO_2 40%, rate of 17 with PEEP of 5, and PFV of 15. Gastrointestinal: Soft with positive bowel sounds; nondistended. Nasogastric tube residuals of 10 cc and 10 cc, respectively. GU: Foley in place. Good urine output: 1396/3100. Endocrine: Serum glucose 152. Accu-Cheks of 137/145 today. No insulin necessary. Electrolytes: Sodium 135, potassium 3.2, chloride 102, CO_2 21.8, BUN 27, creatinine 1.1, and calcium 7.2. The patient had 40 mEq of potassium chloride in the NG tube ×2 doses this morning. Potassium will be redrawn at noon. Hematologic: White blood cells 15.5, down from a high of 17.3. Hemoglobin 15.8, hematocrit 45.6, and platelet count 178. PT is 12.8. INR 1.1 and PTT 24.9. Infectious Disease: Continue antibiotics until sensitivity is back on the sputum culture. Blood culture and urine culture shows no growth. The patient is afebrile. White blood cell count is dropping. Neurologic: The patient is sedated, but minimally responsive. Integumentary: Normal.

DISPOSITION: Change the vent settings to rate of 10 and draw ABG in 30 minutes. Begin weaning the patient from the vent. Anticipate extubation this afternoon. Will see the patient after extubation. Await identification and sensitivity on sputum culture. Cardiology is following the cardiomyopathy. Discontinue Versed drip.

9-3D:

SERVICE CODE(S): ____________________

DX CODE(S): ____________________

9-3E THORACIC MEDICINE/CRITICAL CARE PROGRESS NOTE

LOCATION: Inpatient, Hospital

PATIENT: Kurt Troy

ATTENDING PHYSICIAN: Gregory Dawson, M.D.

The patient is doing well. He had no major events during the night. He was extubated yesterday and transferred out to the floor. He has been walking and eating. His main complaint was back pain, which seems to have been helped by Tylenol.

He denies nausea or vomiting. He is having bowel movements.

PHYSICAL EXAMINATION: He is afebrile. Blood pressure 150/46, heart rate 87 per minute. Respirations 18 per minute. Saturations 100% on 3L. LUNGS: Clear bilaterally. Regular rate and rhythm; no murmur. Soft and nontender abdomen. No sacral or lower extremity edema, no clubbing. The patient is awake, alert, and oriented times three. No focal neurologic deficit.

IMPRESSION:

1. Congestive heart failure and respiratory failure, improved, status post extubation
2. Pulmonary edema
3. Back pain from questionable vertebral fractures without neurologic deficits

PLAN:
1. Taper oxygen
2. Discontinue Triamterene
3. Tylenol 650 mg p.o. q.6h.
4. Possible discharge tomorrow. Will discuss with Dr. Elhart in the morning

Patient and his family who accompany him today agree with this plan.

9-3E:

SERVICE CODE(S): ____________________

DX CODE(S): ____________________

9-3F RADIOLOGY REPORT, CHEST

LOCATION: Inpatient, Hospital

PATIENT: Kurt Troy

ATTENDING PHYSICIAN: Gregory Dawson, M.D.

EXAMINATION OF: Chest

CLINICAL SYMPTOMS: Follow-up congestive heart failure, pulmonary edema, respiratory failure

REFERRING DR: None stated

ONE-VIEW CHEST: 7:50 P.M. Single AP view was obtained of the chest yesterday at 7:50 P.M. Comparison study is the previous day. Endotracheal tube and nasogastric tube have been removed. There is again cardiac enlargement. Pulmonary vascularity is mildly prominent. Along the perihilar and infrahilar regions, there are some hazy density and increased markings. Suspect these findings relate to congestive changes. These findings are generally similar compared with the previous day. Suggest continued progress studies.

9-3F:

SERVICE CODE(S): ____________________

DX CODE(S): ____________________

9-3G DISCHARGE SUMMARY

LOCATION: Inpatient, Hospital

PATIENT: Kurt Troy

ATTENDING PHYSICIAN: Gregory Dawson, M.D.

The patient was admitted with acute respiratory distress secondary to pulmonary edema. His course included intubation and being on the ventilator. He was extubated after the pulmonary edema came under control. He has severe cardiac disease, and ejection fraction was quite diminished. He was able to be discharged.

DISCHARGE DIAGNOSES:
1. Acute respiratory failure secondary to acute pulmonary edema
2. Congestive cardiomyopathy
3. Congestive heart failure

DISCHARGE MEDICATIONS:
1. Tylenol 650 mg q.6h.p.r.n.
2. Furosemide 40 mg q.d.
3. Cozaar 100 mg b.i.d.
4. Protonix 40 mg q.d.

He was to resume his Imdur, Lanoxin, Glucovance, Atrovent, Maxair, Serevent, and Lipitor as he was taking at home prior to admission.

Follow-up was arranged with his primary care physician, Dr. Green, Thursday after discharge to get a basic metabolic panel before that visit. He is to see Dr. Elhart in a month after discharge for medication review. Dr. Elhart will probably elect to use Coreg later when he is stable and use a graduated increasing dose as is customary for severe congestive heart failure. I also advised him not to use ibuprofen because it has some salt retention properties and can aggravate the underlying congestive heart failure by the salt and water retention properties and is also nephrotoxic, especially in low cardiac output states, and he should probably stay off of all nonsteroidal antiinflammatory drugs (*NSAIDs*). I will be glad to see him as necessary, but my duty was mainly for ICU critical care while he was in the hospital.

9-3G:

SERVICE CODE(S): ____________________

DX CODE(S): ____________________

CASE 9-4
9-4A ENT Consultation

CASE 9-4

Dr. Dawson requested an ENT consultation to assess the viability of tracheostomy for a ventilator-dependent patient.

9-4A ENT CONSULTATION

LOCATION: Inpatient, Hospital

PATIENT: Bea Fore

ATTENDING PHYSICIAN: Gregory Dawson, M.D.

CONSULTANT: Jeff King, M.D.

Thank you for asking me to see the patient in consultation.

CHIEF COMPLAINT: Respiratory failure

HISTORY: The patient is a 60-year-old who suffered a left hip fracture 2 weeks ago. She underwent an open reduction internal fixation and required intubation. Postoperatively, she developed pneumonia and some ARDS. She has been ventilated since that time. Any attempts to wean her have been unsuccessful, and it is recommended that she have a tracheostomy to facilitate weaning and tracheal pulmonary toileting.

PAST MEDICAL HISTORY:

1. Hypertension
2. CVA
3. Diabetes
4. Bronchitis
5. Cellulitis of the lower extremity
6. Coronary artery disease
7. Coronary catheter
8. Renal artery stenosis
9. Right carotid stenosis
10. Obesity
11. Chronic obstructive pulmonary disease.

MEDICATIONS:

1. Albuterol
2. Colace
3. Insulin
4. Multi-vites
5. Vasotec
6. Procrit
7. Morphine PCA
8. Protonix

HABITS: She smokes one pack per day and has an approximately 30+-pack-year history. She does not drink alcohol. She has been off work on disability.

ALLERGIES: No known drug allergies

SOCIAL HISTORY: She is married. I was able to speak to her husband today. I understand she has six children.

PHYSICAL EXAMINATION: She is intubated and ventilated. She is not responding to me today. She has an NG tube in place for feeding. Blood pressure is 140/50. Pulse is 99. Respiratory rate is 15 on the vent. She is saturating at 92%. She is afebrile. Examination of her neck reveals a very thick short neck with a lot of adipose tissue. Landmarks are very difficult to palpate.

LABORATORY: She had some increased LFTs. Her hemoglobin was 8.8, red blood cell count 292, hematocrit 28.2, and platelets 264.

IMPRESSION: Chronic respiratory failure

PLAN: We will arrange to perform a tracheostomy procedure for her tomorrow or Wednesday. We will need to arrange for her to be n.p.o. and to have her insulin adjusted appropriately. Thank you again for allowing me to participate in her care.

9-4A:

SERVICE CODE(S): ____________________

DX CODE(S): ____________________

CASE 9-5

Dr. Elhart requested a consultation from Dr. Dawson due to bouts of V. tach, wheezing, chest pain, and possible pulmonary edema.

9-5A CONSULTATION/TRANSFER OF CARE

LOCATION: Inpatient, Hospital

PATIENT: Arlo Dockray

ATTENDING PHYSICIAN: Marvin Elhart, M.D.

CONSULTANT: Gregory Dawson, M.D.

The patient is a 71-year-old Caucasian male who was admitted 6 days ago for severe shortness of breath, which was thought to be related to pneumonia. During his hospitalization, the patient has been complaining of chest pain across his chest, radiating to his jaw and right neck. He had a cardiac perfusion scan that was normal, with an ejection fraction of 70%. He had a neck CT, which was negative for any abscesses.

The patient was doing well. Today he was walking in his room, and suddenly everybody was rushing in the room because he was in V. tach for 30 seconds; however, the patient did not lose his pulse and was totally asymptomatic. His heart rate stayed at around 110 to 130 per minute.

The patient complained of chest pain across his chest later, which was radiating to the shoulders and to the jaw. He received two doses of sublingual nitroglycerin with resolution of the pain. He continues to wheeze, however.

He has been progressively short of breath over the last 2 or 3 weeks. He cannot walk across the room without feeling short-winded. He also has orthopnea and PND.

Apparently the patient had coronary artery disease and had an angiogram in the past, probably 2 years ago or so, by Dr. Elhart. According to the patient, there was some coronary artery disease, but he was not amenable to any intervention.

PAST MEDICAL HISTORY:

1. COPD
2. Type 2 diabetes since 1957
3. Coronary artery disease as mentioned
4. Pancreatic insufficiency, on pancreatic enzymes
5. Benign prostatic hyperplasia
6. Depression
7. History of pulmonary hypertension
8. Gastroesophageal reflux disease
9. Fibromyalgia and osteoarthritis
10. Status post pacemaker placement
11. Partial resection of the colon, appendectomy, and cholecystectomy
12. History of CVA
13. Hyperlipidemia
14. History of mitral and tricuspid regurgitation on echocardiogram
15. History of tuberculosis in the past
16. Left upper lobectomy for tuberculosis
17. Rotator cuff repair
18. Two back surgeries
19. Hypertension

ALLERGIES: No known drug allergies.

SOCIAL HISTORY: The patient never smoked. He lives with his wife in Manytown. He does not use alcohol or drugs.

FAMILY HISTORY: Brother had a heart attack at age 36. Mother had enlarged heart. Father died of natural causes.

REVIEW OF SYSTEMS: General: No fever, chills, or night sweats. Respiratory: Dry cough with wheezing. Cardiovascular: Orthopnea, PND, exertional dyspnea, and generalized edema. GI: No heartburn, abdominal pain, constipation, diarrhea, hematemesis, or hematochezia, but he has been feeling bloated. ENT: Tinnitus bilaterally, which is chronic. Eyes: Negative. Skin: Negative. Neuro: Headache, but that is nonfocal. No neurologic deficits. No motor weakness, numbness, or tingling. Musculoskeletal: Arthralgias. No arthritis. GU: No frequency, urgency, hesitancy, hematuria, or dysuria.

CURRENT MEDICATIONS include the following:

1. Albuterol ipratropium treatments
2. Serevent
3. Amlodipine 5 mg q.d.
4. Pancreatic enzymes
5. Aspirin 325 mg q.d.
6. Sinemet q.h.s.
7. Lasix 40 mg b.i.d.
8. Isosorbide 50 mg q.d.
9. Metoprolol XL 50 mg q.d.
10. Protonix 40 mg q.d.
11. Paxil 20 mg q.d
12. Actos 45 mg q.d.
13. Prednisone 30 mg q.d.
14. Vitamin E
15. Lovenox 40 mg daily
16. Regular insulin and Lantus insulin
17. Bumex 0.5 mg was given stat at 6:00 P.M.
18. Zithromax 500 mg q.d.
19. Claforan 1g q.8h.

EXAMINATION: He is wheezing. His wheezing is audible. His blood pressure is in the 120s to 130s systolic and 60s diastolic. Heart rate is 137, atrial fibrillation with PVCs. He has engorged neck vein distention. I cannot see his JVP because of the engorgement in his neck veins. He is pleasant and talkative and responds nicely. Respiratory rate is probably 25 to 27 per minute. Lungs: Bilateral wheezes, decreased air entry in the left side but no obvious crackles. He has generalized edema, 2+ in the lower extremities, no clubbing. He had some sacral and abdominal wall edema. No organomegaly. The patient is awake and oriented ×3. No focal neurological deficits. Motor power 5/5 bilaterally. He has trace pulses in the extremities.

ECG shows PVC and atrial fibrillation. No Q waves. No ST elevations or T-wave inversions.

Potassium from this morning was 4.5, with bicarb of 34.

IMPRESSION:
1. Wheezing, probably chronic obstructive pulmonary disease and questionable pneumonia
2. Questionable pulmonary edema
3. Engorged neck veins, probably secondary to pulmonary hypertension and right ventricular hypertrophy
4. Diastolic dysfunction on previous echocardiogram with mitral regurgitation
5. Normal cardiac perfusion
6. Multiple PVCs and nonsustained V. tach, which all precipitated after Bumex therapy; this could be related to hypomagnesemia or hypokalemia.
7. Status post pacemaker
8. Generalized edema, which could be related to the diastolic dysfunction. I suspect that the prednisone and Actos have exacerbated that.

PLAN:
1. The patient was transferred to the intensive care unit.
2. Stat x-ray has been ordered.
3. Stat labs including troponin, CPK, magnesium, potassium, and phosphorus were ordered.
4. We will plan to control his heart rate with Cardizem.
5. Will get albuterol nebulizers.
6. We will repeat troponins in the morning.
7. We will consult cardiology in the morning.
8. Per discussion with the patient, he is code level I. In case of cardiopulmonary compromise, he will be fully resuscitated. If he stays on the ventilator more than 4 to 5 days and if we decide that the chances of his survival are minimal, the patient will be withdrawn from life support.

The patient seems to understand and agrees with the above plan.

9-5A:

SERVICE CODE(S): ____________________

DX CODE(S): ____________________

CASE 9-5A DISCUSSION

There are a number of questionable and probable diagnoses listed under the Impression section of the report, such as probable chronic obstructive pulmonary disease and questionable pneumonia. Outpatient coders do not report probable, suspected, questionable, "rule out," or working diagnoses (see Official Guidelines for Coding and Reporting, Section IV, I). Only code symptoms or confirmed diagnoses: wheezing (786.07) and edema (782.3—this is the generalized edema indicated in point 8 of the Impression section of the report, not the questionable pulmonary edema indicated in point 2). Also in point 4 of the Impression section, the physician indicates the patient has mitral regurgitation. When referencing the Index of the ICD-9-CM, under the term "Regurgitation, mitral valve," a cross-reference directs the coder to "Insufficiency, mitral, 424.0," so the regurgitation is not reported separately as it is included in 424.0.

Medicine Services

The pulmonary specialty uses laboratory procedures to diagnose and treat patients with respiratory problems. Codes in the range 94010-94621, 94680-94720, and 94770-94772 are for **diagnostic procedures,** and codes 94640-94668 are for **therapeutic or diagnostic treatments.** It is helpful to the coder to note treatment or procedure next to the code in the margin of the CPT manual to help distinguish easily between the diagnostic and therapeutic codes. Usually these procedures are conducted by a technician that is trained in administration of the test or the treatment. The technician provides these services under the supervision of a physician, usually a pulmonologist.

Many of the codes in the Pulmonary subsection (94010-94799) are **component codes,** which means that both the professional and technical component are included in the code unless the code description specifies otherwise. If the code description is for the entire procedure and only the technical component of the procedure was provided, use the -TC modifier with the code; if only the professional component was provided, you would use -26 modifier with the code.

Pulmonary function tests are performed to evaluate the mechanical ability of the respiratory system and the effectiveness with which the system can exchange carbon dioxide and oxygen. The components of the pulmonary function tests are **spirometry** (94010), lung volume determinations (94240-94370), and diffusion capacity (94720).

Spirometry

A common procedure that has many variations is a **spirometry** (94010-94070), which measures breathing capacity.

Spirometry is one of the best tests available for early detection of many lung disorders. The spirometer takes readings (spirogram) of the patient's breathing and then compares the readings to normal values. The tests are usually administered by a technician under the supervision of a physician. A printout of the results (strip) is then produced for interpretation by the physician. The physician analyzes the results and prepares a written report.

Spirometry can be performed in the laboratory or patient-initiated. For procedures performed in the pulmonary laboratory, the technician measures the patient's breathing capacities. **Patient-initiated spirometry**(94014-94016) results in the same measurements but involves the submission of the data via telephone transmission from the patient's location to the pulmonary laboratory. The data are then reviewed for any signs of problems. The patient-initiated procedure represented in 94014 includes the technician instructing the patient on the use of the machine, graphic recordings, analysis of the data, periodic recalibration of the machine, and physician review and interpretation of results for a 30-day period. 94015 represents only the recording component for the patient-initiated procedure, and 94016 is for only the physician review and interpretation of the results. Patient-initiated spirometry is used to measure the strength of the lung function.

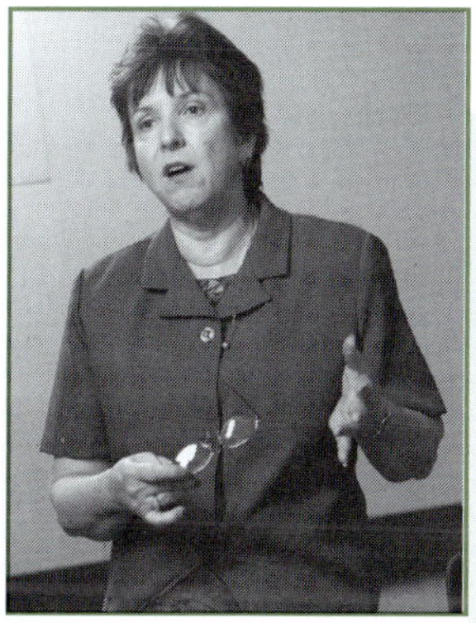

FROM THE TRENCHES

Maryann

"Coding is being widely recognized... being an accredited certified coder is really something that institutions and physician practices are looking for, because they want to do it correctly, and they want to be reimbursed adequately. [Also], they want to be in compliance... because the implications of compliance can be very grave if coding is not done correctly. You want them to understand you know exactly what you are talking about and you are not giving out incorrect information."

The spirometry report uses many assessments, such as the following:

- Forced vital capacity (FVC)—the maximum volume a patient can exhale after a maximum inspiration (volume the patient breathes out)
- Forced expiratory volume (FEV1)—volume that can be expired at the first second after a maximum inhalation
- Forced expiration ratio (FEV1/FVC%)—Forced expiratory volume divided by forced vital capacity. Normal would be that the patient could exhale about 75% to 80% of the air the patient inhaled.
- Peak expiratory flow rate (PEFR)—the fastest speed at which the patient can expel air from the lungs at a maximum effort
- Total lung capacity (TLC)—lung volume following a maximum inspiration

Bronchospasm is the constriction of airways of the lung by a spastic contraction of the muscles of the bronchial area. These contractions obstruct airflow and are an indicator of lung disorders, such as asthma and allergy. There are many bronchospasm agents, such as histamine, methacholine, antigen, or gas. A spirometry is administered before and after a bronchodilator to measure the patient's lung capacities before the bronchodilator and after the bronchodilator and is reported with 94060. The bronchodilators are reported separately with 94070.

A complete spirometry (94060) includes:

1. Flow volume loop (as in 94010)
2. Prebronchodilator flow rates
3. Postbronchodilator values
4. Maximal (ventilation) values [MVV] as in 94200

The bronchospasm is not to be confused with an inhalation bronchial challenge test. An **inhalation bronchial challenge test** (95070, 95071) is the inhalation of various substances to which the patient is thought to be allergic. The patient's bronchial response is then measured. The test does not include the pulmonary function tests necessary to assess the patient's response, only the inhalation of the substance. The function test that would subsequently be administered would be reported separately.

Although each physician establishes what is to be included in his or her complete pulmonary function test, it would include spirometry, lung volume determination, and diffusing capacity. A complete pulmonary function test would often include the following:

94060 PRE-/POST-SPIROMETRY INCLUDES (SPIROMETRY)

flow volume loop

Flow volume loop (FVL) is spirometry that assesses lung function by measuring the amount of air in the lungs and the rate at which the patient can inhale and exhale the air. During the assessment, the patient is exposed to various irritants, such as cold air or methacholine, or during exercise. If an FVL is conducted as part of a pulmonary function test, it is not reported separately with 94010; but if it is conducted separately it is reported with 94375.

prebronchodilator flow
postbronchodilator values

Prebronchodilator and postbronchodilator values are assessments of lung function before a bronchodilator (such as albuterol or Ventolin, the facility reports these separately with 99070) and after a bronchodilator to determine if the lung function is significantly improved after administration of medication to expand the lumina of the air passages of the lungs.

94240 FRC (FUNCTIONAL RESIDUAL CAPACITY), ALSO KNOWN AS A NITROGEN WASHOUT (LUNG VOLUME DETERMINATION)

Functional residual capacity is also known as a *nitrogen washout* and measures the lung volume at the end of normal exhalation. The residual volume (RV) cannot be measured by spirometry because that is the air that remains in the lungs after exhalation. The determination of the residual (remaining) air is calculated by subtracting the expiratory reserve volume (ERV) from the functional residual capacity. Not being able to adequately exhale the air in the lungs is a sign of pulmonary disorder, such as emphysema. The physician interpretation of the results and preparation of the report are included in the services.

94260 TGV (THORACIC GAS VOLUME), ALSO KNOWN AS PLETHYSMOGRAPHY LUNG VOLUME OR LUNG VOLUMES INCLUDES (SPIROMETRY)

single-breath lung volumes
airway collapse or air trapping

Thoracic gas volume (TGV) is a pulmonary function test that is known as *plethysmography lung volume* or *lung volumes*. The test uses various methods to assess the lung function and includes the residual volume or the amount of air that remains in the patient's lungs after exhaling. The assessment includes the volume of a single breath, air trapping (air caught in a collapsed bronchial branch), and airway collapse (closure of a branch or branches of the bronchial tree). The collapse or trapping is caused by bronchial walls that have been weakened by disease.

A nitrogen washout measures residual capacity or residual volume, air remaining in the lungs after exhalation. If a nitrogen washout is performed, do not report 94260 (thoracic gas volume), rather report 94070, methacholine challenge.

94720 DLCO (DIFFUSION CAPACITY OF CARBON MONOXIDE), ALSO KNOWN AS TRANSFER FACTOR (DIFFUSING CAPACITY)

A DLCO is a diffusion spirometry. The DLCO is also referred to as *transfer factor*. A spirometry measures the mechanical properties of the lungs, but the DLCO measures the ability of the lungs to perform gas exchange. The patient inhales a gas that usually consists of helium and carbon monoxide with air. The mixture is held in the lungs for a few seconds. During that time, the lungs diffuse the mixture into the pulmonary blood. The patient then exhales and a sample is taken and the resulting measurement indicates the diffusing capacity of the lungs. This assessment is especially useful in diagnosing interstitial lung disease, which occurs in the interspaces of the lung.

94360 AIRWAY RESISTANCE (LUNG VOLUME DETERMINATION)

Airflow in the respiratory tract encounters resistance when the air molecules are slowed because of collisions with the sides of the ducts. Bronchial constriction or obstruction results in a decrease in the size of the bronchial airway and increases airway resistance. A determination of the resistance to airflow is measured by the air exhaled from the lungs in a single breath.

CASE 9-6
9-6A Pulmonary Function Study

CASE 9-6

You will be reporting only the physician portion of the service. In this case, the diagnoses that you are to report have been bolded. The five reportable services of this study are indicated for you by the name of the study having been placed after each element in the Interpretation section of the report. Note that the components of the spirometry are not indicated in consecutive order in this report and often are not in order; rather, items 1, 2, 7, 8, and 9 are all parts of the spirometry. You will be coding another pulmonary function study in Case 9-9A without any indicators, so study this report carefully to ensure that you can identify the various elements of the study without the indicators.

9-6A PULMONARY FUNCTION STUDY

LOCATION: Outpatient, Clinic

PATIENT: Hag Ulrich

PHYSICIAN: Gregory Dawson, M.D.

ENTRANCE DIAGNOSIS: **Dyspnea** in a patient who has a 67.5-pack-year **history of smoking** and has a nonproductive cough. Gave good consistent effort.

INTERPRETATION:

1. Flow volume loop has mild concavity toward the volume axis, well-preserved inspiratory limb, reduced flow rates. (***spirometry***)
2. No significant change after bronchodilator. (***spirometry***)
3. Lung volumes are normal without evidence of hyperinflation (also known as: functional residual capacity). (***functional residual capacity***)
4. Single-breath lung volumes are also normal without hyperinflation. (***functional residual capacity***)
5. There is significant dynamic airway collapse. (***gas volume***)
6. Transfer factor is reduced to 52% of predicted, suggesting reduced alveolar capillary membrane surface area and/or V/Q mismatching. (***carbon monoxide, diffusion capacity***)
7. Prebronchodilator flow rates have a pattern consistent with mild chronic obstructive pulmonary disease. (***spirometry***)
8. Postbronchodilator values show no significant change, and the same conclusion can be reached. (***spirometry***)
9. The MVV is abnormal prebronchodilator and postbronchodilator. Between that and a normal FEV1, I expect a reasonably normal exercise tolerance. (***spirometry***)
10. Airway resistance is normal. (***resistance to airflow***)

OVERALL IMPRESSION: **COPD** of mild degree; no significant reversibility. It does not explain this patient's complaint of being short of breath after any exertion, and it would probably be reasonable to get a methacholine challenge after the patient quit smoking to see whether he has bronchospastic disorder. One can assume that kind of complaint with his smoking history and that he probably already does have a bronchospastic component.

9-6A:

SERVICE CODE(S): ____________________

DX CODE(S): ____________________

Sleep Studies

Sleep studies are performed to assist the physician in diagnosing sleep disorders. These tests are conducted for 6 or more hours, and the physician reviews and interprets the results and prepares a written report. Polysomnography (many sleep recordings) differs from sleep studies in that they include an electroencephalogram, electrooculogram, and an electromyogram. Other sleep study components (parameters) may be electrocardiography, airflow, ventilation and respiration effort, gas exchanges, extremity muscle activity, snoring, and other parameters as outlined in the Sleep Testing notes (95805-95811) in the CPT.

Somnolence is an unnatural sleepiness or drowsiness that is often an entrance diagnosis for patients who undergo sleep studies.

Symptoms, Signs, and Ill-Defined Conditions

Subjective observations are those that are reported by the patient to the physician, such as drowsiness. The physician has not, at the point when the patient presents with the complaint, diagnosed the reason for the drowsiness. The physician may order a sleep study to assist in the diagnosis process. Reporting the diagnoses for these types of subjective observations leads the coder to either the chapter specific to the body area or to Chapter 16 of the ICD-9-CM, Symptoms, Signs, and Ill-Defined Conditions (780-799). If the reason for the symptom has been identified by the physician, the Chapter 16 codes cannot be used as the primary diagnosis because these codes report symptoms, signs, and ill-defined conditions; but if the reason for the symptoms has not been identified by the physician, the Chapter 16 codes can be assigned as the primary diagnosis. If the physician indicates contrasting or comparative conditions may be responsible for the condition, the symptom is reported as the primary diagnosis, because at that point no more definitive diagnosis has been stated. Once the cause or related condition is identified, the symptom cannot be reported as the primary diagnosis, since a more definitive diagnosis is then known.

Symptoms as Diagnoses

General symptoms are located in the 780 category, with subcategories for altered consciousness (including drowsiness) (780.0x), hallucinations (780.1x), syncope (fainting) and collapse (780.2), convulsions (780.3x), dizziness and giddiness (780.4x), sleep disturbances (780.5x), fever (780.6x), malaise and fatigue (780.7), hyperhidrosis (excessive sweating) (780.8), and other general symptoms (fussy baby, memory loss, etc.) (780.9x).

Symptoms involving the nervous and musculoskeletal systems are reported with 781.x.

For example, abnormal involuntary movements (781.0) or lack of coordination (781.3).

Symptoms involving the skin and other integumentary tissue is reported with 782.x.

For example, localized edema (782.3) or cyanosis (782.5).

Symptoms concerning nutrition, metabolism, and development are reported with 783.x.

For example, anorexia (783.0) or polyphagia (excessive eating) (783.6).

Symptoms involving the head and neck are reported with 784.x.

For example, headache (784.0) or swelling, mass or lump in neck (784.2).

Symptoms involving the cardiovascular system are reported with 785.x.

For example, unspecified tachycardia (785.0) or gangrene (785.4).

Symptoms involving the respiratory system and other chest symptoms are reported with 786.xx.

For example, tachypnea (786.06) or chest pain (786.5x).

Symptoms involving the digestive system are reported with 787.x.

For example, nausea and vomiting (787.0) or dysphagia (difficulty swallowing) (787.2).

Symptoms involving the urinary system are reported with 788.x.

For example, dysuria (788.1) or incontinence (788.3).

Other symptoms involving the abdomen and pelvis are reported with 789.xx.

For example, abdominal pain (789.0x) with a fifth digit for the specific abdominal location, such as right upper quadrant (1) or left upper quadrant (2) and abdominal tenderness (789.6).

Nonspecific Abnormal Findings

Codes in the 790-796 range are used to report abnormal findings that are nonspecific. For example, 790.xx is assigned to nonspecific findings on examination of the blood, such as abnormal red blood cell count (790.x). Sometimes the physician will indicate that the red blood cell count is abnormal but has not indicated what the abnormality is due to, or may document a differential diagnosis (such as, "either iron deficiency anemia [280.9] or pernicious anemia [281.0]"). It is with these types of diagnostic statements that the 790-796 codes are assigned. Review the categories within the 790-796 range now so you are familiar with the types of codes contained there.

CASE 9-7
9-7A Overnight Oxygen Desaturation Study
9-7B Nocturnal Polysomnogram
9-7C Multiple Sleep Latency Study

CASE 9-7

Report the physician services for the follow oxygen saturation levels during a 7-hour sleep study that was attended by a technologist.

9-7A OVERNIGHT OXYGEN DESATURATION STUDY

LOCATION: Outpatient, Hospital

PATIENT: Sheldon Boucher

PHYSICIAN: Gregory Dawson, M.D.

ENTRANCE DIAGNOSIS: Somnolence.

The patient began the study at 2114 hours on 1 L with a baseline O_2 saturation of 91%. Between 2300 and 2330 hours, the patient had a significant period of time when the O_2 saturation was as low as 80%. The continuous printout is not really very helpful. At that time, oxygen was then turned up to 1 L and remained there through the rest of the night; the rest of the night his O_2 saturation was above 90%.

It appears that this patient needs 1 L via nasal prongs to control oxygenation.There was only one episode through the night, but it was for quite some time as you can see by the printout.

9-7A:

SERVICE CODE(S): 95807-26 (Sleep Study

DX CODE(S): 780.09 (somnolence)

9-7B NOCTURNAL POLYSOMNOGRAM

At a later date, the patient also has a nocturnal polysomnogram but one without CPAP (continuous positive airway pressure).

LOCATION: Outpatient, Hospital

PATIENT: Sheldon Boucher

PHYSICIAN: Gregory Dawson, M.D.

ENTRANCE DIAGNOSIS: Somnolence

PROCEDURE PERFORMED: Nocturnal polysomnogram without CPAP titration.

The study began at approximately 2200 hours, continued through to about 0615 hours the next morning for a total of 480.5 minutes in bed, 411 minutes asleep, sleep latency of 26.5 minutes, and 92 arousals. Heart rate of 60 while awake and 50 while asleep. Had only four respiratory events throughout the night. This gives him a respiratory disturbance index of much less than 5; anything over 5 is considered significant, but this is less one. After a total of four episodes, they were all hypopnea; the longest duration was 18 seconds. The lowest saturation was 89%. Heart rate was 45. We did measure some sinus bradycardia. He had no myoclonic leg jerks noted. He had grade 3 snoring that was intermittent, most prominent on his back and the first third of the night.

Because he did not have a significant enough problem, no CPAP was titrated. He had a UPPP in 2000 and that seems to have been effective.

9-7B:

SERVICE CODE(S): 95810-26

DX CODE(S): 780.09

9-7C MULTIPLE SLEEP LATENCY STUDY

Sheldon presents to the clinic 3 days later for a multiple sleep latency study.

LOCATION: Outpatient, Hospital

PATIENT: Sheldon Boucher

PHYSICIAN: Gregory Dawson, M.D.

ENTRANCE DIAGNOSIS: Somnolence

This was performed this morning. He had four separate naps, each of 20 minutes' duration. The first two naps he had a sleep latency of 5 minutes for the first one, 9 minutes for the second time, and did not go to sleep at all the third and fourth time. He had no REM stages with any of these naps.

This is a negative study for narcolepsy. It does show the patient is sleep deprived, however (*sleep deprivation is reported with a V code*).

9-7C:

SERVICE CODE(S): 95805-26

DX CODE(S): 780.09
V69.4 (Deprivation, sleep)

CASE 9-8
9-8A Sleep Study

CASE 9-8

Charlie Grove presents to the clinic for a sleep study.

9-8A SLEEP STUDY

LOCATION: Outpatient, Hospital

PATIENT: Charlie Grove

PHYSICIAN: Gregory Dawson, M.D.

STUDY PERFORMED: Nocturnal polysomnogram with CPAP titration.

ENTRANCE DIAGNOSIS: Daytime somnolence and obstructive sleep apnea.

The study began at about 2230 hours and continued to about 0530 hours the next morning, for a total of 444 minutes in bed, 271 minutes of sleep, with a sleep latency of 26.5 minutes. He had 275 arousals. He had a heart rate of 80 while awake, 78 while asleep, and it took 2 hours to document the severity of the disease. During that first 2 plus hours, he had a total of 46 respiratory events, for a respiratory disturbance index of 31.7; anything over 5 is considered significant. He had a heart rate of 90 while awake and 78 while asleep. The longest duration of any of these events was 39 seconds. The lowest O_2 saturation was 83%, and the lowest heart rate was 70, showing hypoxic and some cardiac effect of these events. He also had 109 myoclonic leg jerks, 97 associated with arousal. He had grade 3 to 4 snoring in all sleep positions, but on his back was much more significant.

Once it was decided that the patient had severe significant sleep apnea, CPAP was titrated with a nasal mask and was not tolerated; full-face mask not tolerated for more than 5 minutes; BiPAP was also not tolerated. The patient experienced nasal obstruction with a claustrophobic feeling and just could not tolerate the masks.

The patient was also up to the bathroom about five times, which may be a direct effect of the significant obstructive sleep apnea.

During the rest of the night he had many more events. The patient has obvious severe significant obstructive apnea.

The patient is intolerant of BiPAP and CPAP, so I would recommend referral to ENT for their consideration of a surgical procedure.

9-8A:

SERVICE CODE(S): 95811-26

DX CODE(S): 780.09
327.23 (Sleep apnea)

95811-26 polysomnography w/CPAP

CASE 9-9

9-9A Pulmonary Function Study
9-9B Cardiothoracic Consultation
9-9C Operative Report, Lung Mass
9-9D Pathology Report
9-9E Thoracic Medicine/Critical Care Note
9-9F Radiology Report, Chest
9-9G Thoracic Medicine/Critical Care Progress Report
9-9H Radiology Report, Chest
9-9I Pulmonary Function Study
9-9J Discharge Summary

CASE 9-9

In the following case, you will be reporting services that include pulmonary function study, consultation, operation, pathology, radiology, and several types of evaluation and management services.

9-9A PULMONARY FUNCTION STUDY

Ellen Zutz is a patient who presents to the pulmonary function laboratory for an assessment for her dyspnea. Dr. Dawson will supervise and interpret the results of this testing.

LOCATION: Outpatient, Clinic

PATIENT: Ellen Zutz

PHYSICIAN: Gregory Dawson, M.D.

ENTRANCE DIAGNOSIS: Dyspnea in a patient who smokes 67.5 packs a year and has a nonproductive cough. Gave good consistent effort.

INTERPRETATION:

1. Flow volume loop has mild concavity toward the volume axis, well-preserved inspiratory limb, and reduced flow rates.
2. No significant change after bronchodilator.
3. Lung volumes are normal without evidence of hyperinflation.
4. Single-breath lung volumes are also normal without hyperinflation.
5. There is no significant dynamic airway collapse (air trapping).
6. Transfer factor is quite reduced to 52% of predicted, suggesting reduced alveolar capillary membrane surface area and/or V/Q mismatching.
7. Prebronchodilator flow rates have a pattern consistent with mild chronic obstructive pulmonary disease/emphysema.
8. Postbronchodilator values show no significant change, and the same conclusion can be reached.
9. The MVV is abnormal prebronchodilator, normal postbronchodilator. Between that and a normal FEV1, I expect a reasonably normal exercise tolerance.
10. Airway resistance is normal.

OVERALL IMPRESSION: Chronic obstructive pulmonary disease/emphysema of mild degree, no significant reversibility. It does not explain this patient's complaint of being short of breath after any exertion, and it would probably be reasonable to get a methacholine challenge after the patient quits smoking to see whether she has bronchospastic disorder. One can assume with that kind of complaint and with her smoking history that she probably already does have a bronchospastic component.

DX: 492.8, 305.1

9-9A:

SERVICE CODE(S): 94060-26 94720-26

~~DX CODE(S)~~: 94240-26 94360-26
94260-26

9-9B CARDIOTHORACIC CONSULTATION

LOCATION: Outpatient, Clinic

PATIENT: Ellen Zutz

PRIMARY CARE PHYSICIAN: Gregory Dawson, M.D.

CONSULTANT: Gary Sanchez, M.D.

REASON FOR CONSULTATION: Right lung lesion

HISTORY OF PRESENT ILLNESS: This 62-year-old long-term smoker was seen by Dr. Elhart last October for angina. At that time, a chest x-ray showed an ill-defined density in the right mid-lung, which prompted a CT scan, which confirmed the lesion. There also appeared to be some hilar and subcarinal adenopathy. The patient has had progressive shortness of breath over the last 6 months with a dry cough. She has not had any hemoptysis at this juncture; however, she did have hemoptysis during episodes of pulmonary embolism several years ago. The patient uses four pillows for her gastroesophageal reflux disease and has some ankle edema. Skin testing four years ago for tuberculosis was negative. She has not had any other exposures of which she is aware. The patient has a 54-year history of smoking up to two to three packs a day and is currently smoking one-half pack of cigarettes per day. She does have some night sweats.

PAST MEDICAL HISTORY:

1. Numerous pulmonary emboli resulting in vena caval ligation.
2. Previous coronary angioplasties, the last angiogram being done last October, which showed total occlusion of the right coronary artery with good left ventricular function but with inferior dyskinesis.
3. Hypercholesterolemia.

PREVIOUS OPERATIONS: Two lumbar laminectomies with vena caval ligation, appendectomy, and hysterectomy.

ALLERGIES: Morphine, which causes swelling, and to penicillin, which causes a rash.

CURRENT MEDICATIONS:

1. Aspirin 325 mg q.d.
2. Combivent 2 puffs b.i.d. to t.i.d.
3. Lipitor 10 mg q.d.
4. Covera HS 240 mg q.d.
5. Nitroglycerin as needed. She states that she takes the nitroglycerin one or two times per month.

SOCIAL HISTORY: The patient is married and lives in Manytown, where she is a postal clerk. She does not drink.

FAMILY HISTORY: Positive for emphysema and coronary artery disease.

REVIEW OF SYSTEMS: Cardiovascular: See above. Respiratory: See above. GI: See above. Musculoskeletal: Normal. Other than noted above is noncontributory.

PHYSICAL EXAMINATION: The patient is a 186-pound, 5 feet 5 inch female in no apparent distress. Blood pressure is 130/72. Heart rate is 90. The jugular venous pressure is normal. Carotids are 2+, equal, and quiet. CHEST is clear and equal. The patient does have an occasional dry cough during conversation. HEART has a regular rhythm with a rate of 90 without murmur, rub, or gallop. ABDOMEN is obese without organomegaly, masses, or tenderness. EXTREMITIES show no clubbing, cyanosis, or edema. There are no varicosities. Pulses are intact peripherally. The patient is grossly neurologically intact.

Chest x-ray shows normal cardiothoracic ratio. There is an ill-defined mass in the right mid-lung field that extends nearly to the parietal pleura. This is confirmed by CT scan, which also shows some borderline adenopathy in the subcarinal area and right hilar area. Pulmonary function tests show a mid-expiratory flow rate of 109% of predicted with a mid-expiratory flow rate of 65% of predicted, and a maximal ventilatory volume of 78% of predicted. Her DLCO is 52%. Echocardiogram done in October showed an ejection fraction of 55% with moderate LV hypertrophy somewhat asymmetric in the septal area along with inferior dyskinesis.

LABORATORY done today showed a pO_2 of 72.6 with a pCO_2 of 41.9. Metabolic panel was essentially normal. PT was 10.8 and PTT was 31.5. Hematocrit was 42.2 with 214,000 platelets.

IMPRESSION: Ill-defined mass in the right mid-lung field not amenable to bronchoscopy or CT-guided needle biopsy diagnosis.

DISPOSITION: The patient will be admitted in 2 days for elective right thoracoscopy and possible right thoracotomy and biopsy. Operation complications including blood transfusion, risks, and alternatives were discussed with the patient and her family.

9-9B:

SERVICE CODE(S): ____________________

DX CODE(S): ____________________

9-9C OPERATIVE REPORT, LUNG MASS

Up until this report, the patient's diagnosis was that of a chest mass, but the pathology report that accompanies 9-9C indicates neoplasm of the middle and upper lobes of the lung. Rather than reporting one diagnosis code for the middle lobe neoplasm and another code for the upper lobe neoplasm, use the code for the lung neoplasm of contiguous sites, because the upper and middle lobe are connected or contiguous.

LOCATION: Inpatient, Hospital

PATIENT: Ellen Zutz

ATTENDING PHYSICIAN: Gregory Dawson, M.D.

SURGEON: Gary Sanchez, M.D.

PREOPERATIVE DIAGNOSIS: Right lung mass

POSTOPERATIVE DIAGNOSIS: Right lung mass

PROCEDURE PERFORMED: Right upper and right middle lobectomy with biopsy of four hilar lymph nodes

INDICATIONS: This 62-year-old female with a recent cough and shortness of breath was noted on chest x-ray to have a vague right mid-lung field lesion, which was confirmed by CT scan. There was some hilar adenopathy as well.

FINDINGS AT SURGERY: Lymph nodes from the hilum were biopsied times four, all of which were negative on frozen section. The inferior pulmonary ligament area, the azygous area, and the paratracheal area were all devoid of lymph nodes. The lesion was deep within the confines of the right upper lobe and appeared to cross the minor fissure into the right middle lobe.

DESCRIPTION OF PROCEDURE: The patient was brought to the operating room and placed in the supine position under general intubation anesthesia with a double-lumen tube. The patient was rolled in her left lateral decubitus position with the right side up. The chest was entered through the sixth intercostal space anterior axillary line with a thoracoscope. Gentle exploration of the right hemithorax showed no evidence of gross tumor implants on the parietal pleura. Retraction of the right lower lobe, however, did show evidence of what appeared to be tumor under the visceral pleura in the right upper lobe. A portion of the right middle lobe had been incorporated into this tumor mass. General exploration of all the lymph node–bearing areas really disclosed only mildly enlarged lymph nodes in the hilum. These were biopsied and sent for frozen section; all were benign. A standard right upper and right middle lobectomy utilizing the arterial first technique was carried out. The arteries were encircled with 0 silk, ligated, and clipped. The pulmonary vein was ligated distally and stapled proximally. The fissures between the upper and lower lobe were divided by several applications of the GIA automatic stapling machine. The bronchus was then skeletonized and clamped. Forced insufflation of the endotracheal tube produced good expansion of the right lower lobe. Following this, the staples were fired, and the right upper and right middle lobes were removed in one piece. These were submitted for frozen-section diagnosis, which showed adenocarcinoma. The chest was then checked for hemostasis and irrigated thoroughly with antibiotic solution and closed over two 36-French atrium chest tubes in the usual fashion. Sterile compression dressings were applied, and the patient returned to the postanesthesia care unit recovery room in satisfactory condition after application of an epidural anesthetic by Dr. Larson. Sponge count and needle count correct ×2.

Dr. Dawson will be assuming all post operative care for this patient.

Pathology Report Later Indicated: See Report 9-9D

9-9C:

SERVICE CODE(S): 32482-54-RT (Lobectomy)

DX CODE(S): 162.8

9-9D PATHOLOGY REPORT

PATIENT: Ellen Zutz

ATTENDING PHYSICIAN: Gregory Dawson, M.D.

SURGEON: Gary Sanchez, M.D.

PATHOLOGIST: Grey Lonewolf, M.D.

CLINICAL HISTORY: Lung mass, right side

SPECIMEN RECEIVED:
A. Hilar lymph nodes, right with FS
B. Hilar lymph node, right no. 2 with FS
C. Right upper and middle lobe with FS

GROSS DESCRIPTION:

A. The specimen is labeled with the patient's name and "right hilar lymph nodes" and consists of three red-brown lymph nodes, 1.0 cm, 1.0 cm, and 1.4 cm in greatest dimension. These were submitted in one cassette.

INTRAOPERATIVE FROZEN SECTION DIAGNOSIS: Right hilar lymph nodes, (3): Benign lymph nodes as per Dr. Greywolf.

B. The specimen is labeled with the patient's name and "right hilar lymph nodes" and consists of 0.5 cm, 0.8 cm, and 1.0 cm in greatest dimension red-brown lymph nodes. Submitted in one cassette.

INTRAOPERATIVE FROZEN SECTION DIAGNOSIS: Right hilar lymph nodes, (3): Benign lymph nodes as per Dr. Greywolf.

C. The specimen is labeled with the patient's name and "right upper and middle lobe" and consists of a 360-g upper and middle lobe segment. Suture marks the location of tumor, and this area is inked black. Cut sections show a scirrhous gray-tan mass, 2.5 × 2.0 × 2.0 cm. Remaining lung tissue is red-brown. Surgical margins are grossly uninvolved by tumor. Possible lymph nodes are submitted in cassettes C2-3. Tumor is submitted in cassettes C4-8. Random section of red-brown lung is submitted in C9, and pleural surface is submitted in C10. Representative sections are submitted in 10 cassettes.

INTRAOPERATIVE FROZEN SECTION DIAGNOSIS: Right upper and middle lobe tumor: Adenocarcinoma as per Dr. Greywolf.

MICROSCOPIC DESCRIPTION:

A. Permanent sections confirm the frozen-section diagnosis of three perihilar lymph nodes negative for metastatic tumor.
B. Permanent sections confirm the frozen-section diagnosis of adenocarcinoma. Sections show infiltrating sheets of neoplastic cells with rudimentary gland formation. The neoplastic cells contain enlarged pleomorphic vesicular nuclei with prominent nucleoli and mitoses scattered throughout. There is surrounding fibrosis with chronic inflammation and anthracotic pigment and hemosiderin deposition. Tumor cells also follow the outline of the alveolar walls in areas. Tumor extends to the pleural surface, which is inked black. Additional perihilar lymph nodes are examined and are all negative for metastatic tumor. Tumor does not involve the surgical margin.

Adjacent lung shows dilated alveoli containing extravasated red cells and hemosiderin-laden macrophages. There is anthracotic pigment deposition in some areas.

DIAGNOSIS:

A. Right hilar lymph nodes, (3): Benign lymph nodes, negative for metastatic tumor.

B. Right upper and middle lobe, lung:
Infiltrating adenocarcinoma, moderately differentiated, forming a mass approximately 2.5 × 2.0 × 2.5 cm, extending to the pleural surface. Tumor does not involve the surgical margin.
Twelve perihilar lymph nodes are negative for metastatic tumor.

9-9D:

SERVICE CODE(S): 88309 88307 X3 88331 88332 X2

DX CODE(S): 162.8 229.0

9-9E THORACIC MEDICINE/CRITICAL CARE NOTE

LOCATION: Inpatient, Hospital

PATIENT: Ellen Zutz

CONSULTANT: Ronald Green, M.D.

ATTENDING PHYSICIAN: Gregory Dawson, M.D.

I have been asked to give an opinion on this patient regarding the care of her emphysema and to assist in weaning the patient off the ventilator. I have seen the patient as an outpatient, the first time in February at the request of Dr. Dawson because of abnormal chest x-ray. That was worked up and thought to be a cancer of the lung. Eventually we sent the patient to Dr. Sanchez, and he operated on her, taking her right upper lobe and her right middle lobe.

The patient is alert and oriented postoperatively and doing well.

For details of all the past medical history, social history, family history, and review of systems, please refer to my physician's assistant note where it is outlined in detail. The patient has also had a pulmonary function study, which showed obstructive disease of a mild degree. She is doing fine at this point just with a bilobectomy.

PHYSICAL EXAMINATION/REVIEW OF SYSTEMS:

CARDIAC SYSTEM REVIEW: Blood pressures are good at 120s-110s/60s. Pulse rate of 90.

PULMONARY SYSTEM REVIEW: Chest is clear. Chest x-ray looks pretty good. The PO_2 is 80.8 on 40%, pH 7.34, and PCO_2 48.

GI SYSTEM REVIEW: Abdomen is soft and benign. I heard one bowel sound, so they are really quite hypoactive. Nontender. No hepatosplenomegaly.

GU SYSTEM REVIEW: She weighs 200 pounds. Baseline weight was 184 pounds taken from our scale in the clinic. No edema. BUN 10, creatinine 0.7, and her fluid input yesterday was 4348 in and 510 out.

ELECTROLYTES: Sodium 140, potassium 4.9, and chloride 104.

HEMATOLOGY: White count 11,560, hemoglobin 12.6, and platelets 246,000.

ENDOCRINOLOGY: Glucose 141.

INFECTIOUS DISEASE: She is afebrile. Sputum is nonexistent. I do not think we have any evidence of active infection at this point.

DISPOSITION: I will try to wean her off the ventilator, and with any luck we can get her extubated later this afternoon. We will have to watch her electrolytes. I would be glad to monitor along if so requested. This looks like it might be relatively easy to get the patient off the ventilator.

9-9E:

SERVICE CODE(S): ____________

DX CODE(S): ____________

9-9F RADIOLOGY REPORT, CHEST

Atelectasis is incomplete expansion of the lung.

LOCATION: Inpatient, Hospital

PATIENT: Ellen Zutz

ATTENDING PHYSICIAN: Gregory Dawson, M.D.

RADIOLOGIST: Morton Monson, M.D.

EXAMINATION OF: Chest x-ray

CLINICAL SYMPTOMS: Follow-up atelectasis

PORTABLE AP CHEST, SINGLE VIEW, 5:00 A.M.: FINDINGS: Comparison is made with yesterday morning's portable AP chest. Right ileojejunal catheter with tip in the right atrium. The patient has been extubated (*ventilator status discontinued*). Two right chest tubes are again seen. Small amount of subcutaneous emphysema has resolved. No appreciable change was seen in the heart size and pulmonary vascularity given the difference in technique. Area of atelectasis in the left lower lobe is somewhat more prominent. There may be a left mid-lung infiltrate, which is more prominent. This could be due to patient rotation. The left costophrenic angle is not included on the film. Strand of fibrosis or linear atelectasis, right perihilar region, is unchanged. Postoperative change is right thoracotomy.

9-9F:

SERVICE CODE(S): ______________________

DX CODE(S): ______________________

9-9G THORACIC MEDICINE/CRITICAL CARE PROGRESS REPORT

Dr. Dawson was called out of town and has asked Dr. Green to assume the postoperative care for this patient. The official transfer was documented in the medical record. When reporting the postoperative care services for Dr. Green, you would report the CPT code for the surgical procedure (lung lobectomy) along with modifier -55, Postoperative Management Only.

LOCATION: Inpatient, Hospital

PATIENT: Ellen Zutz

ATTENDING PHYSICIAN: Ronald Green, M.D.

The patient was extubated yesterday from her surgery. She had a bilobe lobectomy for cancer of the middle lobe and lower lobe and underlying emphysema. This morning, on a simple mask, her pO_2 was 58, pCO_2 was up to 66.5, pH 7.26. Just from using BiPAP 40%, her PO_2 was 54, PCO_2 was down to 58, and the pH was better at 7.31.

PHYSICAL EXAMINATION/REVIEW OF SYSTEMS: The patient was a bit sleepy but sitting on the edge of the bed, cooperating well with the mask; so we do not have to worry about intubation, at least at this time. Pulse, 90.

CARDIAC SYSTEM REVIEW: Blood pressures are excellent, I have 120s to 140s over diastolic of 60s. No S3 or S4. I do not appreciate any murmurs.

PULMONARY SYSTEM REVIEW: Please see above. On exam, she has a few rales scattered about. Chest, symmetrical. Chest x-ray shows increased vascular markings, more on the left than the right.

GI SYSTEM REVIEW: She does have some bowel sounds. She has been started on a clear liquid diet. Abdomen is nontender.

GU SYSTEM REVIEW: BUN 8, creatinine 0.6. She had 2992 in yesterday and 1720 out. She weighs 194.3 pounds today. Her baseline weight is 186 pounds.

ENDOCRINOLOGY: Glucose 142.

ELECTROLYTES: Sodium 134, potassium 4.2, chloride 97, CO_2 32.2, calcium 8.1, magnesium 1.8, and phosphorus 3.2.

HEMATOLOGY: White count is 16,280, hemoglobin 12, and platelets 137.

INFECTIOUS DISEASE: She is afebrile. So far the cultures are negative, and she remains on cefazolin at this point. Chest tube output is 140 over the last 8 hours.

DISPOSITION: Use the BiPAP mask. Adjust it for eating, and if she is more awake she can just have the prongs on. Otherwise, if she is asleep, will have to use the BiPAP mask. Check her labs in the morning. She is just a little bit volume overloaded, so I will try just a little bit of Bumex today and cut down her IV fluids.

9-9G:

SERVICE CODE(S): ______________________

DX CODE(S): ______________________

9-9H RADIOLOGY REPORT, CHEST

LOCATION: Inpatient, Hospital

PATIENT: Ellen Zutz

ATTENDING PHYSICIAN: Ronald Green, M.D.

RADIOLOGIST: Morton Monson, M.D.

EXAMINATION OF: Chest

CLINICAL SYMPTOMS: Follow-up left lower lobe pneumonia

PORTABLE UPRIGHT SITTING CHEST, 5:00 A.M.: Previous is from yesterday 5 A.M. There is cardiomegaly as there has been. The vascular markings on the right are normal. On the left, there are some accentuated perihilar markings and some peripheral lung markings that are decreasing compared with yesterday and likely represent resolving failure pattern. They do not have the appearance of pneumonia. No atelectatic change is seen on left and no pleural effusion on left. In the interval since yesterday, the two chest tubes have been removed from the right hemithorax. There is small apical pneumothorax on the right. There is elevation of right hemidiaphragm. There is no atelectatic change or effusion. There is some prominence of the right paratracheal tissue, stable.

IMPRESSION:

1. Interval removal of right chest tubes. Small apical pneumothorax seen currently.
2. Right paratracheal soft tissue remains.

3. Cardiomegaly.
4. Accentuated parahilar markings on the left and some in the left lung periphery indicating this is respiratory failure rather than a pneumonia or pneumonitis. Overall there is improvement, left aeration, since previous examination of yesterday.

9-9H:

SERVICE CODE(S): ____________________

DX CODE(S): ____________________

Pulmonary Stress Test

There are two versions of the pulmonary stress test: simple (94620, also known as a walking O_2 desaturation) and complex (94621). The simple pulmonary stress test measures the workload and heart rate while also measuring the oxygen desaturation level. This type of test is conducted to measure the degree of hypoxemia that occurs with exertion. The complex pulmonary stress test measures the oxygen uptake and production. This type of test is used to distinguish between cardiac and pulmonary causes of shortness of breath **(dyspnea),** to determine the level of ambulatory oxygen a patient requires, and to develop a safe exercise program for a patient with cardiac or pulmonary conditions as well as other conditions in which this more complex measurement is required.

Pulmonary stress tests are usually conducted with electrocardiographic monitoring. Because they are performed both at the outpatient clinic setting and the outpatient hospital setting, the use of modifier -26 is a consideration. When the clinic physician performs the study at the clinic, the global procedure is reported; but when the physician performs the study in an outpatient department at the hospital, the physician's services are reported with -26.

9-9I PULMONARY FUNCTION STUDY

LOCATION: Inpatient, Hospital

PATIENT: Ellen Zutz

ATTENDING PHYSICIAN: Ronald Green, M.D.

PROCEDURE PERFORMED: Walking O_2 saturation study because of dyspnea

Study began with an O_2 saturation of 90%, 89% on room air. With just a small exercise of up to 0.5 minutes, she had an O_2 saturation of 87, 86, 84, and 85%. In fact, it took 4L per minute by nasal prongs to move the O_2 saturation above 89%. The highest I got was 92. Borg scale was rated as 1. Highest heart rate was 91. She was able to walk 500 feet. The patient walked at a good pace.

The patient does have reasonable exercise tolerance for so soon after a lobectomy, but she has significant oxygen desaturation and requires 4L/min, by nasal prongs with minimal exertion.

9-9I:

SERVICE CODE(S): 94620-26

DX CODE(S): 786.09

9-9J DISCHARGE SUMMARY

LOCATION: Inpatient, Hospital

PATIENT: Ellen Zutz

ATTENDING PHYSICIAN: Ronald Green, M.D.

HOSPITAL COURSE: This 62-year-old white female was noted on chest x-ray to have a lesion in her right lung. It was followed up for a short time and appeared to be somewhat denser. She was therefore submitted for a thoracic surgical consultation. After extensive preoperative evaluation by Dr. Sanchez, she was considered to be a suitable candidate for a thoracotomy.

She underwent a right upper and right middle lobectomy for a stage I adenocarcinoma that appeared to be in the right upper lobe with extension across the fissure to the right middle lobe. The patient was maintained overnight in the ICU, after which she was extubated and transferred to the ambulatory ward. The epidural was removed on the second postoperative day, and the chest tubes were removed on the fourth postoperative day. From that point on, with an episode of atrial fibrillation occurring the fifth day postoperatively, she was treated with digoxin and diltiazem with resolution. She did have short bursts of atrial fibrillation, however, the day prior to discharge; therefore, she was begun on oral anticoagulation, anticipating that she may continue to have episodes of atrial fibrillation after discharge. On the seventh postoperative day, the patient was discharged home and given a return appointment to see me in 2 weeks for a chest x-ray, rhythm strip, and prothrombin time.

MEDICATIONS at the time of discharge:
1. Digoxin 0.25 mg p.o. q.d.
2. Diltiazem 120 mg p.o. q.6h.
3. Ipratropium bromide inhalers.
4. Coumadin 5 mg p.o. q.d.
5. Percodan as needed for pain

FINAL DIAGNOSIS:
1. Stage I adenocarcinoma, right upper and middle lobe
2. Atrial Fibrillation
3. Emphysema

9-9J:

SERVICE CODE(S): ______________________

DX CODE(S): ______________________

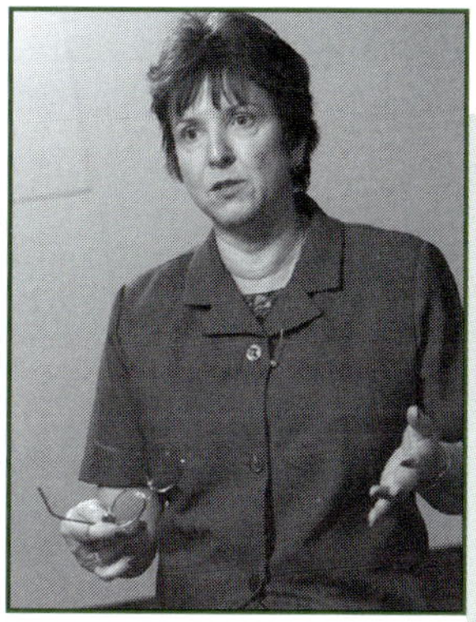

FROM THE TRENCHES

Maryann

"Don't be too hard on yourself. Understand that when you become a certified coder it's like getting a driver's license. You actually learn to drive when you're behind the wheel after you have the license in place… The most important thing is have the support of your physicians, as teachers of the procedures… the more you understand about what procedure it is they are doing the more accurately you can code. I think a real partnership with your physicians is essential."

Septoplasty and Turbinates

The nasal septum divides one side of the nose from the other and is often deviated (crooked). **Septoplasty** is the surgical treatment for a deviated septum to relieve obstruction. The surgeon incises the mucous membrane inside the nose that covers the septum. The cartilage and bone are then elevated and portions of the septum are removed, straightened, or repaired. The mucous membrane is then returned to the normal position, and the nose is splinted and or packed.

A septoplasty may be combined with a turbinate reduction or resection. Turbinates are the bones on the outside of the nose; they are divided into three sections—inferior, middle, and superior as illustrated in Figure 9-1. A resection is removal of an inferior turbinate bone and is reported with 30140. Turbinate reduction is performed to return the normal nasal airway by removal of turbinate tissue and is reported with 30140-52. Note the parenthetical information following 30140 (turbinate resection) that states "(For reduction of turbinates, use 30140 with modifier '-52')." Turbinate tissue will again develop after reduction and as such the reduction may need to be repeated.

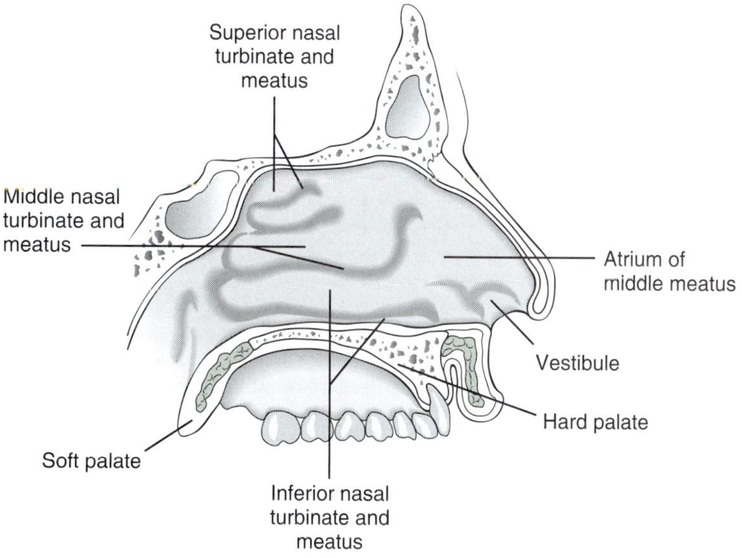

FIGURE 9-1 Superior, inferior, and middle nasal turbinates.

CASE 9-10
9-10A Operative Report, Septoplasty, Turbinate Reduction, and Tonsillectomy

CASE 9-10

9-10A OPERATIVE REPORT, SEPTOPLASTY, TURBINATE REDUCTION, AND TONSILLECTOMY

This report is an excellent example of the need to correlate the CPT procedure code with a diagnosis code that supports the reason for the service. In the following case, the surgeon performed a septoplasty, turbinate reduction, and tonsillectomy. There must be a diagnosis code to support the reason each was performed; for example the septoplasty (CPT code) was performed due to a deviated septum (diagnosis code); the turbinates were reduced (CPT code, this was bilateral), due to hypertrophy of the turbinates (diagnosis code), and the tonsillectomy (CPT code) was performed due to tonsil hypertrophy (diagnosis code). Each service has a supporting diagnosis and therefore substantiates why the procedure was performed (medical necessity). You may also code the sleep apnea as it indicates respiratory difficulties.

LOCATION: Inpatient, Hospital

PATIENT: Art Schear

PHYSICIAN: Gregory Dawson, M.D.

PREOPERATIVE DIAGNOSES:
1. Obstructive sleep apnea
2. Nasal obstruction
3. Septal deviation
4. Bilateral inferior turbinate hypertrophy
5. Hypertrophic tonsils

POSTOPERATIVE DIAGNOSES:
1. Obstructive sleep apnea
2. Nasal obstruction
3. Septal deviation
4. Bilateral inferior turbinate hypertrophy
5. Hypertrophic tonsils

PROCEDURES PERFORMED:
1. Septoplasty
2. Bilateral inferior turbinate mucosal reduction with radiofrequency
3. Tonsillectomy

ANESTHESIA: General endotracheal anesthesia

INDICATION: The patient is a 16-year-old male with documented obstructive sleep apnea. He also has a prior history of severe nasal obstruction due to a traumatic injury to his nose. Examination reveals a significant septal deviation with inferior turbinate hypertrophy. He also has very hypertrophic tonsils. At this point, we will correct his nasal airway and also increase his oral airway by removing his tonsils and see if that will help his sleep apnea. If there is any residual sleep apnea, he may be treated with nasal CPAP or if is unable to tolerate that, further airway expansion surgery.

DESCRIPTION OF PROCEDURE: After parental consent was obtained, the patient was taken to the operating room and placed on the operating table in the supine position. After an adequate level of general endotracheal anesthesia was obtained, the patient was turned and draped in the appropriate manner for nasal surgery. The patient's nose was packed with cotton pledgets and soaked with 4% cocaine. After several minutes, 1% Xylocaine with 1:100,000 units epinephrine was infiltrated into the septum bilaterally. It was also infiltrated into the inferior turbinates bilaterally. The nasal hairs were trimmed. Then, utilizing a right hemitransfixion incision, the mucoperichondrium and mucoperiosteal flaps were elevated. The deviated portion of the cartilaginous bony septum was then removed. Spurs off the maxillary crest were also removed. Hemostasis was achieved with suction cautery along the maxillary crest and then with FloSeal. Attention was then focused on the inferior turbinate. The anterior mucosa was treated with a radiofrequency needle to 500J on each side. The hemitransfixion incision was then closed with interrupted 4-0 chromic suture. A quilting suture of 4-0 plain gut was the performed. Silastic splints were then placed on both sides of the nasal septum and secured with nylon suture. The nose was then packed bilaterally with nasal packs, which consisted of Merocel sponge covered with a gloved finger coated with Bacitracin ointment. This was inflated with local solution. The patient was then repositioned for tonsillectomy. The McIvor mouth gag was placed, allowing visualization of the tonsil. Attention was first focused on the left tonsil. The Dean retractor was placed in the superior pole, and tonsil was retracted toward the midline. Then, utilizing a harmonic scalpel at power level III, the tonsil was removed in its entirety from a superior-to-inferior direction. Hemostasis was achieved from spot suction cautery. The similar procedure was then performed on the right tonsil. The tonsillar fossa was then irrigated with saline. There was no bleeding. Tension of the mouth gag was then released. Reinspection showed no active bleeding. The anterior and posterior pillars of the superior aspect of the tonsillar fossa were then reapproximated with interrupted 3-0 chromic suture and figure-of-eight closure. Subsequent reinspection showed no active bleeding. Mouth gag was then removed. Prior to removal of mouth gag, 1% Xylocaine with 1:100,000 units epinephrine was infiltrated into the retromolar and soft palate areas bilaterally. The patient tolerated the procedure well.

There was no break in technique. The patient was extubated and taken to the postanesthesia care unit in good condition.

FLUIDS ADMINISTERED: 1800 cc of RL

ESTIMATED BLOOD LOSS: Less than 50 cc

PREOPERATIVE MEDICATION: 1 g Ancef and 12 mg Decadron IV

9-10A:

30520 (Septoplasty)

SERVICE CODE(S): 30140-52-50 (Turbinate excision)

DX CODE(S): 30140-51-52

42826-51 (Tonsillectomy)

470, 478.0, 474.11, 327.23

Thoracentesis

Thoracentesis is accomplished by having the patient sit with arms supported, as illustrated in Figure 9-2; local anesthesia is administered, a needle is inserted (Figure 9-3) between the ribs, and fluid is withdrawn. Thoracentesis is performed to withdraw from the pleural space fluid that has accumulated as a result of a variety of conditions, such as congestive heart failure, pneumonia, tuberculosis, or carcinoma.

Thoracentesis may also be performed to insert a chest tube as an indwelling method of draining the accumulated fluid in the pleural space (pleural effusion), as illustrated in Figure 9-4. Local anesthesia is administered, and a small incision is made through the skin, fat, and muscle. The hole is then enlarged by using an instrument, and the tube is inserted into the pleural space. A suture is placed through the skin and tied to the tube. The tube is then secured with tape. The fluid is withdrawn by means of a suction device called a multichamber water-seal suction tube. This therapeutic procedure may be performed when the patient's pleural space contains air or gas (pneumothorax), blood (hemothorax), or a large amount of fluid (pleural effusion). These conditions can be caused by trauma, can be secondary to another disease process, or can occur spontaneously.

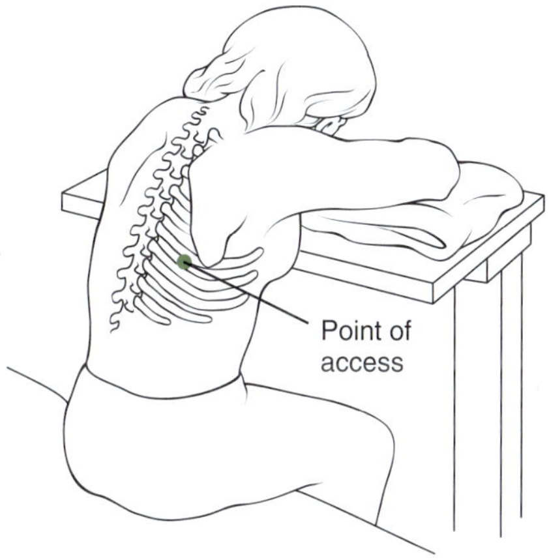

FIGURE 9-2 Patient in position for a thoracentesis.

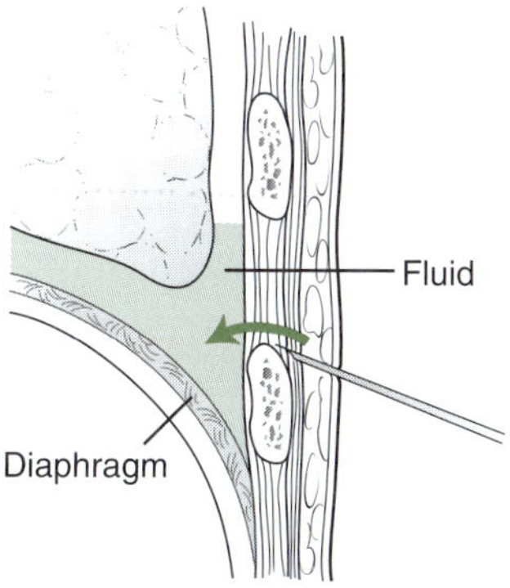

FIGURE 9-3 After administration of local anesthesia, a needle is inserted between the ribs, and fluid is withdrawn (thoracentesis).

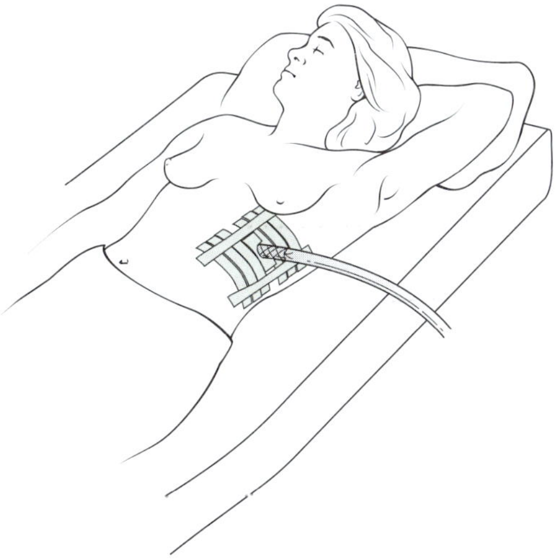

FIGURE 9-4 A chest tube may be inserted after thoracentesis to allow further drainage of fluid.

CASE 9-11
9-11A Operative Report, Thoracentesis

CASE 9-11

9-11A OPERATIVE REPORT, THORACENTESIS

The physician in this report performed not only the thoracentesis but also the professional portion of the ultrasound guidance.

LOCATION: Inpatient, Hospital

PATIENT: Rod Foster

ATTENDING PHYSICIAN: Ronald Green, M.D.

SURGEON: Gregory Dawson, M.D.

EXAMINATION OF: Thoracentesis

CLINICAL SYMPTOMS: Possible infected pleural effusion

THORACENTESIS: The patient is a 57-year-old male with extensive medical history including persistent fevers of unknown etiology. The patient also has pneumococcal pneumonia, right middle lobe, and COPD. Thoracentesis was requested by Dr. Green.

Prior to start of the study, the procedure was explained to the patient's brother, including the risks, complications, and alternatives. The patient's brother understood and consented to the exam.

The patient was prepped and draped in the usual sterile fashion. Using sterile technique under ultrasound guidance following administration of local anesthesia (1% lidocaine), a 19-gauge Yueh sheath needle was advanced into the inferior aspect of the right pleural space. Approximately 750 cc of clear yellow fluid was removed, and a specimen was sent to the lab for analysis. There is no evidence of pneumothorax.

IMPRESSION: Pleural effusion. Removed was 750 cc of clear fluid from the right pleural space as described above.

9-11A:

SERVICE CODE(S): 32550 (Thoracentesis) 76942-26 (Ultrasound)

DX CODE(S): 511.9, 481

Tracheostomy

A tracheostomy is a procedure that can be performed as an emergency procedure, or it may be planned. A planned tracheostomy is performed to provide the patient with ventilation support. There are two approaches to a tracheostomy—transtracheal or cricothyroid, based on the location of the incision. The incision for the transtracheal tracheostomy goes across the trachea, and the incision for the cricothyroid tracheostomy goes vertically over the cricothyroid.

Tracheostomies are reported based on whether the procedure was a planned or an emergency procedure. The emergency procedure codes are further divided based on the approach. The planned procedure codes are divided based on the age of the patient as under 2 or 2 or over.

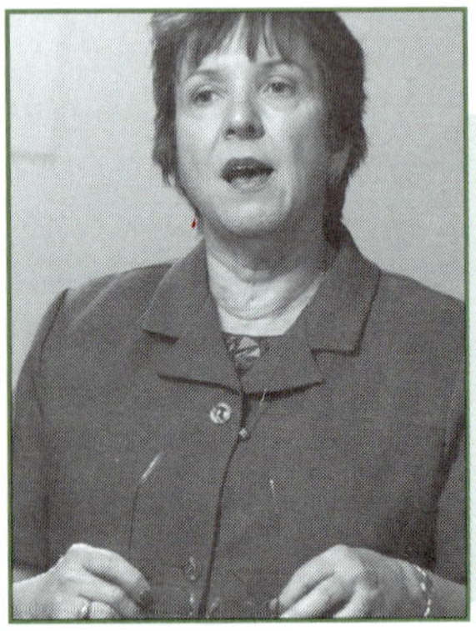

FROM THE TRENCHES

Maryann

"What makes me take the most pride is that I have done a good service both to the physician and to the patient. That I have coded it properly and correctly so that the physician is reimbursed in a way that compensates him ... By the same token, also being sure to code in a way that doesn't incorrectly label the patient to insurance companies and bills adequately, so I'm doing justice to the patient."

CASE 9-12

This patient is 58 years old.

9-12A OPERATIVE REPORT, TRACHEOSTOMY

LOCATION: Inpatient, Hospital

PATIENT: Sally Gross

PHYSICIAN: Gregory Dawson, M.D.

PREOPERATIVE DIAGNOSIS: Failure to extubate, prolonged intubation

POSTOPERATIVE DIAGNOSIS: Chronic respiratory failure

PROCEDURE PERFORMED: Tracheostomy, planned

ANESTHESIA: General endotracheal

PROCEDURE IN DETAIL: Following informed consent from the patient's daughter, Charlene, the patient was taken to the operating room and placed supine on the operating room table. The appropriate monitoring devices were placed on the patient, and general anesthesia was induced. She was already orally intubated with a size 8 endotracheal tube. The neck was prepped and draped in the usual sterile fashion. The patient had a shoulder roll placed beneath her shoulders, and her neck was extended. Great care was taken so that there was not too much tension on the neck, and there was not.

The neck was marked. It was then injected with approximately 3 cc of 1% Xylocaine with 1:100,000 epinephrine. A scalpel was used to incise in a horizontal fashion through the skin. Cautery dissection was used to cauterize between the strap muscles down to the level of the thyroid isthmus. The patient had a very thin neck but surprisingly wide and thick thyroid isthmus, approximately 1 inch wide. Blunt dissection was used to dissect between the thyroid isthmus, and it was divided and tied off. Bleeders were all well controlled before proceeding further.

The cricoid cartilage was identified. A cricoid hook was placed into it. The inner space between the second and third thyroid cartilage was then incised with a no. 15 blade scalpel. Metzenbaum scissors were then used to enlarge this incision. A size no. 8 cuffed Shiley trach tube was then placed into the trachea following partial removal of the endotracheal tube. The cuff was then inflated. A good CO_2 return was then appreciated on the monitor. The Shiley trach tube was then sutured in position. A piece of Xeroform gauze was then placed beneath the flange of the Shiley. The patient tolerated the procedure well. She was transferred to recovery in good condition. Estimated blood loss was less than 5 cc.

9-12A:

SERVICE CODE(S): 31600

DX CODE(S): 518.83

Endoscopic Procedures

Endoscopic procedures utilize a scope that is placed through an existing body opening, or a small incision is made into the body through which the scope is passed. Endoscopic procedures are often used in the diagnosis and treatment of respiratory conditions. When coding endoscopic procedures, be certain you code to the full extent of the procedure and the correct approach. The full extent is the farthest point to which the scope is passed. When multiple procedures are performed, the surgeon may do one procedure with a scope and another procedure without a scope.

When multiple endoscopic procedures are performed through the scope during the same operative session, place the most resource-intensive procedure first and the subsequent procedure(s) to follow with modifier -51. There are, however, many bundled procedures in the respiratory codes, so be certain not to unbundle services that can be reported with one code.

CASE 9-13
9-13A Operative Report, Septoplasty, Turbinoplasty, and Ethmoidectomy

CASE 9-13

This report has several procedures performed during one operative session, which is not uncommon. Code each of the services while watching for bundled surgical services. Just because there are six items under the Procedure Performed section of the report does not mean there were six separate procedures performed. Only by reading the report can you correctly code the operative procedures. The ethmoidectomy is the most resource-intensive procedure performed during this operative session.

9-13A OPERATIVE REPORT, SEPTOPLASTY, TURBINOPLASTY, AND ETHMOIDECTOMY

LOCATION: Outpatient, Hospital

SURGEON: Gregory Dawson, M.D.

PATIENT: Lucy Chang

PREOPERATIVE DIAGNOSES:
1. Septal deviation
2. Hypertrophic inferior turbinates
3. Enlarged (hypertrophic) ethmoid air cells

POSTOPERATIVE DIAGNOSES:
1. Septal deviation
2. Hypertrophic inferior turbinates
3. Enlarged ethmoid air cells

PROCEDURE PERFORMED:
1. Septoplasty
2. Turbinoplasty
3. Left intranasal anterior ethmoidectomy
4. Left intranasal posterior ethmoidectomy
5. Left intranasal removal of middle turbinate
6. Bilateral inferior turbinoplasty

OPERATIVE NOTE: The patient is a 39-year-old woman who was seen in the office and diagnosed with the above condition. She had a significant septal deviation to the right. The ethmoid air cells had overgrown on the opposite side, which meant that they had to be removed to allow the septum to assume a more midline position. She was admitted through the same-day surgery department and taken to the operating room, where she was administered general anesthetic by intravenous injection. She was then intubated endotracheally. The patient was draped in the usual fashion. Pledgets were placed in the nose with 4 cc of 4% cocaine solution. After a short interval, the pledgets were removed and the 4-mm scope (*indicates endoscopic procedure*) was inserted in the left side. The roots of middle turbinate and uncinate were injected with 1% lidocaine with epinephrine. The middle turbinate was medialized. The large anterior ethmoid bulla was taken down, and we went posteriorly into the ethmoid cells and removed a medial portion of the anterior and posterior ethmoid cells (*indicates ethmoidectomy*). The root of the middle turbinate was identified, and the turbinate scissors were used to resect (*left turboplasty*) this, creating space for the septum to move over. We then packed this with some Afrin-soaked strip gauze. The left side of the septum was injected with 1% lidocaine with epinephrine. A left hemitransfixion incision was created, and a mucoperichondrial flap was elevated on this side. This extended posteriorly over the perpendicular place of ethmoid and vomer. We then separated the cartilaginous bony septum with the Freer elevator. We removed the deviated portion of the bony septum posteriorly, and then the cartilaginous portion was removed, leaving the dorsal strip and caudal portion of 1 cm inside for tip support (*indicates septoplasty*). Flap was laid back into position and sewed up with interrupted 4-0 chromic suture, and plain gut sutures were then used to quilt the septum in multiple places. Silastic stents were then placed on either side of the septum and secured with a single 3-0 nylon suture. The inferior turbinates were then medialized; these were large and redundant (*left turbinate*). Approximately two thirds of the turbinate was left in place. The mucosa overlying this turbinate was then treated with electrocautery in several locations, and effective blanching was achieved. The Afrin gauze was then removed, from the ethmoid area, and this side of the nose was packed with Bacitracin-soaked strip gauze. The inferior turbinate on the right side was then medialized, and again the inferior portion was resected (*right turboplasty*). The mucosal portion of the remaining turbinate was then treated with electrocautery, and effective blanching was achieved. This side of the nose was then packed with the same Bacitracin-soaked strip gauze. The patient was then allowed to recover from the general anesthetic and taken to the postanesthesia care unit in stable condition. There were no complications from this procedure.

9-13A:

SERVICE CODE(S): 31255-LT

DX CODE(S): 30520-51

30140-51

~~30140-51~~-50

478.0, 478.1

CASE 9-14

9-14A OPERATIVE REPORT, ETHMOIDECTOMY AND ANTROSTOMY

In this surgical session, the surgeon performed three procedures, each of which is underlined in the Procedure Performed section of the report.

LOCATION: Outpatient, Hospital

PATIENT: Inez Epley

PHYSICIAN: Gregory Dawson, M.D.

PREOPERATIVE DIAGNOSIS: Recurrent acute left-sided sinusitis and left conchal bullosa, left nasal obstruction

POSTOPERATIVE DIAGNOSIS: Recurrent acute left-sided sinusitis and left conchal bullosa, left nasal obstruction

PROCEDURE PERFORMED: Left functional endoscopic sinus surgery and **removal of left conchal bullosa** (*this is a concha bullosa resection*). The patient also had left anterior **ethmoidectomy** and left maxillary **antrostomy**.

ANESTHESIA: General endotracheal anesthesia

PROCEDURE IN DETAIL: Following informed consent from the patient, she was taken to the operating room and placed supine on the operating room table. The appropriate monitoring devices were placed on the patient, and general anesthesia was induced. She was orally intubated without difficulty. The left nasal cavity was packed with Afrin-soaked gauze. This was removed after 5 minutes. The patient was draped in the usual sterile fashion. The lateral nasal wall on the left-hand side was injected with approximately 2 cc of 1% Xylocaine with 1:100,000 epinephrine. The widened left middle turbinate was also injected with 1 cc of the same. Following adequate time for the injection to take effect, a sickle knife was used to incise through the central portion of the left middle turbinate. The lateral half of the conchal bullosa was removed using Wilde forceps. A nice left maxillary sinus antrostomy was then created. The shaver was used to trim the mucosal edges. The anterior ethmoid air cells were opened using the Wilde forceps. The shaver was used to trim some of the mucosa within the left anterior ethmoid air cells. The area was then packed with Afrin-soaked gauze. After 5 minutes it was removed. There was no further bleeding. A stent was then placed into the left ostial meatal complex. The nasopharynx was then suctioned of blood.

The patient was then allowed to recover from general anesthetic and was transferred to the recovery room in good condition. She tolerated the procedure well.

ESTIMATED BLOOD LOSS: Less than 50 cc

9-14A:

SERVICE CODE(S): 31267-LT
31254-51-LT
31240-51-LT (concha bullosa)

DX CODE(S): 473.9
478.0

CASE 9-15
9-15A Thoracic Medicine and Critical Care Consultation
9-15B Thoracic Medicine and Critical Care Progress Report
9-15C Thoracic Medicine and Critical Care Progress Report
9-15D Radiology Report, Chest
9-15E Operative Report, Esophagogastroduodenoscopy
9-15F CT-Guided Lung Biopsy
9-15G Pathology Report
9-15H Ultrasound Marking for Thoracentesis
9-15I Operative Report, Thoracentesis
9-15J Pathology Report
9-15K Oxygen Desaturation Study
9-15L Radiology Report, Chest
9-15M Operative Report, Thoracostomy

CASE 9-15

This case contains many reports for a patient who was admitted to the hospital and received a wide variety of services to diagnose and treat his condition.

9-15A THORACIC MEDICINE AND CRITICAL CARE CONSULTATION

LOCATION: Inpatient, Hospital

PATIENT: Virgil Zejdlek

ATTENDING PHYSICIAN: Ronald Green, M.D.

CONSULTANT: Gregory Dawson, M.D.

This is a patient who is well known to me from the past. I was asked to see the patient again today to comment on his abnormal chest x-ray; actually the patient has already had a biopsy taken. I went to pathology, and we saw on preliminary results poorly differentiated carcinoma. They are having a lot of trouble determining whether it is a non–small cell or small cell. I think we have to wait for the special stains and the core biopsy to come out for a better diagnostic label. The patient does describe dysphagia and shortness of breath. He may need drainage of the pleural fluid again, but we will see how that goes in the future. Right now I think we will let Dr. Green know what is going on with the abnormal CT scan and take a look at the esophagus. He may have actually a lung cancer that has spread through the esophagus. I will let oncology know that they should see whether he could be started on a chemotherapy program of radiation, depending on the final diagnosis.

For a detailed review of the past medical history, social history, family history, and review of systems, please refer to my notes from last time just a little less than a month ago and Dr. Green's note where it is outlined in detail.

PHYSICAL EXAMINATION: On examination, the patient is alert and able to give his own history. Neck is supple. Lungs have diminished breath sounds, in fact more so on the left than the right. Heart shows a regular rhythm without an S3. Abdomen is benign. Extremities show some trace edema. Chest, symmetrical. Back, straight.

IMPRESSION: Poorly differentiated carcinoma of the lung with pleural effusion that may have to be drained again because of the shortness of breath, although he says it is better today than it has been. He is lying flat on his side at this time. I did talk to Dr. Green, who is his primary care physician at this point. We will get in touch with oncology and Dr. White to see what we can offer this patient. He may have some real problems here. I would be happy to follow along if so requested.

CYTOLOGY REPORT of the aspirate confirmed the pleural effusion was not malignant.

9-15A:

SERVICE CODE(S): ____________________

DX CODE(S): ____________________

9-15B THORACIC MEDICINE AND CRITICAL CARE PROGRESS REPORT

Dr. Green transferred care of Virgil Zejdlek to Dr. Dawson, who now is the attending physician. Dr. Dawson continues to update Dr. Green regarding the patient's care by indicating that Dr. Green is the primary care physician, and as such Dr. Green will receive copies of Dr. Dawson's documentation regarding Mr. Zejdlek. Note that for the diagnosis for this report, Dr. Dawson has indicated that the carcinoma is of either the lung or esophagus. As such, as an outpatient coder you cannot report the carcinoma, rather you will report the shortness of breath as the primary diagnosis.

LOCATION: Inpatient, Hospital

PATIENT: Virgil Zejdlek

PRIMARY CARE PHYSICIAN: Ronald Green, M.D.

ATTENDING PHYSICIAN: Gregory Dawson, M.D.

The patient is here with a poorly differentiated carcinoma of either the lung or esophagus. The patient has been experiencing shortness of breath for some time now. Dr. Friendly is going to be scoping the patient today to see what the distal esophagus looks like, and we have some CT scan evidence that there may be some involvement of that. We still do not have a final pathology of the poorly differentiated carcinoma; that will be coming hopefully today or tomorrow. He still has shortness of breath. I think the fluid has reaccumulated. I will check on that today with PA and lateral and left lateral decubitus, and if he has more fluid coming back down, perhaps CT surgery can place a chest tube at this time. We will see if we cannot get it drained more. Chest is barrel-shaped. The chest today sounds like there may be more fluid in there, at least the level of diminished breath sounds seems to be higher, so we will get that ordered today. I am basically waiting for laboratory results to come back.

9-15B:

SERVICE CODE(S): ____________

DX CODE(S):

9-15C THORACIC MEDICINE AND CRITICAL CARE PROGRESS REPORT

LOCATION: Inpatient, Hospital

PATIENT: Virgil Zejdlek

PRIMARY CARE PHYSICIAN: Ronald Green, M.D.

ATTENDING PHYSICIAN: Gregory Dawson, M.D.

The patient has cancer of the lung. We were not sure originally whether it was cancer of lung to esophagus or esophagus to lung, but this is lung to esophagus and has a pleural effusion with it. The patient is still experiencing shortness of breath. Yesterday I received chest x-rays looking for extensive left pleural effusion. I think it is a small amount of fluid that is freely flowing as you can tell by the lateral decubitus. Most of what we see of tumor mass, and atelectatic lung surrounding the tumor mass extends into the mediastinum. I do not think a thoracentesis would be of much help at this point. There was some controversy whether or not the patient had free air in the abdomen, but after consulting with our radiologist, I do not believe that is the problem. I do not think it exists. I think we are just being fooled by the air bubble in either the colon or the stomach. The patient is too out of shape for that. The patient does have some chest pain, but I think it is the same chest discomfort he had when he came in that was pleuritic associated with the mass. ECG done this morning shows sinus rhythm, LVH, and no acute changes anyway. Cardiac enzymes are pending. I did contact Dr. Eagle. He says the patient needs radiation therapy and chemotherapy. I will let the radiation therapists and Dr. Eagle work out who does what to whom first. At this point, unless a pleural effusion becomes larger, I do not think a repeat thoracentesis would be of much help at this point. If it does become larger, I think at that time perhaps a chest tube might be of some help because I think there is going to be a recurrent problem. I talked to the patient about this. I stated that I would be out of town and I would have to sign off the case until I get back. I would be glad to see him again in the future if so requested.

9-15C:

SERVICE CODE(S): ____________

DX CODE(S): ____________

9-15D RADIOLOGY REPORT, CHEST

Note in this report that the reason for the service is primarily the pleural effusion, not the carcinoma of the lung. This means that you should report the pleural effusion code first and the neoplasm code second.

LOCATION: Inpatient, Hospital

PATIENT: Virgil Zejdlek

PRIMARY CARE PHYSICIAN: Ronald Green, M.D.

ATTENDING PHYSICIAN: Gregory Dawson, M.D.

EXAMINATION OF: Chest

CLINICAL SYMPTOMS: Follow-up of pleural effusion. Primary carcinoma lung

PA AND LATERAL CHEST WITH A LEFT LATERAL DECUBITUS VIEW OF THE CHEST: FINDINGS: This examination is compared to a prior chest radiograph. The heart size appears prominent but unchanged compared with the prior examination. The pulmonary vascular markings appear within normal limits. Left-sided pleural effusion is present at this examination. On the decubitus views, at least a portion of this is believed to layer out. There is focal opacity present within the left mid and left lower lung zones, which is similar in appearance to the prior examination. There is radiographic evidence of COPD. Mild patchy right infrahilar opacity is also noted. There is an unusual lucency seen to overlie the central portion of the epigastric region of the upper abdomen. This may be within bowel; however, the possibility of free intraperitoneal air cannot be excluded, and further evaluation with decubitus, supine, and upright views of the abdomen is recommended.

IMPRESSION:

1. Left-sided pleural effusion as described above. At least a portion of this is felt to layer out.
2. Focal opacity is seen within the left mid and left lower lung zone, which is similar to the prior examination. This may relate to atelectasis or infiltrate with underlying lesions not excluded.
3. Unusual lucency seen in the epigastric region. Additional evaluation with dedicated abdominal films is recommended.

9-15D:

SERVICE CODE(S): ____________________

DX CODE(S): ____________________

9-15E OPERATIVE REPORT, ESOPHAGOGASTRODUODENOSCOPY

In this report, the surgeon passes an endoscope through the patient's mouth and obtains a duodenal biopsy. However, note that in addition to this procedure, the surgeon also dilates the esophagus. This is a manual dilation using a Maloney (rubber tube filled with tungsten or mercury) dilator. There are two types of mechanical bougies used for esophageal dilation: Savary dilator (stiff, yet somewhat flexible plastic) and the Maloney. Both types are graded in millimeters (mm) and French (1F = 3 mm). The goal of the dilation is to disrupt any strictures by stretching them. Modifier -59 is added to indicate that the dilation was performed manually rather than via the endoscope as a distinct procedure, because an endoscopic dilation would be bundled into the endoscopy code and is not usually reported separately.

LOCATION: Inpatient, Hospital

PATIENT: Virgil Zejdlek

PRIMARY CARE PHYSICIAN: Ronald Green, M.D.

ATTENDING PHYSICIAN: Gregory Dawson, M.D.

SURGEON: Larry Friendly, M.D.

PREOPERATIVE DIAGNOSIS: Dysphagia

POSTOPERATIVE DIAGNOSIS: An ulcerated stricture area in the upper esophagus consistent with either squamous cell carcinoma of the esophagus or consistent with extrinsic metastases or local invasion.

PROCEDURE PERFORMED: Esophagogastroduodenoscopy with biopsy and esophageal dilation with Maloney dilator.

INDICATIONS: This 77-year-old white male was referred by Dr. Dawson for endoscopy. The patient has poorly differentiated carcinoma of the lung just diagnosed. He has had dysphagia, anorexia, and 30-pound weight loss.

PREOPERATIVE MEDICATION: Demerol 50 mg IV; Versed 2 mg IV

FINDINGS: The Pentax video pediatric endoscope was passed without difficulty into the oropharynx. Immediately seen at 30 cm was what looked like the gastroesophageal junction. At about 31 cm there was an ulcerated strictured area to 34 cm. The area did allow passage of the pediatric endoscope. The patient had discomfort as we passed through the area. The gastroesophageal junction was actually seen at 42 cm. Inspection of the esophagus at this level did not reveal erythema, ulceration, exudate, friability, or other mucosal abnormalities. The stomach proper was entered, and the endoscope advanced into the stomach. There was a large amount of food present, but the patient was fasting post midnight. We were able to advance through the pylorus; however, we did not see any obstruction, and I did not pass beyond the duodenum. The retroflexion revealed a large amount of food. Inspection of the antrum and body from what we could see did not show any abnormalities except the large amount of food. We then, on withdrawal, reviewed the area again in the upper esophagus and performed multiple biopsies. We then removed the endoscope and passed a no. 46 French-Maloney dilator with only minimal resistance noted. The patient tolerated the procedure well.

IMPRESSION: Ulceration in the upper third of esophagus *[This "upper third" is necessary to correctly assign the diagnosis code]*, distance at about 3 cm with some stricturing dilated with a Maloney dilator no. 46 French. This lesion could be the primary source, or it could be secondary with metastases or extrinsic involvement of the esophagus. We will await biopsies.

Pathology Report Later Indicated: Secondary squamous cell carcinoma

9-15E:

SERVICE CODE(S): ____________________

DX CODE(S): ____________________

9-15F CT-GUIDED LUNG BIOPSY

LOCATION: Inpatient, Hospital

PATIENT: Virgil Zejdlek

PRIMARY CARE PHYSICIAN: Ronald Green, M.D.

ATTENDING PHYSICIAN: Gregory Dawson, M.D.

INTERVENTIONAL RADIOLOGIST: Edward Riddle, M.D.

EXAMINATION OF: CT-guided lung biopsy

CLINICAL SYMPTOMS: Lung mass

CT-GUIDED LUNG BIOPSY: The patient is a 77-year-old male with mediastinal and left lung mass. CT-guided lung biopsy was requested by Dr. Dawson.

The patient was prepped and draped in the usual sterile fashion. The mass in the left lobe was again localized. Using sterile technique from a left posterolateral standpoint, three separate core biopsies were obtained utilizing an 18-gauge ASAP Medi-Tech biopsy device. Suspicious cells were noted, and a definite diagnosis is pending.

The patient tolerated the procedure well. The patient denied shortness of breath or chest pain. There is no evidence of pneumothorax on the immediate post-biopsy CT study or on the 3-hour and 5-hour post-biopsy chest x-rays.

IMPRESSION: Three separate core biopsies of the left lung mass utilizing an 18-gauge ASAP Medi-Tech biopsy device as described above.

Pathology Report Later Indicated: See report 9.15G.

9-15F:

SERVICE CODE(S): 32405 (Biopsy, Lung)

DX CODE(S): 76360-51-26 (CAT Scan)

162.9

9-15G PATHOLOGY REPORT

You will be coding not only the pathology examination but also the cytology noted in the last line of the report. Cytology is the study of cells that have been obtained by brushing or washing. Find direction to the correct code for this service by referencing the index of the CPT manual under the heading Cytopathology, Fluid.

LOCATION: Inpatient, Hospital

PATIENT: Virgil Zejdlek

PRIMARY CARE PHYSICIAN: Ronald Green, M.D.

ATTENDING PHYSICIAN: Gregory Dawson, M.D.

PATHOLOGIST: Grey Lonewolf, M.D.

CLINICAL HISTORY: Large mass left lung mediastinal area, concurrent

GROSS DESCRIPTION: Pleural effusion, two diff quiks, six prepared smears

SPECIMEN RECEIVED: Lung touch prep, left, mass

SPECIMEN ADEQUACY: Specimen satisfactory for cytologic evaluation

DIAGNOSIS: Malignant cells suggestive of undifferentiated neoplasm

COMMENTS: The malignant cells show some subjective features reminiscent of small cell carcinoma, but nuclear size is more compatible with non–small cell carcinoma. Cytology correlates with accompanying histology specimen.

9-15G:

SERVICE CODE(S): ____________________

DX CODE(S): ____________________

9-15H ULTRASOUND MARKING FOR THORACENTESIS

LOCATION: Inpatient, Hospital

PATIENT: Virgil Zejdlek

PRIMARY CARE PHYSICIAN: Ronald Green, M.D.

ATTENDING PHYSICIAN: Gregory Dawson, M.D.

RADIOLOGIST: Morton Monson, M.D.

EXAMINATION OF: Ultrasound marking for thoracentesis

CLINICAL SYMPTOMS: Pleural fluid

ULTRASOUND MARKINGS FOR THORACENTESIS: Left hemithorax was marked in the visualized area of the largest amount of pleural fluid on the left. Distance from the skin surface to the central portion of the fluid equals 6 cm.

9-15H:

SERVICE CODE(S): 76942-26 (Ultrasound)

DX CODE(S): 511.9

9-15I OPERATIVE REPORT, THORACENTESIS

LOCATION: Inpatient, Hospital

PATIENT: Virgil Zejdlek

PRIMARY CARE PHYSICIAN: Ronald Green, M.D.

ATTENDING PHYSICIAN: Gregory Dawson, M.D.

PREOPERATIVE DIAGNOSIS: Right pleural effusion with unknown cause

POSTOPERATIVE DIAGNOSIS: Right pleural effusion with unknown cause

PROCEDURES PERFORMED:

1. Diagnostic thoracentesis
2. Four quadrant pleural biopsy *[Note that this indicates the number of biopsies you will be reporting.]*
3. Pleural drainage with a small-caliber temporary chest tube

PROCEDURE: With the usual Betadine scrub to the area previously marked by ultrasound, the area was anesthetized with approximately 15 cc of 1% lidocaine, and then a 21-gauge needle was inserted into the space. Fluid was removed for appropriate bacteriologic, hematologic, and chemical analysis.

Once this was accomplished, a larger tube using a Cope pleural biopsy needle was inserted into the space and four quadrants were biopsied and sent for appropriate pathological specimens. Once that was accomplished, using a small-caliber temporary chest tube from the Cook as well as the pneumothorax set, the space was entered and 1.5 L of bloody fluid was removed. A small bandage was attached afterward. There was no pain involved, and the chest x-ray will be taken afterward to assure ourselves we had a reasonable effect without any ill consequences.

Pathology Report Indicated: See Report 9-8I

9-15I:

SERVICE CODE(S): 32002

DX CODE(S): 32400 X4

162.9

9-15J PATHOLOGY REPORT

Report the cytopathology services provided by Dr. Lonewolf.

LOCATION: Inpatient, Hospital

PATIENT: Virgil Zejdlek

PRIMARY CARE PHYSICIAN: Ronald Green, M.D.

ATTENDING PHYSICIAN: Gregory Dawson, M.D.

PATHOLOGIST: Grey Lonewolf, M.D.

CLINICAL HISTORY: Large mass, left lung and mediastinum, pleural effusion, concurrent cytology

SPECIMEN RECEIVED: Left-lung fine needle biopsy *[This is a fine needle aspiration (FNA).]*

GROSS DESCRIPTION: Submitted in formalin, labeled with patient's name and "left lung FNB" are core needle fragments of white to brown tissue measuring less than 0.25 cc in aggregate. Submitted in toto.

MICROSCOPIC DESCRIPTION: Sections show tiny core needle fragments of fibrous tissue featuring nests of infiltrating poorly differentiated neoplastic cells. There is a surrounding desmoplastic response. The tumor cells show high nuclear/cytoplasmic (N/C) ratios and moderate nuclear enlargement. Focal nests demonstrate cells with a small to moderate amount of pink cytoplasm and vesicular nuclei.

DIAGNOSIS: Lung, left, fine needle biopsy: Invasive poorly differentiated non–small cell carcinoma, fragments of.

9-15J:

SERVICE CODE(S): 88173 (fine needle

DX CODE(S): 162.9

9-15K OXYGEN DESATURATION STUDY

This is an oxygen sleep study being performed to diagnose somnolence.

LOCATION: Inpatient, Hospital

PATIENT: Virgil Zejdlek

PRIMARY CARE PHYSICIAN: Ronald Green, M.D.

ATTENDING PHYSICIAN: Gregory Dawson, M.D.

ENTRANCE DIAGNOSIS: Somnolence

The patient started the study at 2100 and was continued until 0515 the next morning. He was on room air at the beginning, but his O_2 saturation dropped to 87%, and he was started on 1 L. I cannot tell from the tracing how long he was at 87% before starting 1 L per minute. This was continued through the rest of the night, and his O_2 saturation stayed about 90%. He was intermittently observed. (*This indicates attendance by technology.*) No apneas were seen. No snoring was noted on intermittent observations. Lowest O_2 saturation recorded looks like 83%, and it appears that 3% of his time was spent with O_2 saturations in the 80s, and 97% of his time was spent with O_2 saturations 90% or better. That is because most of the night was done with 1 L per minute by nasal prongs.

It appears that the patient does desaturate significantly with sleep, and it appears that it is 87%. The lowest was 83%.

9-15K:

SERVICE CODE(S): ____________________

DX CODE(S): ____________________

9-15L RADIOLOGY REPORT, CHEST

LOCATION: Inpatient, Hospital

PATIENT: Virgil Zejdlek

PRIMARY CARE PHYSICIAN: Ronald Green, M.D.

ATTENDING PHYSICIAN: Gregory Dawson, M.D.

EXAMINATION OF: Chest

CLINICAL SYMPTOMS: Pneumothorax, pleural effusion

ONE-VIEW CHEST, 4:00 P.M.: AP portable view obtained of the chest at 4:00 P.M. Comparison study is from 5 days prior. Pleural effusion on the left appears decreased. There now appears to be left pneumothorax seen superiorly and laterally. This is as marked on the film. There is left basilar/retrocardiac opacity. There appears to be some patient rotation. There are superimposed cardiac leads. Cardiac silhouette is not appreciably changed. There is volume loss on the left.

IMPRESSION:

1. Left pleural effusion appears decreased since prior study. There appears to be residual pleural fluid and there is left basilar opacity. There now appears to be pneumothorax on the left. There is volume loss of the left.
2. Cardiac silhouette appears stable.
3. Not mentioned above, there is some oral contrast noted in the upper abdomen.

9-15L:

SERVICE CODE(S): ____________________

DX CODE(S): ____________________

9-15M OPERATIVE REPORT, THORACOSTOMY

LOCATION: Inpatient, Hospital

PATIENT: Virgil Zejdlek

PRIMARY CARE PHYSICIAN: Ronald Green, M.D.

ATTENDING PHYSICIAN: Gregory Dawson, M.D.

SURGEON: Gary Sanchez, M.D.

PREOPERATIVE DIAGNOSIS: Left pleural effusion

POSTOPERATIVE DIAGNOSIS: Left pleural effusion

NAME OF OPERATION: Left tube thoracostomy

HISTORY OF PRESENT ILLNESS: The patient is a 77-year-old man who was recently admitted with right-sided chest pain and shortness of breath. Chest x-ray revealed a moderate- to large-sized left pleural effusion. A CT scan revealed the presence of a large left pulmonary mass as well as significant subcarinal adenopathy or mass effect. Thoracentesis was performed and the left pleural effusion was drained; however, it recurred after only 24 hours. Cardiothoracic surgery was consulted to discuss the option of tube thoracostomy. The above findings were explained to the patient. The prognosis as well as the risks and benefits of continued observation versus repeat thoracentesis versus tube thoracotomy were discussed at length. His questions concerning his options for therapy were answered. He appeared to understand the above findings, and after our discussion expressed a desire to proceed with tube thoracostomy and gave written consent to proceed.

OPERATIVE FINDINGS: Approximately 700 cc of clear, yellow-red fluid was removed from the left pleural cavity.

DESCRIPTION OF PROCEDURE: The patient was brought to the procedure room and placed on a cart in the decubitus position. The left side was up. The left side of the chest was then prepped and draped in the usual sterile fashion. Local anesthesia was accomplished using 15 cc of 1% Xylocaine. A 2-cm incision was made in the mid-axillary line in approximately the seventh intercostal space. Using a Kelly clamp, subcutaneous tunnel was created. Additional lidocaine was injected and the intercostal muscles separated, and the left pleural cavity was entered. A 32-French chest tube was then inserted into the left pleural cavity and secured in place with a 2-0 silk stitch. The chest tube was placed on 20 cm of water suction, and a sterile dressing was applied. The patient tolerated the procedure quite well. A postprocedure chest x-ray was ordered.

9-15M:

SERVICE CODE(S): 32020-LT (Thoracost

DX CODE(S): 511.9

CASE 9-15 DISCUSSION

This was an excellent case to learn how choosing the diagnoses changes from one report to another based on the service being provided to the patient. Inpatient coders would consider all of the diagnoses stated by all of the physicians when reporting the inpatient hospital services for this patient upon discharge. The outpatient coder reports the diagnosis(es) that was/were the primary reason(s) for the encounter.

CASE 9-16
9-16A Emergency Department Report
9-16B Thoracic Medicine/Critical Care Consultation
9-16C Radiology Report, Chest
9-16D Radiology Report, Chest
9-16E Thoracic Medicine/Critical Care Progress Report
9-16F Discharge Summary

CASE 9-16

9-16A EMERGENCY DEPARTMENT REPORT

Dr. Sutton provides not only the E/M service but also places this patient on a ventilator. The intubation (placing the tube into the trachea) is included in the initial ventilator services and not reported separately. You can locate the directions to the ventilator codes in the index of the CPT under "Ventilation Assist."

LOCATION: Inpatient, Hospital

PATIENT: Reen Hesse

PHYSICIAN: Paul Sutton, M.D.

SUBJECTIVE: The patient is an 80-year-old male in acute respiratory distress. He is from the New York City area and was just about to take a train to go there today. He had sudden onset of shortness of breath and presents now because of it. He denies any chest pain or tightness. He has had no recent cough. He is bringing up frothy sputum as he arrives here.

PAST MEDICAL HISTORY:

Surgical:
1. Bypass surgery
2. Angioplasty and stent
3. Pacemaker

Illnesses: The patient has a previous history of congestive heart failure and has been intubated in the past, most recently 4 months ago with this same problem.

FAMILY HISTORY, SOCIAL HISTORY, and REVIEW OF SYSTEMS were not obtainable for this patient.

OBJECTIVE: This alert 80-year-old male appears to be in acute respiratory distress. Oxygen saturation is 72%. Blood pressure is 210/107. Respirations are 36. Pulse is 120. Telemetry shows a paced wide complexed rhythm. HEENT: Frothy pink sputum coming out of his mouth. NECK is supple without lymphadenopathy. His jugular veins are full. Respirations are labored. LUNGS: Rales throughout. HEART: Rapid rate and rhythm. ABDOMEN: Soft and nontender with normal bowel sounds. EXTREMITIES: No peripheral edema is noted. No clubbing.

ASSESSMENT: Pulmonary edema

PLAN: He was immediately given Lasix 80 mg IV, given Nitro spray, and started on a Nitro drip. We gave him a few minutes to try to turn around. He was on 100% oxygen. He did not turn around and, in fact, he looked worse. We then talked about intubation with him and his wife and proceeded with it. He was bagged. He was given Versed IV, and he then was given succinylcholine 100 mg IV. He was then intubated without difficulty with an 8.0 ET tube to 24 cm. Breath sounds were heard bilaterally. CO_2 monitoring device confirmed placement. The patient was placed on the ventilator and transported to ICU in reasonably stable condition.

9-16A:

SERVICE CODE(S): ____________________

DX CODE(S): ____________________

9-16B THORACIC MEDICINE/CRITICAL CARE CONSULTATION

Reen was admitted to the hospital onto Dr. Elhart's service. Dr. Elhart immediately requested a consultation from Dr. Dawson regarding the patient's respiratory condition.

LOCATION: Inpatient, Hospital

PATIENT: Reen Hesse

ATTENDING PHYSICIAN: Marvin Elhart, M.D.

CONSULTANT: Gregory Dawson, M.D.

I have been asked by Dr. Elhart to see the patient for ICU care. The patient was admitted with pulmonary edema, respiratory failure; he has chronic renal disease and is on Dr. Elhart's service, I would assume for the chronic renal disease as well as respiratory failure but that was secondary. The patient looks like he had a myocardial infarction with elevated troponins, CK-MBs, CPKs, and CKs. His pulmonary edema has started to clear. He was adjusted on the ventilator this morning. The CPAP went from 6 o'clock to 8 o'clock, and then he got too short of breath and went back on the ventilator. Since then he has diuresed more, and I have him on CPAP at present. He is doing quite well with a respiratory rate of 19 with good oxygenation. I think we have a fair chance of getting him extubated today.

The patient was visiting with relatives here in Manytown. He was trying to move some luggage, started to get diaphoretic, and did not feel well, and it started to become difficult to breathe. The wife felt he was gurgling, and he was sent to the emergency room, where he was found to be in pulmonary edema, intubated, and placed on a ventilator.

The patient is intubated and on a ventilator, so I do not have a good family history, social history, past medical history, past surgical history, or review of systems. I got some things from the chart and some things from his wife. The patient's wife is fairly sure that he had stenting of the LAD done last year. We will send for those records. He had a coronary artery bypass graft done before that. It sounds fairly extensive. It seems to have been in 1989. He had at least three grafts, and the cardiologist has this outlined pretty well and what was done at that point. He also had a pacemaker. He has a history of renal artery disease status post renal artery stenosis, history of hypertension, dyslipidemia, bradycardia, and chronic renal disease. He apparently has had some trouble with dye toxicity from angiogram done a year ago and did not quite get over it. I guess there was partial clearing. It is difficult to tell without the records what went on.

PHYSICAL EXAMINATION at the time I saw the patient reveals a patient who is alert, on a ventilator, and able to answer questions, yes and no anyway. He certainly cannot verbalize it. HEENT: Benign. No blood was found in the posterior pharynx or the nose. NECK is supple. No JVD. LUNGS actually show rales bilaterally but in the bases, not in the rest of the areas. HEART shows S1 and S2 are regular without an S3 or S4. There is a systolic murmur at the fourth interspace midclavicular line that is somewhat difficult to hear. It is somewhat vague and soft, but I think it is present. ABDOMEN is soft and benign without hepatosplenomegaly. Normal bowel sounds are present. No bruits heard in either flank; no masses palpable; nontender. EXTREMITIES show no edema, rashes, clubbing, cyanosis, or tremor. LYMPHATIC SYSTEM: No nodes in the neck, clavicular, or axillary area.

IMPRESSION:

1. Acute myocardial infarction with acute pulmonary edema and acute respiratory failure.
2. Chronic renal failure. You can see that on today's material his BUN and creatinine levels are climbing. I am not sure what the plan is at this point. I am waiting for cardiology to come by, but I think I can get him extubated later this afternoon. I will check his sputum. He does have a fair amount to suction and it is somewhat thick, so I will make sure he does not have an infection. He is already on Unasyn for any sort of aspiration that might have occurred, although it is not well documented. We will check a 24-hour urine for creatinine clearance, get the records from the Manytown hospital to see what actually was done there, and then check on his lab in the morning. I will wait for Dr. Elhart to come by before we have any other plans, but hopefully the patient will be extubated here shortly.

9-16B:

SERVICE CODE(S): ____________________

DX CODE(S): ____________________

9-16C RADIOLOGY REPORT, CHEST

This x-ray was taken the day after admission.

LOCATION: Inpatient, Hospital

PATIENT: Reen Hesse

ATTENDING PHYSICIAN: Marvin Elhart, M.D.

RESPIRATORY CARE: Gregory Dawson, M.D.

RADIOLOGIST: Morton Monson, M.D.

EXAMINATION OF: Chest

CLINICAL SYMPTOMS: Follow-up pulmonary edema

PORTABLE AP CHEST, 5:00 A.M.: FINDINGS: Comparison is made with yesterday morning's portable AP chest. Sternotomy with mediastinal clips. No appreciable change in the heart size or pulmonary vascularity given the difference in technique. Lungs are clear.

9-16C:

SERVICE CODE(S): ____________________

DX CODE(S): ____________________

9-16D RADIOLOGY REPORT, CHEST

LOCATION: Inpatient, Hospital

PATIENT: Reen Hesse

ATTENDING PHYSICIAN: Marvin Elhart, M.D.

RESPIRATORY CARE: Gregory Dawson, M.D.

RADIOLOGIST: Morton Monson, M.D.

EXAMINATION OF: Chest

CLINICAL SYMPTOMS: Acute MI, pulmonary edema, acute respiratory failure, and renal disease

PORTABLE AP CHEST X-RAY: FINDINGS: The cardiac silhouette is upper normal to mildly prominent but stable. Mild interstitial prominence remains in the infrahilar areas, but no other significant interval change is noted.

9-16D:

SERVICE CODE(S): ______________________

DX CODE(S): ______________________

9-16E THORACIC MEDICINE/CRITICAL CARE PROGRESS REPORT

LOCATION: Inpatient, Hospital

PATIENT: Reen Hesse

ATTENDING PHYSICIAN: Marvin Elhart, M.D.

RESPIRATORY CARE: Gregory Dawson, M.D.

This is a follow-up for this patient with acute respiratory failure. He was extubated yesterday. He apparently had a cardiac catheterization in the past, and his kidneys were bad enough that they thought he might need dialysis, but then he recovered; but he certainly recovered incompletely because BUN today is 72, creatinine 2.6, and creatinine clearance is pending. Interestingly enough, potassium is low at 2.8, so we will replace that with oral potassium. We will check his basic metabolic panel in the morning and transfer him to the floor on telemetry. He does not want anything done here. He wants to go home by train, which is probably not the best idea because there is no guarantee that what happened to him this time will not happen again.

PHYSICAL EXAMINATION: CHEST: Clear. Chest x-ray looks pretty good too. HEART: Regular rhythm. ABDOMEN: Benign. EXTREMITIES: No edema. No clubbing.

LABORATORY DATA: All in good shape. Sputum showed greater than 25 white cells, less 10 squamous. No bugs were seen, so it may be just inflammation rather than true infection.

MEDICATIONS: He is on Unasyn at this point. We stopped the Unasyn today and put him on Augmentin. There is some question about whether he aspirated on it, but I certainly do not see anything on x-ray right now.

He is going to be talking to Dr. Elhart later today to decide what to do about whether to discharge or have the study done here. The patient is really 4+ positive that he wants to go back to home in case things go wrong with his kidneys. At least he is at home and can undergo the dialysis closer to home. He is most comfortable with the situation there as well as with his surroundings there, so we will leave that up to Dr. Elhart and the patient. But I still think it is a somewhat risky idea, so I imparted that to the patient of those particular ideas. Otherwise, he can be discharged at cardiology's leisure.

9-16E:

SERVICE CODE(S): ______________________

DX CODE(S): ______________________

9-16F DISCHARGE SUMMARY

Dr. Elhart discharges the patient.

LOCATION: Inpatient, Hospital

PATIENT: Reen Hesse

ATTENDING PHYSICIAN: Marvin Elhart, M.D.

RESPIRATORY CARE: Gregory Dawson, M.D.

The patient was admitted with pulmonary edema, respiratory failure, and chronic renal disease. The patient looked like he has had myocardial infarction with elevated troponins. The patient was extubated after the pulmonary edema. Discussions with the patient and his family indicated that he did not want anything further done. He wanted further cardiac care done at home. We arranged for him to be discharged, and he was discharged Tuesday. It was advised that he have a cardiac catheterization to determine the extent of his myocardial infarction and whether anything could be fixed, but this is on top of somebody with chronic renal disease who most likely would suffer from the toxic effects of the dye and would probably have some difficulty with renal failure post cardiac catheterization if everything went wrong. Please see my drug note that outlined the drugs the patient was on when he was sent home.

DISCHARGE DIAGNOSES:
1. Subendocardial infarction
2. Congestive heart failure
3. Pulmonary edema with acute respiratory failure

9-16F:

SERVICE CODE(S): ______

DX CODE(S): ______

CASE 9-17
9-17A Operative Report, Bronchoscopy

CASE 9-17

9-17A OPERATIVE REPORT, BRONCHOSCOPY

There are only two services for this report—a bronchial brushing and a lavage. The washing is designated as a "(separate procedure)" and is only reported if it is the only procedure performed. Note that the diagnosis is going to be an abnormal radiological examination of the lung.

LOCATION: Inpatient, Hospital

PATIENT: Mary Ellen Gavisconi

ATTENDING PHYSICIAN: Marvin Elhart, M.D.

RESPIRATORY CARE: Gregory Dawson, M.D.

PREOPERATIVE DIAGNOSIS: Abnormal chest/lung x-ray

POSTOPERATIVE DIAGNOSIS: Inflammatory secretions

PROCEDURE PERFORMED: Fiberoptic bronchoscopy, cell washings, cell brushings, and bronchoalveolar lavage.

PROCEDURE: For details of the drugs used and the amounts of drugs used, please refer to the bronchoscopy report sheet. The patient was already intubated and on the ventilator. She was sedated as per ICU protocol. She was also given some drugs prior to that. Please refer, again, to the bronchoscopy report sheet.

The patient was monitored throughout the procedure with electrocardiography, O_2 saturations, and ventilator monitoring. These were all within parameters, and no real adverse effects were noted with those various monitoring services.

Once the patient had been sedated, the bronchoscope was introduced into the endotracheal tube. The distal portion of the trachea, the carina, and all the airways were examined both right and left. All the airways were patent and entered. The trachea and the carina were basically normal. The trachea is about 2 cm above the carina. The right and left lungs were also examined. All segments were patent and entered, and no masses were seen. The right lower lobe had some crowding and swelling and some inflammatory changes, but they were relatively mild. I did not see any obvious purulent material. There were excess secretions, but they did not appear thick and discolored. This area was brushed and washed and was also subjected to bronchoalveolar lavage in the right lower lobe. (*This procedure now has become a surgical procedure, and is no longer an exploratory procedure.*) These specimens were sent for appropriate pathological, cytologic, and bacterial studies. Hopefully the results will be back tomorrow. The patient suffered no ill effects from this procedure. She was left in the ICU for monitoring.

9-17A:

SERVICE CODE(S): 3623 (Bronchoscopy)

DX CODE(S): 31624-51 ("")

793.1
V46.11

CASE 9-18
9-18A Operative Report, Bronchoscopy
9-18B Pathology Report, Cytology

CASE 9-18

9-18A OPERATIVE REPORT, BRONCHOSCOPY

LOCATION: Outpatient, Hospital

PATIENT: Greg Encore

PHYSICIAN: Gregory Dawson, M.D.

PREOPERATIVE DIAGNOSIS: Abnormal chest x-ray. We are considering, by history, coccidioidomycosis pneumonia. So far, we are not getting much back for confirmation of this, and this procedure is being done to confirm that diagnosis.

POSTOPERATIVE DIAGNOSIS: Abnormal superior segment, left lower lobe, consistent with either inflammation or tumor or both.

PROCEDURE PERFORMED: Fiberoptic bronchoscopy, transbronchial biopsies, bronchial biopsies, cell washings, cell brushings, and bronchoalveolar lavage superior segment of left lower lobe.

For details of drugs used and the amounts of drugs used, please refer to the bronchoscopy report sheet. The patient was intubated already on a Vaughn cycle ventilator (*ventilator dependent*), sedated, and paralyzed per ICU protocol for the respiratory failure. An additional drug was given with atropine 0.5. The patient was monitored throughout the procedure with electrocardiographically, O_2 saturations, blood pressure, and the usual ICU monitoring with no real adverse problems. The ventilator was monitored by one of the respiratory therapists to ensure that we had adequate volume and adequate oxygenation.

Once the patient was firmly sedated with the usual ICU medications for his respiratory failure, the bronchoscope was introduced through the endotracheal tube. The part of the trachea we saw in the carina appeared to be within normal limits. In the right lung, all segments were patent and entered, and no masses were seen. The left upper lobe was also patent, and all segments were entered and no masses were seen. In the left lower lobe, the superior segment was deformed, closed, had blood in it, and was friable consistent with inflammation, tumor, or both. Multiple biopsies, brushings, and washings were done in the area as well as sheath brushings looking specifically for coccidioidomycosis and not only that, a BAL was performed on this segment with a "mini-BAL" apparatus. Biopsies were then done in this same area: the superior segment of the left lower lobe, both transbronchially and bronchially.

The patient tolerated the procedure well. No adverse effects were noted. We will check a chest x-ray shortly to assure ourselves that there are no problems there. Follow-up will be a little later, when we get the results back.

Pathological Findings: See Report 9-18B.

9-18A:

SERVICE CODE(S): 31628

DX CODE(S): 31623-51, 31624-51

162.5, V46.11

9-18B PATHOLOGY REPORT, CYTOLOGY

LOCATION: Outpatient, Hospital

PATIENT: Greg Encore

PHYSICIAN: Gregory Dawson, M.D.

PATHOLOGIST: Morton Monson, M.D.

CLINICAL HISTORY: Possible coccidia

SPECIMEN RECEIVED:
A. Bronch brush tip, left lower lobe
B. Bronchial biopsy, left lower lobe

GROSS DESCRIPTION:
A. Received in a container labeled "brush tip" is a brush tip with a scant amount of tan-red material. The specimen is totally submitted as A.
B. Received in a container labeled "biopsy" are four fragments of tan-gray tissue measuring 0.2 to 0.3 cm in greatest dimension. The specimen is totally submitted as B.

MICROSCOPIC DESCRIPTION:
A. The bronchial brushings contain rare scattered large atypical cells with hyperchromatic angulated nuclei. Some contain prominent nucleoli. Very small scattered areas show glands lined by similar cells.
B. The bronchial biopsies of the left lower lobe contain irregularly outlined and complex glands lined by enlarged pleomorphic cells. The cells contain hyperchromatic irregularly outlined and angulated nuclei. There is a dense supporting fibrous stroma that shows multiple foci of coagulation necrosis.

DIAGNOSIS:
A. Bronchial brushings, left lower lobe: Malignant cells are present, consistent with adenocarcinoma.
B. Bronchial and transbronchial biopsies, left lower lobe: Adenocarcinoma, well to moderately differentiated.

9-18B:
SERVICE CODE(S): 88104 (Cytopathology)
DX CODE(S): 162.5)

Glossary

atelectasis incomplete expansion of the lung or a portion of the lung.

bronchospasm spasmodic contraction of the muscle of the bronchi causing constriction of the airway.

dyspnea shortness of breath; difficult or painful breathing.

effusion the escape of fluid from blood vessels into a part or tissue.

hemoptysis the expectoration of blood in sputum.

pharyngitis inflammation of the pharynx (i.e., sore throat).

pulmonologist physician specializing in treatment of diseases and disorders of the respiratory system.

septoplasty surgical repair of the nasal septum.

spirometry measurement of breathing capacity.

thoracentesis surgical puncture of the thoracic cavity, usually using a needle, to remove fluids.

Chapter 10

Urinary, Male Genital, and Endocrine Systems

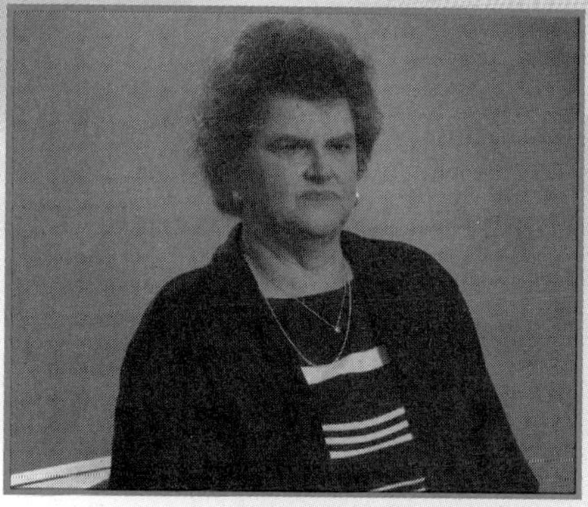

Dorothy D. Steed, CPC-H, CHCC, CPUR, CPAR
Medicare Specialist
Northside Hospital
Atlanta, Georgia

ABBREVIATIONS

ca	cancer
cc	cubic centimeter
cm	centimeter
CMG	cystometrogram
CRF	chronic renal failure
CT	computed tomography scan
ECG	electrocardiogram
EEG	electroencephalogram
EKG	electrocardiogram
EMG	electromyelography
ESRD	end-stage renal disease
ESWL	extracorporeal shockwave lithotripsy
HEENT	head, eyes, ears, nose, throat
IVP	intravenous pyelogram
KUB	kidney, ureter, bladder
mg	milligram
ml	milliliter
PERRLA	pupils equal, round, reactive to light and accommodation
p.o.	by mouth
p.r.n.	as needed
PSA	prostate-specific antigen
q.d.	everyday
QRS	Q wave, R wave, S wave
S1	first heart sound
S2	second heart sound
T&A	tonsillectomy and adenoidectomy
VCUG	voiding cystourethrography

Urinary System

Common urinary symptoms are nocturia, polyuria, hematuria, proteinuria, dysuria, oliguria, urinary **incontinence**, and enuresis. Often treated urinary conditions include hypercalciuria (urinary stones caused by the body's inability to process calcium properly), renal failure, pyelonephritis, and infections as well as kidney and bladder cancer. A physician who specializes in the diagnosis and treatment of conditions of the urinary system is a **urologist**. A **urologist** also specializes in male genitourinary conditions and as such often treats patients with prostatitis, benign prostatic hyperplasia, and prostate cancer. Urology is classified as a surgical subspecialty. A **nephrologist** specializes in the treatment of conditions of the kidney and has special education and training in kidney disease and transplantation as well as dialysis therapy. Nephrology is a subspecialty of internal medicine.

Chronic Renal Failure

Chronic renal failure is a progressive loss of kidney function that causes the kidneys to overcompensate by excessive straining (hyperfiltration) within the remaining **nephrons** (filtering units). In time, this leads to further loss of function. When 70% or more of the kidney function is lost, the patient begins to experience renal failure. One of the diagnostic methods used to determine the cause of the failure or the extent of damage is a biopsy in which a fine needle is percutaneously inserted into the kidney and a sample is withdrawn for analysis.

Diagnosis Coding

For a refresher on diagnosis coding for renal failure, refer back to the information that appears before Case 1-8 in Chapter 1.

Urologist
urinary system
male genitourinary
surgical subspeciality

Nephrology
kidney
internal medicine subspeciality

CASE 10-1
10-1A Operative Report, Kidney Biopsy

CASE 10-1

The patient in this case was in chronic renal failure with blood (hematuria) and excess protein (proteinuria) in her urine. Dr. Avilla performs a percutaneous kidney biopsy. Report only Dr. Avilla's service.

10-1A OPERATIVE REPORT, KIDNEY BIOPSY

LOCATION: Outpatient, Hospital

PATIENT: Maria Ace

SURGEON: Ira Avilla, M.D.

RADIOLOGIST: Morton Monson, M.D.

PROCEDURE PERFORMED: Kidney biopsy

INDICATIONS: Chronic renal failure, hematuria, and proteinuria

DESCRIPTION OF PROCEDURE: The patient was placed in the prone position. The right kidney was visualized using ultrasound provided by Dr. Monson. The skin was prepped in the usual fashion. One-percent lidocaine was used for local anesthesia. Multiple core biopsies were obtained under real ultrasound guidance using an 18-gauge biopsy gun without difficulty. Multiple core biopsies were obtained and were sent for light electromicroscopy and immune fluorescence.

The patient tolerated the procedure well and without immediate complications. She will be sent back to the procedure area to be monitored in 6 hours with repeat hemoglobin on her.

Pathology Report Later Indicated: Renal cell adenocarcinoma, primary

10-1A:

SERVICE CODE(S):________________________

DX CODE(S):________________________

CASE 10-1 DISCUSSION

Note how in this case the hematuria and proteinuria was not reported because a more definitive diagnosis was stated as a primary, malignant neoplasm of the kidney. Also remember that the kidney is a paired organ, and as such needs the -RT modifier to indicate the kidney on the right side.

Nephrostomy Tube

A nephrostomy tube is a small, flexible tube that is placed into one or both kidneys to drain urine when the kidney is not filtering properly. The tube can be placed temporarily, such as when a patient is being prepared for removal of a large kidney stone, or permanently, such as when the kidney is unable to excrete urine on its own. The **ureter** may also be blocked by a stone, tumor, infection, or scarring. In some settings, the interventional radiologist would conduct these placements or replacements of nephrostomy tubes using ultrasound or x-ray to locate the kidney.

CASE 10-2
10-2A Radiology Report, Nephrostogram
10-2B Operative Report, Nephrostomy Tube Exchange

CASE 10-2

10-2A RADIOLOGY REPORT, NEPHROSTOGRAM

At times, the kidney of a patient with a nephrostomy tube will require examination by means of contrast being injected into the kidney using the existing nephrostomy tube. Dr. Avilla referred Richard Arco to Dr. Monson for an x-ray due to a bloody discharge from Richard's nephrostomy tube. Dr. Monson provided the injection procedure and supervision or interpretation. The diagnoses codes for this case will be for a complication of a urinary catheter and ureter obstruction.

LOCATION: Outpatient, Hospital

PATIENT: Richard Arco

SURGEON: Ira Avilla, M.D.

RADIOLOGIST: Morton Monson, M.D.

EXAMINATION OF: Nephrostogram

CLINICAL SYMPTOMS: Bloody drainage from nephrostomy tube

NEPHROSTOGRAM: HISTORY: A 69-year-old man presents with a longstanding right nephrostomy tube. Recently he has had blood drainage from the nephrostomy tube (*this indicates a complication of the catheter*). The patient's creatinine is 2.5, PT 23.1, INR 4.0, and PTT 52.9. Hemoglobin is stable at 10.7 (last Monday it was 10.6).

FINDINGS: Nephrostogram was performed and compared with the prior study of last month. The patient had been doing well until several days ago, when he started to experience bloody discharge. The patient describes a situation where the tube may have been retracted while he was sleeping. INR is 4.0. Nephrostogram was performed and is basically unremarkable. There continues to be distal right ureter obstruction (*This is the indication of the ureter obstruction.*), and the lower pole calyces are not well identified, and they were not present previously as well. There may be a single calyx (*not a reported diagnosis as it is not confirmed*), which is not seen today. The locking pigtail mechanism is at the edge of the renal pelvis and was advanced several centimeters into a more secure position in the mid to distal renal pelvis. There is no evidence of extravasation or clot within the collecting system. With the patient's coagulation times as abnormal (*this is a diagnosis of abnormal blood chemistry, but it is not reported because it is not the reason the service is being provided; rather, it is an incidental finding*) as they currently are, I felt it was not worth any risk of losing access, and we would just leave the current tube in position. We agree that discontinuing Coumadin at least for a time is worthwhile in hopes of normalizing his coagulation times so that we could discontinue the current problem. The bloody discharge is a serosanguineous fluid. It is mixed with both urine and blood. There were really only a few minimal clots that came with gravity drainage from this. Once the patient's coagulation times are normalized, we will follow this closely, and perhaps at that time we will plan to do other interventions. Again, the patient's hemoglobin is stable. It is 10.7 today and was 10.6 on last Monday.

IMPRESSION: Nephrostogram is basically unremarkable. See above comments.

10-2A:

SERVICE CODE(S): ____________________

DX CODE(S): ____________________

10-2B OPERATIVE REPORT, NEPHROSTOMY TUBE EXCHANGE

The patient in this case requires replacement of a previously placed nephrostomy tube. The diagnosis is the reason for the service, which in this case will be a V code for attention to an artificial opening. No guidance is mentioned in this report.

LOCATION: Outpatient, Hospital

PATIENT: Richard Arco

SURGEON: Ira Avilla, M.D.

EXAMINATION OF: Right nephrostomy tube exchange

CLINICAL SYMPTOMS: Routine exchange of nephrostomy tube

RIGHT NEPHROSTOMY TUBE EXCHANGE: HISTORY: An 82-year-old man presents for routine exchange of nephrostomy tube.

FINDINGS: The patient was prepped and draped in the standard fashion. Through the existing no. 8 French nephrostomy tube, contrast was infused (*injection procedure done by radiologist*) and demonstrated sharp calyces and a well-formed renal pelvis with normal flow of control into the distal right ureter to the level of the uterovesical junction, which is the known site of obstruction. There is no evidence of contrast extending into the bladder. No filling defects or calculi were evident. Then, with standard wire and catheter exchange techniques, the no. 8 French nephrostomy tube was exchanged for a new no. 8 French nephrostomy tube. The locking mechanism pigtail was in the right renal pelvis. There were no complications. The patient tolerated the procedure well. The patient did not receive conscious sedation.

IMPRESSION: Successful exchange of no. 8 French right nephrostomy tube. The patient requires routine 3-month exchanges of right nephrostomy tube.

10-2B:

SERVICE CODE(S):____________________

DX CODE(S):____________________

Nephrectomy

A **nephrectomy** is the partial or total removal of the kidney that may be performed due to disease or in those instances when the patient is donating a kidney (a total removal). The procedure can be performed as an open approach (50220-50240) or as a laparoscopic (50543 or 50545) procedure.

Urinary System Subcategories

Open the CPT manual to the Urinary System category. There are the following categories:

Kidney
Ureter(s) (kidney to bladder)
Bladder
Urethra (bladder to external body)

It is very important to know the anatomy of the urinary system when coding from the subsection. It is all too easy to report the wrong code as all of the categories have many of the same types of subcategories. For example, it is easy to report the wrong code when reporting a procedure of the ureter(s) or the urethra. So, make certain you are in the correct category and subcategory before assigning a code. Also, write in your CPT next to Ureter (50600-50980) "kidney(s) to bladder" and next to Urethra (53000-53899) "bladder to external body." These types of notes will personalize your coding manuals and make them easier to use.

Urinary System Cysts

753.1x is assigned to **congenital cysts** of the urinary system. 593.2 is assigned to **acquired cysts** of the kidney (peripelvic [lymphatic] cyst), and a ureteral polyp and ureterocele is reported with 593.89. If there is no diagnostic statement as to whether the cyst is congenital or acquired, assign a **congenital** diagnosis code. This is because in the Index under the term "Cyst, kidney" the term "(congenital)" is a nonessential modifier, so the cyst does not need to be stated as "congenital" for the code to be assigned.

Further congenital abnormalities of the urinary system include:

753.0x	Renal agenesis (absence of an organ) or dysgenesis
753.1x	Cystic kidney disease (cysts of kidney)
753.2x	Obstructive defects of the renal pelvis and ureter
753.3	Other specified anomalies of the kidney or ureter (includes calculus) and kidney abnormalities (horseshoe kidney)
753.5	Exstrophy (turning inside out) of the urinary bladder
753.6	Atresia (absence of external opening) and stenosis of urethra and bladder neck,
753.7	Anomalies of urachus (connects urinary bladder with umbilicus in fetus)
753.8	Other anomalies of the bladder and urethra (such as hernia of bladder and prolapse of bladder)

If the condition is an acquired calculus of the kidney or ureter, code 592.x is assigned. If the calculus is a congenital condition, assign 753.3. If there is no diagnostic statement as to whether the cyst is congenital or acquired, assign an **acquired** diagnosis code. This is because in the Index, under the main term "Calculus, kidney," there is a subterm for "congenital," so unless the stone was specifically stated as congenital, it would be coded as acquired, even though there is no acquired terminology in the Index under the term calculus.

Cyst – no diagnostic statement – code as congenital
Calculus, kidney – code as acquired if no diagnostic statement

CASE 10-3
10-3A Operative Report, Nephrectomy

CASE 10-3

10-3A OPERATIVE REPORT, NEPHRECTOMY

LOCATION: Inpatient, Hospital

PATIENT: Rosa Alvarado

SURGEON: Ira Avilla, M.D.

PREOPERATIVE DIAGNOSIS: Multicystic, dysplastic left kidney

POSTOPERATIVE DIAGNOSIS: Multicystic, dysplastic left kidney

PROCEDURE PERFORMED: Left laparoscopic radical nephrectomy

CLINICAL NOTE: The patient was found to have a multicystic, dysplastic kidney on investigation for abdominal pain. There are multiple complex cysts of this kidney. It is grossly enlarged. There is no way to determine whether there are malignant changes. It is decided to proceed with attempt at laparoscopic nephrectomy for removal of this. Renogram showed the primary dominant kidney to be the right kidney.

OPERATIVE NOTE: The patient was given a general endotracheal anesthetic, prepped, and draped in the left flank position. Foley catheter was placed, and an orogastric tube was placed. Hassan trocar was placed two fingerbreadths above and lateral to the umbilicus at the lateral margin of the rectus fascia. Two further 12-mm ports were placed in the right lower quadrant under visual guidance, and a 5-mm port was placed in the subcostal position in the anterior axillary line.

The colon was mobilized off the kidney. The kidney was grossly enlarged. Cysts could be seen bulging through perirenal fat.

The kidney was mobilized, and the renal hilum was identified. The ureter was identified just below the lower pole of the renal kidney, where it was doubly clipped and divided and used for retraction. A single renal vein and renal artery were identified. The renal artery was in a posterior superior position. This was triply clipped on the patient's side and doubly on the specimen side and divided. The linear GIA was then utilized to clip the renal vein. It was decided to try to spare the adrenal gland, and therefore Gerota's fascia superior to the kidney was taken, but the adrenal gland was left in situ. A harmonic scalpel was used for mobilization. Multiple collateral vessels were around the kidney and desmoplastic reaction. At one point during mobilization, the cyst was entered and the contents spilled. These were evacuated during suction. Then the wound was irrigated at this point and then subsequently. The specimen was ultimately mobilized and freed. It was placed in a large lap sac, and the lap sac was brought through the Hassan trocar site. The wound was draped with clean towels, and the kidney was morselized using the sponge forceps. All cyst fluid was suctioned from the bag and sent for cytologic evaluation. A total of 600 cc of fluid was obtained. The specimen was also sent for pathology. A small pale nodule was identified during the morselization, and this was sent separately as the renal mass.

Gown and gloves were changed; green towels were removed and Hassan trocar reintroduced. The wound was thoroughly irrigated using 1L of Kefzol/heparin in normal saline. Hemostasis was ensured. The 12-mm trocar sites were closed using a GraNee needle and 2-0 Vicryl. Peritoneum and external oblique fascia were closed in the Hassan trocar site using 2-0 Vicryl. Skin was closed with subcuticular Dexon. Sponge and needle counts were reported correct. The patient tolerated the procedure well and was transferred to the recovery room in good condition.

ESTIMATED BLOOD LOSS: 100 cc

Pathology Report Later Indicated: Multiple, benign renal cysts

10-3A:

SERVICE CODE(S):____________________

DX CODE(S):____________________

Renal Calculus

Renal calculus is a kidney stone and often causes excruciating pain. Stones form due to structural disorders, metabolic abnormalities, or recurrent urinary tract infections. Structural abnormalities such as cysts of the kidney (polycystic kidney disease), obstructions, and malformed kidneys predispose stone formation. Metabolic conditions (e.g., hypercalciuria and hyperuricemia) that increase the body's production of calcium increase the chances of kidney stone. Most stones are composed of calcium and magnesium, although stones of other constituents are not uncommon. Stones are very small, with a usual diameter of 1.5 cm or smaller. X-ray (KUB), CT scan, or ultrasound may be useful to visualize the stone. Stones usually pass spontaneously but on occasion may require intervention. Methods of removal include pharmaceuticals that dissolve calcium-based stones, percutaneous removal, transurethral ureteroscopy, extracorporeal shock wave lithotripsy (ESWL), or even open surgical removal. ESWL is the use of ultrasound to shatter the stone so the fragments will then usually pass spontaneously.

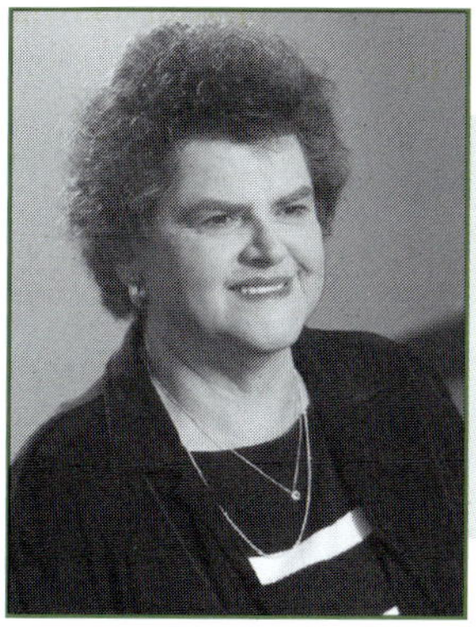

FROM THE TRENCHES

Dorothy

Has being certified made a difference in your job?

"Yes. I don't code on a daily basis, but I'm a Medicare Specialist, so codes matter. Proper reimbursement [is important] as far as fraud and abuse, medical necessity—I work with all of that... I need to know what the codes say."

CASE 10-4

10-4A OPERATIVE REPORT, ESWL

LOCATION: Outpatient, Hospital

PATIENT: Juan Santos

SURGEON: Ira Avilla, M.D.

PREOPERATIVE DIAGNOSIS: Left renal calculus

POSTOPERATIVE DIAGNOSIS: Left renal calculus

PROCEDURE PERFORMED: Left ESWL (extracorporeal shock wave lithotripsy)

CLINICAL NOTE: This gentleman came in with renal colic, and a stent was placed. He had his anticoagulation reversed and presents now for ESWL.

The patient was given a general laryngeal mask anesthetic, prepped, and draped in the supine position. Stone was targeted and shock head engaged. A total of 2400 shocks at maximum KV and stone partial fragmentation and dissolution could be seen. The patient tolerated the procedure well and transferred to the recovery room in good condition. He will be seen in follow-up in 2 weeks' time for KUB.

10-4A:

SERVICE CODE(S):____________________

DX CODE(S):____________________

Urodynamics

Urodynamics is used to study how the bladder stores and releases urine, such as the bladder capacity and ability of the bladder to empty completely. Circular muscle (**sphincters**) close tightly around the urethra to prevent the leakage of urine (incontinence). If the urinary problem is related to nerve damage, electrodes (electromyographic electrodes) may be placed into the urethra and rectum to assess the response of these muscles. When EMG electrodes are used as a part of the urodynamic study, they are reported separately. Another component of the urodynamic assessment may be a cystometrogram (CMG) in which a small catheter is placed into the bladder and warm water is placed into the bladder to measure the capacity of the bladder. Leak point pressure can also be assessed by means of the CMG when the patient coughs with a full bladder. The CMG can also measure the pressure required to urinate with a voiding pressure study (VCUG) that is reported separately. X-ray or ultrasound (video urodynamics) may also be used to image the filling and emptying of the bladder. Contrast material is added to the liquid that is used to fill the bladder to enhance the image.

The notes preceding the Urodynamic category of codes 51725-51798 indicate that if the physician interprets the results or operates the equipment, modifier -26 is to be added to identify that only the professional component of the service was provided. When codes in this category are reported without -26, that use indicates that the professional and technical components of the service were provided. If, for example, the urodynamic assessment was provided by a clinic physician in the outpatient department of the hospital, the hospital would report the technical component and the physician would report the professional component with the -26 modifier.

voiding pressure study (VCUG)

CASE 10-5

The following report indicates the components that are to be coded with bold typeface. You are reporting the professional component of the service, so remember to use the correct modifier (-26) to indicate only the professional component of the service. Because there are multiple procedures, you will need to indicate that with a modifier. Remember to place the modifiers on the code in ascending order with the lowest numbered modifier first followed by the higher numbered modifier.

10-5A URODYNAMIC ASSESSMENT

LOCATION: Outpatient, Hospital

PATIENT: Elva Sexton

SURGEON: Ira Avilla, M.D.

DIAGNOSIS: Chronic renal failure

This lady is referred for urodynamic assessment prior to renal transplantation. Previous attempts were unsuccessful in that she was having what appeared to be a significant hypoglycemic episode and was referred to the emergency room. I have not heard of any follow-up from our emergency department in this regard. The patient presents now.

Uroflow: *(This is the uroflowmetry service.)*

Maximum flow: 17 ml/sec
Average flow: 5.4 ml/sec
Voided volume: 64 cc
Voiding pattern is normal.

Cystometrogram: *(This is the cystometrogram service.)*

Urethral and rectal catheters were placed. EMG electrodes applied. The patient was placed in a semisitting position.

The first sensation of bladder filling after 161 cc
Normal desire to void 289 cc
Strong desire to void 369 cc
Maximum cystometrogram capacity 520 cc

No evidence of uninhibited bladder contractions was seen. **Leak point pressure** *(This is the voiding pressure study of the bladder.)* was not established with Valsalva in excess of 80 cm of water. The patient could not void with the Foley catheter in situ. She did void by Valsalva. Pressure flow showed no evidence of obstruction. EMG activity was normal.

Once the catheter was removed, the patient was able to void easily without evidence of Valsalva and voided to completeness.

ASSESSMENT: No evidence of uninhibited bladder contractions. Normal bladder capacity. The patient was unable to void with catheter in situ, but normal uroflow study and post EMG voiding suggest normal detrusor function.

10-5A:

SERVICE CODE(S):____________________

DX CODE(S):____________________

Stress Incontinence

Stress incontinence is involuntary loss of urine that is usually associated with activities that increase the bladder pressure, such as coughing, sneezing, or exercising. This is a condition that most often occurs in women due to physical changes resulting from pregnancy, childbirth, and menopause. The pelvic floor muscles that support the bladder become weakened and the bladder moves downward (prolapses), preventing the muscles (sphincters) that would force the urethra shut from contracting properly, resulting in leakage. After more conservative treatments have failed, surgery may be used to alleviate the incontinence, such as a wing sling that holds the bladder up and returns it to normal position.

CASE 10-6
10-6A Operative Report, Urethropexy

CASE 10-6

10-6A OPERATIVE REPORT, URETHROPEXY

LOCATION: Outpatient, Hospital

PATIENT: Jan Barens

SURGEON: Ira Avilla, M.D.

PREOPERATIVE DIAGNOSIS: Stress incontinence

POSTOPERATIVE DIAGNOSIS: Stress incontinence

PROCEDURE PERFORMED: Anterior urethropexy

CLINICAL NOTE: The patient is a 59-year-old woman who has stress incontinence. She is undergoing oophorectomy and colposuspension for enterocele. She also has stress incontinence and a hypermobile urethra.

PROCEDURE: The patient was already open and had undergone bilateral oophorectomy by Dr. Sanchez. Prior to apical suspension, I was asked to perform her anterior urethropexy.

The Foley catheter was in situ. With a finger in the vagina, the urethra was identified and sutures were placed bilaterally at the mid-portion of the urethra 1 cm lateral and at the bladder neck 2 cm lateral. These sutures were then suspended to Cooper's ligament bilaterally. The sutures were tied down to elevate the urethra to the horizontal position. One finger could be passed between the urethra and the symphysis anteriorly. Hemostasis was ensured.

10-6A:

SERVICECODE(S):________________________________

DX CODE(S):________________________________

Bladder Rupture

The bladder is ruptured when pressure is placed on a distended bladder. This type of injury is often associated with seatbelt injury in which extreme force results in a compression rupture and most often results in a laceration of the dome of the bladder. The bladder is repaired by means of suture repair (cystorrhaphy) of the resulting lacerations either by percutaneous or open abdominal surgical approach.

CASE 10-7
10-7A Operative Report, Intraperitoneal Bladder Rupture

CASE 10-7

10-7A OPERATIVE REPORT, INTRAPERITONEAL BLADDER RUPTURE

This is an internal injury to the bladder as a result of a fall from a ladder that required a complicated repair. The injury is the primary diagnosis followed by an E code to indicate how the injury happened.

LOCATION: Inpatient, Hospital

PATIENT: Racio Ruiz

SURGEON: Ira Avilla, M.D.

PREOPERATIVE DIAGNOSIS: Intraperitoneal bladder rupture

POSTOPERATIVE DIAGNOSIS: Intraperitoneal bladder rupture

PROCEDURE PERFORMED: Repair of retroperitoneal bladder rupture

INDICATIONS: This is a 22-year-old who sustained an intraperitoneal bladder rupture secondary to a fall from a ladder.

ANESTHESIA: General

PROCEDURE: The patient was brought to the operative theater and placed in the supine position on the operating table. After receiving a general anesthetic, he was prepped and draped in a sterile fashion. A vertical midline incision was made from a little above the umbilicus down to the pubis. Dissection was carried down through the subcutaneous tissues and through the anterior fascia. The peritoneal cavity was entered sharply. Some blood clots down in the pelvis were seen overlying the bladder. This area was packed off. We then examined the rest of the abdomen. There were no blood or fluid collections elsewhere. We did not extend the incision all the way up to the top, so it was difficult to get good visualization of the liver and the spleen; however, there was no blood in this area, and palpation of them revealed no abnormalities. The stomach felt normal. Orogastric tube showed good placement. The small bowel was run from the ligament of Treitz to the terminal ileum. This was fine. The appendix was present and normal. The colon was grossly normal throughout its length. Some stool was present. No gross abnormalities were seen down to the pelvis. We had to remove the packing. There were some blood clots setting in the bladder itself. He had a fairly long laceration (*indicates complexity*) that was for the most part vertical and went fairly close to the superior anterior aspect and continued about two thirds of the way down, pretty much right over the dome (*indicates complexity*). We inspected the inside of the bladder. No other lesions or lacerations could be identified. We then closed this in two layers (*indicates complexity*). The inner layer was a 3-0 Vicryl in a running fashion. We then imbricated all of this with interrupted sutures of 3-0 Vicryl through the serosa/peritoneum. There was another bit of lateral laceration that was not full thickness but involving just the serosa. This was also repaired with interrupted sutures of 3-0 Vicryl in a Lembert fashion. This was to the left side, and there was also another short one to the right side. We made sure that each of the corners/apexes had a three-corner stitch placed. We then gently filled the bladder with 250 cc of methylene blue/normal saline solution. No leaks were identified. We then allowed everything to flush back out and irrigated out the pelvis and the abdomen. Clear returns were present. We again looked down the pelvis to be sure there were no other injuries. He currently has a no. 18 French three-way catheter in place. Instead of placing a suprapubic tube, I think it would be easier to manage him with this Foley catheter, and we will plan to take this out in 2 to 3 weeks' time. He will be allowed to go home with a leg bag. We then pulled down the omentum over the small bowel. We closed the fascia with no. 1 looped PDS in a running fashion. The wound was irrigated out. The skin was then closed with staples. Sterile dressings were applied. The patient tolerated the procedure well and went to the recovery room in stable condition.

10-7A:

SERVICE CODE(S):____________________

DX CODE(S):____________________

Hydronephrosis

Hydronephrosis is an increase in the size of the renal pelvis and calyces and may have a variety of causes, such as obstruction by tumor or stricture in the urinary system. This is a serious condition that, if unattended, can lead to infection and subsequent sepsis. A cystoscopic examination of the urinary system may be performed to ensure that the collection system is free of obstruction. Fluoroscopic examination may also be performed during the procedure and is reported separately on an hourly basis.

CASE 10-8
10-8A Operative Report, Cystoscopy

CASE 10-8

In the following case Dr. Avilla provided ***both*** *the cystoscopic and fluoroscopic examination of the kidney. The physician also reports the bilateral retrograde pyelogram.*

10-8A OPERATIVE REPORT, CYSTOSCOPY

LOCATION: Outpatient, Hospital

PATIENT: Beth Childs

SURGEON: Ira Avilla, M.D.

PREOPERATIVE DIAGNOSIS:
1. Right hydronephrosis
2. Hematuria

POSTOPERATIVE DIAGNOSIS:
1. Mild hydronephrosis
2. No evidence of obstruction
3. Possible old vesicoureteral reflux

PROCEDURE PERFORMED: Cystoscopy, bilateral retrograde pyelogram under fluoroscopic control

CLINICAL NOTE: The patient is a 79-year-old woman who presented with microhematuria (*blood seen with microscope*). Ultrasound showed mild right hydronephrosis.

OPERATIVE NOTE: The patient was prepped and draped in the lithotomy position, given IV sedation, and the urethra was anesthetized with 2% Xylocaine generally. The patient was cystoscoped. The urethra was normal. There was no evidence of bladder neoplasia. Ureteric orifices and ureters were fairly lateral but appeared normal in shape and size. Bilateral retrograde pyelogram was performed, which showed normal collecting system on the left-hand side. The right system was indeed hydronephrotic, but no evidence of filling defect or calculi was identified. The system drained well on fluoroscopic images. I wonder if she may have had mild reflux at a younger age because of this appearance. At any rate, there was no evidence of inflammation or neoplasia or other significant abnormality. The patient tolerated the procedure well. She will be followed up in the clinic in 3 months' time.

10-8A:

SERVICE CODE(S):____________________

DX CODE(S):____________________

Bladder Stones

There are several types of bladder stones: secondary, migrant, and endemic. Secondary stones are those that are formed due to a bladder condition, such as obstruction or infections. Migrant stones originate in the kidney and pass out through the bladder, sometimes becoming lodged in the bladder or ureter. Endemic stones are caused by nutritional deficiencies and are uncommon in the United States. Symptoms of a bladder stone are pain and hematuria.

CASE 10-9
10-9A Operative Report, Ureteroscopic Stone Extraction

CASE 10-9

*The following case involves the removal of a ureteral calculus by means of ureteroscope and insertion of a stent using fluoroscopic imaging. Dr. Avilla provided **both** the scoping procedure and the fluoroscopic imaging supervision and interpretation.*

10-9A OPERATIVE REPORT, URETEROSCOPIC STONE EXTRACTION

LOCATION: Outpatient, Hospital

PATIENT: Oscar Adkins

SURGEON: Ira Avilla, M.D.

PREOPERATIVE DIAGNOSIS: Left ureteral calculus

POSTOPERATIVE DIAGNOSIS: Left ureteral calculus

PROCEDURE PERFORMED: Left ureteroscopic stone extraction and stent insertion under fluoroscopic control

CLINICAL NOTE: The patient is a 37-year-old man with a 3½-week history of intermittent left renal colic. He now has significant urinary frequency.

PROCEDURE: The patient was prepped and draped in the lithotomy position after being given a general endotracheal anesthetic. A 21-French cystoscope was passed per urethra under direct vision. The urethra was normal. The prostate showed mild lateral lobe enlargement and mild outlet obstruction with mild bladder trabeculation. The bladder mucosa was normal without evidence of inflammation or neoplasia. The left ureteral orifice appeared quite narrow. A Terumo guide wire was advanced up the left ureter under fluoroscopic control and beyond the stone in the distal left ureter. Again, attempts to pass the rigid ureteroscope without prior ureteral dilation were unsuccessful because of significant ureteral stenosis. A 6-French balloon dilation catheter was then placed, and the distal ureter was dilated under fluoroscopic control. This was withdrawn, and then the patient was ureteroscoped using 6- and 7-French rigid ureteroscopes. The stone was visualized, grasped with a helical basket, and withdrawn intact. Because of significant ureteral edema from stone impaction, it was decided to stent the patient. A 6-French 28-cm Bard inlay stent was then placed under fluoroscopic control in the usual fashion. The guide wire was withdrawn and the bladder drained. A B and O suppository was placed rectally. The patient tolerated the procedure well and was transferred to the recovery room in good condition.

Pathology Report Later Indicated: Ureteral calculus

10-9A:

SERVICE CODE(S):__________

DX CODE(S):__________

CASE 10-10
10-10A Operative Report, Stent Insertion and TURP

CASE 10-10

Radi Riley has metastatic prostate cancer with liver metastases. There is concern that the cancer is blocking his ureters and has resulted in hydronephrosis. Dr. Avilla is going to open the ureter by means of cystoscope and place a stent to improve his kidney function. Dr. Avilla places the cystoscope into the meatus, through the urethra, and into the bladder with guidance and attempts to correct the obstruction of the left and right ureters. Dr. Avilla provided ***both*** *the guidance and procedure portions of this service.*

10-10A OPERATIVE REPORT, STENT INSERTION AND TURP

LOCATION: Inpatient, Hospital

PATIENT: Radi Riley

SURGEON: Ira Avilla, M.D.

PREOPERATIVE DIAGNOSIS: Left ureteral obstruction

POSTOPERATIVE DIAGNOSIS: Recurrent prostate cancer with bilateral ureteral obstruction. (*Ureter obstruction is the third listed diagnosis.*) Liver metastasis.

PROCEDURE PERFORMED: Cystoscopy. (*Cystourethroscopy with resection of the prostate is the primary procedure*). Attempted left ureteral stent insertion. Right ureteral stent insertion (*Cystourethroscopic insertion of ureteral stent is the second procedure.*) under fluoroscopic control. (*The professional component of the fluoroscopic guidance is the third procedure.*) Transurethral resection of recurrent prostate cancer.

CLINICAL NOTE: The patient has known extensive prostate cancer (*primary neoplasm*) with multiple liver metastases (*secondary neoplasm*). He has responded well to initial antiandrogens but now is on Decadron for androgen resistant prostate cancer. He is noted to have left hydronephrosis, and it was decided to try to stent the left ureter after discussion with the daughter and patient. Obviously, his disease is progressing and his long-term outcome is dismal, but over the short term, we had hoped to preserve some renal function.

OPERATIVE NOTE: The patient was given IV sedation and prepped and draped in the lithotomy position. The flexible cystoscope was passed per urethra. The urethra was normal. Prostate fossa was open. There was increased size in the lesions over the left ureteric orifices from just a couple weeks ago when he was last cystoscoped. I could not identify the orifice; several attempts were unsuccessful. The rigid cystoscope was then employed, and again I was unable to identify the orifice. A guide wire was advanced up the right ureteric orifice under fluoroscopic control. The cancer seemed to be encroaching quite quickly on the right orifice, and therefore it was thought best to stent it.

The patient was stented using a 6-French 26-cm stent under fluoroscopic control in the usual fashion. The rectoscope was then introduced into the bladder under direct vision. The area of recurrent tumor overlying the left ureteral orifice was resected. Careful inspection was carried out down to the point where I could just begin to see paravesicle fat. A ureteric orifice and ureter could not be identified, and therefore the procedure was terminated at this time. The area was cauterized and chips were evacuated from the bladder. Hemostasis was achieved. A 22 three-way catheter was inserted into the bladder and placed for continuous bladder irrigation.

I will have to have a straightforward discussion with the patient and his daughter with regard to any further intervention. We could proceed with left nephrostomy tube insertion and subsequent antegrade stenting or just leave him with this solitary ureteral stent and change this on a regular basis.

10-10A:

SERVICE CODE(S):______________________________

DX CODE(S):______________________________

Urethral Strictures

Urethral strictures (narrowing) result in frequent, slow urination and can lead to infection. The treatment of a stricture is based on the type and duration of the stricture. The narrowing can be alleviated by means of excision using a cystoscopic knife or dilation (stretching). For example, a cystourethroscopy with ureteral meatotomy is when the surgeon inserts a scope through the urethra and bladder and makes an **incision** of the ureter into the bladder (52290). Compare this procedure to 52281, which is also a cystourethroscopy but one that widens the urethra by dilating a urethral stricture/stenosis by means of a **balloon** catheter. Note 52281 specifies "male or female."

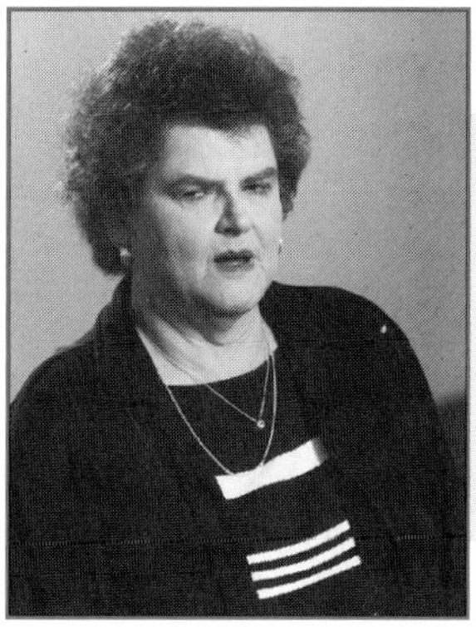

FROM THE TRENCHES

Dorothy

"I have to look at a lot of codes...that have been rejected for some reason and see if it was a coding issue. Was the coder not as knowledgeable as he or she should have been—or was it a matter of the physician not giving her what he or she needed to do a better job? These are the things that I look into."

CASE 10-11
10-11A Operative Report, Meatotomy

CASE 10-11

Keith Hanshaw is a 5-year-old boy who has been diagnosed with urethral stenosis (narrowing) and requires a meatotomy to open the urethral area to allow normal urine flow.

10-11A OPERATIVE REPORT, MEATOTOMY

LOCATION: Outpatient, Hospital

PATIENT: Keith Hanshaw

SURGEON: Ira Avilla, M.D.

PREOPERATIVE DIAGNOSIS: Urethral meatal stenosis

POSTOPERATIVE DIAGNOSIS: Urethral meatal stenosis

PROCEDURE PERFORMED: Urethral meatotomy and cystoscopy

ANESTHESIA: General mask

PROCEDURE: The patient was given a general mask anesthetic as well as a caudal block for postoperative pain control. He was prepped and draped in the lithotomy position. The meatus was calibrated and found to be tight at the 8-French level. A meatotomy was then performed in a ventral position in the standard fashion. Then 4-0 chromic sutures were placed to reapproximate urethral and penile skin. The patient was then cystoscoped using a 9-French instrument. Urethra was normal. Sphincter was intact. The prostate was not obstructed. There were no posterior urethral valves. The ureteric orifices were normal. The trigone was normal. The bladder mucosa was normal. The bladder was drained and the cystoscope withdrawn. The patient tolerated the procedure well and was transferred to the recovery room in good condition.

10-11A:

SERVICE CODE(S):____________________

DX CODE(S):____________________

Male Genital System

A urologist is also a specialist in the diagnosis and treatment of male genital system conditions. Common conditions are benign prostatic hyperplasia, neoplasm of the prostate, and testicular **hydrocele**. Services include procedures of the penis, testis, epididymis, tunica vaginalis, scrotum, vas deferens, spermatic cord, seminal vesicles, and prostate.

Hemangioma

A **hemangioma** is a common benign tumor that commonly occurs in infants and children, although it may occur in patients of any age. The tumor is formed of blood vessels and can be difficult to remove because of the vascularity of the mass. The mass may be removed by means of electrodesiccation, application of chemicals, application of liquid nitrogen, cryothermal instrument, laser beam, or blunt excision. Codes for destruction of lesions of the penis, such as condyloma, papilloma, and herpetic vesicle, are included in the Destruction category of codes (54050-54065). These codes can be located in the Index of the CPT manual under the heading of "Penis" or "Destruction, Penis."

Diagnosis Coding of Hemangioma

Hemangiomas are reported with 228.xx based on the site (such as skin, intracranial, retina, intra-abdominal, other, or unspecified) and includes congenital hemangiomas. You can locate the direction to the codes for hemangioma in the Index of the ICD-9-CM under the main term "Hemangioma" and subtermed by location.

CASE 10-12
10-12A Operative Report, Resection

CASE 10-12

Report Dr. Avilla's surgical services.

10-12A OPERATIVE REPORT, RESECTION

LOCATION: Outpatient, Hospital

PATIENT: Harold Arin

SURGEON: Ira Avilla, M.D.

PREOPERATIVE DIAGNOSIS: Penile mass

POSTOPERATIVE DIAGNOSIS: Probable large hemangioma with vascular malformation and superficial dorsal venous complex, penis

PROCEDURE PERFORMED: Resection of large penile vascular mass

CLINICAL NOTE: This 23-year-old gentleman presents with a 1-month history of increased tender dorsal penile mass. Ultrasound, CT, and MRI have all shown this to be a solid lesion. No flow has been documented within it, and it is suggested that it might be a sarcoma. It is fluctuant and soft, and I wonder whether it might be vascular, but this has not been confirmed on previous imaging.

OPERATIVE NOTE: The patient was given a general endotracheal anesthetic, prepped, and draped in a supine position. An incision was made overlying this large dorsal penile mass at the base of the penis. Just beneath the skin, a large vein was encountered that bled and was dealt with by isolating it and ligating it with 3-0 chromic ligatures. The mass was large, approximately 10 cm in greatest diameter. There was extensive neovascularity, and on further dissection, it was noted that this appeared to be a large hemangioma rising from superficial veins outside Buck's fascia. Extensive care and mobilization were undertaken. This, again, was a very vascular lesion, and I took care to identify all perforating vessels and individually ligated them with chromic ligature. Intraoperative photographs were obtained of the mass showing its extensive vascularity and its location. Frozen section of the mass was obtained that showed no malignant cells. Once the mass was resected, there was a very large cavity. Subcutaneous tissues were closed with 4-0 chromic and skin ultimately with subcuticular Dexon. Compression dressing was applied. The patient tolerated the procedure well and was transferred to the recovery room in good condition.

Pathology Report Later Indicated: Benign hemangioma

10-12A:

SERVICE CODE(S):____________________

DX CODE(S):____________________

Balanitis and Circumcision

Balanitis is an inflammation of the glans penis, and **phimosis** is a constriction of the prepucial orifice that does not allow for the foreskin to fold back over the glans. **Circumcision** is incision of the foreskin and removal of a portion of the foreskin.

The CPT codes for circumcision (54150-54161) are divided based on the method of circumcision (clamp or surgical excision) and whether the patient is a newborn or other than a newborn.

CASE 10-13
10-13A Operative Report, Circumcision

CASE 10-13

10-13A OPERATIVE REPORT, CIRCUMCISION

LOCATION: Outpatient, Hospital

PATIENT: Harlen Mata

SURGEON: Ira Avilla, M.D.

PREOPERATIVE DIAGNOSIS: Recurrent candidiasis, balanitis, and phimosis

POSTOPERATIVE DIAGNOSIS: Recurrent candidiasis, balanitis, and phimosis

PROCEDURE PERFORMED: Circumcision

PROCEDURE: This 2-year-old male child was given general mask anesthetic as well as caudal block for postoperative pain control. He was prepped and draped in the supine position, foreskin retracted, and prepucial adhesions broken down. Circumcision was performed using a dorsal slit technique. Hemostasis was achieved with judicious use of electrocautery and chromic ties. Prepuce was re-anastomosed to the penile skin using 5-0 chromic catgut. Vaseline gauze dressing was applied. The patient tolerated the procedure well and was transferred to the recovery room in good condition.

Pathology Report Later Indicated: Benign penile tissue

10-13A:

SERVICE CODE(S):____________________

DX CODE(S):____________________

CASE 10-14
10-14A Operative Report, Biopsy

CASE 10-14

Azoospermia, sometimes documented as male infertility, is the absence of sperm and can be caused by many conditions, including neoplasm of the testes. Biopsies of the testis can be accomplished by means of percutaneous biopsy or open incision biopsy. Code the following services provided to John Ibarra.

10-14A OPERATIVE REPORT, BIOPSY

LOCATION: Outpatient, Hospital

PATIENT: John Ibarra

SURGEON: Ira Avilla, M.D.

PREOPERATIVE DIAGNOSIS: Azoospermia

POSTOPERATIVE DIAGNOSIS: Azoospermia

PROCEDURE PERFORMED: Bilateral testicular biopsies

PROCEDURE: The patient was given a general mask anesthetic and prepped and draped in the supine position. Bilateral testicular cord blocks were performed with a 50% mixture of 0.5% Marcaine and 2% Xylocaine with epinephrine. Beginning on the right side, a scrotal incision was made. The tunica vaginalis was identified and opened, and a stay stitch was placed in the testis. A small incision was made, and tubules delivered, resected, and sent for permanent resection. The testis was closed with 3-0 Vicryl, the tunica vaginalis with 3-0 chromic, and skin with 3-0 chromic.

The procedure was repeated in identical fashion on the contralateral side. The patient tolerated the procedure well. Dressings were applied. Scrotal support was applied. He will be contacted when the results are available. A discharge prescription for Tylenol no. 3 was given.

Pathology Report Later Indicated: Benign testicular tissue

10-14A:

SERVICE CODE(S):____________________________

DX CODE(S):____________________________

Vasectomy

A **vasectomy** is a method of permanent birth control for men that is nearly 100% effective. Sperm are produced in the testicles and mix with seminal fluid to form semen. A vasectomy intersects (cuts) the vas deferens and blocks the sperm from mixing with the seminal fluid. During ejaculation the sperm-free seminal fluid is ejected. If a vasectomy is an incidental procedure conducted at the time of a more major procedure of the area, the vasectomy is not reported separately but is bundled into the more major procedure.

If the only reason the patient presents is for sterilization, a V code is assigned to indicate an encounter for the purpose of sterilization.

CASE 10-15

10-15A OPERATIVE REPORT, VASECTOMY

LOCATION: Outpatient, Hospital

PATIENT: Jessy Arley

SURGEON: Ira Avilla, M.D.

PROCEDURE NOTE: The patient is in for a vasectomy having undergone counseling earlier today. He was placed in a supine position, and the scrotal area was shaved. Under sterile technique, the scrotal area was prepped with Betadine, and the sterile drapes were applied. The right vas was localized and under sterile technique was infiltrated with 1% Xylocaine. The vas was externalized, and 1.5-cm portion of the tube was removed. Proximal and distal stumps were doubly ligated with 4-0 silk. A small blood vessel in the skin was oozing and was clamped. Attention was directed to the left side, where a similar procedure was performed. With hemostasis intact, the proximal and distal stumps on the left were retracted into the scrotum, and attention was directed to the right side, where there was slight oozing from the skin edge. With pressure, this did resolve, and the proximal and distal stumps were retracted into the scrotum.

ASSESSMENT: Vasectomy

PLAN: The patient had been given the postvasectomy instruction sheet, and Bacitracin and gauze dressing were applied. He is to apply antibiotics a couple of times a day with gauze. He was given an instruction sheet to have sperm counts done in 2 months' time and to take contraceptive precautions in the meantime.

Pathology Report Later Indicated: Benign vas deferens tissue

10-15A:

SERVICE CODE(S):____________________

DX CODE(S):____________________

Hydrocele

Hydrocele is an accumulation of fluid caused by trauma, infection, or tumor; treatment can include surgical excision of the hydrocele. **Epididymitis** is inflammation of the epididymis (**Figure 10-1**); treatment can include surgical excision of the epididymis.

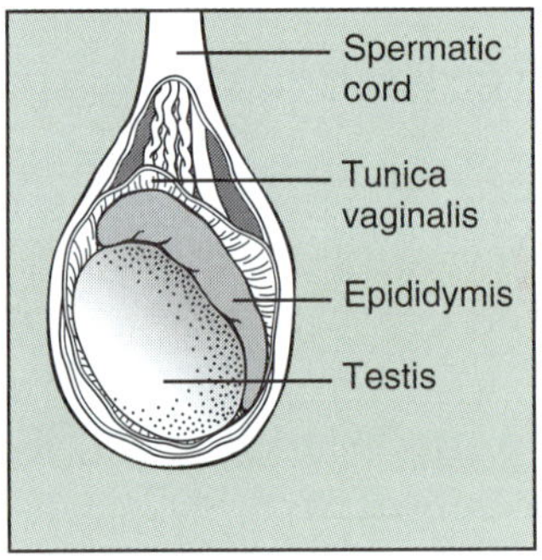

FIGURE 10-1 Scrotal contents.

CASE 10-16
10-16A Operative Report, Resection Hydrocele and Epididymectomy

CASE 10-16

10-16A OPERATIVE REPORT, RESECTION HYDROCELE AND EPIDIDYMECTOMY

This service includes a unilateral excision of epididymis and a unilateral excision of hydrocele. Remember to use the correct HCPCS modifier to indicate on which side the surgery was performed. The diagnoses codes must support the reason for each of these two services. See Figure 10-2 for illustration.

LOCATION: Outpatient, Hospital

PATIENT: Dwain Frost

SURGEON: Ira Avilla, M.D.

PREOPERATIVE DIAGNOSIS: Recurrent left hydrocele, chronic epididymitis

POSTOPERATIVE DIAGNOSIS: Recurrent left hydrocele, chronic epididymitis

PROCEDURE PERFORMED: Resection of left hydrocele and left epididymectomy

CLINICAL NOTE: This gentleman has a recurrent left hydrocele and chronic epididymal pain. On examination, he is very tender in his epididymis. I have discussed options with him. He has requested a left epididymectomy and repair of the hydrocele.

He is aware of the potential risks associated with this procedure, including infection, chronic pain, and testicular atrophy.

PROCEDURE: The patient was given general endotracheal anesthetic and prepped and draped in the supine position. A left ilioinguinal nerve block was performed with a 50% mixture of 2% Xylocaine and 0.5% Marcaine with epinephrine. A scrotal incision was made and the testis delivered. There were dense adhesions of the pseudohydrocele sac around the scrotum; these were liberated using electrocautery. The sac was then opened and resected. The epididymis was buried beneath scar tissue. With electrocautery and sharp and blunt technique, the epididymis was identified and resected, and hemostasis was ensured. I could not identify the testicular artery, but I do not believe it was involved. Hemostasis was ensured, and the testis returned to the scrotum. A 1/4-inch Penrose drain was left through a separate stab wound and sutured to the skin with 3-0 Prolene. The scrotum was closed in two layers with 3-0 chromic. A supportive dressing was applied. The patient tolerated the procedure well and was discharged in good condition. He will be seen next week in the clinic for drain removal.

Pathology Report Later Indicated: Benign epididymis tissue

10-16A:

SERVICE CODE(S):______________________________

DX CODE(S):______________________________

Prostate-Specific Antigen

Prostate-specific antigen (PSA) is secreted by the epithelial cells of the prostate gland (including cancerous cells), and an elevation in the levels of PSA in the blood indicates an abnormality of the prostate gland. The screening test is used to detect potential problems in the prostate gland and to follow the progress of prostate cancer. A reading greater than 4 ng/ml is abnormal and generally indicates that a prostate biopsy would be performed. A biopsy may be obtained transrectally and often includes the use of ultrasound to ensure correct placement of the biopsy forceps. The ultrasound is reported in addition to the biopsy code. The biopsy may also be obtained by an incisional approach.

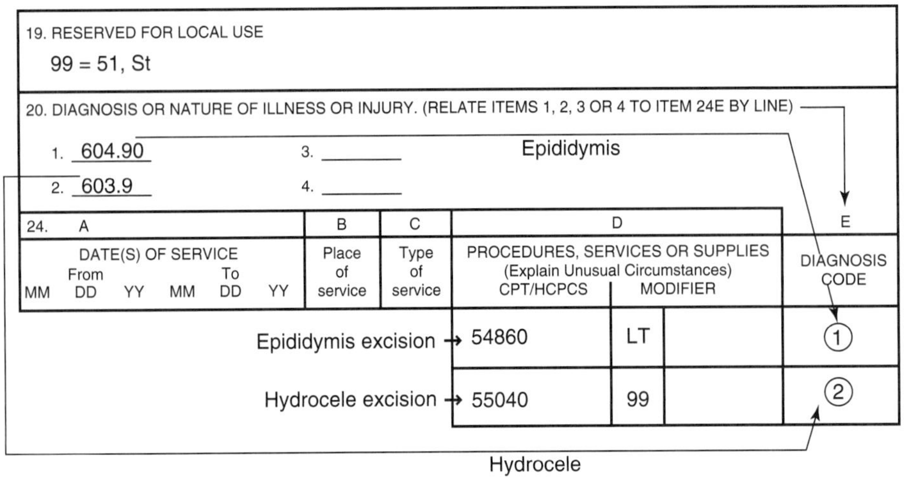

FIGURE 10-2 Diagnosis supports medical necessity for each service.

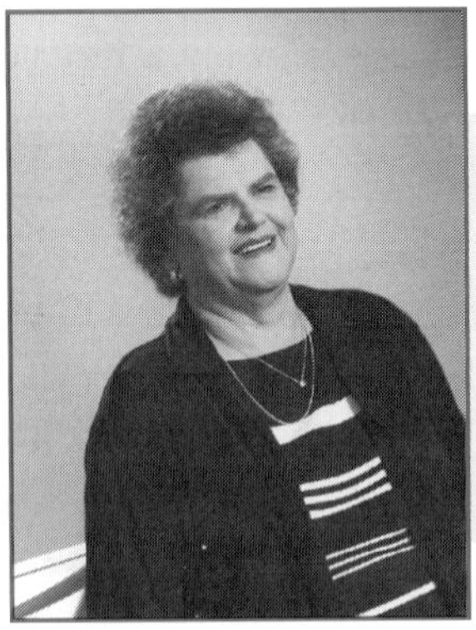

FROM THE TRENCHES

Dorothy

"I think coding has a lot of value and a lot of staying power... You can have a pretty good feeling about job security. Coders—if they're good at what they do and they have the desire for more education, more credentials, there will be a place for them. I like that about the industry, overall."

CASE 10-17

10-17A TRANSRECTAL ULTRASOUND FOR PROSTATE VOLUME DETERMINATION AND BIOPSY

The surgeon provides both the biopsy of the prostate and the professional component of the ultrasonic determination of the prostate size. The diagnosis for this service is an elevated PSA. You can find direction to the code in the Index of the ICD-9-CM under the main term "Elevated" and subterm "prostate specific antigen" or under the main term "Finding, abnormal, without diagnosis" and subterm "prostate specific antigen." Often these abnormal findings diagnoses are the most challenging to locate, so review these two headings in the ICD-9-CM and you will be directed to codes in Chapter 16, Symptoms, Signs, and Ill-Defined Conditions.

LOCATION: Outpatient, Hospital

PATIENT: Ray Engert

SURGEON: Ira Avilla, M.D.

PREOPERATIVE DIAGNOSIS: Elevated PSA

POSTOPERATIVE DIAGNOSIS: Elevated PSA

CLINICAL NOTE: The patient has a PSA of 6.5 and a benign-feeling prostate.

PROCEDURE NOTE: The patient was placed in the left lateral position, and the ultrasound probe was introduced. Prostate volume was determined at 50.7 g. Some calcifications are found in the right lobe, with no obvious hypoechogenic abnormality. The base of the prostate was infiltrated with 1% Xylocaine, and random biopsies were performed in the usual fashion. The patient tolerated the procedure well. He was discharged in good condition and will be contacted when results are available.

Pathology Report Later Indicated: Benign prostate tissue

10-17A:

SERVICE CODE(S):____________________

DX CODE(S):____________________

Prostate Cancer

Prostate cancer is the second most common malignancy in men (skin cancer is first), and it is also the second leading cause of death (lung cancer is first). PSA screening and transrectal ultrasound with biopsy are two important diagnostic tools in early diagnosis of prostate cancer. Staging for cancer is a process of assigning a stage (level of invasion) to a cancer. Two staging methods are the Whitmore-Jewett method and the TNM (tumor, nodes, metastases) method, as illustrated in **Figures 10-3** and **10-4.** A prostatectomy is the surgical removal of a portion of or the entire prostate, and reporting of the procedure is based on the extent of the procedure and the approach used. A retropubic approach (55831-55845) is one in which the incision is made in the lower abdomen behind the pubic arch. With a perineal approach (55801-55815), the incision is made in the skin between the scrotum and the anus. A suprapubic approach (55821) is above the pubic arch.

WHITMORE-JEWETT STAGES:

Stage A is clinically undetectable tumor confined to the gland and is an incidental finding at prostate surgery.
A1: well-differentiated with focal involvement
A2: moderately or poorly differentiated or involves multiple foci in the gland
Stage B is tumor confined to the prostate gland.
B0: nonpalpable, PSA-detected
B1: single nodule in one lobe of the prostate
B2: more extensive involvement of one lobe or involvement of both lobes
Stage C is a tumor clinically localized to the periprostatic area but extending through the prostatic capsule; seminal vesicles may be involved.
C1: clinical extracapsular extension
C2: extracapsular tumor producing bladder outlet or ureteral obstruction
Stage D is metastatic disease.
D0: clinically localized disease (prostate only) but persistently elevated enzymatic serum acid phosphatase
D1: regional lymph nodes only
D2: distant lymph nodes, metastases to bone or visceral organs
D3: D2 prostate cancer patients who relapse after adequate endocrine therapy

FIGURE 10-3 Whitmore-Jewett stages.

TNM STAGES:

Primary Tumor (T)

TX: Primary tumor cannot be assessed
T0: No evidence of primary tumor
T1: Clinically inapparent tumor not palpable or visible by imaging
- T1a: Tumor incidental histologic finding in 5% or less of tissue resected
- T1b: Tumor incidental histologic finding in more than 5% of tissue resected
- T1c: Tumor identified by needle biopsy (e.g., because of elevated PSA)

T2: Tumor confined within the prostate
- T2a: Tumor involves half a lobe or less
- T2b: Tumor involves more than half of a lobe, but not both lobes
- T2c: Tumor involves both lobes; extends through the prostatic capsule

T3a: Unilateral extracapsular extension
T3b: Bilateral extracapsular extension
T3c: Tumor invades the seminal vesicle(s)
T4: Tumor is fixed or invades adjacent structures other than the seminal vesicle(s)
- T4a: Tumor invades any of bladder neck, external sphincter, or rectum
- T4b: Tumor invades levator muscles and/or is fixed to the pelvic wall

Regional lymph nodes (N)

NX: Regional lymph nodes cannot be assessed
N0: No regional lymph node metastasis
N1: Metastasis in a single lymph node, 2 cm or less in greatest dimension
N2: Metastasis in a single lymph node, more than 2 cm but not more than 5 cm in greatest dimension; or multiple lymph node metastases, none more than 5 cm in greatest dimension
N3: Metastasis in a single lymph node more than 5 cm in greatest dimension

Distant metastases (M)

MX: Presence of distant metastasis cannot be assessed
M0: No distant metastasis
M1: Distant metastasis
- M1a: Nonregional lymph node(s)
- M1b: Bone(s)
- M1c: Other site(s)

FIGURE 10-4 TNM stages.

In the index of the CPT manual, locate the main term "Prostate" and subterm "Excision." Note that there are subterms for partial, perineal, radical, retropubic, subrapubic, and transurethral. Partial and radical are the **extent of the procedure.** Perineal, retropubic, and subprapubic are **surgical approaches** that can be either laparoscopic or by means of an open surgical site. Transurethral is a surgical **technique** by means of an endoscope. This means the coder has to identify the correct approach or technique as well as the extent of the procedure. For example, 55831-55845 are for radical (extent) retropubic (approach) prostatectomies. If a laparaoscopic retropubic (surgical approach) radical (extent) prostatectomy was performed, the service is reported with 55866.

- Extent:
  Partial
  Radical
- Surgical approaches:
  Perineal
  Retropubic
  Suprapubic
  -by either laparoscopic or open surgical site
- Technique:
  Transurethral
  -by means of endoscope

CASE 10-18
10-18A Operative Report, Prostatectomy

CASE 10-18

Donald Berry's prostate biopsy indicated carcinoma of the prostate. Dr. Avilla has scheduled a bilateral pelvic lymphadenectomy and prostatectomy.

10-18A OPERATIVE REPORT, PROSTATECTOMY

LOCATION: Inpatient, Hospital

PATIENT: Donald Berry

SURGEON: Ira Avilla, M.D.

PREOPERATIVE DIAGNOSIS: Carcinoma of the prostate

POSTOPERATIVE DIAGNOSIS: Carcinoma of the prostate

OPERATIVE PROCEDURE: Bilateral pelvic lymph node dissection and radical retropubic prostatectomy

CLINICAL NOTE: This 65-year-old man presented with a PSA of 8.1. He has a 100-g prostate, and 1 of 10 cores was positive for a Gleason's 6/10 carcinoma and T4A on the TNM.

PROCEDURE NOTE: The patient was given a spinal anesthetic with epidural assist. He was prepped and draped in the supine position. A no. 20 French Foley catheter was then inserted into the bladder and placed to straight drainage. A lower abdominal midline incision was made. The retropubic space was entered. The Omni retractor was used for exposure. Bilateral pelvic lymphadenectomy was performed in the usual fashion. Obturator nerves were identified and spared. The lymph nodes were small and benign in palpation and therefore were sent for permanent resection. The endopelvic fascia was opened bilaterally. The prostate was extremely large, and the parapelvis very narrow, which made it difficult for mobilization. There was not much of a superficial venous complex. Dorsal venous complex was surrounded with a McDougall clamp, doubly ligated distally with no. 1 silk, and oversewn proximally with 0 chromic. Puboprostatic ligaments were divided sharply. The dorsal venous complex was then divided with electrocautery. The urethra was identified and divided anteriorly with a scalpel. The catheter was withdrawn, clamped, and divided, and the urethra was divided posteriorly. The prostate was densely adherent to the Denonvilliers fascia. A small tear in the prostate was created at the apex. This was recognized and repaired. The prostate was then mobilized using blunt dissection technique. Bilateral nerve-sparing technique was employed. Neurovascular bundles were dissected off the prostate using sharp dissection techniques and 2-0 chromic suture ligatures for hemostasis. Denonvilliers fascia was opened posteriorly to identify the seminal vesicles and ampulla. These were dissected near the base of the seminal vesicles in which they were individually clipped and divided. Lateral pedicles were taken with 0 chromic suture ligatures. The bladder neck was opened anteriorly. The bladder, ureteric orifices, and then trigone were identified, and the bladder neck was divided posteriorly and the specimen removed. Hemostasis was ensured with 2-0 chromic suture ligatures. The bladder neck was closed in a tennis racquet fashion using 2-0 chromic. Mucosa was inverted using 4-0 chromic and urethra to re-anastomose the bladder neck over a 20-French Foley catheter using 2-0 Monocryl sutures. A 10-mm Jackson-Pratt drain was left through a right lower quadrant stab wound and sutured to the skin using 2-0 Prolene. The fascia was closed with clips with no. 1 Vicryl, subcutaneous tissues with 2-0 chromic, and the skin with 4-0 subcuticular Dexon. Dressings were applied. The patient tolerated the procedure well. Estimated blood loss was 450 cc. Sponge and needle counts were reported as correct. The patient was transferred to the recovery room in good condition.

(Biopsy)

Pathology Report Later Indicated: Adenocarcinoma prostate, primary

10-18A:

SERVICE CODE(S):____________________

DX CODE(S):____________________

Staging

Staging is assigning a level of invasion to cancer patients based on the information available. Staging is used in the development of a treatment plan. There are two staging methods: Whitmore-Jewett staging, developed in 1956, and the TNM, developed in 1992. The TNM is more detailed than the Whitmore-Jewett (see Figures 10-3 and Figure 10-4).

CASE 10-19
10-19A Operative Report, Lymphadenectomy, Prostatectomy, and Plastic Repair

CASE 10-19

This prostatectomy includes an additional element of plastic repair of the bladder neck (cystourethroplasty), which is reported separately.

10-19A OPERATIVE REPORT, LYMPHADENECTOMY, PROSTATECTOMY, AND PLASTIC REPAIR

LOCATION: Inpatient, Hospital

PATIENT: Rex Kaat

SURGEON: Ira Avilla, M.D.

PREOPERATIVE DIAGNOSIS: Carcinoma of the prostate

POSTOPERATIVE DIAGNOSIS: Carcinoma of the prostate

PROCEDURE: Bilateral pelvic lymphadenectomy with frozen section, radical retropubic prostatectomy, and plastic repair of bladder neck.

CLINICAL NOTE: This man was found to have poorly differentiated diffuse adenocarcinoma of the prostate after presenting with a PSA of 7.8 and an abnormal digital rectal examination.

PROCEDURAL NOTE: The patient was given a spinal anesthetic and prepped and draped in the supine position. A 20-French Foley catheter was inserted into the bladder and placed to straight drainage. A lower abdominal midline incision was made. The Omni retractor was used for exposure. The retropubic space was entered. Bilateral pelvic lymphadenectomy was performed, and obturator nerves were identified and spared. There were palpable abnormalities in the right pelvic lymph nodes; therefore, both sets of nodes were sent for frozen section, and results were benign.

Endopelvic fascia was then opened bilaterally. Puboprostatic ligaments were divided. Dorsal venous complex surrounded with no. 1 silk distally and oversewn proximally with 0 chromic. This was then divided using electrocautery. Urethra was identified and divided anteriorly; catheter was withdrawn, clamped, and divided; and then the urethra was divided posteriorly. There was significant fibrotic reaction at the prostatic apex with adhesions to Denonvilliers fascia. A non–nerve-sparing technique was used, and neurovascular bundles were taken widely, particularly on the left. During dissection of the apex, a small piece of the prostate was torn, and this was sent separately, labeled as prostatic apex.

Neurovascular bundles were controlled with 0 chromic suture ligatures. Lateral pedicles were taken of 0 chromic suture ligatures. Seminal vesicles were dissected to the base, where they were clipped and divided along with the ampulla of the vas. Bladder neck was opened anteriorly, ureteric orifice identified, and the bladder neck divided posteriorly. The specimen was sent for permanent resection. Hemostasis was achieved with 2-0 chromic. The bladder neck was closed in a tennis racquet fashion using 2-0 chromic and mucosa inverted using 4-0 chromic. Urethra was reanastomosed to the bladder neck using five 2-0 Monocryl sutures in the usual fashion. Fresh 20-French Foley catheter was placed prior to closure of the bladder neck. A 10-mm Jackson-Pratt drain was left through a right lower quadrant stab wound and sutured to the skin with 2-0 Prolene. Fascia was closed with no. 1 Vicryl in a running fashion, subcutaneous tissues with 2-0 chromic, and skin with 4-0 subcuticular Dexon. Steri-Strips were applied. Estimated blood loss was 500 cc. Sponge and needle counts were reported as correct.

Pathology Report Later Indicated: N3 metastasis and T4a primary adenocarcinoma of the bladder neck. (Refer to Figure 10-4, entries "T4a" and "N3" to determine the results of the pathologic examination.)

10-19A:

SERVICE CODE(S):________________________________

DX CODE(S):________________________________

Cryoablation

Cryoablation (use of super-cold liquid) is used to freeze the prostate, destroying all living tissue of the gland. Ultrasound guidance in included in the procedure and is not reported separately for the placement of the cryoprobes into the prostate. Several probes are inserted using guidance, and then a substance such as nitrogen is inserted through the probes. The area may be allowed to thaw and then is refrozen (termed *cycles*) one or more times to ensure that no viable prostatic tissue remains. The probes are removed and the puncture sites closed with stitches.

CASE 10-20
10-20A Operative Report, Cryoablation of Prostate

CASE 10-20

10-20A OPERATIVE REPORT, CRYOABLATION OF PROSTATE

This case demonstrates the use of cryoablation. In the index of CPT manual, locate direction to the codes under the main term "Ablation" or "Destruction."

LOCATION: Outpatient, Hospital

PATIENT: Dean Jailor

SURGEON: Ira Avilla, M.D.

PREOPERATIVE DIAGNOSIS: Recurrent primary prostate cancer

POSTOPERATIVE DIAGNOSIS: Recurrent primary prostate cancer

PROCEDURE PERFORMED: Cryoablation of prostate, insertion of suprapubic catheter, and cystoscopy

CLINICAL NOTE: This gentleman had radiation therapy for adenocarcinoma of the prostate. Unfortunately, he has developed a recurrence and has a biopsy-proven adenocarcinoma. Biopsies from the right mid-region of the prostate were positive. Options were discussed. The patient was cleared preoperatively for surgery. He decided to proceed with cryoablation. He is aware of the risks of incontinence and rectal injury.

ANESTHESIA: General

PROCEDURE: The patient was given a general endotracheal anesthetic and was prepped and draped in the lithotomy position. An 18-French Foley catheter was placed in the bladder to straight drainage. A transrectal probe was introduced. Prostate volume was returned at 28.5 g. A six-probe freeze was selected. Using the quick stick method, sheaths were placed under ultrasound guidance. Following placement of the sheaths, temperature probes were then placed in the left and right neurovascular bundles, apex, external sphincter, and Denonvilliers fascia. The patient then underwent cystoscopy after removal of the Foley catheter with the flexible instrument. The urethra was normal. The external sphincter probe appeared to be in good position. The bladder was inspected, and no evidence of violation of the bladder was seen. A 12-French Cook suprapubic catheter was then placed in trocar fashion under endoscopic guidance and secured to the skin.

A guide wire was left in the bladder, and over this guide wire the urethra-warming catheter was placed. Continuous bladder irrigation was achieved by running warm saline through the suprapubic and out through the urethra-warming catheter.

A two-cycle probe freeze was undertaken. The first cycle had a very rapid freeze, and the second cycle was more prolonged. (Please see operative note for detailed records of freeze times and temperature.) The external sphincter temperature never reached less than 0° C. The freeze was monitored both digitally as well as radiographically with ultrasound.

The probes were withdrawn after full thaw. Two active thaw cycles were undertaken. The perineal incisions were then closed with 3-0 plain catgut subcuticular sutures. The suprapubic catheter was left in situ. Urethral catheter was not placed at the end of the case. The patient tolerated the procedure well and was transferred to the recovery room in good condition.

10-20A:

SERVICE CODE(S):____________________

DX CODE(S):____________________

Endocrine System

An **endocrinologist** is a physician who specializes in the diagnosis and treatment of conditions of the endocrine system. Conditions include goiter, diabetes mellitus, ketoacidosis, hypothyroidism, thyroiditis, adrenal insufficiencies, calcemia, kalemia, natremia, and various fluid imbalances. Endocrine conditions that require surgery may be diagnosed by an endocrinologist, but usually a general surgeon performs the surgical procedure, which is often excision of a lesion.

The CPT codes for the thyroid gland include only one code for an incision (60000). The remaining codes are for excisions (60001-60281) based on the extent of the procedure, except for 60001 (aspiration or injection of thyroid cyst) and

60100 (thyroid biopsy by core needle). If the aspiration of the thyroid is performed by fine needle, report with 10021 or 10022. The codes in the range 60500-60699 are primarily for excision of the parathyroid, thymus, adrenal, pancreas, and carotid body, with two codes for laparoscopic procedures (60650-60659). Often the diagnosis will be a neoplasm or mass of the gland, pancreas, or carotid body, which explains the predominance of the excision codes.

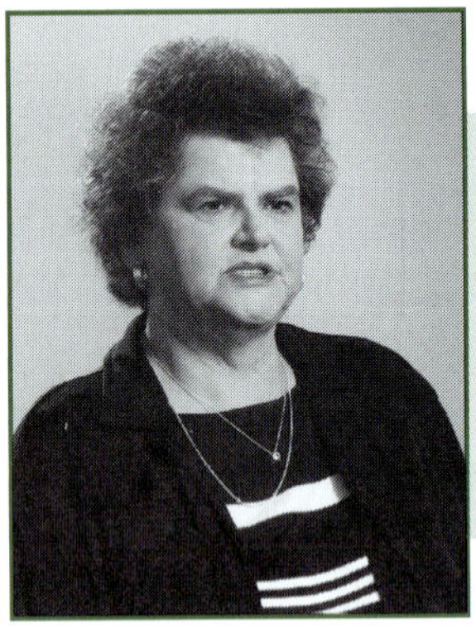

FROM THE TRENCHES

Dorothy

"You have to be dedicated to details ... I think attention to details and integrity that you're going to do a good job are the most important qualities. You won't make something 'fit.' You have to be dedicated to doing the best job that you can, and if the information is not there, go make the extra step to get it."

CASE 10-21
10-21A Operative Report, Left Thyroid Mass

CASE 10-21

Yolonda Saldivar had an enlarged thyroid gland that biopsy showed was benign. She continues to have edema, and Dr. Avilla referred her to Dr. Sanchez for a possible thyroidectomy.

10-21A OPERATIVE REPORT, LEFT THYROID MASS

LOCATION: Inpatient, Hospital

PATIENT: Yolanda Saldivar

PRIMARY CARE PHYSICIAN: Ira Avilla, M.D.

SURGEON: Gary Sanchez, M.D.

PREOPERATIVE DIAGNOSIS: Left thyroid mass

POSTOPERATIVE DIAGNOSIS: Left thyroid mass, right thyroid nodules (Nodule, Thyroid)

PROCEDURE PERFORMED: Total thyroidectomy

OPERATIVE NOTE: The patient is a 29-year-old woman who was seen in the office and diagnosed with the above-named condition. The decision was made in consultation with the patient to undergo the above-named procedure. The risks and benefits of surgery were discussed prior to the operation. Informed consent was obtained. The patient had a history of previous lymphoma. She has undergone mantle radiation. She was concerned that the masses could represent cancer.

She was admitted through the inpatient surgery program and taken to the operating room, where she was administered a general anesthetic by intravenous injection. She was then intubated endotracheally. She was prepped and draped in the usual sterile fashion. The anterior neck was injected with 1% lidocaine with epinephrine. An 8-cm transverse skin incision was created with a no. 15 blade through the skin and subcutaneous tissue. We dissected down to the platysma, which was also incised sharply with the no. 15 blade. Subplatysma flaps were elevated superiorly to the thyroid notch and inferiorly to the sternal notch. Gelpi retractor was then placed in the wound and expanded. The midline straps were grasped on either side of the midline using electrocautery. The straps were divided from the thyroid notch down to the sternal notch area. We then retracted the straps on the left side and dissected over the gland and identified a large mass. The trachea was identified midline above and below the isthmus. We then identified the superior pole, the vessels were clamped and ligated, and 2-0 and silk sutures were used to tie off the pole vessels. The gland was then rotated medially, and the inferior pole was identified. These vessels were then ligated and tied with the same 2-0 silk suture. We dissected in a subscapular fashion and identified the superior and inferior parathyroid glands. These were reflected down. The recurrent laryngeal nerve was then identified and traced medially to its insertion. The gland was then elevated off this area. The isthmus was divided midline with Kelly clamps and tied with the same 2-0 silk suture. Once the gland was pedicled on the thyroid, the remaining Berry's ligament was removed, and the gland was sent to the pathologist for tissue identification. The quick section identification suggested an adenomatous lesion. We then elevated the straps off the right side of the thyroid, and there were at least two prominent nodules on this side. These nodules were quite firm, and both were about 1 cm large. The decision was made at this point, given the aforementioned history and the patient's previous expressed desire to have these lesions removed, to go ahead with removal of the right thyroid gland. We dissected in a subcapsular fashion on this side. Superior vessels were again identified, clamped, and ligated. Silk ties (2-0) were used to tie off the superior pole vessels. Again, the inferior vessels were identified and tied off. We rotated the gland medially and dissected in a subcapsular fashion to identify the superior parathyroid gland. The recurrent laryngeal nerve was somewhat difficult to find. We dissected carefully along its usual course and identified it, tucked underneath the trachea. We were able to dissect this clearly, and it was preserved right to its entrance way into the larynx. We then removed the remaining thyroid off this area and incised the remaining Berry's ligament. The gland was then sent to the pathologist for identification. The wound was thoroughly irrigated. Careful hemostasis was achieved. Two pieces of Surgicel were placed on either side in the gutter areas. We then placed two medium Hemovac drains through separate stab incisions. These were secured with 2-0 silk suture. The straps were then re-approximated with interrupted 4-0 Vicryl suture. The skin was then closed in two layers; the first layer was an interrupted 4-0 Vicryl suture, and the second layer was a running subcuticular 5-0 Prolene suture. The wound was then reinforced with Steri-Strips. The patient was then allowed to recover from the general anesthetic and taken to the post-anesthesia care unit in a stable condition. No complications occurred during this procedure.

Pathology Report Later Indicated: Benign colloid nodule

10-21A:

SERVICE CODE(S):____________________

DX CODE(S):____________________

CASE 10-22
10-22A Operative Report, Excision of Right Carotid Body Tumor
10-22B Pathology Report

CASE 10-22

10-22A OPERATIVE REPORT, EXCISION OF RIGHT CAROTID BODY TUMOR

The excision is of a tumor of the carotid body. Electroencephalography (EEG) is used during this procedure and is reported separately.

LOCATION: Inpatient, Hospital

PATIENT: Delores Janus

SURGEON: Gary Sanchez, M.D.

PREOPERATIVE DIAGNOSIS: Right carotid body tumor

POSTOPERATIVE DIAGNOSIS: Frozen section confirmed a right carotid body tumor with tortuous internal and external carotids that have been displaced by tumor mass with multiple blood vessels feeding this tumor mass, rising from the external carotid, all ligated individually. The tumor was highly vascularized.

OPERATIVE PROCDURE: Excision of right carotid body tumor

ANESTHESIA: General endotracheal with EEG monitoring.

The patient tolerated the procedure well.

COMPLICATIONS: None

NEEDLE AND SPONGE COUNTS: Needle and sponge counts appear correct. No adverse EEG changes were noted during the procedure.

ESTIMATED BLOOD LOSS: 125 cc. No drains were placed. Incision was closed.

INDICATION FOR PROCEDURE: The patient, on a workup for another problem, was dubiously noted to have what looked like a carotid body tumor on CT scan. Subsequently an angiogram was done to examine this further. This confirmed our suspicions and also showed that the blood supply was derived mostly from the external carotid. Consent was obtained for operative intervention. The procedure, indication, risks, benefits, and alternatives were discussed at length with the patient. She understood and wished to proceed.

OPERATIVE TECHNIQUE: The patient was brought to the operating room and placed supine on the operating room table. General endotracheal anesthesia was administered under EEG monitoring. We then proceeded to prep the neck, lower face, and upper chest with Betadine and draped off in a sterile fashion. We proceeded with proper placement of her neck, somewhat extended to provide adequate exposure. We proceeded with her incision anterior to the sternocleidomastoid. We extended this through skin and subcutaneous tissues and the platysma muscle down to the sternocleidomastoid and then subsequently retracted the sternocleidomastoid laterally and exposed the jugular vein, which was quite large and had many tributaries. These tributaries were doubly ligated on the large ones and also retracted laterally. The common carotid was identified, dissected down onto the common carotid, and a vessel loop placed around the common carotid dissection, subsequently carried distally. We identified the internal and external carotids and also placed vessel loops around this. On the external carotid, we identified the superior thyroid, placed a vessel loop around this, and followed this further. Another branch of the external carotid was noted to be feeding the tumor mass between external and internal carotid; multiple small feeding vessels were also identified and were individually ligated. We used bipolar cautery to dissect some of the tissue because this was very hypervascular. The tumor was well circumscribed, although it caused a lot of hypervascularity around it. We were able to dissect this off, identified and preserved the hypoglossal nerve, and identified and preserved the vagus nerve posteriorly. Also, after taking the mass out and sending it for frozen section, we had confirmation that this was a carotid body tumor. We will await permanent sections. Hemostasis was good. We then irrigated. Once we were satisfied with this procedure, we closed the platysma muscles with running 3-0 Vicryl sutures and closed the skin with 4-0 Vicryl subcuticular running sutures. We applied Steri-Strips and sterile dressings. The patient tolerated the procedure well without complications. On awakening in the operating room, she was able to move all extremities. She will be transferred to the surgical critical care unit for further observation and recovery.

Pathology Report Later Indicated: See 10-23B.

10-22A:

SERVICE CODE(S):____________________

DX CODE(S):____________________

10-22B PATHOLOGY REPORT

LOCATION: Outpatient, Hospital

PATIENT: Delores Janus

SURGEON: Gary Sanchez, M.D.

PATHOLOGIST: Grey Lonewolf, M.D.

CLINICAL HISTORY: Patient has right carotid body mass. She has a history of thyroid cancer.

SPECIMEN RECEIVED: Carotid body tumor with FS

GROSS DESCRIPTION: The specimen is labeled with the patient's name and "right carotid body mass" and consists of a 3.5 × 2.8 × 1.4cm red-brown tissue weighing 8.5 g. The tumor is inked black. Cut sections show a solid red-brown center. The specimen is submitted in five cassettes.

INTRAOPERATIVE FROZEN-SECTION DIAGNOSIS: Right carotid body tumor. Paraganglioma (carotid body tumor)

MICROSCOPIC DESCRIPTION: Permanent sections confirm the frozen-section diagnosis of carotid body tumor. The lesion appears relatively well circumscribed, partially surrounded by a hyalinized fibrous capsule. The tumor is composed of nests (Zellballen) of polygonal cells with areas of trabeculae of fibrous tissue. The tumor cells have abundant granular eosinophilic cytoplasm and predominantly round to ovoid nuclei showing some focal pleomorphism and hyperchromatism. Mitoses are scant. Vascular invasion is not seen. (1)

DIAGNOSIS: Right carotid body mass: carotid body paraganglioma

COMMENT: It is almost impossible histologically to judge the clinical course of a carotid body tumor by its histology, even though these tumors are seldom malignant. Mitoses, nuclear pleomorphism, and even vascular invasion are unreliable markers of malignancy. Close clinical follow-up needed because these tumors may recur.

10-22B:

SERVICE CODE(S):______________________

DX CODE(S):______________________

Glossary

balanitis inflammation of the glans penis.

circumcision removal of all or part of the foreskin.
cryoablation removal of tissue by destroying it with extreme cold.

endocrinologist a physician who specializes in the diagnosis and treatment of conditions of the endocrine system.
epididymitis inflammation of the epididymis.

hemangioma benign tumor formed of blood vessels; common in infants and children.
hydrocele sac or accumulation of fluid.

incontinence inability to control excretory functions, such as urination.

nephrectomy excision of a kidney, either entirely or partially.
nephrologist physician who specializes in the diagnosis and treatment of conditions of the kidney.

nephrons filtering units in the kidneys.

phimosis constriction of the prepucial orifice that does not allow the foreskin to fold back over the glans.

sphincters circular bands of muscles that constrict a passage or close a natural orifice.

ureter tube that carries urine from the kidneys to the bladder.
urodynamics pertaining to the flow and motion of liquids in the urinary tract.
urologist physician who specializes in the diagnosis and treatment of conditions of the urinary system.

vasectomy male sterilization procedure in which the vas deferens is cut, preventing the sperm from mixing with the seminal fluid.

cystourethroplasty - plastic repair of bladder neck

Carotid body - neurovascular structure found in ~~the~~ the bifurcation of the right & left carotid artery

Chapter 11

Female Genital System and Maternity Care/Delivery

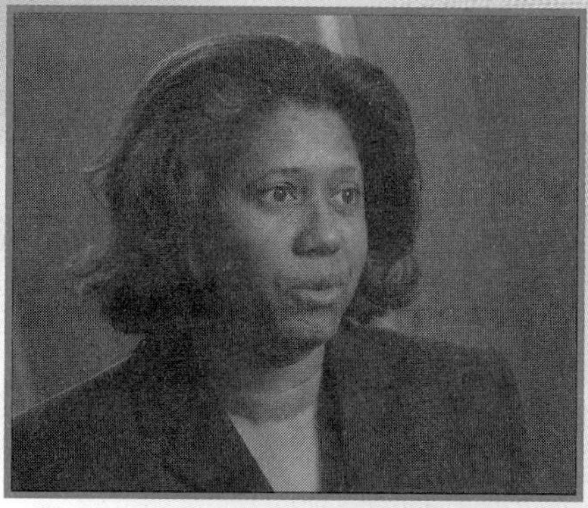

Charlene Smith Isaacs, CPC, CPC-H, CCS
Executive Officer
The National Insurance Board of the Bahamas
Nassau, Bahamas

ABBREVIATIONS

AC	abdominal circumference
AFI	amniotic fluid index
AFT	atrial flutter
AMA	advanced maternal age
AROM	artificial rupture of membranes
BBOW	bulging bag of water
BCP	birth control pills
BSO	bilateral salpingo-oophorectomy
BTL	bilateral tubal ligation
BUS	Bartholin's, urethra, and Skene's glands
cc	cubic centimeter
CD	cesarean delivery
cm	centimeter
CW	clockwise
Cx	cervix
D and C	dilatation and curettage
D&C	dilatation and curettage
D&E	dilatation and evacuation
DUB	dysfunctional uterine bleeding
DVT	deep vein thrombosis
ECC	endocervical curettage
ECOG	Eastern cooperative oncology group
EDC	estimated date of conception
EDC	estimated date of confinement
EDD	estimated date of delivery
EKG	electrocardiogram
EMB	endometrial biopsy
EP	ectopic pregnancy
FHR	fetal heart rate
FHT	fetal heart tones
FIGO	Federation of Gynecology and Obstetrics (an organization that establishes staging classification for grading cancer of female genitalia)
FM	fetal movements
g	gram
GI	gastrointestinal
gm	gram
gravida	pregnant woman
GU	genitourinary
H and P	history and physical
H/C	head circumference
HEENT	head, eye, ears, nose, throat
ICN	intensive care; neonatal
ICU	intensive care unit
IM	intermuscular
INR	international normalized ratio
IUGR	intrauterine growth retardation
IUP	intrauterine pregnancy
JVD	jugular vein distention
LDH	lactate dehydrogenase
LMP	last menstrual period
LT C/S	low transverse C section
mg	milligram
mm	millimeter
NICU	neonatal intensive care unit
npo	nothing by mouth; (Lat.) *nihil per os*
NSVD	normal spontaneous vaginal delivery
OB	obstetrics
OCP	oral contraceptive pill
os	mouth
PCO	polycystic ovaries
para	to bring forth
PERRLA	pupils, equal, round reactive to light and accommodation
PID	pelvic inflammatory disease
PIH	pregnancy induced hypertension
p.o.	by mouth; (Lat.) *per os*
POC	products of conception
PR	pulse rate
prn	as needed; (Lat.) *pro re nata*
PROM	premature rupture of membrane
PT	prothrombin
PTL	preterm labor
q	each, every; (Lat.) *quaque*
q.d.	every day; (Lat.) *quaque die*
RDS	respiratory distress syndrome
S1	first heart sound
S2	second heart sound
SAB	spontaneous abortion
SROM	spontaneous rupture of membrane
STD	sexually transmitted disease
SVD	spontaneous vaginal delivery
TA	therapeutic abortion
TAH	total abdominal hysterectomy
UC	uterine contraction
URI	upper respiratory infection
V tach	ventral tachycardia
VB	vaginal bleeding
VBAC	vaginal birth after C-section
WPW	Wolf-Parkinson-White Syndrome

FEMALE GENITAL SYSTEM

Female genital disorders are treated by all types of physicians, such as family medicine, internal medicine, and other types of primary care physicians. A **gynecologist** specializes in female genital diagnoses and treatment. Often, the gynecologist is an obstetric and gynecology specialist (OB/GYN), and patients are referred to the specialist for more complex diagnosis, treatment, and/or delivery. For example, an established patient presents to her primary care physician with complaints of spotting between menstrual cycles. The physician examines the patient, obtains a Pap smear, and based on abnormal test results refers the patient to a gynecologist with a request for a cervical biopsy.

Common reproductive presenting complaints are dysmenorrhea (painful menstruation), abnormal vaginal bleeding, abnormal Pap smears, nipple discharge, vaginal discharge, and pelvic pain. Conditions often treated are fibrocystic breast disease, female genital system cancer, vaginitis, cervicitis, sexually transmitted diseases, endometriosis, menopause, premenstrual syndrome, infertility, and pregnancy. Frequently performed office procedures are the Pap smear, **colposcopy**, and cervical biopsy, as well as implantation of contraceptives such as an intrauterine device, Norplant, and diaphragm fitting.

Evaluation and Management

OB/GYN physicians provide the same types of E/M services as other physicians, such as office visits, hospital services, and consultations, and these services are reported with E/M codes.

Pains and Other Female Genital Organ Symptoms

Pains and other symptoms associated with the female genital organs (**625**) includes dyspareunia (difficult or painful sexual intercourse, 625.0), vaginismus (painful vaginal spasms due to involuntary contractions, 625.1), mittelschmerz (painful ovulation, 625.2), dysmenorrhea (painful menstruation, 625.3), premenstrual tension syndrome (premenstrual syndrome [PMS], 625.4), pelvic congestion syndrome (chronic pelvic pain, 625.5), stress incontinence (urine leakage on stress, such as coughing or sneezing, 625.6), other specified symptoms associated with the female genital organs (625.8) (symptoms such as perineal swelling, palpable uterus, etc.), and unspecified symptoms (625.9) (such as generalized pain).

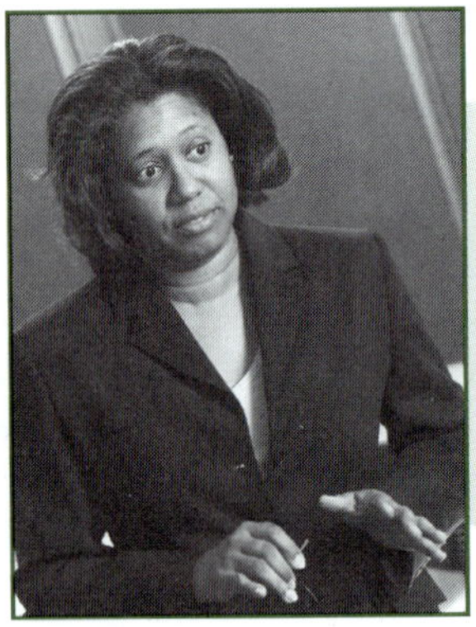

FROM THE TRENCHES

Charlene

"Coding is an international thing. It's a way we can link everyone together in the world. We can get statistics on global trends and global health problems. If we have coders all over the world putting that information in, then we have a better body of knowledge."

CASE 11-1
11-1A Emergency Department Services

CASE 11-1

Dr. Sutton provided an emergency department service for Rachel Grey.

11-1A EMERGENCY DEPARTMENT SERVICES

LOCATION: Outpatient, Hospital

PATIENT: Rachel Grey

PHYSICIAN: Paul Sutton, M.D.

SUBJECTIVE: The patient is a 26-year-old female with complaint of low abdominal pain. In reality, she points to the right adnexal region. She states that she had excruciating pain earlier today that caused her to bend over in discomfort. She states that the pain was bad; it was like spasm. She was unable to straighten up. At the time she felt like there was a bump at the site, and the pain at this time went away after she took ibuprofen. She denies any pain at this time. With further questioning she denies any vaginal discharge or itching. No dysuria. She does state that in August she quit taking contraceptive pills because she would not quit smoking; so this was discontinued. She had her period September 15. With further questioning she does admit to having a similar pain almost 4 weeks ago at the same site. She denies any fever or chills.

OBJECTIVE: On examination, this is a pleasant female in no acute distress. She is afebrile (98.5). Vital signs are stable. HEENT is unremarkable. Lungs are clear. Cardiovascular is regular. Abdomen is soft. Normotensive bowel sounds. No organomegaly. On palpation over the right adnexal region, there is mild tenderness. No palpable masses. No suprapubic tenderness. No costovertebral angle.

Pregnancy test declined. Urinalysis unremarkable.

ASSESSMENT: Right adnexal pain, rule out mittelschmerz.

PLAN: Reassurance is given. After talking to the patient regarding ovulatory pain, she does feel that this possibly may be the etiology. She feels comfortable right now without any pain whatsoever. Instructions for her to take ibuprofen 600 to 800 mg every 8 hours as needed should the pain return. If it is ovulatory pain, this may dissipate when her menstrual cycle kicks in off the contraceptive pill. If she continues to have problems, she is to follow-up with her primary care physician. Patient is agreeable to this.

11-1A:

SERVICE CODE(S): ______________________

DX CODE(S): ______________________

Surgical Procedures

The gynecologist may prefer to perform the surgical procedures required himself or herself, whereas other gynecologists diagnose and treat patients but prefer to have a general surgeon perform surgical procedures, such as a hysterectomy. Because the reproductive system is so closely related to the urinary system, urologists also work closely with gynecologists. For example, an older female patient with prolapsing uterus may have a bladder displacement in which the bladder is not the supporting the uterus. A gynecologist would repair the prolapsing uterus, and the urologist would return the bladder to the original position.

A **hysterectomy** is the surgical removal of the uterus. The CPT hysterectomy codes are divided based on the approach (abdominal or vaginal) and the secondary procedures that are performed at the same time, such as surgical removal of the ovaries or fallopian tubes. For the **abdominal approach** hysterectomy, the abdomen is incised and opened to the view of the surgeon. For a **vaginal approach** hysterectomy, the surgeon makes an incision in the vagina around the cervix and removes the uterus and/or ovaries/fallopian tubes (salpingo-oophorectomy) through the incision. The cuff of the vagina is then closed with sutures. **Laparoscopic approach** is the insertion of a scope through the abdomen, and the surgical procedure is completed by means of surgical instrumentation manipulated through ports. A **hysteroscope** can also be used in conjunction with a laparoscope, as illustrated in **Figure 11-1.**

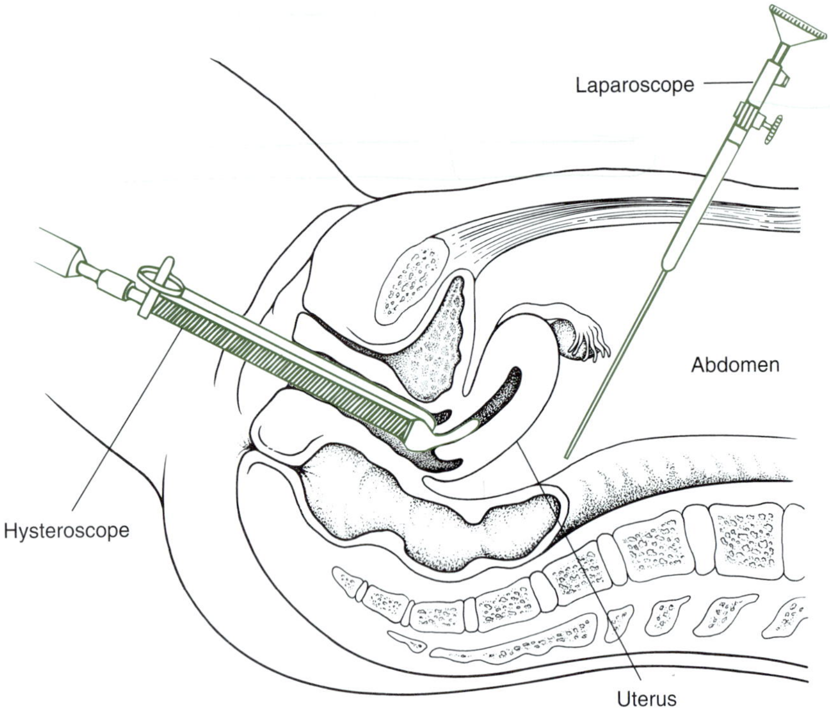

FIGURE 11-1 Hysteroscopy/laparoscopy.

Menopausal and Postmenopausal Disorders

Menopausal and postmenopausal disorders (627) include premenopausal menorrhagia (excessive bleeding associated with onset of menopause, 627.0), postmenopausal bleeding (menstrual bleeding after menopause, 627.1), symptomatic or female climacteric state (irregular ovarian and estrogen level fluctuation, 627.2), postmenopausal atrophic vaginitis (decreased levels of estrogen resulting in inflammation of the vagina, 627.3), symptoms associated with artificial menopause (result of drug-induced or surgical menopause, 627.4), other specified disorders (627.8), and unspecified menopausal or postmenopausal disorders (627.9).

CASE 11-2
11-2A Consultation, Postmenopausal Bleeding
11-2B Operative Report, Hysteroscopy
11-2C Operative Report, Cholecystectomy
11-2D Oncology Consultation
11-2E Discharge Summary

CASE 11-2

Dr. Green's patient, Gladys Hardy, is seen in consultation by Dr. Martinez for postmenopausal bleeding.

11-2A CONSULTATION, POSTMENOPAUSAL BLEEDING

LOCATION: Outpatient, Clinic

PATIENT: Gladys Hardy

ATTENDING PHYSICIAN: Ronald Green, M.D.

CONSULTANT: Andy Martinez, M.D.

This is a 72-year-old white female gravida 2, para 2, 0, 0, 2, who is postmenopausal and is referred by Dr. Green to render an opinion regarding postmenopausal bleeding. Papanicolaou smear last year in July. Mammograms unknown.

REASON FOR THE VISIT: The patient has a chief complaint of postmenopausal bleeding.

Evaluation by Dr. Green, including pelvic ultrasound, demonstrates the uterus to be enlarged for age with multiple calcifications suggesting residuals of prior fibroid and thickened endometrium with what appears to be a 3.2 × 3.3 × 2.3-cm solid mass endometrium with some surrounding fluid.

Differential diagnoses are endometrial polyp, localized hyperplasia, and even malignancy. Endometrial sampling for further evaluation is highly recommended.

The right ovary is normal in size and texture. The left ovary is not well visualized, probably due to atrophy.

MEDICATIONS: Multivitamins and calcium

MEDICAL PROBLEMS:

Illnesses: None
Injuries: None
Surgeries: None

ALLERGIES: No known drug allergies

TOBACCO: None. ALCOHOL: None.

SOCIAL HISTORY: The patient is a retired bookkeeper.
The above was discussed with the patient.

FAMILY HISTORY: Positive for colon cancer, breast cancer, and heart disease. Negative for hypertension, cholesterol, diabetes, osteoporosis, and ovarian cancer.

REVIEW OF SYSTEMS: The patient is positive for eyeglasses, arthritis of the left shoulder, the above genitourinary symptoms, pelvic relaxation, stress urinary incontinence, and postmenopausal bleeding.

GYNECOLOGY EXAMINATION: Blood pressure is 110/68. Height $63\frac{1}{2}$ inches. Weight is 138 pounds. Neck: Supple. Nonpalpable thyroid. Breasts: Negative for masses, discharge, or tenderness. Breasts are symmetrical. Pelvic: Adult female genitalia, marital vagina, cervix multiparous, and uterus 6 weeks. Midline adnexa negative. Rectal: Deferred. Musculoskeletal, within normal limits.

IMPRESSION: Postmenopausal bleeding with abnormal pelvic ultrasound and symptomatic pelvic relaxation.

PLAN: Hysteroscopy with fractional D&C. Subsequent to the D&C, the patient will probably require a total abdominal hysterectomy with bilateral salpingo-oophorectomy and Burch urethrovesical neck suspension in conjunction with Dr. Sanchez (surgery) with possible staging for malignancy. The risks, benefits, indications, and alternatives to surgery have been discussed with the patient and her daughter. The patient gives informed consent and elects to proceed with surgery. The patient is scheduled for surgery 3 days from now. Dr. Green's preoperative history and physical are reviewed, and he feels she is "okay" for anesthesia and procedure as planned. The patient does have advanced directives.

11-2A:

SERVICE CODE(S): ______________________

DX CODE(S): ______________________

Colposcopy

A **colposcope** is illustrated in **Figure 11-2** and is used to examine the vagina and cervix as illustrated in **Figure 11-3.** A **colposcopy** is an examination and/or biopsy of the vaginal and cervical areas and is most often an office procedure.

A **hysteroscope** is a scope that is inserted through the vagina and cervix and into the uterus. A **hysteroscopy** is a procedure performed in an operating room because of the danger for possible uterine perforation and/or hemorrhage.

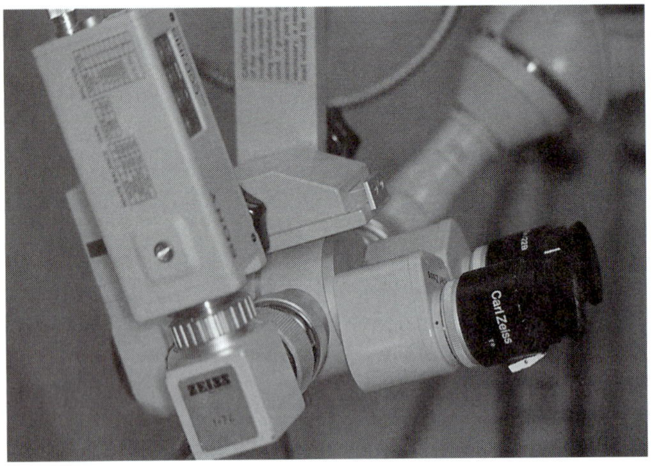

FIGURE 11-2 Office colposcope with beam splitter. *(From Baggish MS:* Colposcopy of the cervix, vagina, and vulva: a comprehensive textbook. *Philadelphia, 2003, Mosby.)*

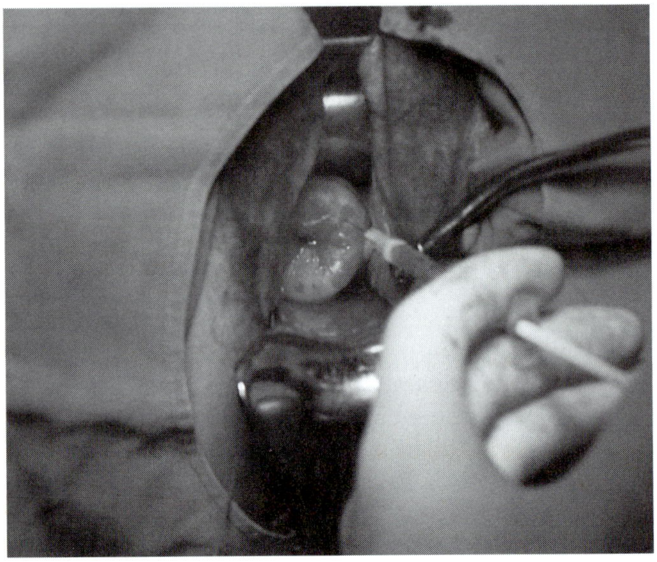

FIGURE 11-3 Colposcopy. *(From Baggish MS:* Colposcopy of the cervix, vagina, and vulva: a comprehensive textbook. *Philadelphia, 2003, Mosby.)*

11-2B OPERATIVE REPORT, HYSTEROSCOPY

Dr. Martinez schedules a hysteroscopy for Gladys. During the procedure, it is found that Gladys has extensive gallbladder calcification. Dr. Sanchez is called into the operating room to assess the gallbladder, and he recommends that the gallbladder be removed during this operative session (Operative Report 11-2C). Before surgery, the patient had signed a consent form to proceed with the cholecystectomy if it were warranted. Report the services of Dr. Martinez for the following:

LOCATION: Inpatient, Hospital

PATIENT: Gladys Hardy

ATTENDING PHYSICIAN: Ronald Green, M.D.

SURGEON: Andy Martinez, M.D.

PREOPERATIVE DIAGNOSIS: Postmenopausal bleeding with abnormal pelvic ultrasound

POSTOPERATIVE DIAGNOSIS: Grade 1, stage I endometrial cancer and porcelain gallbladder

PROCEDURE PERFORMED: Hysteroscopy with fractional dilation and curettage by Dr. Martinez. Exploratory laparotomy with lysis by Dr. Sanchez. Total hysterectomy and bilateral salpingo-oophorectomy by Dr. Martinez. Cholecystectomy by Dr. Sanchez.

ANESTHESIA: General laryngeal mask

ESTIMATED BLOOD LOSS: 350

URINE OUTPUT: 220

FLUIDS: 2700

COMPLICATIONS: Perforation of uterus at time of hysteroscopy and D&C

PROCEDURE: The patient was prepped and draped in a lithotomy position under general laryngeal mask anesthesia. The weighted speculum was placed in the vagina. The anterior lip of the cervix was grasped with a single-tooth tenaculum. The Kevorkian curet was then used to obtain endocervical curettings. There was thick brown mucous material present. The uterus then sounded to a depth of 8 cm. The cervical os was then serially dilated to allow passage of a hysteroscope. The hysteroscope was then passed into the uterine cavity. With poor visualization of the uterine contents, it became apparent that there was a perforation (*Report accidental puncture during surgery based on this comment.*) in the posterior uterine cavity. The instruments were removed from the vagina. The patient was then placed in a supine position, and a Foley catheter was placed. The abdomen was prepped and draped. A vertical incision was made in the lower abdomen (*this is where the procedure converted to a TAH*). The fascia was divided in the midline. The peritoneum was entered in a sharp, and the incision was extended vertically. Palpation of the abdominal cavity revealed an abnormally hard, fixed lesion in the right upper quadrant by the liver that was suspicious for metastatic malignancy. The incision was extended. The bowel was packed out of the operative field using a self-retaining retractor and laparotomy sponges. An adhesiolysis was required to mobilize the sigmoid off the posterior uterine wall. The uterus was grasped and elevated. The round ligaments were cross-clamped, divided, and ligated with 0 Vicryl suture ligature. The bladder flap was created using sharp and blunt dissection and reflected inferiorly. The ureters were attempted to be visualized bilaterally. The right ovary was adherent to the pelvic sidewall, and then the utero-ovarian ligament was clamped, divided, and ligated with 0 Vicryl suture ligature. The left infundibulopelvic ligament was doubly clamped, divided, and ligated with 0 Vicryl free tie and 0 Vicryl suture ligatures. The uterine vessels were skeletonized. The bladder was advanced from the operative field. The broad ligaments were stepwise fashioned down to the uterosacral-cardinal ligament complex using 0 Vicryl suture. (*Although not mentioned elsewhere in the report, this describes a bladder suspension [Burch colposuspension] and would be considered when choosing a hysterectomy code*). The vaginal cuff was reapproximated using 0 Vicryl figure-of-eight sutures times three. The operative was inspected and was hemostatic. The right adnexa was then grasped, and adhesiolysis was performed to allow mobilization of the left adnexa. The infundibulopelvic ligament was then doubly clamped, divided, and ligated and then surgically excised from the pelvic sidewall. Operative sites were inspected and were hemostatic. The pelvis and abdomen were liberally irrigated. See Dr. Sanchez's dictation for cholecystectomy. At completion of this procedure, hemostasis was observed in the operative site. The omentum was brought down anteriorly. The fascia and peritoneum were closed with 0 Vicryl internal interrupted retention sutures and 0 PDS continuous suture. The incision was irrigated. The skin was closed with staples. All sponges and needles were accounted for at completion of the procedure. The patient left the operating room in apparent good condition having tolerated the procedure well. The Foley catheter was patent and draining clear yellow urine at completion of the procedure.

Pathology Report Later Indicated: Grade I, endometrial cancer with minimal myometrial invasion. Focal areas of FIGO grade 2 and 3 with focal invasion limited to the inner one third of the myometrium.

11-2B:

SERVICE CODE(S): ______________________

DX CODE(S): ______________________

11-2C OPERATIVE REPORT, CHOLECYSTECTOMY

Dr. Sanchez removes the diseased gallbladder of this patient during the same operative session as the hysterectomy performed by Dr. Martinez. Report the services of Dr. Sanchez in the following:

LOCATION: Inpatient, Hospital

PATIENT: Gladys Hardy

ATTENDING PHYSICIAN: Ronald Green, M.D.

SURGEON: Gary Sanchez, M.D.

PREOPERATIVE DIAGNOSIS: Porcelain gallbladder

POSTOPERATIVE DIAGNOSIS: Porcelain gallbladder

PROCEDURE PERFORMED: Open cholecystectomy

INDICATION: This is a 72-year-old female on whom Dr. Martinez had performed a hysterectomy. This was done in regard to endometrial cancer. Please see his operative note for specific details. Briefly, it had been a D&C and hysteroscopy, but a perforation of the uterus had occurred. He then converted to an open procedure for the hysterectomy. During this time, on exploration of the abdomen, it was noted that she had a contracted, rock-hard porcelain gallbladder present. I was called in for evaluation of this. Please see my intraoperative consult dictation regarding this. I recommended removal of her porcelain gallbladder because of the potential malignancy being present.

PROCEDURE: The abdomen had already been opened through a vertical midline incision. This went from a little way above the umbilicus down to the pubic symphysis. To get adequate exposure of the gallbladder and liver, we had to extend the incision superiorly some. Then, with the use of a Balfour retractor and the upper arm, we were able to get good exposure. Laps were packed on top of the liver to bring it down. We were able to dissect out the neck of the gallbladder, the cystic duct, and the cystic artery. The cystic artery was ligated with 4-0 silks. It was then transected. We then dissected all the way around the cystic duct. We then took down the gallbladder out of the gallbladder fossa using cautery. We clamped the cystic duct just above the common duct. We identified the junction. It was transected and handed off the table as specimen. We doubly ligated the cystic duct stump then with 3-0 Vicryl. Hemostasis was achieved. Dr. Martinez then came back in to finish the closure of the wound. Again, this is an abbreviated dictation.

I met with the patient's family member postoperatively and did discuss the removal of her gallbladder and the reason for the decision regarding this. Her questions were answered. She understood and was glad that the gallbladder was removed at this time.

Pathology Report Later Indicated: Extensive calcification of gallbladder, benign

11-2C:

SERVICE CODE(S): ____________________

DX CODE(S): ____________________

11-2D ONCOLOGY CONSULTATION

Dr. Green requests that Dr. White, oncologist, provide his opinion about the patient's uterine cancer.

LOCATION: Inpatient, Hospital

PATIENT: Gladys Hardy

ATTENDING PHYSICIAN: Ronald Green, M.D.

CONSULTANT: Rapheal White, M.D., ONCOLOGY

REASON FOR CONSULTATION: Endometrial uterine carcinoma

HISTORY OF PRESENT ILLNESS: The patient is a 72-year-old white lady who had been seen at the beginning of May by Dr. Martinez for vaginal bleeding. Evaluation included D&C. She has had perforation of the uterus. Surgery of total abdominal hysterectomy had been performed for tumor of the uterus. Porcelain gallbladder had been found and this had been also removed. Postoperatively, she has recovered relatively promptly, started feeding, and has had bowel movements. She required fluid support and because of this probably she has developed tachycardia in the range of 175 with blood pressure dropped from 160 systolic to 120. She had been treated with digoxin and diltiazem and had been transferred to the surgical ICU and started on esmolol. Electrolytes also had been replaced. At this point, she gives no specific complaints. She feels somewhat depressed and scared by the whole situation.

PAST MEDICAL HISTORY: Past medical history has been insignificant. She has had no illnesses, injuries, or surgeries.

Her only medications have been multivitamins and calcium.

SOCIAL HISTORY: She is a retired bookkeeper. Lives together with her husband in Manytown. There is no history of tobacco abuse or alcohol abuse.

She has no known allergies.

FAMILY HISTORY: Notable above for colon cancer and breast cancer. There is also heart disease in the family. No significant history of dyslipidemia, diabetes, osteoporosis, or history of ovarian cancer.

REVIEW OF SYSTEMS: Except for the events in the hospital associated with tachyarrhythmia, she has had no chest pain, cough, shortness of breath, nausea, or vomiting. Constitutional: There is no history of any significant weight loss. Appetite has been good. There is no history of fevers. HEENT: She uses glasses. No significant change in vision. No blurred or double vision. No change in hearing or swallowing problems. No new headaches. No new neck stiffness. She has arthritis of the left shoulder that has been present for a long time. Respiratory: She has had no history of exposure to tuberculosis. No pneumonia. No chronic history of any shortness of breath, cough, or expectoration. No hemoptysis. Cardiovascular: No significant prior history. No palpitations or chest pain. Gastrointestinal: No history of abdominal pain. No history of gastroesophageal reflux, regurgitation, peptic ulcer disease, or recent change significant of bowel habits. No melena or hematochezia. No mucus in the stool. Genitourinary: She has had complaints of stress urinary incontinence. Gynecologic: There is postmenopausal bleeding for which she had surgery. She is para 2. She has had uncomplicated deliveries. She has a son and daughter who are living close by and essentially healthy. She has not been on hormonal replacement treatment. Musculoskeletal: She has complaints consistent with osteoarthritis, pain mainly in the left shoulder that had been present for a long time. Neurologic: No history of stroke, seizures, loss of consciousness, paresis, tingling, or numbness. Hematologic: No history of easy bruising or bleeding prior to the postmenopausal bleeding. No history of blood transfusions. Lymphatic: No history of lymph node enlargement. Endocrine: No history of polydipsia. No cold or heat intolerance. Immunologic: No history of hives or recurrent frequent infections. Psychiatric: No history of major depression or psychosis.

PHYSICAL EXAMINATION: She is alert and oriented times three; was in apparent distress while in the ICU. Blood pressure at present in the range of 122-150/70-80. Pulse is in the range of 79; it reaches 120-130 at times. Respiratory rate is 16. She is afebrile. Normocephalic and atraumatic. Eyes: PERRLA. No jaundice. No extraocular muscle movement. No sinus tenderness. Clear oral and nasal mucosa. Tongue and uvula midline. No pharyngeal exudates, erythema, or thrush. The ear canals are clear. The neck is supple. No JVD. Trachea midline. Nonpalpable thyroid. No palpable cervical, supraclavicular, axillary, or inguinal lymph nodes. Lungs are clear to auscultation and percussion bilaterally. Heart: S1 and S2. No gallop or rub. No significant murmur. Breast exam: No palpable mass or nipple discharge. The abdomen is soft and nondistended. Bowel sounds are present, hypoactive. Difficult to examine, she has had recent surgery but no palpable masses or organomegaly. Extremities: There is no cyanosis, clubbing, or edema.

Pulses are present. Neurologic: There are no focal motor, sensory, or cranial nerves II-XII deficits. Muscle tone and reflexes are grossly within normal range. She shows appropriate insight and judgment. Mood is somewhat depressed. Affect is grossly normal.

Her ECG and monitor slips have shown episodes of V-tach, episodes of atrial fibrillation, and some slowed PR intervals. Dr. Martinez has considered WPW.

LABORATORY DATA: White blood cell 15.27, hemoglobin 12.4, hematocrit 35.2, platelets 186, and normal red cell indices. Differential: Increased neutrophils 88.6%, decreased lymphocytes 5.7%, monocytes 5%, eosinophils 0.6, and basophils 0.1%. Basic metabolic panel: potassium 3.5, glucose 123, and calcium 7.4. The rest is within normal range. PT/INR today has been 13 and 1.2. Magnesium was normal at 1.7, and phosphorus decreased to 0.3. Urine culture has been done but is not available yet. LDH was 143. Troponin had been 0.08. The pathology result from the surgery has concluded with endocervical curettings and benign endocervical mucosa; the uterus has shown endometrial adenocarcinoma endometrioid-type, predominantly grade 1 with focal areas of FIGO grade 2 and 3 with focal invasion limited to the one third of the myometrium. Left ovary, fallopian tube, no pathologic diagnosis. Multiple intramural and subserosal leiomyomata showing the myometrium, benign, right ovary and fallopian tube portion of benign ovary and fallopian tube. The gallbladder has shown extensive calcification.

ASSESSMENT: A 72-year-old patient has had recent surgery at this point and is in critical condition namely because of cardiac arrhythmias probably related to fluid overload, related also to medications. She has been started in the hospital on Peri-Colace, Zoloft, azithromycin, cefotaxime, and Zofran, and Tylenol has been given. In terms of the uterine cancer, the cancer seems to be early stage. As per the available data, the tumor is T1B, N0, M0, the stage is IB endometrioid carcinoma, low grade in most of the tumor. No evidence of any intravascular, perineural spread. These are also associated, most likely, with stress leukocytosis as well as electrolyte abnormalities. The patient at this point is still in critical condition in terms of her cardiac function. She has been monitored. Anticoagulation has been planned considering relatively prolonged hospital stay, and at this point she is bedridden in the ICU. Dr. Green has started replacement of electrolytes and anticoagulation. She has been kept n.p.o. with consideration of possible ileus. Aside from this, her immediate problems, which will be managed by Dr. Green in terms of the uterine cancer, the only disturbing factor is the fact that there was perforation of the uterus during D&C, which may have caused some spilling of tumor cells in the pelvic area. Still this is not a justifiable consideration for any additional adjuvant treatment. The recommendation in her case would be after stabilization of her condition in several weeks to perform CT scans to evaluate for any pelvic, periaortic, possible adenopathy, which at her stage of cancer is not very likely. As there was tumor spilling, the risk for recurrence of such an early stage uterine cancer is minimal, and studies would be indicated in less than 10% over 5 years. Considering these facts, no additional treatment would be recommended; yet a cautious approach with obtaining of imaging studies, CT scan of pelvis and abdomen could be considered once she is stable, and if those are negative further follow-up could be done on a clinical basis. The patient herself is not willing to proceed with any aggressive treatment, which again in her case is not recommended and most likely will not be needed in the future either. She will need regular gynecological follow-up as well as mammograms as per guidelines. I would be glad to follow with her in 1 to 2 months when she would be able to have the CT scans done. I appreciate the opportunity to see this pleasant lady, who in terms of her uterine cancer would have very likely good prognosis.

11-2D:

SERVICE CODE(S): ______________________

DX CODE(S): ______________________

11-2E DISCHARGE SUMMARY

LOCATION: Inpatient, Hospital

PATIENT: Gladys Hardy

PRIMARY CARE PHYSICIAN: Ronald Green, M.D.

ATTENDING PHYSICIAN: Ronald Green, M.D.

PRINCIPAL DIAGNOSES:

1. Endometrial uterine adenocarcinoma
2. Porcelain gallbladder

POSTOPERATIVE DIAGNOSIS: Wolff-Parkinson-White syndrome

OPERATIVE PROCEDURE: Hysteroscopy with fractional dilatation and curettage converted to a total abdominal hysterectomy with bilateral salpingo-oophorectomy, open cholecystectomy, lysis of adhesions, open biopsy frozen section of ovary and fallopian tube, arterial line insertion, and postoperative fluid overload.

CONSULTANTS: Drs. Martinez, Sanchez, White, and Orbitz.

IDENTIFICATION HISTORY OF PRESENT ILLNESS: The patient had preoperative history and physical by Dr. Green.

PREOPERATIVE GYN NOTE: The patient is a 72-year-old white female, gravida 2, para 2, who is postmenopausal with postmenopausal bleeding. Pap smear 11/03. Mammogram unknown.

REASON FOR THE VISIT: The patient had a chief complaint of postmenopausal bleeding. Evaluation by Dr. Monson (radiology) including pelvic ultrasound demonstrates the uterus to be enlarged for age with multiple calcifications suggesting residuals of prior fibroid and thickened endometrium with what appears to be a 3.2 × 3.3 × 2.3-cm solid mass in the endometrium with some surrounding fluid. Differential diagnoses are endometrial polyp, localized hyperplasia, and even malignancy. Endometrial sample for further evaluation is highly recommended. The right ovary is normal size and texture. The left ovary is not well visualized, probably due to atrophy.

MEDICATIONS: Multivitamins and calcium

MEDICAL PROBLEMS: None

ILLNESSES: None

INJURIES: None

SURGERY: None

ALLERGIES: No known drug allergies

TOBACCO: None. ALCOHOL: None.

SOCIAL HISTORY: The patient is a retired bookkeeper.

FAMILY HISTORY: Positive for colon cancer, breast cancer, and heart disease.

REVIEW OF SYSTEMS: The patient is positive for eyeglasses, arthritis of left shoulder, the above genitourinary findings, pelvic relaxation, stress urinary incontinence, and postmenopausal bleeding.

EXAMINATION: Blood pressure is 110/68. Height: 63½ inches. Weight: 138 pounds. Neck is supple. Nonpalpable thyroid. Breasts negative for masses, discharge, or tenderness. Breasts are symmetrical. Pelvic: Adult female genitalia, marital clean vagina. Cervix multiparous. Adnexa negative. Rectal: Deferred. BUS within NORMAL LIMITS. Some pelvic relaxation is noted.

IMPRESSION: Postmenopausal bleeding with abnormal pelvic ultrasound and symptomatic pelvic relaxation.

HOSPITAL COURSE: During the hysteroscopy and D&C, it was noted that there was perforation of the uterus, at which time the procedure was converted to a total abdominal hysterectomy and bilateral salpingo-oophorectomy. During that time there was noted to be a gelatinous mass posterior to the uterus, which was sent to pathology. At the time of frozen-section pathologic evaluation, it was determined that the endocervical curettings were benign endocervical mucosa. Uterus, left fallopian tube, and ovary resection with endometrial adenocarcinoma endometrioid-type: Predominantly grade 1 with focal areas of FIGO grade 2 and 3 with focal invasion limited to the inner one third of the myometrium. Left ovary and fallopian tube resection: No pathologic diagnosis. Multiple intramural and subserosal leiomyomata showing extensive hyalinization with focal calcification. Focal adenomyosis: Myometrium, benign. Right ovary and fallopian tube: Portion of benign ovary and fallopian tube. Gallbladder excision: Extensive calcification of the gallbladder. The cytologic washings returned atypical cells; cannot rule out malignancy.

The hospital course continued with the patient developing problems with fluid overload, at which time Dr. Orbitz (nephrology) was consulted, and he determined that the patient had Wolff-Parkinson-White syndrome, which was aggravated by the stress of surgery. The patient also had frequent episodes of atrial fibrillation and was anticoagulated, and he thought she should remain anticoagulated until she was further evaluated in 4 to 6 weeks. She was discharged on Toprol XL 100 daily, and he thought she should stay on the beta-blocker indefinitely. She should also have a Holter monitor done in 4 to 6 weeks. Then if she is in sustained sinus rhythm at that time, it would be reasonable to remove the anticoagulation. The patient was discharged postoperative day 8 with instructions to return to the clinic in 1 week for incision check and in 4 weeks for postoperative evaluation. A consultation was arranged with oncology, who felt that she would not require additional treatment; yet they recommend a cautious approach with obtaining imaging studies, CT scan of the pelvis and abdomen every 3 months times one year. The patient was not willing to proceed with any aggressive treatment at the time of discharge.

DISCHARGE MEDICATIONS:

1. Metoprolol 50 mg q.12h.
2. Coumadin 1 tablet q.d. at 1 P.M.
3. Tylenol p.r.n.

This narrative discharge summary is being sent to Dr. White to render an opinion regarding recommendations about further treatment for this cancer relative to perforation of the uterus at time of D&C hysteroscopy (*tumor cells spilled into abdomen*). We will also send copies of the cytology and slides for that evaluation. I spent a total of 45 minutes providing this discharge service for this patient.

11-2E:

SERVICE CODE(S): ____________________

DX CODE(S): ____________________

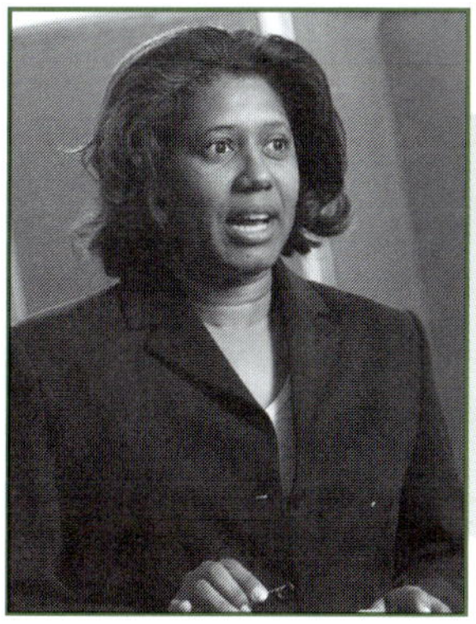

FROM THE TRENCHES

Charlene

"Coding is also about quality—about the patient getting the best care... You don't want the patients to pay more than they need to pay. But you also want to reimburse doctors at the proper fee. So you have this tension between the cost benefits to patients and physicians."

Pelvic Pain

Pelvic pain is a common gynecologic complaint and can have many origins, for example, pregnancy-related pelvic pain, pelvic inflammatory disease (PID), dysmenorrhea (painful menstruation), endometriosis, and pelvic adhesions. The pelvic pain can also indicate a nongynecologic etiology, and so the OB/GYN physician is alert to differential diagnoses from other organ systems. Gastrointestinal-related pelvic pain could indicate appendicitis, irritable bowel syndrome, or inflammatory bowel disease. Urology-related pelvic pain could indicate urinary tract infection or renal stones. Musculoskeletal-related pelvic pain could indicate strain, contusion, fracture, or radiating pain from a herniated disk or arthritic condition of the spine.

CASE 11-3

11-3A History and Physical Examination
11-3B Operative Report, Ureteral Stents
11-3C Operative Report, Hysterectomy
11-3D Pathology Report
11-3E Discharge Summary

CASE 11-3

The patient in this case, Gloria Rhodes, has been experiencing pelvic pain and dysmenorrhea. She is admitted by Dr. Martinez for a hysterectomy.

11-3A HISTORY AND PHYSICAL EXAMINATION

LOCATION: Inpatient, Hospital

PATIENT: Gloria Rhodes

ATTENDING PHYSICIAN: Andy Martinez, M.D.

CHIEF COMPLAINT: Pelvic pain and pain with periods

HISTORY: This lady is a 39-year-old married white female, gravida 2, para 2. Her LMP was May 14, and she received an injection of Depo-Provera at 200 mg IM on May 17. The patient has a longstanding history of endometriosis dating back 10 years ago when she had bilateral ovarian cystectomies for endometriosis. She was then treated with danazol for 6 months. She had a laparoscopy with lysis of adhesions 8 years ago, at which time the right ovary was mildly adherent to the pelvic side wall but was broken up somewhat with dissection, and she had some small bowel adherent to the left ovary. She was then treated on multiple cycles of Klonopin citrate because of luteal-phase deficiency but failed to conceive. She has undergone repeat laparoscopy with exploratory laparotomy and pelvic adhesiolysis having had bowel and pelvic adhesions, and she had resection of several areas of endometriosis. At that point, the patient continued to try to get pregnant but was having more problems with pain, and therefore it was treated with oral contraceptives and nonsteroidal anti-inflammatory drugs. The patient did spontaneously conceive and delivered her second child. She was not having much success in alleviating her symptoms of dysmenorrhea and dyspareunia; therefore, she was begun on continuous oral contraceptives in the form of Demulen 1/50. This did result in the expected amenorrhea, and her symptoms were initially controlled fairly well. She then started having more in the way of cramping and pain; however, dyspareunia had improved. At this point, she is being brought in for definitive surgery because of persistent pelvic pain and cramping.

CURRENT MEDICATIONS: Calcium 1000 mg q.d.

ALLERGIES: None

REVIEW OF SYSTEMS: She has occasional lower abdominal cramping, but this is improved somewhat since her injection of Depo-Provera on May 17. She has no URI symptoms of cough. No GI or GU symptoms. No vaginal discharge. Cardiovascular, negative.

FAMILY HISTORY: Her dad has maturity-onset diabetes, coronary artery disease, and hypertension, but he is living. Paternal grandfather and grandmother had heart problems. Her mom is in good health. She had two maternal aunts with breast cancer, and there are other types of cancer in her mother's siblings, the specifics of which are unknown.

SOCIAL HISTORY: Habits: Occasional alcohol. Very rarely does she smoke a cigarette.

PAST SURGICAL HISTORY:

1. Eight years prior, laparoscopy, exploratory laparotomy with adhesiolysis
2. Ovarian cystectomy and appendectomy
3. Diagnostic laparoscopy

PHYSICAL EXAMINATION: Weight is 148 pounds. Blood pressure is 100/60. HEENT unremarkable. Neck has no masses. Lungs are clear to auscultation. Heart has a regular rhythm without audible murmurs or gallops. Breasts are negative. Abdomen shows a laparoscopy scar and Pfannenstiel scar. Vulva and vagina are normal. Cervix is parous. Uterus is anterior and normal size. Adnexa reveal tenderness on the left but not on the right. On rectovaginal examination, there is some extreme nodularity on the left side of the cul-de-sac. Extremities show no phlebitis.

LABORATORY STUDIES: Preop laboratory work taken on the date of examination shows the urinalysis to be normal. White count is 5440. Hemoglobin is 13.6 g.

PREOPERATIVE DIAGNOSIS: Endometriosis with chronic dysmenorrhea and pelvic pain.

OPERATIVE PLAN: Total abdominal hysterectomy and bilateral salpingo-oophorectomy. The patient will receive a mechanical and antibiotic bowel prep, and she will also have ureteral catheters placed preoperatively by Dr. Avila. The patient understands the potential complications, infections, bleeding, bowel, bladder, and ureteral injury. Potential complications of blood clot formation and pulmonary emboli are also discussed with the patient. She understands the necessity of the operation, its intended outcome, and risks and agrees to proceed as planned.

11-3A:

SERVICE CODE(S): ____________________

DX CODE(S): ____________________

Endometriosis

Endometriosis is a condition for which no clear cause has been identified. Endometrial tissue is expelled from the uterus into the body and can implant onto a variety of organs. Classification is based on the site of implant of the endometrial tissue. Category **617** is used to classify the condition based on the specific site of implantation. For example, 617.1 is endometriosis of the ovary, and 617.5 is endometriosis of the intestine. Often the endometriosis is of several locations and these multiple locations, if documented, are reported.

11-3B OPERATIVE REPORT, URETERAL STENTS

Report Dr. Avila's services.

LOCATION: Inpatient, Hospital

PATIENT: Gloria Rhodes

ATTENDING PHYSICIAN: Andy Martinez, M.D.

SURGEON: Ira Avila, M.D.

PREOPERATIVE DIAGNOSES:

1. Expressed desire of the operating gynecologist to insert indwelling ureteral stents for ease of dissection of the anticipated enlarged adherent uterus
2. Gynecologic diagnosis of uterine endometriosis

POSTOPERATIVE DIAGNOSIS: Same

PROCEDURE PERFORMED: Cystourethroscopy, insertion of bilateral ureteral catheters

TECHNIQUE OF THE PROCEDURE: After general anesthesia, and after the abdomen and genitalia had been prepped and draped in the usual fashion, the patient was placed in the dorsolithotomy position. The genitalia were examined and proved to be essentially unremarkable. The urethra was instrumented with a no. 24 French Panendoscope sheath, and, using the Foroblique and right-angle lenses, inspection of the entire cavity showed no indication of any pathologic lesion. There is slight indention on some of the bladder incident to the uterine impression. The two ureteral orifices appear to be essentially unremarkable. The left ureteral orifice was catheterized with a no. 6 French Whistle Tip catheter with ease. The catheter was advanced to approximately 25 cm on the left side. Attention was then directed to the right side, and the right ureteral orifice was catheterized with a no. 6 French Whistle Tip catheter. The catheter was placed at approximately 24 cm. The bladder was then entered, and the Panendoscope sheath was withdrawn. A no. 18 French 5-ml balloon Foley catheter was then inserted into the bladder and left indwelling to the Foley catheter. The two ureteral catheters were anchored with no. 1 black silk. The two ureteral catheters and the Foley catheters were then connected to straight drainage, and the patient was removed from the dorsolithotomy position. Dr. Martinez, the patient's gynecologist, then proceeded with a total abdominal hysterectomy and bilateral salpingo-oophorectomy.

Pathology Report Later Indicated: See report 11-3D.

11-3B:

SERVICE CODE(S): ____________________

DX CODE(S): ____________________

11-3C OPERATIVE REPORT, HYSTERECTOMY

Report the services of Dr. Martinez.

LOCATION: Inpatient, Hospital

PATIENT: Gloria Rhodes

ATTENDING PHYSICIAN: Andy Martinez, M.D.

SURGEON: Andy Martinez, M.D.

PREOPERATIVE DIAGNOSIS: Endometriosis with resultant chronic pelvic pain

POSTOPERATIVE DIAGNOSIS: Same with mild pelvic adhesions

PROCEDURES PERFORMED:

1. Total abdominal hysterectomy with bilateral salpingo-oophorectomy
2. Cystoscopy with placement of ureteral catheters (Dr. Avila)

ANESTHESIA: General endotracheal

SURGICAL INDICATIONS: This lady is a 39-year-old, gravida 2, para 2, who has had multiple operations in the past for endometriosis. She had recently been tried on hormonal suppression for her symptoms of pain, and this initially worked; however, she has had breakthrough bleeding and quite bothersome discomfort. At this point in time, she had elected definitive surgery.

OPERATIVE FINDINGS: The uterus was normal size. There were a lot of anterior cul-de-sac adhesions over the bladder and anterior surface of the uterus. There were some adhesions between the left tube and ovary and the posterior aspect of the left broad ligament. The right adnexa was free of any significant adhesions. Both ovaries were small, but she had been on hormonal suppression for the past several months.

PROCEDURE: After Dr. Avila did a cystoscopy and placed ureteral catheters, the patient was placed in the supine position and the abdominal area was prepped and draped. The abdomen was opened through a Pfannenstiel incision. A Balfour retractor was placed. The adhesions in the anterior cul-de-sac and left adnexa were separated with Metzenbaum scissors. The bowel was packed off out of the pelvis with wet lap sponges. The uterus was elevated with Pean clamps. The left round ligament was clamped, divided, and suture ligated. All sutures heretofore are 1-0 Vicryl unless otherwise indicated. The round ligament was suture ligated and tagged. The peritoneum lateral to the left infundibulopelvic ligament was opened with Metzenbaum scissors, isolating the left ovarian vasculature. This pedicle was then clamped, divided and doubly tied, first with a free tie and then a stick tie medial to the free tie. The anterior leaf of the left broad ligament was opened with Metzenbaum scissors. These structures were treated identically on the right side. The bladder was dissected free from the lower uterine segment and cervix with blunt and sharp dissection. The uterine artery pedicles were skeletonized on both sides with Metzenbaum scissors. The uterine artery pedicles were clamped with curved Rogers clamps, cut and suture ligated with fixation sutures of a Heaney type. The cardinal ligaments were taken with straight Heaney-Ballantine clamps, cut, and suture ligated. The vaginal angles were clamped with curved Rogers clamps and incised, and then the apex of the vagina was incised across with right-angle scissors, removing the uterus, which was then handed off. Kocher clamps were placed in the vaginal apex and mucosa for identification. Angle sutures at both right and left angles were placed and then the middle of the vagina closed with several figure-of-eight sutures of 1-0 Vicryl. There was a small bit of oozing on the underside of the bladder, and this was isolated and oversewn with 3-0 Vicryl on a GI needle. A small piece of Hemopad was then placed over the vaginal cuff. The bladder flap was loosely approximated over the vaginal cuff with a mattress suture of 3-0 Vicryl. The pelvis was irrigated with saline. There was no bleeding noted at this time. The sponges were removed and, with sponge and needle counts correct, attention was directed toward closure. The peritoneum was closed with a running 2-0 Vicryl. A medium Hemovac drain was placed subfascially to exit below the right side of the incision. The fascia was then closed with running locked 1-0 Vicryl using two strands, one from either side to the middle. The skin was closed with staples and the drain sutured to the skin with Prolene. Blood loss estimated by Anesthesia was 175 ml. Specimen to pathology was the uterus with attached tubes and ovaries. Final sponge and needle counts were correct.

Pathology Report Later Indicated: See report 11-3D.

11-3C:

SERVICE CODE(S): ____________________

DX CODE(S): ____________________

11-3D PATHOLOGY REPORT

LOCATION: Inpatient, Hospital

PATIENT: Gloria Rhodes

ATTENDING PHYSICIAN: Andy Martinez, M.D.

SURGEONS: Ira Avila, M.D., and Andy Martinez, M.D.

PATHOLOGIST: Grey Lonewolf, M.D.

CLINICAL HISTORY: Endometriosis

TISSUE RECEIVED: UTO

GROSS DESCRIPTION:
The specimen is labeled with the patient's name and "uterus, tubes, and ovaries" and consists of a 143-g chordate uterus with attached fallopian tubes and ovaries. The serosal surface is smooth pink-tan. The cervix is white-tan, patent, and transverse. The endometrium is 0.2 cm thick and light tan. The myometrium is 1.8 cm deep and trabeculated pink-tan.

The right ovary is 4.0 × 2.7 × 2.2 cm. Attached is a 6.0-cm segment of fallopian tube, which includes the distal fimbriated end. Cut sections show multiple fluid-filled cysts ranging from 0.3 to 1.0 cm in greatest dimension. An occasional cyst is filled with blood. The ovarian parenchyma is pink-tan. Cut sections of fallopian tube show cylindrical white-tan tissue. Representative sections of right ovary and fallopian tube are submitted in cassettes 8-10.

The left ovary is 3.5 × 3.1 × 1.3 cm. Attached is a 5.2-cm segment of fallopian tube, which includes the distal fimbriated end. Cut sections of ovary show pink-tan parenchyma and two fluid-filled cysts, 0.3 and 1.0 cm in greatest dimension. Representative sections of left ovary and fallopian tube are submitted in cassettes 11-13.

Representative sections of the entire specimen are submitted in 13 cassettes.

MICROSCOPIC DESCRIPTION:
Sections of cervix show benign squamous metaplasia overlying cervical glands, some of which are cystically dilated. The cervical stroma contains foci of lymphocyte and plasma cell infiltrates. There is a small focus of microglandular hyperplasia. The endometrium appears relatively thin and inactive and contains small tubular glands lined by a single layer of cuboidal epithelium. Occasional glands are cystically dilated. The surrounding endometrial stroma appears focally edematous but is otherwise unremarkable. The superficial myometrium contains a rare focus of endometrial glands and stroma. The remaining myometrium is histologically unremarkable.

Sections of the right ovary and left ovary contain multiple follicular cysts, some of which are focally hemorrhagic. Other cysts are also present and are lined by a flattened epithelium. The right ovary contains a large hemorrhagic cyst lined by one to three layers of cuboidal epithelium. The wall contains numerous decidualized cells. The remaining ovarian parenchyma contains a spindled stroma with corpora albicantia scattered throughout. Foci of hemosiderin-laden macrophages are present. The serosal surface of the right ovary shows attached fibrous adhesions. The serosal surface of the left and right ovary also contains occasional foci of small endometrial glands and stroma. Some show hemorrhage with hemosiderin-laden macrophages. Cross-sections of left and right fallopian tube are unremarkable.

DIAGNOSIS:
Uterus, bilateral fallopian tubes and ovaries, excision:
1. Mild chronic cervicitis with squamous metaplasia
2. Benign nonsecretory endometrium
3. Adenomyosis
4. Left and right fallopian tubes: No diagnostic abnormality
5. Left and right ovaries: Endometriosis

11-3D:

SERVICE CODE(S): ______________________

DX CODE(S): ______________________

11-3E DISCHARGE SUMMARY

LOCATION: Inpatient, Hospital

PATIENT: Gloria Rhodes

ATTENDING PHYSICIAN: Andy Martinez, M.D.

DISCHARGING SERVICE: Gynecology

HISTORY: This lady is a 39-year-old gravida 2, para 2, who has had multiple surgical treatments as well as medical treatment for endometriosis. Despite treatment with oral contraceptives and nonsteroidal anti-inflammatories, she continued to have pelvic pain and dyspareunia. At this time, she is brought in for definitive surgery because of persistent pelvic pain and cramping.

PAST SURGICAL HISTORY revealed laparoscopy 6 years ago with an exploratory laparotomy and adhesional lysis. Ten years ago, she had an ovarian cystectomy and an appendectomy. Five years ago, she had a diagnostic laparoscopy. Preoperative hemoglobin was 13.6 g.

PERTINENT FINDINGS ON ADMISSION were limited to the pelvis. The vulva and vagina were normal. The cervix was parous. The uterus was anterior and normal in size. Adnexa revealed tenderness on the left side, but not on the right. On rectovaginal exam, there was some extreme nodularity on the left side of the cul-de-sac. This area was quite tender.

HOSPITAL COURSE: On the day of admission, the patient underwent a total abdominal hysterectomy with bilateral salpingo-oophorectomy after placement of ureteral catheters by Dr. Avila. At the time of surgery, she had a lot of adhesions in the anterior cul-de-sac over the bladder and adhesions between the left tube and ovary and the posterior aspect of the left broad ligament. The right adnexum was free of any significant adhesions. Pathology revealed adenomyosis in the uterus and endometriosis on both left and right ovaries. Postoperatively, she had no significant problems. She had a singular temperature elevation at 38.2 on the evening of surgery but after that remained essentially afebrile (*no fever*). Hemoglobin postoperatively on the first day was 12.2 g. She was discharged on the third postoperative day to return to the clinic in 2 weeks for follow-up.

DISCHARGE DIAGNOSES:
1. Endometriosis of uterus and ovaries
2. Chronic pelvic pain secondary to endometriosis
3. Pelvic adhesions secondary to endometriosis
4. Adenomyosis
5. Cervicitis

PRINCIPAL PROCEDURE: Abdominal hysterectomy with bilateral salpingo-oophorectomy

ADDITIONAL PROCEDURE: Cystoscopy with placement of ureteral catheters

11-3E:

SERVICE CODE(S): ______________________

DX CODE(S): ______________________

Dysfunctional Uterine Bleeding

Dysfunctional uterine bleeding (DUB) is bleeding manifestations of the menstruation cycle. In the normal cycle, the endometrial lining builds up during the proliferation phase due primarily to estrogen until ovulation. The secretory phase of the cycle follows with sloughing of the endometrial lining. With a dysfunctional cycle, the estrogen can continue to stimulate the buildup of the endometrial lining, causing an abnormal thickening that can lead to intermittent sloughing of the endometrial lining or DUB. Polycystic ovarian disease (PCOD or Stein-Leventhal syndrome) is a condition that can lead to DUB. This dysfunctional bleeding can also be caused by low levels of estrogen in relationship to the progesterone, for example, with low-estrogen oral contraceptive pills (OCP). The dysfunction can be irregular and/or unpredictable and/or heavy bleeding.

The constant stimulation of the **endometrium** with estrogen can lead to **hypertrophy** of the endometrium and then to endometrial cancer. A hysterectomy is the treatment of last resort for chronic DUB. The dysfunctional bleeding may also be caused by polyps, ovulation, fibroids, cancer, cervicitis, PID (pelvic inflammatory disease), or certain bleeding conditions.

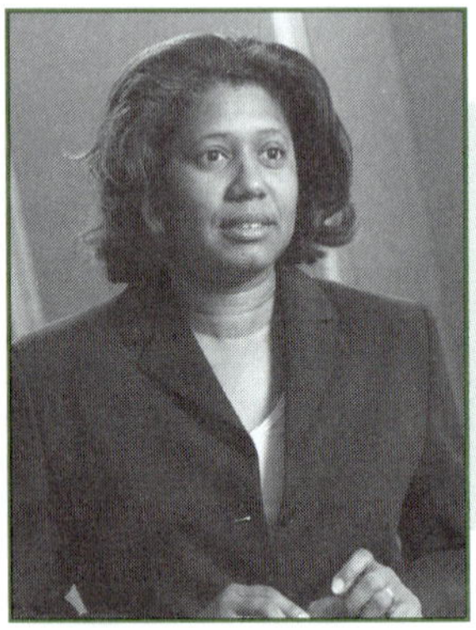

FROM THE TRENCHES

Charlene

"Get certified… Certification will enhance you, your job, your understanding. When you have knowledge behind what you do, it makes it fuller. You know what you're doing. You're sure of what you're doing… Read your books. Sacrifice. Make the time."

CASE 11-4
11-4A Operative Report, Hysterectomy
11-4B Pathology Report

CASE 11-4

11-4A OPERATIVE REPORT, HYSTERECTOMY

LOCATION: Inpatient, Hospital

PATIENT: Charlotte Sweet

ATTENDING PHYSICIAN: Andy Martinez, M.D.

SURGEON: Andy Martinez, M.D.

PREOPERATIVE DIAGNOSIS: Dysfunctional uterine bleeding

POSTOPERATIVE DIAGNOSIS: Dysfunctional uterine bleeding

PROCEDURE PERFORMED: Subtotal abdominal hysterectomy

PREAMBLE: The patient is a 32-year-old gravida 4, para 3, SA 1 who presented with a history of irregular menstrual bleeding. The patient had tried oral contraceptive pills to see if this would cause any improvement in her menses, but no improvement was noted. Trial of Provera also failed to cause any improvement in the cycles. The patient stated that she was done with her childbearing, and she requested definitive therapy in the form of abdominal hysterectomy. The ovaries were to be conserved given the patient's age. The patient did have prior surgeries, including repair of a bicornuate uterus, as well as two cesarean sections in the past.

PROCEDURE NOTE: The patient was taken to the operating room, and spinal anesthetic was administered. The patient was then prepped and draped in the usual manner in supine position. A Foley catheter was inserted.

A Pfannenstiel incision was made through the preexisting scar. There was lots of scarring of the fascia, and this was taken down sharply. The peritoneal cavity was then entered without incident. Upon inspection of the pelvis, the bladder was noted to be quite firmly adherent to the uterus anteriorly. Bicornuate shape of the uterus was noted. Both fallopian tubes and ovaries appeared normal to inspection.

The uterus was grasped, and round ligaments were identified bilaterally. These were then suture ligated using 0 Vicryl. The anterior release of the broad ligament was then sharply entered to create the bladder flap. This was quite adherent mostly on the left-hand side. Bladder was then taken down away from the front of the cervix using sharp dissection. Again, the bladder was found to be quite densely adherent to the cervix, particularly on the left-hand side. Bleeding was encountered while trying to take the bladder down. At this point then, attention was directed toward the adnexa. Blunt finger dissection was used to create a hole in the broad ligaments to allow for placement of Heaney clamps bilaterally across the fallopian tubes and utero-ovarian ligaments. These pedicles were then cut and suture ligated with 0 Vicryl. Free tie was placed around each pedicle first so that these pedicles would be doubly ligated. At this point then, the uterine arteries were skeletonized bilaterally. Heaney clamps were then used to clamp the uterine arteries bilaterally, and pedicles were cut and suture ligated with 0 Vicryl. At this point, the cervix was palpated, and it was quite long and deep into the pelvis. Since the bladder was so adherent anteriorly given the patient's previous surgeries, the decision was made just to complete a subtotal hysterectomy and leave the cervix in place to minimize patient morbidity. The fundus of the uterus was therefore sharply excised. The remaining cervical stump was then grasped using Kochers. Any remaining endometrium was cauterized at the level of the cervix. The cervical stump was then oversewn using 0 Vicryl. Good hemostasis was ensured. At this point, the pelvis was washed with sterile water. Bleeding site was identified on the right utero-ovarian pedicle, and this was suture ligated with 0 Vicryl. Good hemostasis was then ensured aside from a small amount of oozing, which persisted from the bladder. A small piece of Surgicel was therefore placed at the level of the bladder flap for this. The packs and retractors were then removed. The fascia was closed using running 0 Vicryl. The skin was then reapproximated using staples.

The patient tolerated the procedure well and went to the recovery room in good condition. There were no complications. The estimated blood loss was 250 cc.

Pathology Report Later Indicated: See report 11-4B.

11-4A:

SERVICE CODE(S): ______________________

DX CODE(S): ______________________

11-4B PATHOLOGY REPORT

LOCATION: Inpatient, Hospital

PATIENT: Charlotte Sweet

ATTENDING PHYSICIAN: Andy Martinez, M.D.

SURGEON: Andy Martinez, M.D.

PATHOLOGIST: Grey Lonewolf, M.D.

CLINICAL HISTORY: Dysfunctional uterine bleeding. Concurrent case exists.

TISSUE RECEIVED: Uterus

GROSS DESCRIPTION:
The specimen is labeled with the patient's name and "uterus" and consists of a 70-g, heart-shaped uterus, 7.5 × 5.0 × 3.2 cm. The cervix is not attached. The serosa surface is a smooth pink-tan. The endometrium appears hemorrhagic and is 0.4 cm thick. The myometrium is pink-tan and 2.4 cm in thickness. Representative sections are submitted in four cassettes.

MICROSCOPIC DESCRIPTION:
The endometrial lining consists of tubular glands lined by stratified columnar epithelium. Foci of endometrial glands and stroma are present within the myometrium.

DIAGNOSIS:
Bicornuate uterus, subtotal hysterectomy:
1. Proliferative phase endometrium (endometriosis of uterus)
2. Adenomyosis

11-4B:

SERVICE CODE(S): ______________________

DX CODE(S): ______________________

CASE 11-5

11-5A OPERATIVE REPORT, DILATATION AND CURETTAGE

LOCATION: Inpatient, Hospital

PATIENT: Mary Moore

ATTENDING PHYSICIAN: Andy Martinez, M.D.

SURGEON: Andy Martinez, M.D.

PREOPERATIVE DIAGNOSIS: Irregular uterine bleeding

POSTOPERATIVE DIAGNOSIS: Irregular uterine bleeding

OPERATIVE PROCEDURE: Hysteroscopy and dilatation and curettage of the uterus

ANESTHESIA: General

SURGICAL INDICATIONS: This patient is a 41-year-old multiparous female who had been having irregular, abnormal, and prolonged bleeding since June of this year. Ultrasound suggested a small myoma on the right side of her uterus.

OPERATIVE FINDINGS: The uterus was 7.5 cm deep. The cavity was symmetrical without evidence of polyps or submucous myomas.

DESCRIPTION OF PROCEDURE: After introduction of general anesthesia, the patient was placed in the dorsolithotomy position, after which the perineum and vagina were prepped and bladder straight catheterized. The patient was then draped. The cervix was grasped with a single-tooth tenaculum, and sharp endocervical curettage was done. The endocervical canal was then dilated to 7 cm with Hegar dilators. A 5.5-mm Olympus hysteroscope was introduced and the cavity inspected. The hysteroscope was withdrawn, and then a sharp endometrial curettage was done. Blood loss was 5-10 cc. Specimen to pathology: Endocervical and endometrial curettings. The patient tolerated the procedure well and returned to the recovery room in stable condition.

Pathology Report Later Indicated: Primary endometrial cancer

11-5A:

SERVICE CODE(S): ______________________

DX CODE(S): ______________________

Maternity Care/Delivery

The gestation of a fetus takes approximately 266 days or 40 weeks; but when the **estimated date of delivery (EDD)** is calculated, 280 days are often used, counting the time from the **last menstrual period (LMP).** The gestation is divided into three time periods, called trimesters. The trimesters are as follows:

- First — LMP to week 12
- Second — Weeks 13-27
- Third — Weeks 28-EDD

When a maternity case is uncomplicated, the service codes normally include the **antepartum** care, delivery, and **postpartum** care in the global package. **Antepartum care** is considered to include both the initial and subsequent history and physical examinations, blood pressures, patient's weight, routine urinalysis, fetal heart tones, and monthly visits to 28 weeks of gestation, biweekly visits from gestation weeks 29 through 36, and weekly visits from week 37 to delivery when these services are provided by the same physician. If the patient is seen by the same physician for a service other than those identified as part of antepartum care, you would report that service separately (59425-59426).

Delivery includes admission to the hospital, which includes the admitting history and examination, management of an uncomplicated labor, and delivery that is either vaginal or by cesarean section (including any episiotomy and use of forceps). If the labor or delivery is complicated, you would report those services separately (59411).

Included in **postpartum care** are the hospital visits and/or office visits for 6 weeks after a delivery. If the postpartum care is complicated or if services are provided to the patient during the postpartum period, but the services are not generally part of the postpartum care, you would report those services separately.

Routine Obstetric Care

There are four codes that describe the global routine obstetric care that includes the antepartum care, delivery, and postpartum care based on the delivery:

59400	Vaginal delivery
59510	Cesarean delivery
59610	Vaginal delivery after a previous cesarean delivery
59618	Cesarean delivery following an attempted vaginal delivery after previous cesarean delivery

If the physician provided only a portion of the global routine obstetric care, the service is reported with codes that describe that portion of the service as delivery only or postpartum care only based on the delivery method. For example, if the physician provided only the delivery portion of the service, you would report the service with the following:

59409	Vaginal delivery only
59514	Cesarean delivery only
59612	Vaginal delivery only, after previous cesarean delivery
59620	Cesarean delivery only, following an attempted vaginal delivery after previous cesarean delivery

If the global obstetric care is provided and twins are delivered vaginally, the same codes are used, but, depending on the third-party payer, modifier -22 (Unusual Procedural Services) or -51 (Multiple Procedures) is added. If a global obstetric care is provided and both twins are delivered by cesarean, most payers will allow only one code (59510) to report both deliveries. If the global obstetric care is provided when one twin is delivered vaginally and then the second twin is delivered cesarean, you would report the cesarean delivery with the global code (59510 or 59618) for the first twin and the second twin with a code for vaginal delivery only (59409 or 59612).

At the time of delivery, the patient may request permanent sterilization, such as a tubal ligation. These procedures may be conducted at the time of delivery (such as when a cesarean is performed) or shortly after the delivery during the same hospitalization. These procedures may be performed by the OB/GYN or by another physician, such as a general surgeon.

Third-party payers would usually include a tubal ligation at the time of delivery in the surgical bundle for the delivery.

Admission for Normal Delivery

Admission for normal delivery is reported with **650** but is only assigned when a single liveborn is the outcome of a completely normal (**V27.0**), spontaneous vaginal delivery after the completion of 38 to 42 weeks of gestation. The newborn presents head first (cephalic presentation) with only minimal or with no assistance. No instrumentation (forceps) or fetal manipulation (such as rotation to cephalic presentation) would be required during a normal delivery. An episiotomy (surgical incision into the perineum and vagina to prevent tearing during delivery) may be performed, and the delivery can still be assigned to 650. There were no antepartum or postpartum complications when assigned to 650. So, a completely normal, spontaneous vaginal delivery with no complications before, during, or after delivery (650) and the outcome of which is a single liveborn (V27.0) must be reported together.

CASE 11-6
11-6A Operative Report, Sterilization
11-6B Discharge Summary

CASE 11-6

Susan requests a tubal ligation shortly after delivering her child. Report Dr. Sanchez's services. A V code is assigned to report the sterilization.

11-6A OPERATIVE REPORT, STERILIZATION

LOCATION: Inpatient Hospital

PATIENT: Susan Hillard

ATTENDING PHYSICIAN: Andy Martinez, M.D.

SURGEON: Gary Sanchez, M.D.

PREOPERATIVE DIAGNOSIS: Desire for sterilization

POSTOPERATIVE DIAGNOSIS: Desire for sterilization

PROCEDURE PERFORMED: Postpartum tubal ligation (bilateral ampullofimbriectomies)

ANESTHESIA: General

SURGICAL INDICATIONS: This patient is a 43-year-old lady who delivered her fourth child yesterday by vaginal delivery and desired permanent sterilization by tubal interruption.

PROCEDURE: After induction of general anesthesia, the patient was in the supine position, and the abdomen was prepped and draped. A transverse subumbilical incision was made, and then dissection was carried down bluntly to the fascia, which was picked up with small Kocher clamps, nicked in the midline with a scalpel, and then incised vertically with Mayo scissors. Army-Navy retractors were placed inside the fascial edges, and the peritoneum was identified and entered without incident. A vein retractor was used to elevate the right fallopian tube, which was then grasped with Babcock clamps and marched to its fimbriated end. The mesosalpinx underneath the ampullary portion was opened with Bovie cautery, and then the tube was cross-clamped across the ampullary portion. Then the mesosalpinx underneath this was cross-clamped. The lateral portion of the tube, including the fimbriated end, was excised. Pedicles were doubly tied with 2-0 Vicryl. An identical procedure was carried out on the left tube. The fascia was closed with a running locked 2-0 Vicryl and the skin with subcuticular 4-0 Vicryl. Blood loss was less than 5 cc. Specimens to pathology—segments of right and left fallopian tubes. The patient tolerated the procedure well and returned to the recovery room in stable condition.

Pathology Report Later Indicated: Benign right and left fallopian tubes

11-6A:

SERVICE CODE(S): ______________________

DX CODE(S): ______________________

11-6B DISCHARGE SUMMARY

Susan was subsequently discharged 3 days after admission by her attending physician, Dr. Martinez.

LOCATION: Inpatient Hospital

PATIENT: Susan Hillard

ATTENDING PHYSICIAN: Andy Martinez, M.D.

SUMMARY OF HOSPITALIZATION: The patient was admitted with a history of 37 weeks' pregnancy. She was having some leaking membranes and some contractions. The patient was stable on admission. She had a spontaneous vaginal delivery 3 days ago. Both baby and mother were healthy. On postnatal day 1, the patient had a tubal ligation done by Dr. Sanchez. The postoperative and postpartum period was uneventful. The patient was stable. Vital signs: Temperature 36 degrees, pulse 72, respirations 20, blood pressure 105/72. The patient was discharged today.

DISCHARGE INSTRUCTIONS: Activity level: Pelvic rest for 6 weeks; no heavy weight lifting for 6 weeks. Diet: Regular.

MEDICATIONS: Pain control medication p.r.n.

FOLLOW-UP in 6 weeks.

CONDITION ON DISCHARGE: Patient's condition was improved. Bleeding and pain were minimal. Vital signs were stable.

DISCHARGE DIAGNOSIS: Postpartum day 2 with postoperative tubal ligation day 1.

11-6B:

SERVICE CODE(S): ______________________

DX CODE(S): ______________________

Echography

Ultrasound and sonography both describe echography, which is often used in the care of pregnancies. Radiology codes 76801-76828 describe transabdominal ultrasound of the obstetrical pelvis. Codes 76801 and 76802 describe ultrasound using real-time imaging documentation that is performed during the first trimester. 76802 is an add-on code that is used to report each additional gestation, which means that if the ultrasound detected twins, both 76801 and 76802 would be reported. These codes indicate a survey of the fetus, placenta, amniotic fluid, gestational sac, maternal uterus, and adnexa. Although a trimester is 12 weeks, these codes describe the first trimester as less than 14 weeks, so pay special attention to reporting these trimester-specific codes. 76805 and 76810 are similar to 76801 and 76802 but for echography after the first trimester (as described by CPT as 14 weeks). Included in 76805 and 76810 is an assessment of the number of fetuses, measurement of the amniotic sac, fetal anatomy, umbilical cord insertion, placenta, and amniotic fluid, which is a more detailed assessment than the 14-weeks-or-less codes. Note that 76810 is an add-on code used only with 76805.

An examination focused on taking a quick ultrasound to assess one or more elements is described in 76815. For example, if the fetal heart beat is being assessed, 76815 would be reported. Note that the code is reported only once even though multiple elements noted in the code description are provided. So, if the fetal heartbeat and the fetal position were assessed, 76815 would be reported only once for both of the assessments.

Be certain to read the notes for the Pelvis, Obstetrical subheading (76801-76828), before coding echographic services provided to the obstetrical patient.

Cesarean Section

Cesarean delivery is referred to as C-section, cesarean, or CD and is the surgical removal of the fetus through an abdominal incision. Cesarean is used when a vaginal delivery would endanger either the mother or the child. A vaginal birth may be possible on subsequent deliveries and referred to as VBAC, vaginal birth (or delivery) after a previous cesarean delivery. Cesarean delivery codes are divided in the CPT manual based on whether the procedure is a cesarean (59510-59515) or a vaginal delivery after a previous cesarean or a cesarean delivery after an attempted vaginal delivery when the mother previously delivered a baby by means of cesarean (59610-59622). The codes are subdivided based on the type of services provided, such as postpartum care or delivery only, etc.

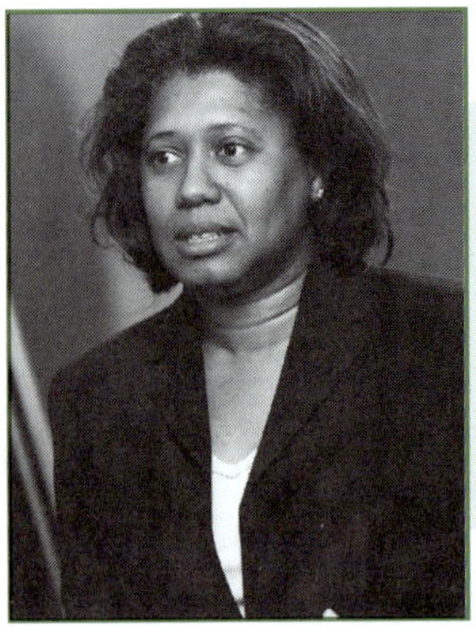

FROM THE TRENCHES

Charlene

"You have to be detail-oriented. You need to think about the value of coding to everybody—the payer, the patient, the physician. It's needed everywhere, and the details are so helpful."

CASE 11-7
11-7A Real-Time Ultrasound
11-7B Sonogram
11-7C Operative Report, Cesarean Section
11-7D Discharge Summary

CASE 11-7

This case will give you an opportunity to better understand how the ultrasound is used in obstetrical care as this patient has a variety of ultrasound services.

11-7A REAL-TIME ULTRASOUND

Beth is sent to Dr. Martinez for maternity/delivery care based on abnormal echography by her hometown physician. Dr. Martinez has assumed the patient's care for the duration of her pregnancy and has seen Beth in the clinic where he scheduled her for an ultrasound at the radiology department at the hospital.

LOCATION: Outpatient, Hospital

PATIENT: Beth Lariat

PRIMARY CARE PHYSICIAN: Andy Martinez, M.D.

RADIOLOGIST: Morton Monson, M.D.

OBSTETRICAL ULTRASOUND: I have a report from an outside ultrasound from Denver Clinic dated 8 weeks ago. I do not have those films, however. That report states "a 2-cm isoechoic 'mass' with a hypoechoic rim seen along the external aspect of the placenta." A single living intrauterine pregnancy is identified in breech presentation. Average sonographic gestational age is 22 weeks 6 days. Since the previous examination, there has been 8 weeks 1 day, with interval growth of 8 weeks. Fetal cardiac activity identified at 140 beats per minute. Fetal motion is identified. Examination is technically difficult and fetal screen is limited. This is due to fetal lie and patient body habitus. No images were submitted of the fetal heart since this cannot be adequately visualized. There is limited visualization of the posterior fossa/cisterna magna region. The placenta is noted to be anterior. There is an approximately 6-cm hyperechoic area seen at the junction of the uterus and placenta anteriorly and measures up to 6 cm in greatest length. This is worrisome for an area of hemorrhage/abruption. I do not have any color flow of this area, however. No placenta previa is identified.

IMPRESSION:

1. A single living intrauterine pregnancy is identified with average sonographic gestational age 22 weeks 6 days. Suggest the patient return to complete fetal anatomic survey (i.e., fetal four-chamber heart and posterior fossa/cisterna magna).
2. Hyperechoic area seen, a malformation of the placenta (*this is the diagnosis*) along the junction along the anterior aspect of the placenta and uterus measuring up to 6 cm in greatest dimension. This is worrisome for an area of hemorrhage/abruption. Other etiologies are not completely excluded. Suggest the patient return for reassessment of this area over a short interval. Per outside report, there was a 2-cm isoechoic lesion reported previously. Dr. Martinez was not immediately available, and a preliminary report was given to his nurse.

11-7A:

SERVICE CODE(S): ____________________

DX CODE(S): ____________________

11-7B SONOGRAM

Approximately 7 weeks after the ultrasound in 11-7A, Dr. Martinez orders a sonogram to assess fetal development.

LOCATION: Outpatient, Hospital

PATIENT: Beth Lariat

PRIMARY CARE PHYSICIAN: Andy Martinez, M.D.

RADIOLOGIST: Morton Monson, M.D.

FOLLOW-UP OB SONOGRAM:

HISTORY: Interval growth, placental mass. Last menstrual period is uncertain; estimated menstrual age is 29 weeks 5 days. There is a comparison, which is not the latest, but is used for calculating interval growth. The latest comparison to the ultrasound of 7 weeks prior to follow up the "placental mass."

FINDINGS: Anterior to the placenta is a thin, more linear, hyperechoic focus anterior to the placenta at the placental uterine interface, which is not measured on today's examination, although grossly appears less prominent. Etiology as previously mentioned is uncertain. This could be due to a focus of resolving hemorrhage. The current biparietal diameter, head circumference, abdominal circumference, and femur length measurements correspond to an average estimated gestational age of 33 weeks 4 days. Estimated fetal weight 2002 g. Fetal motion and cardiac activity are demonstrated with a heart rate of 141 beats per minute. Adequate interval growth.

11-7B:

SERVICE CODE(S): ______________________

DX CODE(S): ______________________

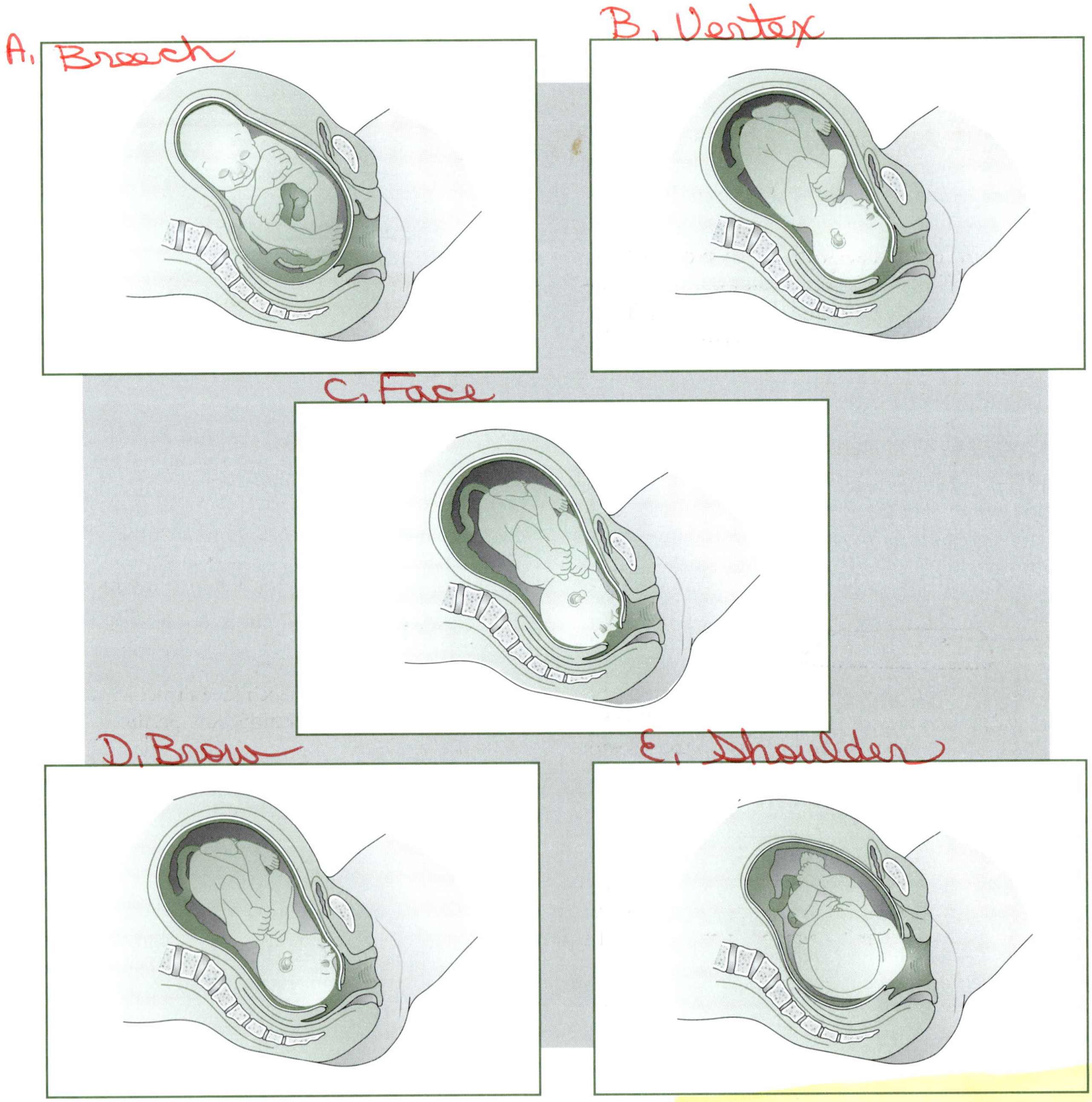

FIGURE 11-4 Five types of malposition and malpresentation of the fetus: **A,** Breech. **B,** Vertex. **C,** Face. **D,** Brow. **E,** Shoulder.

11-7C OPERATIVE REPORT, CESAREAN SECTION

Dr. Martinez admits Beth to the hospital and schedules a cesarean section.

LOCATION: Inpatient, Hospital

PATIENT: Beth Lariat

ATTENDING PHYSICIAN: Andy Martinez, M.D.

SURGEON: Andy Martinez, M.D

PREOPERATIVE DIAGNOSIS: Previous cesarean section

POSTOPERATIVE DIAGNOSES:
1. Previous cesarean section
2. Macrosomia
3. Breech presentation

PROCEDURE PERFORMED: Repeat low transverse cesarean section

FINDINGS: Viable infant male with Apgars of 8 and 9. The infant's weight is 4206 g. Maternal anatomy normal, including uterus, ovaries, and tubes. She did have significant scarring and adhesions in the subcutaneous tissue as well as subfascially.

ESTIMATED BLOOD LOSS: Approximately 800 cc

COMPLICATIONS: None

ANESTHESIA: Spinal anesthetic with Duramorph

TECHNIQUE: The patient was prepped and draped in the usual fashion. A Pfannenstiel incision was made. I did remove a nevus that looked somewhat inflamed and was oozing. It was right on the incision. The nevus was removed at that time. (*This nevus is also reported as a diagnosis.*) This was to be sent to pathology. I sharply dissected down to the rectus fascia. The fascia was then incised in the midline. I used sharp and cautery for dissection of this subcutaneous tissue laterally and anteriorly in a U-shape. The fascia was also incised with Mayo scissors laterally and anteriorly in a U-shape. Kocher clamps were placed on the superior and inferior aspect of the fascia, removing it from the underlying rectus muscles in the midline. The fascia was removed both sharply and with cautery. I entered the peritoneum sharply by tenting the peritoneum. The peritoneal incision was extended superiorly and inferiorly by blunt lateral traction. At this point, the lower uterine segment was identified. The anterior serosa of the lower uterine segment was incised. The incision was extended laterally and anteriorly in a U-shape with Metzenbaum scissors. Bladder flap was developed at this time.

The lower uterine segment was incised. The incision was extended laterally and anteriorly in a U-shape with bandage scissors. The infant was found to be in a breech presentation with double footling presentation. (*This will have an affect on the diagnosis code.*) The infant was delivered through the uterine incision without problems or complications. The cord was clamped and cut. The infant was handed to the nursery team standing by. The placenta was manually removed intact with three vessels. On inspection, the placenta had appeared normal. The uterus was exteriorized and wiped clean with a moist lap. The fascial incision was then repaired in a running locking layer. There was good hemostasis. The posterior cul-de-sac was irrigated. The uterus was placed back into the abdomen. Both right and left gutters were irrigated. On inspection of the uterine incision, there was good hemostasis. The fascia was then closed in a running fashion with 0 Vicryl. The subcutaneous tissue was irrigated, and the skin was closed with staples. All needle, sponge, and instrument counts were correct. The patient was stable in the recovery room. She will be transferred to floor status when she meets criteria.

Pathology Report Later Indicated: Benign nevus

11-7C:

SERVICE CODE(S): ______________________

DX CODE(S): ______________________

CASE DISCUSSION 11-7C

The mother who has previously delivered by cesarean section (654.2X, fifth digits 0, 1, or 3) is assigned the fifth digit 0 for unspecified episode of care, 1 to indicate delivered with or without antepartum condition, or 3 to indicate antepartum complication or condition. Notice that in report 11-7C the Preoperative Diagnosis and the Postoperative Diagnosis sections of the report indicate a previous cesarean section delivery.

The presentation was breech (See Figure 11-4) which is a malposition or wrong position. Any position other than cephalic is a malposition or malpresentation. Malpositions are reported with **652.XX**, with a fourth digit to indicate the position and a fifth digit 1 to indicate delivered with or without antepartum condition or 2 to indicate delivery with postpartum complication.

Macrosomia is excessive birth weight. There is no clear definition of the exact weight of the newborn that defines the status of excessive birth weight, but birth weight of 4000-4500 g (8 lb 13 oz to 9 lb 15 oz) is usually classified as excessive. Excessive fetal growth is reported with **656.6X** with a fifth digit 1 to indicate delivered with or without antepartum condition or 2 to indicate delivery with postpartum complication.

The outcome of delivery, single liveborn, is reported with V27.0.

11-7D DISCHARGE SUMMARY

LOCATION: Inpatient, Hospital

PATIENT: Beth Lariat

ATTENDING PHYSICIAN: Andy Martinez, M.D.

REASON FOR ADMISSION: Low transverse C-section
The patient had a low transverse C-section secondary to breech and macrosomia. Patient had a previous C-section a few years ago. The patient's hospital course was unremarkable. On postoperative day 3, the patient was tolerating diet, having good urine output, but with mild pain that was well controlled. The patient had flatus and bowel movements. Vital signs remained stable.

Physical examination remained unremarkable.

The patient was discharged on postoperative day 3. Hemoglobin 10.6.

INSTRUCTIONS TO PATIENT ON DISCHARGE: The patient is to follow up with me in 6 weeks' time.

DISCHARGE MEDICATIONS:
1. Peri-Colace 100 mg 2 p.o. q.d., #20 given
2. Ibuprofen 200 mg q.6h. p.r.n.
3. Percocet 1 tablet q.4h.

Prior to discharge, patient's staples were removed.

FINAL DIAGNOSIS: Status post low transverse cesarean section secondary to macrosomia and breech presentation.

DISPOSITION ON DISCHARGE: Stable

11-7D:

SERVICE CODE(S): ______________________

DX CODE(S): ______________________

CASE 11-8
11-8A Admission History and Physical
11-8B Operative Report, Cesarean Section
11-8C Discharge Summary

CASE 11-8

Dr. Martinez admits a patient who will undergo a cesarean section. The diagnoses for this patient will include the gestation code to indicate twins, a V code for the premature rupture of the membrane, and a V code for the pregnancy that is affected by the previous abortions.

11-8A ADMISSION HISTORY AND PHYSICAL

LOCATION: Inpatient, Hospital

PATIENT: Joan Corcoran

ATTENDING PHYSICIAN: Andy Martinez, M.D.

CHIEF COMPLAINT: Spontaneous rupture of membranes

HPI: This is a 24-year-old female with twin gestation, who now presents to labor and delivery with spontaneous rupture of membranes. The patient has had essentially an uneventful twin gestation and is currently at 34-3/7 weeks. Yesterday evening, she started having contractions. At 4 o'clock this morning, she had spontaneous rupture of membranes. Rupture produced clear fluids. There was no meconium or blood noted. After rupture, the patient's contractions intensified and frequency increased. She presented to labor and delivery in active labor. Cervical exam revealed dilation of 3 cm with 100% effacement and breech presentation of the first twin. The patient was immediately notified of the risks, benefits, consequences, and alternatives to delivery by cesarean section. The patient is a consenting adult and elected to go forth with the procedure immediately. Dr. Sanchez was notified and will be performing the procedure.

OB HISTORY:
1. 07/89 male, 8 pounds 2 ounces, 41 weeks, 17 hours labor, SVD
2. 07/94 male 8 pounds 1 ounce, 40 weeks, 24 hours labor, SVD
3. 10/98 SAB at 10 weeks
4. 02/01 SAB at 11 weeks

PAST MEDICAL HISTORY:
1. D&C

ALLERGIES: SULFA, develops a rash.

FAMILY HISTORY: Father had an MI at age 65. He also had bladder cancer. Mother was noted to have ovarian cancer. No known birth defects in the family. She has three brothers and two sisters, all healthy.

SOCIAL HISTORY: Unremarkable. Nonsmoker. Nondrinker.

MEDICATIONS: Prenatal vitamins

REVIEW OF SYSTEMS: As above

PHYSICAL EXAM: Afebrile at 98°. Vital signs are stable. BP is 120/80. General: Mild distress with contractions. Skin: Warm, dry, and pink. HEENT: Unremarkable. No nystagmus. Acuity is normal. Peripheral vision normal. Lungs are clear. CVS: S1 and S2, regular rate and rhythm without murmur, rub, or gallop. Abdomen: Soft and nontender. Gravida. Palpable contractions. Cervix: 3 cm/100%/-1/breech. Extremities: No edema. No rash. No calf tenderness. Neurologic: Nonfocal.

LABORATORY AND TESTS: A positive, antibody negative, rubella immune, hepatitis B surface antigen negative, HIV negative, Pap smear negative, hemoglobin 12.2, and group B negative.

ASSESSMENT:
1. A 34-3/7 weeks' twin gestation in active labor.
2. Breech presentation.
3. Prior history of spontaneous abortions.

PLAN: The patient will be admitted to labor and delivery. Dr. Sanchez has been notified, and a cesarean section will be performed. The patient has been notified of the risks, benefits, consequences, and alternatives to the treatment. She is a consenting adult and elects to go forth with the procedure. She will have a permit signed and does wish to have a tubal ligation as well. This was also discussed in great depth.

another physician called in to perform C-section

11-8A:

SERVICE CODE(S): ____________________

DX CODE(S): ____________________

SVD – spontaneous vaginal delivery
SAB – spontaneous abortion

11-8B OPERATIVE REPORT, CESAREAN SECTION

In this report, you will report the diagnoses of the twin pregnancy, breech delivery due to the malposition of the first infant, twins as the outcome of delivery (V code), and sterilization (V code).

LOCATION: Inpatient, Hospital

PATIENT: Joan Corcoran

ATTENDING PHYSICIAN: Andy Martinez, M.D.

SURGEON: Gary Sanchez, M.D.

PREOPERATIVE DIAGNOSIS: Uterine pregnancy at 34 weeks 4 days with twin gestation, spontaneous rupture of membranes, in active labor with breech presentation of the first twin. Multiparity, desires permanent sterilization.

POSTOPERATIVE DIAGNOSIS: Uterine pregnancy at 34 weeks 4 days with twin gestation, spontaneous rupture of membranes, in active labor with breech presentation of the first twin. Multiparity, desires permanent sterilization.

PROCEDURE PERFORMED: Primary low transverse cervical segment cesarean section with postpartum tubal ligation.

ANESTHESIA: Spinal

ESTIMATED BLOOD LOSS: 800 cc

URINE OUTPUT: 125

FLUIDS: 2000

COMPLICATIONS: None

FINDINGS: Two viable female infants with breech presentation of Infant B. Infant A weighed 5 pounds 6.2 ounces with Apgar of 9 at one minute and 9 at five minutes. Infant B had Apgar of 9 at one minute and 9 at five minutes weighing 4 pounds 12 ounces.

PROCEDURE: The patient was prepped and draped in the supine position with left lateral displacement of the uterine fundus under spinal anesthesia with Foley catheter indwelling. A transverse incision was made in the lower abdomen. The fascia was divided laterally. The rectus muscles were divided in the midline. The peritoneum was entered in a sharp manner. The incision was extended vertically. The bladder flap was created using sharp and blunt dissection and reflected inferiorly. The uterus was entered in a sharp manner in the lower uterine segment. The incision was extended laterally with blunt traction. The membranes were ruptured, and the buttocks of the first infant was grasped and delivered. The infant was delivered to the chest, the arms were swept forward, and the head was delivered spontaneously. The infant was bulb suctioned while the cord was doubly clamped and divided. The infant was given to the intensive nursery staff in apparent good condition. Palpation of the second infant revealed that it was breech. The hips were grasped; membranes were ruptured. The infant was delivered to the chest, the arms were swept forward, and the head was delivered spontaneously. The infant was bulb suctioned while the cord was being doubly clamped and divided. The infant was given to the intensive nursery staff in apparent good condition. The placenta was manually expressed. The uterus was delivered from the abdominal cavity and placed on a wet lap sponge. A dry lap sponge was used to ensure that the remaining products of conception were removed. The cervical os was ensured to be patent with ring forceps. The uterine incision was closed with 0 Vicryl interlocking suture in two layers with the second layer imbricating the first. Figure-of-eight sutures were also placed as required for hemostasis. The operative site was irrigated and hemostatic. The bladder flap was reapproximated using 2-0 Vicryl continuous sutures. The left tube was then identified in its entirety, including fimbriated end. It was grasped in its midportion and elevated. The mesosalpinx was transected using the Bovie. Approximately 3 cm of tube was isolated and excised. The proximal end of the distal portion and the distal end of the proximal portion were ligated with 0 chromic suture. Operative sites were inspected and were hemostatic. The uterus was placed back within the abdominal cavity. Pelvic gutters were irrigated. Operative sites were inspected and were hemostatic. The anterior peritoneum was reapproximated using 2-0 Vicryl continuous suture. The incision was irrigated. The skin was closed with staples. All sponges and needles were accounted for at the completion of the procedure. The patient left the operating room in apparent good condition having tolerated the procedure well. The Foley catheter was patent and draining clear yellow urine at completion of the procedure.

11-8B:

SERVICE CODE(S): ______________________

DX CODE(S): ______________________

11-8C DISCHARGE SUMMARY

In this discharge report, you will report the diagnoses of the twin pregnancy, breech delivery due to the malposition of the first infant, twins as the outcome of delivery (V code), and sterilization (V code).

LOCATION: Inpatient, Hospital

PATIENT: Joan Corcoran

ATTENDING PHYSICIAN: Andy Martinez, M.D.

HOSPITAL COURSE: The patient had a low transverse C-section secondary to a twin gestation as well as bilateral tube ligation. The patient's hospital course was unremarkable. The patient tolerated a diet well, had flatus. Lochia was minimal. Pain was well controlled.

Vital signs remained stable. Physical examination was unremarkable and unchanged. The patient was sent home on postoperative day 3. Prior to discharge staples were removed.

Hemoglobin 12.4.

DISCHARGE INSTRUCTIONS: The patient is to follow up in 2 weeks' and 6 weeks' time with Dr. Sanchez.

DISCHARGE MEDICATIONS: Percocet and ibuprofen

FINAL DIAGNOSES:

1. Status post low transverse cesarean section secondary to twin gestation.
2. Bilateral tubal ligation.

CONDITION ON DISCHARGE: The patient is discharged in stable condition.

11-8C:

SERVICE CODE(S): ______________________

DX CODE(S): ______________________

According to the Guidelines, Section 1, C11, A2, codes from Chapter 11 of the ICD-9-CM, Chapter 11 codes in the range 630-677 are assigned to report complications of pregnancy, childbirth, and the puerperium. It is the physician's responsibility to document if the condition being treating is **not** complicating pregnancy and if no such documentation is present to indicate the condition is not complicating the pregnancy, the condition is considered to be complicating the pregnancy. For sequencing, the pregnancy complication codes take priority over codes from other chapters. The complication codes 630-677 are only used on the mother's record, not on the newborn's record.

Additional codes from other chapters may be used in conjunction with the pregnancy complication codes from Chapter 11 to further specify the condition. For example, if the pregnant patient has diabetes, you assign a 648.0X (pregnancy complicated by diabetes); but this code alone does not indicate the type of diabetes and as such a 250.XX code would give further specificity to the type of diabetes and should be assigned. Another example of the need for a diagnosis code in addition to the pregnancy complication code would be if the pregnant patient presented with nausea with vomiting. There is a complication code for pregnancy complicated by vomiting (643.8X), but that code does not describe the nausea, so 787.01, nausea with vomiting, would be assigned in addition to the pregnancy complication code. Some codes from Chapter 11 are very specific and the use of further codes would be redundant. For example, if the patient had chronic hypertension during pregnancy, there is a pregnancy complication code (642.03, hypertension complicating pregnancy, childbirth, or puerperium; chronic) to describe the condition fully and further code(s) would be redundant.

Some of the pregnancy complication codes (640-648 and 651-676) require the use of a fifth digit to indicate whether the encounter is antepartum or postpartum and whether a delivery has occurred during that encounter. Not all fifth digits can be used with all pregnancy complication codes. For example, the fifth digits of 0 (unspecified) and 3 (antepartum) can be assigned to 641.1, false labor. The fifth digits that indicate delivery occurred (1, 2) or a postpartum condition (4) could not be assigned as false labor is one in which labor did not commence and no birth took place. The fifth digits that are appropriate for each code are listed in brackets under each code.

In an episode of care in which no delivery occurs, the principal diagnosis should correspond to the principal complication of the pregnancy that was the reason for the encounter. If there is more than one complication, and all were **treated or monitored,** all complications are listed before codes from other chapters and any one may be sequenced first.

If the pregnancy was incidental to the encounter, V22.2, incidental pregnancy state, is reported.

CASE 11-9
11-9A OB/GYN Consultation
11-9B Duplex Venous Examination
11-9C Ultrasound
11-9D Biophysical Profile
11-9E Doppler Umbilical Arterial
11-9F OB Ultrasound
11-9G OB Ultrasound
11-9H Operative Report, Amniocentesis
11-9I OB Ultrasound
11-9J Operative Report, Cesarean Section
11-9K Pathology Report

CASE 11-9

This complex case will be quite detailed and provide you an opportunity to code many services that are provided to this patient. The patient is pregnant and presents for care because of nausea with vomiting and diarrhea, which is a complication of pregnancy. The patient also has diabetes with nephropathy that will be reported. The diabetes is another complication of this pregnancy as is the chronic hypertension.

11-9A OB/GYN CONSULTATION

(not a consultation per brackets below)

LOCATION: Inpatient, Hospital

PATIENT: Patricia Garrison

ATTENDING PHYSICIAN: George Orbitz, M.D.

CONSULTANT: Andy Martinez, M.D.

CHIEF COMPLAINT: Nausea, vomiting (*complication of pregnancy*), and diarrhea

HISTORY OF PRESENT ILLNESS: This patient is pregnant and has been followed by Dr. Orbitz. I got a message to see the patient by orders from the ward secretary. However, [I was not sure exactly the reason for the consultation since there had been no direct contact from the admitting physician as to what I was expected to do at this time.] She had an insulin reaction 2 days ago, came to the emergency room, and then was discharged. She then had some nausea, vomiting, and diarrhea. She has had no vaginal bleeding or cramping. She is around 30 weeks' gestation.

PHYSICAL EXAMINATION: On examination, the fundus is palpable, slightly above the symphysis pubis. I cannot hear tones with the Doppler; however, there is a lot of static electricity interference. An ultrasound was obtained, which showed the baby to be viable gestational size.

The patient's pregnancy is complicated by insulin-dependent diabetes (*complication of pregnancy*) with diabetic nephropathy and chronic hypertension (*complication of pregnancy*).

DIAGNOSES:
1. Intrauterine pregnancy
2. Probable gastroenteritis
3. Type 1 diabetes mellitus with diabetic nephropathy

PLAN: I have been asked by Dr. Orbitz to assume attending for this patient, to which I have agreed.

11-9A:

SERVICE CODE(S): ____________________

DX CODE(S): ____________________

11-9B DUPLEX VENOUS EXAMINATION

Because you are reporting outpatient services, you do not consider the diagnoses from the previous report. This report, 11-9B, is assigned diagnoses based on the documentation within this one report. The first-listed diagnosis is, therefore, the complication of pregnancy (other specified complication) followed by the code for the leg swelling, which gives specifics to the type of complication. The thrombophlebitis cannot be reported as it is a "rule out" diagnosis that was not confirmed.

LOCATION: Inpatient, Hospital

PATIENT: Patricia Garrison

ATTENDING PHYSICIAN: Andy Martinez, M.D.

INTERVENTIONAL RADIOLOGIST: Edward Riddle, M.D.

EXAMINATION OF: Duplex venous examination

CLINICAL SYMPTOMS: Rule out deep venous thrombosis

DUPLEX VENOUS EXAMINATION: Patient is a 28-year-old with leg swelling *(complication of pregnancy)* and possible DVT. She is an OB patient.

Both legs were examined with the duplex scanner in CW and imaging modes. We checked the veins at the common femoral, superficial femoral, popliteal, saphenous, and posterior tibial levels. We checked for spontaneous flow, phasicity, augmentation, and compressibility. The above were all normal.

CONCLUSION: No evidence of thrombophlebitis

11-9B:

SERVICE CODE(S): ____________________

DX CODE(S): ____________________

11-9C ULTRASOUND

The reason for this service is an antenatal screening reported with a V code.

LOCATION: Inpatient, Hospital

PATIENT: Patricia Garrison

ATTENDING PHYSICIAN: Andy Martinez, M.D.

RADIOLOGIST: Morton Monson, M.D.

EXAMINATION OF: Limited obstetrical ultrasound *(this is a fetal testing ultrasound)*

CLINICAL SYMPTOMS: Amniotic fluid volume

LIMITED OBSTETRICAL ULTRASOUND: Comparison is made with the previous study outlined in 11-9B. Estimated gestational age by last menstrual period is 29 weeks 2 days.

A single intrauterine pregnancy is seen in cephalic presentation with longitudinal lie. Amniotic fluid index is at the upper norm. The amniotic fluid index is 22.6. The placenta is posterior and grade 1 with no indication of previa. Detailed measurements were not obtained. Detailed anatomical survey was not performed. Fetal heart rate is 129 beats per minute and fetal motion is noted.

CONCLUSION:

1. Limited obstetrical sonogram for amniotic fluid index only. A single intrauterine pregnancy is seen in cephalic presentation with longitudinal lie.
2. Amniotic fluid volume is at the upper norm. The amniotic fluid index is also at the upper norm at 22.6.
3. Fetal heart rate is 129 beats per minute and fetal motion is noted.

11-9C:

SERVICE CODE(S): ____________________

DX CODE(S): ____________________

11-9D BIOPHYSICAL PROFILE

The documentation indicates the reason for this service is the diabetes that is complicating the pregnancy (See Clinical Symptoms section). A code is also required to indicate the type of diabetes.

LOCATION: Inpatient, Hospital

PATIENT: Patricia Garrison

ATTENDING PHYSICIAN: Andy Martinez, M.D.

INTERVENTIONAL RADIOLOGIST: Edward Riddle, M.D.

CLINICAL SYMPTOMS: Fetal biophysical profile, based on mother's diabetes, type 1.

BIOPHYSICAL PROFILE: FINDINGS: Single active intrauterine gestation is identified in longitudinal lie and cephalic presentation. Placenta is predominantly posterior in location and, as visualized, appears within normal limits. Cervical os area is difficult to visualize due to fetal head position. Please see previous dictations. The non-stress testing revealed fetal heart rate recorded at 126 beats per minute. Fetus receives scores of 2 for fetal breathing movements, fetal movements, fetal tone, and amniotic fluid volume. AFI on today's exam is 21.8, which places this between the 50th and 95th percentile but closer to 95th percentile; 95th percentile would be 23.8 cm. The amniotic fluid index has been mildly prominent for the last several readings. Please see previous dictations.

IMPRESSION: Biophysical profile score is 8 out of 9. Please see additional above comments.

11-9D:

SERVICE CODE(S): ____________________

DX CODE(S): ____________________

11-9E DOPPLER UMBILICAL ARTERIAL

There are two complications of pregnancy codes needed for this case, as well as codes to describe the diabetes in more detail.

LOCATION: Inpatient, Hospital

PATIENT: Patricia Garrison

ATTENDING PHYSICIAN: Andy Martinez, M.D.

RADIOLOGIST: Morton Monson, M.D.

EXAMINATION OF: Umbilical arterial Doppler

CLINICAL SYMPTOMS: History of renal nephropathy due to diabetes type 1 and chronic hypertension, complicating pregnancy. The initial report talks about chronic hypertension, so I believe she had hypertension before she was pregnant.

UMBILICAL ARTERIAL DOPPLER: FINDINGS: Limited evaluation was performed. A single active intrauterine gestation is identified in longitudinal lie in cephalic presentation with fetal heart rate recorded at 121 beats per minute. Relatively normal-appearing umbilical arterial waveform is present. Three umbilical artery Doppler tracings were done with systolic-to-diastolic ratio would be less than 4.2. Previous umbilical arterial ratios were 3.2, 3.7, 2.5, and 4 days prior. The AFI on today's exam is measured at 50th percentile.

11-9E:

SERVICE CODE(S): ______________________

DX CODE(S): ______________________

11-9F OB ULTRASOUND

LOCATION: Inpatient, Hospital

PATIENT: Patricia Garrison

ATTENDING PHYSICIAN: Andy Martinez, M.D.

RADIOLOGIST: Morton Monson, M.D.

EXAMINATION OF: Limited OB ultrasound

CLINICAL SYMPTOMS: Estimated fetal weight; preterm labor

LIMITED OB ULTRASOUND: FINDINGS: A single active intrauterine gestation in longitudinal lie and cephalic presentation is identified. Average gestational age is 32 weeks 4 days. This represents interval growth of 23 weeks 1 day and chronological growth of 22 weeks 3 days. Fetal heart rate is recorded at 128 beats per minute. Systolic/diastolic ratios of the umbilical artery on today's exam were measured at 4, 3.4, and 3.4, which is within normal limits. Normal for 33 weeks would be 4.2 or less.

IMPRESSION: Normal interval growth and normal umbilical arterial ratio.

11-9F:

SERVICE CODE(S): ______________________

DX CODE(S): ______________________

11-9G OB ULTRASOUND

LOCATION: Inpatient, Hospital

PATIENT: Patricia Garrison

ATTENDING PHYSICIAN: Andy Martinez, M.D.

RADIOLOGIST: Morton Monson, M.D.

EXAMINATION OF: OB ultrasound for amniocentesis

CLINICAL SYMPTOMS: Check lung maturity; follow-up

OB ULTRASOUND FOR AMNIOCENTESIS: Numerous comparisons are available, including umbilical arterial Doppler from 2 days ago and biophysical profiles from 5 days ago. Fetal motion is noted by the technologist. Fetal heart rate prior to the procedure is 129 beats per minute. After the procedure, it was 143 beats per minute. It is noted by the technologist that Dr. Riddle retrieved approximately 20 cc of clear amniotic fluid. No immediate complications were encountered. Incidental note of a nuchal cord. Umbilical arterial ratios are 2.9, 2.8, and 2.6. Normal for a 34-week fetus is less than 4.1.

11-9G:

SERVICE CODE(S): ______________________

DX CODE(S): ______________________

11-9H OPERATIVE REPORT, AMNIOCENTESIS

Note how in this report the patient's chronic hypertension is not documented. In the outpatient setting, you report only those diagnoses that are stated in the documentation and only those that are being treated or monitored.

LOCATION: Inpatient, Hospital

PATIENT: Patricia Garrison

SURGEON: Andy Martinez, M.D.

PREOPERATIVE DIAGNOSES:
1. Intrauterine pregnancy at 32 plus weeks
2. Insulin-dependent diabetes, type 1
3. Diabetic nephropathy

POSTPROCEDURE DIAGNOSES:
1. Intrauterine pregnancy at 32 plus weeks
2. Insulin-dependent diabetes, type 1
3. Diabetic nephropathy

DATE OF PROCEDURE:

PROCEDURE PERFORMED: Amniocentesis

ANESTHESIA: None

INDICATIONS: The patient is a 28-year-old with a complicated pregnancy who has been on bedrest because of diabetic nephropathy. Due to the fact that the fetus might be in a hostile environment, we felt that accelerated pulmonary maturity might be a possibility. Therefore, at this time we elected to go with amniocentesis to help us manage her pregnancy. She had been fully informed of the risks and benefits of the procedure prior to proceeding.

DESCRIPTION OF PROCEDURE: Ultrasound scanning was done by the technologist, and placenta was posterior. We prepped the abdomen and draped it. We used a sterile covered ultrasound transducer with guide and located a pocket of fluid. The 20-gauge needle was inserted. As we got into the uterus, the baby moved into the area; therefore the needle was immediately withdrawn. The fetus was palpated a little bit, and we stimulated the baby and it moved out of the area. We then repositioned the transducer and we were able to drop into the pocket of amniotic fluid and withdrew 20 cc of clear yellow amniotic fluid. The fluid was sent for maturity studies. The patient tolerated the procedure without difficulty.

11-9H:

SERVICE CODE(S): ____________________

DX CODE(S): ____________________

11-9I OB ULTRASOUND

LOCATION: Inpatient, Hospital

PATIENT: Patricia Garrison

ATTENDING PHYSICIAN: Andy Martinez, M.D.

RADIOLOGIST: Morton Monson, M.D.

EXAMINATION OF: Obstetric ultrasound follow-up

CLINICAL SYMPTOMS: Fetal weight, umbilical artery Doppler, estimated menstrual age 34 weeks 2 days

OBSTETRICAL ULTRASOUND FINDINGS: Single active intrauterine gestation, cephalic presentation, longitudinal lie. Average sonographic gestational age is 34 weeks 4 days. Estimated fetal weight is 2345 g. Fetal cardiac activity at 158 beats per minute. Fetal motion was present during this study. Since the previous study, where the estimated sonographic gestational age was 9 weeks 3 days, there has been interval growth of 25 weeks 1 day in a 23-week 2-day interval. Umbilical arterial Doppler shows normal waveform with systolic/diastolic ratios of 2.1, 3.5, and 3.5. Normal-appearing amount of amniotic fluid. Amniotic fluid index measures 12.3 cm, which is within normal limits. Placenta is in a posterior location with no evidence of placenta previa seen.

11-9I:

SERVICE CODE(S): ____________________

DX CODE(S): ____________________

11-9J OPERATIVE REPORT, CESAREAN SECTION

When this patient was admitted, Dr. Orbitz was the attending physician. Dr. Martinez was brought in as a consultant and then care was transferred from Dr. Orbtiz to Dr. Martinez, who then became the attending. Dr. Martinez is performing the cesarean section and the necessary postpartum care. For the diagnoses, the record indicates there were complications of pregnancy, diabetic nephropathy, a cesarean delivery in addition to V codes for the outcome of delivery and sterilization.

PREOPERATIVE DIAGNOSES:
1. Intrauterine pregnancy, 33 weeks
2. Insulin-dependent diabetes with diabetic nephropathy
3. Desire for sterilization
4. Previous cesarean section

POSTOPERATIVE DIAGNOSES:
1. Intrauterine pregnancy, 33 weeks
2. Insulin-dependent diabetes with diabetic nephropathy
3. Desire for sterilization
4. Previous cesarean section

PROCEDURE PERFORMED:
1. Repeat low transverse cervical cesarean section
2. Bilateral tubal ligation

SURGEON: Andy Martinez, M.D.

ANESTHESIA: Subarachnoid block

SURGICAL INDICATIONS: The patient is a 28-year-old gravida 2, para 1 with an EDC of 08/01 who had been hospitalized for the past several weeks with hypertension and diabetes. Her condition appeared to be worsening, her diabetes was suddenly poorly controlled, and she having epigastric pain. Her platelet count and AST was normal preoperatively. She had a previous C-section. She also desired permanent sterilization by tubal interruption.

OPERATIVE DESCRIPTION: After induction of subarachnoid block anesthesia, a Foley catheter was placed and the Venodynes were placed as well. The abdomen was prepped and draped. The abdomen was opened through a Pfannenstiel incision. When we separated the rectus muscles, it became apparent that there was very little room as there was so much scarring of the fascia; therefore, a Maylard incision was done by separating the bellies of the rectus muscles transversely. Retractors were placed over the bladder. There was a poor bladder flap, but we dissected some of the bladder downward. An incision was made in the low transverse part of the uterus and entering the uterus was accomplished by blunting with a Kelly clamp. A finger was introduced into the uterus to guide a bandage scissors for a low transverse incision. The infant's head was delivered through the incision, and the muscles were so tight that we were having a little difficulty extracting the head; therefore, I removed my hand and put a Murless retractor behind the head and then the baby was easily delivered. The cord was clamped and cut, and then a segment of cord was sent off for gases. The placenta was then delivered manually. The uterus was closed in two layers, first with a running locked 0 Vicryl, followed by a running horizontal Lembert 0 Vicryl. The pelvis was then irrigated with saline. A few small bleeders were bovie coagulated. The right fallopian tube was elevated and the fimbriated end identified. The mesosalpinx underneath the ampullary portion was opened with bovie, and then the lateral mesosalpinx was cross-clamped on the lateral tube. The lateral portion of the tube, including the fimbriated end, was then excised and pedicles were doubly tied with 2-0 Vicryl. An identical procedure was carried out on the left tube. With sponge and needle counts correct, attention was directed toward closure. The rectus muscles were closed with a series of mattress sutures of 0 Vicryl. A medium Hemovac drain was placed subfascially. The fascia was closed with running locked 0 Vicryl using two strands, one from either side to the middle and tied independently. The skin was then closed with staples, and the drain was sutured to the skin with silk.

BLOOD LOSS ESTIMATION: 400-500 cc

SPECIMEN TO PATHOLOGY: Placenta

FINAL SPONGE AND NEEDLE COUNTS: Correct

The patient tolerated the procedure well and returned to the recovery room in stable condition. After the child was extracted, we did start some magnesium sulfate.

Pathology Report Later Indicated: See 11-9K.

11-9J:

SERVICE CODE(S): ____________________

DX CODE(S): ____________________

11-9K PATHOLOGY REPORT

LOCATION: Inpatient, Hospital

PATIENT: Patricia Garrison

ATTENDING PHYSICIAN: Andy Martinez, M.D.

PATHOLOGIST: Grey Lonewolf, M.D.

CLINICAL HISTORY: Diabetic nephropathy, 33 weeks, unstable; hypertension, unstable; repeat C-section; desires sterilization

SPECIMEN RECEIVED: A: Placenta, third trimester. B: Left fallopian tube. C: Right fallopian tube.

GROSS DESCRIPTION: The specimens were received in three containers:

A. In the container labeled "placenta" is a discoid-shaped placenta measuring 17 × 17 × 3 cm in greatest dimension and weighing 410 g. An umbilical cord measuring 7 cm in length inserts 4 cm from the closest margin. The membranes are smooth, shiny, tan-gray, and translucent. The chorionic surface is unremarkable. On the maternal surface, lacerations extend from short distance into the parenchyma. The parenchyma is uniformly spongy and pink-red on sectioning. On sectioning, the umbilical cord demonstrates three vessels. Multiple representative sections of placenta, umbilical cord, and membranes are submitted.
B. In the container labeled "left tube" is a cylindrical tan tissue segment measuring 2.8 cm in length and 0.6 cm in diameter. The specimen is step-sectioned and totally submitted as "B."
C. In the container labeled "right tube" is a cylindrical tan tissue segment measuring 2.8 cm in length and 0.8 cm in diameter. The specimen is step-sectioned and totally submitted as "C."

MICROSCOPIC DESCRIPTION:

A. The umbilical cord demonstrates three vessels within a normal supporting Wharton's jelly. The placenta demonstrates well-vascularized third-trimester villi. The membranes show normal morphology.

B. The left fallopian tube demonstrates normal morphology. (*1 specimen*)

C. The right fallopian tube demonstrates normal morphology. (*1 specimen*)

DIAGNOSIS:

A. Placenta, umbilical cord, and membranes: No pathologic diagnosis.

B. Left fallopian tube segment: No pathologic diagnosis.

C. Right fallopian tube segment: No pathologic diagnosis.

11-9K:

SERVICE CODE(S): ______________________

DX CODE(S): ______________________

Glossary

antepartum before childbirth.

colposcope scope used to examine the cervix and vagina.

colposcopy examination of the cervix and vagina by means of a colposcope.

endometrium the inner mucous membrane of the uterus.

gynecologist a physician specializing in the diagnosis, treatment, and management of female genital diseases and disorders.

hypertrophy the enlargement or overgrowth of an organ due to the increase in size of its cells.

hysterectomy surgical removal of the uterus.

hysteroscope scope used to examine the uterus.

hysteroscopy visualization of the canal of the uterine cervix and uterine cavity using a scope placed through the vagina.

postpartum after childbirth.

Chapter 12

Nervous System

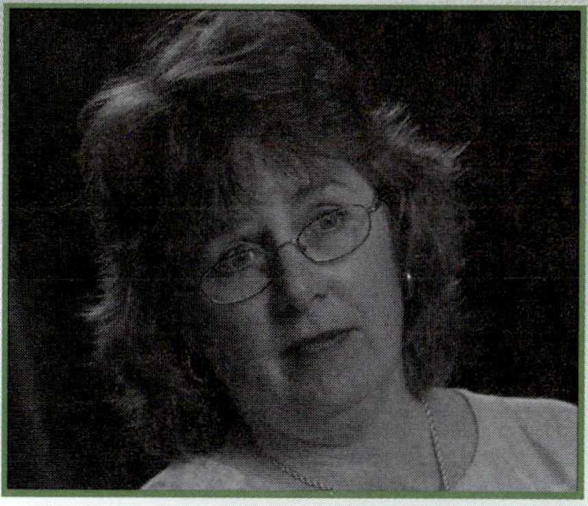

Jeanice Porta, CPC
Administrative Medical Programs
Lee County High Tech Center North
Cape Coral, Florida

ABBREVIATIONS

ANS	autonomic nervous system
C1-C5	cervical vertebra
CSF	cerebrospinal fluid
CNS	central nervous system
CVA	stroke/cerebrovascular accident
EEG	electroencephalogram
L1-L5	lumbar vertebra
LFT	liver function test
LP	lumbar puncture
PAR	postanesthesia recovery
PNS	peripheral nervous system
S1-S5	sacral vertebra
T1-T12	thoracic vertebra
TENS	transcutaneous electrical nerve stimulator
TIA	transient ischemic attack

The nervous system is divided into the sympathetic nervous system and the parasympathetic nervous system, as illustrated in **Figures 12-1** and **12-2.** A **neurologist** is a physician who treats and diagnoses conditions of the nervous system, including the spinal cord, brain, nerves, and muscles. Common neurologic disorders are dizziness, tremor, paresthesia (abnormal touch sensation), stroke, altered mental states, headache, seizure, sleep disorders, and neuralgia. The neurologist uses a variety of diagnostic tools, including magnetic resonance imaging (MRI), computed axial tomography (CAT or CT), electroencephalography (EEG), and EMG/NCV (electromyography/nerve conduction velocity). A **neurosurgeon** is a surgeon who specializes in surgical procedures or treatment of conditions of the nervous system, such as lumbar puncture, brain tumor, head injury, **hematoma,** and disk herniation.

Twist Drill or Burr Holes

Twist drill or burr holes are the opening of the brain to relieve pressure, to insert monitoring devices, or to place tubing or inject contrast material. The placement of these holes leaves the skull intact except for the hole, which is repaired at a later time. This procedure is also termed *trephine.* The CPT codes for these procedures (61105-61253) are based on the reason for the hole (such as implantation of catheter or pressure device, biopsy, aspiration of hematoma, etc.) and, in some instances, the location of the hole (such as supratentorial or infratentorial). The tentorium is a tented sheet of dura mater or covering that covers the cerebellum. **Supratentorial** is above the tentorium of the cerebellum and **infratentorial** is beneath the tentorium of the cerebellum. For the purposes of coding, the supratentorial is the part of the brain above the cerebellum, and infratentorial is the part of the brain beneath the cerebellum.

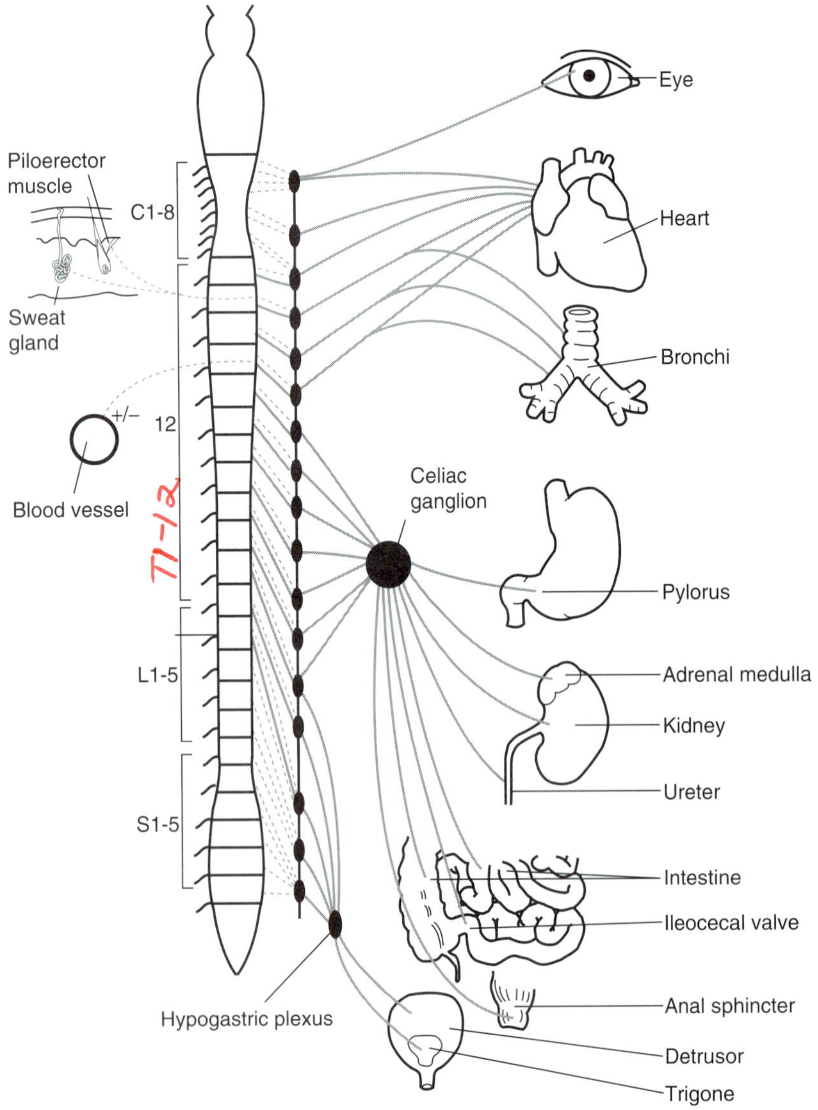

FIGURE 12-1 Sympathetic nervous system.

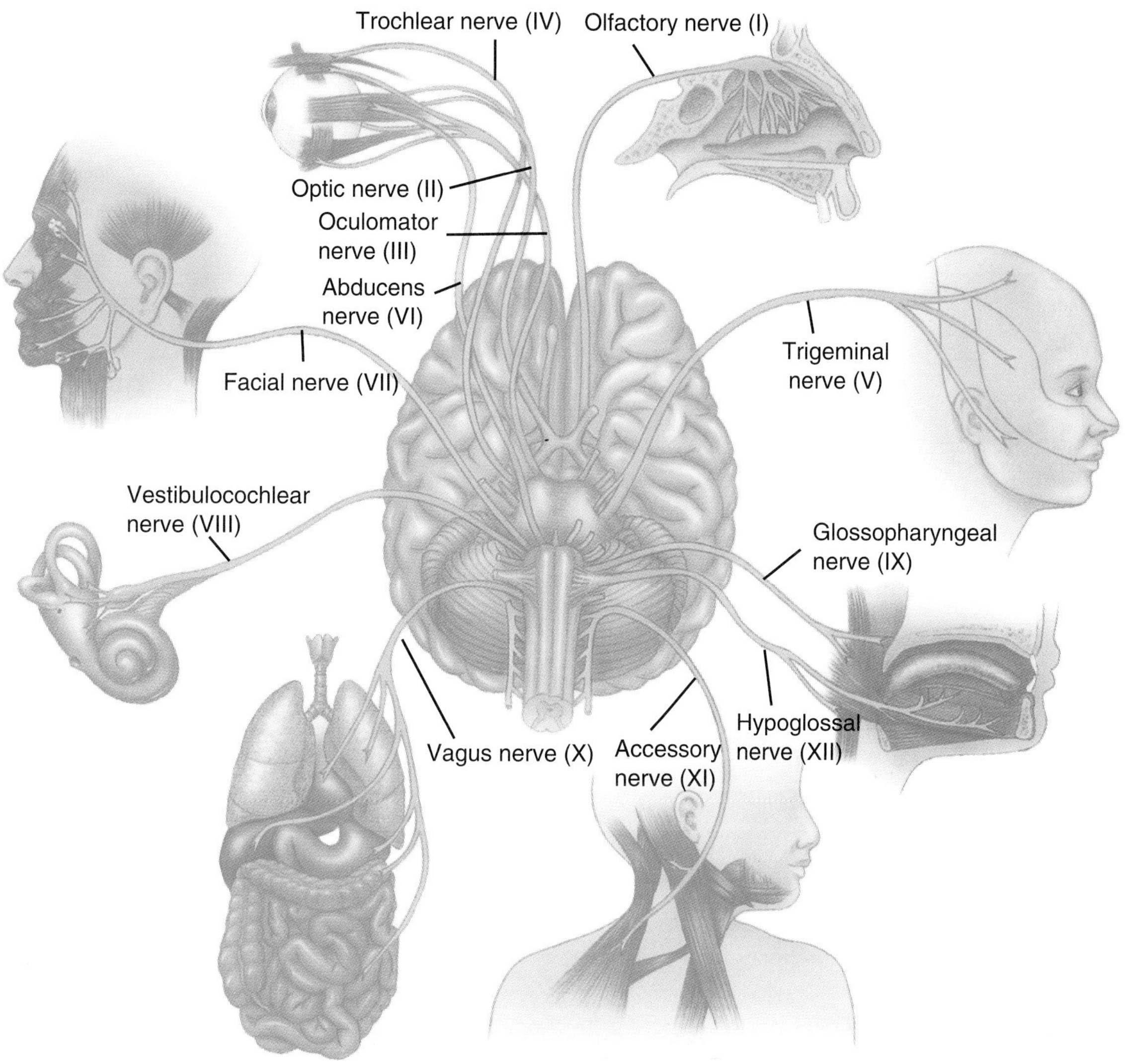

FIGURE 12-2 Parasympathetic nervous system. *(From Thibodeau GA, Patton KI:* Anatomy and physiology, *ed 4, St. Louis, 1999, Mosby.)*

CASE 12-1
12-1A Operative Report, Ventriculostomy

CASE 12-1

Dick is a patient in the intensive care unit of the hospital. He has an obstructive hydrocephalus as a result of an intracerebral hemorrhage. Report the services of Dr. Pleasant.

12-1A OPERATIVE REPORT, VENTRICULOSTOMY

LOCATION: Inpatient, Hospital

PATIENT: Dick Dawn

ATTENDING PHYSICIAN: Timothy Pleasant, M.D.

SURGEON: Timothy Pleasant, M.D.

PREPROCEDURE DIAGNOSIS: Obstructive hydrocephalus, secondary to intracerebral hemorrhage

POSTPROCEDURE DIAGNOSIS: Obstructive hydrocephalus, secondary to intracerebral hemorrhage

PROCEDURE PERFORMED: Ventriculostomy

OPERATIVE NOTE: While in the intensive care unit, the patient was noted to be deteriorating neurologically and suffering from obstructive hydrocephalus. The right side of the scalp was shaved, prepped, and draped in the usual sterile manner. A small incision was made in the midpupillary line approximately 10 cm behind the supraorbital rim. The standard hole was then fashioned. The dura was then punctured, and a catheter was inserted uneventfully into the right lateral ventricle. Bloody CSF was immediately obtained and was noted to be under high pressure. It was then externalized through the subcutaneous tissue and through another wound. The original wound was then sutured, and a sterile dressing was applied. There were no operative complications.

12-1A:

SERVICE CODE(S): ____________________

DX CODE(S): ____________________

Craniotomy

A **craniotomy** is the surgical removal of a section of bone and is referred to as a *bone flap*. Removal of the bone is done in preparation for an operative procedure of the brain. The removed bone is returned to the original site at the end of the procedure. If tissue or bone is removed and not returned to the original site, the procedure is a **craniectomy**. For example, when a blood clot is removed and the bone flap is replaced, that is a craniotomy. If, however, a portion of the brain was removed due to a disease or condition, the procedure is a craniectomy. The craniotomy or craniectomy is performed for conditions such as trauma, infection, tumor, and aneurysm.

Codes 61510-61530 report the removal or treatment of brain tumor(s), abscess, or cyst in which a portion of the skull bone is removed, procedure performed, bone replaced, and the bone then stabilized in place. (Figure 12-3.)

- 61510-61516 are used to report these types of procedures when they are performed supratentorially (above the tentorium of the cerebellum).
- 61518-61524 are used when performed infratentorially (below the tentorium of the cerebellum).
- 61526-61530 are used when performed transtemporally (across the temporal lobe).

If stealth is used during the procedure, it is reported in addition to the procedure with 61795. A full description of stealth is presented before Case 12-3.

Subdural Hematoma

A *subdural hematoma* is a hemorrhage characterized by a collection of blood between the dura mater and the arachnoid membrane. A subdural hematoma is often a result of contusion with the source of the bleeding being an artery or vein. If the hematoma ruptures the arachnoid membrane, the condition is termed *subdural hygroma*. Subdural hematomas caused by trauma (such as head injuries) are categorized according to the presentation after injury: hyperacute (less than 24 hours), acute (1-3 days), early subacute (3-7 days), late subacute (more than 7 days), or chronic (more than 3 weeks). Other causes of subdural hematoma are artery or vein abnormalities (arteriovenous malformation) as a result of shunting procedures or a lumbar puncture, neoplasm, hypertension, hemodialysis, intracranial operations, infections, or as a result of bleeding disorder (such as hemophilia).

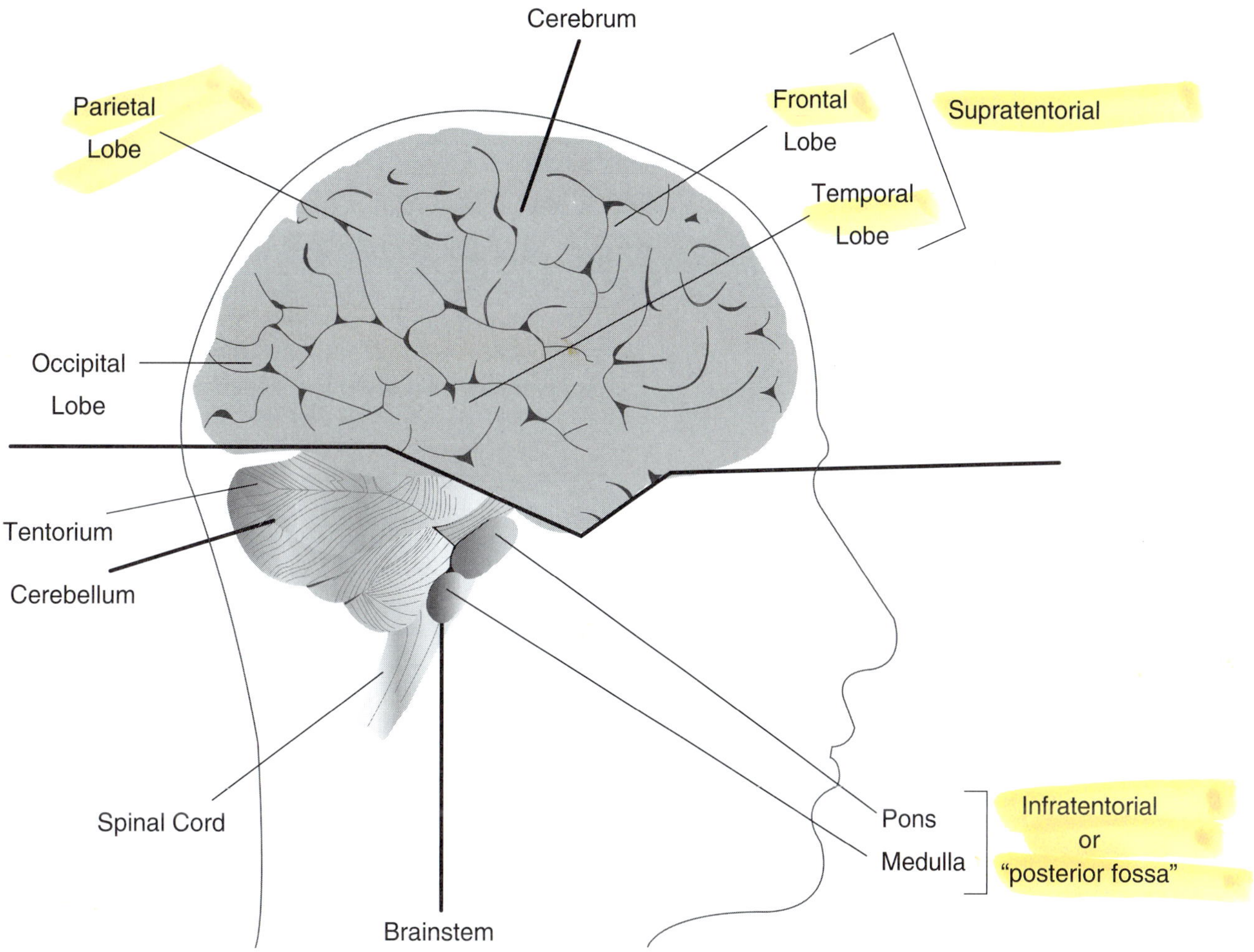

FIGURE 12-3 Cerebral hemisphere and tentorium.

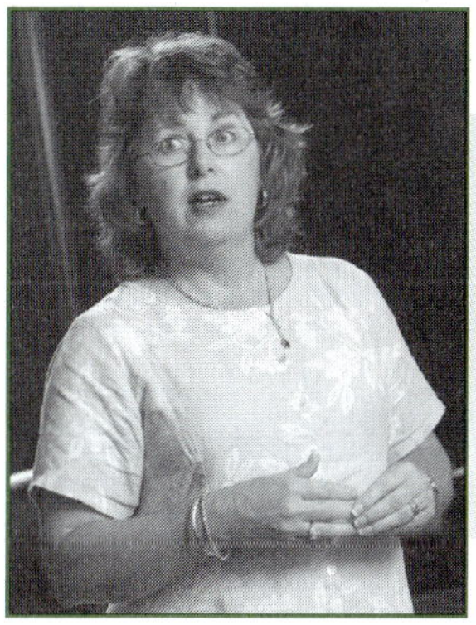

FROM THE TRENCHES

Jeanice

"The hardest things for my students to do is to code directly from a patient record. A lot of them want something that's black and white, and the records are hard for them because there is so much 'gray.' But that's what you have to learn how to do. That is real life—that's what it's all about."

CASE 12-2
12-2A Operative Report, Osteoplastic Craniotomy

CASE 12-2

The following craniotomy is for the purpose of removal of a subdural hematoma.

12-2A OPERATIVE REPORT, OSTEOPLASTIC CRANIOTOMY

LOCATION: Inpatient, Hospital

PATIENT: Larry Colter

ATTENDING PHYSICIAN: Timothy Pleasant, M.D.

SURGEON: Timothy Pleasant, M.D.

PREOPERATIVE DIAGNOSIS: Acute subdural hematoma, left side

POSTOPERATIVE DIAGNOSIS: Acute subdural hematoma, left side

PROCEDURE PERFORMED: Osteoplastic craniotomy

ANESTHESIA: General anesthesia

PROCEDURE: Under general anesthesia, the left head was prepped and draped in the usual manner after having been placed in Mayfield pins. Hemoclips and Dandy clips were utilized on the scalp edges. Part of the temporalis muscle was taken down. Two burr holes and a circumferential flap were made. The bone was elevated. The dura was incised in an inverted U-shaped fashion. We saw acute clot; probably 45-50 cc of clot was irrigated from the frontal, temporal, and posterior parietal areas (*indicates supratentorial; see Figure 12-2*). Having cleaned it out, there was no free bleeder that I saw. I placed a piece of Gelfoam on the brain and then began closure of the dura with 3-0 Vicryl; this was done. A little patch was necessary; we used temporalis fascia. We tacked up the dura, replaced the bone flap, utilized Wurzburg plates and burr hole cover. Having secured this, we then closed the scalp with 2-0 Vicryl on the galea with surgical staples on the skin, with a Hemovac drain having been applied prior to closure.

12-2A:

SERVICE CODE(S): ______________________

DX CODE(S): ______________________

Stealth Surgery

Stealth surgery is computer-assisted surgery that produces three-dimensional images and uses infrared intraoperative guidance that enables location of tumors of the brain and spinal cord with great accuracy. The technology is the same as the B22 Stealth Bomber. A CT of the patient's brain is fed into the stealth computer to use as a road map during surgery. The computer tracks the surgical instruments being used by the surgeon during the operation by means of an infrared sensor that is located over the operating table. The computer then translates these instrument movements into a three-dimensional image for the surgeon to view. There is a red *x* located on the screen indicating the location of the tumor or area of damage. The technology is accurate to within 1 mm and greatly decreases damage to the brain during these invasive procedures. When stealth technology is utilized during a procedure (and the technology is used with a wide variety of procedures, not just brain surgery), you report the use of the technology in addition to the primary procedure. This technology is referred to in the CPT as stereotaxis, which is the precise positioning in space. The code for stereotaxis is located in the CPT index under "Stereotaxis, Computer Assisted, Brain Surgery."

CASE 12-3
12-3A Operative Report, Craniectomy
12-3B Patthology Report

CASE 12-3

The label of a procedure (such as, craniectomy or craniotomy) does not mean that the title is the exact procedure. The following procedure is the removal of a tumor and an intracranial clot by means of a craniectomy. Sometimes, the report title might state craniotomy when a craniectomy was performed. Only careful reading of the entire report will reveal the exact procedure and ensure accurate coding. See Figure 12-4 for location of ventricle.

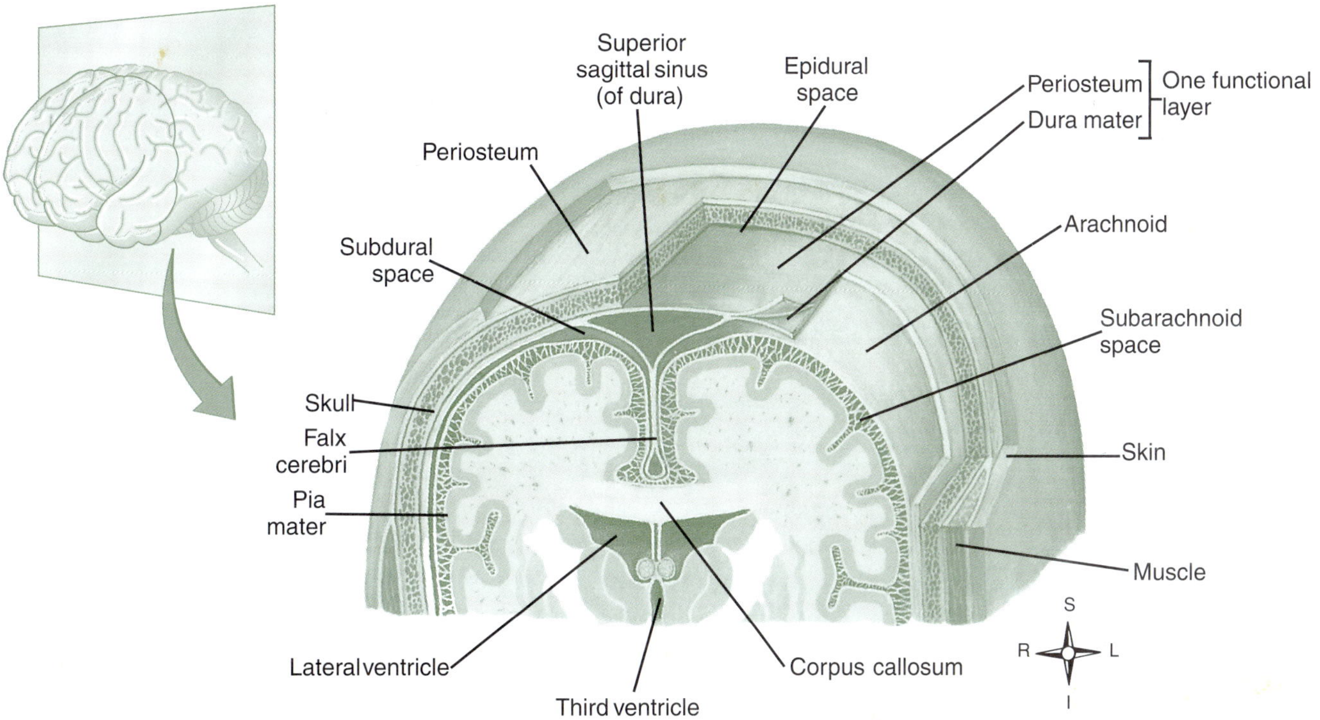

FIGURE 12-4 Frontal section of the superior portion of the head, as viewed from the front. Both the bony and the membranous coverings of the brain can be seen. (From Thibodeau GA, Patton KI: *Anatomy and physiology, St. Louis, 1999, Mosby.*)

12-3A OPERATIVE REPORT, CRANIECTOMY

LOCATION: Inpatient, Hospital

PATIENT: Erika Witt

ATTENDING PHYSICIAN: Timothy Pleasant, M.D.

SURGEON: Timothy Pleasant, M.D.

PREOPERATIVE DIAGNOSIS: Recurrent tumor, intracranial clot

POSTOPERATIVE DIAGNOSIS: Recurrent tumor, intracranial clot

PROCEDURE PERFORMED: Craniotomy, removal of tumor, and removal of intracranial clot. ②

ANESTHESIA: General

PREOPERATIVE NOTE: This patient has been forewarned about her condition and that we are operating on a marginally reserve patient, that we do not know what the results will be but will certainly try to remove the tumor and the clot to improve the situation.

This case was done under Stealth protocol (reported separately). We utilized a localizer, and we were able to show that the tumor cavity was totally entered and the tumor and clot were removed.

PROCEDURE: Under general anesthesia, the patient was placed in Mayfield pins. The head was prepped and draped in the usual manner. An inverted U-shaped incision was made. The previous craniotomy was opened up, and the dura was incised. We got into the ventricle. We removed what looked like yellow tumor, which was necrotic tissue. We removed a large intracranial clot as well and cleaned out the ventricular area. There was tumor or clot in the temporal lobe as well as in the lateral ventricle. I could see the foramen of Monro. I could clean out the entire cavity. This wound was irrigated; on the raw surface a piece of Gelfoam was placed after coagulation was achieved. The dura was then closed with Duragen. The bone flap was replaced with 22 wires, and the scalp wound was then closed in layers with 3-0 Vicryl on the galea and surgical staples on the skin. A dressing was applied. The patient was discharged to the recovery area.

Pathology Report Later Indicated: See 12-3B.

12-3A: ① Neoplasm, brain, ventricle (benign)

SERVICE CODE(S): 61510

DX CODE(S): ____________

12-3B PATHOLOGY REPORT

LOCATION: Inpatient, Hospital

PATIENT: Erika Witt

ATTENDING PHYSICIAN: Timothy Pleasant, M.D.

SURGEON: Timothy Pleasant, M.D.

PATHOLOGIST: Grey Lonewolf, M.D.

CLINICAL HISTORY: Recurrent meningioma with intracerebral hemorrhage

SPECIMEN RECEIVED: Meningioma

GROSS DESCRIPTION:
The specimen is labeled with the patient's name and "meningioma" and consists predominantly of blood clot with a few fragments of gray-tan lobulated tissue, 1 and 5 cm in greatest dimension. Representative sections are submitted in 6 cassettes.

MICROSCOPIC DESCRIPTION:
Sections of brain show areas of reactive gliosis with associated focal fibrosis, hemosiderin-laden macrophages, and foamy macrophages. Areas of recent hemorrhage with blood clot and focal areas of necrosis are also seen. A neoplastic infiltrate is not identified.

DIAGNOSIS:
Brain, frontal cortex, excision: Benign brain showing reactive gliosis with areas of fibrosis, foamy macrophages, and foci of necrosis and accompanying blood clot.

12-3B:

SERVICE CODE(S): ____________

DX CODE(S): ____________

CASE 12-4

The removal of this tumor is conducted through a bone flap.

12-4A OPERATIVE REPORT, CRANIOTOMY

LOCATION: Inpatient, Hospital

PATIENT: Arlene Samuels

ATTENDING PHYSICIAN: Timothy Pleasant, M.D.

SURGEON: Timothy Pleasant, M.D.

PREOPERATIVE DIAGNOSIS: Right temporal parietal frontal brain tumor

POSTOPERATIVE DIAGNOSIS: Glioblastoma multiforme

PROCEDURE PERFORMED: Osteoplastic craniotomy with removal of tumor in temporal lobe, frontal lobe, and middle cerebral artery complex (*contiguous [adjoining] sites*).

ANESTHESIA: General

PROCEDURE: Under general anesthesia, the patient's head was prepped and draped in the usual manner. A question mark incision was made in the front of the ear up to the frontal area. The skin flap was turned down. The temporalis muscle was incised. We then did an osteoplastic craniotomy with burr holes and craniotome. The flap was turned. The dura was incised. We then made an incision into the superior temporal lobe. The plan was to resect the temporal lobe to get into the tumor and stay away from the middle cerebral complex and also to decompress her on the frontal lobe as well since the tumor was going into the frontal lobe. I got into the tumor and sent specimen for biopsy and then began the gradual dissection. I encountered some bleeding, probably from middle cerebral artery branches. I had to take a few with silver clips, perhaps two to three. Otherwise, we left the sylvian vein intact and decompressed the area (*decompression is bundled into tumor removal*). We got into the tumor cavity and took as much visual tumor as we could. The bed was then dried. I irrigated the wound well. I placed a piece of Gelfoam over the raw surface of the brain and began closure of the dura with 3-0 Vicryl. The bone flap was replaced with two straight four-holed Wurzburg plates. Hemovac was placed, and the scalp was closed in layers utilizing 3-0 Vicryl on the galea with surgical staples on the skin. Dressing was applied. The patient was discharged to PAR.

Pathology Report Later Indicated: Glioblastoma multiforme

12-4A:

SERVICE CODE(S): 61510-RT

DX CODE(S): ______________________

CASE 12-5

12-5A Operative Report, Pterygocraniotomy and Cranioplasty

CASE 12-5

(1) aneurysm, brain
(2) Hemorrhage, subarachnoid)

An operating microscope is used in this procedure and is reported separately. Simple aneurysms are any that are 15 millimeters or less.

12-5A OPERATIVE REPORT, PTERYGOCRANIOTOMY AND CRANIOPLASTY

LOCATION: Inpatient, Hospital

PATIENT: Brett Richards

ATTENDING PHYSICIAN: Timothy Pleasant, M.D.

SURGEON: Timothy Pleasant, M.D. (2)

PREOPERATIVE DIAGNOSIS: Subarachnoid hemorrhage secondary to right posterior communicating artery aneurysm (1)

POSTOPERATIVE DIAGNOSIS: Subarachnoid hemorrhage secondary to right posterior communicating artery aneurysm, 12 mm

PROCEDURE PERFORMED: Right pterygocraniotomy with microsurgical clipping of right posterior communicating artery aneurysm and cranioplasty

DESCRIPTION OF PROCEDURE: The patient was taken to the operating room and placed under general endotracheal anesthesia. The right scalp (*This indicates an intracranial approach as versus a cervical approach.*) was then shaved, prepped, and draped in the usual sterile manner. A modified Souttar bicoronal incision was then outlined in the skin and subcutaneous tissue and was infiltrated with lidocaine with epinephrine. The skin was incised, and sharp dissection was carried through subcutaneous tissue. LeRoy-Raney clips were then applied to the skin edges and the galeacutaneous flap was elevated and reflected anteriorly. Temporalis muscle was then incised and reflected anteriorly, and a free bone flap was fashioned using a Midas burr. A generous craniectomy was carried out on the squamous portion of the temporal bone and the lateral sphenoid wing. Twenty-five grams of mannitol had been given prior to skin incision, and dura was noted to be moderately tense. A horseshoe-shaped dural flap was then fashion based inferiorly. Great care was taken to preserve the Sylvian vein. Only a small amount of cerebral edema was noted at this point. The anterior inferior aspect of the Sylvian fissure was then split, and the CSF was released. This portion of the procedure was somewhat tedious and allowed for brain retraction. The right olfactory nerve was then visualized and protected. The optic nerve was then identified as well as the proximal portion of the intercranial carotid artery. Fixed retractors were then placed, and the remainder of the procedure was carried out using microsurgical technique. (69990 microscope) The carotid cistern was opened using an arachnoid knife. The proximal portion of the intracranial carotid was then dissected free with thickened hemorrhagic arachnoid. Great care was exercised to minimize retraction on the temporal lobe. An aneurysm was noted in the proximal third of the intracranial and carotid artery immediately proximal to the bifurcation. (*This indicates the intracranial aneurysm was in the carotid circulation.*) Carefully dissecting the neck of the aneurysm revealed the origin of the anterior choroidal artery immediately distal to the neck. The dome of the aneurysm appeared to be immersed in scar and was largely immobile. After adequately dissecting the neck (*This "neck" is the neck of the aneurysm, not the patient's neck.*) and allowing for passage of microdissectors along the tract of the clip, the straight clip was selected. Clipping of the aneurysm then proceeded uneventfully. Post clipping, the internal carotid artery was noted to be widely patent, and the anterior choroidal artery was also visualized and noted to be unaffected by the aneurysm clip. Hemostasis was then ensured. The exposed brain was lined with a single layer of Surgicel. The area was generously irrigated with a body-temperature saline. The dura was closed using a running silk suture. The dural tacking sutures were also applied. The bone cap was secured and a cranioplasty was carried out for the squamous portion of the temporal bone and the lateral sphenoid wing. Muscle flap of the temporalis muscle was then repaired using interrupted Vicryl sutures. The galea was closed using interrupted Vicryl sutures, and sutures were utilized for the skin. Steri-Strips and sterile dressing were applied to the wound. The patient tolerated the procedure well. The patient was noted to be moving all extremities in the operating room and was transferred to the recovery room in satisfactory condition.

12-5A:

SERVICE CODE(S): ______________________

DX CODE(S): ______________________

CASE 12-6
12-6A Operative Report, Craniectomy

CASE 12-6

12-6A OPERATIVE REPORT, CRANIECTOMY

LOCATION: Inpatient, Hospital

PATIENT: Suzanne Tracy

ATTENDING PHYSICIAN: Timothy Pleasant, M.D.

SURGEON: Timothy Pleasant, M.D.

PREOPERATIVE DIAGNOSIS: Brain tumor

POSTOPERATIVE DIAGNOSIS: Brain tumor

PROCEDURE PERFORMED: Craniectomy and removal of temporal lobe tumor

ANESTHESIA: General

Stealth protocol was utilized in doing this tumor. It was utilized in localizing the tumor.

PROCEDURE: Under general anesthesia, the patient was placed in the supine position. The head was turned to the right. The head was prepped and draped. The phaser was utilized to localize the tumor and to place it into the Stealth machine. Having done this, we then prepped and draped the patient. We made a linear incision extending from the temporal pole, having localized the tumor on the surface of the skin with the pointer. I then incised the skin and incised the temporalis fascia and muscle. I divided it. I then proceeded to perform a burr hole and a small craniectomy over the right temporal lobe tip. This having been done, we then incised the dura. This tumor was attached to the dura, and I removed the tumor; it was the size of a walnut. This was undermined from the surrounding brain with patties. There was no bleeding. This came out very easily. We then utilized Duraplast to repair the dura. We were utilizing 4-0 Nurolon. The bone edges were packed with some beeswax, and the dural edges were cauterized. The Duraplast having been placed, I then put a piece of Gelfoam on this, and I approximated the temporalis muscle and temporalis fascia with 0 Vicryl. I utilized 2-0 Vicryl on the galea. Surgical staples on the skin. Tight dressing was applied, and the patient was discharged to recovery.

Pathology Report Later Indicated: Benign neoplasm, meninges

12-6A:

SERVICE CODE(S): ____________________

DX CODE(S): ____________________

Cranioplasty

Cranioplasty is the repair of a cranial defect. The surgeon uses autograft (from the patient) bone that is shaped and grafted into the defect area. If the defect is larger or more complicated than the surgeon can repair by bone grafting, a prosthetic plate may be used. Sometimes the plate is used as the foundation on which the surgeon places surgical cement to fill in an area of defect. The CPT codes in the cranial repair category (62000-62148) are divided based on the type of repair and in some codes the extent of the repair (see 62140 for defects up to 5 cm in diameter).

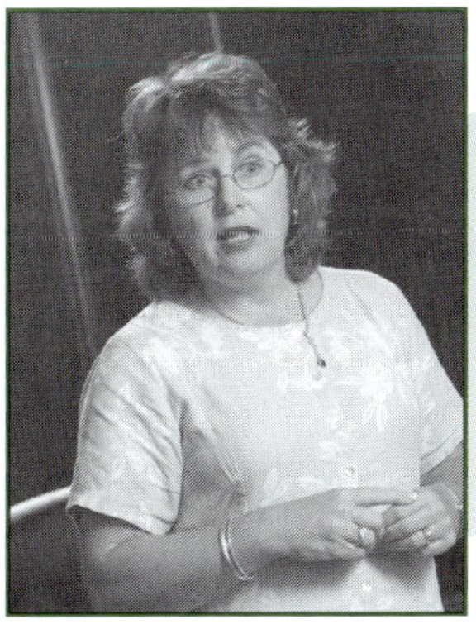

FROM THE TRENCHES

Jeanice

"Over the last 10 years, coding has become a profession… I've seen a big change in the physician's respect for coding knowledge and that's what we have to keep working on. There's a value there that coders know what they're doing and they're there to help the physicians."

CASE 12-7
12-7A Operative Report, Cranioplasty

CASE 12-7

12-7A OPERATIVE REPORT, CRANIOPLASTY

LOCATION: Inpatient, Hospital

PATIENT: Sylvia Reagan

ATTENDING PHYSICIAN: Timothy Pleasant, M.D.

SURGEON: Timothy Pleasant, M.D.

PREOPERATIVE DIAGNOSIS: Cranial deformity

POSTOPERATIVE DIAGNOSIS: Cranial deformity

PROCEDURE PERFORMED: Cranioplasty

PREOPERATIVE NOTE: This is a patient who has had a cranial defect because she had a bone removed. She was in cerebral swelling post aneurysm clipping and she survived. Now she is set up to have repair of the 10-cm cranial defect. An expander had been placed in this defect before.

PROCEDURE: The patient's head was prepped and draped in the usual manner. An incision was made in the skin. The expander was removed. There was a plate in there. We were able to use this as a base to pour the methylmethacrylate cement. This was fashioned over the steel mesh. Afterward, this was formed to fill the defect out. We utilized the burr to shape it to the defect. We then closed the wound in one layer utilizing 2-0 Prolene on the scalp. A dressing was applied, and the patient was discharged to the PAR.

12-7A:

SERVICE CODE(S): ______________________

DX CODE(S): ______________________

Shunts

A **shunt** is a passage from one area to another that diverts fluid from one area to another. There are many different types of shunts. A ventricular shunt is a catheter that is placed into the ventricle of the brain to drain cerebrospinal fluid (CSF) into the peritoneal cavity. **Figure 12-5** illustrates a ventriculoperitoneal shunt. If the catheter becomes damaged or otherwise obstructed, the shunt is replaced. The diagnosis is a complication of a catheter device.

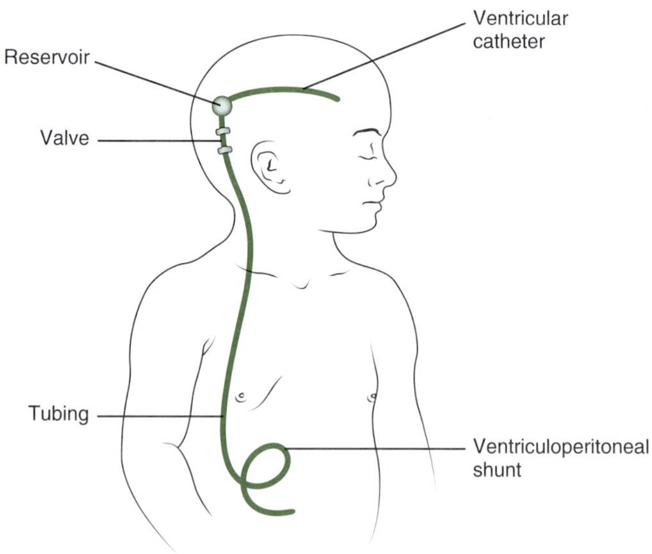

FIGURE 12-5 Ventriculoperitoneal shunt.

CASE 12-8
12-8A Operative Report, Shunt Repair

CASE 12-8

12-8A OPERATIVE REPORT, SHUNT REPAIR

This is a report of a shunt obstruction which represents a diagnosis of a complication of a shunt, specifically a ventricular catheter device (996.X).

LOCATION: Inpatient, Hospital

PATIENT: Dean Rob

ATTENDING PHYSICIAN: Timothy Pleasant, M.D.

SURGEON: Timothy Pleasant, M.D.

PREOPERATIVE DIAGNOSIS: Shunt obstruction

POSTOPERATIVE DIAGNOSIS: Fracture of shunt

PROCEDURE PERFORMED: Repair of shunt. Replacement of ventricular catheter and valve.

ANESTHESIA: General

Under general anesthesia, the patient's right head was prepped and draped in the usual manner. The entire abdomen and neck were draped. We were planning to possibly replace the entire shunt. After incising over the head and the shunt in the right posterior parietal area, it was obvious what the problem was. I incised the skin, turned down the flap, and the ventricular end of shunt had fractured from the shunt valve. I removed the valve. I removed the ventricular end and replaced it with a Delta One valve and 6 cm of ventricular shunt tubing and connected it up to the peritoneal catheter. It flowed easily. We did not inspect the peritoneal end, hoping that this would do and solve the problem. The fluid flowed freely into the peritoneal cavity. What I think happened here was the child probably hit his head and fractured the tube.

PROCEDURE: After reconnecting the shunt, we then closed the galea with 2-0 Vicryl interrupted and 4-0 nylon sutures on the skin. A dressing was applied. The patient was discharged to the PAR.

12-8A:

SERVICE CODE(S): ______________________

DX CODE(S): ______________________

Lumbar Puncture

A lumbar puncture is also termed a spinal tap. This procedure obtains cerebrospinal fluid by means of a needle inserted into the subarachnoid space in the lumbar region as illustrated in **Figure 12-6.** The patient is positioned so the space between the vertebra is as wide as possible. Any interspace can be used for the procedure, but L5-S1 is the largest and is most often used as the site of withdrawal. The CSF fluid is used for diagnoses of various conditions. Commonly assessed are the appearance, protein, sugar, serology, cell count, and at times bacterial and fungal cultures of fluid.

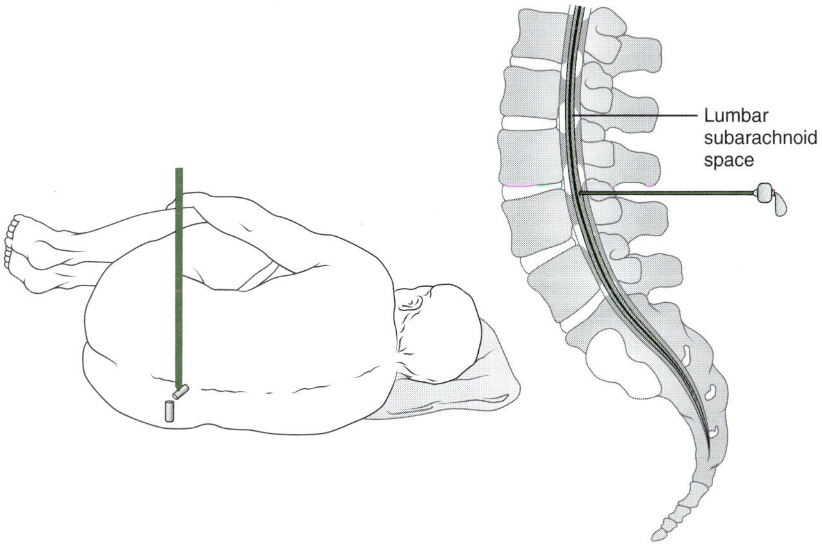

FIGURE 12-6 Lumbar puncture.

CASE 12-9
12-9A Operative Report, Lumbar Puncture

CASE 12-9

12-9A OPERATIVE REPORT, LUMBAR PUNCTURE

LOCATION: Inpatient, Hospital

PATIENT: Larry Swope

ATTENDING PHYSICIAN: Timothy Pleasant, M.D.

SURGEON: Timothy Pleasant, M.D.

INDICATION: Vascular headache

PROCEDURE PERFORMED: Diagnostic lumbar puncture

PROCEDURE: Following Betadine prep, local anesthetic was instilled in the L3-4 interspace. A #20-gauge needle was then inserted in this interspace and advanced until it entered the subarachnoid space on the second pass. Opening pressure was 110 mm of water. Five centimeters of crystal-clear fluid was obtained and sent to the laboratory for routine diagnostic studies, including viral culture. The patient tolerated the procedure well. He was given instructions as to how to avoid postlumbar tap headache.

12-9A:

SERVICE CODE(S): ________________

DX CODE(S): ________________

Pump Implantation

Pumps are implanted into the body to dispense various drugs. For example, in Case 12-10A, a baclofen pump is being implanted. Baclofen is a drug that decreases the frequency and severity of muscle spasms, which can be administered orally or intrathecally. Intrathecal baclofen therapy (ITB therapy) is a long-term delivery of baclofen via a titanium disk that is 3 inches in diameter and delivers the baclofen directly into the spinal fluid (intrathecal). The pump is programmable with a telemetry wand that is used on the outside of the body, as illustrated in **Figure 12-7,** to adjust the dosage. There are two procedures performed when implanting a pump—the implantation of the pump (62360-62368) and the catheter that leads from the pump to the spinal column or brain (62350-62355). The pump is refillable, and the refilling and maintenance are reported separately with 95990. A **laminectomy** (excision of a posterior arch of a vertebra) may be performed when implanting the pump system and requires the selection of a code to indicate the dual procedures of implantation and excision (62351).

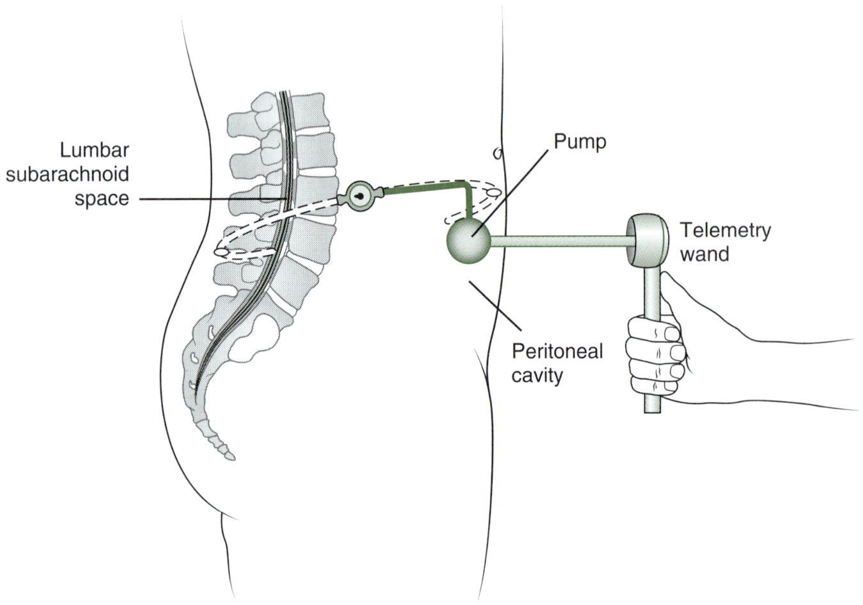

FIGURE 12-7 Lumbo-peritoneal shunt.

CASE 12-10
12-10A Operative Report, Pump Implantation

CASE 12-10

12-10A OPERATIVE REPORT, PUMP IMPLANTATION

LOCATION: Inpatient, Hospital

PATIENT: Ross Lowell

ATTENDING PHYSICIAN: Timothy Pleasant, M.D.

SURGEON: Timothy Pleasant, M.D.

PREOPERATIVE DIAGNOSIS: Spasticity secondary to multiple sclerosis

POSTOPERATIVE DIAGNOSIS: Spasticity secondary to multiple sclerosis

PROCEDURE PERFORMED: Implantation of Medtronic baclofen pump

ANESTHESIA: General

PROCEDURE: Under general anesthesia, the patient's spine, side, and right abdomen were prepped and draped in the usual manner. The procedure started as follows: Having draped the patient, we then incised the skin over the spinous processes of L2, L3, and L4 paramedian and got down to the fascia; here I was able, with a spinal needle, to insert the needle into the subarachnoid space, got good backflow, and placed the catheter into the subarachnoid space, obtaining good CSF flow. I put a clamp on it, and then began the anchoring of the tubing in the paramedian area by securing the tubing to the plastic insert, which holds the tubing to the fascia. We secured this with 2-0 silk. I then went to the anterior right quadrant and made an incision there for acceptance of the pump. This pump was placed into the pocket after using blunt dissection. I then passed the tubing from the posterior to the anterior incision using the trocar. I then had good CSF flow. I connected this to the baclofen pump utilizing the prescribed technique for doing same, that is, anchoring it with sutures. I anchored the pump with two sutures to the fascia and then began closure of the wounds. Both wounds were closed watertight with 2-0 Vicryl in the subcutaneous tissue, 2-0 plain in the subcuticular tissue, and surgical staples on the skin. A dressing was applied. The patient was discharged to PAR.

12-10A:

SERVICE CODE(S): ____________________

DX CODE(S): ____________________

CASE 12-11
12-11A Preoperative Consultation
12-11B Operative Report, Intrathecal Catheter Placement
12-11C Operative Report, Removal of Bard Port
12-11D Discharge Summary

CASE 12-11

The patient in this case is scheduled to have a baclofen infusion pump implanted, and Dr. Pleasant has requested a consultation prior to surgery by Dr. Green to ensure that there are no contraindications to the procedure. The reason for this service is the cerebral palsy.

12-11A PREOPERATIVE CONSULTATION

LOCATION: Inpatient, Hospital

PATIENT: Foy Crow

ATTENDING PHYSICIAN: Timothy Pleasant, M.D.

CONSULTATION: Ronald Green, M.D.

PROCEDURE: Intrathecal catheter placement for baclofen infusion

MEDICATIONS: None

ALLERGIES: None

PAST MEDICAL HISTORY: Cerebral palsy. No previous surgeries. No medical problems.

FAMILY HISTORY: Heart disease in grandparents. There is no diabetes or cancer.

SOCIAL HISTORY: He just recently moved back to Manytown. He is living in his own townhouse. He does have disabilities related to his cerebral palsy. He has been having more problems with speech.

REVIEW OF SYSTEMS: The patient is denying any fevers, chills, cough, sore throat, or allergy problems. He sleeps well except the pain that he gets from the left arm. He is not having any constipation or diarrhea. He denies any dysuria or change in urinary frequency. He is not bothered by a rash. He has no history of blood clots or bleeding disorder.

PHYSICAL EXAMINATION: The patient appears in no acute distress. His speech is very difficult to understand. There is some drooling when trying to talk. His blood pressure is 140/94. HEENT: The oropharynx membranes are moist. There is no exudate. The ears have normal landmarks. Nares are pink. Neck is supple. No tenderness. No adenopathy. No carotid bruits. Heart is regular; S1 and S2. Lungs: He has good aeration. No wheezes. No crackles. Abdomen is soft and nontender. The left arm is prompted forward and has minimal motion. Extremities do not reveal any pedal edema. There is no cyanosis.

Chest x-ray does not reveal any infiltrate. Urinalysis is pending. CBC is pending.

ASSESSMENT: Cerebral palsy

PLAN: The patient has no contraindications to the planned surgery. He has average surgical risks. We are awaiting the laboratory results.

12-11A:

SERVICE CODE(S): ______________________

DX CODE(S): ______________________

12-11B OPERATIVE REPORT, INTRATHECAL CATHETER PLACEMENT

Even though you know from previous reports that this patient has cerebral palsy, this specific report does not indicate that. You therefore report the reason for the service as the dystonia as documented in the report. In this operative report, the surgeon is implanting a temporary, non-programmable Bard pump. It is not uncommon for a temporary pump that cannot be programmed to be implanted and then if the patient responds well to the temporary pump, the pump is removed and replaced with a permanent, programmable pump.

A programmable pump can be adjusted to deliver a set amount of medication.

LOCATION: Inpatient, Hospital

PATIENT: Foy Crow

ATTENDING PHYSICIAN: Timothy Pleasant, M.D.

SURGEON: Timothy Pleasant, M.D.

PREOPERATIVE DIAGNOSIS: Symptomatic torsion dystonia

POSTOPERATIVE DIAGNOSIS: Symptomatic torsion dystonia

PROCEDURE PERFORMED: Placement of a Bard port with intrathecal placement of catheter

ANESTHESIA: General anesthesia

PROCEDURE: Under general anesthesia, the patient's back was prepped and draped. The C-arm was introduced. We then placed a needle into the subarachnoid space. This was with a Tuohy needle. We then threaded the catheter in up to T1-T2, got good back flow, removed the needle, and then undercut by the plastic tubing so that we could place a trocar, which would come around the right flank. This was done. The path of least resistance was made, and the incision was made over the right quadrant. The plastic catheter was then connected to the Bard port and secured. The wound was then closed. The patient was to have a trial at infusion of medications in the Bard pump, to be brought back at a later date for removal and placement of a Synchro pump. The wound was closed in layers utilizing 4-0 nylon sutures on the skin, and a dressing was applied.

12-11B:

SERVICE CODE(S): ____________________

DX CODE(S): ____________________

12-11C OPERATIVE REPORT, REMOVAL OF BARD PORT

The temporary Bard port was replaced with a programmable Medtronic pump. This was a staged procedure, which alerts you to the need for a modifier.

LOCATION: Inpatient, Hospital

PATIENT: Foy Crow

ATTENDING PHYSICIAN: Timothy Pleasant, M.D.

SURGEON: Gary Sanchez, M.D.

PREOPERATIVE DIAGNOSIS: Symptomatic torsion dystonia

POSTOPERATIVE DIAGNOSIS: Symptomatic torsion dystonia

PROCEDURE PERFORMED: Removal of Bard; placement of Sofamor-Danek Medtronic pump delivery system for intrathecal medication.

PROCEDURE: The skin over the abdomen was prepped and draped. The previous incision was incised. The Bard pump was removed. A pocket was made in the right quadrant of the abdomen by undermining the subcutaneous fat. The pump was then anchored and connected to the catheter securely with 4-0 nylon sutures. Having done this, we then closed the wound in layers utilizing 3-0 Vicryl on the subcutaneous tissue with 2-0 plain in the subcuticular tissue and 4-0 nylon sutures, interrupted mattress, on the skin. A dressing was applied.

12-11C:

SERVICE CODE(S): ____________________

DX CODE(S): ____________________

12-11D DISCHARGE SUMMARY

In this discharge report, the documentation indicates both the cerebral palsy and the dystonia and is therefore reported as the diagnoses.

LOCATION: Inpatient, Hospital

PATIENT: Foy Crow

ATTENDING PHYSICIAN: Timothy Pleasant, M.D.

PRINCIPAL DIAGNOSES:

1. Cerebral palsy secondary to encephalopathy
2. Severe symptomatic torsion dystonia and spasticity
3. Now status post intrathecal catheter placement with intrathecal baclofen pump

NEUROSURGEON: Timothy Pleasant, M.D.

PREOPERATIVE CONSULTATION: Ronald Green, M.D.

ALLERGIES: None

PRINCIPAL PROCEDURE: Placement of Bard with intrathecal placement of catheter by Dr. Sanchez under general anesthesia.

Removal of Bard, placement of Medtronic pump delivery system for intrathecal medication, model #87, serial #L550, and #063, implanted catheter length 30 inches, implanted catheter volume 0.168, internal implanted tubing in baclofen pump 0.26.

HOSPITAL COURSE: The patient has done well during his hospitalization. An intrathecal catheter and a Bard were placed intraoperatively. Catheter tip T1 to T2. The catheter was attached to the Bard. The patient was started on his intrathecal baclofen test dose with an initial dose of 100 mcg per 24 hours. He tolerated this well without complications. He noted improvement in dystonia. On day 2 of his hospital stay, his total daily dose of baclofen was increased to 175 mcg per 24 hours at 9:40 A.M. He had no difficulties with this. At 5:28 P.M., on day 2, the dose was increased to 225 mcg per 24 hours with continued positive benefits. On day 3, the total daily dose was increased to 300 mcg per 24 hours with continued positive results and no side effects. On day 4, the Bard was surgically removed and a definitive intrathecal baclofen pump was placed. The patient was given a priming bolus and started on 360 mcg per day. He had no difficulties with this, and on day 5, the total dose was increased to 375 mcg per day. Overall, he has noted a marked decrease in dystonia. He is now able to feel his left fingertips and has decreased pain in his left elbow and resolution of pain in his left shoulder. He does have some mild discomfort across the anterior aspect of the right elbow that may be secondary to position during surgery.

He has had difficulty with urinary retention post both operations and required straight catheter. Volumes have been significant at greater than 700-900 cc. Once he is able to stand, this does improve. He had some initial difficulties with abdominal distention secondary to gas. This has resolved. He does use a Dulcolax suppository p.r.n. Initial pain management was with Demerol. When given 75 mg IV, he was slightly sedated and required a small amount of O_2. When given only 25 mg this did not control his pain but for 45 minutes, when given 35-50, this was sufficient. He also took additional Toradol p.r.n. for pain, and pain management has been good.

He did have initial headache post the initial surgery felt to be spinal leak of CSF in origin as occurred when he sat up, resolved when he laid down. A blood patch was done on day 5, and this is much better. Today he did have some mild light-headedness after straight catheter for urinary residual, and this is resolving with supine position.

The patient has participated in dystonia monitoring by physical therapy and occupational therapy, and they noted an improvement.

The patient will be transferred to the Manytown Rehabilitation Hospital today for continued rehab services status post intrathecal baclofen pump placement and to monitor and increase dosage. Will continue with occupational therapy, physical therapy, and speech evaluation. Will increase dose as necessary.

DISCHARGE DIET: Regular

DISCHARGE MEDICATIONS:

1. Intrathecal baclofen, currently 375 mcg per day
2. IV has been discontinued
3. Tylenol 650 mg q.4-6h. p.o. p.r.n.
4. Bisacodyl suppository 10 mg p.r.n.
5. Ibuprofen 600 mg p.o. p.r.n.
6. Physostigmine to take at bedside 0.7 to 2 mg if needed for inadvertent overdose of baclofen.

PHYSICAL EXAMINATION: Lungs are clear to auscultation. Regular rate and rhythm. Abdomen is soft and nontender. Abdominal incision site is good. No redness or warmth is noted. Neurologically, marked decrease in dystonia.

12-11D:

SERVICE CODE(S): ______________________

DX CODE(S): ______________________

Laminotomy and Foraminotomies

Laminotomies and laminectomies are two of the most frequently performed surgeries used in treatment of herniated discs, spinal trauma, aneurysm correction, and removal of spinal cord tumors. The procedures involve an incision over the operative area and removal of a portion of the bone of the vertebrae (**lamina**). The bulging or damaged portion of the disc is then removed. Foraminotomy is removal of a portion of the vertebra to relieve pressure on the **foramina** (that area of the channel in which the nerves are located). If a laminotomy and foraminotomy are performed at the same session, the laminotomy is reported because the code descriptions for the laminectomies include foraminotomy. If the procedures are performed on both sides of the vertebra, modifier -50 is used to indicate a bilateral procedure was performed.

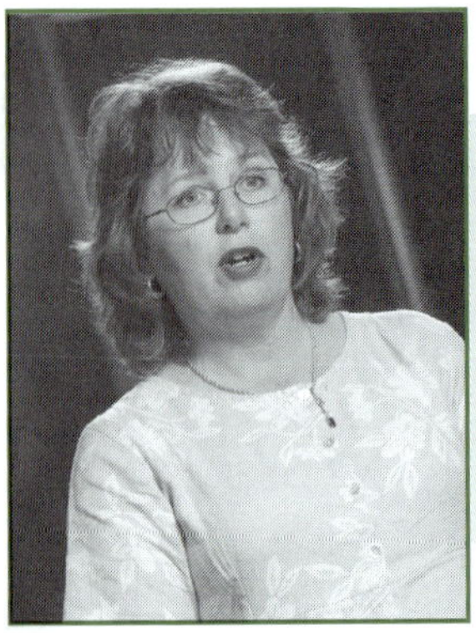

FROM THE TRENCHES

Jeanice

"Have integrity. Have honesty and integrity because that's your profession. To do it right. Do it the right way, even if it's a struggle, because that's what gives you credibility."

CASE 12-12
12-12A Radiology Report, Lumbar Spine
12-12B Operative Report, Laminotomies and Foraminotomies
12-12C Discharge Summary

CASE 12-12

Prior to surgery for laminectomies and foraminotomies, Dr. Pleasant orders an x-ray. The reason for this service is the herniation (displacement) of an intervertebral disc.

12-12A RADIOLOGY REPORT, LUMBAR SPINE

LOCATION: Inpatient, Hospital

PATIENT: Todd Osmond

ATTENDING PHYSICIAN: Timothy Pleasant, M.D.

RADIOLOGIST: Grey Lonewolf, M.D.

EXAMINATION OF: Lumbar spine

CLINICAL SYMPTOMS: Lumbar laminectomy, herniated disk L3-4, L5-S1

LATERAL TWO VIEW OF LUMBAR SPINE: COMPARISON: Comparison is made to a previous lateral view of the lumbar spine dated 2 months ago. For the purposes of this examination, it will be assumed that there are five lumbar-type vertebral bodies. There is evidence of previous fusion of the L4 and L5. Surgical instruments are seen posterior to the L4 vertebral segment. A surgical probe is seen to extend anteriorly from the surgical instruments. The distal tip lies posterior to the superior endplate of L4.

12-12A:

SERVICE CODE(S): ____________________

DX CODE(S): ____________________

12-12B OPERATIVE REPORT, LAMINOTOMIES AND FORAMINOTOMIES

LOCATION: Inpatient, Hospital

PATIENT: Todd Osmond

ATTENDING PHYSICIAN: Timothy Pleasant, M.D.

SURGEON: Timothy Pleasant, M.D.

PREOPERATIVE DIAGNOSIS: Herniated disk L3-4 on the right and the left

POSTOPERATIVE DIAGNOSIS: Herniated disk L3-4 on the right and the left

PROCEDURE PERFORMED: Bilateral laminotomies and foraminotomies at L3-4 with removal of the disk from the right and left side. Application of Gleotec 2.5 cc on each side.

ANESTHESIA: General

PROCEDURE: The patient was placed in a prone position. The back was prepped and draped in the usual manner. The previous incision was incised. The erector spinae muscles were dissected from the lamina. About three or four retractors were placed in the wound. We isolated the L3-4 interspace via x-ray. Laminotomies were performed with foraminotomies on the left and the right side. The ligamentum flavum was very hypertrophic. The facets were hypertrophic. We took these down. Retracted on the nerve root and got the disk space. Here is what happened on the left side: There was a disk material on the body of L4. I took this down, went into the disk space, and removed much degenerating material. On the right side, did the same thing. The disk here was on the body of L3. We took it down, took the midline fragments down. I was satisfied that I had cleaned out the disk space. There was no compression on the nerve roots. Passed a hockeystick up and medially and down and medially into the foramen. The dura was well compressed. Irrigated the wound well. After this, we then put Gleotec about 2.5 cc on the right and on the left side. No drains were utilized. The lumbodorsal fascia was approximated with double knotted 0 chromic, 0 Vicryl as well, 2-0 plain in the subcutaneous tissue, and surgical staples on the skin. A dressing was applied. The patient was discharged to the PAR.

12-12B:

SERVICE CODE(S): ____________________

DX CODE(S): ____________________

12-12C DISCHARGE SUMMARY

LOCATION: Inpatient, Hospital

PATIENT: Todd Osmond

ATTENDING PHYSICIAN: Timothy Pleasant, M.D.

SURGEON: Timothy Pleasant, M.D.
The patient presented with unbearable left leg pain. He apparently had stopped smoking, stopped drinking and had a herniated L3-L4 disk. He wanted to go ahead with surgery. He was preoperatively prepped by Dr. Green. Cardiovascular system had a heart murmur.

HOSPITAL COURSE: The patient underwent a bilateral laminectomy, foraminotomy, and removal of disk at L3-4. His postoperative course is uneventful. He has a little drainage from the wound, but I think that will seal; it is clear. His leg pain is gone. I will see him on Thursday for a wound check. He is discharged with Percocet for pain.

FINAL DIAGNOSIS: Herniated disk at L3-4

PROCEDURE PERFORMED: Bilateral laminotomy, foraminotomy, and removal of disk.

12-12C:

SERVICE CODE(S): ____________________

DX CODE(S): ____________________

CASE 12-13
12-13A Operative Report, Hemilaminectomy and Foraminotomy

CASE 12-13

One type of nerve pain is radiculopathy, which is pain emanating from the root of the nerve, that is, the part of the nerve that exits the spinal cord and enters the body. In this case the surgeon performs a hemilaminectomy, which is the removal of only one side of the vertebral lamina due to radiculopathy (nerve disease).

12-13A OPERATIVE REPORT, HEMILAMINECTOMY AND FORAMINOTOMY

LOCATION: Inpatient, Hospital

PATIENT: Tana Thrall

ATTENDING PHYSICIAN: Timothy Pleasant, M.D.

SURGEON: Timothy Pleasant, M.D.

PREOPERATIVE DIAGNOSIS: Intractable left S1 radiculopathy

POSTOPERATIVE DIAGNOSIS: Intractable left S1 radiculopathy

PROCEDURE PERFORMED: Left L4-5 and L5-S1 redo hemilaminectomy and foraminotomy

PROCEDURE: The patient was taken to the operating room and placed under general endotracheal anesthesia. She was then rotated into the prone position on chest rolls with the arms extended over the head. The lumbar region was shaved, prepped, and draped in the usual sterile manner. The proposed vertical midline incision was then infiltrated with lidocaine with epinephrine. The skin was incised, and sharp dissection was carried through the subcutaneous tissue. The fascia was then incised and subperiosteal dissection was undertaken on the left. X-ray localization confirmed the proper position. There was a generous amount of scar noted at L4-5 that was gradually removed, dissecting along the bone. Dissection proceeded until the left L-4 nerve root could be safely identified, tracking through the neural foramen. The L4 nerve root was well decompressed. The next level was then approached. A generous amount of fusion mass was noted at L5-S1. This was removed with a drill and then with #45-Kerrison punch. The L5-S1 nerve roots were then identified. The L5-S1 foramen was noted to be moderately stenotic, and a generous decompression was undertaken. In addition, the left S1 nerve root appeared to be slightly compromised by bone, displacing it slightly medially. This nerve was then fully decompressed. On completion, the L4, L5, and S1 nerve roots had all been visualized and were noted to be well decompressed. Hemostasis was then ensured. The epidural space was lined with a single layer of Surgicel and fat graft. The wound was closed with interrupted layers of 4-0 Vicryl subcuticular stitch for skin. Steri-Strips and sterile dressing were applied to the wound. The patient tolerated the procedure well and was transferred to the recovery room in good condition.

12-13A:

SERVICE CODE(S): ______________________

DX CODE(S): ______________________

CASE 12-14
12-14A Radiology Report, Disk Repair
12-14B Operative Report, Diskectomies and Foraminotomies
12-14C Pathology Report
12-14D Radiology Report, Lumbar Spine MRI
12-14E Radiology Report, Lumbar Spine MRI

CASE 12-14

12-14A RADIOLOGY REPORT, DISK REPAIR

LOCATION: Inpatient, Hospital

PATIENT: Sara Vasek

ATTENDING PHYSICIAN: Timothy Pleasant, M.D.

RADIOLOGIST: Grey Lonewolf, M.D.

EXAMINATION OF: Four lumbar films for lumbar laminectomy

CLINICAL SYMPTOMS: Disk herniation (herniated disk)

FOUR LUMBAR FILMS FOR LUMBAR LAMINECTOMY: FINDINGS: No comparisons. On the image labeled #1, there is a metallic marker seen posteriorly at the L2 level superior endplate, assuming there are five lumbar-type vertebral bodies. On the image labeled #2, there is a metallic density seen posteriorly with the thin metallic rod pointing at the L1 level and the other metallic hardware at the L1-2 level. On the film labeled #3, a posterior metallic hardware is again noted. The most cephalad metallic density is at the L2-3 level, and the thinner caudal metallic density is at the L3-4 level. Film labeled #4 demonstrates metallic densities, and they are located at the L1-2 and L4-5 levels.

12-14A:

SERVICE CODE(S): ____________________

DX CODE(S): ____________________

12-14B OPERATIVE REPORT, DISKECTOMIES AND FORAMINOTOMIES

LOCATION: Inpatient, Hospital

PATIENT: Sara Vasek

ATTENDING PHYSICIAN: Timothy Pleasant, M.D.

SURGEON: Timothy Pleasant, M.D.

PREOPERATIVE DIAGNOSIS: Herniated nucleus pulposus, L1-2 and herniated nucleus pulposus, L4-5 with back pain, left-sided leg pain, and corresponding radiculopathies.

POSTOPERATIVE DIAGNOSIS: Herniated nucleus pulposus, L1-2 and herniated nucleus pulposus, L4-5 with back pain, left-sided leg pain, and corresponding radiculopathies and left L2-3 disk herniation.

PROCEDURE PERFORMED: Left L1-2, L2-3, and L4-5 diskectomies with foraminotomies, and a left L3-4 foraminotomy.

ANESTHESIA: General endotracheal

COMPLICATIONS: Nil
A Hemovac drain was placed.

HISTORY: This is a 32-year-old white female who underwent previous left-sided laminotomies and foraminotomies by me. This was for left-sided neurogenic claudication and spinal stenosis. She did extremely well with this operation; however, she developed a sudden onset of back pain and left-sided leg pain. An MRI scan was obtained, and it revealed a large disk herniation eccentric to the left at L1-2. It also showed some disk degeneration and foraminal stenosis eccentric to the left, interestingly at all levels of the lumbar spine, L2-3, L3-4, and L4-5. She also had a disk herniation with facet hypertrophy and circumferential stenosis at L4-5. Her symptoms were only on the left.

Indications, alternatives, risks, and benefits of surgery were discussed in detail. The patient was consented for a left-sided L1-2 and a left L4-5 diskectomy with lumbar exploration.

The patient was brought to the operating theater and identified. General endotracheal anesthesia was induced. Intravenous antibiotics were given. The region in the low back was prepped and draped in a sterile fashion. A localizing x-ray was obtained after placement of a spinal needle. The old incision was utilized and marked using a skin marker. The region of the incision was infiltrated with 1.5% Xylocaine with epinephrine. A vertical midline incision was made through the old incision using #10 blade scalpel. Hemostasis was achieved using Bovie electrocautery. Subcutaneous and subcuticular tissues were divided using Bovie electrocautery. The self-retaining retractors were placed. The dorsal lumbar fascia was incised using Bovie electrocautery. The paraspinal musculature and multifidi were reflected off of the spinous process and laminae of L1-2, L2-3, L3-4, and L4-5 using Bovie electrocautery, Cobb elevators, and sponges.

Our attention was directed at entry into the L1-2 space on the left. Using the straight and curved curettes, ligamentum flavum and scar tissue was resected from the superior edge of the inferior lamina of L1 and the inferior edge of the superior lamina of L2. There was a lot of dense scar adherent to the bone. I then redirected and went to the L2-3 space and did a general foraminotomy.

Ligamentum flavum and scar tissue were resected and removed and curetted from the superior edge of the inferior lamina of L3 and the inferior edge of the superior lamina of L2. A general foraminotomy was then fashioned using a 3- and 5-mm Kerrison punch. The disk seemed to be humped up, and there was an extruded fragment compressing the nerve from below. This disk fragment was removed, and disk material was removed in a piecemeal fashion and handed off as specimen. Copious amounts of saline irrigation were utilized until the supernatant was clear. We had entry into the L2-3 space. A large laminotomy was fashioned. The scar adhesions were resected. I then readdressed the L1-2 interspace. A foraminotomy was fashioned using 3- and 5-mm Kerrison punches. The ball-ended probe could pass without let or hindrance. Copious amounts of saline irrigation were utilized. The exiting nerve root and thecal sac were retracted medially. The disk was incised. A large disk fragment presented itself once the annulus was incised. This was handed off as specimen. We alternated between curettes and pituitary punches and handed disk material off as specimen. Copious amounts of saline irrigation were utilized until the supernatant was clear.

Our attention was directed at the L4-5 interspace on the left. A foraminotomy was fashioned. The superior edge of the inferior lamina of L5 and the inferior edge of the superior lamina of L4 were curetted and scar tissue was resected. We entered into the space created with resection of the soft tissue and performed a generous foraminotomy and laminotomy. The thecal sac and exiting nerve root were retracted off as specimen. I directed my attention to L3-4 and proceeded to perform a small foraminotomy. The ball-ended probe could pass without let or hindrance. This lady tolerated surgery well. There were no intraoperative complications. A Hemovac drain was placed.

Hemostasis was achieved using Bovie electrocautery and bipolar electrocautery. Dorsal lumbar fascia and the paraspinal musculature were reapproximated using double-knotted chromic suture. Subcutaneous tissues were reapproximated using 2-0 Vicryl. Hemovac drain was placed and carried out through a separate stab incision. The skin was reapproximated using staples. All counts were correct and verified.

Pathology Report Later Indicated: See 12-14C.

12-14B:

SERVICE CODE(S): ______________________

DX CODE(S): ______________________

12-14C PATHOLOGY REPORT

LOCATION: Inpatient, Hospital

PATIENT: Sara Vasek

ATTENDING PHYSICIAN: Timothy Pleasant, M.D.

SURGEON: Timothy Pleasant, M.D.

PATHOLOGIST: Grey Lonewolf, M.D.

CLINICAL HISTORY: Disk herniation

SPECIMEN RECEIVED: Lumbar disk

GROSS DESCRIPTION: The specimen is labeled with the patient's name and "disk" and consists of approximately 5 g of fibrous fragments.

MICROSCOPIC DESCRIPTION: Sections show disk tissue.

DIAGNOSIS: Disk tissue, benign

12-14C:

SERVICE CODE(S): ______________________

DX CODE(S): ______________________

12-14D RADIOLOGY REPORT, LUMBAR SPINE MRI

LOCATION: Inpatient, Hospital

PATIENT: Sara Vasek

ATTENDING PHYSICIAN: Timothy Pleasant, M.D.

SURGEON: Timothy Pleasant, M.D.

RADIOLOGIST: Grey Lonewolf, M.D.

EXAMINATION OF: Lumbar spine MRI

CLINICAL SYMPTOMS: Herniated disc

LUMBAR SPINE MRI WITH and WITHOUT CONTRAST: TECHNIQUE: T1, T2, and fat-saturated postcontrast T1 sagittal images were acquired. T1, T2, and postcontrast T1 axial images were acquired from L1 to S1. No prior studies are provided for comparison.

FINDINGS: The conus is normal.
The T11-12 disk space is desiccated with an inferior endplate Schmorl's node and mild anterior spurring.

The T12-L1 disk space is unremarkable.

At L1-2, there is a peripherally enhancing left anterolateral epidural soft-tissue process. A left laminotomy with a peripherally enhancing fluid collection is noted. The disk space is desiccated with bulging. There is no enhancement abnormality within the disk space.

At L2-3, there is a left laminotomy, facetectomy, and foraminotomy with a peripherally enhancing fluid collection in the surgical bed. Enhancing epidural and perineural tissues are noted. Sagittal images show some bright enhancing T2 signal in the left hemisphere of the disk space, without associated endplate changes. Within the left lateral recess of L3 is a peripherally enhancing collection having long T1/long T2 signal. For example, compare postcontrast axial image #16 with T2-weighted axial image #16 and precontrast image #16.

At L3-4, there is a left laminectomy and inferior facetectomy with enhancing granulation tissue in the surgical bed. The disk space is desiccated with bulge and mild spurring.

At L4-5, there is a left laminectomy and partial facetectomy with enhancing epidural granulation tissue. Right ligamentum flavum is redundant. Right lateral recess is moderately to markedly stenotic. Moderate to marked degenerative disease is present in the right facet joint. Right neural foramen is moderately to markedly stenotic. The left neural foramen is amply patent.

At L5-S1, there is advanced bilateral degenerative facet disease with disk desiccation with bulge.

IMPRESSION:

1. Left laminectomies and/or facet postoperative changes including L1-2 through L4-5.
2. Peripherally enhancing mass in the left L3 lateral recess has indeterminate etiology. Given findings of recent surgery, packing material or postoperative fluid collection is considered. A free fragment of peripherally enhancing disk material could have a similar appearance.
3. Enhancing in the left hemisphere of the L2-3 disk space in conjunction with bright T2 signal intensity may represent postoperative change.
4. Multilevel degenerative disk disease.
5. Moderate to marked right L4-5 foraminal stenosis.
6. Peripherally enhancing soft tissue at the dorsal aspect of the L1-2 disk space has uncertain significance. This finding likely represents acute postoperative change; however, clinical correlation is suggested. Acute postoperative change has been described in the literature as mimicking residual or recurrent disk herniation.

12-14D:

SERVICE CODE(S): ____________________

DX CODE(S): ____________________

12-14E RADIOLOGY REPORT, LUMBAR SPINE MRI

LOCATION: Inpatient, Hospital

PATIENT: Sara Vasek

ATTENDING PHYSICIAN: Timothy Pleasant, M.D.

SURGEON: Timothy Pleasant, M.D.

RADIOLOGIST: Grey Lonewolf, M.D.

EXAMINATION OF: Lumbar MR

CLINICAL SYMPTOMS: Herniated disc, recent surgery

MAGNETIC RESONANCE EXAMINATION OF THE LUMBAR SPINE was performed utilizing a combination of T1, gradient echo, and fast spin-echo (fat suppressed) T2-weighted sequences. Appropriate sequences were also performed following intravenous infusion of contrast material.

The patient has had multiple surgical procedures with surgery at almost every level in the lumbar region from L1-2 to L4-5.

Unfortunately, the patient was moving during the acquisition of some sequences.

At L1-2, there does appear to be abnormal soft-tissue mass to the left of midline, with compression on the dural sac. It certainly has the appearance of disk herniation. However, one also needs to realize that large disk herniation can appear very similarly following surgery as it did prior to surgery, even with removal of the disk.

At L2-3 and L3-4, I believe there has been entry to the spinal canal on the left. There is bulging of the intervertebral disk, and there are underlying bone bars at both levels, and there is indentation of the dural sac, but I doubt that there is evidence of overt disk herniation at this time. I do not feel there is significant stenosis, although the dural sac is small at both levels. I believe there has been previous satisfactory decompression.

At L4-5, I believe there is significant spinal stenosis circumferentially. There might also be a small disk herniation at L4-5 to the left of midline.

I do not believe there is significant abnormality directly at L5-S1.

IMPRESSION: The patient has had multiple surgical procedures. She had recent very extensive surgery. Essentially, there does appear to be residual disk herniation at L1-2 to the left of midline. As noted above, it needs to be remembered that an appearance of large disk herniation might not change in the immediate postoperative period, even though the disk has been removed. This would not explain the right lower extremity pain.

Continued spinal stenosis at L4-5 with possible small disk herniation to the left of midline.

Previous decompression at L2-3 and L3-4. I believe decompression is satisfactory. I do not believe there is evidence of disk herniation at these levels.

I do not believe there is significant abnormality at L5-S1.

12-14E:

SERVICE CODE(S): ____________________

DX CODE(S): ____________________

Spinal Fusion

Spinal fusion is the fixation of two or more vertebrae together that is performed to provide stabilization to the spinal column. The fusion may be done for degenerative conditions such as spondylolisthesis in which one disk slips over the one below (slipped disk) or for congenital abnormalities. Fusions are reported with codes from the Musculoskeletal System, Spine (Vertebral Column), Arthrodesis (22548-22632) based on the approach used. The approach is the access location, such as anterior (front), posterior (back), anterolateral (to one side of the front), or posterolateral (to one side of the back). Often a spinal evoked potential monitoring, which is an electroencephalogram (EEG) and monitors the electrical activity of the brain, will be conducted intraoperatively and is reported separately.

If a biomechanical device, such as bone dowel or cage, is applied at the time of surgery, the application of the device is reported separately with add-on code 22851.

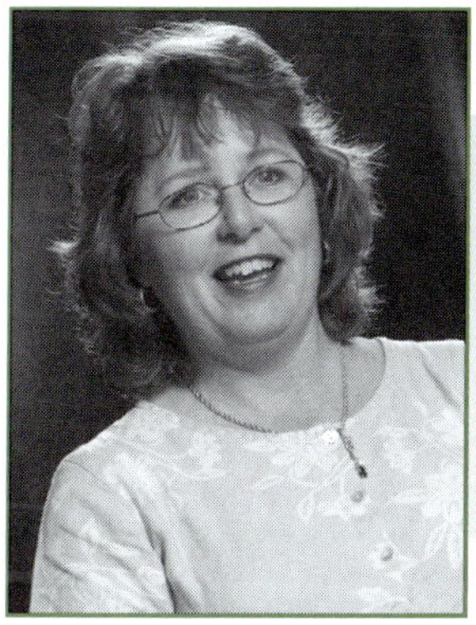

FROM THE TRENCHES

Jeanice

"Coding is always changing...It is a difficult but interesting profession. You are not going to get bored with it. It is going to change all the time. And there are so many different avenues you can [specialize in] as a coder—from the insurance side to the physician side. It's a great field to be in."

CASE 12-15
12-15A Operative Report, Cage Fusion

CASE 12-15

This patient has a degeneration of an intervertebral disk.

12-15A OPERATIVE REPORT, CAGE FUSION

LOCATION: Inpatient, Hospital

PATIENT: Carmen Schultz

ATTENDING PHYSICIAN: Timothy Pleasant, M.D.

SURGEON: Timothy Pleasant, M.D.

PREOPERATIVE DIAGNOSIS: Severe degenerative disk disease at L5-S1

POSTOPERATIVE DIAGNOSIS: Severe degenerative disk disease at L5-S1

PROCEDURE PERFORMED: L5-S1 anterior intervertebral cage fusion with spinal evoked potential monitoring (*evoked potential somatosensory study is reported separately*)

ANESTHESIA: General endotracheal anesthesia

OPERATIVE NOTE: The patient was taken to the operating room and placed under general endotracheal anesthesia. The abdomen was then prepped and draped in the usual sterile manner. Anterior exposure was obtained. After exposure had been obtained and x-ray localization was provided, anterior intervertebral cage fusion was performed using standard technique. A 13 × 20 BAK cage was placed uneventfully between the L5 and S1 vertebral bodies under x-ray guidance. Cancellous bone was packed into the BAK cages in the standard fashion. Hemostasis was ensured, and the wound was closed in standard fashion.

12-15A:

SERVICE CODE(S): ______

DX CODE(S): ______ Spine insertion, instrument

22558 (Spine, fusion, anterior approach)
22851 (Spine, insertion, instrumentation)
95927-26 (Evoked potential, somatosensory testing)

CASE 12-16
12-16A Operative Report, Halo Vest Placement and Repair

CASE 12-16

Now here is a case to challenge your coding abilities. Reference the "Procedure Performed" section of the report to identify the number of procedures to be coded, noting that there are two segments to report for the fixation and fusion. Then read the report and ensure that the procedures are those identified in the "Procedure Performed" section. Assume this is the initial care of this fracture. There will be a CPT for the fracture treatment, arthrodesis, autograft, skeletal fixation, cranial halo, and the evoked potentials. Assign a diagnosis code for the fracture and an E code for the fracture circumstances.

12-16A OPERATIVE REPORT, HALO VEST PLACEMENT AND REPAIR

LOCATION: Inpatient, Hospital

PATIENT: Tim Brent

ATTENDING PHYSICIAN: Timothy Pleasant, M.D.

SURGEON: Timothy Pleasant, M.D.

PREOPERATIVE DIAGNOSIS: Unstable C5 fracture with spinal deformity and upper extremity weakness

POSTOPERATIVE DIAGNOSIS: Unstable C5 fracture with spinal deformity and upper extremity weakness

PROCEDURE PERFORMED:
1. Halo vest placement
2. Posterior segmental fixation C4 through C6 with Halifax clamps
3. Open correction of cervical fracture
4. Posterior cervical fusion C4 through C6 using bone autograft and right iliac crest graft
5. Evoked potential monitoring of upper extremity

ANESTHESIA: General endotracheal anesthesia

OPERATIVE NOTE: The patient was taken to the operating room and placed under general endotracheal anesthesia. This was done fiberoptically. On completion of the successful intubation, the patient was then placed in a four-pin halo vest. This was done maintaining an in-line cervical traction using standard technique after neutral position on chest rolls. The posterior cervical region as well as the area surrounding the left iliac crest were then shaved, prepped, and draped in the usual sterile manner. The left iliac crest graft was harvested first. This was done through a standard incision. The split-thickness graft with a generous amount of cancellous bone was harvested. The wound was then closed in interrupted layers after hemostasis had been ensured. The posterior cervical region was then incised. Sharp dissection was carried out through the subcutaneous tissue. The fascia was incised and a subperiosteal dissection was undertaken from C4 through C6. Great care was utilized to avoid stripping the muscle from C3 and C7 in an attempt to minimize any chance of incorporating growing fusion at these levels. The superior aspect of the hemilamina of C4 and the inferior aspect of the hemilamina of C6 were then carefully exposed using curettes. Halifax clamps were then fashioned and secured from C4 through C6. The area of C5 was noted to be fractured in multiple places, including the facet joints bilaterally and the lamina. The Halifax clamp construct was then assembled uneventfully and was noted to be secure. The lamina was then decorticated with a cutting burr, and the cancellous and cortical bones were utilized to complete the posterior cervical fusion. Halifax clamping ensured proper correction of the slight cervical deformity, and throughout the procedure, the evoked potential monitoring *(Electrodes are placed on the scalp, electrically stimulates nerves, and records results. Reported separately.)* was noted to be normal. Hemostasis was then ensured. The wound was closed in interrupted layers with staples for the skin.

12-16A:

SERVICE CODE(S): ______________________

DX CODE(S): ______________________

CASE 12-17
12-17A Operative Report, Diskectomy

CASE 12-17

This case is another challenge for you to take on. Read the report carefully to ensure that you are reporting all the various components of the service. There will be a code for each of the diskectomies, decompression of the spinal cord, allograft, spinal fusion, arthrodesis, skeletal fixation, and evoked potentials.

12-17A OPERATIVE REPORT, DISKECTOMY

LOCATION: Inpatient, Hospital

PATIENT: Liz Neil

ATTENDING PHYSICIAN: Timothy Pleasant, M.D.

SURGEON: Timothy Pleasant, M.D.

PREOPERATIVE DIAGNOSIS: Cervical disk displacement, C4-5 and C5-6

POSTOPERATIVE DIAGNOSIS: Spinal stenosis, cervical disk displacement, C4-5 and C5-6

PROCEDURES PERFORMED:
1. Cervical diskectomy, C4-5 and C5-6
2. Corpectomy, C5
3. Placement of allograft from C4 to C6
4. Placement of arthrodesis 34-mm plate from C4 to C6

ANESTHESIA: General

This case was done under sensory evoked potential monitoring.

PROCEDURE: Under general anesthesia, the patient was placed in the supine position. The head was turned to the left. The neck was prepped and draped in the usual manner.

An incision was made in a linear fashion along the medial border of the sternocleidomastoid, and then dissecting the platysma, we got by the omohyoid and onto the prevertebral fascia. We then localized the C4-5 and C5-6 interspace and took an x-ray (*reported by radiologist*). I then sectioned the anterior longitudinal ligament and prepared myself for the diskectomy, in which I incised the C4-5 disk space and the C5-6 disk space and removed as much disk material as I could. Then, with an air drill, I did a corpectomy, made a trough in this middle of C5 about 3 mm above the anterior longitudinal ligament. Having done this, I worked with curets and various Kerrison rongeurs to remove all the disk and to take the ridges off C4 and C5 as well as complete the corpectomy. This having been done, I was satisfied that I could see the dura and took out the disk fragments. There was no penetration to see the posterior longitudinal ligament, but we cleaned out this area well so that we could provide acceptance of the graft. I then fashioned a graft from the bone bank. (*Literally, a bank of donated bone that is used to reduce the trauma to the patient that is receiving the bone. This is an allograft. Bone is the second most transplanted tissue [blood is first]*). With gentle extraction on the neck, I was able to place the bone graft so that the surfaces of C4 and C6 having been curreted and that cancellous bone was applied to the cancellous bone. Having done this, at this point, we then did the Synthes plate. We placed a 34-mm plate onto the body of C4 and C6 utilizing screws. We put screws into the body of C6 as well as C4 and into the graft. We took an x-ray (*reported by radiologist*) and felt it was secure and adequate. We irrigated the wound, placed a Hemovac drain in the wound, and closed the wound in layers utilizing a 2-0 chromic on the platysma, 2-0 plain on the subcutaneous tissue, and 3-0 interrupted mattress sutures on the skin. A dressing was applied. The patient was discharged to the PAR.

12-17A:

SERVICE CODE(S): ______________________

DX CODE(S): ______________________

Neurology and Neuromuscular Procedures

Electroencephalography (EEG) is an important and frequent diagnostic tool used in neurology, as is EMG/NCV (electromyography/nerve conduction velocity). You have coded the EEG in several of the cases in the chapter, but the following reports will give you an additional opportunity to code these reports. The nerve conduction velocity study is one in which electrical impulses are applied to one end of the nerve and the time it takes to travel to the other end of the nerve is measured. Damaged peripheral nerves can be identified by means of this study. When these studies are done at the hospital, remember to use the professional component only modifier.

CASE 12-18
12-18A Electroencephalogram Report

CASE 12-18

12-18A ELECTROENCEPHALOGRAM REPORT

LOCATION: Outpatient, Hospital

PATIENT: Reed Tolbert

REQUESTING PHYSICIAN: Ronald Green, M.D.

INDICATION: Convulsions (1)

PHYSICIAN: Timothy Pleasant, M.D.

The patient was drowsy and asleep during much of this bedside EEG. The recording was requested for follow-up of a seizure, which occurred 2 months ago.

MEDICATIONS:
1. Albuterol
2. Atrovent
3. Epoetin
4. Bacitracin
5. Flagyl
6. Nystatin
7. Diflucan
8. Fosphenytoin
9. Gentamicin
10. Piperacillin
11. Protonix

While the patient was awake, the background activity was somewhat poorly organized and consisted of varying mixtures of 15-16Hz beta and some 8-10Hz alpha, with amplitudes of 25-35uV.

Stages I and II of sleep were observed; vertex waves and sleep spindles appear normal.

Hyperventilation and photic stimulation were not performed.

IMPRESSION: This is a minimally abnormal EEG because of somewhat poor organization of the background while the patient was awake. No epileptogenic activity was seen.

12-18A:

SERVICE CODE(S): ______________________

DX CODE(S): ______________________

CASE 12-19
12-19A Electroencephalogram Report

CASE 12-19

12-19A ELECTROENCEPHALOGRAM REPORT

LOCATION: Outpatient, Hospital

PATIENT: Brian Wheaton

REQUESTING PHYSICIAN: Ronald Green, M.D.

PHYSICIAN: Timothy Pleasant, M.D.

TECHNICAL STATEMENT: This is a 21-channel digital recording using the International 10-20 electrode placement system. Three channels were devoted to monitoring the eye movements and EEG. The patient was unresponsive. (*reported diagnosis*)

ELECTROGRAPHIC DATA: Background is low amplitude 4 to 5 Hz theta activity. A more prominent high amplitude, polymorphic delta rhythm of 2 to 3 Hz persists throughout the record. This delta activity is more prominent throughout the frontal regions.

During activation with tactile and sound stimuli, delta activity is accentuated and the background frequency increases minimally to 7 Hz. Theta activity is slightly more developed over the right hemisphere. In the absence of activation, background amplitude declines considerably.

The heart rate was 114 per minute.

CLINICAL INFORMATION: Severe head trauma 19 days prior. Episodes of seizure-like activity (*convulsions are a reported diagnosis*) in the last few days; treated with Dilantin.

CLINICAL INTERPRETATION: This is an abnormal record (*reported diagnosis*) due to markedly slow background with continuous delta activity. The symmetry of stimulus-induced frequency is not significant. No epileptiform activity is detected.

OPINION: Although epileptiform activity is not present in this record, the episodes of tremulousness are highly suggestive of autonomic overflow phenomenon. I recommend continued anti-seizure medications on a prophylactic basis.

The findings seem to be consistent with severe encephalopathy.

12-19A:

SERVICE CODE(S): ______________________

DX CODE(S): ______________________

"Unresponsive" means coma.

CASE 12-20

This is a nerve conduction study in which each study (motor nerve and sensory nerve) is reported separately.

12-20A ELECTRODIAGNOSTIC EVALUATION SUMMARY REPORT

LOCATION: Outpatient, Hospital

PATIENT: Lynn Jie

REQUESTING PHYSICIAN: Ronald Green, M.D.

PHYSICIAN: Timothy Pleasant, M.D.

CLINICAL SYMPTOM: Arm pain

Motor Nerve Study

Left Median Nerve

Rec Site: APB	Lat (ms)	Norm Lat	Amp (mV)	Dist (mm)	C.V. (m/s)	Norm C.V.
STIM SITE						
Wrist	3.7	4.2	3.8	60		
Elbow	7.7		.167	220	55.0	49

Left Ulnar Nerve

Rec Site: ADM	Lat (ms)	Norm Lat	Amp (mV)	Dist (mm)	C.V. (m/s)	Norm C.V.
STIM SITE						
Wrist	2.7	3.6	12.0	60		
B. Elbow	6.5		4.7	230	60.0	48
A. Elbow	8.3		.667	120	68.5	

Sensory Nerve Study

Left Median Nerve

Rec Site: Index	Lat (ms)	Norm Lat	Amp (uV)	Dist (mm)	C.V. (m/s)	Norm C.V.
STIM SITE						
Wrist	3.1	3.6	25.3	130	42.6	48

Left Ulnar Nerve

Rec Site: 5th digit						
STIM SITE						
Wrist	3.0	3.1	1.3	110	37.0	48

Left Median-MP Nerve

Rec Site: Wrist						
STIM SITE						
Midpalm	1.6	1.9	40.0	60	37.8	

SUMMARY/INTERPRETATION:

FINDINGS:

1. Normal left median nerve sensory conduction studies including both antidromic and orthodromic techniques
2. Normal left median nerve sensory conduction study
3. Normal left ulnar nerve sensory conduction study
4. Normal left ulnar nerve motor conduction study

IMPRESSION: Normal left upper extremity nerve conduction study per standard interpretation criteria

Thanks for the opportunity to have provided you this information. The findings have been briefly reviewed with the patient in the clinic today. Please let me know if you have further questions or if I might be able to provide further information.

12-20A:

SERVICE CODE(S): ______________________

DX CODE(S): ______________________

Glossary

cranioplasty surgical correction of defects in the skull.
craniotomy the surgical removal of (or an incision into) the cranium.

foramina a natural opening or passage.

hematoma a localized collection of blood in any body space.

lamina either of the pair of broad plates of bone flaring out from the pedicles of the vertebral arches.
laminectomy surgical excision of the lamina.

neurologist a physician who specializes in the diagnosis and treatment of conditions of the nervous system.
neurosurgeon a physician who specializes in surgical procedures of the nervous system.

shunt a device that diverts fluids the body cannot drain properly from one body area to another.

Chapter 13

Eye and Auditory Systems

EYE

Eye Examinations

Cataracts

Photocoagulation

Ectropion and Entropion

EAR

Office Services

Myringotomy and Tympanostomy

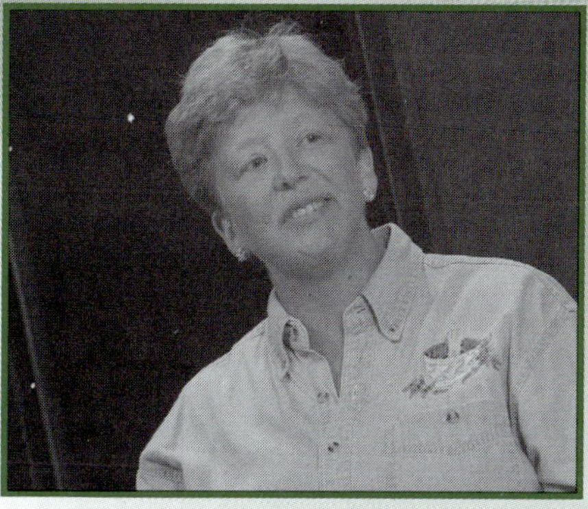

Ruth Brockmann, RN, CCS-P
Clinical Documentation Specialist
Rochester, Minnesota

ABBREVIATIONS

ABR	auditory brainstem response
CBC	complete blood cell count
cc	cubic centimeter
CPAP	continuous positive airway pressure
CT	cat scan
ENT	ear, nose, throat
ER	emergency department
INR	International Normalized Ratio
IV	intravenous
MAC	maximum allowable concentrate
mg	milligram
mmHg	millimeters of mercury
OD	right eye, (Lat.) oculus dexter
OR	operating room
OS	left eye (Lat.) oculus sinister
OU	both eyes
PE	pressure equalization
PTT	partial prothrombin time
TA	tonsillectomy and adenoidectomy
TMJ	temporomandibular joint
UV	ultraviolet

Eye

An **ophthalmologist** is a physician who specializes in medical and surgical care of the eye and visual system. The ophthalmologist provides a full spectrum of care, including the diagnosis and medical treatment of eye disorders and diseases, prescription of eyeglasses, routine eye exams, a variety of eye and visual system surgery, and management of eye problems that are caused by systemic illnesses, such as diabetic retinopathy. Ophthalmologists can be doctors of osteopathy (D.O.) or medical doctors (M.D.). Optometrists and opticians perform eye examinations, but they are not physicians and cannot perform surgery.

Common conditions diagnosed and treated by an ophthalmologist are conjunctivitis, corneal ulceration, corneal foreign body removal, optic neuritis, retinopathy, refractive error correction, macular degeneration, glaucoma, **cataracts**, and blepharitis.

Eye Examinations

During an eye examination, the physician assesses the visual acuity of the patient. This is accomplished by using a hanging wall chart that the patient reads from a distance of 20 feet. The patient covers one eye and reads the smallest character on the chart. Each eye is tested independently (i.e., one is covered while the other is used to read). The charts are marked with a number at the end of each line (e.g., 100, 200) that provides a comparison of that patient's vision with that of persons with normal vision. The larger the number, the worse the acuity. For example 20/100 means that the patient can see at 20 feet what a normal patient could see at 100 feet. A visual acuity chart displaying the classification and descriptions of visual acuity is illustrated in **Figure 13-1**.

The definitions of a new patient and established patient are the same as for all patients (less than 3 years since being treated by that physician or another physician of the same specialty who belongs to the same practice group, new; more than 3 years, established). There are two new patient codes and two established patient codes for eye examinations (92002-92014). There are extensive notes before the codes that must be read before coding eye examinations. These notes describe the intermediate, comprehensive, and special ophthalmologic services and should be read prior to coding ophthalmologic services.

FIGURE 13-1 Visual acuity chart.

Classification: "Legal"	Classification: WHO*	Levels of Visual Impairment: Visual Acuity and/or Visual Field Limitation (Whichever Is Worse)	Additional Descriptors Which May Be Encountered
	(Near-) normal vision	Range of Normal Vision 20/10 2.0; 20/13 1.6; 20/16 1.25; 20/20 1.0; 20/25 0.8	
		Near-Normal Vision 0.7; 20/30 0.6; 20/40 0.5; 20/50 0.4; 20/60 0.3	
	Low vision	Moderate Visual Impairment 20/70; 20/80 0.25; 20/100 0.20; 20/125 0.16; 20/160 0.12	Moderate low vision
Legal Blindness (U.S.A.) both eyes		Severe Visual Impairment 20/200 0.10; 20/250 0.03; 20/320 0.06; 20/400 0.05 Visual field: 20 degrees or less	Severe low vision, "Legal" blindness
	Blindness (WHO) one or both eyes	Profound Visual Impairment 20/500 0.04; 20/630 0.03; 20/800 0.025; 20/1000 0.02 Count fingers at: less than 3 m (10 ft) Visual field: 10 degrees or less	Profound low vision, Moderate blindness
		Near-Total Visual Impairment Visual acuity: less than 0.02 (20/1000) Count fingers: 1 m (3 ft) or less Hand movements: 5 m (15 ft) or less Light projection, light perception Visual field: 5 degrees or less	Severe blindness, Near-total blindness
		Total Visual Impairment No light perception (NLP)	Total blindness

**WHO = World Health Organization*
Visual acuity refers to best achievable acuity with correction.
Non-listed Snellen fractions may be classified by converting to the nearest decimal equivalent, e.g., 10/200 = 0.05, 6/30 = 0.20.
CF(count fingers) without designation of distance, may be classified to profound impairment.
HM (hand motion) without designation of distance, may be classified to near-total impairment.
Visual field measurements refer to the largest field diameter for a 1/100 white test object.

CASE 13-1
13-1A Clinic Progress Note, Eye Examination

CASE 13-1

The cataract is determined to be a "juvenile" cataract, (as opposed to "senile") based on the age of the patient at the time of onset.

13-1A CLINIC PROGRESS NOTE, EYE EXAMINATION

LOCATION: Outpatient, Clinic

PATIENT: Jay Bender

PHYSICIAN: Rita Wimer, M.D.

Today I saw Jay, who is now 21 years old. I last saw him 6 years ago when he had a corneal ulcer in his right eye. This is now cleared, and he has noticed that he cannot see well. He can read well, but he cannot see down the road. The last time I saw him, he was 20/30 in the right and 20/25 in the left. Now he is 20/80 in the right and 20/50 in the left, and this cannot be improved with refraction. His near-vision correction is still 20/25OU. The pressures are 12OU.

The patient has a normal corneal anterior chamber and iris but with very slow dilating pupils. There is no pseudoexfoliation, but there are dense juvenile nuclear cataracts in both eyes, the right greater than the left. From what I can see in the retina, the macula, optic nerve, and peripheral retina, they are normal. I counseled him for cataract surgery of his right eye first and then the left eye, the need for postoperative correction, a 4- to 6-week recovery time, and the type of procedure; we will see him in surgery on the last Monday of the month.

1

Decision for surgery

13-1A:

SERVICE CODE(S): ______________________

DX CODE(S): ______________________

CASE 13-2
13-2A Clinic Progress Note, Eye Examination

CASE 13-2

Dr. Wimer uses a B-scan ultrasound to assess the status of Rex's retina while doing an eye examination. The ultrasound is reported in addition to the examination. There is an E code that will be assigned to this case. Report the medications given to the patient intramuscularly and intravenously with HCPCS codes. Do not report the drops that were placed in the patient's eye, ointment, or patch.

13-2A CLINIC PROGRESS NOTE, EYE EXAMINATION

LOCATION: Outpatient, Clinic

PATIENT: Rex Dagg

PHYSICIAN: Rita Wimer, M.D.

Today, I saw Rex, a 68-year-old, a new patient to me, who was wrapping a couch with a bungee cord in preparation for moving the couch, when the cord snapped and the metal fitting hit him in his left eye squarely. He has pain and loss of vision and was seen in the ER; there was no light perception, and there was blood in the anterior chamber and a nonmoving pupil.

He was sent to me, and I saw that he was 20/20 in the right and had bare light perception in the left. The pressure was 33, and there was 25% hyperemia and a vitreous hemorrhage. B-scan showed no detachment or separation of the optic nerve. I gave him 60 of Toradol IM for pain and started him on Cosopt 2 drops and Iopidine 1% two drops and gave him 500 of Diamox IV push. Within a few minutes his pressure had reduced to 22, and the vision improved to finger counting and facial features. I placed atropine ointment, TobraDex patch, and Telfa over his eye and had him on strict bedrest without work. We will see him again in 24 hours.

13-2A:

SERVICE CODE(S): ______________________

DX CODE(S): ______________________

Cataracts

There are various types of cataracts, such as senile cataracts linked to the aging process, and many location areas for formation of a cataract, such as anterior or posterior polar cataracts. **Figure 13-2** illustrates a mature senile cataract.

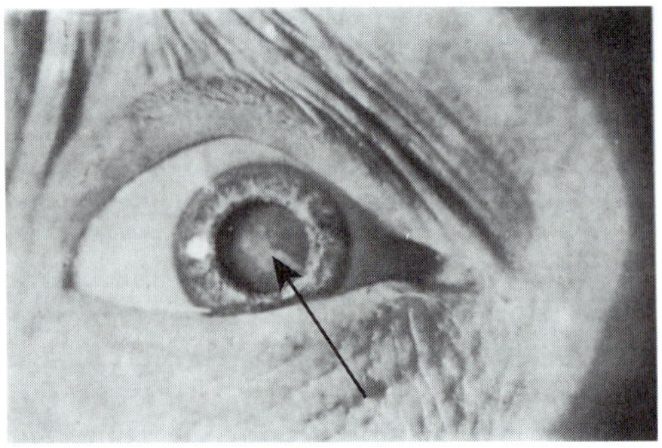

FIGURE 13-2 Mature cataract with gray fissures. *(From Pau H: Differential diagnosis of eye diseases. Philadelphia, 1978, WB Saunders.)*

Reference the term *cataract* in a medical dictionary to see the various types of cataracts. Cataract removal and lens replacement (66830-66990) use three different approaches:

- Extracapsular cataract extraction (ECCE): partial removal, which removes the hard nucleus in one piece, then removal of the soft cortex in multiple pieces. Extracapsular is on the outside of the eyeball chamber.
- Intracapsular cataract extraction (ICCE): total removal, which removes the cataract in one piece. Intracapsular is inside the eyeball chamber.
- Phacoemulsification: dissolves the hard nucleus by means of ultrasound and then the soft cortex is removed in one piece.

CASE 13-3
13-3A Clinic Progress Note, Senile Cataracts

CASE 13-3

As you code the services for this report, the choice of code for the cataract will be based on the age of the patient.

13-3A CLINIC PROGRESS NOTE, SENILE CATARACTS

LOCATION: Outpatient, Clinic

PATIENT: Margo Himon

PHYSICIAN: Rita Wimer, M.D.

DIAGNOSIS: Senile cataracts.

FINDINGS: This 69-year-old established patient is in for an exam. Vision is 20/50 and 20/70. Failed driver's license eye examination. See visual findings as noted. Glass Rx as encircled. Slight improvement in right eye can be obtained by increasing Rx by 0.50 to 0.75 sphere. Applanation reading is 16 bilateral. Medications are listed. Drives daytime only.

TREATMENT: Six to eight months' fundus. Copy of glass Rx for right lens change. Driver's license form filled out.

13-3A:

SERVICE CODE(S): ______________________________

DX CODE(S): ______________________________

CASE 13-4
13-4A Operative Report, Senile Cataracts

CASE 13-4

Phacoemulsification is used in the following cataract surgery.

13-4A OPERATIVE REPORT, SENILE CATARACTS

LOCATION: Outpatient, Hospital

PATIENT: Ingrid Cady

ATTENDING PHYSICIAN: Rita Wimer, M.D.

SURGEON: Rita Wimer, M.D.

PREOPERATIVE DIAGNOSIS: Senile nuclear cataract, right eye

POSTOPERATIVE DIAGNOSIS: Senile nuclear cataract, right eye

PROCEDURE PERFORMED: Extracapsular cataract extraction by phacoemulsification, right eye (model SI40RB, +14.5 diopters, serial no. 38982) and implantation of intraocular lens.

ANESTHESIA: Topical

ESTIMATED BLOOD LOSS: Minimal

COMPLICATIONS: None

PROCEDURE: In the operating room, a drop of lidocaine 4%-MPF was applied to the eye. The patient was prepped and draped in the usual sterile fashion for an intraocular procedure of the right eye. A lid speculum was placed. A Weck-cel soaked with lidocaine 4%-MPF was placed at the limbus, both in the area of the planned phaco incision and planned side port incision. A keratome was used to enter the chamber at the arcade. A small amount of preservative-free lidocaine 1% was injected in the anterior chamber. The aqueous was exchanged with viscoelastic material, and a side port incision was made with a 15-degree angle blade. A continuous tear capsulotomy was made with a bent needle and the Utrata forceps. The nucleus was hydrodissected and removed with phacoemulsification using an ultrasound time of 2.4 minutes and a phaco percentage of 15%. The remaining cortical material was removed with irrigation and aspiration. The capsule was polished and vacuumed as indicated. A small additional amount of lidocaine 1% was again injected into the anterior chamber. Viscoelastic was used to deepen the chamber, and the posterior chamber intraocular lens was unfolded into the capsular bag and dialed into position. Irrigation and aspiration were used to remove the remaining viscoelastic. The globe was pressurized and the cornea hydrated to ensure a good seal. The wound was tested and found to be watertight. TobraDex drops were placed on the surface of the eye. The patient left the operating room in stable condition without complications, having tolerated the procedure well.

13-4A:

SERVICE CODE(S): ______________________

DX CODE(S): ______________________

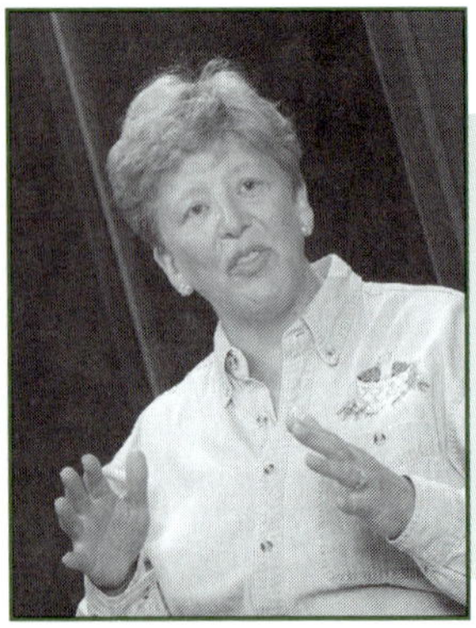

FROM THE TRENCHES

Ruth

What advice would you give an entry-level coder?

"I think it's very important to get the anatomy and terminology versus trying to go directly into coding... I think it's beneficial to take an anatomy class and a terminology class to have a good understanding... And keep the reference books on [your] desk. Don't be afraid to use them!"

Photocoagulation

Photocoagulation is the use of laser to seal leaky blood vessels, destroy abnormal blood vessels, destroy abnormal tissue at the back of the eye, and seal retinal tears. The procedure is an office procedure that does not usually require anesthesia other than eyedrops.

Diabetic retinopathy is a condition that manifests by leakage from blood vessels in the retina, causing swelling, which results in decreased vision. Photocoagulation is the treatment of choice for sealing off the leaking vessels. When reporting the diagnoses for diabetic retinopathy, the Index of the ICD-9-CM will indicate diabetes (250.5X) followed by a retinopathy code in brackets *[362.01]*, which directs the coder to list the diabetes first followed by the retinopathy. Diabetes is the etiology, and retinopathy is the manifestation.

CASE 13-5
13-5A Clinic Progress Note, Eye Examination
13-5B Clinic Progress Note, Photocoagulation

CASE 13-5

13-5A CLINIC PROGRESS NOTE, EYE EXAMINATION

LOCATION: Outpatient, Clinic

PATIENT: Carl Kerrie

PHYSICIAN: Rita Wimer, M.D.

Today I saw this new patient, who is nearly completely blind and deaf. The patient is accompanied by his son, who translated. The patient had glasses at one time but ceased to wear them because they did not help. He noticed that his vision has come down some but noticed no flurries. He has had type 1 diabetes for about 10 years.

Today, when I saw him, he was 20/40OU with a pressure of 9 on the right and 11 on the left. There was normal pupillary time and a question of rubeosis on the left. The lens and vitreous were clear on both eyes. The patient had extensive preproliferative and frank neovascularization elsewhere but not on the disk of the left eye only. There are numerous exudates and abortive efforts at neovascularization nasal and superior to the disk. The peripheral retinas are flat, and the macula shows some wrinkle on the left but is free on the right. The optic nerve is normal on the right, and there is no proliferative neuropathy in the right eye. This patient is insulin dependent.

We are dealing with a preproliferative diabetic retinopathy that needs panretinal photocoagulation as soon as possible. We have set up the treatment soon, and this will be started and commenced within the next few days.

13-5A:

SERVICE CODE(S): ______________________________

DX CODE(S): ______________________________

13-5B CLINIC PROGRESS NOTE, PHOTOCOAGULATION

Refer to Report 13-5A for the diagnosis information on this patient.

LOCATION: Outpatient, Clinic

PATIENT: Carl Kerrie

PHYSICIAN: Rita Wimer, M.D.

PROCEDURE: Photocoagulation, left eye

DIAGNOSIS: Diabetic retinopathy, insulin-dependent

The patient presents today for a photocoagulation treatment: VA 20/60-2, SC 20/30-1, OP 608, 0.1 sec, 200, 400. Follow-up is in 2 weeks in the office.

13-5B:

SERVICE CODE(S): ______________________________

DX CODE(S): ______________________________

Ectropion and Entropion

Ectropion is a condition in which the lower eyelid **droops** due to age, excessive exposure to the sun, or gravity that relaxes the structures that hold the eyelid in place. **Figure 13-3A** illustrates a patient with ectropion. The punctum is the drain hole on each lid, near the nose, that drains the tears. However, when the eyelid droops, the tears do not drain naturally into the nose. This leads to deterioration of the protective covering of the eye and results in burning, itching, irritation, and discomfort. Repair of ectropion is reported with codes from the 67914-67917 range. The ectropion repair codes include repair of one eye; if two eyes are done, report the service with modifier -50 to indicate bilateral.

Entropion is a condition in which the lower eyelid turns **inward. Figure 13-3B** illustrates a patient with entropion. The eyelashes and skin of the eyelid then rub against the

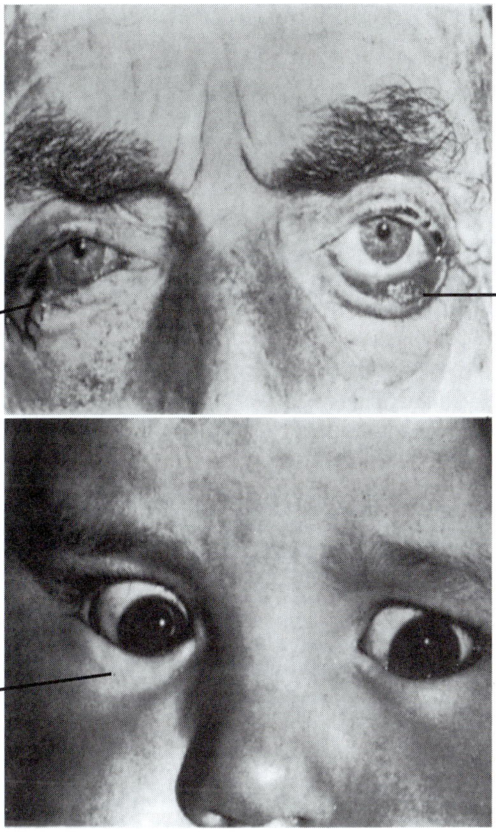

FIGURE 13-3 **A,** A 72-year-old male with senile ectropion on the left and postsurgical correction on the right. **B,** Entropion in a 6-month-old male infant. *(From Pau H: Differential diagnosis of eye diseases. Philadelphia, 1978, WB Saunders.)*

cornea and conjunctiva, which leads to excessive tearing crusting eyelid, discharge, impaired vision, and irritation of the cornea. Repair of entropion is reported with codes from the 67921-67924 range. The entropion repair codes include repair of one eye; if two eyes are done, report the service with modifier -50 to indicate bilateral.

Some third-party payers require the use of the HCPCS modifiers on the service codes:

E1 upper-left eyelid
E2 lower-left eyelid
E3 upper-right eyelid
E4 lower-right eyelid

CASE 13-6
13-6A Operative Report, Entropion and Ectropion Repair

CASE 13-6

Use the HCPCS and CPT modifiers when reporting the services for this patient.

13-6A OPERATIVE REPORT, ENTROPION AND ECTROPION REPAIR

LOCATION: Outpatient, Hospital

PATIENT: Robert Vobr

ATTENDING PHYSICIAN: Rita Wimer, M.D.

PREOPERATIVE DIAGNOSIS:
1. Upper lid entropion, both eyes; lower lid ectropion, both eyes
2. Graves' disease
3. Status post chemical decompression for Graves' disease
4. Chronic exposure, keratitis secondary to diagnoses 1, 2, and 3
5. Chronic conjunctivitis secondary to diagnoses 1, 2, 3, and 4

POSTOPERATIVE DIAGNOSIS:
1. Upper lid entropion, both eyes; lower lid ectropion, both eyes
2. Graves' disease
3. Status post chemical decompression for Graves' disease
4. Chronic exposure, keratitis secondary to diagnoses 1, 2, and 3
5. Chronic conjunctivitis secondary to diagnoses 1, 2, 3, and 4

OPERATIONS PERFORMED:
1. Upper lid entropion repair, both eyes
2. Lower lid ectropion repair, both eyes

ANESTHESIA: MAC

INDICATION: The patient has had progressive increase of upper lid entropion and lower lid ectropion, ptosis, and a number of other problems secondary to eye disease related to thyroid disease. The excess tissue is now interfering with his vision.

DESCRIPTION OF PROCEDURE: After the patient was placed on the operating room table, the skin to be resected on the upper lid was marked out with a blue sterile marking pen, as was the lower lid. There was a fishtail superiorly and lateral oblique inferiorly. This was infiltrated with Xylocaine 2%, 0.75% Marcaine, and bicarbonate. It was on a 25-gauge needle, and a total of 40 cc was used throughout the procedure. The 15 Bard-Parker blade then dissected the skin to be resected superiorly on the upper lids. This was freehand dissected, and a 2-mm strip of orbicularis was removed. The lateral, central, and medial fat pads were isolated, clamped, cut, and cauterized on the upper lids. The wound was reapproximated without supratarsal fixation using 6-0 nylon black suture to create a 2-mm ectropion of the upper lids. The lower lids were cut out with a 15 Bard-Parker blade through the marked incision. The fat pads centrally, medially, and laterally were identified, clamped, cut, cauterized, and allowed to retract. The amount of skin to be resected inferiorly was determined by the up-eye/open-mouth position, and this was mainly a lateral resection. The wounds were then closed with 6-0 nylon sutures. Maxitrol ointment and Telfa strips were laid on all four lids and half patches so the eyes remained open. There were no complications.

13-6A:

SERVICE CODE(S): ____________________

DX CODE(S): ____________________

Epiphora

Epiphora is a condition in which there is excessive production of tears. Acute epiphora is caused by allergies, foreign bodies, obstruction, or another associated condition. This type of epiphora resolves with treatment. Chronic epiphora is the excessive tearing that does not resolve with treatment. The chronic condition is most commonly caused by a malaligned eyelid, an obstructed lacrimal duct, or an ocular surface disorder. Surgical intervention sometimes is required to open the lacrimal duct by means of a nasal probe.

CASE 13-7
13-7A Operative Report, Nasolacrimal Duct Probing

CASE 13-7

Use HCPCS modifiers when reporting the service for this patient. Epiphora is excessive tearing that is mainly due to obstruction of the lacrimal passage.

13-7A OPERATIVE REPORT, NASOLACRIMAL DUCT PROBING

LOCATION: Outpatient, Hospital

PATIENT: Peggy Crase

ATTENDING PHYSICIAN: Rita Wimer, M.D.

PREOPERATIVE DIAGNOSIS:
1. Epiphora, both eyes
2. Nasolacrimal duct obstruction, both eyes

POSTOPERATIVE DIAGNOSIS:
1. Epiphora, both eyes
2. Nasolacrimal duct obstruction, both eyes

PROCEDURE PERFORMED: Nasolacrimal duct probing, both eyes

ANESTHESIA: Anesthesia

INDICATIONS: This 32-month-old white female was referred by Dr. Peterson after an allergy workup to investigate her chronic otitis media, PE tubes times two, and the chronic epiphora that she has had in both eyes since birth. The mother was counseled as to the success of probing at this age and the possible reoperations that may be needed.

PROCEDURE: After the patient was placed under suitable anesthesia via the mask, a small punctum dilator was used to dilate the punctum inferiorly and superiorly. These were found to be very tight and occluded. A 2-0 Bowman probe could be passed only through the inferior system with difficulty on both sides. The C-loop could not be irrigated. Probing could not be attempted because of a large bony obstruction that resisted all efforts to pass the tube. There was no fluorescein removed in the nose. TobraDex drops were placed in the eyes. The procedure was complete, and the patient was sent to the recovery room. The patient will be referred for further ENT consultation and to Dr. Lorabi for the possibility of a white cell deficiency that is causing these chronic infections or other immune problems. There were no complications.

13-7A:

SERVICE CODE(S): ______________________

DX CODE(S): ______________________

Ear

Office Services

Otolaryngologists are physicians trained in the medical and surgical management and treatment of patients with diseases and disorders of the ear, nose, and throat (ENT) and are often referred to as ENT physicians. There are many subspecialty areas in otolaryngology, such as pediatric otolaryngology, otology or neurotology (ears, balance, and tinnitus), allergy, facial plastic and reconstructive surgery, head and neck, laryngology, and rhinology. Some otolaryngologists limit their practices to one area, and others practice across all areas.

Because an otolaryngologist specializes in the ears, nose, and throat, there is a wide range of conditions that are treated, such as ear infections, sinusitis, septal deviation, laryngitis, and pharyngitis.

CASE 13-8
13-8A Clinic Progress Note, Sore Throat
13-8B Clinic Progress Note, Well Child Care

CASE 13-8

Report both the E/M and lab service. A hint for looking up the strep screen in the CPT index is that it is a bacterial culture.

13-8A CLINIC PROGRESS NOTE, SORE THROAT

LOCATION: Outpatient, Clinic

PATIENT: Leah Charles

PHYSICIAN: Rita Wimer, M.D.

SUBJECTIVE: The patient is a 3½-year-old girl who was seen by me 4 months ago, and today presents with her parents to the clinic. Her mother states that both her brother and sister have been on medication for the second time because of being positive for strep. The patient started complaining of a sore throat 2 days ago. She is also complaining of some ear pain. She does have an ALLERGY to SULFA. Mother noticed a rash on the side of her lips just the other day.

OBJECTIVE: On general appearance, the patient is alert. She does not appear to be in acute distress. Temperature is 99.9. Weight is 13.6 kg. HEENT: Both TMs are clear. Her PE tube is out in the canal on the left. Oropharynx is erythematous. Also, along her lip she does have some erythematous lesions with golden crust and consistent with impetigo. Neck has shotty (*like a pellet*) cervical nodes bilaterally but is supple. Heart reveals a regular rate and rhythm without murmur. Lungs are clear to auscultation bilaterally. Her abdomen is soft.

IMPRESSION:
1. Pharyngitis, rule out strep
2. Impetigo

PLAN:
1. Keflex 250 mg/5cc ¾ teaspoon orally, three times daily × 10 days.
2. We will also do a strep screen as well, today.

13-8A:

SERVICE CODE(S):____________________

DX CODE(S):____________________

13-8B CLINIC PROGRESS NOTE, WELL CHILD CARE

Three months later, Leah again is brought to the clinic by her mother. The first-listed diagnosis is the otitis media, but you will also need to report a V code to indicate that the purpose of this visit was a medical examination for admission to preschool.

LOCATION: Outpatient, Clinic

PATIENT: Leah Charles

PHYSICIAN: Rita Wimer, M.D.

SUBJECTIVE: The patient is an almost 4-year-old girl who presents to the clinic with her parents for well child care and Head Start physical. Mother states that she was seen 1 month ago when they noted fluid in one of her ears. Mother does not notice any problems with the patient's hearing or speech development. She has not had a runny nose, cough, or fever. She eats well from the four food groups and has no problems with constipation or diarrhea.

OBJECTIVE: On general appearance, the patient is alert and does not appear to be in any acute distress. Temperature is 97.7. Weight is 15.8 kg, which places her right at the 50th percentile. Height is 97.8 cm, which places her right beneath the 25th percentile. Blood pressure is 90/60. HEENT: PERRLA. EOMI. Disks are sharp. Right TM does have some fluid present behind it. The left TM is nice and clear. Oropharynx is unremarkable. Neck is supple. Heart reveals a regular rate and rhythm. Lungs are clear to auscultation bilaterally, and her abdomen is soft. GU: Normal female genitalia. Extremities have full range of motion. Back reveals a straight spine. Hearing was checked and is normal bilaterally. Vision is 20/25 bilaterally.

IMPRESSION: Female almost 4 years old with right serous otitis media

PLAN: I recommended following up with the patient in 2 months to ensure that the fluid has gone. Prescribed amoxicillin, 20 mg, q8h. If it has not at that point, we may need to look into further ways of management. Mother was in agreement with this.

13-8B:

SERVICE CODE(S):____________________

DX CODE(S):____________________

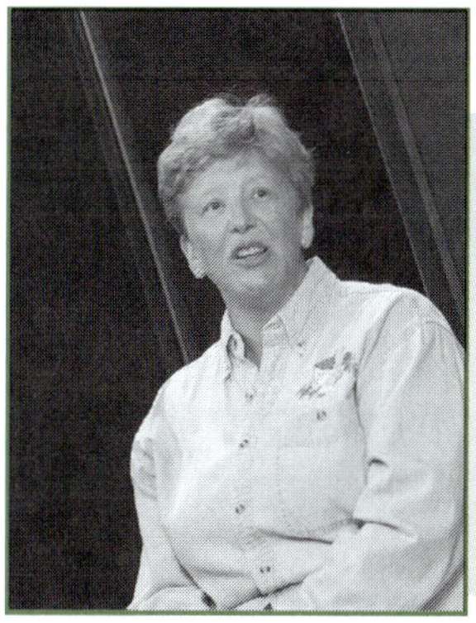

FROM THE TRENCHES

Ruth

"I meet with physicians and educate them on the codes they're selecting. When a new transmittal comes out that affects their practice, I let them know about the change. The physicians are dependent on us to do that kind of 'watching' for guideline changes. It's an opportunity for revenue, and of course they always want to be in compliance. If there's a change, they expect us to let them know of that change."

Myringotomy and Tympanostomy

The eustachian tube connects the middle ear to the back of the throat and allows for drainage of any fluid that may collect there. When a eustachian tube dysfunctions, fluid collects in the middle ear. The tube can become inflamed from allergies or infection. Eustachian tube dysfunction is a fairly common condition in children because the eustachian tube has not always matured to the level of normal function and therefore does not work as well as it does in an adult. The condition prevents air from entering the middle ear, and pressure builds up in the middle ear. Surgical intervention is a **myringotomy** (incision into the tympanic membrane) and reinflation of the eustachian tube or insertion of a small plastic or metal tube (PE [pressure equalization] tube) that allows the fluid to drain (**tympanostomy**). See **Figure 13-4** for an illustration of the placement of a PE tube. The tubes may later be removed, fall out naturally, or sometimes are just left in place.

A myringotomy is the incision and draining of fluid from the middle ear. A tympanostomy is the incision and placement of tubes to drain fluid from the middle ear. If the ventilation tubes are removed due to a complication, the diagnosis is reported based on the reason for the complication, such as an infection.

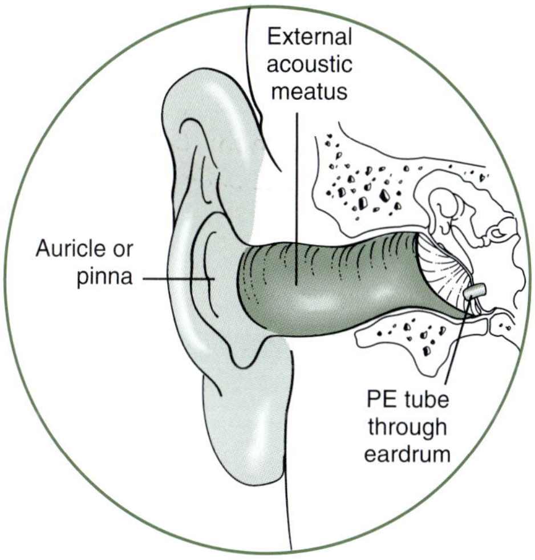

FIGURE 13-4 Placement of pressure equalization (PE) tube.

CASE 13-9
13-9A Operative Report, Pressure Equalization Tube Removal

CASE 13-9

13-9A OPERATIVE REPORT, PRESSURE EQUALIZATION TUBE REMOVAL

LOCATION: Outpatient, Hospital

PATIENT: Ann Sjol

ATTENDING PHYSICIAN: Jeff King, M.D.

PREOPERATIVE DIAGNOSIS:
1. Retained PE tubes
2. Obstructed PE tubes

POSTOPERATIVE DIAGNOSIS:
1. Retained PE tubes
2. Obstructed PE tubes

complication

PROCEDURE PERFORMED: Removal of bilateral PE tubes

OPERATIVE NOTE: The patient is a 7-year-old female who has had PE tubes in for a prolonged period. Recently, she has had problems with recurrent infections and persistent fluid. She has granulation on both tubes. A decision was made to remove these in the operating room. She was admitted through the same-day surgery program and taken to the operating room, where a general anesthetic was administered via inhalation. A 4-mm speculum was inserted in the right ear. Wax was removed from the canal. The tube was visualized. Using cup forceps, this tube was removed. There was granulation tissue around the opening. Two drops of Cortisporin were applied. The speculum was removed and inserted on the opposite side. Again, wax was removed from the canal. The PE tube was removed with cup forceps. Again, granulation tissue seemed to close the perforation nicely. Two drops of Cortisporin were applied here. The speculum was removed. The patient was allowed to recover from the general anesthetic and taken to the postanesthesia care unit in stable condition. There were no complications during this procedure.

13-9A:

SERVICE CODE(S):____________________

DX CODE(S):____________________

CASE 13-10
13-10A Operative Report, Tonsillectomy, Adenoidectomy, and Myringotomy

CASE 13-10

In the following case, a myringotomy and a tonsillectomy/adenoidectomy (the most resource-intense) are performed.

13-10A OPERATIVE REPORT, TONSILLECTOMY, ADENOIDECTOMY, AND MYRINGOTOMY

LOCATION: Outpatient, Hospital

PATIENT: Dustin Boyle

ATTENDING PHYSICIAN: Jeff King, M.D.

PREOPERATIVE DIAGNOSES:
1. Chronic adenotonsillitis
2. Adenotonsillar hypertrophy
3. Chronic serous otitis media

POSTOPERATIVE DIAGNOSES:
1. Chronic adenotonsillitis
2. Adenotonsillar hypertrophy
3. Chronic serous otitis media

PROCEDURE PERFORMED:
1. Myringotomy bilaterally
2. Tonsillectomy and adenoidectomy

OPERATIVE NOTE: The patient is a 15-year-old boy seen in the office and diagnosed with the above condition. The decision was made in consultation with his family to take him to the operating room to undergo the above-named procedures.

PROCEDURE: The patient was admitted through the same-day surgery program and taken to the operating room, where he was administered general anesthetic by intravenous injection. He was then intubated endotracheally. A 4-mm speculum was inserted into the right ear, and wax was removed from the canal. An anterior/inferior incision was created, and a small amount of fluid was removed. The speculum was removed and inserted in the opposite ear. Again, wax was removed from the canal. An anterior/inferior incision was created. This middle ear cavity was dry. The speculum was removed.

The patient was turned 90 degrees. The Jennings gag was placed into the mouth and expanded. This was secured to a Mayo stand. Two red rubber catheters were placed through the nose, brought out through the mouth, and secured with snaps. A laryngeal mirror was placed into the nasopharynx, and the adenoid tissue was identified. This was removed with a suction cautery in a systematic fashion. Once this was completed, the red rubbers were released and brought out through the mouth. The right tonsil was grasped with an Allis forceps and retracted medially. Using the harmonic scalpel, the capsule was identified laterally. The tonsil was removed from its fossa in an inferior-to-superior fashion. Once this was completed, the bed was inspected. One small area was cauterized. The left tonsil was grasped with an Allis forceps and retracted medially. Again, the capsule was identified laterally with the harmonic scalpel. The tonsil was removed from its fossa in a superior-to-inferior fashion. Once this was completed, the bed was inspected. No bleeding was noted. Three tonsil sponges were then soaked with 1% Marcaine and epinephrine; one was placed in the nasopharynx and one in each tonsil bed. These were left in position for 5 minutes. At the end of the interval, they were removed. The beds were inspected, and no further bleeding was noted. The gag was released and removed from the mouth. The TMJ was checked. The patient was allowed to recover from the general anesthetic and taken to the postanesthesia care unit in stable condition. There were no complications during this procedure.

Pathology Report Later Indicated: Benign tonsil and adenoid tissue.

13-10A:

SERVICE CODE(S):________________________

DX CODE(S):________________________

CASE 13-11
13-11A Operative Report, Tube Removal

CASE 13-11

In this case, both a removal of impacted PE tube and tympanostomy are performed.

13-11A OPERATIVE REPORT, TUBE REMOVAL

LOCATION: Outpatient, Hospital

PATIENT: Will Boyle

ATTENDING PHYSICIAN: Jeff King, M.D.

PREOPERATIVE DIAGNOSIS: Impacted left PE tube

POSTOPERATIVE DIAGNOSIS: Impacted left PE tube

PROCEDURE PERFORMED:
1. REMOVAL OF IMPACTED PE TUBE, LEFT EAR
2. PLACEMENT OF NEW PE TUBE, LEFT EAR

OPERATIVE NOTE: Will is a patient who was seen in the office with a diagnosis of the above-named condition. A decision was made in consultation with the family for the above-named procedure.

The patient was admitted through same-day surgery department and taken to the operating room, where he was administered a general anesthetic by inhalation. A 3.5-mm speculum was inserted into the right ear. A small amount of wax was removed. The speculum was removed and inserted into the left ear. The impacted PE tube was then removed. There was some granulation tissue around this site. We created a new site posteriorly within some tympanosclerotic plaque. A new PE tube was inserted. The patient was then allowed to recover from the general anesthetic and taken to the postanesthesia care unit in stable condition. There were no complications during this procedure.

13-11A:

SERVICE CODE(S):________________

DX CODE(S):________________

CASE 13-12
13-12A Operative Report, Myringotomy and Tympanostomy

CASE 13-12

Report Dr. King's portion only.

13-12A OPERATIVE REPORT, MYRINGOTOMY AND TYMPANOSTOMY

LOCATION: Outpatient, Hospital

PATIENT: Karen Vince

SURGEON: Jeff King, M.D.

PREOPERATIVE DIAGNOSIS:
1. Bilateral nasolacrimal duct obstruction
2. Bilateral cerumen impaction
3. Right otitis media with effusion with nonfunctional pressure equalization tube

POSTOPERATIVE DIAGNOSIS:
1. Bilateral nasolacrimal duct obstruction
2. Bilateral cerumen impaction
3. Acute right otitis media with effusion with nonfunctional pressure equalization tube

PROCEDURE PERFORMED:
1. Bilateral nasolacrimal duct endoscopy
2. Left endoscopic nasal examination with inferior turbinate fracture
3. Bilateral microscopic ear examination with cleaning of the left and right ear
4. Right myringotomy with tympanostomy tube placement

ANESTHESIA: General endotracheal anesthesia

INDICATION: A 10-year-old female with bilateral nasolacrimal duct obstruction. The patient is now here for treatment. She has very narrow nasal anatomy. She also has bilateral cerumen impactions that do not allow for ease of access for examination of her ears for the status of her PE tubes.

DESCRIPTION OF PROCEDURE: After consent was obtained, the patient was taken to the operating room and placed on the operating table in a supine position. After an adequate level of general endotracheal anesthesia was obtained, the patient was draped in an appropriate manner and the nasolacrimal duct dilation performed, bilaterally. The nose was packed with cotton pledgets soaked with 0.25% Neo-Synephrine. Attention was first focused on the left eye. The left nasal cavity was examined endoscopically. The turbinate was infractured to allow access to the inferior meatus. The turbinate was then repositioned to its normal position and the nose packed with the pledgets soaked with the Neo-Synephrine solution. Attention was then focused on the right. A similar procedure was performed; however, endoscopic examination and turbinate outfracture were not necessary on that side. The right side was then packed with the pledgets soaked with the Neo-Synephrine solution. Attention was then focused on the ears. Using the ear speculum and microscope, the left ear canal was cleared of cerumen. It was functional, and there were no abnormalities on that side. Attention was then focused on the right side, where the ear canal was again cleared of cerumen impaction. Subsequent examination showed an extruded PE tube lying on the tympanic membrane with surrounding cerumen and squamous debris. This was removed. Subsequently, a myringotomy incision was placed in the anterior-inferior quadrant. A large amount of mucoid effusion was suctioned. A bobbin tympanostomy tube was then placed without difficulty. Cortisporin Otic suspension and a cotton ball were then placed in the right ear. The nasal packs were then removed. There was no bleeding. The patient tolerated the procedure well. There was no break in technique. The patient was extubated and taken to the post anesthesia care unit in good condition.

FLUIDS ADMINISTERED: 50 cc of RL

ESTIMATED BLOOD LOSS: Less than 20 cc

PREOPERATIVE MEDICATION: 4 mg of Decadron IV

13-12A:

SERVICE CODE(S):__________

DX CODE(S):__________

(1) 69436-RT (Tympanostomy)
(2) 68801-51-50 (Dilation, nasolacrimal)
(3) 30930-51-LT (Fracture, nasal turbinate)

CASE 13-13
13-13A Operative Report, Tympanoplasty

CASE 13-13

The patient in this case has a history of chronic otitis media and cholesteatoma and presents for reconstruction of the tympanic membrane. Use an HCPCS modifier.

13-13A OPERATIVE REPORT, TYMPANOPLASTY

LOCATION: Inpatient, Hospital

PATIENT: Neil Fraser

ATTENDING PHYSICIAN: Jeff King, M.D.

PREOPERATIVE DIAGNOSES:
1. Right moderate conductive hearing loss
2. History of right ear cholesteatoma, status post tympanoplasty and mastoidectomy

POSTOPERATIVE DIAGNOSES:
1. Right moderate conductive hearing loss [Discontinuity of ear ossicles]
2. History of right ear cholesteatoma, status post tympanoplasty and mastoidectomy

PROCEDURE PERFORMED: Right tympanoplasty with ossicular reconstruction using a Kurt titanium partial ossicular replacement prosthesis

ANESTHESIA: General endotracheal anesthesia

INDICATION: A 12-year-old male with history of right chronic otitis media and cholesteatoma. He has undergone tympanoplasty and mastoidectomy. This resulted in a moderate conductive hearing loss. The patient has not shown any evidence of recurrent disease, and the patient is in now for reexploration and reconstruction if no cholesteatoma is found.

DESCRIPTION OF PROCEDURE: After parental consent was obtained, the patient was taken to the operating room and placed on the operating table in a supine position. After an adequate level of general endotracheal anesthesia was obtained, the patient was positioned for surgery on the right ear. The patient's right ear was prepped with Betadine prep and draped in a sterile manner. One-percent Xylocaine with 1:100,000 U of epinephrine was infiltrated into the preauricular, tragus, postauricular area, and then in the ear canal. The speculum was secured with a speculum holder. The mastoid cavity was clean. A tympanomeatal flap was then elevated. The chorda tympani nerve was identified and preserved. There was no evidence of recurrent cholesteatoma. The posterior aspect of the tympanic membrane was thin. This was elevated off the head of the stapes. No incus was present. The long process of the malleus was present, but there was no head of the malleus. The stapes was mobile, and there was a round window reflex. Attention was then focused on the tragus, where a cartilage and perichondrium graft was harvested in standard fashion. That incision was closed with interrupted 6-0 rapid absorbing gut suture. The Kurz titanium partial replacement prosthesis was selected. Sizers were placed to determine the appropriate length. This was determined to be 2.5 mm. Dry Gelfoam was placed in the middle ear. The prosthesis was then placed on top of the stapes superstructure. Cartilage and perichondrium were then placed on top of this to act as an interface between the titanium and the thin drum remnant and also to reinforce the drum remnant. The tympanomeatal flap was then brought back over this and brought onto the canal wall and facial ridge. Gelfoam soaked with PhysioSol was then placed on this. The proximal ear canal was then filled with Bacitracin ointment. A cotton ball coated with Bacitracin ointment was placed in the conchal bowl area, and then a Band-Aid dressing was applied. The patient tolerated the procedure well, and there was no break in technique. The patient was extubated and taken to the postanesthesia care unit in good condition.

FLUIDS ADMINISTERED: 1600 cc of RL

ESTIMATED BLOOD LOSS: Less than 10 cc

13-13A:

SERVICE CODE(S):____________________

DX CODE(S):____________________

Glossary

blepharoplasty corrective surgery on the eyelid.

cataract opaque covering on or in the lens.

ectropion a condition in which the lower eyelid sags or turns outward.

entropion a condition in which the eyelid, usually the lower lid, rolls inward toward the eye.

epiphora abnormal overflow of tears, sometimes due to a blockage of the lacrimal passages.

extruded pushing out.

impacted wedged in.

myringotomy the creation of a hole and/or incision in the tympanic membrane.

ophthalmologist physician specializing in medical and surgical care of the eye and visual system.

otolaryngologist physician specializing in the management and treatment of diseases and disorders of the ear, nose, and throat; often referred to as an ENT physician.

phacoemulsification emulsification (making liquid) and aspiration of a cataract.

photocoagulation procedure that uses a controlled laser to treat leaky retinal blood vessels and destroy abnormal vessels or tissues at the back of the eye.

tympanostomy excision of the tympanic membrane to insert a PE tube for fluid drainage.

Chapter 14
Anesthesia

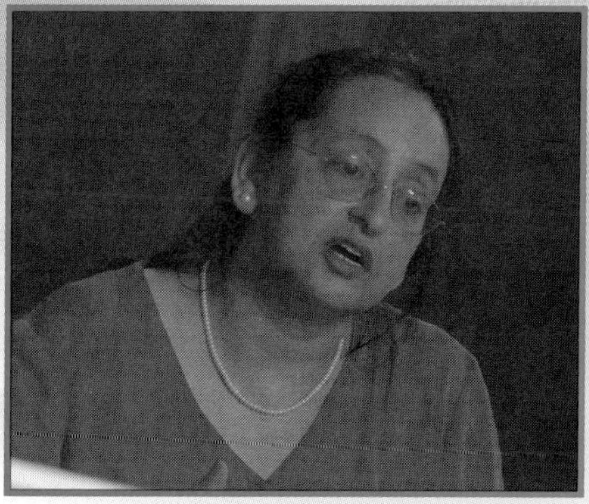

Deepa Malhotra, MS, CPC
President
Healthcare Educational Resource Services, Inc.
Aurora, Illinois

ABBREVIATIONS

ABD	Adriamycin, bleomycin, dacarbazine
cc	cubic centimeter
cm	centimeter
CPAP	continuous positive airway pressure
CRNA	certified registered nurse anesthetist
CT	computed tomography
EEG	electroencephalogram
ENT	ear, nose, throat
g	gram
mg	milligram
mm	millimeter
OR	operating room
PAR	postanesthesia recovery
PCA	patient-controlled analgesia
PE	pressure equalization

An **anesthesiologist** is a specialist in Perioperative Medicine who specializes in care of a patient prior to, during, and immediately after surgery, including the evaluation and preparation of a patient for anesthesia service. The anesthesiologist plans the anesthetic for the patient and then cares for the patient during the surgical procedure by monitoring blood pressure, heart rate, breathing, temperature, and level of consciousness and **analgesia.** They can also administer drugs for analgesia (pain relief) before, during, and after the procedure.

The anesthesiologist is responsible for any adjustments to the anesthetic plan, medications, fluids (blood volume and electrolytes), and other parameters to provide a pain-free and safe surgical experience for the patient. In the event of an emergency, it is the anesthesiologist who is responsible for the management of cardiac and respiratory resuscitation should the need arise during the surgery. The anesthesiologist also provides **postoperative** care while the patient is in the recovery room.

An anesthesiologist is also a specialist in the control of chronic pain. They staff and manage pain clinics to treat patients with terminal illnesses (such as cancer), chronic pain, or injury.

Anesthesia Section Format

The Anesthesia section of the CPT manual is used by the anesthesiologist or **anesthetist** to report the provision of anesthesia services. Anesthesia procedure codes are divided first by anatomic site and then by specific type of procedure. The last four subsections in Anesthesia—Radiologic Procedures, Burn Excisions or Debridement, Obstetric, and Other Procedures—are *not* by anatomic division. The CPT codes in the Radiologic Procedures subsection of the Anesthesia section are used to report anesthesia services when radiologic services are provided to the patient for diagnostic or therapeutic reasons. The radiologic services are reported separately.

Moderate (Conscious) Sedation

Moderate or **conscious sedation** is a type of sedation that can be provided by any physician performing a procedure; it provides a decreased level of consciousness that does not put the patient completely to sleep. This level of consciousness allows the patient to breathe without assistance and to respond to stimulation and verbal commands. A trained observer is required to be present during the use of the conscious sedation to assist the physician in monitoring the patient. The codes used to report this type of conscious sedation (moderate) are located in the Medicine section (99143-99150), not in the Anesthesia section. If the sedation is provided by an anesthesiologist other than the physician performing the procedure, you would use the appropriate anesthesia code.

The conscious sedation codes in the Medicine section are divided based on the age of the patient (under 5 or 5 or over), time (first 30 minutes and each additional 15 minutes), and if the service is provided by the physician or other than the physician. These sedation methods are much less debilitating than is the complete loss of consciousness. For example, for a colonoscopy, a physician could administer an intravenous sedation, such as meperidine (Demerol), morphine, or diazepam (Valium). The patient would be monitored closely as the medication is administered so that the appropriate level of sedation is reached. After the procedure, the physician may administer a drug such as naloxone (Narcan) intravenously to reverse the effects of the sedation. The patient would have this procedure in an outpatient setting and be able to go home after the procedure.

Some types of anesthesia are named for the site of anesthesia administration, such as sacral, lumbar, or caudal. Other types of anesthesia are named for the category, such as frost or cryoanesthesia. Some of the more commonly used terms are endotracheal, epidural, and regional. Endotracheal anesthesia is accomplished by inserting a tube through the mouth or nose into the trachea, and then administering a gaseous drug to achieve general anesthesia. Epidural anesthesia is the injection of an anesthetic agent into the spaces between the vertebrae. This type of anesthesia is also known as peridural, epidural block, spinal, intraspinal, or subarachnoid anesthesia.

General anesthesia is a state of unconsciousness that is achieved by means of inhalation, intramuscular, rectal, or intravenous. Regional is also known as a field block that anesthetizes a specific region or area of the body. A nerve block is a type of regional anesthesia. Local anesthesia is the application of an anesthetic agent directly to the area involved, such as lidocaine that is subcutaneously injected for repair of a laceration.

Patient-controlled analgesia (PCA) is a system that allows the patient to self-administer an analgesic drug by depressing a button on a pump that holds the drug. In this way the patient controls the amount of drug and the frequency of administration.

Qualifying Circumstances

At times, anesthesia is provided in situations that make the administration of the anesthesia more difficult. These types of cases include those that are performed in emergency situations and those dealing with patients of extreme age; they also include services performed during the use of controlled **hypotension** or the use of **hypothermia.**

Medicine section

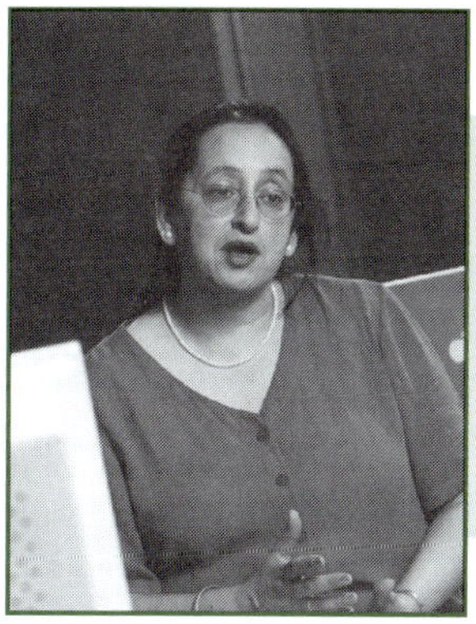

FROM THE TRENCHES

Deepa

"You can't be in the healthcare industry without the language of coding. Go ahead and learn the language—it's a beautiful language... You have to understand what we are talking about with these numbers. The numbers mean so much."

The **Qualifying Circumstances** codes begin with the number 99 and are considered add-on codes. Add-on codes cannot be used alone but must be used in addition to another code, and are used to provide additional information only.

The Qualifying Circumstances code is used in addition to the anesthesia procedure code. The Qualifying Circumstances codes are located in two places in the CPT manual: the Medicine section and the Anesthesia section guidelines. In both locations the plus symbol is located next to the codes (99100-99140), indicating their status as add-on codes only.

In some cases, more than one qualifying circumstances code may apply and can be coded. For example, a surgical procedure performed on a patient of extreme age (99100) in which the anesthesia is complicated by an emergency condition (99140).

Physical Status Modifiers

The second type of modifying unit used in the Anesthesia section is the **physical status modifier**. These modifiers are used to indicate the patient's condition at the time anesthesia was administered. The physical status modifier not only indicates the patient's condition at the time of anesthesia but also serves to identify the level of complexity of services provided to the patient. For instance, anesthesia service to a gravely ill patient is much more complex than the same type of service to a normal, healthy patient. The physical status modifier is not assigned by the coder but is determined by the anesthesiologist and documented in the anesthesia record. The physical status modifier begins with the letter *P* and contains a number from 1 to 6. Note that the relative value for -P1, -P2, and -P6 is zero because these conditions are considered not to affect the service provided.

Every anesthesia code billed must have an accompanying physical status modifier. Qualifying circumstances codes may or may not apply.

Concurrent Care Modifiers

Some third-party payers require additional modifiers to indicate how many cases an anesthesiologist is performing or supervising at one time. Certified registered nurse anesthetists (CRNAs) may administer anesthesia to patients under the direction of a licensed physician, or they may work independently according to state law. When an anesthesiologist is directing the provision of anesthesia in more than one case at a time, modifiers are used to indicate the context and number of cases that are being reported concurrently. The following modifiers are among the most commonly used:

-AA	Anesthesia services performed personally by anesthesiologist
-AD	Medical supervision by a physician: more than four concurrent anesthesia procedures
-GC	This service has been performed in part by a resident under the direction of a teaching physician
-QK	Medical direction of two, three, or four concurrent anesthesia procedures involving a qualified individual
-QX	Certified registered nurse anesthetist (CRNA) service, with medical direction by a physician
-QY	Anesthesiologist medically directs one CRNA
-QZ	CRNA service, without medical direction by a physician

Anesthesia Services in the Hospital Setting

If a hospital bills for anesthesiologists and/or CRNA services, it would bill the **professional service component** on a separate bill (CMS1500). The codes assigned for the professional component of the anesthesia services would be the same if the anesthesia staff were employed by the facility or were independent. The UB-92 (CMS1450) would include all the charges for the OR, laboratory, supplies, drugs, recovery room, room and board, etc. The hospital bill may or may not include a line item billing for anesthesia. The charges that would be included under this charge would most likely be for drugs and anesthetic gases. Routine nonbillable supplies and anesthesia equipment charges are combined with the operating room charges. As a result, no anesthesia CPT codes are used on the UB-92, and the ICD-9 codes that are assigned by the hospital coders are related to the actual surgical procedure.

You have assigned service and diagnoses codes to the following procedures throughout this text; therefore, no service or diagnosis codes need be assigned in this chapter. Assign the anesthesia codes and modifiers to the following cases:

CASE 14-1

This anesthesia service is being provided for a 76-year-old patient who has severe hypertension that the physician is having difficulty managing at the time of this procedure.

14-1A OPERATIVE REPORT, FLAPS AND GRAFTS

LOCATION: Inpatient, Hospital

PATIENT: Josh Peterson

SURGEON: Gary Sanchez, M.D.

PREOPERATIVE DIAGNOSIS: Open wound, left lower extremity, with exposed tibia and exposed plate

POSTOPERATIVE DIAGNOSIS: Ulcer, left lower extremity, with exposed tibia and exposed plate

PROCEDURES PERFORMED:

1. Soleus muscle flap
2. Split-thickness skin graft 2.5 × 2.5 cm from the left thigh to the left lower extremity

ANESTHESIA: General endotracheal (a

ESTIMATED BLOOD LOSS: 130 cc

DRAINS: One #10 Jackson-Pratt

SURGICAL FINDINGS: There was an open wound extending from the lower third of the tibia up into the middle third of the leg with an exposed plate, but tissue loss of the lower third of the leg was evident. Dr. Almaz, Orthopedics, had previously inserted antibiotic beads.

PROCEDURE: An incision was made 2.5 cm medial to the tibial border. We developed a bilobed flap and identified the separation of the soleus muscle and the gastrocnemius medial head following incision of the deep fascia. I dissected the soleus muscle free distally as far as possible and then cut it distally at the Achilles tendon insertion, transposing it through a tunnel of the bilobed flap and covering the area of soft-tissue loss by using bolsters that were tied in place with 0 Prolene. This effectively covered the open area, and then we closed the remainder of the area with 0 Prolene, closing the donor area also with 0 Prolene. We put nitro paste along the edges where there was some skin blanching and put a #10 Jackson-Pratt drain in the distal end of the wound, bringing it out through a separate stab wound incision. A split-thickness skin graft about 2.5 × 2.5 cm was taken from the left thigh, meshed with 1:1.5 mesher, and applied to the defect area measuring 2.5 × 2.5 cm with 2-0 Prolene sutures and staples. We dressed the wound with Xeroform, Kerlix fluffs, Kerlix roll, Kling, and Sof-Rol, and then a cast was applied by the orthopedic technician. The donor site was dressed with scarlet red and an ABD pad. The patient tolerated the procedure well and left the area in good condition.

14-1A:

ANESTHESIA CODE(S): ______________________

Anesthesia, leg, lower

CASE 14-2
14-2A Operative Report, Perirectal Fistulectomies

CASE 14-2A
Unless stated otherwise, assume "normal, healthy patient."

14-2A OPERATIVE REPORT, PERIRECTAL FISTULECTOMIES

LOCATION: Outpatient, Hospital

PATIENT: George Papenfuss

SURGEON: Larry Friendly, M.D.

PREOPERATIVE DIAGNOSIS: Chronic perirectal fistulas

POSTOPERATIVE DIAGNOSIS: Perirectal fistulas

PROCEDURE PERFORMED: Perirectal fistulectomies

ANESTHESIA: General anesthetic

INDICATIONS FOR SURGERY: The patient is a 61-year-old Caucasian male who had draining perirectal fistulas, which had been incised and drained in the past. The patient is now being seen for excision of these fistulas.

DESCRIPTION OF PROCEDURE: The patient was placed in a jackknife position. He was prepped and draped in the usual manner. The patient was given a general anesthetic. The fistulous tracts were in the 2 and 11 o'clock positions. The fistulous tracts were excised; one of them had an abscessed pocket, and this was excised in its entirety. The tracts continued over the 12 o'clock midline position over into about the 2 o'clock position. All these tracts were combined into one large incision, and all of the inflammatory tissue was excised sharply. The rectum was also dilated up and examined. There was no evidence of any tract that could be seen directly draining into the rectum at this time and no induration. The inflammatory tissue that was present on the outer skin area was completely excised. The operative area was thoroughly irrigated. Hemostasis was obtained using Bovie cautery. The wounds were left open, drain was placed, and dressings were applied. The patient tolerated the operation and returned to recovery in stable condition.

14-2A:

ANESTHESIA CODE(S): ____________________

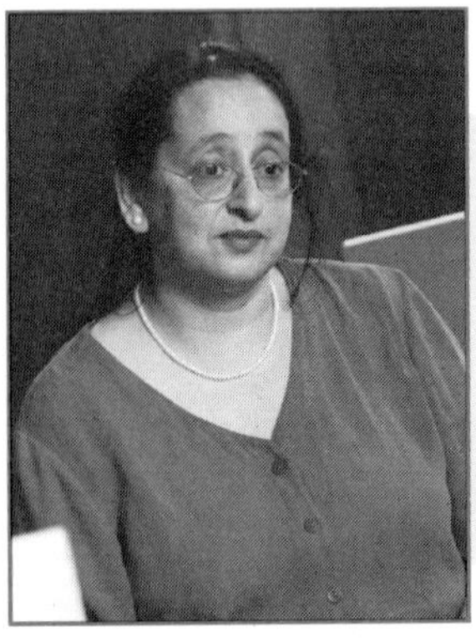

FROM THE TRENCHES

Deepa

"You have to be totally open. Your mind has to absorb things... I find the more I teach, the more I learn. I expect [you], as a coder or a coding student, to not only be a self-start person, but to also be an educator for the person next to you. You can't go wrong with that. The more you share, the more you get."

CASE 14-3

The most costly procedure is the arthrodesis.

14-3A OPERATIVE REPORT, FUSION WITH AUTOGRAFT

LOCATION: Outpatient, Hospital

PATIENT: Rose Stich

SURGEON: Mohomad Almaz, M.D.

PREOPERATIVE DIAGNOSIS: Posttraumatic subtalar osteoarthritis, left hindfoot, due to old calcaneal fracture

POSTOPERATIVE DIAGNOSIS: Posttraumatic subtalar osteoarthritis, left hindfoot, due to old calcaneal fracture

PROCEDURE PERFORMED: Left subtalar fusion using moldable autograft obtained from the left iliac crest

ANESTHESIA: General

OPERATIVE PROCEDURE: The patient is a 32-year-old female. After suitable general anesthesia had been achieved, the patient's left iliac crest and left foot and ankle were prepped and draped in the usual manner. Prior to prepping, a thigh tourniquet was applied, but initially it was not inflated. Bone graft was harvested from the left iliac crest. A 10-cm incision was made and carried down through the subcutaneous fat. The fascia was incised in line with the crest starting about 2 cm back from the anterior-superior iliac spine. Cortical cancellous bone graft was then harvested from the inner table. Defect was packed with Gelfoam. The wound was closed in layers. The skin was closed with staples.

The leg was then elevated. The tourniquet was inflated. The incision was made from the tip of the fibula to the base of the fourth metatarsal. Distally based flap of the extensor digitorum brevis was elevated off the lateral aspect of the calcaneus. Fat pad and the sinus tarsi were split in line with the skin incision. Anterior process of the calcaneus was excised. The capsule was incised. A lot of thickened synovial tissue was removed. The joint surfaces were noted to be substantially damaged from the old calcaneal fracture. The remaining articular cartilage and scar tissue were removed with curet and rongeur. The subchondral bone was then carefully burred down to a bleeding surface. Autograft from the iliac crest was then packed in between the bone surfaces. Using image intensifier, a large fragment cannulated screw was then placed starting at the talar neck across the posterior face of the subtalar joint into the central aspect of the calcaneal body. Further gap in the fusion at the sinus tarsi area was filled with autograft and allograft. The wound was then closed. Skin was closed with 4-0 nylon. Dressing and a Robert Jones dressing with a posterior fiberglass splint were then applied. The tourniquet was released. Following tourniquet release, good circulation was noted to return to the foot. The patient tolerated the procedure well and returned to the recovery room in stable condition.

14-3A:

ANESTHESIA CODE(S): ______________________

CASE 14-4
14-4A Operative Report, Septoplasty, Turbinate Reduction, Tonsillectomy

CASE 14-4

The septoplasty is the most resource-intensive procedure.

14-4A OPERATIVE REPORT, SEPTOPLASTY, TURBINATE REDUCTION, TONSILLECTOMY

LOCATION: Inpatient, Hospital

PATIENT: Art Schear

ATTENDING PHYSICIAN: Gregory Dawson, M.D.

SURGEON: Loren White, M.D.

PREOPERATIVE DIAGNOSES:
1. Obstructive sleep apnea
2. Nasal obstruction
3. Septal deviation
4. Bilateral inferior turbinate hypertrophy
5. Hypertrophic tonsils

POSTOPERATIVE DIAGNOSES:
1. Obstructive sleep apnea
2. Nasal obstruction
3. Septal deviation
4. Bilateral inferior turbinate hypertrophy
5. Hypertrophic tonsils

PROCEDURES PERFORMED:
1. Septoplasty
2. Bilateral inferior turbinate mucosal reduction with radiofrequency
3. Tonsillectomy

ANESTHESIA: General endotracheal

INDICATION: The patient is a 16-year-old male with documented obstructive sleep apnea. He also has a prior history of severe nasal obstruction due to a traumatic injury to his nose. Examination reveals a significant septal deviation with inferior turbinate hypertrophy. He also has very hypertrophic tonsils. At this point, we will correct his nasal airway and also increase his oral airway by removing his tonsils and see if that will help his sleep apnea. If there is any residual sleep apnea, he may be treated with nasal CPAP; or if he is unable to tolerate that, further airway expansion surgery will be considered.

DESCRIPTION OF PROCEDURE: After consent was obtained, the patient was taken to the operating room and placed on the operating table in the supine position. After an adequate level of general endotracheal anesthesia was obtained, the patient was turned and draped in the appropriate manner for nasal surgery. The patient's nose was packed with cotton pledgets and soaked with 4% cocaine. After several minutes, 1% Xylocaine with 1:100,000 units of epinephrine was infiltrated into the septum bilaterally. It was also infiltrated into the inferior turbinates bilaterally. The nasal hairs were trimmed. Then, utilizing a right hemitransfixion incision, the mucoperichondrium and mucoperiosteal flaps were elevated. The deviated portion of the cartilaginous bony septum was then removed. Spurs off the maxillary crest were also removed. Hemostasis was achieved with suction cautery along the maxillary crest and then with FloSeal. Attention was then focused on the inferior turbinate. The anterior mucosa was treated with a radiofrequency needle to 500J on each side. The hemitransfixion incision was then closed with interrupted 4-0 chromic suture. A quilting suture of 4-0 plain gut was then performed. Silastic splints were then placed on both sides of the nasal septum and secured with nylon suture. The nose was then packed bilaterally with nasal packs. Packs consisted of Merocel sponge covered with a gloved finger coated with Bacitracin ointment. This was inflated with local solution. The patient was then repositioned for tonsillectomy. The McIvor mouth gag was placed allowing visualization of the tonsil. Attention was first focused on the left tonsil. The Dean retractor was placed in the superior pole, and tonsil was retracted toward the midline. Then, utilizing a harmonic scalpel at power level III, the tonsil was removed in its entirety from a superior-to-inferior direction. Hemostasis was achieved from spot suction cautery. The similar procedure was then performed on the right tonsil. The tonsillar fossa was then irrigated with saline. There was no bleeding. Tension of the mouth gag was then released. Reinspection showed no active bleeding. The anterior and posterior pillar of the superior aspect of the tonsillar fossa was then reapproximated with interrupted 3-0 chromic suture and figure-of-eight closure. Subsequent reinspection showed no active bleeding. Mouth gag was then removed. Prior to removal of mouth gag, 1% Xylocaine with 1:100,000 units of epinephrine was infiltrated into the retromolar and soft palate areas bilaterally. The patient tolerated the procedure well. There was no break in technique. The patient was extubated and taken to the post anesthesia care unit in good condition.

FLUIDS ADMINISTERED: 1800 cc of RL

ESTIMATED BLOOD LOSS: Less than 50 cc

PREOPERATIVE MEDICATION: 1g Ancef and 12 mg Decadron IV

14-4A:

ANESTHESIA CODE(S): ____________________

CASE 14-5
14-5A Operative Report, Excision of Right Carotid Body Tumor

CASE 14-5

This patient has a mild systemic disease and is 82 years old.

14-5A OPERATIVE REPORT, EXCISION OF RIGHT CAROTID BODY TUMOR

LOCATION: Inpatient, Hospital

PATIENT: Delores Janus

SURGEON: Gary Sanchez, M.D.

PREOPERATIVE DIAGNOSIS: Right carotid body tumor

POSTOPERATIVE DIAGNOSIS: Frozen section confirmed a right carotid body tumor with tortuous internal and external carotids that have been displaced by tumor mass with multiple blood vessels feeding this tumor mass, rising from the external carotid, all ligated individually. The tumor was highly vascularized.

OPERATIVE PROCEDURE: Excision of right carotid body tumor

ANESTHESIA: General endotracheal with EEG monitoring

COMPLICATIONS: Nil

NEEDLE AND SPONGE COUNTS: Needle and sponge counts appear correct. No adverse EEG changes were noted during the procedure.

ESTIMATED BLOOD LOSS: 125 cc

No drains were placed. Incision was closed.

INDICATION FOR PROCEDURE: The patient, an 82-year-old female, upon a workup for another problem, was dubiously noted on CT scan to have what looked like a carotid body tumor; subsequently, an angiogram was done to examine this further and confirmed our suspicions and also showed that the blood supply was derived mostly from the external carotid. Consent was obtained for operative intervention. The procedure, indication, risks, benefits, and alternatives have been discussed at length with the patient. She understood and wished to proceed.

OPERATIVE TECHNIQUE: The patient was brought to the operating room and placed supine on the operating room table. General endotracheal anesthesia was administered under EEG monitoring. We then proceeded to prep the neck, lower face, and upper chest with Betadine and draped off in a sterile fashion. We proceeded with proper placement of her neck, somewhat extended to provide adequate exposure. We then proceeded with her incision anterior to the sternocleidomastoid. We extended this through skin and subcutaneous tissues and the platysma muscle down to the sternocleidomastoid and then subsequently retracted the sternocleidomastoid laterally and exposed the jugular vein, which was quite large and had many tributaries. These tributaries were doubly ligated on the large ones and also retracted laterally. The common carotid was identified, dissection carried down onto the common carotid, and a vessel loop placed around the common carotid dissection and subsequently carried distally. We identified the internal and external carotids and also placed vessel loops around this. On the external carotid, we identified the superior thyroid, placed a vessel loop around this, and followed this further. Another branch of the external carotid was noted to be feeding the tumor mass between external and internal carotid, and multiple small feeding vessels were also identified. These were individually ligated. We used bipolar cautery to dissect some of the tissues off because this was very hypervascular. The tumor was well circumscribed, although it caused a lot of hypervascularity around it. We were able to dissect this off, identified and preserved the hypoglossal nerve, and identified and preserved the vagus nerve posteriorly. Also, after taking the mass out and sending it for frozen section, this confirmed that it was a carotid body tumor. We will await permanent sections. Hemostasis was good. We then irrigated. Once satisfied with this procedure, we closed the platysma muscles with running 3-0 Vicryl sutures. We closed the skin with 4-0 Vicryl subcuticular running sutures. We applied Steri-Strips and sterile dressings. The patient tolerated the procedure well without complications. On waking up in the operating room, she was able to move all extremities. She will be transferred to the surgical critical care unit for further observation and recovery.

14-5A:

ANESTHESIA CODE(S): ____________________

CASE 14-6
14-6A Operative Report, Circumcision

CASE 14-6

Sometimes one or more combinations of anesthesia types will be used during a procedure. Note that in this procedure both general anesthesia and a caudal block are used.

14-6A OPERATIVE REPORT, CIRCUMCISION

LOCATION: Outpatient, Hospital

PATIENT: Harlen Mata

SURGEON: Ira Avilla, M.D.

PREOPERATIVE DIAGNOSIS: Recurrent balanitis and phimosis

POSTOPERATIVE DIAGNOSIS: Recurrent balanitis and phimosis

PROCEDURE PERFORMED: Circumcision

PROCEDURE: The 2-year-old male child was given general mask anesthetic as well as caudal block for postoperative pain control. He was prepped and draped in the supine position, foreskin retracted, preputial adhesions broken down. Circumcision was performed using a dorsal slit technique. Hemostasis was achieved with judicious use of electrocautery and chromic ties. Prepuce was re-anastomosed to the penile skin using 5-0 chromic catgut. Vaseline gauze dressing was applied. The patient tolerated the procedure well and transferred to the recovery room in good condition.

Pathology Report Later Indicated: Benign penile tissue

14-6A:

ANESTHESIA CODE(S): ____________________

CASE 14-7

Unless stated otherwise, assume "normal, healthy patient." Assume the anesthesia service was performed personally by the anesthesiologist unless stated otherwise on the anesthesia record.

14-7A OPERATIVE REPORT, HYSTEROSCOPY, DILATATION, AND CURETTAGE

LOCATION: Outpatient, Hospital

PATIENT: Mary Moore

ATTENDING PHYSICIAN: Andy Martinez, M.D.

SURGEON: Andy Martinez, M.D.

PREOPERATIVE DIAGNOSIS: Irregular uterine bleeding

POSTOPERATIVE DIAGNOSIS: Irregular uterine bleeding

OPERATIVE PROCEDURE: Hysteroscopy and dilatation and curettage of the uterus

ANESTHESIA: General

SURGICAL INDICATIONS: This patient is a 41-year-old multiparous female who had been having irregular, abnormal, and prolonged bleeding since June of this year. Ultrasound had suggested a small myoma on the right side of her uterus.

OPERATIVE FINDINGS: The uterus was 7.5 cm deep. The cavity was symmetrical without evidence of polyps or submucous myomas.

DESCRIPTION OF PROCEDURE: After introduction of general anesthesia, the patient was placed in the dorsolithotomy position, after which the perineum and vagina were prepped and bladder straight catheterized. The patient was then draped. The cervix was grasped with a single-tooth tenaculum, and sharp endocervical curettage was done. The endocervical canal was then dilated to 7 cm with Hegar dilators. A 5.5-mm Olympus hysteroscope was introduced, and the cavity was inspected. The hysteroscope was withdrawn, and then a sharp endometrial curettage was done. Blood loss was 5-10 cc. Specimen to pathology: Endocervical and endometrial curettings. The patient tolerated the procedure well and returned to the recovery room in stable condition.

Pathology Report Later Indicated: Primary endometrial carcinoma

14-7A:

ANESTHESIA CODE(S): ______________________

CASE 14-8
14-8A Operative Report, Osteoplastic Craniotomy

CASE 14-8

This patient is in a constant threat of loss of life, and this procedure was performed under emergency circumstances that the operative report does not document.

14-8A OPERATIVE REPORT, OSTEOPLASTIC CRANIOTOMY

LOCATION: Inpatient, Hospital

PATIENT: Arlene Samuels

ATTENDING PHYSICIAN: Timothy Pleasant, M.D.

SURGEON: Timothy Pleasant, M.D.

PREOPERATIVE DIAGNOSIS: Right temporal parietal frontal brain tumor

POSTOPERATIVE DIAGNOSIS: Glioblastoma multiforme

PROCEDURE PERFORMED: Osteoplastic craniotomy with removal of tumor in temporal lobe, frontal lobe, and middle cerebral artery complex

ANESTHESIA: General

PROCEDURE: Under general anesthesia, the patient's head was prepped and draped in the usual manner. A question mark incision was made in the front of the ear up to the frontal area. The skin flap was turned down. The temporalis muscle was incised. We then did an osteoplastic craniotomy with burr holes and craniotome. The flap was turned. The dura was incised. We then made an incision into the superior temporal lobe. The plan was to resect the temporal lobe to get into the tumor and stay away from the middle cerebral complex and also to decompress on her on the frontal lobe as well because the tumor was going into the frontal lobe. I got into the tumor and sent specimen for biopsy and then began the gradual dissection. I encountered some bleeding, probably from middle cerebral artery branches. I had to take a few with silver clips, perhaps two to three. Otherwise, we left the sylvian vein intact and decompressed the area. We got into the tumor cavity and took as much visual tumor as we could. The bed was then dried. I irrigated the wound well. I placed a piece of Gelfoam over the raw surface of the brain and began closure of the dura with 3-0 Vicryl. The bone flap was replaced with two straight four-holed Wurzburg plates. Hemovac was placed, and the scalp was closed in layers utilizing 3-0 Vicryl on the galea with surgical staples on the skin. Dressing was applied. The patient was discharged to PAR.

Pathology Report Later Indicated: Glioblastoma multiforme

14-8A:

ANESTHESIA CODE(S): ______________________

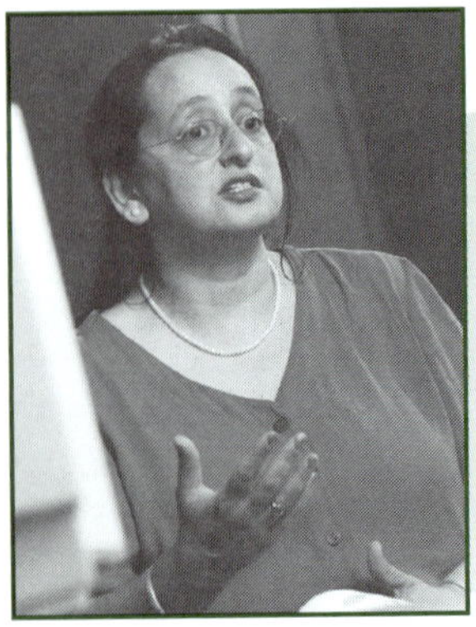

FROM THE TRENCHES

Deepa

"Learning coding doesn't mean that you are just going to sit and code...We are the educators. We are the resource people... We can work with so many different people and make a difference... That's the kind of passion I want in people once they get this knowledge. They should use that knowledge to make a difference in the healthcare industry... You can't just keep it to yourself."

CASE 14-9

A certified registered nurse anesthetist provided the anesthesia service under the supervision of an anesthesiologist who was supervising three procedures at the same time. Report the CRNA and the anesthesiologist's services.

14-9A OPERATIVE REPORT, NASOLACRIMAL DUCT PROBING

LOCATION: Outpatient, Hospital

PATIENT: Peggy Crase

ATTENDING PHYSICIAN: Rita Wimer, M.D.

SURGEON: Loren White, M.D.

PREOPERATIVE DIAGNOSIS:
1. Epiphora, both eyes
2. Nasolacrimal duct obstruction, both eyes

POSTOPERATIVE DIAGNOSIS:
1. Epiphora, both eyes
2. Nasolacrimal duct obstruction, both eyes

PROCEDURE PERFORMED: Nasolacrimal duct probing, both eyes

ANESTHESIA: General

INDICATIONS: This 32-month-old white female was referred by Dr. Peterson after an allergy workup to investigate her chronic otitis media, PE tubes times two, and the chronic epiphora that she has had in both eyes. The mother was counseled as to the success of probing at this age and the possible reoperations that may be needed.

PROCEDURE: After the patient was placed under suitable anesthesia via the mask, a small punctum dilator was used to dilate the punctum inferiorly and superiorly. These were found to be very tight and occluded. A 2-0 Bowman probe could be passed only through the inferior system with difficulty on both sides. The C-loop was not irrigatable. Probing could not be attempted because there was a large bony obstruction that resisted all efforts to pass the tube. There was no fluorescein inserted in the nose. TobraDex drops were placed in the eyes. The procedure was complete, and the patient was sent to the recovery room. The patient will be referred for further ENT consultation and to Dr. Lorabi for the possibility of a white cell deficiency that is causing these chronic infections or other immune problems. There were no complications.

14-9A:

ANESTHESIA CODE FOR CRNA: ____________________

CODE FOR ANESTHESIOLOGIST: ____________________

CASE 14-10
14-10A Operative Report, Hemithoracic Cavity Packing

CASE 14-10

The anesthesiologist was supervising a CRNA during this procedure.

14-10A OPERATIVE REPORT, HEMITHORACIC CAVITY PACKING

LOCATION: Outpatient, Hospital

PATIENT: LoriLee Putman

ATTENDING PHYSICIAN: Rita Wimer, M.D.

SURGEON: Loren White, M.D.

PREOPERATIVE DIAGNOSIS: Right empyema with bronchopleural fistula

POSTOPERATIVE DIAGNOSIS: Right empyema with bronchopleural fistula

PROCEDURE PERFORMED: Changing packing, right hemithoracic cavity

ANESTHESIA: IV sedation

PROCEDURE: The patient was brought to the operating room and sedated. The old packing was removed; the wound was examined and repacked with two vaginal packings soaked in 0.5% Flagyl solution. The patient tolerated the procedure well and was sent to recovery in satisfactory condition. Sponge count and needle count were correct.

14-10A:

ANESTHESIA CODE FOR CRNA: ____________________

CODE FOR ANESTHESIOLOGIST: ____________________

Glossary

analgesia absence of sensibility to pain.

anesthesiologist a physician who specializes in the care of a patient before, during, and after surgery, including the evaluation and preparation of a patient for anesthesia service.

anesthetist a nurse or technician trained to administer anesthetics.

conscious sedation a decreased level of consciousness in which the patient is not completely asleep.

hypotension abnormally low blood pressure.

hypothermia low body temperature; sometimes induced during surgical procedures.

physical status modifier used to indicate patient's condition at the time anesthesia was administered.

postoperative period of time after a surgical procedure.

professional component term used in describing services provided by a physician.

Qualifying Circumstances five-digit CPT codes that describe situations or conditions that make the administration of anesthesia more difficult than normal.

Appendix A
E/M Audit Form

A blank E/M audit form is included in this appendix. The coder is to photocopy the audit form for each E/M case in the worktext and for the tests that contain E/M cases. A blank form is also located on the companion web page, http://evolve.elsevier.com/Buck/next.

CHAPTER _______, CASE _______

HISTORY ELEMENTS	Documented
HISTORY OF PRESENT ILLNESS (HPI)	
1. Location (site on body)	
2. Quality (characteristic: throbbing, sharp)	
3. Severity (1/10 or how intense)	
4. Duration (how long for problem or episode)	
5. Timing (when it occurs)	
6. Context (under what circumstances does it occur)	
7. Modifying factors (what makes it better or worse)	
8. Associated signs and symptoms (what else is happening when it occurs)	
TOTAL	
LEVEL	
REVIEW OF SYSTEMS (ROS)	Documented
1. Constitutional (e.g., weight loss, fever)	
2. Ophthalmologic (eyes)	
3. Otolaryngologic (ears, nose, mouth, throat)	
4. Cardiovascular	
5. Respiratory	
6. Gastrointestinal	
7. Genitourinary	
8. Musculoskeletal	
9. Integumentary (skin and/or breasts)	
10. Neurologic	
11. Psychiatric	
12. Endocrine	
13. Hematologic/Lymphatic	
14. Allergic/Immunologic	
TOTAL	
LEVEL	
PAST, FAMILY, AND/OR SOCIAL HISTORY (PFSH)	Documented
1. Past illness, operations, injuries, treatments, and current medications	
2. Family medical history for heredity and risk	
3. Social activities, both past and present	
TOTAL	
LEVEL	

History Level	1	2	3	4
	Problem Focused	Expanded Problem Focused	Detailed	Comprehensive
HPI	Brief 1-3	Brief 1-3	Extended 4+	Extended 4+
ROS		Problem Pertinent	Extended 2-9	Complete 10+
PFSH			Pertinent 1	Complete 2-3
			HISTORY LEVEL	

EXAMINATION ELEMENTS	Documented
CONSTITUTIONAL	
1. Blood pressure, sitting	
2. Blood pressure, lying	
3. Pulse	
4. Respirations	
5. Temperature	
6. Height	
7. Weight	
8. General appearance	
NUMBER	
BODY AREAS (BA)	Documented
1. Head (including face)	
2. Neck	
3. Chest (including breasts and axillae)	
4. Abdomen	
5. Genitalia, groin, buttocks	
6. Back (including spine)	
7. Each extremity	
NUMBER	
ORGAN SYSTEMS (OS)	Documented
1. Integumentary (skin and/or breasts)	
2. Neurologic	
3. Psychiatric	
4. Endocrine	
5. Hematologic/Lymphatic	
6. Allergic/Immunologic	
7. Musculoskeletal	
8. Integumentary	
9. Neurologic	
10. Psychiatric	
11. Hematologic/Lymphatic/Immunologic	
NUMBER	
TOTAL BA/OS	

Exam Level	1	2	3	4
	Problem Focused	Expanded Problem Focused	Detailed	Comprehensive
	Limited to affected BA/OS	Limited to affected BA/OS & other related OSs	Extended of affected BA & other related OSs	General multi-system or complete single OS
# of OS or BA	1	2-7 limited	2-7 extended	8+ or 1 complete single system
			EXAMINATION LEVEL	

MDM ELEMENTS	Documented
# OF DIAGNOSIS/MANAGEMENT OPTIONS	
1. Minimal	
2. Limited	
3. Multiple	
4. Extensive	
LEVEL	
AMOUNT OR COMPLEXITY OF DATA TO REVIEW	Documented
1. Minimal/None	
2. Limited	
3. Moderate	
4. Extensive	
LEVEL	
RISK OF COMPLICATION OR DEATH IF NOT TREATED	Documented
1. Minimal	
2. Low	
3. Moderate	
4. High	
LEVEL	

MDC*	1	2	3	4
	Straightforward	Low	Moderate	High
Number of DX or management options	Minimal	Limited	Multiple	Extensive
Amount or complexity of data	Minimal/None	Limited	Moderate	Extensive
Risks	Minimal	Low	Moderate	High
			MDM LEVEL	

*To qualify for a given type of MDM complexity, 2 of 3 elements in the table must be met or exceeded.

History:

Examination:

MDM:

Number of Key Components:

Code:

Appendix B
CMS AB-01-44

Program Memorandum Intermediaries/Carriers

Transmittal AB-01-144

Department of Health
& Human Services (DHHS)
Centers for Medicare &
Medicaid Services (CMS)
Date: SEPTEMBER 26, 2001
CHANGE REQUEST 1724

SUBJECT: ICD-9-CM Coding for Diagnostic Tests

Introduction

This Program Memorandum (PM) clarifies our current coding guidelines for reporting diagnostic tests. Specifically, this PM clarifies the reporting of the International Classification of Diseases, Ninth Revision, Clinical Modification (ICD-9-CM) codes for diagnostic tests.

As required by the Health Insurance Portability and Accountability Act (HIPAA), the Secretary published a rule designating the ICD-9-CM and its *Official ICD-9-CM Guidelines for Coding and Reporting* as one of the approved code sets for use in reporting diagnoses and inpatient procedures. This final rule requires the use of ICD-9-CM and its official coding and reporting guidelines by most health plans (including Medicare) by October 16, 2002.

The *Official ICD-9-CM Guidelines for Coding and Reporting* provides guidance on coding. The ICD-9-CM Coding Guidelines for Outpatient Services, which is part of the *Official ICD-9-CM Guidelines for Coding and Reporting,* provides guidance on diagnoses coding specifically for outpatient facilities and physician offices.

The ICD-9-CM Coding Guidelines for Outpatient Services (hospital-based and physician office) have instructed physicians to report diagnoses based on test results. The Coding Clinic for ICD-9-CM confirms this longstanding coding guideline. CMS agrees with these longstanding official coding and reporting guidelines.

Following are instructions for contractors, physicians, hospitals, and other health care providers to use in determining the use of ICD-9-CM codes for coding diagnostic test results.

The instructions below provide guidance on the appropriate assignment of ICD-9-CM diagnoses codes to simplify coding for diagnostic tests consistent with the ICD-9-CM Guidelines for Outpatient Services (hospital-based and physician office). Note that physicians are responsible for the accuracy of the information submitted on a bill.

A. Determining the Appropriate Primary ICD-9-CM Diagnosis Code for Diagnostic Tests Ordered Due to Signs and/or Symptoms

1. If the physician has confirmed a diagnosis based on the results of the diagnostic test, the physician interpreting the test should code that diagnosis. The signs and/or symptoms that prompted ordering the test may be reported as additional diagnoses if they are not fully explained or related to the confirmed diagnosis.

   Example 1: A surgical specimen is sent to a pathologist with a diagnosis of "mole". The pathologist personally reviews the slides made from the specimen and makes a diagnosis of "malignant melanoma". The pathologist should report a diagnosis of "malignant melanoma" as the primary diagnosis.

   Example 2: A patient is referred to a radiologist for an abdominal CT scan with a diagnosis of abdominal pain. The CT scan reveals the presence of an abscess. The radiologist should report a diagnosis of "intra-abdominal abscess."

CMS Pub. 60AB

   Example 3: A patient is referred to a radiologist for a chest x-ray with a diagnosis of "cough". The chest x-ray reveals 3 cm peripheral pulmonary nodule. The radiologist should report a diagnosis of "pulmonary nodule" and may sequence "cough" as an additional diagnosis.

2. If the diagnostic test did not provide a diagnosis or was normal, the interpreting physician should code the sign(s) or symptom(s) that prompted the treating physician to order the study.

   Example 1: A patient is referred to a radiologist for a spine x-ray due to complaints of "back pain".

The radiologist performs the x-ray, and the results are normal. The radiologist should report a diagnosis of "back pain" since this was the reason for performing the spine x-ray.

Example 2: A patient is seen in the ER for chest pain. An EKG is normal, and the final diagnosis is chest pain due to suspected gastroesophageal reflux disease (GERD). The patient was told to follow-up with his primary care physician for further evaluation of the suspected GERD. The primary diagnosis code for the EKG should be chest pain. Although the EKG was normal, a definitive cause for the chest pain was not determined.

3. If the results of the diagnostic test are normal or non-diagnostic, and the referring physician records a diagnosis preceded by words that indicate uncertainty (e.g., probable, suspected, questionable, rule out, or working), then the interpreting physician should not code the referring diagnosis. Rather, the interpreting physician should report the sign(s) or symptom(s) that prompted the study. Diagnoses labeled as uncertain are considered by the ICD-9-CM Coding Guidelines as unconfirmed and should not be reported. This is consistent with the requirement to code the diagnosis to the highest degree of certainty.

   Example: A patient is referred to a radiologist for a chest x-ray with a diagnosis of "rule out pneumonia." The radiologist performs a chest x-ray, and the results are normal. The radiologist should report the sign(s) or symptom(s) that prompted the test (e.g., cough).

B. Instruction to Determine the Reason for the Test

As specified in § 4317(b) of the Balanced Budget Act (BBA), referring physicians are required to provide diagnostic information to the testing entity at the time the test is ordered. As further indicated in 42 CFR 410.32 all diagnostic tests "must be ordered by the physician who is treating the beneficiary." As defined in § 15021 of the Medicare Carrier Manual (MCM), an "order" is a communication from the treating physician/practitioner requesting that a diagnostic test be performed for a beneficiary. An order may include the following forms of communication:

a. A written document signed by the treating physician/practitioner, which is hand-delivered, mailed, or faxed to the testing facility;
b. A telephone call by the treating physician/practitioner or his/her office to the testing facility; and
c. An electronic mail by the treating physician/practitioner or his/her office to the testing facility.

NOTE: If the order is communicated via telephone, both the treating physician/practitioner or his/her office and the testing facility must document the telephone call in their respective copies of the beneficiary's medical records.

On the rare occasion when the interpreting physician does not have diagnostic information as to the reason for the test and the referring physician is unavailable to provide such information, it is appropriate to obtain the information directly from the patient or the patient's medical record if it is available. However, an attempt should be made to confirm any information obtained from the patient by contacting the referring physician.

Example: A patient is referred to a radiologist for a gastrografin enema to rule out appendicitis. However, the referring physician does not provide the reason for the referral and is unavailable at the time of the study. The patient is queried and indicates that he/she saw the physician for abdominal pain, and was referred to rule out appendicitis. The radiologist performs the x-ray, and the results are normal. The radiologist should report the abdominal pain as the primary diagnosis.

C. Incidental Findings

Incidental findings should never be listed as primary diagnoses. If reported, incidental findings may be reported as secondary diagnoses by the physician interpreting the diagnostic test.

Example 1: A patient is referred to a radiologist for an abdominal ultrasound due to jaundice. After review of the ultrasound, the interpreting physician discovers that the patient has an aortic aneurysm. The interpreting physician reports jaundice as the primary diagnosis and may report the aortic aneurysm as a secondary diagnosis because it is an incidental finding.

Example 2: A patient is referred to a radiologist for a chest x-ray because of wheezing. The x-ray is normal except for scoliosis and degenerative joint disease of the thoracic spine. The interpreting physician reports wheezing as the primary diagnosis since it was the reason for the patient's visit, and may report the other findings (scoliosis and degenerative joint disease of the thoracic spine) as additional diagnoses.

Example 3: A patient is referred to a radiologist for a magnetic resonance imaging (MRI) of the lumbar spine with a diagnosis of L-4 radiculopathy. The MRI reveals degenerative joint disease at L1 and L2. The radiologist reports radiculopathy as the primary diagnosis and may report degenerative joint disease of the spine as an additional diagnosis.

D. Unrelated/Co-Existing Conditions/Diagnoses

Unrelated and co-existing conditions/diagnoses may be reported as additional diagnoses by the physician interpreting the diagnostic test.

Example: A patient is referred to a radiologist for a chest x-ray because of a cough. The result of the chest x-ray indicates the patient has pneumonia. During the performance of the diagnostic test, it was determined that the patient has hypertension and diabetes mellitus. The interpreting physician reports a primary diagnosis of pneumonia. The interpreting physician may report the hypertension and diabetes mellitus as secondary diagnoses.

E. Diagnostic Tests Ordered in the Absence of Signs and/or Symptoms (e.g., screening tests)

When a diagnostic test is ordered in the absence of signs/symptoms or other evidence of illness or injury, the physician interpreting the diagnostic test should report the reason for the test (e.g., screening) as the primary ICD-9-CM diagnosis code. The results of the test, if reported, may be recorded as additional diagnoses.

F. Use of ICD-9-CM to the Greatest Degree of Accuracy and Completeness

NOTE: This section explains certain coding guidelines that address diagnoses coding. These guidelines are long-standing coding guidelines that have been part of the *Official ICD-9-CM Guidelines for Coding and Reporting.*

The interpreting physician should code the ICD-9-CM code that provides the highest degree of accuracy and completeness for the diagnosis resulting from the test, or for the sign(s)/symptom(s) that prompted the ordering of the test.

In the past, there has been some confusion about the meaning of "highest degree of specificity," and in "reporting the correct number of digits." In the context of ICD-9-CM coding, the "highest degree of specificity" refers to assigning the most precise ICD-9-CM code that most fully explains the narrative description of the symptom or diagnosis.

Example 1: A chest x-ray reveals a primary lung cancer in the left lower lobe. The interpreting physician should report the ICD-9-CM code as 162.5 for malignancy of the left "lower lobe, bronchus or lung", not the code for a malignancy of "other parts of bronchus or lung" (162.8) or the code for "bronchus and lung unspecified" (162.9).

Example 2: If a sputum specimen is sent to a pathologist and the pathologist confirms growth of "streptococcus, type B," which is indicated in the patient's medical record, the pathologist should report a primary diagnosis as 482.32 (Pneumonia due to streptococcus, Group B). However, if the pathologist is unable to specify the organism, then the pathologist should report the primary diagnosis as 486 (Pneumonia, organism unspecified).

In order to report the correct number of digits when using ICD-9-CM, refer to the following instructions:

ICD-9-CM diagnosis codes are composed of codes with 3, 4, or 5 digits. Codes with 3 digits are included in ICD-9-CM as the heading of a category of codes that may be further subdivided by the use of fourth and/or fifth digits to provide greater specificity. Assign three-digit codes only if there are no four-digit codes within that code category. Assign four-digit codes only if there is no fifth-digit subclassification for that category. Assign the fifth-digit subclassification code for those categories where it exists.

Example 3: A patient is referred to a physician with a diagnosis of diabetes mellitus. However, there is no indication that the patient has diabetic complications or that the diabetes is out of control. It would be incorrect to assign code 250 since all codes in this series have 5 digits. Reporting only three digits of a code that has 5 digits would be incorrect. One must add two more digits to make it complete. Because the type (adult onset/juvenile) of diabetes is not specified, and there is no indication that the patient has a complication or that the diabetes is out of control, the correct ICD-9-CM code would be 250.00. The fourth and fifth digits of the code would vary depending on the specific condition of the patient. One should be guided by the code book.

For the latest ICD-9-CM coding guidelines, please refer to the following website: http://www.cdc.gov/nchs/datawh/ftpserv/ftpicd9/ftpicd9.htm#guide.

Refer to the attachment for further guidance on determining the appropriate ICD-9-CM diagnoses codes. The attachment is a listing of questions and answers that appeared in the American Hospital Association's (AHA) Coding Clinic for ICD-9-CM (1st Qtr 2000).

NOTE: Contractors are advised to make this PM available to physicians and other health care professionals. If available, immediately place this PM on your website. This PM should be distributed with your next regularly scheduled bulletin.

Attachment

The *effective date* for this PM is January 1, 2002.
The *implementation date* for this PM is January 1, 2002.
These instructions should be implemented within your current operating budget.
This PM may be discarded after January 1, 2003.
If you have any questions, contact your regional office.

Appendix C

ICD-9-CM Official Guidelines for Coding and Reporting

Effective October 1, 2002

The Centers for Medicare and Medicaid Services (CMS) formerly the Health Care Financing Administration (HCFA) and the National Center for Health Statistics (NCHS), two departments within the Department of Health and Human Services (DHHS), present the following guidelines for coding and reporting using the International Classification of Diseases, 9th Revision, Clinical Modification (ICD-9-CM). These guidelines should be used as a companion document to the official version of the ICD-9-CM as published on CD-ROM.

These guidelines for coding and reporting have been developed and approved by the Cooperating Parties for ICD-9-CM: the American Hospital Association, the American Health Information Management Association, CMS, and the NCHS. These guidelines, published by the Department of Health and Human Services, have also appeared in the Coding Clinic for ICD-9-CM, published by the American Hospital Association.

These guidelines have been developed to assist the user in coding and reporting in situations where the ICD-9-CM does not provide direction. Coding and sequencing instructions in volumes I, II, and III of ICD-9-CM take precedence over any guidelines. The conventions, general guidelines and chapter-specific guidelines apply to the proper use of ICD-9-CM, regardless of the health care setting. A joint effort between the attending physician and coder is essential to achieve complete and accurate documentation, code assignment, and reporting of diagnoses and procedures. These guidelines have been developed and approved by the Cooperating Parties to assist both the physician and the coder in identifying those diagnoses that are to be reported. The importance of consistent, complete documentation in the medical record cannot be overemphasized. Without such documentation the application of all coding guidelines is a difficult, if not impossible, task.

These guidelines are not exhaustive. The cooperating parties are continuing to conduct reviews of these guidelines and develop new guidelines as needed. Users of the ICD-9-CM should be aware that only guidelines approved by the cooperating parties are official. Revision of these guidelines and new guidelines will be published by the U.S. Department of Health and Human Services when they are approved by the cooperating parties. The term "admitted" is used generally to mean a health care encounter in any setting.

The guidelines have been reorganized into several new sections including an enhanced introduction that provides more detail about the structure and conventions of the classification usually found in the classification itself. The other new section, General Guidelines, brings together overarching guidelines that were previously found throughout the various sections of the guidelines. The new format of the guidelines also includes a resequencing of the disease-specific guidelines. They are sequenced in the same order as they appear in the tabular list chapters (Infectious and Parasitic diseases, Neoplasms, etc.).

These changes will make it easier for coders, experienced and beginners, to more easily find the specific portion of the coding guideline information they seek.

Table of Contents

Section I Conventions, General Coding Guidelines and Chapter-Specific Guidelines

The conventions, general guidelines and chapter-specific guidelines are applicable to all health care settings unless otherwise indicated.

A. Conventions for the ICD-9-CM

The conventions for the ICD-9-CM are the general rules for use of the classification independent of the guidelines. These conventions are incorporated within the index and tabular of the ICD-9-CM as instructional notes. The conventions are as follows:

1. Format: The ICD-9-CM uses an indented format for ease in reference
2. Abbreviations
   a. Index Abbreviations
      NEC "Not elsewhere classifiable"
      This abbreviation in the index represents "other specified". When a specific code is not available for a condition the index directs the coder to the "other specified" code in the tabular.
   b. Tabular Abbreviations
      NEC "Not elsewhere classifiable"
      This abbreviation in the tabular represents "other specified". When a specific code is not available for a condition the tabular includes an NEC entry under a code to identify the code as the "other specified" code. (see "Other" codes)
      NOS "Not otherwise specified" This abbreviation is the equivalent of unspecified. (see "Unspecified" codes)
3. Punctuation
   [ ] Brackets are used in the tabular list to enclose synonyms, alternative wording or explanatory phrases. Brackets are used in the index to identify manifestation codes. (see etiology/manifestations)

( ) Parentheses are used in both the index and tabular to enclose supplementary words which may be present or absent in the statement of a disease or procedure without affecting the code number to which it is assigned. The terms within the parentheses are referred to as nonessential modifiers.

: Colons are used in the Tabular list after an incomplete term which needs one or more of the modifiers following the colon to make it assignable to a given category.

4. Includes and Excludes Notes and Inclusion terms

Includes: This note appears immediately under a three-digit code title to further define, or give examples of, the content of the category.

Excludes: An excludes note under a code indicates that the terms excluded from the code are to be coded elsewhere. In some cases the codes for the excluded terms should not be used in conjunction with the code from which it is excluded. An example of this is a congenital condition excluded from an acquired form of the same condition. The congenital and acquired codes should not be used together. In other cases, the excluded terms may be used together with an excluded code. An example of this is when fractures of different bones are coded to different codes. Both codes may be used together if both types of fractures are present.

Inclusion terms: List of terms are included under certain four and five digit codes. These terms are the conditions for which that code number is to be used. The terms may be synonyms of the code title, or, in the case of "other specified" codes, the terms are a list of the various conditions assigned to that code. The inclusion terms are not necessarily exhaustive. Additional terms found only in the index may also be assigned to a code.

5. Other and Unspecified codes

a. "Other" codes

Codes titled "other" or "other specified" (usually a code with a 4th digit 8 or fifth-digit 9 for diagnosis codes) are for use when the information in the medical record provides detail for which a specific code does not exist. Index entries with NEC in the line designate "other" codes in the tabular. These index entries represent specific disease entities for which no specific code exists so the term is included within an "other" code.

b. "Unspecified" codes

Codes (usually a code with a 4th digit 9 or 5th digit 0 for diagnosis codes) titled "unspecified" are for use when the information in the medical record is insufficient to assign a more specific code.

6. Etiology/manifestation convention ("code first", "use additional code" and "in diseases classified elsewhere" notes)

Certain conditions have both an underlying etiology and multiple body system manifestations due to the underlying etiology. For such conditions the ICD-9-CM has a coding convention that requires the underlying condition be sequenced first followed by the manifestation. Wherever such a combination exists there is a "use additional code" note at the etiology code, and a "code first" note at the manifestation code. These instructional notes indicate the proper sequencing order of the codes, etiology followed by manifestation.

In most cases the manifestation codes will have in the code title, "in diseases classified elsewhere." Codes with this title are a component of the etiology/manifestation convention. The code title indicates that it is a manifestation code. "In diseases classified elsewhere" codes are never permitted to be used as first listed or principal diagnosis codes. They must be used in conjunction with an underlying condition code and they must be listed following the underlying condition.

There are manifestation codes that do not have "in diseases classified elsewhere" in the title. For such codes a "use additional code" note will still be present and the rules for sequencing apply.

In addition to the notes in the tabular, these conditions also have a specific index entry structure. In the index both conditions are listed together with the etiology code first followed by the manifestation codes in brackets. The code in brackets is always to be sequenced second.

The most commonly used etiology/manifestation combinations are the codes for Diabetes mellitus, category 250. For each code under category 250 there is a use additional code note for the manifestation that is specific for that particular diabetic manifestation. Should a patient have more than one manifestation of diabetes more than one code from category

250 may be used with as many manifestation codes as are needed to fully describe the patient's complete diabetic condition. The 250 diabetes codes should be sequenced first, followed by the manifestation codes.

"Code first" and "Use additional code" notes are also used as sequencing rules in the classification for certain codes that are not part of an etiology/manifestation combination. See—Other multiple coding for a single condition in the General Guidelines section.

B. General Coding Guidelines

1. Use of Both Alphabetic Index and Tabular List
   Use both the Alphabetic Index and the Tabular List when locating and assigning a code. Reliance on only the Alphabetic Index or the Tabular List leads to errors in code assignments and less specificity in code selection.
2. Locate each term in the Alphabetic Index and verify the code selected in the Tabular List. Read and be guided by instructional notations that appear in both the Alphabetic Index and the Tabular List.
3. Level of Detail in Coding
   Diagnosis and procedure codes are to be used at their highest number of digits available.

   ICD-9-CM diagnosis codes are composed of codes with 3, 4, or 5 digits. Codes with three digits are included in ICD-9-CM as the heading of a category of codes that may be further subdivided by the use of fourth and/or fifth digits, which provide greater detail.

   A three-digit code is to be used only if it is not further subdivided. Where fourth-digit subcategories and/or fifth-digit subclassifications are provided, they must be assigned. A code is invalid if it has not been coded to the full number of digits required for that code. For example, Acute myocardial infarction, code 410, has fourth digits that describe the location of the infarction (e.g., 410.2, Of inferolateral wall), and fifth digits that identify the episode of care. It would be incorrect to report a code in category 410 without a fourth and fifth digit.

   ICD-9-CM Volume 3 procedure codes are composed of codes with either 3 or 4 digits. Codes with two digits are included in ICD-9-CM as the heading of a category of codes that may be further subdivided by the use of third and/or fourth digits, which provide greater detail.
4. The appropriate code or codes from 001.0 through V83.89 must be used to identify diagnoses, symptoms, conditions, problems, complaints or other reason(s) for the encounter/visit.
5. The selection of codes 001.0 through 999.9 will frequently be used to describe the reason for the admission/encounter. These codes are from the section of ICD-9-CM for the classification of diseases and injuries (e.g., infectious and parasitic diseases; neoplasms; symptoms, signs, and ill-defined conditions, etc.).
6. Codes that describe symptoms and signs, as opposed to diagnoses, are acceptable for reporting purposes when a related definitive diagnosis has not been established (confirmed) by the physician. Chapter 16 of ICD-9-CM, Symptoms, Signs, and Ill-defined conditions (codes 780.0-799.9) contain many, but not all codes for symptoms.
7. Conditions that are an integral part of a disease process
   Signs and symptoms that are integral to the disease process should not be assigned as additional codes.
8. Conditions that are not an integral part of a disease process
   Additional signs and symptoms that may not be associated routinely with a disease process should be coded when present.
9. Multiple coding for a single condition
   In addition to the etiology/manifestation convention that requires two codes to fully describe a single condition that affects multiple body systems, there are other single conditions that also require more than one code. "Use additional code" notes are found in the tabular at codes that are not part of an etiology/manifestation pair where a secondary code is useful to fully describe a condition. The sequencing rule is the same, "use additional code" indicates that a secondary code should be added.

   For example, for infections that are not included in chapter 1, a secondary code from category 041, Bacterial infection in conditions classified elsewhere and of unspecified site, may be required to identify the bacterial organism causing the infection. A "use additional code" note will normally be found at the infection code indicates a need for the organism code to be added as a secondary code.

   "Code first" notes are also under certain codes that are not specifically manifestation codes but may be due to an underlying cause. When a "code first" note is present and an underlying condition is present the underlying condition should be sequenced first.

   "Code, if applicable, any causal condition first", notes indicate that this code may be assigned as a principal diagnosis when the causal condition is unknown or not applicable. If a causal condition is known, then the code for that condition should be sequenced as the principal or first-listed diagnosis.

Multiple codes may be needed for late effects, complication codes and obstetric codes to more fully describe a condition. See the specific guidelines for these conditions for further instruction.

10. Acute and Chronic Conditions

If the same condition is described as both acute (subacute) and chronic, and separate subentries exist in the Alphabetic Index at the same indentation level, code both and sequence the acute (subacute) code first.

11. Combination Code

A combination code is a single code used to classify: two diagnoses, or

A diagnosis with an associated secondary process (manifestation) A diagnosis with an associated complication.

Combination codes are identified by referring to subterm entries in the Alphabetic Index and by reading the inclusion and exclusion notes in the Tabular List.

Assign only the combination code when that code fully identifies the diagnostic conditions involved or when the Alphabetic Index so directs. Multiple coding should not be used when the classification provides a combination code that clearly identifies all of the elements documented in the diagnosis. When the combination code lacks necessary specificity in describing the manifestation or complication, an additional code may be used as a secondary code.

12. Late Effects

A late effect is the residual effect (condition produced) after the acute phase of an illness or injury has terminated. There is no time limit on when a late effect code can be used. The residual may be apparent early, such as in cerebrovascular accident cases, or it may occur months or years later, such as that due to a previous injury. Coding of late effects generally requires two codes sequenced in the following order: The condition or nature of the late effect is sequenced first. The late effect code is sequenced second.

An exception to the above guidelines are those instances where the code for late effect is followed by a manifestation code identified in the Tabular List and title, or the late effect code has been expanded (at the fourth and fifth-digit levels) to include the manifestation(s). The code for the acute phase of an illness or injury that led to the late effect is never used with a code for the late effect.

13. Impending or Threatened Condition

Code any condition described at the time of discharge as "impending" or "threatened" as follows:

If it did occur, code as confirmed diagnosis.

If it did not occur, reference the Alphabetic Index to determine if the condition has a subentry term for "impending" or "threatened" and also reference main term entries for "Impending" and for "Threatened."

If the subterms are listed, assign the given code.

If the subterms are not listed, code the existing underlying condition(s) and not the condition described as impending or threatened.

C. Chapter-Specific Coding Guidelines

In addition to general coding guidelines, there are guidelines for specific diagnoses and/or conditions in the classification. Unless otherwise indicated, these guidelines apply to all health care settings.

C1. Infectious and Parasitic Diseases

A. Human Immunodeficiency Virus (HIV) Infections

1. Code only confirmed cases of HIV infection/illness. This is an exception to the hospital inpatient guideline Section II, H.

In this context, "confirmation" does not require documentation of positive serology or culture for HIV; the physician's diagnostic statement that the patient is HIV positive, or has an HIV-related illness is sufficient.

2. Selection and sequencing

a. If a patient is admitted for an HIV-related condition, the principal diagnosis should be 042, followed by additional diagnosis codes for all reported HIV-related conditions.

b. If a patient with HIV disease is admitted for an unrelated condition (such as a traumatic injury), the code for the unrelated condition (e.g., the nature of injury code) should be the principal diagnosis. Other diagnoses would be 042 followed by additional diagnosis codes for all reported HIV-related conditions.

c. Whether the patient is newly diagnosed or has had previous admissions/encounters for HIV conditions is irrelevant to the sequencing decision.

d. V08 Asymptomatic human immunodeficiency virus [HIV] infection, is to be applied when the patient without any documentation of symptoms is listed as being

"HIV positive," "known HIV," "HIV test positive," or similar terminology. Do not use this code if the term "AIDS" is used or if the patient is treated for any HIV-related illness or is described as having any condition(s) resulting from his/her HIV positive status; use 042 in these cases.

e. Patients with inconclusive HIV serology, but no definitive diagnosis or manifestations of the illness, may be assigned code 795.71, Inconclusive serologic test for Human Immunodeficiency Virus [HIV].

f. Previously diagnosed HIV-related illness
Patients with any known prior diagnosis of an HIV-related illness should be coded to 042. Once a patient had developed an HIV-related illness, the patient should always be assigned code 042 on every subsequent admission/encounter. Patients previously diagnosed with any HIV illness (042) should never be assigned to 795.71 or V08.

g. HIV Infection in Pregnancy, Childbirth and the Puerperium
During pregnancy, childbirth or the puerperium, a patient admitted (or presenting for a health care encounter) because of an HIV-related illness should receive a principal diagnosis of 647.6X, Other specified infectious and parasitic diseases in the mother classifiable elsewhere, but complicating the pregnancy, childbirth or the puerperium, followed by 042 and the code(s) for the HIV-related illness(es). Codes from Chapter 15 always take sequencing priority.
Patients with asymptomatic HIV infection status admitted (or presenting for a health care encounter) during pregnancy, childbirth, or the puerperium should receive codes of 647.6X and V08.

h. Encounters for Testing for HIV
If a patient is being seen to determine his/her HIV status, use code V73.89, Screening for other specified viral disease. Use code V69.8, Other problems related to lifestyle, as a secondary code if an asymptomatic patient is in a known high risk group for HIV. Should a patient with signs or symptoms or illness, or a confirmed HIV related diagnosis be tested for HIV, code the signs and symptoms or the diagnosis. An additional counseling code V65.44 may be used if counseling is provided during the encounter for the test.
When a patient returns to be informed of his/her HIV test results use code V65.44, HIV counseling, if the results of the test are negative.
If the results are positive but the patient is asymptomatic use code V08, Asymptomatic HIV infection. If the results are positive and the patient is symptomatic use code 042, HIV infection, with codes for the HIV related symptoms or diagnosis. The HIV counseling code may also be used if counseling is provided for patients with positive test results.

B. Septicemia and Septic Shock

1. When the diagnosis of septicemia with shock or the diagnosis of general sepsis with septic shock is documented, code and list the septicemia first and report the septic shock code as a secondary condition. The septicemia code assignment should identify the type of bacteria if it is known.
2. Sepsis and septic shock associated with abortion, ectopic pregnancy, and molar pregnancy are classified to category codes in Chapter 11 (630-639).
3. Negative or inconclusive blood cultures do not preclude a diagnosis of septicemia in patients with clinical evidence of the condition.

C2. Neoplasms

Chapter 2 of the ICD-9-CM contains the code for most benign and all malignant neoplasms. Certain benign neoplasms, such as prostatic adenomas, may be found in the specific body system chapters. To properly code a neoplasm it is necessary to determine from the record if the neoplasm is benign, in-situ, malignant, or of uncertain histologic behavior. If malignant, any secondary (metastatic) sites should also be determined.

The neoplasm table in the Alphabetic Index should be referenced first. If the histological term is documented, that term should be referenced first, rather than going immediately to the Neoplasm Table, in order to determine which column in the Neoplasm Table is appropriate. For example, if the documentation indicates "adenoma," refer to the term in the Alphabetic Index to review the entries under this term and the instructional note to "see also neoplasm, by site, benign." The table provides the proper code based on the type of neoplasm and the site. It is important to select the proper column in the table that corresponds to the type of neoplasm. The tabular should then be referenced to verify that the correct code has been selected from the table and that a more specific site code does not exist.

A. If the treatment is directed at the malignancy, designate the malignancy as the principal diagnosis.
B. When a patient is admitted because of a primary neoplasm with metastasis and treatment is directed toward the secondary site only, the secondary neoplasm is designated as the principal diagnosis even though the primary malignancy is still present.
C. Coding and sequencing of complications associated with the malignant neoplasm or with the therapy thereof are subject to the following guidelines:
   1. When admission/encounter is for management of an anemia associated with the malignancy, and the treatment is only for anemia, the anemia is designated at the principal diagnosis and is followed by the appropriate code(s) for the malignancy.
   2. When the admission/encounter is for management of an anemia associated with chemotherapy or radiotherapy and the only treatment is for the anemia, the anemia is sequenced first followed by the appropriate code(s) for the malignancy.
   3. When the admission/encounter is for management of dehydration due to the malignancy or the therapy, or a combination of both, and only the dehydration is being treated (intravenous rehydration), the dehydration is sequenced first, followed by the code(s) for the malignancy.
   4. When the admission/encounter is for treatment of a complication resulting from a surgical procedure performed for the treatment of an intestinal malignancy, designate the complication as the principal or first-listed diagnosis if treatment is directed at resolving the complication.
D. When a primary malignancy has been previously excised or eradicated from its site and there is no further treatment directed to that site and there is no evidence of any existing primary malignancy, a code from category V10, Personal history of malignant neoplasm, should be used to indicate the former site of the malignancy. Any mention of extension, invasion, or metastasis to another site is coded as a secondary malignant neoplasm to that site. The secondary site may be the principal or first-listed with the V10 code used as a secondary code.
E. Admissions/Encounters involving chemotherapy and radiation therapy
   1. When an episode of care involves the surgical removal of a neoplasm, primary or secondary site, followed by chemotherapy or radiation treatment, the neoplasm code should be assigned as principal or first-listed diagnosis. When an episode of inpatient care involves surgical removal of a primary site or secondary site malignancy followed by adjunct chemotherapy or radiotherapy, code the malignancy as the principal or first-listed diagnosis, using codes in the 140-198 series or where appropriate in the 200-203 series.
   2. If a patient admission/encounter is solely for the administration of chemotherapy or radiation therapy code V58.0, Encounter for radiation therapy, or V58.1, Encounter for chemotherapy, should be the first-listed or principal diagnosis. If a patient receives both chemotherapy and radiation therapy both codes should be listed, in either order of sequence.
   3. When a patient is admitted for the purpose of radiotherapy or chemotherapy and develops complications such as uncontrolled nausea and vomiting or dehydration, the principal or first-listed diagnosis is V58.0, Encounter for radiotherapy, or V58.1, Encounter for chemotherapy.
F. When the reason for admission/encounter is to determine the extent of the malignancy, or for a procedure such as paracentesis or thoracentesis, the primary malignancy or appropriate metastatic site is designated as the principal or first-listed diagnosis, even though chemotherapy or radiotherapy is administered.
G. Symptoms, signs, and ill-defined conditions listed in Chapter 16 characteristic of, or associated with, an existing primary or secondary site malignancy cannot be used to replace

the malignancy as principal or first-listed diagnosis, regardless of the number of admissions or encounters for treatment and care of the neoplasm.

C3. Endocrine, Nutritional, and Metabolic Diseases and Immunity Disorders
Reserved for future guideline expansion

C4. Diseases of Blood and Blood Forming Organs
Reserved for future guideline expansion

C5. Mental Disorders
Reserved for future guideline expansion

C6. Diseases of Nervous System and Sense Organs
Reserved for future guideline expansion

C7. Diseases of Circulatory System

A. Hypertension

The Hypertension Table, found under the main term, "Hypertension", in the Alphabetic Index, contains a complete listing of all conditions due to or associated with hypertension and classifies them according to malignant, benign, and unspecified.

1. Hypertension, Essential, or NOS Assign hypertension (arterial) (essential) (primary) (systemic) (NOS) to category code 401 with the appropriate fourth digit to indicate malignant (.0), benign (.1), or unspecified (.9). Do not use either .0 malignant or .1 benign unless medical record documentation supports such a designation.

2. Hypertension with Heart Disease
Heart conditions (425.8, 429.0-429.3, 429.8, 429.9) are assigned to a code from category 402 when a causal relationship is stated (due to hypertension) or implied (hypertensive). Use an additional code from category 428 to identify the type of heart failure in those patients with heart failure. More than one code from category 428 may be assigned if the patient has systolic or diastolic failure and congestive heart failure.

The same heart conditions (425.8, 428, 429.0-429.3, 429.8, 429.9) with hypertension, but without a stated causal relationship, are coded separately. Sequence according to the circumstances of the admission/encounter.

3. Hypertensive Renal Disease with Chronic Renal Failure
Assign codes from category 403, Hypertensive renal disease, when conditions classified to categories 585-587 are present. Unlike hypertension with heart disease, ICD-9-CM presumes a cause-and-effect relationship and classifies renal failure with hypertension as hypertensive renal disease.

4. Hypertensive Heart and Renal Disease
Assign codes from combination category 404, Hypertensive heart and renal disease, when both hypertensive renal disease and hypertensive heart disease are stated in the diagnosis. Assume a relationship between the hypertension and the renal disease, whether or not the condition is so designated. Assign an additional code from category 428, to identify the type of heart failure. More than one code from category 428 may be assigned if the patient has systolic or diastolic failure and congestive heart failure.

5. Hypertensive Cerebrovascular Disease
First assign codes from 430-438, Cerebrovascular disease, then the appropriate hypertension code from categories 401-405.

6. Hypertensive Retinopathy
Two codes are necessary to identify the condition. First assign the code from subcategory 362.11, Hypertensive retinopathy, then the appropriate code from categories 40-05 to indicate the type of hypertension.

7. Hypertension, Secondary
Two codes are required: one to identify the underlying etiology and one from category 405 to identify the hypertension. Sequencing of codes is determined by the reason for admission/encounter.

8. Hypertension, Transient
Assign code 796.2, Elevated blood pressure reading without diagnosis of hypertension, unless patient has an established diagnosis of hypertension. Assign code 642.3x for transient hypertension of pregnancy.

9. Hypertension, Controlled
Assign appropriate code from categories 401-405. This diagnostic statement usually refers to an existing state of hypertension under control by therapy.

10. Hypertension, Uncontrolled
Uncontrolled hypertension may refer to untreated hypertension or hypertension not responding to current therapeutic regimen. In either case, assign the appropriate code from categories 401-405 to designate the stage and type of hypertension. Code to the type of hypertension.

11. Elevated Blood Pressure
    For a statement of elevated blood pressure without further specificity, assign code 796.2, Elevated blood pressure reading without diagnosis of hypertension, rather than a code from category 401.

B. Late Effects of Cerebrovascular Disease
   Category 438 is used to indicate conditions classifiable to categories 430-437 as the causes of late effects (neurologic deficits), themselves classified elsewhere. These "late effects" include neurologic deficits that persist after initial onset of conditions classifiable to 430-437. The neurologic deficits caused by cerebrovascular disease may be present from the onset or may arise at any time after the onset of the condition classifiable to 430-437.

   Codes from category 438 may be assigned on a health care record with codes from 430-437, if the patient has a current cerebrovascular accident (CVA) and deficits from an old CVA. Assign code V12.59 (and not a code from category 438) as an additional code for history of cerebrovascular disease when no neurologic deficits are present.

C8. Diseases of Respiratory System
    Reserved for future guideline expansion

C9. Diseases of Digestive System
    Reserved for future guideline expansion

C10. Diseases of Genitourinary System
     Reserved for future guideline expansion

C11. Complications of Pregnancy, Childbirth, and the Puerperium

A. General Rules for Obstetric Cases

1. Obstetric cases require codes from chapter 11, codes in the range 630-677, Complications of Pregnancy, Childbirth, and the Puerperium. Should the physician document that the pregnancy is incidental to the encounter, then code V22.2 should be used in place of any chapter 11 codes. It is the physician's responsibility to state that the condition being treated is not affecting the pregnancy.
2. Chapter 11 codes have sequencing priority over codes from other chapters. Additional codes from other chapters may be used in conjunction with chapter 11 codes to further specify conditions. For example, sepsis and septic shock associated with abortion, ectopic pregnancy, and molar pregnancy are classified to category codes in Chapter 11 (630-639).
3. Chapter 11 codes are to be used only on the maternal record, never on the record of the newborn.
4. Categories 640-648, 651-676 have required fifth-digits, which indicate whether the encounter is antepartum, postpartum and whether a delivery has also occurred.
5. The fifth-digits, which are appropriate for each code number, are listed in brackets under each code. The fifth-digits on each code should all be consistent with each other. That is, should a delivery occur all of the fifth-digits should indicate the delivery.
6. For prenatal outpatient visits for patients with high-risk pregnancies, a code from category V23, Supervision of high-risk pregnancy, should be used as the principal or first-listed diagnosis. Secondary chapter 11 codes may be used in conjunction with these codes if appropriate. A thorough review of any pertinent excludes note is necessary to be certain that these V codes are being used properly.
7. An outcome of delivery code, V27.0-V27.9, should be included on every maternal record when a delivery has occurred. These codes are not to be used on subsequent records or on the newborn record.
8. For routine outpatient prenatal visits when no complications are present codes V22.0, Supervision of normal first pregnancy, and V22.1, Supervision of other normal pregnancy, should be used as the first-listed diagnoses. These codes should not be used in conjunction with chapter 11 codes.

B. Selection of OB Principal or First-listed Diagnosis

1. In episodes when no delivery occurs, the principal diagnosis should correspond to the principal complication of the pregnancy, which necessitated the encounter. Should more than one complication exist, all of which are treated or monitored, any of the complications codes may be sequenced first.
2. When a delivery occurs, the principal diagnosis should correspond to the main circumstances or complication of the delivery.
   In cases of cesarean delivery, the selection of the principal diagnosis should correspond to the reason the cesarean delivery was performed unless the reason for admission/encounter was unrelated to the condition resulting in the cesarean delivery.

C. Fetal Conditions Affecting the Management of the Mother
Codes from category 655, Known or suspected fetal abnormality affecting management of the mother, and category 656, Other fetal and placental problems affecting the management of the mother, are assigned only when the fetal condition is actually responsible for modifying the management of the mother, i.e., by requiring diagnostic studies, additional observation, special care, or termination of pregnancy. The fact that the fetal condition exists does not justify assigning a code from this series to the mother's record.

D. HIV Infection in Pregnancy, Childbirth and the Puerperium
During pregnancy, childbirth or the puerperium, a patient admitted because of an HIV-related illness should receive a principal diagnosis of 647.6X, Other specified infectious and parasitic diseases in the mother classifiable elsewhere, but complicating the pregnancy, childbirth or the puerperium, followed by 042 and the code(s) for the HIV-related illness(es). This is an exception to the sequencing rule found in above.

Patients with asymptomatic HIV infection status admitted during pregnancy, childbirth, or the puerperium should receive codes of 647.6X and V08.

E. Normal Delivery, 650
1. Code 650 is for use in cases when a woman is admitted for a full-term normal delivery and delivers a single, healthy infant without any complications antepartum, during the delivery, or postpartum during the delivery episode.
2. Code 650 may be used if the patient had a complication at some point during her pregnancy but the complication is not present at the time of the admission for delivery.
3. Code 650 is always a principal diagnosis. It is not to be used if any other code from chapter 11 is needed to describe a current complication of the antenatal, delivery, or perinatal period. Additional codes from other chapters may be used with code 650 if they are not related to or are in any way complicating the pregnancy.
4. V27.0, Single liveborn, is the only outcome of delivery code appropriate for use with 650.

F. The Postpartum Period
1. The postpartum period begins immediately after delivery and continues for six weeks following delivery.
2. A postpartum complication is any complication occurring within the six-week period.
3. Chapter 11 codes may also be used to describe pregnancy-related complications after the six-week period should the physician document that a condition is pregnancy related.
4. Postpartum complications that occur during the same admission as the delivery are identified with a fifth digit of "2." Subsequent admissions/encounters for postpartum complications should identified with a fifth digit of "4."
5. When the mother delivers outside the hospital prior to admission and is admitted for routine postpartum care and no complications are noted, code V24.0, Postpartum care and examination immediately after delivery, should be assigned as the principal diagnosis.
6. A delivery diagnosis code should not be used for a woman who has delivered prior to admission to the hospital. Any postpartum procedures should be coded.

G. Code 677, Late effect of complication of pregnancy, childbirth, and the puerperium
1. Code 677, Late effect of complication of pregnancy, childbirth, and the puerperium is for use in those cases when an initial complication of a pregnancy develops a sequelae requiring care or treatment at a future date.
2. This code may be used at any time after the initial postpartum period.
3. This code, like all late effect codes, is to be sequenced following the code describing the sequelae of the complication.

H. Abortions
1. Fifth-digits are required for abortion categories 634-637. Fifth-digit 1, incomplete, indicates that all of the products of conception have not been expelled from the uterus. Fifth-digit 2, complete, indicates that all products of conception have been expelled from the uterus prior to the episode of care.
2. A code from categories 640-648 and 651-657 may be used as additional codes with an abortion code to indicate the complication leading to the abortion.

Fifth digit 3 is assigned with codes from these categories when used with an abortion code because the other fifth digits will not apply. Codes from the 660-669 series are not to be used for complications of abortion.

3. Code 639 is to be used for all complications following abortion. Code 639 cannot be assigned with codes from categories 634-638.
4. Abortion with Liveborn Fetus.
   When an attempted termination of pregnancy results in a liveborn fetus assign code 644.21, Early onset of delivery, with an appropriate code from category V27, Outcome of Delivery. The procedure code for the attempted termination of pregnancy should also be assigned.
5. Retained Products of Conception following an abortion.
   Subsequent admissions for retained products of conception following a spontaneous or legally induced abortion are assigned the appropriate code from category 634, Spontaneous abortion, or legally induced abortion, with a fifth digit of "1" (incomplete). This advice is appropriate even when the patient was discharged previously with a discharge diagnosis of complete abortion.

C12. Diseases Skin and Subcutaneous Tissue
Reserved for future guideline expansion

C13. Diseases of Musculoskeletal and Connective Tissue
Reserved for future guideline expansion

C14. Congenital Anomalies
Reserved for future guideline expansion

C15. Newborn (Perinatal) Guidelines
For coding and reporting purposes the perinatal period is defined as birth through the 28th day following birth. The following guidelines are provided for reporting purposes. Hospitals may record other diagnoses as needed for internal data use.

A. General Perinatal Rule
All clinically significant conditions noted on routine newborn examination should be coded.
A condition is clinically significant if it requires:
clinical evaluation; or
therapeutic treatment; or
diagnostic procedures; or
extended length of hospital stay; or
increased nursing care and/or monitoring; or
has implications for future health care needs.
Note: The perinatal guidelines listed above are the same as the general coding guidelines for "additional diagnoses," except for the final point regarding implications for future health care needs. Whether or not a condition is clinically significant can only be determined by the physician.

B. Use of Codes V30-V39
When coding the birth of an infant, assign a code from categories V30-V39, according to the type of birth. A code from this series is assigned as a principal diagnosis, and assigned only once to a newborn at the time of birth.

C. Newborn Transfers
If the newborn is transferred to another institution, the V30 series is not used at the receiving hospital.

D. Use of Category V29
1. Assign a code from category V29, Observation and evaluation of newborns and infants for suspected conditions not found, to identify those instances when a healthy newborn is evaluated for a suspected condition that is determined after study not to be present. Do not use a code from category V29 when the patient has identified signs or symptoms of a suspected problem; in such cases, code the sign or symptom.
2. A V29 code is to be used as a secondary code after the V30, Outcome of delivery, code. It may also be assigned as a principal code for readmissions or encounters when the V30 code no longer applies. It is for use only for healthy newborns and infants for which no condition after study is found to be present.

E. Maternal Causes of Perinatal Morbidity
Codes from categories 760-763, Maternal causes of perinatal morbidity and mortality, are assigned only when the maternal condition has actually affected the fetus or newborn. The fact that the mother has an associated medical condition or experiences some complication of pregnancy, labor or delivery does not justify the routine assignment of codes from these categories to the newborn record.

F. Congenital Anomalies
Assign an appropriate code from categories 740-759, Congenital Anomalies, as an additional diagnosis when a specific abnormality is diagnosed for an infant. Congenital anomalies may also be the principal or first listed diagnosis for admissions/encounters subsequent to the newborn admission. Such abnormalities may occur as a set of symptoms or multiple malformations. A code should be assigned for each presenting

manifestation of the syndrome if the syndrome is not specifically indexed in ICD-9-CM.

G. Coding of Additional Perinatal Diagnoses

1. Assign codes for conditions that require treatment or further investigation, prolong the length of stay, or require resource utilization.
2. Assign codes for conditions that have been specified by the physician as having implications for future health care needs.

   Note: This guideline should not be used for adult patients.
3. Assign a code for Newborn conditions originating in the perinatal period (categories 760-779), as well as complications arising during the current episode of care classified in other chapters, only if the diagnoses have been documented by the responsible physician at the time of transfer or discharge as having affected the fetus or newborn.

H. Prematurity and Fetal Growth Retardation

Codes from category 764 and subcategories 765.0 and 765.1 should not be assigned based solely on recorded birthweight or estimated gestational age, but on the attending physician's clinical assessment of maturity of the infant. NOTE: Since physicians may utilize different criteria in determining prematurity, do not code the diagnosis of prematurity unless the physician documents this condition.

A code from subcategory 765.2, Weeks of gestation, should be assigned as an additional code with category 764 and codes from 765.0 and 765.1 to specify weeks of gestation as documented by the physician.

C16. Signs, Symptoms and Ill-Defined Conditions

Reserved for future guideline expansion

C17. Injury and Poisoning

A. Coding of Injuries

When coding injuries, assign separate codes for each injury unless a combination code is provided, in which case the combination code is assigned. Multiple injury codes are provided in ICD-9-CM, but should not be assigned unless information for a more specific code is not available. These codes are not to be used for normal, healing surgical wounds or to identify complications of surgical wounds.

The code for the most serious injury, as determined by the physician, is sequenced first.

1. Superficial injuries such as abrasions or contusions are not coded when associated with more severe injuries of the same site.
2. When a primary injury results in minor damage to peripheral nerves or blood vessels, the primary injury is sequenced first with additional code(s) from categories 950-957, Injury to nerves and spinal cord, and/or 900-904, Injury to blood vessels. When the primary injury is to the blood vessels or nerves, that injury should be sequenced first.

B. Coding of Fractures

The principles of multiple coding of injuries should be followed in coding fractures. Fractures of specified sites are coded individually by site in accordance with both the provisions within categories 800-829 and the level of detail furnished by medical record content. Combination categories for multiple fractures are provided for use when there is insufficient detail in the medical record (such as trauma cases transferred to another hospital), when the reporting form limits the number of codes that can be used in reporting pertinent clinical data, or when there is insufficient specificity at the fourth-digit or fifth-digit level. More specific guidelines are as follows:

1. Multiple fractures of same limb classifiable to the same three-digit or four-digit category are coded to that category.
2. Multiple unilateral or bilateral fractures of same bone(s) but classified to different fourth-digit subdivisions (bone part) within the same three-digit category are coded individually by site.
3. Multiple fracture categories 819 and 828 classify bilateral fractures of both upper limbs (819) and both lower limbs (828), but without any detail at the fourth-digit level other than open and closed type of fractures.
4. Multiple fractures are sequenced in accordance with the severity of the fracture and the physician should be asked to list the fracture diagnoses in the order of severity.

C. Coding of Burns

Current burns (940-948) are classified by depth, extent and by agent (E code). Burns are classified by depth as first degree (erythema), second degree (blistering), and third degree (full-thickness involvement).

1. Sequence first the code that reflects the highest degree of burn when more than one burn is present.

2. Classify burns of the same local site (three-digit category level, (940-947)) but of different degrees to the subcategory identifying the highest degree recorded in the diagnosis.
3. Non-healing burns are coded as acute burns. Necrosis of burned skin should be coded as a non-healed burn.
4. Assign code 958.3, Posttraumatic wound infection, not elsewhere classified, as an additional code for any documented infected burn site.
5. When coding burns, assign separate codes for each burn site. Category 946 Burns of Multiple specified sites, should only be used if the location of the burns are not documented. Category 949, Burn, unspecified, is extremely vague and should rarely be used.
6. Assign codes from category 948, Burns classified according to extent of body surface involved, when the site of the burn is not specified or when there is a need for additional data. It is advisable to use category 948 as additional coding when needed to provide data for evaluating burn mortality, such as that needed by burn units. It is also advisable to use category 948 as an additional code for reporting purposes when there is mention of a third-degree burn involving 20 percent or more of the body surface.

   In assigning a code from category 948:

   Fourth-digit codes are used to identify the percentage of total body surface involved in a burn (all degree).

   Fifth-digits are assigned to identify the percentage of body surface involved in third-degree burn.

   Fifth-digit zero (0) is assigned when less than 10 percent or when no body surface is involved in a third- degree burn.

   Category 948 is based on the classic "rule of nines" in estimating body surface involved: head and neck are assigned nine percent, each arm nine percent, each leg 18 percent, the anterior trunk 18 percent, posterior trunk 18 percent, and genitalia one percent. Physicians may change these percentage assignments where necessary to accommodate infants and children who have proportionately larger heads than adults and patients who have large buttocks, thighs, or abdomen that involve burns.
7. Encounters for the treatment of the late effects of burns (i.e., scars or joint contractures) should be coded to the residual condition (sequelae) followed by the appropriate late effect code (906.5-906.9). A late effect E code may also be used, if desired.
8. When appropriate, both a sequelae with a late effect code, and a current burn code may be assigned on the same record.

D. Coding of Debridement of Wound, Infection, or Burn

Excisional debridement may be performed by a physician and/or other health care provider and involves an excisional, as opposed to a mechanical (brushing, scrubbing, washing) debridement.

For coding purposes, excisional debridement, 86.22.

Nonexcisional debridement is assigned to 86.28.

Modified based on *Coding Clinic*, 2nd Quarter 2000, p. 9.

E. Adverse Effects, Poisoning and Toxic Effects

The properties of certain drugs, medicinal and biological substances or combinations of such substances, may cause toxic reactions. The occurrence of drug toxicity is classified in ICD-9-CM as follows:

1. Adverse Effect

   When the drug was correctly prescribed and properly administered, code the reaction plus the appropriate code from the E930-E949 series. Codes from the E930-E949 series must be used to identify the causative substance for an adverse effect of drug, medicinal and biological substances, correctly prescribed and properly administered. The effect, such as tachycardia, delirium, gastrointestinal hemorrhaging, vomiting, hypokalemia, hepatitis, renal failure, or respiratory failure, is coded and followed by the appropriate code from the E930-E949 series.

   Adverse effects of therapeutic substances correctly prescribed and properly administered (toxicity, synergistic reaction, side effect, and idiosyncratic reaction) may be due to (1) differences among patients, such as age, sex, disease, and genetic factors, and (2) drug-related factors, such as type of drug, route of administration, duration of therapy, dosage, and bioavailability.

2. Poisoning
   a. When an error was made in drug prescription or in the administration of the drug by physician, nurse, patient, or other person, use the appropriate poisoning code from the 960-979 series.
   b. If an overdose of a drug was intentionally taken or administered and resulted in drug toxicity, it would be coded as a poisoning (960-979 series).
   c. If a nonprescribed drug or medicinal agent was taken in combination with a correctly prescribed and properly administered drug, any drug toxicity or other reaction resulting from the interaction of the two drugs would be classified as a poisoning.
   d. When coding a poisoning or reaction to the improper use of a medication (e.g., wrong dose, wrong substance, wrong route of administration) the poisoning code is sequenced first, followed by a code for the manifestation. If there is also a diagnosis of drug abuse or dependence to the substance, the abuse or dependence is coded as an additional code.

C18. Classification of Factors Influencing Health Status and Contact with Health Service "V codes"

A. ICD-9-CM provides codes to deal with encounters for circumstances other than a disease or injury. The Supplementary Classification of Factors Influencing Health Status and Contact with Health Services (V01.0-V83.89) is provided to deal with occasions when circumstances other than a disease or injury (codes 001-999) are recorded as a diagnosis or problem.

   There are four primary circumstances for the use of V codes:

   1. When a person who is not currently sick encounters the health services for some specific reason, such as to act as an organ donor, to receive prophylactic care, such as inoculations or health screenings, or to receive counseling on health related issue.
   2. When a person with a resolving disease or injury, or a chronic, long-term condition requiring continuous care, encounters the health care system for specific aftercare of that disease or injury (e.g., dialysis for renal disease; chemotherapy for malignancy; cast change). A diagnosis/symptom code should be used whenever a current, acute, diagnosis is being treated or a sign or symptom is being studied.
   3. When circumstances or problems influence a person's health status but are not in themselves a current illness or injury.
   4. For newborns, to indicate birth status.

B. V codes are for use in both the inpatient and outpatient setting but are generally more applicable to the outpatient setting. V codes may be used as either a first listed (principal diagnosis code in the inpatient setting) or secondary code depending on the circumstances of the encounter. Certain V codes may only be used as first listed, others only as secondary codes.

C. V Codes indicate a reason for an encounter. They are not procedure codes. A corresponding procedure code must accompany a V code to describe the procedure performed.

D. Categories of V Codes
   1. Contact/Exposure
      Category V01 indicates contact with or exposure to communicable diseases. These codes are for patients who do not show any sign or symptom of a disease but have been exposed to it by close personal contact with an infected individual or are in an area where a disease is epidemic. These codes may be used as a first listed code to explain an encounter for testing, or, more commonly, as a secondary code to identify a potential risk.
   2. Inoculations and vaccinations
      Categories V03-V06 are for encounters for inoculations and vaccinations. They indicate that a patient is being seen to receive a prophylactic inoculation against a disease. The injection itself must be represented by the appropriate procedure code. A code from V03-V06 may be used as a secondary code if the inoculation is given as a routine part of preventive health care, such as a well-baby visit.
   3. Status
      Status codes indicate that a patient is either a carrier of a disease or has the sequelae or residual of a past disease or condition. This includes such things as the presence of prosthetic or mechanical devices resulting from past treatment. A status code is informative because the status may affect the course of treatment and its outcome. A status code is distinct from a history code. The history

code indicates that the patient no longer has the condition.

The status V codes/categories are:

V02 Carrier or suspected carrier of infectious diseases

Carrier status, indicates that a person harbors the specific organisms of a disease without manifest symptoms and is capable of transmitting the infection.

V08 Asymptomatic HIV infection status

This code indicates that a patient has tested positive for HIV but has manifested no signs or symptoms of the disease.

V09 Infection with drug-resistant microorganisms

This category indicates that a patient has an infection which is resistant to drug treatment. Sequence the infection code first.

V21 Constitutional states in development

V22.2 Pregnant state, incidental

This code is a secondary code only for use when the pregnancy is in no way complicating the reason for visit. Otherwise, a code from the obstetric chapter is required.

V26.5x Sterilization status

V42 Organ or tissue replaced by transplant

V43 Organ or tissue replaced by other means

V44 Artificial opening status

V45 Other postsurgical states

V46 Other dependence on machines

V49.6 Upper limb amputation status

V49.7 Lower limb amputation status

V48.81 Postmenopausal status

V49.82 Dental sealant status

V58.6 Long-term (current) drug use

This subcategory indicates a patient's continuous use of a prescribed drug (including such things as aspirin therapy) for the long-term treatment of a condition or for prophylactic use. It is not for use for patients who have addictions to drugs.

V83 Genetic carrier status

Categories V42-V46, and subcategories V49.6, V49.7 are for use only if there are no complications or malfunctions of the organ or tissue replaced, the amputation site or the equipment on which the patient is dependent. These are always secondary codes.

4. History (of)

There are two types of history V codes, personal and family. Personal history codes explain a patient's past medical condition that no longer exists and is not receiving any treatment but that has the potential for recurrence, and, therefore, may require continued monitoring. The exceptions to this general rule are category V14, Personal history of allergy to medicinal agents and subcategory V15.0, Allergy, other than to medicinal agents. A person who has had an allergic episode to a substance or food in the past should always be considered allergic to the substance.

Family history codes are for use when a patient has a family member(s) who has had a particular disease that causes the patient to be at higher risk of also contracting the disease.

Personal history codes may be used in conjunction with follow-up codes and family history codes may be use in conjunction with screening codes to explain the need for a test or procedure. History codes are also acceptable on any medical record regardless of the reason for visit. A history of an illness, even if no longer present, is important information that may alter the type of treatment ordered.

The history V code categories are:

V10 Personal history of malignant neoplasm

V12 Personal history of certain other diseases

V13 Personal history of other diseases

Except: V13.4, Personal history of arthritis, and V13.6, Personal history of congenital malformations. These conditions are life-long so are not true history codes.

V14 Personal history of allergy to medicinal agents

V15 Other personal history presenting hazards to health

Except: V15.7, Personal history of contraception.

V16 Family history of malignant neoplasm
V17 Family history of certain chronic disabling diseases
V18 Family history of certain other specific diseases
V19 Family history of other conditions

5. Screening
Screening is the testing for disease or disease precursors in seemingly well individuals so that early detection and treatment can be provided for those who test positive for the disease. Screenings that are recommended for many subgroups in a population include: routine mammograms for women over 40, a fecal occult blood test for everyone over 50, an amniocentesis to rule out a fetal anomaly for pregnant women over 35, because the incidence of breast cancer and colon cancer in these subgroups is higher than in the general population, as is the incidence of Down's syndrome in older mothers.

The testing of a person to rule out or confirm a suspected diagnosis because the patient has some sign or symptom is a diagnostic examination, not a screening. In these cases, the sign or symptom is used to explain the reason for the test.

A screening code may be a first listed code if the reason for the visit is specifically the screening exam. It may also be used as an additional code if the screening is done during an office visit for other health problems. A screening code is not necessary if the screening is inherent to a routine examination, such as a pap smear done during a routine pelvic examination.

Should a condition be discovered during the screening then the code for the condition may be assigned as an additional diagnosis.

The V code indicates that a screening exam is planned. A procedure code is required to confirm that the screening was performed.

The screening V code categories:
V28 Antenatal screening
V73-V82 Special screening examinations

6. Observation
There are two observation V code categories. They are for use in very limited circumstances when a person is being observed for a suspected condition that is ruled out. The observation codes are not for use if an injury or illness or any signs or symptoms related to the suspected condition are present. In such cases the diagnosis/symptom code is used with the corresponding E code to identify any external cause.

The observation codes are to be used as principal diagnosis only. The only exception to this is when the principal diagnosis is required to be a code from the V30, Live born infant, category. Then the V29 observation code is sequenced after the V30 code. Additional codes may be used in addition to the observation code but only if they are unrelated to the suspected condition being observed.

The observation V code categories:
V29 Observation and evaluation of newborns for suspected condition not found
A code from category V30 should be sequenced before the V29 code.
V71 Observation and evaluation for suspected condition not found

7. Aftercare
Aftercare visit codes cover situations when the initial treatment of a disease or injury has been performed and the patient requires continued care during the healing or recovery phase, or for the long-term consequences of the disease. The aftercare V code should not be used if treatment is directed at a current, acute disease or injury, the diagnosis code is to be used in these cases. Exceptions to this rule are codes V58.0, Radiotherapy, and V58.1, Chemotherapy. These codes are to be first listed, followed by the diagnosis code when a patient's encounter is solely to receive radiation therapy or chemotherapy for the treatment of a neoplasm. Should a patient receive both chemotherapy and radiation therapy during the same encounter code V58.0 and V58.1 may be used together on a record with either one being sequenced first.

The aftercare codes are generally first listed to explain the specific reason for the encounter. An aftercare code may be used as an additional code when some type of aftercare is provided in addition to the reason for admission and no diagnosis code is applicable. An example of this would be the closure of a colostomy during an encounter for treatment of another condition.

Certain aftercare V code categories need a secondary diagnosis code to describe the resolving condition or sequelae, for others, the condition is inherent in the code title.

Additional V code aftercare category terms include, fitting and adjustment, and attention to artificial openings.

The aftercare V category/codes:

V52	Fitting and adjustment of prosthetic device and implant
V53	Fitting and adjustment of other device
V54	Other orthopedic aftercare
V55	Attention to artificial openings
V56	Encounter for dialysis and dialysis catheter care
V57	Care involving the use of rehabilitation procedures
V58.0	Radiotherapy
V58.1	Chemotherapy
V58.3	Attention to surgical dressings and sutures
V58.41	Encounter for planned post-operative wound closure
V53.42	Aftercare, surgery, neoplasm
V53.43	Aftercare, surgery, trauma
V58.49	Other specified aftercare following surgery
V53.71-V53.78	Aftercare following surgery
V58.81	Fitting and adjustment of vascular catheter
V58.82	Fitting and adjustment of non-vascular catheter
V53.83	Monitoring therapeutic drug
V58.89	Other specified aftercare

8. Follow-up

The follow-up codes are for use to explain continuing surveillance following completed treatment of a disease, condition, or injury. They infer that the condition has been fully treated and no longer exists. They should not be confused with aftercare codes which explain current treatment for a healing condition or its sequelae. Follow-up codes may be used in conjunction with history codes to provide the full picture of the healed condition and its treatment. The follow-up code is sequenced first, followed by the history code.

A follow-up code may be used to explain repeated visits. Should a condition be found to have recurred on the follow-up visit, then the diagnosis code should be used in place of the follow-up code.

The follow-up V code categories:

V24	Postpartum care and evaluation
V67	Follow-up examination

9. Donor

Category V59 is the donor codes. They are for use for living individuals who are donating blood or other body tissue. These codes are only for individuals donating for others, not for self donations. They are not for use to identify cadaveric donations.

10. Counseling

Counseling V codes are for use for when a patient or family member receives assistance in the aftermath of an illness or injury, or when support is required in coping with family or social problems. They are not necessary for use in conjunction with a diagnosis code when the counseling component of care is considered integral to standard treatment.

The counseling V categories/codes:

V25.0	General counseling and advice for contraceptive management
V26.3	Genetic counseling
V26.4	General counseling and advice for procreative management
V61	Other family circumstances
V65.1	Person consulted on behalf of another person
V65.3	Dietary surveillance and counseling
V65.4	Other counseling, not elsewhere classified

11. Obstetrics and related conditions

See the Obstetrics guidelines for further instruction on the use of these codes.

V codes for pregnancy are for use in those circumstances when none of the problems or complications included in the codes from the Obstetrics chapter exist (a routine prenatal visit or postpartum care) V22.0, Supervision of normal first pregnancy, and V22.1, Supervision of other normal pregnancy, are always first listed and are not to be used with any other code from the OB chapter.

The outcome of delivery, category V27, should be included on all maternal delivery records. It is always a secondary code.

V codes for family planning (contraceptive) or procreative management and counseling should be included on an obstetric record either during the pregnancy or the postpartum stage, if applicable.

Obstetrics and related conditions V code categories:

V22 Normal pregnancy

V23 Supervision of high-risk pregnancy

Except: V23.2, Pregnancy with history of abortion. Code 646.3, Habitual aborter, from the OB chapter is required to indicate a history of abortion during a pregnancy.

V24 Postpartum care and evaluation

V25 Encounter for contraceptive management

Except V25.0x (See counseling above)

V26 Procreative management

Except V26.5x, Sterilization status, V26.3 and V26.4 (Counseling)

V27 Outcome of delivery

V28 Antenatal screening

See Screening- see section 5 of this article

12. Newborn, infant and child

See the newborn guidelines for further instruction on the use of these codes.

Newborn V code categories:

V20 Health supervision of infant or child

V29 Observation and evaluation of newborns for suspected condition not found—see Observation, section 6 of this article.

V30-V39 Liveborn infant according to type of birth

13. Routine and administrative examinations

The V codes allow for the description of encounters for routine examinations, such as, a general check-up, or, examinations for administrative purposes, such as, a pre-employment physical. The codes are for use as first listed codes only and are not to be used if the examination is for diagnosis of a suspected condition or for treatment purposes. In such cases the diagnosis code is used. During a routine exam, should a diagnosis or condition be discovered, it should be coded as an additional code. Pre-existing and chronic conditions, and history codes may also be included as additional codes as long as the examination is for administrative purposes and not focused on any particular condition.

Pre-operative examination V codes are for use only in those situations when a patient is being cleared for surgery and no treatment is given.

The V codes categories/code for routine and administrative examinations:

V20.2 Routine infant or child health check

Any injections given should have a corresponding procedure code.

V70 General medical examination

V72 Special investigations and examinations

Except V72.5 and V72.6

14. Miscellaneous V codes

The miscellaneous V codes capture a number of other health care encounters that do not fall into one of the other categories. Certain of these codes identify the reason for the encounter, others are for use as additional codes which provide useful information on circumstances which may affect a patient's care and treatment.

Miscellaneous V code categories/codes:

V07 Need for isolation and other prophylactic measures

V50 Elective surgery for purposes other than remedying health states

V58.5 Orthodontics

V60 Housing, household, and economic circumstances

V62 Other psychosocial circumstances

V63 Unavailability of other medical facilities for care

V64 Persons encountering health services for specific procedures, not carried out

V66 Convalescence and Palliative Care

V68 Encounters for administrative purposes

V69 Problems related to lifestyle

15. Nonspecific V codes

Certain V codes are so non-specific, or potentially redundant with other codes in the classification that there can be little justification for their use in the inpatient setting. Their use in the outpatient setting should be limited to those instances when there is no further documentation to permit more precise coding. Otherwise, any sign or symptom or any other reason for visit which is captured in another code should be used.

Nonspecific V code categories/codes:

V11 Personal history of mental disorder
A code from the mental disorders chapter, with an in remission fifth-digit, should be used.

V13.4 Personal history of arthritis

V13.6 Personal history of congenital malformations

V15.7 Personal history of contraception

V23.2 Pregnancy with history of abortion

V40 Mental and behavioral problems

V41 Problems with special senses and other special functions

V47 Other problems with internal organs

V48 Problems with head, neck, and trunk

V49 Problems with limbs and other problems
Exceptions:

V49.6 Upper limb amputation status

V49.7 Lower limb amputation status

V49.81 Postmenopausal status

V49.82 Dental sealant status

V51 Aftercare involving the use of plastic surgery

V58.2 Blood transfusion, without reported diagnosis

V58.9 Unspecified aftercare

V72.5 Radiological examination, NEC

V72.6 Laboratory examination
Codes V72.5 and V72.6 are not to be used if any sign or symptoms, or reason for a test is documented. See section K and L of the outpatient guidelines.

C19. Supplemental Classification of External Causes of Injury and Poisoning (E-codes)

Introduction: These guidelines are provided for those who are currently collecting E codes in order that there will be standardization in the process. If your institution plans to begin collecting E codes, these guidelines are to be applied. The use of E codes is supplemental to the application of ICD-9-CM diagnosis codes. E codes are never to be recorded as principal diagnosis (first-listed in noninpatient setting) and are not required for reporting to CMS.

External causes of injury and poisoning codes (E codes) are intended to provide data for injury research and evaluation of injury prevention strategies. E codes capture how the injury or poisoning happened (cause), the intent (unintentional or accidental; or intentional, such as suicide or assault), and the place where the event occurred. Some major categories of E codes include:

transport accidents
poisoning and adverse effects of drugs, medicinal substances and biologicals
accidental falls
accidents caused by fire and flames
accidents due to natural and environmental factors
late effects of accidents, assaults or self injury
assaults or purposely inflicted injury
suicide or self inflicted injury

These guidelines apply for the coding and collection of E codes from records in hospitals, outpatient clinics, emergency departments, other ambulatory care settings and physician offices, and nonacute care settings, except when other specific guidelines apply. (See Section III, Reporting Diagnostic Guidelines for Hospital-based Outpatient Services/Reporting Requirements for Physician Billing.)

A. General E Code Coding Guidelines

1. An E code may be used with any code in the range of 001-V83.89, which indicates an injury, poisoning, or adverse effect due to an external cause.
2. Assign the appropriate E code for all initial treatments of an injury, poisoning, or adverse effect of drugs.
3. Use a late effect E code for subsequent visits when a late effect of the initial injury or poisoning is being treated. There is no late effect E code for adverse effects of drugs.
4. Use the full range of E codes to completely describe the cause, the intent and the place of occurrence, if applicable, for all injuries, poisonings, and adverse effects of drugs.
5. Assign as many E codes as necessary to fully explain each cause. If only one E code can be recorded, assign the E code most related to the principal diagnosis.
6. The selection of the appropriate E code is guided by the Index to External Causes, which is located after the alphabetical index to diseases and by Inclusion and Exclusion notes in the Tabular List.
7. An E code can never be a principal (first listed) diagnosis.

B. Place of Occurrence Guideline

Use an additional code from category E849 to indicate the Place of Occurrence for injuries and poisonings. The Place of Occurrence describes the place where the event occurred and not the patient's activity at the time of the event.

Do not use E849.9 if the place of occurrence is not stated.

C. Adverse Effects of Drugs, Medicinal and Biological Substances Guidelines

1. Do not code directly from the Table of Drugs and Chemicals. Always refer back to the Tabular List.
2. Use as many codes as necessary to describe completely all drugs, medicinal or biological substances.
3. If the same E code would describe the causative agent for more than one adverse reaction, assign the code only once.
4. If two or more drugs, medicinal or biological substances are reported, code each individually unless the combination code is listed in the Table of Drugs and Chemicals. In that case, assign the E code for the combination.
5. When a reaction results from the interaction of a drug(s) and alcohol, use poisoning codes and E codes for both.
6. If the reporting format limits the number of E codes that can be used in reporting clinical data, code the one most related to the principal diagnosis. Include at least one from each category (cause, intent, place) if possible.

   If there are different fourth digit codes in the same three digit category, use the code for "Other specified" of that category. If there is no "Other specified" code in that category, use the appropriate "Unspecified" code in that category.

   If the codes are in different three digit categories, assign the appropriate E code for other multiple drugs and medicinal substances.
7. Codes from the E930-E949 series must be used to identify the causative substance for an adverse effect of drug, medicinal and biological substances, correctly prescribed and properly administered. The effect, such as tachycardia, delirium, gastrointestinal hemorrhaging, vomiting, hypokalemia, hepatitis, renal failure, or respiratory failure, is coded and followed by the appropriate code from the E930-E949 series.

D. Multiple Cause E Code Coding Guidelines

If two or more events cause separate injuries, an E code should be assigned for each cause. The first listed E code will be selected in the following order:

E codes for child and adult abuse take priority over all other E codes—see Child and Adult abuse guidelines.

E codes for terrorism events take priority over all other E codes except child and adult abuse.

E codes for cataclysmic events take priority over all other E codes except child and adult abuse and terrorism.

E codes for transport accidents take priority over all other E codes except cataclysmic events and child and adult abuse and terrorism.

The first-listed E code should correspond to the cause of the most serious diagnosis due to an assault, accident, or self-harm, following the order of hierarchy listed above.

E. Child and Adult Abuse Guideline

1. When the cause of an injury or neglect is intentional child or adult abuse, the first listed E code should be assigned from categories E960-E968, Homicide and injury purposely inflicted by other persons, (except category E967). An E code from category E967, Child and adult battering and other maltreatment, should be added as an additional code to identify the perpetrator, if known.
2. In cases of neglect when the intent is determined to be accidental E code E904.0, Abandonment or neglect of infant and helpless person, should be the first listed E code.

F. Unknown or Suspected Intent Guideline

1. If the intent (accident, self-harm, assault) of the cause of an injury or poisoning is unknown or unspecified, code the intent as undetermined E980-E989.
2. If the intent (accident, self-harm, assault) of the cause of an injury or poisoning is questionable, probable or suspected, code the intent as undetermined E980-E989.

G. Undetermined Cause

When the intent of an injury or poisoning is known, but the cause is unknown, use codes: E928.9, Unspecified accident, E958.9, Suicide and self-inflicted injury by unspecified means, and E968.9, Assault by unspecified means.

These E codes should rarely be used, as the documentation in the medical record, in both the inpatient outpatient and other settings, should normally provide sufficient detail to determine the cause of the injury.

H. Late Effects of External Cause Guidelines
   1. Late effect E codes exist for injuries and poisonings but not for adverse effects of drugs, misadventures and surgical complications.
   2. A late effect E code (E929, E959, E969, E977, E989, or E999.1) should be used with any report of a late effect or sequela resulting from a previous injury or poisoning (905-909).
   3. A late effect E code should never be used with a related current nature of injury code.

I. Misadventures and Complications of Care Guidelines
   1. Assign a code in the range of E870-E876 if misadventures are stated by the physician.
   2. Assign a code in the range of E878-E879 if the physician attributes an abnormal reaction or later complication to a surgical or medical procedure, but does not mention misadventure at the time of the procedure as the cause of the reaction.

J. Terrorism Guidelines
   1. When the cause of an injury is identified by the Federal Government (FBI) as terrorism, the first-listed E-code should be a code from category E979, Terrorism. The definition of terrorism employed by the FBI is found at the inclusion note at E979. The terrorism E-code is the only E-code that should be assigned. Additional E codes from the assault categories should not be assigned.
   2. When the cause of an injury is suspected to be the result of terrorism a code from category E979 should not be assigned. Assign a code in the range of E codes based circumstances on the documentation of intent and mechanism.
   3. Assign code E979.9, Terrorism, secondary effects, for conditions occurring subsequent to the terrorist event. This code should not be assigned for conditions that are due to the initial terrorist act.
   4. For statistical purposes these codes will be tabulated within the category for assault, expanding the current category from E960-E969 to include E979 and E999.1.

Section II Selection of Principal Diagnosis(es) for Inpatient, Short-term, Acute Care Hospital Records

The circumstances of inpatient admission always govern the selection of principal diagnosis. The principal diagnosis is defined in the Uniform Hospital Discharge Data Set (UHDDS) as "that condition established after study to be chiefly responsible for occasioning the admission of the patient to the hospital for care."

The UHDDS definitions are used by acute care short-term hospitals to report inpatient data elements in a standardized manner. These data elements and their definitions can be found in the July 31, 1985, Federal Register (Vol. 50, No, 147), pp. 31038-40.

In determining principal diagnosis the coding conventions in the ICD-9-CM, Volumes I and II take precedence over these official coding guidelines. (See Section IA).

The importance of consistent, complete documentation in the medical record cannot be overemphasized. Without such documentation the application of all coding guidelines is a difficult, if not impossible, task.

A. Codes for symptoms, signs, and ill-defined conditions
   Codes for symptoms, signs, and ill-defined conditions from Chapter 16 are not to be used as principal diagnosis when a related definitive diagnosis has been established.

B. Two or more interrelated conditions, each potentially meeting the definition for principal diagnosis.
   When there are two or more interrelated conditions (such as diseases in the same ICD-9-CM chapter or manifestations characteristically associated with a certain disease) potentially meeting the definition of principal diagnosis, either condition may be sequenced first, unless the circumstances of the admission, the therapy provided, the Tabular List, or the Alphabetic Index indicate otherwise.

C. Two or more diagnoses that equally meet the definition for principal diagnosis.
   In the unusual instance when two or more diagnoses equally meet the criteria for principal diagnosis as determined by the circumstances of admission, diagnostic workup and/or therapy provided, and the Alphabetic Index, Tabular List, or another coding guidelines does not provide sequencing direction, any one of the diagnoses may be sequenced first.

D. Two or more comparative or contrasting conditions.
   In those rare instances when two or more contrasting or comparative diagnoses are documented as "either/or"

(or similar terminology), they are coded as if the diagnoses were confirmed and the diagnoses are sequenced according to the circumstances of the admission. If no further determination can be made as to which diagnosis should be principal, either diagnosis may be sequenced first.

E. A symptom(s) followed by contrasting/comparative diagnoses.
When a symptom(s) is followed by contrasting/comparative diagnoses, the symptom code is sequenced first. All the contrasting/comparative diagnoses should be coded as additional diagnoses.

F. Original treatment plan not carried out.
Sequence as the principal diagnosis the condition, which after study occasioned the admission to the hospital, even though treatment may not have been carried out due to unforeseen circumstances.

G. Complications of surgery and other medical care.
When the admission is for treatment of a complication resulting from surgery or other medical care, the complication code is sequenced as the principal diagnosis. If the complication is classified to the 996-999 series, an additional code for the specific complication may be assigned.

H. Uncertain Diagnosis.
If the diagnosis documented at the time of discharge is qualified as "probable", "suspected", "likely", "questionable", "possible", or "still to be ruled out", code the condition as if it existed or was established. The bases for these guidelines are the diagnostic workup, arrangements for further workup or observation, and initial therapeutic approach that correspond most closely with the established diagnosis.

Section III Reporting Additional Diagnoses for Inpatient, Short-term, Acute Care Hospital Records

GENERAL RULES FOR OTHER (ADDITIONAL) DIAGNOSES

For reporting purposes the definition for "other diagnoses" is interpreted as additional conditions that affect patient care in terms of requiring:

clinical evaluation; or
therapeutic treatment; or
diagnostic procedures; or
extended length of hospital stay; or
increased nursing care and/or monitoring.

The UHDDS item #11-b defines Other Diagnoses as "all conditions that coexist at the time of admission, that develop subsequently, or that affect the treatment received and/or the length of stay. Diagnoses that relate to an earlier episode which have no bearing on the current hospital stay are to be excluded." UHDDS definitions apply to inpatients in acute care, short-term, hospital setting The UHDDS definitions are used by acute care short-term hospitals to report inpatient data elements in a standardized manner. These data elements and their definitions can be found in the July 31, 1985, Federal Register (Vol. 50, No, 147), pp. 31038-40.

The following guidelines are to be applied in designating "other diagnoses" when neither the Alphabetic Index nor the Tabular List in ICD-9-CM provide direction. The listing of the diagnoses in the patient record is the responsibility of the attending physician.

A. Previous conditions
If the physician has included a diagnosis in the final diagnostic statement, such as the discharge summary or the face sheet, it should ordinarily be coded. Some physicians include in the diagnostic statement resolved conditions or diagnoses and status-post procedures from previous admission that have no bearing on the current stay. Such conditions are not to be reported and are coded only if required by hospital policy.
However, history codes (V10-V19) may be used as secondary codes if the historical condition or family history has an impact on current care or influences treatment.

B. Abnormal findings
Abnormal findings (laboratory, x-ray, pathologic, and other diagnostic results) are not coded and reported unless the physician indicates their clinical significance. If the findings are outside the normal range and the attending physician has ordered other tests to evaluate the condition or prescribed treatment, it is appropriate to ask the physician whether the abnormal finding should be added.

Please note: This differs from the coding practices in the outpatient setting for coding encounters for diagnostic tests that have been interpreted by a physician.

C. Uncertain Diagnosis
If the diagnosis documented at the time of discharge is qualified as "probable", "suspected", "likely", "questionable", "possible", or "still to be ruled out", code the condition as if it existed or was established. The bases for these guidelines are the diagnostic workup, arrangements for further workup or observation, and initial therapeutic approach that correspond most closely with the established diagnosis.

Section IV Diagnostic Coding and Reporting Guidelines for Outpatient Services

These coding guidelines for outpatient diagnoses have been approved for use by hospitals/physicians in coding and reporting hospital-based outpatient services and physician office visits.

Information about the use of certain abbreviations, punctuation, symbols, and other conventions used in the ICD-9-CM Tabular List (code numbers and titles), can be found in Section IA of these guidelines, under "Conventions Used in the Tabular List." Information about the correct sequence to use in finding a code is also described in Section I.

The terms encounter and visit are often used interchangeably in describing outpatient service contacts and, therefore, appear together in these guidelines without distinguishing one from the other.

Though the conventions and general guidelines apply to all settings, coding guidelines for outpatient and physician reporting of diagnoses will vary in a number of instances from those for inpatient diagnoses, recognizing that:

> The Uniform Hospital Discharge Data Set (UHDDS) definition of principal diagnosis applies only to inpatients in acute, short-term, general hospitals.
> Coding guidelines for inconclusive diagnoses (probable, suspected, rule out, etc.) were developed for inpatient reporting and do not apply to outpatients.

A. Selection of first-listed condition
In the outpatient setting, the term first-listed diagnosis is used in lieu of principal diagnosis.
In determining the first-listed diagnosis the coding conventions of ICD-9-CM, as well as the general and disease specific guidelines take precedence over the outpatient guidelines.
Diagnoses often are not established at the time of the initial encounter/visit. It may take two or more visits before the diagnosis is confirmed.
The most critical rule involves beginning the search for the correct code assignment through the Alphabetic Index. Never begin searching initially in the Tabular List as this will lead to coding errors.

B. The appropriate code or codes from 001.0 through V83.89 must be used to identify diagnoses, symptoms, conditions, problems, complaints, or other reason(s) for the encounter/visit.

C. For accurate reporting of ICD-9-CM diagnosis codes, the documentation should describe the patient's condition, using terminology which includes specific diagnoses as well as symptoms, problems, or reasons for the encounter. There are ICD-9-CM codes to describe all of these.

D. The selection of codes 001.0 through 999.9 will frequently be used to describe the reason for the encounter. These codes are from the section of ICD-9-CM for the classification of diseases and injuries (e.g., infectious and parasitic diseases; neoplasms; symptoms, signs, and ill-defined conditions, etc.).

E. Codes that describe symptoms and signs, as opposed to diagnoses, are acceptable for reporting purposes when a diagnosis has not been established (confirmed) by the physician. Chapter 16 of ICD-9-CM, Symptoms, Signs, and Ill-defined conditions (codes 780.0-799.9) contain many, but not all codes for symptoms.

F. ICD-9-CM provides codes to deal with encounters for circumstances other than a disease or injury. The Supplementary Classification of factors Influencing Health Status and Contact with Health Services (V01.0-V83.89) is provided to deal with occasions when circumstances other than a disease or injury are recorded as diagnosis or problems.

G. Level of Detail in Coding
1. ICD-9-CM is composed of codes with either 3, 4, or 5 digits. Codes with three digits are included in ICD-9-CM as the heading of a category of codes that may be further subdivided by the use of fourth and/or fifth digits, which provide greater specificity.
2. A three-digit code is to be used only if it is not further subdivided. Where fourth-digit subcategories and/or fifth-digit subclassifications are provided, they must be assigned. A code is invalid if it has not been coded to the full number of digits required for that code. See also discussion under Section I, General Coding Guidelines, Level of Detail.

H. List first the ICD-9-CM code for the diagnosis, condition, problem, or other reason for encounter/visit shown in the medical record to be chiefly responsible for the services provided. List additional codes that describe any coexisting conditions.

I. Do not code diagnoses documented as "probable", "suspected," "questionable," "rule out," or "working diagnosis". Rather, code the condition(s) to the highest degree of certainty for that encounter/visit, such as symptoms, signs, abnormal test results, or other reason for the visit.

Please note: This differs from the coding practices used by hospital medical record departments for coding the diagnosis of acute care, short-term hospital inpatients.

J. Chronic diseases treated on an ongoing basis may be coded and reported as many times as the patient receives treatment and care for the condition(s).

K. Code all documented conditions that coexist at the time of the encounter/visit, and require or affect patient care treatment or management. Do not code conditions that were previously treated and no longer exist. However, history codes (V10-V19) may be used as secondary codes if the historical condition or family history has an impact on current care or influences treatment.

L. For patients receiving diagnostic services only during an encounter/visit, sequence first the diagnosis, condition, problem, or other reason for encounter/visit shown in the medical record to be chiefly responsible for the outpatient services provided during the encounter/visit. Codes for other diagnoses (e.g., chronic conditions) may be sequenced as additional diagnoses.

For outpatient encounters for diagnostic tests that have been interpreted by a physician, and the final report is available at the time of coding, code any confirmed or definitive diagnosis(es) documented in the interpretation. Do not code related signs and symptoms as additional diagnoses.

Please note: This differs from the coding practice in the hospital inpatient setting regarding abnormal findings on test results.

M. For patients receiving therapeutic services only during an encounter/visit, sequence first the diagnosis, condition, problem, or other reason for encounter/visit shown in the medical record to be chiefly responsible for the outpatient services provided during the encounter/visit. Codes for other diagnoses (e.g., chronic conditions) may be sequenced as additional diagnoses.

The only exception to this rule is that when the primary reason for the admission/encounter is chemotherapy, radiation therapy, or rehabilitation, the appropriate V code for the service is listed first, and the diagnosis or problem for which the service is being performed listed second.

N. For patient's receiving preoperative evaluations only, sequence a code from category V72.8, Other specified examinations, to describe the pre-op consultations. Assign a code for the condition to describe the reason for the surgery as an additional diagnosis. Code also any findings related to the pre-op evaluation.

O. For ambulatory surgery, code the diagnosis for which the surgery was performed. If the postoperative diagnosis is known to be different from the preoperative diagnosis at the time the diagnosis is confirmed, select the postoperative diagnosis for coding, since it is the most definitive.

P. For routine outpatient prenatal visits when no complications are present codes V22.0, Supervision of normal first pregnancy, and V22.1, Supervision of other normal pregnancy, should be used as principal diagnoses. These codes should not be used in conjunction with chapter 11 codes.

Appendix D
Abbreviations

A1 pulley	tendon on anterior surface of finger
ABD	Adriamycin, bleomycin, dacarbazine
ABG	arterial blood gases
ABO	three main blood types
AC	abdominal circumference
ACL	anterior cruciate ligament
ACLS	Advanced Cardiac Life Support
ACTH	adrenocorticotropic hormone
AF	atrial fibrillation (also A Fib)
AFB	acid-fast bacillus
AFI	amniotic fluid index
A Fib	atrial fibrillation (also AF)
AFT	atrial flutter
AIC	amino-imidazole carboxamide anti-inflammatory corticoid
AKA	above-knee amputation
Alb	albumin
Alk phos	alkaline phosphatase
ALT	alanine transaminase (formerly SGPT)
AM	acute marginal (branch of RCA)
AMA	advanced maternal age
ANA	antinuclear antibodies
ANS	autonomic nervous system
AP	anterior posterior
APTT	activated partial thromboplastin time
AR	aortic regurgitation
ARDS	acute or adult respiratory distress syndrome
AROM	artificial rupture of membranes
AS	aortic stenosis
ASCVD	arteriosclerotic cardiovascular disease
ASHD	arteriosclerotic heart disease
ASO	antistreptolysin O
AST	aspartate aminotransferase (formerly SGOT)
ASVD	arteriosclerotic vascular disease
ATN	acute tubular necrosis
AU	both ears
AV	arteriovenous
BBOW	bulging bag of water
BCP	birth control pills
b.i.d.	twice a day
Bili tot	direct bilirubin, total and direct
BiPAP	bilevel positive airway pressure
BKA	below-knee amputation
BOOP	bronchiolitis obliterans organizing pneumonia
BPG	bypass graft
BSO	bilateral salpingo-oophorectomy
BTL	bilateral tubal ligation
BUN	blood urea nitrogen
BUS	Bartholin's, urethra, and Skene's glands

C	Celsius
C1-C7	cervical vertebrae
C1	first cervical vertebra
C2	second cervical vertebra
C3	third cervical vertebra
C4	fourth cervical vertebra
C5	fifth cervical vertebra
C6	sixth cervical vertebra
C7	seventh cervical vertebra
ca	cancer
Ca	calcium
CABG	coronary artery bypass graft
CAD	coronary artery disease
CAPD	chronic peritoneal dialysis
CBC	complete blood count
Cc;cc	cubic centimeter
CCU	coronary care unit
CD	cesarean delivery
C. difficile	*Clostridium difficile*
CEA	carcinoembryonic antigen
CHD	congenital heart disease
CHF	congestive heart failure
Chol tot	total serum cholesterol
Cl	chloride
CK	creatine kinase
cm	centimeter
CMP	cardiomyopathy
CMT	chiropractic manipulative treatment
CMV	Cytomegalovirus
CNS	central nervous system
CO	cardiac output
CO2	carbon dioxide
COPD	chronic obstructive pulmonary disease
COX2	cyclooxygenase-2 inhibitors
CPAP	continuous positive airway pressure
CPB	cardiopulmonary bypass
CPK	creatine phosphokinase
CPR	cardiopulmonary resuscitation
Creat	creatinine
CRNA	certified registered nurse anesthetist
CSF	cerebrospinal fluid
CT	computerized tomography; CAT scan
CTS	carpal tunnel syndrome
CVA	stroke/cardiovascular accident
CVD	cerebrovascular disease
CVP	central venous pressure
CW	clock-wise
CX	circumflex artery
Cx	cervix

D&C	dilatation and curettage (also D and C)
D&E	dilatation and evacuation
D1	diagonal branch of the LAD artery
D2	diagonal branch of the LAD artery
D5	dextrose 5% water
D and C	dilatation and curettage (also D&C)
DAT	direct antiglobulin test
DC	doctor of chiropractic
dl	deciliter
DLCO	diffuse capacity of lungs for carbon monoxide
DMI	diabetes mellitus
DO	doctor of osteopathy
DOLV	double outlet left ventricle
DORV	double outlet right ventricle
DTPA	diethylene-triamine penta-acetic acid
DUB	dysfunctional uterine bleeding
DVT	deep vein thrombosis
ECA	external carotid artery
ECC	endocervical curettage; extracorporeal circulation (or circuit)
ECG	electrocardiogram (also EKG)
ECHO	echocardiogram (also ECHO-C)
ECHO-C	echocardiogram (also ECHO)
ECOG	Eastern Cooperative Oncology Group
EDC	estimated date of confinement; estimated date of conception
EEG	electroencephalogram
EF	ejection fraction; the percent of the left ventricular volume ejected in a cardiac contraction
EIA	enzyme immunoassay
EKG	electrocardiogram (also ECG)
EMB	endometrial biopsy
ENA	extractable nuclear antigen
ENT	ear, nose, throat
EOM, EOMs	extraocular movement(s)
EOMI	extraocular movement intact
EP	ectopic pregnancy
ER	emergency department
ESRD	end-stage renal disease
ESRF	end-stage renal failure
FEF	forced expiratory flow
FEV1	forced expiratory volume in one second
FEV1:FVC	forced expiratory volume in one second to forced vital capacity ratio
FHR	fetal heart rate
FHT	fetal heart tones
FI	forced inspiration
FIGO	International Federated Gynecological Oncology (staging classification for grading cancer of female genitalia)
FM	fetal movements
FRC	functional residual capacity
FSH	follicle stimulating hormone
FVC	forced vital capacity
g	gram (also gm)
g/dl	gram/deciliter
GERD	gastroesophageal reflux
GGT	gamma glutamyl transferase
GI	gastrointestinal
Glu	glucose
gm	gram
GU	genitourinary
GYN	gynecology
h	hour
H/C	head circumference
H&H	hemoglobin and hematocrit (also stated HH)
H_2	histamine-2
H and P	history and physical
HB3Ag	lipoprotein
HCG	human chorionic gonadotropin
HCT; Hct	hematocrit
HDL	high-density lipoprotein
HEENT	head, ears, eyes, nose, throat
HIDA	hydroxy iminodiacetic acid (imaging test)
HGB; Hgb	hemoglobin
HH	hemoglobin and hematocrit (also stated H&H)
HHN	hand-held nebulizer
HIV	human immunodeficiency virus
HR	heart rate
Hs	at bedtime
HTN	hypertension
I&D	incision and drainage
I&O	intake and output
IABP	intraaortic balloon pump
IBC	iron-binding capacity
ICA	internal carotid artery
ICN	intensive care; neonatal
ICU	intensive care unit
ICS	intercostal space
IgM	immunoglobulin M
IM	intramuscular
INR	International Normalized Ratio
INT	osteal ramus intermedius
IPAP	inspiratory positive airway pressure
IUGR	intrauterine growth retardation
IUP	intrauterine pregnancy
IV	intravenous
IVC	inferior vena cava
IVCD	interventricular conduction defect
IVP	intravenous pyelogram
JP	jugular process, jugular pulse
JVD	jugular vein distention
K	potassium
kg	kilogram
KUB	Kidney, ureter, bladder
L1-L5	lumbar vertebrae
L1	first lumbar vertebra
L2	second lumbar vertebra
L3	third lumbar vertebra
L4	fourth lumbar vertebra
L5	fifth lumbar vertebra
LA	left atrium
LAD	left anterior descending coronary artery
LBBB	left bundle branch block
LDH	lactate dehydrogenase
LDL	low-density lipoprotein
LFT	liver function test

LIMA left internal mammary artery
LLL left lower lobe
lm lumen
LM left main coronary artery
LMCA left main coronary artery
LMP last menstrual period
LP lumbar puncture
LT C/S low transverse C section
LV left ventricle
LVET left ventricle
LVH left ventricular hypertrophy
m/sec millisecond
M1 tibial tibial insert
MAA melanoma associated antigen
MAC maximum allowable concentrate; monitored anesthesia care
MAP mean aortic pressure, mean arterial pressure
MB methylene blue, mesio-buccal; cardiac muscle
mc millicurie
mcg microgram
MCHC mean corpuscular hemoglobin
MCV mean corpuscular volume
MDI metered dose inhaler
mEq milliequivalent
mg milligram
mg/dl milligram/deciliter
MI myocardial infarction; mitral insufficiency
mL; ml milliliter
mm millimeter
mm/hr millimeter/hour
mmHg millimeters of mercury
MMPI Minnesota Multiphasic Personality Inventory
MMRV measles, mumps, rubella, varicella
MR mitral regurgitation
MRI magnetic resonance imaging
MS mitral stenosis
MUGA multiple gated acquisition test; a radionuclide test of myocardial performance
MV mitral valve
MVR mitral valve repair
MVV maximum voluntary ventilation
N negative
Na sodium
NC no charge
neb nebula, a spray
NG nasogastric, nitroglycerin
NICU neonatal intensive care unit
n.p.o. nothing by mouth (also NPO)
NPO nothing by mouth (also n.p.o.)
NSAID nonsteroidal antiinflammatory drug
NSVD NI spontaneous vaginal delivery
O_2 oxygen
OA osteoarthritis
OB obstetrics
OBT occult blood test
o.d. right eye
OM1 OM2 obtuse marginal
OMT osteopathic manipulative treatment
OP outpatient
OPC outpatient clinic
OPD outpatient department; obstructive pulmonary disease
OPS outpatient surgery
OPV oral poliovirus vaccine
OR operating room
os mouth
OTC over-the-counter
OU each eye; both eyes
OURQ outer upper right quadrant
OV office visit
PA pulmonary artery
PAC premature atrial contraction
PAD peripheral arterial disease
PAR postanesthesia recovery
para to bring forth
PAWP pulmonary artery wedge pressure
PCA patient-controlled analgesia
PCL posterior cruciate ligament
PCO polycystic ovaries
PCO_2 partial pressure of carbon dioxide
PCWP pulmonary capillary wedge pressure
PD peritoneal dialysis
PDA posterior descending artery, part of the RCA
PE pressure equalization
PEA pulseless electrical activity
PEAP positive end-airway pressure
PEEP positive end-expiratory pressure
PERRLA pupils equal, round, reactive to light and accommodation
PFT pulmonary function test
pH; ph potential of hydrogen
PID pelvic inflammatory disease
PIH pregnancy induced hypertension
PMI point of maximal impulse
PND paroxysmal nocturnal dyspnea
PNS peripheral nervous system
p.o. by mouth
POC products of conception
PR pulse rate
p.r.n. pro re nata, as needed (also prn)
prn pro re nata, as needed (also p.r.n.)
PROM premature rupture of membrane
Prot tot total protein
PSA prostate-specific antigen
PSVT paroxysmal supraventricular tachycardia
PT prothrombin time
PTCA percutaneous transluminal coronary angioplasty
PTH parathyroid hormone, plasma thrombopastin antecendent, post-transfusional hepatitis
PTL preterm labor
PTT partial thromboplastin time
PV pulmonary valve
PVC premature ventricular contraction
PVD peripheral vascular disease
q every
q.2wk every 2 weeks
q.3h every 3 hours
q.4h every 4 hours
q.4wk every 4 weeks

q.a.m.	every morning
q.d.	every day
q.d.s.	four times a day
q.h.	every hour
q.h.s.	each bed time
q.i.d.	four times a day
q.m.	every morning
q.o.d.	every other day
q.os.	as needed
q.p.m.	every afternoon or every evening
q.q.h.	every fourth hour
q.s.	quantity sufficient
qq.	each, every
qq.h	every hour
QRS	Q-wave R-wave S-wave
RA	right atrium; rheumatoid arthritis
RBBB	right bundle branch block
RBC	red blood cell
RCA	right coronary artery
RDS	respiratory distress syndrome
RDW	red cell distribution width
RF	rheumatoid factor
Rh	rhesus factor
Rh(D)	rhesus factor blood typing
RIMA	right internal mammary artery
RLQ	right lower quadrant
RPR	rapid reagin plasma
RV	respiratory volume; right ventricle
RV:TLC	respiratory volume to total lung capacity ratio
RVH	right ventricular hypertrophy
RX	medication
s	*sans* (without), *sigma* (sign, mark), *semis* (half)
S1	first heart sound
S1 S2	sequential 1 and 2 heart sounds
S2	second heart sound
S3	third heart sound
S4	fourth heart sound
Sa	saphenous
SAB	spontaneous abortion
SBE	subacute bacterial endocarditis
SBP	systolic blood pressure
SGOT	serum glutamic oxaloacetic transaminase (AST)
SGPT	serum glutamic pyruvic transaminase (ALT)
SIADH	syndrome of inappropriate antidiuretic hormone
SIMV	synchronized intermittent mandatory ventilation
SPECT	single photon emission tomography
SROM	spontaneous rupture of membrane
S tach	sinus tachycardia (also ST)
ST	sinus tachycardia (also S tach)
SVC	superior vena cava
SVD	spontaneous vaginal delivery
SVG	saphenous vein graft
SV tach	supraventricular tachycardia (also SVT)
SVT	supraventricular tachycardia (also SV tach)
T&A	tonsillectomy and adenoidectomy
T1-T12	thoracic vertebrae
T1	first thoracic vertebra
T2	second thoracic vertebra
T3	third thoracic vertebra
T4	fourth thoracic vertebra; tumor 4
T5	fifth thoracic vertebra
T6	sixth thoracic vertebra
T7	seventh thoracic vertebra
T8	eighth thoracic vertebra
T9	ninth thoracic vertebra
T10	tenth thoracic vertebra
T11	eleventh thoracic vertebra
T12	twelfth thoracic vertebra
T^4	symbol for thyroxine
TA	therapeutic abortion
TAH	total abdominal hysterectomy
Tc-99M	technetium-99m
TCD	transcranial Doppler
TEE	transesophageal echocardiography
TENS	transcutaneous electrical nerve stimulator
TH	tumor 4
TIA	transient ischemic attack
t.i.d.	three times a day
TLC	total lung capacity
TLV	total lung volume
TMJ	temporomandibular joint
TPN	total parenteral nutrition
TR	tricuspid regurgitation
Trig	triglycerides
TS	tricuspid stenosis
TSH	thyroid stimulating hormone
TV	tricuspid valve
u/dl	deciliter
UA	urine analysis
UC	uterine contraction
UPPP	uvulo-palato-pharyngoplasty
URI	upper respiratory infection
UV	ultraviolet
VAD	ventricular assist device
VB	vaginal bleeding
VBAC	vaginal birth after C-section
VBR	ventricular branch
VF	ventricular fibrillation (also V fib)
V fib	ventricular fibrillation (also VF)
V/Q scan	ventilation/perfusion scan
VSD	ventricular septal defect
VT	ventricular tachycardia (also V tach)
V tach	ventricular tachycardia (also VT)
WBC	white blood count
WPW	Wolf-Parkinson-White
ZE	Zollinger-Ellison

Appendix E, Part 1

1995 Documentation Guidelines for Evaluation and Management Services

I. INTRODUCTION

WHAT IS DOCUMENTATION AND WHY IS IT IMPORTANT?

Medical record documentation is required to record pertinent facts, findings, and observations about an individual's health history including past and present illnesses, examinations, tests, treatments, and outcomes. The medical record chronologically documents the care of the patient and is an important element contributing to high quality care. The medical record facilitates:

- the ability of the physician and other health care professional to evaluate and plan the patient's immediate treatment, and to monitor his/her health care over time;
- communication and continuity of care among physicians and other health care professionals involved in the patient's care;
- accurate and timely claims review and payment;
- appropriate utilization review and quality of care evaluations; and
- collection of data that may be useful for research and education.

An appropriately documented medical record can reduce many of the "hassles" associated with claims processing and may serve as a legal document to verify the care provided, if necessary.

WHAT DO PAYERS WANT AND WHY?

Because payers have a contractual obligation to enrollees, they may require reasonable documentation that services are consistent with the insurance coverage provided. They may request information to validate:

- the site of service;
- the medical necessity and appropriateness of the diagnostic and/or therapeutic services provided; and/or
- that services provided have been accurately reported.

II. GENERAL PRINCIPLES OF MEDICAL RECORD DOCUMENTATION

The principles of documentation listed below are applicable to all types of medical and surgical services in all settings. For Evaluation and Management (E/M) services, the nature and amount of physician work and documentation varies by type of service, place of service and the patient's status. The general principles listed below may be modified to account for these variable circumstances in providing E/M services.

1. The medical record should be complete and legible.
2. The documentation of each patient encounter should include:
   - reason for the encounter and relevant history, physical examination findings and prior diagnostic test results;
   - assessment, clinical impression or diagnosis;
   - plan for care; and
   - date and legible identity of the observer.
3. If not documented, the rationale for ordering diagnostic and other ancillary services should be easily inferred.
4. Past and present diagnoses should be accessible to the treating and/or consulting physician.
5. Appropriate health risk factors should be identified.
6. The patient's progress, response to and changes in treatment, and revision of diagnosis should be documented.
7. The CPT and ICD-9-CM codes reported on the health insurance claim form or billing statement should be supported by the documentation in the medical record.

III. DOCUMENTATION OF E/M SERVICES

The publication provides definitions and documentation guidelines for the three ***key*** components of E/M services and for visits which consist predominately of counseling or coordination of care. The three key components–history, examination, and medical decision making–appear in the descriptors for office and other outpatient services, hospital observation services, hospital inpatient services, consultations, emergency department services, nursing facility services, domiciliary care services, and home services. While some of the text of CPT has been repeated in this publication, the reader should refer to CPT for the complete descriptors for E/M services and instructions for selecting a level of service. **Documentation guidelines are identified by the symbol • *DG.***

The descriptors for the levels of E/M services recognize seven components which are used in defining the levels of E/M services. These components are:

- history;
- examination;
- medical decision making;
- counseling;
- coordination of care;
- nature of presenting problem; and
- time

The first three of these components (i.e., history, examination and medical decision making) are the ***key*** components in selecting the level of E/M services. An exception to this rule is the case of visits which consists predominantly of counseling or coordination of care; for these services time is the key or controlling factor to qualify for a particular level of E/M service.

For certain group of patients, the recorded information may vary slightly from that described here. Specifically, the medical records of infants, children, adolescents and pregnant women may have additional or modified information recorded in each history and examination area.

As an example, newborn records may include under history of the present illness (HPI) the details of mother's pregnancy and the infant's status at birth; social history will focus on family structure; family history will focus on congenital anomalies and hereditary disorders in the family. In addition, information on growth and development and/or nutrition will be recorded. Although not specifically defined in these documentation guidelines, these patient group variations on history and examination are appropriate.

A. Documentation of History

The levels of E/M services are based on four types of history (Problem Focused, Expanded Problem Focused, Detailed, and Comprehensive.) Each type of history includes some or all of the following elements:

- Chief complaint (CC);
- History of present illness (HPI);
- Review of systems (ROS); and
- Past, family and/or social history (PFSH).

The extent of history of present illness, review of systems and past, family and/or social history that is obtained and documented is dependent upon clinical judgment and the nature of the presenting problem(s).

The chart below shows the progression of the elements required for type of history. To qualify for a given type of history, all three elements in the table must be met. (A chief complaint is indicated at all levels.)

History of present Illness (HPI)	Review of Systems (ROS)	Past, Family, and/or Social History (PFSH)	Type of History
Brief	N/A	N/A	***Problem Focused***
Brief	Problem Pertinent	N/A	***Expanded Problem Focused***
Extended	Extended	Pertinent	***Detailed***
Extended	Complete	Complete	***Comprehensive***

- DG: The CC, ROS and PFSH may be listed as separate elements of history, or they may be included in the description of the history of the present illness.
- DG: A ROS and/or a PFSH obtained during an earlier encounter does not need to be re-recorded if there is evidence that the physician reviewed and updated the previous information. This may occur when a physician updates his or her own record or in an institutional setting or group practice where many physicians use a common record. The review and update may be documented by:
  - describing any new ROS and/or PFSH information or noting there has been no change in the information; and
  - noting the date and location of the earlier ROS and/or PFSH.
- DG: The ROS and/or PFSH may be recorded by ancillary staff or on a form completed by the patient. To document that the physician reviewed the information, there must be a notation supplementing or confirming the information recorded by others.
- DG: If the physician is unable to obtain a history from the patient or other source, the record should describe the patient's condition or other circumstance which precludes obtaining a history.

Definitions and specific documentation guidelines for each of the elements of history are listed below.

Chief Complaint (CC). The CC is a concise statement describing the symptom, problem, condition, diagnosis, physician recommended return, or other factor that is reason for the encounter.

- DG: The medical record should clearly reflect the chief complaint.

History of Present Illness (HPI). The HPI is a chronological description of the development of the patient's present illness from the first sign and/or symptom or form the previous encounter to the present. It includes the following elements:

- location,
- quality,
- severity,
- duration,
- timing,
- context,
- modifying factors, and
- associated signs and symptoms.

Brief and *extended* HPIs are distinguished by the amount of detail needed to accurately characterize the clinical problem(s).

A ***brief*** HPI consists of one to three element of the HPI.

- DG: The medical record should describe one to three elements of the present illness (HPI)

An ***extended*** HPI consists of four or more elements of the HPI.

- DG: The medical record should describe four or more elements of the present illness (HPI) or associated comorbidities

Review of Systems (ROS). A ROS is an inventory of body systems obtained through a series of questions seeking to identify signs and/or symptoms which the patient may be experiencing or has experienced.

For purpose of ROS, the following systems are recognized:

- Constitutional symptoms (e.g., fever, weight loss)
- Eyes
- Ears, Nose, Mouth, Throat
- Cardiovascular
- Respiratory
- Gastrointestinal
- Genitourinary
- Musculoskeletal
- Integumentary (skin and/or breast)
- Neurological
- Psychiatric
- Endocrine
- Hematologic/Lymphatic
- Allergic/Immunologic

A ***problem pertinent*** ROS inquires about the system directly related to the problem(s) identified in the HPI.

- DG: The patient's positive responses and pertinent negatives for the system related to the problem should be documented.

A ***extended*** ROS inquires about the system directly related to the problem(s) identified in the HPI and a limited number of additional systems.

- DG: The patient's positive responses and pertinent negatives for two to nine systems should be documented.

A ***complete*** ROS inquires about the system(s) directly related to the problem(s) identified in the HPI plus all additional body systems.

- DG: At least ten organ systems must be reviewed. Those systems with positive or pertinent negative responses must be individually documented. For the remaining systems, a notation indicating all other systems are negative is permissible. In the absence of such a notation, at least ten system must be individually documented.

Past, Family and/or Social History (PFSH). The PFSH consists of review of three areas:

- past history (the patient's past experiences with illnesses, operations, injuries and treatments);
- family history (a review of medical events in the patient's family, including diseases which may be hereditary or place the patient at risk); and
- social history (an age appropriate review of past and current activities).

For the categories of subsequent hospital care, follow-up inpatient consultations and subsequent nursing facility care, CPT requires only an "interval" history. It is not necessary to record information about the PFSH.

A ***pertinent*** PFSH is a review of the history area(s) directly related to the problem(s) identified in the HPI

- DG: At least one specific item from any of the three history areas must be documented for a pertinent PFSH.

A ***complete*** PFSH is of a review of two or all three of the PFSH history areas, depending on the category of the E/M service. A review of all three history areas is required for services that by their nature include a comprehensive assessment or reassessment of the patient. A review of two of the three history areas is sufficient for other services.

- DG: At least one specific item from two of the three history areas must be documented for a complete PFSH for the following categories of E/M services: office or other outpatient services, established patient; emergency department; subsequent nursing facility care; domiciliary care, established patient; and home care, established patient.
- DG: At least one specific item from each of the three history areas must be documented for a complete PFSH for the following categories of E/M services: office or other outpatient services, new patient; hospital observation services; hospital inpatient services, initial care; consultations; comprehensive nursing facility assessments; domiciliary care, new patient; and home care new patient.

B. Documentation of Examination

The levels of E/M services are based on four types of examination that are defined as follows:

- ***Problem Focused***–a limited examination of the affected body area or organ system.
- ***Expanded Problem Focused***–a limited examination of the affected body area or organ system and other symptomatic or related organ system(s).
- ***Detailed***–an extended examination of the affected body area(s) and other symptomatic or related organ system(s).
- ***Comprehensive***–a general multi-system examination or complete examination of a single organ system.

For purpose of examination, the following ***body areas*** are recognized:

- Head, including the face
- Neck
- Chest, including breasts and axillae
- Abdomen
- Genitalia, groin, buttocks
- Back, including spine
- Each extremity

For purpose of examination, the following ***organ systems*** are recognized:

- Constitutional (e.g., vital signs, general appearance)
- Eyes
- Ears, nose, mouth and throat
- Cardiovascular
- Respiratory
- Gastrointestinal
- Genitourinary
- Musculoskeletal
- Skin
- Neurologic
- Psychiatric
- Hematologic/lymphatic/immunologic

The extent of examinations performed and documented is dependent upon clinical judgement and the nature of the presenting problem(s). They range from limited examination of single body areas to general multi-system or complete single organ system examinations.

- DG: Specific abnormal and relevant negative findings of the examination of the affected or symptomatic body area(s) or organ system(s) should be documented. A notation of "abnormal" without elaboration is insufficient.
- DG: Abnormal or unexpected findings of the examination of the unaffected or asymptomatic body area(s) or organ system(s) should be described.
- DG: A brief statement or notation indication "negative" or "normal" is sufficient to document normal findings related to unaffected area(s) or asymptomatic organ system(s).
- DG: The medical record for a general multi-system examination should include findings about 8 or more of the 12 organ systems.

C. Documentation of the Complexity of Medical Decision making

The levels of E/M services recognize four types of medical decision making (straight-forward, low complexity, moderate complexity and high complexity). Medical decision making refers to the complexity of establishing a diagnosis and/or selecting a management option as measured by:

- the number of possible diagnoses and/or the number of management options that must be considered;
- the amount and/or complexity of medical records, diagnostic tests, and/or other information that must be obtained, reviewed and analyzed; and
- the risk of significant complications, morbidity and/or mortality, as well as comorbidities, associated with the patient's presenting problem(s), the diagnostic procedure(s) and/or the possible management options.

The chart below shows the progression of the elements required for each level of medical decision-making. To qualify for a given decision-making, **two of the three elements in the table must be either met or exceeded.**

Number of diagnoses or management options	Amount and/or complexity of data to be reviewed	Risk of complications and/or morbidity or mortality	Type of decision making
Minimal	Minimal or None	Minimal	***Straightforward***
Limited	Limited	Low	***Low Complexity***
Multiple	Moderate	Moderate	***Moderate Complexity***
Extensive	Extensive	High	***High Complexity***

Each of the elements of medical decision making is described below.

Number of Diagnoses or Management Options. The number of possible diagnoses and/or the number of management options that must be considered is based on the number and types of problems addressed during the encounter, the complexity of establishing a diagnosis and the management decisions that are made by the physician.

Generally, decision making with respect to a diagnosed problem is easier than that for an identified but undiagnosed problem. The number and type of diagnostic tests employed may be an indicator of the number of possible diagnoses. Problems which are improving or resolving are less complex than those which are worsening or failing to change as expected. The need to seek advice from others is another indicator of complexity or management problems.

- DG: For each encounter, an assessment, clinical impression, or diagnosis should be documented. It may be explicitly stated or implied in documented decisions regarding management plans and/or further evaluation.
  - For a presenting problem with an established diagnosis the record should reflect whether the problem is: a) improved, well controlled, resolving or resolved; or, b) inadequately controlled, worsening, or failing to change as expected.
  - For a presenting problem without an established diagnosis, the assessment or clinical impression may be stated in the form of a differential diagnoses or as "possible", "probable", or "rule out" (R/O) diagnoses.
- DG: The initiation of, or changes in, treatment should be documented. Treatment includes a wide range of management options including patient instructions, nursing instructions, therapies, and medications.
- DG: If referrals are made, consultations requested or advice sought, the record should indicate to whom or where the referral or consultation is made or from whom the advice is requested.

Amount and/or Complexity of Data to be Reviewed. The amount and complexity of data to be reviewed is based on the types of diagnostic testing ordered or reviewed. A decision to obtain and review old medical records and/or obtain history form sources other than the patient increases the amount and complexity of data to be reviewed.

Discussion of contradictory or unexpected test results with the physician who performed or interpreted the test is an indication of the complexity of data being reviewed. On occasion the physician who ordered a test may personally review the image, tracing or specimen to supplement information form the physician who prepared the test report or interpretation; this is another indication of the complexity of data being reviewed.

- DG: If a diagnostic service (test or procedure) is ordered, planned, scheduled, or performed at the time of the E/M encounter, the type of service, e.g., lab or x-ray, should be documented.
- DG: The review of lab, radiology and/or other diagnostic tests should be documented. An entry in a progress note such as "WBC elevated" or "chest x-ray unremarkable" is acceptable. Alternatively, the review may be documented by initialing and dating the report containing the test results.
- DG: A decision to obtain old record or decision to obtain additional history from the family, caretaker or other source to supplement that obtained from the patient should be documented.
- DG: Relevant finding form the review of old records, and/or the receipt of additional history from the family, caretaker or other source should be documented. If there is no relevant information beyond that already obtained, that fact should be documented. A notation of "Old records reviewed" or "additional history obtained from family" without elaboration is insufficient.
- DG: The results of discussion of laboratory, radiology or other diagnostic tests with the physician who performed or interpreted the study should be documented.
- DG: The direct visualization and independent interpretation of an image, tracing or specimen previously or subsequently interpreted by another physician should be documented.

Risk of Significant Complications, Morbidity, and/or Mortality. The risk of significant complications, morbidity, and/or mortality is based on the risks associated with the presenting problem(s), the diagnostic procedure(s), and the possible management options.

- DG: Comorbidities/underlying diseases or other factors that increase the complexity of medical decision making by increasing the risk of complications, morbidity, and/or mortality should be documented.
- DG: If a surgical or invasive diagnostic procedure is ordered, planned or scheduled at the time of the E/M encounter, the type of procedure, e.g., Laparoscopy, should be documented.
- DG: If a surgical or invasive diagnostic procedure is performed at the time of the E/M encounter, the specific procedure should be documented.
- DG: The referral for or decision to perform a surgical or invasive diagnostic procedure on an urgent basis should be documented or implied.

The following table may be used to help determine whether the risk of significant complications, morbidity, and/or mortality is **minimal, low, moderate,** or **high**. Because the determination of risk is complex and not readily quantifiable, the table includes common clinical examples rather than absolute measures of risk. The assessment of risk of the presenting problem(s) is based on the risk related to the disease process anticipated between the present encounter and the next one. The assessment of risk of selecting diagnostic procedures and management options is based on the risk during and immediately following any procedures or treatment. The highest level of risk in any one category (presenting problem(s), diagnostic procedure(s), or management options) determines the overall risk.

TABLE OF RISK

Level of Risk	Presenting Problem(s)	Diagnostic Procedure(s) Ordered	Management Options Selected
Minimal	• One self-limited or minor problem, eg cold, insect bite, tinea corporis	• Laboratory tests requiring venipuncture • Chest x-rays • EKG/EEG • Urinalysis • Ultrasound, eg, echocardiography • KOH prep	• Rest • Gargles • Elastic bandages • Superficial dressings
Low	• Two or more self-limited or minor problems • One stable chronic illness, eg well controlled hypertension or non-insulin dependent diabetes, cataract, BPH • Acute uncomplicated illness or injury, eg, cystitis, allergic rhinitis, simple sprain	• Physiologic tests not under stress, eg, pulmonary function tests • Non-cardiovascular imaging studies with contrast, eg, barium enema • Superficial needle biopsies • Clinical laboratory tests requiring arterial puncture • Skin biopsies	• Over-the-counter drugs • Minor surgery with no identified risk factors • Physical therapy • Occupational therapy • IV fluids without additives
Moderate	• One or more chronic illnesses with mild exacerbation, progression, or side effects of treatment • Two or more stable chronic illnesses • Undiagnosed new problem with uncertain prognosis, eg, lump in breast • Acute illness with systemic symptoms, eg, pyelonephritis, pneumonitis, colitis • Acute complicated injury, eg head injury with brief loss of consciousness	• Physiologic tests under stress, eg, cardiac stress test, fetal contraction stress test • Diagnostic endoscopies with no identified risk factors • Deep needle or incisional biopsy • Cardiovascular imaging studies with contrast and no identified risk factors, eg arteriogram, cardiac catheterization • Obtain fluid form body cavity, eg lumbar puncture, thoracentesis, culdocentesis	• Minor surgery with identified risk factors • Elective major surgery (open percutaneous or endoscopic) with no identified risk factors • Prescription drug management • Therapeutic nuclear medicine • IV fluids with additives • Closed treatment of fracture or dislocation without manipulation
High	• One or more chronic illness with severe exacerbation, progression, or side effects of treatment • Acute or chronic illnesses or injuries that pose a threat to life or bodily function, eg multiple trauma, acute MI, pulmonary embolus, severe respiratory distress, progressive severe rheumatoid arthritis, psychiatric illness with potential threat to self or others, peritonitis, acute renal failure • An abrupt change in neurologic status, eg seizure, TIA, weakness, or sensory loss	• Cardiovascular imaging studies with contrast with identified risk factors cardiac electrophysiological tests • Diagnostic Endoscopies with identified risk factors • Discography	• Elective major surgery (open percutaneous or endoscopic) with identified risk factors • Emergency major surgery (open, percutaneous or endoscopic) • Parenteral controlled substances • Drug therapy requiring intensive monitoring for toxicity • Decision not to resuscitate or to de-escalate care because of poor prognosis

D. Documentation of an Encounter Dominated by Counseling or Coordination of Care

In the case where counseling and/or coordination of care dominates (more than 50%) of the physician/patient and/or family encounter (face-to-face time in the office or other outpatient setting or floor/unit time in the hospital or nursing facility), time is considered the key or controlling factors to qualify for a particular level of E/M services.

- DG: If the physician elects to report the level of service based on counseling and/or coordination of care, the total length of time of the encounter (face-to-face or floor time, as appropriate) should be documented and the record should describe the counseling and/or activities to coordinate care.

Appendix E, Part 2

Documentation Guidelines for Evaluation and Management Services*

Table of Contents

*Developed jointly by the American Medical Association (AMA) and the Health Care Financing Adminitration (HCFA).

1. INTRODUCTION

What Is Documentation and Why Is It Important?

Medical record documentation is required to record pertinent facts, findings, and observations about an individual's health history including past and present illnesses, examinations, tests, treatments, and outcomes. The medical record chronologically documents the care of the patient and is an important element contributing to high quality care. The medical record facilitates:

- the ability of the physician and other health care professionals to evaluate and plan the patient's immediate treatment, and to monitor his/her health care over time
- communication and continuity of care among physicians and other health care professionals involved in the patient's care;
- accurate and timely claims review and payment;
- appropriate utilization review and quality of care evaluations; and
- collection of data that may be useful for research and education.

An appropriately documented medical record can reduce many of the "hassles" associated with claims processing and may serve as a legal document to verify the care provided, if necessary.

What Do Payers Want and Why?

Because payers have a contractual obligation to enrolees, they may require reasonable documentation that services are consistent with the insurance coverage provided. They may request information to validate:

- the site of service;
- the medical necessity and appropriateness of the diagnostic and/or therapeutic services provided; and/or
- that services provided have been accurately reported.

II. GENERAL PRINCIPLES OF MEDICAL RECORD DOCUMENTATION

The principles of documentation listed below are applicable to all types of medical and surgical services in all settings. For Evaluation and Management (E/M) services, the nature and amount of physician work and documentation varies by type of service, place of service and the patient's status. The following list of general principles may be modified to account for these variable circumstances in providing E/M services.

1. The medical record should be complete and legible.
2. The documentation of each patient encounter should include:
   - reason for the encounter and relevant history, physical examination findings and prior diagnostic test results;
   - assessment, clinical impression or diagnosis;
   - plan for care; and
   - date and legible identity of the observer.
3. If not documented, the rationale for ordering diagnostic and other ancillary services should be easily inferred.
4. Past and present diagnoses shoulod be accessible to the treating and/or consulting physician.
5. Appropriate health risk factors should be identified.
6. The patient's progress, response to and changes in treatment, and revision of diagnosis should be documented.
7. The CPT and ICD-9-CM codes reported on the health insurance claim form or billing statement should be supported by the documentation in the medical record.

III. DOCUMENTATION OF E/M SERVICES

This publication provides definitions and documentation guidelines for the three key components of E/M services and for visits which consist predominantly of counseling or coordination of care. The three *key* components—history, examination, and medical decision making—appear in the descriptors for office and other outpatient services, hospital observation services, hospital inpatient services, consultations, emergency department services, nursing facility services, domiciliary care services, and home services. While some of the text of CPT has been repeated in this publication, the reader should refer to CPT for the complete descriptors for E/M services and instructions for selecting a level of service. Documentation guidelines are identified by the symbol • *DG*

The descriptors for the levels of E/M services recognize seven components which are used in defining the levels of E/M services. These components are:

- history;
- examination;
- medical decision making;
- counseling;
- coordination of care;
- nature of presenting problem; and
- time.

The first three of these components (i.e., history, examination and medical decision making) are the key components in selecting the level of E/M services. In the case of visits which consist *predominantly* of counseling or coordination of care, time is the key or controlling factor to qualify for a particular level of E/M service.

Because the level of E/M service is dependent on two or three key components, performance and documentation of one component (e.g., examination) at the highest level does not necessarily mean that the encounter in its entirety qualifies for the highest level of E/M service.

These Documentation Guidelines for E/M services reflect the needs of the typical adult population. For certain groups of patients, the recorded information may vary slightly from that described here. Specifically, the medical records of infants, children, adolescents and pregnant women may have additional or modified information recorded in each history and examination area.

As an example, newborn records may include under history of the present illness (HPI) the details of mother's pregnancy and the infant's status at birth; social history will focus on family structure; family history will focus on congenital anomalies and hereditary disorders in the family. In addition, the content of pediatric examination will vary with the age and development of the child. Although not specifically defined in these documentation guidelines, these patient group variations on history and examination are appropriate.

A. Documentation of History

The levels of E/M services are based on four types of history (Problem Focused, Expanded Problem Focused, Detailed, and Comprehensive). Each type of history includes some or all of the following elements:

- Chief complaint (CC);
- History of present illness (HPI);
- Review of systems (ROS); and
- Past, family and/or social history (PFSH).

The extent of history or present illness, review of systems and past, family and/or social history that is obtained and documented is dependent upon clinical judgement and the nature of the presenting problem(s).

The chart below shows the progression of the elements required for each type of history. To qualify for a given type of history all three elements in the table must be met. (A chief complaint is indicated at all levels.)

History of present Illness	Review of Systems (ROS)	Past, Family, and/or Social History	Type of History
Brief	N/A	N/A	Problem Focused
Brief	Problem Pertinent	N/A	Expanded Problem Focused
Extended	Extended	Pertinent	Detailed
Extended	Complete	Complete	Comprehensive

- DG: The CC, ROS, and PFSH may be listed as separate elements of history, or they may be included in the description of the history of the present illness.
- DG: A ROS and/or a PFSH obtained during an earlier encounter does not need to be re-recorded if there is evidence that the physician reviewed and updated the previous information. This may occur when a physician updates his or her own record or in an institutional setting or group practice where many physicians use a common record. The review and update may be documented by:
  - describing any new ROS and/or PFSH information or noting there has been no change in the information; and
  - noting the date and location of the earlier ROS and/or PFSH.
- DG: The ROS and/or PFSH may be recorded by ancillary staff or on a form completed by the patient. To document that the physician reviewed the information, there must be a notation supplementing or confirming the information recorded by others.
- DG: If the physician is unable to obtain a history from the patient or other source, the record should describe the patient's condition or other circumstance which precludes obtaining a history.

Definitions and specific documentation guidelines for each of the elements of history are in the following list.

Chief Complaint (CC). The CC is a concise statement describing the symptom, problem, condition, diagnosis, physician recommended return, or other factor that is the reason for the encounter, usually stated in the patient's words.

- DG: The medical record should clearly reflect the chief complaint.

History of Present Illness (HPI). The HPI is a chronological description of the development of the patient's present illness from the first sign and/or symptom or from the previous encounter to the present. It includes the following elements:

- location,
- quality,
- severity,
- duration,
- timing,
- context,
- modifying factors, and
- associated signs and symptoms.

Brief and *extended* HPIs are distinguished by the amount of detail needed to accurately characterize the clinical problem(s).

A *brief* HPI consists of one to three elements of the HPI.

- DG: The medical record should describe one to three elements of the present illness (HPI).

An *extended* HPI consists of at least four elements of the HPI or the status of at least three chronic or inactive conditions.

- DG: The medical record should describe at least four elements of the present illness (HPI), or the status of at least three chronic or inactive conditions.

Review of Systems (ROS). A ROS is and inventory of body systems obtained through a series of questions seeking to identify signs and/or symptoms which the patient may be experiencing or has experienced.

For purposes of ROS, the following systems are recognized:

- Constitutional symptoms (e.g., fever, weight loss)
- Eyes
- Ears, Nose, Mouth, Throat
- Cardiovascular
- Respiratory
- Gastrointestinal
- Genitourinary
- Musculoskeletal
- Integumentary (skin and/or breast)
- Neurological
- Psychiatric
- Endocrine
- Hematologic/Lymphatic
- Allergic/Immunologic

A *problem pertinent* ROS inquires about the system directly related to the problem(s) identified in the HPI.

- DG: The patient's positive responses and pertinent negatives for the system related to the problem should be documented.

An *extended* ROS inquires about the system directly related to the problem(s) identified in the HPI and a limited number of additional systems.

- DG: The patient's positive responses and pertinent negatives for two to nine systems should be documented.

A *complete* ROS inquires about the system(s) directly related to the problem(s) identified in the HPI *plus* all additional body systems.

- DG: At least ten organs systems must be reviewed. Those systems with positive or pertinent negative responses must be individually documented. For the remaining systems, a notation indicating all other systems are negative is permissible. In the absence of such a notation, at least ten systems must be individually documented.

Past, Family and/or Social History (PFSH). The PFSH consists of a review of three areas:

- past history (the patient's past experiences with illnesses, operations, injuries and treatments);
- family history (a review of medical events in the patient's family, including diseases which may be hereditary or place the patient at risk); and
- social history (an age appropriate review of past and current activities).

For certain categories of E/M services that include only an interval history, it is not necessary to record information about the PFSH. Those categories are subsequent hospital care, follow-up inpatient consultations and subsequent nursing facility care.

A *pertinent* PFSH is a review of the history area(s) directly related to the problem(s) identified in the HPI.

- DG: At least one specific item from any of the three history areas must be documented for a pertinent PFSH.

A *complete* PFSH is a review of two or all three of the PFSH history areas, depending on the category of the E/M service. A review of all three history areas is required for services that by their nature include a comprehensive assessment or reassessment of the patient. A review of two of the three history areas is sufficient for other services.

- DG: At least one specific item from two of the three history areas must be documented for a complete PFSH for the following categories of E/M services: office or other outpatient services, established patient; emergency department; domiciliary care, established patient; and home care, established patient.
- DG: At least one specific item from each of the three history areas must be documented for a complete PFSH for the following categories of E/M services: office or other outpatient services, new patient; hospital observation services; hospital inpatient services, initial care; consultations; comprehensive nursing facility assessments; domiciliary care, new patient; and home care, new patient.

B. Documentation of Examination

The levels of E/M services are based on four types of examination:

- *Problem focused*—a limited examination of the affected body area or organ system.
- *Expanded problem focused*—a limited examination of the affected body area or organ system and any other symptomatic or related body area(s) or organ system(s).
- *Detailed*—an extended examination of the affected body area(s) or organ system(s) and any other symptomatic or related body area(s) or organ system(s).
- *Comprehensive*—a general multi-system examination, or complete examination of a single organ system and other symptomatic or related body area(s) or organ system(s).

These types of examinations have been defined for general multi-system and the following single organ systems:

- Cardiovascular
- Ears, Nose, Mouth and Throat
- Eyes
- Genitourinary (Female)
- Genitourinary (Male)
- Hematologic/Lymphatic/Immunologic
- Musculoskeletal
- Neurological
- Psychiatric
- Respiratory
- Skin

A general multi-system examination or a single organ system examination may be performed by any physician regardless of specialty. The type (general multi-system or single organ system) and content of examination are selected by the examining physician and are based upon clinical judgment, the patient's history, and the nature of the presenting problem(s).

The content and documentation requirements for each type and level of examination are summarized following and described in detail in Chapter 1. In the tables, organ systems and body areas recognized by CPT for purposes of describing examinations are shown in the left column. The content, or individual elements, of the examination pertaining to that body area or organ system are identified by bullets (•) in the right column.

Parenthetical examples, "(e.g.,...)," have been used for clarification and to provide guidance regarding documentation. Documentation for each element must satisfy any numeric requirements (such as "Measurement of *any three of the following seven*...") included in the description of the element. Elements with multiple components but with no specific numeric requirement (such as "Examination of *liver* and *spleen*") require documentation of at least one component. It is possible for a given examination to be expanded beyond what is defined here. When that occurs, findings related to the additional systems and/or areas should be documented.

- DG: Specific abnormal and relevant negative findings of the examination of the affected or symptomatic body area(s) or organ system(s) should be documented. A notation of "abnormal" without elaboration is insufficient.
- DG: Abnormal or unexpected findings of the examination of any asymptomatic body area(s) or organ systems(s) should be described.
- DG: A brief statement or notation indicating "negative" or "normal" is sufficient to document normal findings related to unaffected area(s) or asymptomatic organs system(s).

General Multi-System Examinations. General multi-system examinations are described in detail beginning on page 571. To qualify for a given level of multi-system examination, the following content and documentation requirements should be met:

- *Problem Focused Examination*—should include performance and documentation of one to five elements identified by a bullet (•) in one or more organ system(s) or body area(s).
- *Expanded Problem Focused Examination*—should include performance and documentation of at least six elements identified by a bullet (•) is one or more organ system(s) or body area(s).
- *Detailed Examination*—should include at least six organ systems or body areas. For each system/area selected, performance and documentation of at least two elements identified by a bullet (•) is expected. Alternatively, a detailed examination may include performance and documentation of at least twelve elements identified by a bullet (•) in two or more organ systems or body areas.
- *Comprehensive Examination*—should include at least nine organ systems or body areas. For each system/area selected, all elements of the examination identified by a bullet (•) should be performed, unless specific directions limit the content of the examination. For each area/system, documentation of at least two elements identified by a bullet is expected.

Single Organ System Examinations. The single organ system examinations recognized by CPT are described in detail beginning on page 574. Variations among these examinations in the organ systems and body areas identified in the left columns and in the elements of the examinations described in the right columns reflect differing emphases among specialties. To qualify for a given level of single organ system examination, the following content and documentation requirements should be met:

- *Problem Focused Examination*—should include performance and documentation of one to five elements identified by a bullet (•), whether in a box with a shaded or unshaded border.
- *Expanded Problem Focused Examination*—should include performance and documentation of at least six elements identified by a bullet (•), whether in a box with shaded or unshaded border.
- *Detailed Examination*—examinations other than the eye and psychiatric examinations should include performance and documentation of at least twelve elements identified by a bullet (•), whether in box with a shaded or unshaded border.
  Eye and psychiatric examinations should include the performance and documentation of at least nine elements identified by a bullet (•), whether in a box with a shaded or unshaded border.
- *Comprehensive Examination*—should include performance of all elements identified by a bullet (•), whether in a shaded or unshaded box. Documentation of every element in each box with a shaded border and at least one element in each box with an unshaded border is expected.

Content and Document Requirements

GENERAL MULTI-SYSTEM EXAMINATION

System/Body Area	Elements of Examination
Constitutional	• Measurement of any three of the following seven vital signs: 1) sitting or standing pressure, 2) supine blood pressure, 3) pulse rate and regularity, 4) respiration, 5) temperature, 6) height 7) weight (may be measured and recorded by ancillary staff) • General appearance of patient (eg, development, nutrition, body habitus, deformities, attention to grooming)
Eyes	• Inspection of conjunctivae and lids • Examination of pupils and irises (eg, reaction to light and accommodation, size and symmetry) • Opthalmoscopic examination of optic discs (eg, size, C/D ratio, appearance) and posterior segments (eg, vessel changes, exudates, hemorrhages)
Ears, Nose, Mouth and Throat	• External inspection of ears and nose (eg, overall appearance, scars, lesions, masses) • Otoscopic examination of external auditory canals and tympanic membranes • Assessment of hearing (eg, whispered voice, finger rub, tuning fork) • Inspection of nasal mucosa, septum and turbinates • Inspection of lips, teeth and gums • Examination of oropharynx: oral mucosa, salivary glands, hard and soft palates, tongue, tonsils and posterior pharynx
Neck	• Examination of neck (eg, masses, overall appearance, symmetry, tracheal position, crepitus) • Examination of thyroid (eg, enlargement, tenderness, mass)
Respiratory	• Assessment of respiratory effort (eg, intercostal retractions, use of accessory muscles, diaphragmatic movement • Percussions of chest (eg, dullness, flatness, hyperresonance) • Palpation of chest (eg, tactile fremitus) • Ausculatation of lungs (eg, breath sounds, adventitious sounds, rubs)
Cardiovascular	• Palpation of heart (eg, location, size, thrills) • Ausculatation of heart with notation of abnormal sounds and murmurs Examination of: • carotid arteries (eg, pulse amplitude, bruits) • abdominal aorta (eg, size, bruits) • femoral arteries (eg, pulse amplitude, bruits) • pedal pulses (eg, pulse amplitude) • extremities for edema and/or varicosities
Chest (Breasts)	• Inspection of breasts (eg, symmetry nipple discharge) • Palpation of breasts and axillae (eg, masses or lumps, tenderness)
Gastrointestinal (Abdomen)	• Examination of abdomen with notation of presence of masses or tenderness • Examination of liver and spleen • Examination for presence or absence of hernia • Examination (when indicated) of anus, perineum and rectum, including sphincter tone, presence of hemorrhoids, rectal masses • Obtain stool sample for occult blood test when indicated
Genitourinary	**Male:** • Examination of the scrotal content (eg, hydrocele, spermatocele, tenderness of cord, testicular mass) • Examination of the penis • Digital rectal examination of prostate gland (eg, size, symmetry, nodularity, tenderness)

Continued

GENERAL MULTI-SYSTEM EXAMINATION—Cont'd

System/Body Area	Elements of Examination
	Female: Pelvic examination (with or without specimen collection for smears and cultures), including • Examination of external genitalia (eg, general appearance, hair distribution, lesions) and vagina (eg, general appearance, estrogen effect, discharge, lesions, pelvic support, cystocele, rectocele) • Examination of urethra (eg, masses, tenderness, scarring) • Examination of bladder (eg, fullness, masses, tenderness) • Cervix (eg, general appearance, lesions, discharge) • Uterus (eg, size, contour, position, mobility, tenderness, consistency, descent or support) • Adnexa/parametria (eg, masses, tenderness, organomegaly, nodularity)
Lymphatic	Palpation of lymph nodes in two or more areas: • Neck • Axillae • Groin • Other
Musculoskeletal	• Examination of gait and station • Inspection and/or palpation of digits and nails (eg, clubbing, cyanosis,) inflammatory conditions, petechiae, ischemia, infections, nodes Examination of joints, bones and muscles of one or more of the following six areas: 1) head and neck; 2) spine, ribs and pelvis; 3) right upper extremity; 4) left upper extremity; 5) right lower extremity; and 6) left lower extremity. The examination of a given area includes: • Inspection and/or palpation with notation of presence of any misalignment, asymmetry, crepitation, defects, tenderness, masses, effusions • Assessment of range of motion with notation of any pain, crepitation or contracture • Assessment of stability with notation of any dislocation (luxation), subluxation or laxity • Assessment of muscle strength and tone (eg, flaccid, cog wheel, spastic) with notation of any atrophy or abnormal movements
Skin	• Inspection of skin and subcutaneous tissue (eg, rashes, lesions, ulcers) • Palpation of skin and subcutaneous tissue (eg, induration, subcutaneous nodules, tightening)
Neurologic	• Test cranial nerves with notation of any deficits • Examination of deep tendon reflexes with notation of pathological reflexes (eg, Babinski) • Examination of sensation (eg, by touch, pin, vibration, proprioception)
Psychiatric	• Description of patient's judgment and insight Brief assessment of mental status including: • orientation to time, place and person • recent and remote memory • mood and affect (eg, depression, anxiety, agitation)

Content and Documentation Requirements

Level of Exam	Perform and Document
Problem Focused	One to five elements identified by a bullet.
Expanded Problem Focused	At least six elements identified by a bullet.
Detailed	At least two elements identified by a bullet from each of six areas/systems OR at least twelve elements identifted by a bullet in two or more areas/systems.
Comprehensive	Perform all elements identified by a bullet in at least nine organ systems or body areas and document at least two elements identified by a bullet from each of nine areas/systems.

CARDIOVASCULAR EXAMINATION

System/Body Area	Elements of Examination
Constitutional	• Measurement of any three of the following seven vital signs: 1) sitting or standing blood pressure, 2) supine blood pressure, 3) pulse rate and regularity, 4) respiration, 5) temperature, 6) height, 7) weight (may be measured and recorded by ancillary staff) • General appearance of patient (eg, development, nutrition, body habitus, deformities, attention to grooming)
Head and Face	
Eyes	• Inspection of conjunctivae and lids (eg, xanthelasma)
Ears, Nose, Mouth and Throat	• Inspection of teeth, gums and palate • Inspection of oral mucosa with notation of presence of pallor or cyanosis
Neck	Examination of jugular veins (eg, distension; a, v or cannon a waves) • Examination of thyroid (eg, enlargement, tenderness, mass)
Respiratory	• Assessment of respiratory effort (eg, intercostal retractions, use of accessory muscles, diaphragmatic movement) • Auscultation of lungs (eg, breath sounds, adventitious sounds, rubs)
Cardiovascular	• Palpation of heart (eg, location, size and forcefulness of the point of maximal impact; thrills; lifts; palpable S3 or S4) • Auscultation of heart including sounds, abnormal sounds and murmurs • Measurement of blood pressure in two or more extremities when indicated (eg, aortic dissection, coarctation)

Continued

CARDIOVASCULAR EXAMINATION—Cont'd

System/Body Area	Elements of Examination
	Examination of: • Carotid arteries (eg, waveform, pulse amplitude, bruits, apical-carotid delay) • Abdominal aorta (eg, size, bruits) • Femoral arteries (eg, pulse amplitude, bruits) • Pedal pulses (eg, pulse amplitude) • Extremities for peripheral edema and/or varicosities
Chest (Breasts)	
Gastrointestinal (Abdomen)	• Examination of abdomen with notation of presence of masses or Tenderness • Examination of liver and spleen • Obtain stool sample for occult blood from patients who are being considered for thrombolytic or anticoagulant therapy
Genitounnary (Abdomen)	
Lymphatic	
Musculoskeletal	• Examination of the back with notation of kyphosis or scoliosis • Examination of gait with notation of ability to undergo exercise testing and/or participation in exercise programs • Assessment of muscle strength and tone (eg, flaccid, cog wheel, spastic) with notation of any atrophy and abnormal movements
Extremities	• Inspection and palpation of digits and nails (eg, clubbing, cyanosis, inflammation, petechiae, ischemia, infections, Osler's nodes)
Skin	• Inspection and/or palpation of skin and subcutaneous tissue (eg, stasis dermatitis, ulcers, scars, xanthomas)
Neurologic/ Psychiatric	Brief assessment of mental status including • Orientation to time, place and person • Mood and affect (eg, depression, anxiety, agitation)

Content and Documentation Requirements

Level of Exam	Perform and Document
Problem Focused	One to five elements identified by a bullet.
Expanded Problem Focused	At least six elements identified by a bullet.
Detailed	At least twelve elements identified by a bullet.
Comprehensive	Perform all elements identified by a bullet; document every element in each box with a shaded border and at least one element in each box with an unshaded border.

EARS, NOSE AND THROAT EXAMINATION

System/Body Area	Elements of Examination
Constitutional	• Measurement of any three of the following seven vital signs: 1) sitting or standing blood pressure, 2) supine blood pressure, 3) pulse rate and regularity, 4) respiration, *5)* temperature, 6) height, 7) weight (may be measured and recorded by ancillary staff) • General appearance of patient (eg, development, nutrition, body habitus, deformities, attention to grooming) • Assessment of ability to communicate (eg, use of sign language or other communication aids) and quality of voice
Head and Face	• Inspection of head and face (eg, overall appearance, scars, lesions and masses) • Palpation and/or percussion of face with notation of presence or absence of sinus tenderness • Examination of salivary glands • Assessment of facial strength
Eyes	• Test ocular motility including primary gaze alignment
Ears, Nose, Mouth and Throat	• Otoscopic examination of external auditory canals and tympanic membranes including pneumo-otoscopy with notation of mobility of membranes • Assessment of hearing with tuning forks and clinical speech reception thresholds (eg, whispered voice, finger rub) • External inspection of ears and nose (eg, overall appearance, scars, lesions and masses) • Inspection of nasal mucosa, septum and turbinates • Inspection of lips, teeth and gums • Examination of oropharynx: oral mucosa, hard and soft palates, tongue, tonsils and posterior pharynx (eg, asymmetry, lesions, hydration of mucosal surfaces) • Inspection of pharyngeal walls and pyriform sinuses (eg, pooling of saliva, asymmetry, lesions) • Examination by mirror of larynx including the condition of the epiglottis, false vocal cords, true vocal cords and mobility of larynx (use of mirror not required in children) • Examination by mirror of nasopharynx including appearance of the mucosa, adenoids, posterior choanae and eustachian tubes (use of mirror not required in children)
Neck	• Examination of neck (eg, masses, overall appearance, symmetry, tracheal position. crepitus) • Examination of thyroid (eg, enlargement, tenderness, mass)
Respiratory	• Inspection of chest including symmetry expansion and/or assessment of respiratory effort (eg, intercostal retractions, use of accessory muscles, diaphragmatic movement) • Auscultation of lungs (eg, breath sounds, adventitious sounds, rubs)

Continued

EARS, NOSE AND THROAT EXAMINATION—Cont'd

System/Body Area	Elements of Examination
Cardiovascular	• Auscultation of heart with notation of abnormal sounds and murmurs • Examination of peripheral vascular system by observation (eg, swelling, varicosities) and palpation (eg, pulses, temperature, edema, tenderness)
Chest (Breasts)	
Gastrointestinal (Abdomen)	
Genitourinary	
Lymphatic	• Palpation of lymph nodes in neck, axillae, groin and/or other location
Musculoskeletal	
Extremities	
Skin	
Neurological/Psychiatric	• Test cranial nerves with notation of any deficits Brief assessment of mental status including • Orientation to time, place and person • Mood and affect (eg, depression, anxiety, agitation)

Content and Documentation Requirements

Level of Exam	Perform and Document
Problem Focused	One to five elements identified by a bullet.
Expanded Problem Focused	At least six elements identified by a bullet.
Detailed	At least twelve elements identified by a bullet.
Comprehensive	Perform all elements identified by a bullet; document every element in each box with a shaded border and at least one element in each box with an unshaded borde.

EYE EXAMINATION

System/Body Area	Elements of Examination
Constitutional	
Head and Face	
Eyes	• Test visual acuity (does not include determination of refractive error) • Gross visual field testing by confrontation • Test ocular motility including primary gaze alignment • Inspection of bulbar and palpebral conjunctivae • Examination of ocular adnexae including lids (eg, ptosis or lagophthalmos), lacrimal glands, lacrimal drainage, orbits and preauricular lymph nodes • Examination of pupils and irises including shape, direct and consensual reaction (afferent pupil), size (eg, anisocoria) and morphology • Slit lamp examination of the corneas including epithelium, stroma, endothelium, and tear film • Slit lamp examination of the anterior chambers including depth, cells, and flare • Slit lamp examination of the lenses including clarity, anterior and posterior capsule, cortex, and nucleus • Measurement of intraocular pressures (except in children and patients with trauma or infectious disease) • Ophthalmoscopic examination through dilated pupils (unless contraindicated) of • Optic discs including size, C/D ratio, appearance (eg, atrophy, cupping, tumor elevation) and nerve fiber layer • Posterior segments including retina and vessels (eg, exudates and hemorrhages)
Ears, Nose, Mouth and Throat	
Neck	
Respiratory	
Cardiovascular	
Chest (Breasts)	
Gastrointestinal (Abdomen)	
Genitourinary	
Lymphatic	
Musculoskeletal	
Extremities	
Skin	
Neurological/Psychiatric	Brief assessment of mental status including • Orientation to time, place and person • Mood and affect (eg, depression, anxiety, agitation)

Content and Documentation Requirements

Level of Exam	Perform and Document
Problem focused	One to five elements identified by a bullet.
Expanded Problem Focused	At least six elements identified by a bullet.
Detailed	At least nine elements identified by a bullet.
Comprehensive	Perform all elements identified by a bullet; document every element in each box with shaded border and at least one element in each box with an unshaded border.

GENITOURINARY EXAMINATION

System/body Area	Elements of Examination
Constitutional	• Measurement of **any three of the following seven** vital signs: 1) sitting or standing blood pressure, 2) supine blood pressure, 3) pulse rate and regularity, 4) respiration, 5) temperature, 6) height, 7) weight (may be measured and recorded by ancillary staff) • General appearance of patient (eg, development, nutrition, body habitus, deformities, attention to grooming)
Head and Face	
Eyes	
Ears, Nose, Mouth and Throat	
Neck	• Examination of neck (eg, masses, overall appearance, symmetry, tracheal position, crepitus) • Examination of thyroid (eg, enlargement, tenderness, mass)
Respiratory	• Assessment of respiratory effort (eg, intercostal retractions, use of accessory muscles, diaphragmatic movement) • Auscultation of lungs (eg, breath sounds, adventitious sounds rubs)
Cardiovascular	• Auscultation of heart with notation of abnormal sounds and murmurs • Examination of peripheral vascular system by observation (eg, swelling, varicosities) and palpation (eg, pulses, temperature, edema, tenderness)
Chest (Breasts)	[see genitourinary (female).]
Gastrointestinal (Abdomen)	• Examination of abdomen with notation of presence of masses or tenderness • Examination for presence or absence of hernia • Examination of liver and spleen • Obtain stool sample for occult blood test when indicated
Genitourinary	**Male:** • Inspection of anus and perineum Examination (with or without specimen collection for smears and cultures) of genitalia including: • Scrotum (eg, lesions, cysts, rashes) • Epididymides (eg, size, symmetry, masses) • Testes (eg, size symmetry, masses) • Urethral meatus (eg, size, location, lesions, discharge) • Penis (eg, lesions, presence or absence of foreskin, foreskin retractability, plaque, masses, scarring, deformities) Digital rectal examination including: • Prostate gland (eg, size, symmetry, nodularity, tenderness) • Seminal vesicles (eg, symmetry, tenderness, masses, enlargement) • Sphincter tone, presence of hemorrhoids, rectal masses **Female:** Include **at least seven of the following** eleven elements identified by bullets: • Inspection and palpation of breasts (eg, masses or lumps, tenderness, symmetry, nipple discharge) • Digital rectal examination including sphincter tone, presence of hemorrhoids, rectal masses Pelvic examination (with or without specimen collection for smears and cultures) including: • External genitalia (eg, general appearance, hair distribution, lesions) • Urethral meatus (eg, size, location, lesions, prolapse) • Urethra (eg, masses, tenderness, scarring) • Bladder (eg, fullness, masses, tenderness) • Vagina (eg, general appearance, estrogen effect, discharge, lesions, pelvic support, cystocele, rectocele) • Cervix (eg, general appearance, lesions, discharge) • Uterus (eg, size, contour, position, mobility, tenderness, consistency, decent or support) • Adnexa/parametria (eg, masses, tenderness, organomegaly, nodularity)
Lymphatic	• Palpation of lymph nodes in neck, axillae, groin and/or other location
Musculoskeletal	
Extremities	
Skin	• Inspection and/or palpation of skin and subcutaneous tissue (eg, rashes, lesions, ulcers)
Neurological/Psychiatric	Brief assessment of mental status including • Orientation (eg, time place and person) and • Mood and affect (eg, depression, anxiety, agitation)

Content and Documentation Requirements

Level of Exam	Perform and Document
Problem Focused	One to five elements identify in bullet.
Expanded Problem Focused	At least six elements identified in bullet.
Detailed	At least twelve elements identified by a bullet.
Comprehensive	Perform all elements identified by a bullet; document every element in each box with a shaded border and at least one element in each box with an unshaded border.

HEMATOLOGIC/LYMPHATIC/IMMUNOLOGIC EXAMINATION

System/Body Area	Elements of Examination
Constitutional	• Measurement of any three of the following seven vital signs: 1) sitting of standing blood pressure, 2) supine blood pressure, 3) pulse rate and regularity, 4) respiration, 5) temperature, 6) height, 7) weight (may be measured and recorded by ancillary staff) • General appearance of patient (eg, development, nutrition, body habitus, deformities, attention to grooming

Continued

HEMATOLOGIC/LYMPHATIC/IMMUNOLOGIC EXAMINATION—Cont'd

System/Body Area	Elements of Examination
Head and Face	• Palpation and/or percussion of face with notation of presence or absence of sinus tenderness
Eyes	• Inspection of conjunctive and lids
Ears, Nose, Mouth and Throat	• Otoscopic examination of external auditory canals and tympanic membranes • Inspection of nasal mucosa, septum and turbinates • Inspection of teeth and gums • Examination of oropharynx (eg, oral mucosa, hard and soft palates, tongue, tonsils, posterior pharynx)
Neck	• Examination of neck (eg, masses, overall appearance, symmetry, tracheal position, crepitus) • Examination of thyroid (eg, enlargement, tenderness, mass)
Respiratory	• Assessment of respiratory effort (eg, intercostal retractions, use of accessory muscles, diaphragmatic movement) • Auscultation of lungs (eg, breath sounds, adventitious sounds, rubs)
Cardiovascular	• Auscultation of heart with notation of abnormal sounds and murmurs • Examination of peripheral vascular system by observation (eg, swelling, varicosities) and palpation (eg, pulses, temperature, edema, tenderness)
Chest (Breasts)	
Gastrointestinal (Abdomen)	• Examination of abdomen with notation of presence of masses or tenderness • Examination of liver and spleen
Genitourinary	
Lymphatic	• Palpation of lymph nodes in neck, axillae, groin, and/or other location
Musculoskeletal	
Extremities	• Inspection and palpation of digits and nails (eg, clubbing, cyanosis, inflammation, petechiae, ischemia, infections, nodes)
Skin	• Inspection and/or palpation of skin and subcutaneous tissue (eg, rashes, lesions, ulcers, ecchymoses, bruises)
Neurological/ Psychiatric	Brief assessment of mental status including • Orientation to time, place and person • Mood and affect (eg, depression, anxiety, agitation)

Content and Documentation Requirements

Level of Exam	Perform and Document
Problem Focused	One to five elements identified by a bullet.
Expanded Problem Focused	At least six elements identified by a bullet.
Detailed	At least twelve elements identified by a bullet.
Comprehensive	Perform all elements identified by a bullet; document every element in each box with a shaded border and at least one element in each box with an unshaded border

MUSCULOSKELETAL EXAMINATION

System/Body Area	Elements of Examination
Constitutional	• Measurement of any three of the following seven vital signs: 1) sitting or standing blood pressure, 2) supine blood pressure, 3) pulse rate and regularity, 4) respiration, 5) temperature, 6) height, 7) weight (may be measured and recorded by ancillary staff) • General appearance of patient (eg, development, nutrition, body habitus, deformities, attention to grooming)
Head and Face	
Eyes	
Ears, Nose, Mouth and Throat	
Neck	
Respiratory	
Cardiovascular	• Examination of peripheral vascular system by observation (eg, swelling, varicosities) and palpation (eg, pulses, temperature, edema, tenderness)
Chest (Breasts)	
Gastrointestinal (Abdomen)	
Genitourinary	
Lymphatic	• Palpation of lymph nodes in neck, axillae, groin and/or other location
Musculoskeletal	• Examination of gait and station Examination of joint(s), bone(s) and muscle(s)/tendon(s) of four of the following six areas: 1) head and neck; 2) spine, ribs and pelvis; 3) right upper extremity; 4) left upper extremity; 5) right lower extremity; and 6) left lower extremity. The examination of a given area includes: • Inspection, percussion and/or palpation with notation of any misalignment, asymmetry, crepitation, defects, tenderness, masses or effusions • Assessment of range of motion with notation of any pain (eg, straight leg raising), crepitation or contracture • Assessment of stability with notation of any dislocation (luxation), subluxation or laxity • Assessment of muscle strength and tone (eg, flaccid, cog wheel, spastic) with notation of any atrophy or abnormal movements *Note:* For the comprehensive level of examination, all four of the elements identified by a bullet must be performed and documented for each of four anatomic areas. For the three lower levels of examination, each element is counted separately for each body area. For example, assessing range of motion in two extremities constitutes two elements.

Continued

MUSCULOSKELETAL EXAMINATION—Cont'd

System/Body Area	Elements of Examination
Extremities	[See musculoskeletal and skin.]
Skin	• Inspection and/or palpation of skin and subcutaneous tissue (eg, scars, rashes, lesions, cafe-au-lait spots, ulcers) in four of the following six areas: 1) head and neck; 2) trunk; 3) right upper extremity; 4) left upper extremity; 5) right lower extremity; and 6) left lower extremity. *Note:* For the comprehensive level, the examination of all four anatomic areas must be performed and documented. For the three lower levels of examination, each body area is counted separately. For example, inspection and/or palpation of the skin and subcutaneous tissue of two extremities constitutes two elements.
Neurological/Psychiatric	• Test coordination (eg, finger/nose, heel/knee/shin, rapid alternating movements in the upper and lower extremities, evaluation of fine motor coordination in young children) • Examination of deep tendon reflexes and/or nerve stretch test with notation of pathological reflexes (eg, Babinski) • Examination of sensation (eg, by touch, pin, vibration, proprioception) Brief assessment of mental status including • Orientation to time, place and person • Mood and affect (eg, depression, anxiety, agitation)

Content and Documentation Requirements

Level of Exam	Perform and Document
Problem Focused	One to five elements identified by a bullet.
Expanded Problem Focused	At least six elements identified by a bullet.
Detailed	At least twelve elements identified by a bullet.
Comprehensive	Perform all elements identified by a bullet; document every element in each box with a shaded border and at least one element in each box with an unshaded border.

NEUROLOGICAL EXAMINATION

System/Body Area	Elements of Examination
Constitutional	• Measurement of any three of the following seven vital signs: 1) sitting or standing blood pressure, *2)* supine blood pressure, 3) pulse rate and regularity, 4) respiration, 5) temperature, 6) height, 7) weight (may be measured and recorded by ancillary staff) • General appearance of patient (eg, development, nutrition, body habitus, deformities, attention to grooming)
Head and Face	
Eyes	• Ophthalmoscopic examination of optic discs (eg, size, C/I ratio, appearance) and posterior segments (eg, vessel changes, exudates, hemorrhages)
Ears, Nose, Mouth and Throat	
Neck	
Respiratory	
Cardiovascular	• Examination of carotid arteries (eg, pulse amplitude, bruits) • Auscultation of heart with notation of abnormal sounds and murmurs • Examination of peripheral vascular system by observation (eg, swelling, varicosities) and palpation (eg, pulses, temperature, edema, tenderness)
Chest (Breasts)	
Gastrointestinal (Abdomen)	
Genitourinary	
Lymphatic	
Musculoskeletal	• Examination of gait and station Assessment of motor function including: • Muscle strength in upper and lower extremities • Muscle tone in upper and lower extremities (eg, flaccid, cog wheel, spastic) with notation of any atrophy or abnormal movements (eg, fasciculation, tardive dyskinesia)
Extremities	[See musculoskeletal.]
Skin	
Neurological	Evaluation of higher integrative functions including: • Orientation to time, place and person • Recent and remote memory • Attention span and concentration • Language (eg, naming objects, repeating phrases, spontaneous speech) • Fund of knowledge (eg, awareness of current events, past history vocabulary) Test the following cranial nerves: • 2nd cranial nerve (eg, visual acuity, visual fields, fundi) • 3rd, 4th and 6th cranial nerves (eg, pupils, eye movements) • 5th cranial nerve (eg, facial sensation, corneal reflexes) • 7th cranial nerve (eg, facial symmetry, strength) • 8th cranial nerve (eg, hearing with tuning fork, whispered voice and/or finger rub) • 9th cranial nerve (eg, spontaneous or reflex palate movement) • 11th cranial nerve (eg, shoulder shrug strength) • 12th cranial nerve (eg, tongue protrusion) • Examination of sensation (eg, by touch, pin, vibration, proprioception) • Examination of deep tendon reflexes in upper and lower extremities wish notation of pathological reflexes (eg, Babinski)
Psychiatric	• Test coordination (eg, finger/nose, heel/knee/shin, rapid alternating movements in the upper and lower extremities, evaluation of fine motor coordination in young children)

Content and Documentation Requirements

Level of Exam	Perform and Document
Problem Focused	One to five elements identified by a bullet.
Expanded Problem Focused	At least six elements identified by a bullet.
Detailed	At least twelve elements identified by a bullet.
Comprehensive	Perform all elements identified by a bullet; document every element in each box with a shaded border and at least one element in each box with an unshaded border.

PSYCHIATRIC EXAMINATION

System/Body Area	Elements of Examination
Constitutional	• Measurement of any three of the following seven vital signs: 1)-sitting or standing blood pressure, 2) supine blood pressure, 3) pulse rate and regularity, 4) respiration, 5) temperature, 6) height, *7)* weight (may be measured and recorded by ancillary staff) • General appearance of patient (eg, development, nutrition, body habitus, deformities, attention to grooming)
Head and Face	
Eyes	
Ears, Nose, Mouth and Throat	
Neck	
Respiratory	
Cardiovascular	
Chest (Breasts)	
Gastrointestinal (Abdomen)	
Genitourinary	
Lymphatic	
Musculoskeletal	• Assessment of muscle strength and tone (eg, flaccid, cog wheel, spastic) with notation of any atrophy and abnormal movements • Examination of gait and station
Extremities	
Skin	
Neurological	
Psychiatric	• Description of speech including: rate; volume; articulation; coherence; and spontaneity with notation of abnormalities (eg, perseveration, paucity of language) • Description of thought processes including: rate of thoughts; content of thoughts (eg, logical vs. illogical, tangential); abstract reasoning; and computation • Description of associations (eg, loose, tangential, circumstantial, intact) • Description of abnormal or psychotic thoughts including: hallucinations; delusions; preoccupation with violence; homicidal or suicidal ideation; and obsessions • Description of the patient's judgment (eg, concerning everyday activities and social situations) and insight (eg, concerning psychiatric condition) Complete mental status examination including • Orientation to time, place and person • Recent and remote memory • Attention span and concentration • Language (eg. naming objects, repeating phrases) • Fund of knowledge (eg, awareness of current events, past history, vocabulary) • Mood and affect (eg, depression, anxiety, agitation, hypomania, lability)

Content and Documentation Requirements

Level of Exam	Perform and Document
Problem Focused	One to five elements identified by a bullet.
Expanded Problem Focused	At least six elements identified by a bullet.
Detailed	At least nine elements identified by a bullet.
Comprehensive	Perform all elements identified by a bullet; document every element in each box with a shaded border and at least one element in each box with an unshaded border.

RESPIRATORY EXAMINATION

System/Body Area	Elements of Examination
Constitutional	• Measurement of any three of the following seven vital signs: 1) sitting or standing blood pressure, 2) supine blood pressure, 3) pulse rate and regularity, 4) respiration, 5) temperature, 6) height, *7)* weight (may be measured and recorded by ancillary staff) • General appearance of patient (eg, development, nutrition, body habitus, deformities, attention to grooming)

Continued

RESPIRATORY EXAMINATION—Cont'd

System/Body Area	Elements of Examination
Head and Face	
Eyes	
Ears, Nose, Mouth and Throat	• Inspection of nasal mucosa, septum and turbinates • Inspection of teeth and gums • Examination of oropharynx (eg, oral mucosa, hard and soft palates, tongue, tonsils and posterior pharynx)
Neck	• Examination of neck (eg, masses, overall appearance, symmetry, tracheal position, crepitus) • Examination of thyroid (eg, enlargement, tenderness, mass) • Examination of jugular veins (eg, distension; a, v or cannon a waves)
Respiratory	• Inspection of chest with notation of symmetry and expansion • Assessment of respiratory effort (eg, intercostal retractions, use of accessory muscles, diaphragmatic movement) • Percussion of chest (eg, dullness, flatness, hyperresonance) • Palpation of chest (eg, tactile fremitus) • Auscultation of lungs (eg, breath sounds, adventitious sounds, rubs)
Cardiovascular	• Auscultation of heart including sounds, abnormal sounds and murmurs • Examination of peripheral vascular system by observation (eg, swelling, varicosities) and palpation (eg, pulses, temperature, edema, tenderness)
Chest (Breasts)	
Gastrointestinal (Abdomen)	• Examination of abdomen with notation of presence of masses or tenderness • Examination of liver and spleen
Genitourinary	
Lymphatic	• Palpation of lymph nodes in neck, axillae, groin and/or other location
Musculoskeletal	• Assessment of muscle strength and tone (eg, flaccid, cog wheel, spastic) with notation of any atrophy and abnormal movements • Examination of gait and station
Extremities	• Inspection and palpation of digits and nails (eg, clubbing, cyanosis, inflammation, petechiae, ischemia, infections, nodes)
Skin	• Inspection and/or palpation of skin and subcutaneous tissue (eg, rashes, lesions, ulcers)
Neurological/Psychiatric	Brief assessment of mental status including • Orientation to time, place and person • Mood and affect (eg, depression, anxiety, agitation)

Content and Documentation Requirements

Level of Exam	Perform and Document
Problem Focused	One to five elements identified by a bullet.
Expanded Problem Focused	At least six elements identified by a bullet.
Detailed	At least twelve elements identified by a bullet.
Comprehensive	Perform all elements identified by a bullet; document every element in each box with a shaded border and at least one element in each box with an unshaded border.

SKIN EXAMINATION

System/Body Area	Eiements of Examination
Constitutional	• Measurement of any three of the following seven vital signs: 1) sitting or standing blood pressure, 2) supine blood pressure, 3) pulse rate and regularity, 4) respiration, 5) temperature, 6) height, *7)* weight (may be measured and recorded by ancillary staff) • General appearance of patient (eg, development, nutrition, body habitus, deformities, attention to grooming)
Head and Face	
Eyes	• Inspection of conjunctivae and lids
Ears, Nose, Mouth and Throat	• Inspection of lips, teeth and gums • Examination of oropharynx (eg, oral mucosa, hard and soft palates, tongue, tonsils, posterior pharynx)
Neck	• Examination of thyroid (eg, enlargement, tenderness, mass)
Respiratory	
Cardiovascular	• Examination of peripheral vascular system by observation (eg, swelling, varicosities) and palpation (eg, pulses, temperature, edema, tenderness)
Chest (Breasts)	
Gastrointestinal (Abdomen)	• Examination of liver and spleen • Examination of anus for condyloma and other lesions
Genitourinary	
Lymphatic	• Palpation of lymph nodes in neck, axillae, groin and/or other location
Musculoskeletal	
Extremities	• Inspection and palpation of digits and nails (eg, clubbing, cyanosis, inflammation, petechiae, ischemia, infections, nodes)

Continued

SKIN EXAMINATION—Cont'd

System/Body Area	Elements of Examination
Skin	• Palpation of scalp and inspection of hair of scalp, eyebrows, face, chest, pubic area (when indicated) and extremities • Inspection and/or palpation of skin and subcutaneous tissue (eg, rashes, lesions, ulcers, susceptibility to and presence of photo damage) in eight of the following ten areas • Head, including the face and neck • Chest, including breasts and axillae • Abdomen • Genitalia, groin, buttocks • Back • Right upper extremity • Left upper extremity • Right lower extremity • Left lower extremity *Note:* For the comprehensive level, the examination of at least eight anatomic areas must be performed and documented. For the three lower levels of examination, each body area is counted separately. For example, inspection and/or palpation of the skin and subcutaneous tissue of the right upper extremity and the left upper extremity constitutes two elements. • Inspection of eccrine and apocrine glands of skin and subcutaneous tissue with identification and location of any hyperhidrosis, chromhidroses or bromhidrosis
Neurological/ Psychiatric	Brief assessment of mental status including • Orientation to time, place and person • Mood and affect (eg, depression, anxiety, agitation)

C. Documentation of the Complexity of Medical Decision-Making

The levels of *E/M* services recognize four types of medical decision-making (straightforward, low complexity, moderate complexity and high complexity). Medical decision-making refers to the complexity of establishing a diagnosis and/or selecting a management option as measured by:

- the number of possible diagnoses and/or the number of management options that must be considered;
- the amount and/or complexity of medical records, diagnostic tests, and/or other information that must be obtained, reviewed and analyzed; and
- the risk of significant complications, morbidity and/or mortality, as well as comorbidities, associated with the patient's presenting problem(s), the diagnostic procedure(s) and/or the possible management options.

The following chart shows the progression of the elements required for each level of medical decision-making. To qualify for a given type of decision-making, two of the three elements in the table must be either met or exceeded.

Number of diagnoses or management options	Amount and/or complexity of data to be reviewed	Risk of complications and/or morbidity or mortality	Type of decision making
Minimal	Minimal or None	Minimal	*Straightforward*
Limited	Limited	Low	*Low Complexity*
Multiple	Moderate	Moderate	*Moderate Complexity*
Extensive	Extensive	High	*High Complexity*

Each of the elements of medical decision-making is described following.

Number of Diagnoses or Management Options. The number of possible diagnoses and/or the number of management options that must be considered is based on the number and types of problems addressed during the encounter, the complexity of establishing a diagnosis and the management decisions that are made by the physician.

Generally, decision-making with respect to a diagnosed problem is easier than that for an identified but undiagnosed problem. The number and type of diagnostic tests employed may be an indicator of the number of possible diagnoses. Problems which are improving or resolving are less complex than those which are worsening or failing to change as expected. The need to seek advice from others is another indicator of complexity of diagnostic or management problems.

- DG: For each encounter, an assessment, clinical impression, or diagnosis should be documented. It may be explicitly stated or implied in documented decisions regarding management plans and/or further evaluation.
  - For a presenting problem with an established diagnosis the record should reflect whether the problem is: a) improved, well controlled, resolving or resolved; or, b) inadequately controlled, worsening, or failing to change as expected.
  - For a presenting problem without an established diagnosis, the assessment or clinical impression may be stated in the form of differential diagnoses or as a "possible," "probable," or "rule out" (R/O) diagnosis.
- DG: The initiation of, or changes in, treatment should be documented. Treatment includes a wide range of management options including patient instructions, nursing instructions, therapies, and medications.
- DG: If referrals are made, consultations requested or advice sought, the record should indicate to whom or where the referral or consultation is made or from whom the advice is requested.

Amount and/or Complexity of Data to Be Reviewed. The amount and complexity of data to be reviewed is based on the types of diagnostic testing ordered or reviewed. A decision to obtain and review old medical records and/or obtain history from sources other than the patient increases the amount and complexity of data to be reviewed.

Discussion of contradictory or unexpected test results with the physician who performed or interpreted the test is an indication of the complexity of data being reviewed. On occasion the physician who ordered a test may personally review the image, tracing or specimen to supplement information from the physician who prepared the test report or interpretation; this is another indication of the complexity of data being reviewed.

- DG: If a diagnostic service (test or procedure) is ordered, planned, scheduled, or performed at the time of the E/M encounter, the type of service, e.g., lab or x-ray, should be documented.
- DG: The review of lab, radiology and/or other diagnostic tests should be documented. A simple notation such as "WBC elevated" or "chest x-ray unremarkable" is acceptable. Alternatively, the review may be documented by initialing and dating the report containing the test results.
- DG: A decision to obtain old records or decision to obtain additional history from the family, caretaker or other source to supplement that obtained from the patient should be documented.
- DG: Relevant findings from the review of old records, and/or the receipt of additional history from the family, caretaker or other source to supplement that obtained from the patient should be documented. If there is no relevant information beyond that already obtained, that fact should be documented. A notation of "Old records reviewed" or "additional history obtained from family" without elaboration is insufficient.
- DG: The results of discussion of laboratory, radiology or other diagnostic tests with the physician who performed or interpreted the study should be documented.
- DG: The direct visualization and independent interpretation of an image, tracing or specimen previously or subsequently interpreted by another physician should be documented.

Risk of Significant Complications, Morbidity, and/or Mortality. The risk of significant complications, morbidity, and/or mortality is based on the risks associated with the presenting problem(s), the diagnostic procedure(s), and the possible management options.

- DG: Comorbidities/underlying diseases or other factors that increase the complexity of medical decision making by increasing the risk of complications, morbidity, and/or mortality should be documented.
- DG: If a surgical or invasive diagnostic procedure is ordered, planned or scheduled at the time of the E/M encounter, the type of procedure, e.g., laparoscopy, should be documented.
- DG: If a surgical or invasive diagnostic procedure is performed at the time of the E/M encounter, the specific procedure should be documented.
- DG: The referral for or decision to perform a surgical or invasive diagnostic procedure on an urgent basis should be documented or implied.

The following table may be used to help determine whether the risk of significant complications, morbidity, and/or mortality is *minimal, low, moderate,* or *high.* Because the determination of risk is complex and not readily quantifiable, the table includes common clinical examples rather than absolute measures of risk. The assessment of risk of the presenting problem(s) is based on the risk related to the disease process anticipated between the present encounter and the next one. The assessment of risk of selecting diagnostic procedures and management options is based on the risk during and immediately following any procedures or treatment. **The highest level of risk in any one category (presenting problem(s), diagnostic procedure(s), or management options) determines the overall risk.**

TABLE OF RISK

Level of Risk	Presenting Problem(s)	Diagnostic Procedure(s) Ordered	Management Options Selected
Minimal	• One self-limited or minor problem, eg, cold, insect bite, tinea corporis	• Laboratory tests requiring venipuncture • Chest x-rays • EKG/EEG • Urinalysis • Ultrasound, eg, echocardiography • KOH prep	• Rest • Gargles • Elastic bandages • Superficial dressings
Low	• Two or more self-limited or minor problems • One stable chronic illness, eg, well controlled hypertension, non-insulin dependent diabetes, cataract, BPH • Acute uncomplicated illness or injury, eg, cystitis, allergic rhinitis, simple sprain	• Physiologic tests not under stress, eg, pulmonary function tests • Non-cardiovascular imaging studies with contrast, eg, barium enema • Superficial needle biopsies • Clinical laboratory tests requiring arterial puncture • Skin biopsies	• Over-the-counter drugs • Minor surgery with no identified risk factors • Physical therapy • Occupational therapy • IV fluids without additives
Moderate	• One or more chronic illnesses with mild exacerbation, progression, or side effects of treatment • Two or more stable chronic illnesses • Undiagnosed new problem with uncertain prognosis, eg, lump in breast • Acute illness with systemic symptoms, eg, pyelonephritis, pneumonitis, colitis • Acute complicated injury, eg, head injury with brief loss of consciousness	• Physiologic tests under stress, eg, cardiac stress test, fetal contraction stress test • Diagnostic endoscopies with no identified risk factors • Deep needle or incisional biopsy • Cardiovascular imaging studies with contrast and no identified risk factors, eg, arteriogram, cardiac catheterization • Obtain fluid from body cavity, eg, lumbar puncture, thoracentesis, culdocentesis	• Minor surgery with identified risk factors • Elective major surgery (open, percutaneous or endoscopic) with no identified risk factors • Prescription drug management • Therapeutic nuclear medicine • IV fluids with additives • Closed treatment of fracture or dislocation without manipulation

Continued

TABLE OF RISK—Cont'd

Level of Risk	Presenting Problem(s)	Diagnostic Procedure(s) Ordered	Management Options Selected
High	• One or more chronic illnesses with Severe exacerbation, progression, or side effects of treatment • Acute or chronic illnesses or injuries that pose a threat to life or bodily function, eg, multiple trauma, acute MI, pulmonary embolus, severe respiratory distress, progressive severe rheumatoid arthritis, psychiatric illness with potential threat to self or others, peritonitis, acute renal failure • An abrupt change in neurologic status, eg, seizure, TIA, weakness, sensory loss	• Cardiovascular imaging studies with contrast with identified risk factors • Cardiac electrophysiological tests • Diagnostic, endoscopies with identified risk factors • Discography	• Elective major surgery (open, percutaneous or endoscopic) with identified risk factors • Emergency major surgery (open, percutaneous or endoscopic) • Parenteral controlled substances • Drug therapy requiring intensive monitoring for toxicity • Decision not to resuscitate or to deescalate care because of poor prognosis

D. Documentation of an Encounter Dominated by Counseling or Coordination of Care

In the case where Counseling and/or coordination of care dominates (more than 50%) of the physician/patient and/or family encounter (face-to-face time in the office or other or outpatient setting, floor/unit time in the hospital or nursing facility), time is considered the key or controlling factor to qualify for a particular level of E/M services.

- DG: If the physician elects to report the level of service based on counseling and/or coordination of care, the total length of time of the encounter (face-to-face or floor time, as appropriate) should be documented and the record should describe the counseling and/or activities to coordinate care.

Appendix F

List of Physicians

Physicians by Name

Alanda, MD, Leslie	Internal Medicine and Vascular
Aljabar, MD, Alfa	Nuclear Medicine
Almaz, MD, Mohomad	Orthopaedics
Avila, MD, Ira	Urology
Barneswell, MD, Mary	Physical Therapy
Barton, MD, David	Cardiothoracic Surgery
Brown, MD, Robert	Critical Care
Dawson, MD, Gregory	Respiratory Care
Doron, MD, Phil	Endocrinology
Eagle, MD, James	Radiation Oncology
Elhart, MD, Marvin	Cardiology
Erickson, MD, Mark	Plastic Surgery
Friendly, MD, Larry P.	Gastroenterology
Gaul, MD, Frank	Family Practice
Green, MD, Ronald	Internal Medicine and Critical Care
Hamilton, MD, Monica J.	Interventional Radiology
Hart, MD, Phillip	Neuroradiology—Hospital Employee
Hodgson, MD, John	Surgical Neurosurgery
Jayco, MD, Gordon	Endocrinology and Nephrology
King, MD, Jeff	Otorhinolaryngology
Larson, MD, Janice E.	Anesthesia
Lauer, MD, Elmer	Dermatology
Lin, MD, Lou	Infectious Diseases
Lonewolf, MD, Grey	Pathology
Lorabi, MD, Gerald	Hematology
Lovejoy, MD, Noah	Dermatology
Martinez, MD, Andy	Obstetrics & Gynecology
Monson, MD, Morton	Radiology
Munoz, MD, Orland	Psychiatry
Naraquist, MD, Alma	Internal Medicine
Nelson, MD, Jerome	Neuropsychology
Noonar, MD, James	Cardiology
Noss, MD, Laddie N.	Diabetes & Internal Medicine
Olanka, MD, Daniel G.	Gastroenterology
Orbitz, MD, George	Nephrology
Ortez, MD, Rolando	Pediatrics & Neonatology
Peterson, MD, Rush K.	Allergy & Immunology
Pleasant, MD, Timothy L.	Neurology
Riddle, MD, Edward	Interventional Radiology
Ripple, MD, Ronald	Thoracic Surgery
Sanchez, MD, Gary I.	General Surgery
Smithson, MD, Paula	Urology
Sutton, MD, Paul	Emergency Medicine-Hospital Employee
Warner, MD, Samuel	Podiatry
White, MD, Loren	General Surgery
White, MD, Rapheal	Oncology
Wimer, MD, Rita	Ophthalmology

Physician by Specialty

Peterson, MD, Rush K.	Allergy & Immunology
Larson, MD, Janice E.	Anesthesia
Noonar, MD, James	Cardiology
Elhart, MD, Marvin	Cardiology
Barton, MD, David	Cardiothoracic Surgery
Brown, MD, Robert	Critical Care
Lauer, MD, Elmer	Dermatology
Lovejoy, MD, Noah	Dermatology
Noss, MD, Laddie N.	Diabetes & Internal Medicine
Sutton, MD, Paul	Emergency Medicine-Hospital Employee
Jayco, MD, Gordon	Endocrinology
Doron, MD, Phil	Endocrinology
Gaul, MD, Frank	Family Practice
Olanka, MD, Daniel G.	Gastroenterology
Friendly, MD, Larry P.	Gastroenterology
Sanchez, MD, Gary I.	General Surgery
White, MD, Loren	General Surgery
Lorabi, MD, Gerald	Hematology
Lin, MD, Lou	Infectious Diseases
Naraquist, MD, Alma	Internal Medicine
Green, MD, Ronald	Internal Medicine and Critical Care
Alanda, MD, Leslie	Internal Medicine and Vascular
Riddle, MD, Edward	Interventional Radiology
Hamilton, MD, Monica J.	Interventional Radiology
Orbitz, MD, George	Nephrology
Jayco, MD, Gordon	Nephrology
Pleasant, MD, Timothy L.	Neurology
Nelson, MD, Jerome	Neuropsychology
Hart, MD, Phillip	Neuroradiology—Hospital Employee
Aljabar, MD, Alfa	Nuclear Medicine
Martinez, MD, Andy	Obstetrics & Gynecology
White, MD, Rapheal	Oncology
Wimer, MD, Rita	Ophthalmology
Almaz, MD, Mohomad	Orthopaedics
King, MD, Jeff	Otorhinolaryngology
Lonewolf, MD, Grey	Pathology
Ortez, MD, Rolando	Pediatrics & Neonatology
Barneswell, MD Mary	Physical Therapy
Erickson, MD, Mark	Plastic Surgery
Warner, MD, Samuel	Podiatry
Munoz, MD, Orland	Psychiatry
Eagle, MD, James	Radiation Oncology
Monson, MD, Morton	Radiology
Dawson, MD, Gregory	Respiratory Care
Hodgson, MD, John	Surgical Neurosurgery
Ripple, MD, Ronald	Thoracic Surgery
Avila, MD, Ira	Urology
Smithson, MD, Paula	Urology

APPENDIX G

Answers to Every Other Case

Chapter 1

Evaluation and Management Services

CASE 1-1

1-1A INITIAL HOSPITAL CARE

Professional Services: 99223 (Evaluation and Management, Hospital); **250.11** (Diabetes, with, ketoacidosis, type I), **493.90** (Asthma)

Facility Services: This is an inpatient stay. The entire record would need to be reviewed before coding. No inpatient codes are assigned in this worktext.

1-1B DISCHARGE SUMMARY

Professional Services: 99238 (Evaluation and Management, Hospital, Discharge); **250.11** (Diabetes, ketoacidosis, type I), **276.51** (Dehydration), **493.90** (Asthma)

Facility Services: This is an inpatient stay. The entire record would need to be reviewed before coding. We will not be assigning codes on inpatients.

CASE 1-3

1-3A INITIAL HOSPITAL SERVICE

Professional Services: 99222 (Evaluation and Management, Hospital); **789.03** (Pain, abdominal), **250.01** (Diabetes), **461.9** (Sinusitis, acute), **493.90** (Asthma)

Facility Services: This is an inpatient stay. The entire record would need to be reviewed before coding. We will not be assigning codes on inpatients.

1-3B CONSULTATION

Professional Services: 99253 (Evaluation and Management, Consultation); ~~**250.00**~~ (Diabetes, type I), **789.03** (Pains, abdominal) 250.01

Facility Services: This is an inpatient stay. The entire record would need to be reviewed before coding. We will not be assigning codes on inpatients.

1-3C RADIOLOGY REPORT

Professional Services: 76705-26 (Ultrasound, Abdomen); **789.03** (Pain, abdominal)

Facility Services: This is an inpatient stay. The entire record would need to be reviewed before coding. We will not be assigning codes on inpatients.

1-3D RADIOLOGY REPORT

Professional Services: 71020-26 (X-Ray, Chest); **786.2** (Cough), **780.6** (Fever)

Facility Services: This is an inpatient stay. The entire record would need to be reviewed before coding. We will not be assigning codes on inpatients.

CASE 1-5

1-5A INITIAL HOSPITAL CARE

Professional Services: 99223 (Evaluation and Management, Hospital); **427.89** (Bradycardia), **285.9** (Anemia), **427.31** (Fibrillation, atrial)

Facility Services: This is an inpatient stay. The entire record would need to be reviewed before coding. We will not be assigning codes on inpatients.

1-5B PROGRESS REPORT

Professional Services: 99233 (Evaluation and Management, Hospital); **427.89** (Bradycardia), **285.9** (Anemia), **427.31** (Fibrillation, atrial)

Facility Services: This is an inpatient stay. The entire record would need to be reviewed before coding. We will not be assigning codes on inpatients.

CASE 1-7

1-7A PROGRESS REPORT

Professional Services: 99232 (Evaluation and Management, Hospital); **584.9** (Failure, renal, acute), **585.9** (Failure, renal, chronic), **285.21** (Anemia, in, chronic kidney disease), **427.31** (Fibrillation, atrial)

Facility Services: This is an inpatient stay. The entire record would need to be reviewed before coding. We will not be assigning codes on inpatients.

CASE 1-9

1-9A DISCHARGE SUMMARY

Professional Services: 99238 (Evaluation and Management, Hospital, Discharge); **532.70** (Ulcer, duodenum, chronic)

Facility Services: This is an inpatient stay. The entire record would need to be reviewed before coding. We will not be assigning codes on inpatients.

CASE 1-11

1-11A CONSULTATION

Professional Services: 99245 (Evaluation and Management, Consultation); **533.90** (Ulcer, peptic), **305.1** (Dependence, tobacco)

Facility Services: No facility services provided.

CASE 1-13

1-13A CRITICAL CARE

Professional Services: 99291, 99292 (Critical Care Services); **786.06** (Tachypnea), **303.02** (Alcoholism, acute), **401.9** (Hypertension, unspecified)

Facility Services: This is an inpatient stay. The entire record would need to be reviewed before coding. We will not be assigning codes on inpatients.

CASE 1-15

1-15A CRITICAL CARE

Professional Services: 99291 (Evaluation and Management, Critical Care), **99292** (Evaluation and Management, Critical Care); **425.5** (Cardiomyopathy, alcoholic), **428.0** (Failure, heart, congestive), **416.0** (Hypertension, pulmonary, primary), **593.9** (Insufficiency, renal)

Facility Services: This is an inpatient stay. The entire record would need to be reviewed before coding. We will not be assigning codes on inpatients.

CASE 1-17

1-17A CRITICAL CARE ADMISSION

Professional Services: 99291 (Critical Care), **99292** × 2 (Critical Care) to report a total of 120 minutes; **458.9** (Hypotension), **518.81** (Failure; respiration, respiratory), **428.0** (Failure, congestive), **584.9** (Failure, renal, acute)

Facility Services: This is an inpatient stay. The entire record would need to be reviewed before coding. We will not be assigning codes on inpatients.

CASE 1-19

1-19A OFFICE VISIT

Professional Services: 99203 (Evaluation and Management, Office and Other Outpatient); **465.9** (Infection, respiratory, upper), **785.6** (Lymphadenopathy)

Facility Services: No facility services provided.

1-19B OFFICE VISIT

Professional Services: 99213 (Evaluation and Management, Office and Other Outpatient); **289.3** (Lymphadenitis)

Facility Services: No facility services provided.

1-19C CLINIC PROGRESS NOTE

Professional Services: 99213 (Evaluation and Management, Office or Other Outpatient); **465.9** (Infection, respiratory, upper), **462** (Pharyngitis)

Facility Services: No facility services provided.

CASE 1-21

1-21A NEWBORN CARE

Professional Services: 1/1 99431, 1/2 99433, 1/3 99433, 1/4 99433 (Evaluation and Management, Newborn Care), **1/3 54150** (Circumcision), **1/5 99238-24** (E/M, Hospital, Discharge); **V31.01** (Newborn, twin, mate liveborn, born in hospital)

Facility Services: This is an inpatient stay. The entire record would need to be reviewed before coding. We will not be assigning codes on inpatients.

CASE 1-23

1-23A OFFICE VISIT

Professional Services: 99395 (E/M Services, Preventive Services); **V72.31** (Examination, gynecological), **244.9** (Hypothyroidism), **278.00** (Obesity)

Facility Services: No facility services provided.

1-23B OFFICE VISIT

Professional Services: 99395 (E/M Services, Preventive Services); **V70.0** (Examination, health, checkup), **244.9** (Hypothyroidism), **278.00** (Obesity)

Facility Services: No facility services provided.

1-23C OFFICE VISIT

Professional Services: 99395 (E/M Services, Preventive Services); **V70.5** (Examination, health, defined sub-population), **V72.31** (Examination, gynecological), **244.9** (Hypothyroidism)

Facility Services: No facility services provided.

CASE 1-25

1-25A OFFICE VISIT

Professional Services: 99392 (E/M, Preventive Services); **V20.2** (Examination; health; child, routine)

Facility Services: No facility services provided.

Chapter 2
Medicine

CASE 2-1

2-1A CHART NOTE

Professional Services:

Substance: 90658 (Vaccine, Influenza)

Administration: G0008 (Vaccination, influenza)

Diagnosis: V04.81 (Influenza, vaccination)

Facility Services: Services were provided at the clinic; no facility (hospital) services were provided.

CASE 2-3

2-3A CHART NOTE

Professional Services:

Substance: 90710 (Vaccines; Measles, Mumps, Rubella, and Varicella)

Administration: 90471 (Administration, Immunization)

Diagnosis: V06.4 (Vaccination, prophylactic; mumps, with measles and rubella), **V05.4** (Vaccination, prophylactic; varicella)

Facility Services: Services were provided at the clinic; no facility (hospital) services were provided.

CASE 2-5

2-5A CHART NOTE

Professional Services: 90772 (Injection, Intramuscular, Antibiotic), **J0120** (Table of Drugs, Tetracycline); **465.9** (Infection, respiratory, upper, acute)

Facility Services: Services were provided at the clinic; no facility (hospital) services were provided.

CASE 2-7

2-7A HEMODIALYSIS PROGRESS REPORT

Professional Services:

90921 (Dialysis, End Stage) (For a full month of service)
V56.0 (Admission /Encounter for dialysis)
403.91 (Hypertension, kidney, with, chronic kidney disease, unspecified)
250.40 (Diabetes, nephropathy)
583.81 (Diabetes, nephropathy)
276.9 (Electrolyte, imbalance)
V45.73 (Absence, kidney, acquired)

Facility Services:

90921 (Dialysis, End Stage Renal Disease)
V56.0 (Admission/Encounter for, dialysis)
403.91 (Hypertension, kidney, with, chronic kidney disease, unspecified)
250.40 (Diabetes, nephropathy)
583.81 (Diabetes, nephropathy)
V45.73 (Absence, kidney, acquired)
275.3 (Hyperphosphatemia)
275.41 (Hypocalcemia)
244.9 (Hypothyroidism)

CASE 2-9

2-9A DUPLEX CAROTID ARTERY STUDY

Professional Services: 93880-26 (Vascular Studies, Arterial Studies [Non-Invasive], Extracranial); **427.1** (Tachycardia, ventricular)

Facility Services: 93880 (Vascular Studies, Arterial Studies [Non-invasive], Extracranial); **427.1** (Tachycardia, ventricular)

CASE 2-11

2-11A ARTERIAL DOPPLER TEST

Professional Services: 93923-26 (Vascular Studies, Arterial Studies [Non-Invasive], Extremities); **729.5** (Pain, leg), **250.00** (Diabetes)

Facility Services: 93923 (Vascular Studies, Arterial Studies [Non-Invasive], Extremities); **729.5** (Pain, leg), **250.00** (Diabetes)

CASE 2-13

2-13A ELECTRICAL CARDIOVERSION

Professional Services: 92960 (Cardioversion); **427.32** (Flutter, atrial)

Facility Services: This is an inpatient stay. The entire record would need to be reviewed before coding.

CASE 2-15

2-15A COGNITIVE FUNCTION ASSESSMENT

Professional Services: 96116 × **2** (Cognitive Function Tests); **290.21** (Dementia, senile, with, depressive features)

Facility Services: Services were provided at the clinic; no facility (hospital) services were provided.

CASE 2-17

2-17A INFUSION

Professional Services: 90765 (Chemotherapy, Intravenous); **J9050** (Table of Drugs, Carmustine); **V58.11** (Admission/Encounter, for Chemotherapy), **203.00** (Myeloma)

Facility Services: Services were provided at the clinic; no facility (hospital) services were provided.

CASE 2-19

2-19A PHYSICAL THERAPY EVALUATION

Professional Services: 97001 (Physical Medicine/Therapy/Occupational Therapy, Evaluation); **715.96** (Arthritis, degenerative), **V58.78** (Aftercare, following surgery NEC, for, of, musculoskeletal system)

Facility Service: Services were provided at the rehab clinic; no facility (hospital) services were provided.

CASE 2-21

2-21A OFFICE PROCEDURE

Professional Services: 11750-TA, 11750-T5 (Nails, Excision); **703.0** (Ingrowing, nail)

Facility Services: Services were provided at the clinic; no facility (hospital) services were provided.

2-21B CLINIC PROGRESS NOTE

Professional Services: 99024 (Post-Op Visit); **V67.09** (Examination following, treatment, for, specified condition, NEC)

Facility Services: Services were provided at the clinic; no facility (hospital) services were provided.

Chapter 3

Radiology

CASE 3-1

3-1A RADIOLOGY REPORT, CHEST

Professional Services: 71010-26 (X-Ray, Chest); **V56.1** (Admission [Encounter] for, dialysis catheter, fitting and adjustment, extracorporeal), **V72.5** (X-ray, of chest, routine)

Facility Services: 71010 (X-ray, Chest); **V56.1** (Admission [Encounter] for, dialysis catheter, fitting and adjustment, extracorporeal), **V72.5** (X-ray, of chest, routine)

CASE 3-3

3-3A RADIOLOGY REPORT, ABDOMEN

Professional Services: 74000-76-26 (X-Ray, Abdomen); **V58.82** (Admission [Encounter], for, adjustment, catheter, non-vascular), **789.00** (Pain, abdominal)

Facility Services: 74000-76 (X-ray, Abdomen); **789.00** (Pain, abdominal)

CASE 3-5

3-5A RADIOLOGY REPORT, FEMUR

Professional Services: 73550-26-LT (X-Ray, Femur); **729.5** (Pain, Leg)

Facility Services: 73550-LT (X-ray, Femur); **729.5** (Pain, Leg)

CASE 3-7

3-7A RADIOLOGY REPORT, SHOULDER

Professional Services: 73030-26-RT (X-Ray, Shoulder); **719.41** (Pain, joint, shoulder)

Facility Services: 73030-RT (X-ray, Shoulder); **719.41** (Pain, joint, shoulder)

CASE 3-9

3-9A VIDEO SWALLOW

Professional Services: 74230 (Swallowing, Evaluation, Video); **787.2** (Dysphagia)

Facility Services: 74230 (Swallowing, Evaluation, Video); **787.2** (Dysphagia)

CASE 3-11

3-11A CT SCAN, SINUSES

Professional Services: 70486-26 (CT Scan, without Contrast, Face), **76377-26** (CT Scan, Other Planes); **428.0** (Congestive, heart), **799.0** (Hypoxemia)

Facility Services: The technical portion of the service would be reported with the other charges from this inpatient stay. The entire record would need to be reviewed before coding. We will not be assigning codes on inpatients.

CASE 3-13

3-13A CT SCAN, CHEST

Professional Services: 71250-26 (CT Scan, without Contrast, Thorax); **277.3** (Amyloidosis)

Facility Services: 71250 (CT Scan, without Contrast, Thorax); **277.3** (Amyloidosis).

CASE 3-15

3-15A CT SCAN, CHEST

Professional Services: 71260-26 (CT Scan, with Contrast, Thorax); **511.9** (Effusion, pleural), **V45.71** (Absence of breast, acquired)

Facility Services: 71260 (CT Scan, with Contrast, Thorax); **511.9** (Effusion, pleural), **V45.71** (Absence of breast, acquired).

CASE 3-17

3-17A CT SCAN, ABDOMEN

Professional Services: 74160-26 (CT Scan, with contrast, Abdomen); **793.6** (Abnormal, radiological examination, Abdomen, NEC)

Facility Services: 74160 (CT Scan, with contrast, Abdomen); **793.6** (Abnormal, radiological examination, Abdomen, NEC).

CASE 3-19

3-19A CT-GUIDED KIDNEY BIOPSY

Professional Services: 50200-50 (Biopsy, Kidney, Bilateral), **76360-26** (CT Scan, Guidance, Needle Placement), **76380-26** (CT Scan, Follow-Up Study); **593.9** (Insufficiency, Kidney), **581.9** (Syndrome, nephrotic), **285.9** (Anemia)

Facility Services: 50200-50 (Biopsy, Kidney [bilateral]), **76360** (CT Scan, Guidance, Needle Placement), **76380** (CT Scan, Follow-Up Study); **593.9** (Insufficiency, kidney), **581.9** (Syndrome, nephrotic), **285.9** (Anemia).

CASE 3-21

3-21A ULTRASOUND, RIGHT LOWER QUADRANT

Professional Services: 76705-26 (Ultrasound, Abdomen); **789.03** (Pain, abdominal), **780.6** (Fever with chills)

Facility Services: 76705 (Ultrasound, Abdomen); **789.03** (Pain, abdominal), **780.6** (Fever with chills).

CASE 3-23

3-23A ULTRASOUND, RENAL

Professional Services: 76770-26 (Ultrasound, Kidney); **581.9** (Nephritis, nephrotic syndrome)

Facility Services: 76770 (Ultrasound, Kidney); **581.9** (Nephritis, nephrotic syndrome).

CASE 3-25

3-25A ULTRASOUND, RENAL

Professional Services: 76770-26 (Ultrasound, Kidney); **585.9** (Failure, renal, chronic), **575.11** (Cholecystitis, chronic), **753.19** (Cyst, kidney, multiple), **789.5** (Ascites, abdominal NEC)

Facility Services: 76770 (Ultrasound, Kidney); **585.9** (Failure, renal, chronic), **575.11** (Cholecystitis, chronic), **753.19** (Cyst, kidney, multiple), **789.5** (Ascites, abdominal NEC).

CASE 3-27

3-27A ULTRASOUND, RETROPERITONEAL

Professional Services: 76775-26 (Ultrasound, retroperitoneal); **590.80** (Pyelonephritis)

Facility Services: 76775 (Ultrasound, retroperitoneal), **590.80** (Pyelonephritis).

CASE 3-29

3-29A RADIATION ONCOLOGY CONSULTATION NOTE

Professional Services: 99244 (E/M, Consultation); **198.2** (Neoplasm, skin NEC, Secondary), **185** (Neoplasm, prostate, Primary)

Facility Services: No facility services were provided.

3-29B RADIATION ONCOLOGY TREATMENT PLANNING NOTE

Professional Services: 77263 (Radiation Therapy, Planning, Complex); **198.2** (Neoplasm, skin NEC, Secondary), **185** (Neoplasm, prostate, Primary)

Facility Services: No facility services were provided.

3-29C RADIATION ONCOLOGY SIMULATION NOTE

Professional Services: 77290 (Radiation Therapy, Field Setup), **77334** (Radiation Therapy, Treatment Device); **198.2** (Neoplasm, skin NEC, Secondary), **185** (Neoplasm, prostate, Primary)

Facility Services: 77290 (Radiation Therapy, Field Setup), **77334** (Radiation Therapy, Treatment Device); **198.2** (Neoplasm, skin, NEC, Secondary), **185** (Neoplasm, prostate, primary).

3-29D RADIATION ONCOLOGY PROGRESS NOTE—WEEK 1, 5 DAYS

Professional Services: 77427 (Radiation Therapy, Treatment Delivery, Weekly); **198.2** (Neoplasm, skin NEC, Secondary), **185** (Neoplasm, prostate, Primary)

Facility Services: 77413 × 5 (Radiation Therapy, Treatment Delivery, Three or More Areas), **77417** (Port Films); **198.2** (Neoplasm, skin, NEC, Secondary), **185** (Neoplasm, prostate, primary)

3-29E RADIATION ONCOLOGY PROGRESS NOTE—WEEK 2, 5 DAYS

Professional Services: 77427 (Radiation Therapy, Treatment Delivery, Weekly); **198.2** (Neoplasm, skin NEC, Secondary), **185** (Neoplasm, prostate, Primary)

Facility Services: 77413 × 5 (Radiation Therapy, Treatment Delivery, Three or More Areas), **77417** (Port Films); **198.2** (Neoplasm, skin, NEC, Secondary), **185** (Neoplasm, prostate, primary)

CASE 3-31

3-31A VENTILATION-PERFUSION LUNG SCAN

Professional Services: 78588-26 (Nuclear Medicine, Lung, Imaging Ventilation); **786.50** (Pain, chest)

Facility Services: 78588 (Nuclear Medicine, Lung, Imaging Ventilation); **786.50** (Pain, chest)

CASE 3-33

3-33A GASTROJEJUNOSTOMY CATHETER PLACEMENT

Professional Services: 43750 (Gastrostomy Tube, Insertion, Percutaneous); **269.9** (Nutrition deficiency)

Facility Services: 43750 (Gastrostomy, Tube, Insertion, Percutaneous), **74350** (Gastrointestinal Tract, X-ray, Guide, Intubation); **269.9** (Nutrition deficient)

CASE 3-35

3-35A GASTROJEJUNOSTOMY CATHETER PLACEMENT

Professional Services: 43750 (Gastrostomy, Tube Insertion, Percutaneous), **74350-26** (X-Ray, Gastrointestinal Tract, Guide Intubation); **434.91** (Stroke), **518.82** (Syndrome, adult respiratory), **V46.11** (Status, ventilator)

Facility Services: This is an inpatient stay. The entire record would need to be reviewed before coding. We will not be assigning codes on inpatients.

Chapter 4

Pathology and Laboratory

CASE 4-1

Panels

4-1A BASIC METABOLIC PANEL

Ca **calcium**
CO_2 **carbon dioxide**
Cl **chloride**
Creat **creatinine**
Glu **glucose**
K **potassium**
Na **sodium**
BUN **blood urea nitrogen**

4-1B COMPREHENSIVE METABOLIC PANEL

Alb **albumin**
Bili tot **bilirubin, total**
Ca **calcium**
CO_2 **carbon dioxide**
Cl **chloride**
Creat **creatinine**
Glu **glucose**
alk phos **alkaline phosphatase**
K **potassium**
Prot tot **protein, total**
Na **sodium**
AST **aspartate aminotransferase**
ALT **alanine aminotransferase**
BUN **blood urea nitrogen**

4-1C HEPATIC FUNCTION PANEL

Prot tot **protein, total**
Alb **albumin**
Bili tot, dir **bilirubin, total and direct** (**these are two separate tests**)
alk phos **alkaline phosphatase**
AST **aspartate aminotransferase**
ALT **alanine aminotransferase**

4-1D LIPID PANEL

Chol tot **cholesterol, total serum**
HDL **lipoprotein, direct measurement, high-density cholesterol**
Trig **triglycerides**

4-1E GENERAL HEALTH PANEL

Comp met **comprehensive metabolic**
CBC **complete blood count**
TSH **thyroid stimulating hormone**

CASE 4-3

4-3A CHEMISTRY TESTS

Terms in parentheses are the CPT index location of the code.

1. **82040**
2. **84075**
3. **84460**
4. **82150**
5. **82803**
6. **84450**
7. **82248**
8. **82247**
9. **84520**
10. **82310**
11. **82374**
12. **82378**
13. **82435**
14. **82465**
15. **82550**
16. **82565**
17. **83001**
18. **82728**
19. **82746**
20. **82977**
21. **82947**
22. **83036**
23. **84703**
24. **84702**
25. **83718**
26. **86334-90**
27. **83540**
28. **83550**

NC % saturated requires iron and IBC to be ordered.

29. **83615**
30. **83002**
31. **83735**
32. **84100**
33. **84132**
34. **84146**
35. **84155**
36. **84165-90**
37. **84153**
38. **84295**
39. **84439**
40. **84443**
41. **84478**
42. **84550**
43. **82607**
44. **83525** (Insulin, Blood)
45. **83540** (Iron)
46. **83550**
47. **84590** (Vitamin, A)
48. **82607** (Vitamin, B_{12})
49. **82565** (Creatinine, Blood)
50. **82248** (Bilirubin, Blood [direct])
51. **82247** (Bilirubin, Blood [total])
52. **84442** (Thyroxine Binding Globulin)
53. **84146** (Prolactin)

CASE 4-5

4-5A COAGULATION

1. **85730** (Thromboplastin, Partial Time)
2. **85610** (Prothrombin Time)
3. **85002** (Bleeding Time)
4. **85002** (Bleeding Time)
5. **85348** (Coagulation Time)
6. **85378** (Fibrin Degradation Products)
7. **85244** (Clotting Factor)
8. **85366** (Fibrin Degradation Products)
9. **85384** (Fibrinogen)
10. **85730** (Thromboplastin, Partial Time)
11. **85610** (Prothrombin Time)

CASE 4-7

The index locations for the codes in 406 appear in the text before the case.

4-7A IMMUNOLOGY

1. **86038**
2. **86225**
3. **86235 × 2**
4. **86235 × 2**
5. **86063**
6. **86430**
7. **86593**
8. **86157**
9. **87340**
10. **87340-90**
11. **86701-90**
12. **86308**
13. **86762**

CASE 4-9

4-9A OFFICE TESTING

1. **81002**

CASE 4-11

4-11A EVOCATIVE/SUPPRESSION TESTING

1. **80434** (Evocative/Suppression Test), **255.4** (Deficiency, corticoadrenal)
2. **80418** (Evocative/Suppression Test), 369.9 (Impaired vision NEC), 784.0 (Headache)

CASE 4-13 MICROBIOLOGY

4-13A MICROBIOLOGY

1. **87086** (Culture, Bacteria, Urine); **788.1** (Dysuria)
2. **87110** (Culture, Chlamydia); **079.88** (Infection, Chlamydia) To code the 079.88, the lab results are needed; otherwise, it would be a screening code or, if symptoms were present, the symptoms would be coded.

CASE 4-15

4-15A CONSULTATIONS (CLINICAL PATHOLOGY)

1. **80500** (Consultation, Clinical Pathology); **V58.83** (Test, blood-drug, for, therapeutic drug monitoring)
2. **88321** (Consultation, Surgical Pathology); **185** (Neoplasm, prostate, malignant, primary)
3. **88329** (Consultation, Surgical Pathology, Intraoperative); **174.0** (Neoplasm, breast, Malignant, Primary)

174.9

CASE 4-17

4-17A SURGICAL PATHOLOGY REPORT

88305 (Pathology, Surgical, Gross and Micro Exam, Level IV); **211.3** (Polyp, colon)

CASE 4-19

4-19A PATHOLOGY AND LABORATORY SECTION REVIEW

1. **86677** (Antibody, Helicobacter pylori) **DX: 530.81** (Reflux, esophageal)
2. **87207** (Smear and Stains, Parasites)
3. **87252** (Culture, Tissue, Virus)
4. **86694** (Antibody, Herpes Simplex) **DX: 054.10** (Herpes, genital)
5. **86689** (Western Blot, HIV)
6. **85027** (Blood Cell Count, Hemogram, Automated)
7. **86038** (Antinuclear Antibodies, ANA); **DX: V73.89** (Screening, disease, viral, specified type NEC), **V69.8** (Problem, lifestyle, specified NEC)
8. **82947** (Glucose, Body Fluid)
9. **82010** (Ketone Body, Acetone)
10. **80051** (Organ or Disease-Oriented Panel, Electrolyte)
11. **82803** (Blood Gases, CO_2) **DX: 250.00** (Diabetes) Ketoacidosis has not been confirmed, so it is not coded.
12. **82465** (Cholesterol, Serum)
13. **83718** (Cholesterol, Testing) **DX: 272.4** (Hyperlipidemia)
14. **85027** (Complete Blood Count, CBC)
15. **84443** (Thyroid Stimulating Hormone, TSH)
16. **84146** (Prolactin)
17. **84402** (Testosterone) **DX: 607.84** (Impotence, organic) By doing the lab tests, they are looking for physical reason for the impotence; therefore, that is the diagnosis code.
18. **85027** (Complete Blood Count, CBC)
19. **85032** (Platelet, Count)
20. **82310** (Calcium, Total)
21. **83735** (Magnesium)
22. **84550** (Uric Acid, Blood)
23. **85610** (Prothrombin time)
24. **85730** (Thromboplastin, Partial Time) **DX: 205.00** (Leukemia, myelocytic)
25. **84520** (Blood Urea Nitrogen)
26. **82565** (Creatinine, Blood)
27. **85027** (Complete Blood Count, CBC)
28. **85060** (Blood Smear) **DX: 289.6** (Polycythemia, benign, familial)
29. **82947** (Glucose, Body Fluid) **DX: 783.21** (Loss, weight), **783.5** (Polydipsia), **V18.0** (History, family, diabetes mellitus) This is not a screening code as there are symptoms present.
30. **82947** (Glucose, Blood Test)
31. **80061** (Organ or Disease-Oriented Panel, Lipid Panel) **DX: 278.01** (Obesity, morbid)
32. **85652** (Sedimentation Rate, Blood Cell, Automated)
33. **85027** (Complete Blood Count, CBC) **DX: 424.90** (Endocarditis)
34. **84520** (Blood Urea Nitrogen)
35. **81003** (Urinalysis, automated) **DX: 617.0** (Endometriosis, uterus)
36. **85027** (Complete Blood Count)
37. **85652** (Sedimentation Rate, Blood Cell, Automated)
38. **82947** (Glucose, Blood Test)
39. **84540** (Urea Nitrogen, Urine)
40. **84520** (Blood Urea Nitrogen)
41. **80076** (Organ or Disease-Oriented Panel, Hepatic Function Panel)
42. **82565** (Creatinine, Blood) **DX: 351.0** (Bell's palsy)
43. **88305** (Pathology, Surgical, Gross and Micro Exam, Level IV), **85097** (Bone Marrow, Smear); **DX: 277.3** (Amyloidosis)
44. **80053** (Organ or Disease-Oriented Panel, Metabolic, Comprehensive); **592.0** (Calculus, renal, recurrent)
45. **85049** (Platelet, Count), **85610** (Prothrombin Time), **85002** (Bleeding Time); **287.5** (Thrombocytopenia)
46. **85652** (Sedimentation Rate, Blood Cell, Automated), **84439** (Thyroxine, Free), **84443** (Thyroid Stimulating

Hormone, TSH); **242.90** (Hyperthyroidism, without mention of complication)

47. **84075** (Alkaline Phosphatase), **84100** (Phosphorus), **84443** (Thyroid Stimulating Hormone, TSH), **85009** (Blood Cell Count, Differential WBC Count), **85652** (Sedimentation Rate), **733.00** (Osteoporosis)
48. **86593** (Syphilis Test), **80061** (Organ or Disease-Oriented Panel [Lipid Panel]), **386.00** (Meniere's disease, syndrome or vertigo)
49. **84153** (Prostate Specific Antigen), **85008** (Blood Cell Count, Blood Smear); **601.0** (Prostatitis, acute)
50. **83001** (Follicle Stimulating Hormone, FSH), **83002** (Luteinizing Hormone, LH), **84439** (Thyroxine, Free), **84443** (Thyroid Stimulating Hormone); **253.1** (Hyperprolactinemia)
51. **84520** (Blood Urea Nitrogen), **82565** (Creatinine, Blood); **585.9** (Failure, renal, chronic)

Chapter 5

Integumentary System

CASE 5-1

5-1A OPERATIVE REPORT, EXCISION FAT NECROSIS

Professional Services: 11042-78 (Debridement, Skin, Subcutaneous Tissue); **709.3** (Degeneration, skin)

Facility Services: This is an inpatient stay. The entire record would need to be reviewed before coding. We will not be assigning codes on inpatients.

CASE 5-3

5-3A OPERATIVE REPORT, SKIN TAGS

Professional Services: 11200 (Skin, Tags, Removal); **701.9** (Tag, skin)

Facility Services: 11200 (Skin, Tags, Removal); **701.9** (Tag, skin)

CASE 5-5

5-5A OPERATIVE REPORT, LESIONS

Professional Services: 11402 × **2** (Excision, Lesion, Skin, Benign); **216.5** (Neoplasm, skin, chest, Benign), **V10.3** (History, personal, malignant neoplasm, breast)

Facility Services: 11402 (Excision, Lesion, Skin, Benign), **11402-59** (Excision, Lesion, Skin, Benign); **216.5** (Neoplasm, skin, chest, benign), **V10.3** (History, personal, malignant neoplasm, breast)

CASE 5-7

5-7A OPERATIVE REPORT, NEVUS

Professional Services: 11424 (Excision, Skin, Lesion, Benign); **216.4** (Neoplasm, skin, neck, Benign)

Facility Services: 11424 (Excision, Skin, Lesion, Benign); **216.4** (Neoplasm, skin, neck, benign).

CASE 5-9

5-9A OPERATIVE REPORT, KERATOSIS EXCISION

Professional Services: 11442 (Excision, Skin, Lesion, Benign); **702.0** (Keratosis, actinic)

Facility Services: 11442 (Excision, Skin, Lesion, Benign); **702.0** (Keratosis, actinic).

CASE 5-11

5-11A OPERATIVE REPORT, SQUAMOUS CELL CARCINOMA

Professional Services: 11643 (Excision, Skin, Lesion, Malignant); **173.3** (Neoplasm, skin, temple, Malignant, Primary)

Facility Services: 11643 (Excision, Skin, Lesion, Malignant); **173.3** (Neoplasm, skin, temple, Malignant, Primary).

CASE 5-13

5-13A CLINIC PROGRESS NOTE

Professional Services: 11750-T5 (Excision, Nails); **703.0** (Onychocryptosis)

Facility Services: No facility services were provided.

CASE 5-15

5-15A OPERATIVE REPORT, LACERATION

Professional Services: 13152 (Wound, Repair, Complex); **873.53** (Wound, open, lip, complicated), **E816.1** (Accident, motor vehicle, not involving collision)

Facility Services: 13152 (Wound, Repair, Complex) A facility E/M code would be assigned for the ER visit. Each facility defines its own E/M levels so this varies from one hospital to the next; **873.53** (Wound, open, lip, complicated), **E816.1** (Accident, motor vehicle, not involving collision, passenger)

CASE 5-17

5-17A OPERATIVE REPORT, UMBILICOPLASTY

Professional Services: 13101 (Wound, Repair, Complex), **11403-51** (Excision, Skin, Lesion, Benign); **709.2** (Scar), **709.3** (Necrosis, fat, skin)

Facility Services: 13101 (Wound, Repair, Complex), **11403** (Excision, Skin, Lesion, Benign); **709.2** (Scar), **709.3** (Necrosis, fat, skin).

CASE 5-19

5-19A OPERATIVE REPORT, DERMABRASION

Professional Services: 13132 (Wound, Repair, Complex), **13133** × 2 (Wound, Repair, Complex); **709.2** (Scar)

Facility Services: 13132 (Wound, Repair, Complex), **13133** × 2 (Wound, Repair, Complex); **709.2** (Scar).

CASE 5-21

5-21A OPERATIVE REPORT, EXCISION GANGLION CYST

Professional Services: 14040 (Skin, Graft and Flap, Tissue); **727.43** (Cyst, ganglion)

Facility Services: 14040 (Skin, Graft and Flap, Tissue); **727.43** (Cyst, ganglion).

CASE 5-23

5-23A OPERATIVE REPORT, SPLIT-THICKNESS AUTOGRAFT

Professional Services: 15100 (Skin, Grafts, Autograft); **998.83** (Wound, open, non-healing surgical)

Facility Services: This is an inpatient stay. The entire record would need to be reviewed before coding. We will not be assigning codes on inpatients.

CASE 5-25

5-25A OPERATIVE REPORT, FULL-THICKNESS SKIN GRAFT

Professional Services: 15240-FA (Skin, Grafts, Free); **883.0** (Wound, open, finger)

Facility Services: 15240-FA (Skin, Grafts, Free); **883.0** (Wound, open, finger) After review of the entire record and determination of the cause of the injury, the appropriate E code can be assigned.

CASE 5-27

5-27A OPERATIVE REPORT, COMPOSITE GRAFT

Professional Services: 15760 (Skin Graft and Flap, Composite); **232.3** (Neoplasm, skin, nose, Ca in situ)

Facility Services: 15760 (Skin Graft and Flap, Composite); **232.3** (Neoplasm, skin, nose, Ca in situ)

CASE 5-29

5-29A OPERATIVE REPORT, POST SKIN GRAFT

Professional Services: 15852-78 (Dressings, Change); **V58.3** (Admission for change of dressing)

Facility Services: 15852 (Dressings, Change); **V58.3** (Admission for change of surgical dressing).

CASE 5-31

5-31A OPERATIVE REPORT, BREAST BIOPSY

Professional Services: 19101-LT (Biopsy, Breast); **217** (Neoplasm, Breast, axillary breast tail, Benign)

Facility Services: This is an inpatient stay. The entire record would need to be reviewed before coding. We will not be assigning codes on inpatients.

5-31B PATHOLOGY REPORT

Professional Services: 88307 (Pathology, Surgical, Gross and Micro Exam), **88331** (Pathology, Surgical, Consultation, Intraoperative); **217** (Neoplasm, Breast, axillary breast tail, Benign)

Facility Services: This is an inpatient stay. The entire record would need to be reviewed before coding. We will not be assigning codes on inpatients.

5-31C PROGRESS NOTE

Professional Services: 99024 (Post-Op Visit); **V58.3** (Aftercare, involving, removal of, dressing)

Facility Services: No facility services were provided.

CASE 5-33

5-33A OPERATIVE REPORT, BREAST BIOPSY WITH NEEDLE LOCALIZATION

Professional Services: 19125-RT (Excision, Breast, Lesion, by Needle Localization); **610.3** (Fibrosis, breast)

Facility Services: 19125-RT (Excision, Breast, Lesion, by Needle Localization), **76096** (Mammogram, Breast, Localization Nodule), **76098** (X-ray, Specimen, Surgical), **88305** (Pathology, Surgical, Gross and Micro Exam); **610.3** (Fibrosis, breast).

5-33B PATHOLOGY REPORT

Professional Services: 88305 (Pathology, Surgical, Gross and Micro Exam); **610.3** (Fibrosis, breast)

Facility Services: See 5-33A.

CASE 5-35

5-35A PREOPERATIVE CONSULTATION

Professional Services: 99242-57 (E/M, Consultation); **611.72** (Mass, Breast), **V10.3** (History, Malignant neoplasm, breast)

Facility Services: No facility services were provided.

5-35B OPERATIVE REPORT, MODIFIED RADICAL MASTECTOMY

Professional Services: 19240-RT (Mastectomy); **174.2** (Neoplasm, breast, upper inner quadrant, Primary)

Facility Services: This is an inpatient stay. The entire record would need to be reviewed before coding. We will not be assigning codes on inpatients.

5-35C PATHOLOGY REPORT

Professional Services: 88309 (Pathology, Surgical, Gross and Micro Exam), **88331** and **88332** (Pathology, Surgical, Consultation, Intraoperative); **174.2** (Neoplasm, breast, upper inner quadrant, Primary)

Facility Services: This is an inpatient stay. The entire record would need to be reviewed before coding. We will not be assigning codes on inpatients.

5-35D DISCHARGE SUMMARY

Professional Services: 99238 (E/M, Hospital, Discharge); **174.2** (Neoplasm, breast, upper inner quadrant, Primary)

Facility Services: This is an inpatient stay. The entire record would need to be reviewed before coding. We will not be assigning codes on inpatients.

5-35E PROGRESS NOTE

Professional Services: 99024 (Post-Op Visit); **V58.42** (Aftercare, following surgery NEC)

Facility Services: No facility services were provided.

CASE 5-37

5-37A OPERATIVE REPORT, MAMMOPLASTY

Professional Services: 19325-50 (Mammoplasty, Augmentation); **V50.1** (Admission for breast augmentation)

Facility Services: This is an inpatient stay. The entire record would need to be reviewed before coding. We will not be assigning codes on inpatients.

Chapter 6
Cardiovascular System

CASE 6-1

6-1A CARDIOTHORACIC SURGERY CONSULTATION

Professional Services: 99252-57 (Consultation, Initial Inpatient); **414.01** (Arteriosclerosis, coronary artery, native artery), **250.00** (Diabetes)

Facility Services: This is an inpatient stay. The entire record would need to be reviewed before coding. We will not be assigning codes on inpatients.

CASE 6-3

6-3A CARDIOLOGY FOLLOW-UP NOTE

Professional Services: 99215 (Evaluation and Management, Office and Other Outpatient); **427.81** (Syndrome, sick, sinus), **294.8** (Dementia)

Facility Services: No facility services were provided.

CASE 6-5

6-5A HOLTER REPORT

Professional Services: 93224 (Echocardiography, 24-hour monitoring); **427.31** (Fibrillation, atrial), **425.4** (Cardiomyopathy)

Facility Services: No facility services were provided.

6-5B RADIOLOGY REPORT, PREIMPLANTATION

Professional Services: 71020-26 (X-Ray, Chest); **427.81** (Syndrome, sick, sinus), **429.3** (Cardiomegaly)

Facility Services: The chest x-ray charge would be included on the bill with the implantation.

6-5C OPERATIVE REPORT, PACEMAKER IMPLANTATION

Professional Services: 33208 (Pacemaker, Heart, Insertion, Electrode); **427.89** (Bradycardia)

Facility Services: 33208 (Pacemaker, Heart, Insertion, Electrode), **71020** (X-ray, Chest), **71010** (X-ray, Chest); **427.89** (Bradycardia)

6-5D RADIOLOGY REPORT, POSTIMPLANTATION

Professional Services: 71010-26 (X-Ray, Chest); **V45.01** (Status, post, pacemaker, cardiac), **427.89** (Bradycardia)

Facility Services: The chest x-ray charge would be included on the bill with the implantation.

CASE 6-7

6-7A CARDIOLOGY CONSULTATION

Professional Services: 99245 (Office and/or Other Outpatient Service, Consultation); **786.59** (Tightness, chest)

Facility Services: No facility services were provided.

6-7B HOSPITAL SERVICE

Professional Services: No E/M code would be assigned (as the level of service was too low to meet the lowest level of initial inpatient admission service.); **414.9** (Ischemia, coronary, heart), **785.2** (Murmur), **424.90** (Disease, vascular)

Facility Services: This is an inpatient stay. The entire record would need to be reviewed before coding. We will not be assigning codes on inpatients.

6-7C RADIOLOGY REPORT, CHEST

Professional Services: 71020-26 (X-ray, chest); **786.50** (Pains, chest), **429.2 (ACVD)**

Facility Services: This is an inpatient stay. The entire record would need to be reviewed before coding. We will not be assigning codes on inpatients.

6-7D CARDIOTHORACIC SURGICAL CONSULTATION

Professional Services: 99254 (Evaluation and Management, Consultation); **414.01** (Arteriosclerosis, coronary, native vessel), **424.0** (Insufficiency, mitral)

Facility Services: This is an inpatient stay. The entire record would need to be reviewed before coding. We will not be assigning codes on inpatients.

6-7E RADIOLOGY REPORT, CHEST

Professional Services: 71020-26 (X-ray, chest); **786.7** (Rales), **786.2** (Cough)

Facility Services: This is an inpatient stay. The entire record would need to be reviewed before coding. We will not be assigning codes on inpatients.

CASE 6-9

6-9A CARDIOLOGY CONSULTATION

Professional Services: 99253 (Consultation, Inpatient); **427.31** (Fibrillation, atrial), **998.11** (Complication, surgical, hemorrhage), **285.1** (Anemia, blood loss, acute), **785.2** (Murmur)

Facility Services: This is an inpatient stay. The entire record would need to be reviewed before coding. We will not be assigning codes on inpatients. The facility charges for the Emergency Room visit would be included on the inpatient billing.

CASE 6-11

6-11A HOSPITAL ADMISSION

Professional Services: 99221 (Evaluation and Management, Hospital); **785.1** (Palpitation)

Facility Services: This is an inpatient stay. The entire record would need to be reviewed before coding. We will not be assigning codes on inpatients. The facility charges for the Emergency Room visit would be included on the inpatient billing.

6-11B GENERAL CHEMISTRY

Professional Services: 80048 (Organ or Disease-Oriented Panel, Metabolic, Basic); **785.1** (Palpitation)

Facility Services: This is an inpatient stay. The entire record would need to be reviewed before coding. We will not be assigning codes on inpatients. The facility charges for the lab panel would be included on the inpatient billing.

6-11C HEMATOLOGY

Professional Services: 85007 (Blood Cell Count, Blood Smear), **85004** (Blood Cell Count, Automated); **785.1** (Palpitation)

Facility Services: This is an inpatient stay. The entire record would need to be reviewed before coding. We will not be assigning codes on inpatients. The facility charges for the lab work would be included on the inpatient billing.

6-11D ELECTROCARDIOGRAPHY

Professional Services: 93000 (Cardiography, Electrocardiogram, Evaluation); **785.1** (Palpitation)

Facility Service: This is an inpatient stay. The entire record would need to be reviewed before coding. We will not be assigning codes on inpatients. The facility charges for the echocardiogram would be included on the inpatient billing.

6-11E RADIOLOGY REPORT, CHEST

Professional Services: 71020-26 (X-Ray, chest); **785.1** (Palpitation), **496** (Disease, pulmonary, obstructive, diffuse)

Facility Services: This is an inpatient stay. The entire record would need to be reviewed before coding. We will not be assigning codes on inpatients. The facility charges for the chest x-ray would be included on the inpatient billing.

CASE 6-13

6-13A CARDIOVERSION

Professional Services: 92960 (Cardioversion); **427.31** (Fibrillation, atrial), **427.32** (Flutter, atrial)

Facility Services: 92960 (Cardioversion); **427.31** (Fibrillation, atrial), **427.32** (Flutter, Atrial).

CASE 6-15

6-15A OPERATIVE REPORT, THROMBOENDARTERECTOMY

Professional Services: 35301-RT (Thromboendarterectomy), **95955-26** (Electroencephalography, Intraoperative); **433.10** (Narrowing, artery, carotid)

Facility Services: 35301-RT (Thromboendarterectomy), **95955** (Electroencephalography, intraoperative); **433.10** (Narrowing, artery, carotid).

CASE 6-17

6-17A OPERATIVE REPORT, ARTERIOVENOUS FISTULA

Professional Services: 36830 (Creation, Arteriovenous); **585.6** (Failure, renal, end stage)

Facility Services: This is an inpatient stay. The entire record would need to be reviewed before coding. We will not be assigning codes on inpatients.

CASE 6-19

6-19A OPERATIVE REPORT, FEMORAL ARTERY LACERATION

Professional Services: 35226 (Repair, Artery, Lower Extremity), **35226-80** (Repair, Artery, Lower Extremity); **998.2** (Complications, accidental puncture or laceration during a procedure)

Facility Services: This is an inpatient stay. The entire record would need to be reviewed before coding. We will not be assigning codes on inpatients.

Chapter 7

Digestive System, Hemic/Lymphatic System, and Mediastinum/Diaphragm

CASE 7-1

7-1A SURGICAL CONSULTATION

Professional Services: 99251 (E/M, Consultation); **560.9** (Obstruction, intestine)

Facility Services: This is an inpatient stay. The entire record would need to be reviewed before coding. We will not be assigning codes on inpatients.

CASE 7-3

7-3A OPERATIVE REPORT, INTERSPHINCTERIC ABSCESS

Professional Services: 46045 (Abscess, Rectum, Incisions and Drainage); **566** (Abscess, perirectal)

Facility Services: This is an inpatient stay. The entire record would need to be reviewed before coding. We will not be assigning codes on inpatients.

CASE 7-5

7-5A OPERATIVE REPORT, HEMORRHOIDECTOMY

Professional Services: 46255 (Hemorrhoidectomy, Simple); **455.2** (Hemorrhoids, internal, bleeding, prolapsed, strangulated or ulcerated)

Facility Services: 46255 (Hemorrhoidectomy, Simple); **455.2** (Hemorrhoids, internal, bleeding, prolapsed, strangulated or ulcerated).

CASE 7-7

7-7A OPERATIVE REPORT, ESOPHAGOGASTRODUODENOSCOPY

Professional Services: 43239 (Endoscopy, Gastrointestinal, Upper, Biopsy); **535.50** (Gastritis), **535.60** (Duodenitis), **531.40** (Ulcer, stomach, chronic, with hemorrhage), **553.3** (Hernia, hiatal)

Facility Services: 43239 (Endoscopy, Gastrointestinal, Upper, Biopsy); **535.50** (Gastritis), **535.60** (Duodenitis), **531.40** (Ulcer, stomach, chronic, with hemorrhage), **553.3** (Hernia, hiatal)

CASE 7-9

7-9A OPERATIVE REPORT, SIGMOIDOSCOPY

Professional Services: 45330 (Endoscopy, Colon-Sigmoid, Exploration); **793.4** (Abnormal, radiological examination, gastrointestinal tract)

Facility Services: 45330 (Endoscopy, Colon-Sigmoid, Exploration); **793.4** (Abnormal, radiological examination, gastrointestinal tract).

CASE 7-11

7-11A OPERATIVE REPORT, COLONOSCOPY

Professional Services: 45380 (Endoscopy, Colon, Biopsy); **153.6** (Neoplasm, intestine, large, colon, ascending, Malignant, Primary)

Facility Services: This is an inpatient stay. The entire record would need to be reviewed before coding. We will not be assigning codes on inpatients.

7-11B SURGICAL CONSULTATION

Professional Services: 99252-57 (E/M, Consultation); **153.6** (Neoplasm, intestine, large, colon, ascending, Malignant, Primary)

Facility Services: This is an inpatient stay. The entire record would need to be reviewed before coding. We will not be assigning codes on inpatients.

7-11C OPERATIVE REPORT, HEMICOLECTOMY

Professional Services: 44160 (Colectomy, Partial, with Ileum Removal); **153.6** (Neoplasm, intestine, large, colon, ascending, Malignant, Primary), **197.6** (Neoplasm, mesentery, Malignant, Secondary)

Facility Services: This is an inpatient stay. The entire record would need to be reviewed before coding. We will not be assigning codes on inpatients.

7-11D PATHOLOGY REPORT

Professional Services: 88309 (Pathology, Surgical, Gross and Micro Exam, Level IV); **153.6** (Neoplasm, intestine, large, colon, ascending), **197.6** (Neoplasm, mesentery, Malignant, Secondary)

Facility Services: This is an inpatient stay. The entire record would need to be reviewed before coding. We will not be assigning codes on inpatients.

CASE 7-13

7-13A OPERATIVE REPORT, APPENDECTOMY

Professional Services: 44950 (Appendectomy); **540.9** (Appendicitis, acute), **998.2** (Complications, surgical accidental puncture or laceration), **863.29** (Injury, internal ileum), **V64.41** (Laparoscopic surgical procedure converted to open procedure)

Facility Services: 44950 (Appendectomy); **540.9** (Appendicitis, acute), **998.2** (Complications, surgical, accidental puncture or laceration), **863.29** (Injury, internal ileum), **V64.41** (Laparoscopic surgical procedure converted to open procedure).

The pathology report would be reviewed prior to coding to make sure that the selection of the acute appendicitis code is the correct code.

CASE 7-15

7-15A SURGICAL CONSULTATION

Professional Services: 99243 (E/M, Consultation); **531.70** (Ulcer, stomach, chronic)

Facility Services: This is an inpatient stay. The entire record would need to be reviewed before coding. We will not be assigning codes on inpatients.

7-15B EMERGENCY AND OUTPATIENT RECORD

Professional Services: 99281 (E/M, Emergency Department); **789.00** (Pain, stomach), **531.90** (Ulcer, abdominal)

Facility Services: 789.00 (Pain, abdominal), **531.90** (Ulcer, stomach) A facility E/M code would be assigned for the ER visit. Each facility defines its own E/M levels, so this varies from one hospital to the next. Many times it will correspond with the same level that is assigned by the physician, but that is not always so.

7-15C CRITICAL CARE

Professional Services: 99245 (E/M, Consultation); **533.70** (Ulcer, peptic, chronic)

Facility Services: No facility services were provided.

7-15D OPERATIVE REPORT, ULCER AND CHOLECYSTITIS

Professional Services: 43632 (Gastrectomy, Partial, with Gastrojejunostomy), **43635** (Vagotomy, with Partial Distal Gastrectomy), **47605** (Cholecystectomy); **532.70** (Ulcer, duodenal, chronic), **575.11** (Cholecystitis, chronic)

Facility Services: This is an inpatient stay. The entire record would need to be reviewed before coding. We will not be assigning codes on inpatients.

7-15E INTRAOPERATIVE CHOLANGIOGRAM

Professional Services: 74300-26 (Cholangiography, Intraoperative); **575.11** (Cholecystitis, chronic)

Facility Services: This is an inpatient stay. The entire record would need to be reviewed before coding. We will not be assigning codes on inpatients.

7-15F PATHOLOGY REPORT

Professional Services:
88305 × 3 (Pathology, Surgical, Gross and Micro Exam, Level IV [lymph node × 1, nerves × 2])
88307 × 2 (Pathology, Surgical, Gross and Micro Exam, Level V [stomach, ulcer])
88304 (Pathology, Surgical, Gross and Micro Exam, Level III [gallbladder])
88331 (Pathology, Surgical, Consultation, Intraoperative)
88332 × 3 (Pathology, Surgical, Consultation, Intraoperative, Each additional segment)
532.30 (Ulcer, duodenal, chronic, acute)

531.30 (Ulcer, stomach, chronic [gastric], acute)
785.6 (Hyperplasia, lymph node)
575.11 (Cholecystitis, chronic)

Facility Services: This is an inpatient stay. The entire record would need to be reviewed before coding. We will not be assigning codes on inpatients.

7-15G DISCHARGE SUMMARY

Professional Services: 99238 (E/M, Hospital, Discharge); **532.70** (Ulcer, duodenal, chronic), **575.11** (Cholecystitis, chronic)

Facility Services: This is an inpatient stay. The entire record would need to be reviewed before coding. We will not be assigning codes on inpatients.

CASE 7-17

7-17A OPERATIVE REPORT, HEMICOLECTOMY

Professional Services: 44160 (Colectomy, Partial, with Ileum Removal); **153.6** (Neoplasm, intestine, colon, ascending, primary), **198.89** (Neoplasm, abdomen cavity, secondary)

Facility Services: This is an inpatient stay. The entire record would need to be reviewed before coding. We will not be assigning codes on inpatients.

CASE 7-19

7-19A OPERATIVE REPORT, GASTROJEJUNOSTOMY/TRACHEOSTOMY

Professional Services: 44604 (Colporrhaphy), **43820-51** (Gastrojejunostomy, without Vagotomy), **31600** (Tracheostomy, Planned); **555.9** (Disease, Crohn's)

Facility Services: This is an inpatient stay. The entire record would need to be reviewed before coding. We will not be assigning codes on inpatients.

CASE 7-21

7-21A HOSPITAL INPATIENT SERVICE

Professional Services: 99221 (E/M, Hospital); **789.33** (Mass, abdominal, RLQ); **599.0** (Infection, urinary), **401.9** (Hypertension, unspecified), **041.4** (Infection, *Escherichia coli,* NEC)

Facility Services: This is an inpatient stay. The entire record would need to be reviewed before coding. We will not be assigning codes on inpatients.

7-21B OPERATIVE REPORT, CECECTOMY

Professional Services: 44160 (Colon, Excision, Partial), **44955** (Appendectomy); **540.0** (Appendicitis, acute with rupture), **789.39** (Mass, abdomen [specified site])

Facility Services: This is an inpatient stay. The entire record would need to be reviewed before coding. We will not be assigning codes on inpatients.

7-21C DISCHARGE SUMMARY

Professional Services: 99238 (E/M, Hospital, Discharge); **540.1** (Appendicitis, with, peritoneal, abscess), **403.91** (Hypertension, with, chronic kidney disease, unspecified), **584.9** (Failure, renal, acute), **518.81** (Failure, respiratory), **997.4** (Complication, surgical procedures, gastrointestinal), **552.8** (Hernia, abdominal, with obstruction), **599.0** (Infection, urinary), **041.4** (Infection, Escherichia coli, NEC), **285.9** (Anemia)

Facility Services: This is an inpatient stay. The entire record would need to be reviewed before coding. We will not be assigning codes on inpatients.

CASE 7-23

7-23A HOSPITAL INPATIENT SERVICE

Professional Services: 99221-57 (E/M, Hospital); **550.91** (Hernia, inguinal)

Facility Services: This is an inpatient stay. The entire record would need to be reviewed before coding. We will not be assigning codes on inpatients.

7-23B OPERATIVE REPORT, RIGHT INGUINAL HERNIA REPAIR

Professional Services: 49505-RT (Hernia, Inguinal); **550.91** (Hernia, inguinal)

Facility Services: This is an inpatient stay. The entire record would need to be reviewed before coding. We will not be assigning codes on inpatients.

7-23C PATHOLOGY REPORT

Professional Services: 88302 (Pathology, Surgical, Gross and Micro Exam, Level II); **550.91** (Hernia, inguinal)

Facility Services: This is an inpatient stay. The entire record would need to be reviewed before coding. We will not be assigning codes on inpatients.

CASE 7-25

7-25A OPERATIVE REPORT, AXILLARY NODE DISSECTION

Professional Services: 38525-LT (Lymph Nodes, Excision); **200.14** (Lymphosarcoma)

Facility Services: This is an inpatient stay. The entire record would need to be reviewed before coding. We will not be assigning codes on inpatients.

7-25B PATHOLOGY REPORT

Professional Services: 88307 (Pathology, Surgical, Gross and Micro Exam, Level V), **88331** (Pathology, Surgical, Consultation, Intraoperative); **200.14** (Lymphosarcoma)

CASE 7-27

7-27A BONE MARROW BIOPSY

Professional Services: 38221 (Biopsy, Bone Marrow), **38220-51** (Aspiration, Bone Marrow); **285.9** (Anemia), **584.9** (Failure, renal, acute), **733.90** (Pain, bone)

Facility Services: This is an inpatient stay. The entire record would need to be reviewed before coding. We will not be assigning codes on inpatients.

Chapter 8

Musculoskeletal System

CASE 8-1

8-1A ORTHOPEDIC CONSULTATION

Professional Services: 99241-25 (E/M, Consultation), **20605-RT** (Arthrocentesis, Intermediate Joint), **J1040** (Injection, Methylprednisolone acetate); **726.32** (Epicondylitis)

Facility Services: No facility services were provided.

CASE 8-3

8-3A OPERATIVE REPORT, HARDWARE REMOVAL

Professional Services: 20680-RT (Removal, Implantation); **V54.01** (Aftercare, fracture, removal of internal, fixation device)

Facility Services: 20680-RT (Removal, Implantation); **V54.01** (Aftercare, fracture, removal of internal, fixation device).

CASE 8-5

8-5A OPERATIVE REPORT, CARBUNCLE REMOVAL

Professional Services: 38525-LT (Excision, Lymph Nodes), **10061-51-LT** (Incision and drainage carbuncle, skin); **289.3** (Inflamed lymph node), **680.3** (Carbuncle, axilla)

Facility Services: 38525-LT (Excision Lymph Node), **10061-LT** (Incision and drainage carbuncle, skin); **289.3** (Inflamed, lymph node), **680.3** (Carbuncle, axilla).

CASE 8-7

8-7A OPERATIVE REPORT, NEVUS REMOVAL

Professional Services: 21555-LT (Excision, Tumor, Thorax); **216.5** (Neoplasm, skin, chest, Benign)

Facility Services: 21555-LT (Excision, Tumor, Thorax); **216.5** (Neoplasm, skin, chest, Benign).

CASE 8-9

8-9A OPERATIVE REPORT, SHOULDER MASS EXCISION

Professional Services: 23076-RT (Excision, Tumor, Shoulder), **214.8** (Lipoma, muscle)

Facility Services: 23076-RT (Excision, Tumor, Shoulder), **88304** (Pathology, Surgical, Gross and Micro exam); **214.8** (Lipoma, muscle).

8-9B PATHOLOGY REPORT

Professional Services: 88304 (Pathology, Surgical, Gross and Micro Exam); **214.1** (Lipoma, Skin)

Facility Services: See reporting in Case 8-9A.

CASE 8-11

8-11A OPERATIVE REPORT, GANGLION CYST

Professional Services: 26160-F1 (Tendon Sheath, Finger, Lesion); **727.43** (Cyst, ganglion)

Facility Services: 26160-F1 (Tendon Sheath, Finger, Lesion); **727.43** (Cyst, ganglion).

CASE 8-13

8-13A CONSULTATION, TENDON RUPTURE

Professional Services: 99221-57 (E/M, Hospital); **840.8** (Rupture, tendon, biceps), **E927** (E code index, overexertion)

Facility Services: No facility services were provided.

8-13B RADIOLOGY REPORT, SHOULDER

Professional Services: 73020-26-RT (X-Ray, Shoulder); **840.8** (Rupture, tendon, biceps), **E927** (E code index, overexertion)

Facility Services: No facility services were provided.

8-13C OPERATIVE REPORT, OPEN TENDON REPAIR

Professional Services: **24342-RT** (Repair, Arm, Muscle); **840.8** (Rupture, tendon, biceps), **E927** (E code index, overexertion)

Facility Services: No facility services were provided.

8-13D DISCHARGE SUMMARY

Professional Services: **99238** (E/M, Hospital Discharge); **840.8** (Rupture, tendon, biceps), **E927** (E code index, overexertion)

Facility Services: No facility services were provided.

CASE 8-15

8-15A OPERATIVE REPORT, ARTHROPLASTY

Professional Services: **27447-RT** (Arthroplasty, Knee); **715.96** (Osteoarthritis)

Facility Services: This is an inpatient stay. The entire record would need to be reviewed before coding. We will not be assigning codes on inpatients.

CASE 8-17

8-17A OPERATIVE REPORT, OPEN REDUCTION

Professional Services: **25628-RT** (Fracture, Scaphoid), **20900-RT** (Bone Graft, Harvesting); **814.01** (Fracture scaphoid, wrist, closed), **E917.9** (E code index, Striking, against object, moving)

Facility Services: **25628-RT** (Fracture, Scaphoid), **20900-RT** (Bone Graft, Harvesting), **73100-RT** (X-Ray, Wrist), **814.01** (Fracture scaphoid, wrist, closed), **E917.9** (E code index, Striking, against object, moving).

8-17B RADIOLOGY REPORT, WRIST

Professional Services: **73100-26-RT** (X-Ray, Wrist); **814.01** (Fracture scaphoid, wrist, closed), **E917.9** (E code index, Striking against object, moving)

Facility Services: The charges for the x-ray would be listed on the same bill as the outpatient operating room charges. See Case 8-17A for CPT code for x-ray.

CASE 8-19

8-19A RADIOLOGY REPORT, RIGHT FEMUR

Professional Services: **73550-26-RT** (X-Ray, Femur); **821.01** (Fracture, femur, shaft), **E888.9** (E code index, Fall, same level NEC)

Facility Services: **73550-RT** (X-ray, Femur); **821.01** (Fracture, femur, shaft), **E888.9** (Fall, same level NEC).

8-19B ORTHOPEDIC CONSULTATION, THIGH PAIN

Professional Services: **99253-57** (E/M, Consultation); **821.01** (Fracture, femur, shaft), **733.00** (Osteoporosis), **E888.9** (E code index, Fall, same level NEC)

Facility Services: This is an inpatient stay. The entire record would need to be reviewed before coding. We will not be assigning codes on inpatients.

8-19C OPERATIVE REPORT, FEMUR REPAIR, INTRAMEDULLARY NAILING

Professional Services: **27506-RT** (Fracture, Femur, Shaft); **821.01** (Fracture, femur, shaft), **E888.9** (E code index, Fall, same level NEC)

Facility Services: This is an inpatient stay. The entire record would need to be reviewed before coding. We will not be assigning codes on inpatients.

8-19D DISCHARGE SUMMARY

Professional Services: **99238** (E/M, Hospital, Discharge), **821.01** (Fracture, femur, shaft), **E888.9** (E code index, Fall, same level NEC)

Facility Services: This is an inpatient stay. The entire record would need to be reviewed before coding. We will not be assigning codes on inpatients.

CASE 8-21

8-21A OPERATIVE REPORT, AMPUTATION

Professional Services: **27880-LT** (Amputation, Leg, Lower); **250.70** (Diabetes, gangrene), **785.4** (Diabetes, gangrene), **443.81** (Angiopathia, Angiopathy; diabetic, peripheral)

Facility Services: This is an inpatient stay. The entire record would need to be reviewed before coding. We will not be assigning codes on inpatients.

CASE 8-23

8-23A OPERATIVE REPORT, DEBRIDEMENT

Professional Services: **29825-LT** (Arthroscopy, Shoulder); **726.0** (Frozen shoulder)

Facility Services: **29825-LT** (Arthroscopy, Shoulder); **726.0** (Frozen shoulder).

CASE 8-25

8-25A OPERATIVE REPORT, ACROMIOPLASTY

Professional Services: 29819-RT (Arthroscopy, Surgical, Shoulder), **29826-51-RT** (Arthroscopy, Surgical, Shoulder), **23412-RT** (Repair, Shoulder, Cuff); **727.61** (Rupture, rotator cuff, nontraumatic), **715.11** (Osteoarthrosis, localized, idiopathic), **718.11** (Loose, body, joint, shoulder), **V64.43** (Conversion, closed surgical procedure to open procedure, arthroscopic)

Facility Services: This is an inpatient stay. The entire record would need to be reviewed before coding. We will not be assigning codes on inpatients.

8-25B OPERATIVE REPORT, DEBRIDEMENT AND IRRIGATION

Professional Services: 10180-78-RT (Incision and Drainage, Wound Infection); **998.6** (Complications, surgical procedure, fistula), **041.11** (Infection, staphylococcal, aureus)

Facility Services: 10180-78-RT (Incision and Drainage, Wound Infection); **998.6** (Complications, surgical procedures, fistula), **041.11** (Infection, staphylococcal, aureus)

CASE 8-27

8-27A OPERATIVE REPORT, KNEE

Professional Services: 29881-RT (Arthroscopy, Surgical, Knee), **27420-51-RT** (Reconstruction, Knee Cap, Instability); **822.0** (Fracture, Knee, Cap), **717.2** (Tear, meniscus, medial, posterior horn, old), **E927** (E code index, Overexertion)

Facility Services: 29881-RT (Arthroscopy, Surgical, Knee), **27420-RT** (Reconstruction, Knee Cap, Instability); **822.0** (Fracture, Knee, Cap), **717.2** (Tear, meniscus, medial, posterior horn, old), **E927** (E code index, Overexertion).

Chapter 9

Respiratory System

CASE 9-1

9-1A EVENING CLINIC, SORE THROAT

Professional Services: 99213 (Evaluation and Management, Office and Other Outpatient); **460** (Rhinopharyngitis)

Facility Services: No facility services were provided.

9-1B LABORATORY, RESPIRATORY CULTURES

Professional Services: 87430 (Antigen Detection, Enzyme Immunoassay, Streptococcus); **460** (Rhinopharyngitis)

Facility Services: No facility services were provided.

CASE 9-3

9-3A THORACIC MEDICINE/CRITICAL CARE CONSULTATION

Professional Services: 99223-25 (E/M, Hospital), **94656** (Ventilation Assist); **518.81** (Failure, Respiratory), **514** (Edema, lung)

Facility Services: This is an inpatient stay. The entire record would need to be reviewed before coding. We will not be assigning codes on inpatients.

9-3B THORACIC MEDICINE/CRITICAL CARE PROGRESS NOTE

Professional Services: 99233-25 (E/M, Hospital), **94657** (Ventilation Assist); **518.81** (Failure, Respiratory), **518.4** (Edema, lung, acute), **425.4** (Cardiomyopathy)

Facility Services: This is an inpatient stay. The entire record would need to be reviewed before coding. We will not be assigning codes on inpatients.

9-3C RADIOLOGY REPORT, CHEST

Professional Services: 71010-26 (X-Ray, Chest); **428.0** (Congestive heart failure), **V46.11** (Dependence, on, ventilator)

Facility Services: This is an inpatient stay. The entire record would need to be reviewed before coding. We will not be assigning codes on inpatients.

9-3D THORACIC MEDICINE/CRITICAL CARE PROGRESS NOTE

Professional Services: 99232-25 (E/M, Hospital), **94657** (Ventilation Assist); **518.81** (Failure, Respiratory), **518.4** (Edema, lung, acute), **425.4** (Cardiomyopathy)

Facility Services: This is an inpatient stay. The entire record would need to be reviewed before coding. We will not be assigning codes on inpatients.

9-3E THORACIC MEDICINE/CRITICAL CARE PROGRESS NOTE

Professional Services: 99232 (E/M, Hospital); **428.0** (Congestive heart failure), **518.81** (Failure, Respiratory), **514** (Edema, lung), **724.5** (Pain, back)

Facility Services: This is an inpatient stay. The entire record would need to be reviewed before coding. We will not be assigning codes on inpatients.

9-3F RADIOLOGY REPORT, CHEST

Professional Services: 71010-26 (X-Ray, Chest); **428.0** (Congestive heart failure), **514** (Edema, lung), **518.81** (Failure, Respiratory)

Facility Services: This is an inpatient stay. The entire record would need to be reviewed before coding. We will not be assigning codes on inpatients.

9-3G DISCHARGE SUMMARY

Professional Services: 99238 (E/M, Hospital, Discharge); **518.81** (Failure, Respiratory), **514** (Edema, lung), **425.4** (Cardiomyopathy), **428.0** (Failure, heart, congestive)

Facility Services: This is an inpatient stay. The entire record would need to be reviewed before coding. We will not be assigning codes on inpatients.

CASE 9-5

9-5A CONSULTATION/TRANSFER OF CARE

Professional Services: 99255 (E/M, Consultation); **786.07** (Wheezing), **424.0** (Insufficiency, mitral), **786.59** (Pain, chest), **782.3** (Edema)

Facility Services: This is an inpatient stay. The entire record would need to be reviewed before coding. We will not be assigning codes on inpatients.

CASE 9-7

9-7A OVERNIGHT OXYGEN DESATURATION STUDY

Professional Services: 95807-26 (Sleep Study), **780.09** (Somnolence)

Facility Services: 95807 (Sleep Study), **780.09** (Somnolence).

9-7B NOCTURNAL POLYSOMNOGRAM

Professional Services: 95810-26 (Polysomnography), **780.09** (Somnolence)

Facility Services: 95810 (Polysomnography), **780.09** (Somnolence).

9-7C MULTIPLE SLEEP LATENCY STUDY

Professional Services: 95805-26 (Sleep Study), **780.09** (Somnolence), **V69.4** (Deprivation, sleep)

Facility Services: 95805 (Sleep Study), 780.09 (Somnolence).

CASE 9-9

9-9A PULMONARY FUNCTION STUDY

Professional Services:

94060-26 (Pulmonology, Diagnostic, Spirometry)
94240-26 (Pulmonology, Diagnostic, Functional Residual Capacity)
94260-26 (Pulmonology, Diagnostic, Thoracic Gas Volume)
94720-26 (Pulmonology, Diagnostic, Carbon Monoxide, Diffusion Capacity)
94360-26 (Pulmonology, Diagnostic, Resistance to Airflow)
492.8 (Emphysema)
305.1 (Tobacco, abuse)

Facility Services: No facility services were provided

9-9B CARDIOTHORACIC CONSULTATION

Professional Services: 99245 (E/M, Consultation); **786.6** (Mass, chest)

Facility Services: No facility services were provided.

9-9C OPERATIVE REPORT, LUNG MASS

Professional Services: 32482-54-RT (Lobectomy, Lung); **162.8** (Neoplasm, lung, contiguous sites, Primary)

Facility Services: This is an inpatient stay. The entire record would need to be reviewed before coding. We will not be assigning codes on inpatients.

9-9D PATHOLOGY REPORT

Professional Services:

88309 (Pathology, Surgical, Gross and Micro Exam, Level VI [lung, lobe, segment])
88307 × **3** (Pathology, Surgical, Gross and Micro Exam, Level V [lymph nodes × 3, regional resection])
88331 (Pathology, Surgical, Consultation, Intraoperative)
88332 × **2** (Pathology, Surgical, Consultation, Intraoperative)
162.8 (Neoplasm, lung, contiguous sites, Malignant, Primary)
229.0 (Neoplasm, lymph gland, hilar, Benign)

Facility Services: This is an inpatient stay. The entire record would need to be reviewed before coding. We will not be assigning codes on inpatients.

9-9E THORACIC MEDICINE/CRITICAL CARE NOTE

Professional Services: 99252 (E/M, Consultation); **492.8** (Emphysema), **V46.11** (Dependence, on, ventilator)

Facility Services: This is an inpatient stay. The entire record would need to be reviewed before coding. We will not be assigning codes on inpatients.

9-9F RADIOLOGY REPORT, CHEST

Professional Services: 71010-26 (X-Ray, Chest); **518.0** (Atelectasis)

Facility Services: This is an inpatient stay. The entire record would need to be reviewed before coding. We will not be assigning codes on inpatients.

9-9G THORACIC MEDICINE/CRITICAL CARE PROGRESS REPORT

Professional Services: 32482-55-RT (Lobectomy, Lung); **162.8** (Neoplasm, lung, contiguous sites), **492.8** (Emphysema)

Facility Services: This is an inpatient stay. The entire record would need to be reviewed before coding. We will not be assigning codes on inpatients.

9-9H RADIOLOGY REPORT, CHEST

Professional Services: 71010-26 (X-Ray, Chest); **518.81** (Failure, respiratory)

Facility Services: This is an inpatient stay. The entire record would need to be reviewed before coding. We will not be assigning codes on inpatients.

9-9I PULMONARY FUNCTION STUDY

Professional Services: 94620-26 (Stress Test, Pulmonary); **786.09** (Dyspnea)

Facility Services: This is an inpatient stay. The entire record would need to be reviewed before coding. We will not be assigning codes on inpatients.

9-9J DISCHARGE SUMMARY

Professional Services: 99238 (E/M, Hospital, Discharge); **162.8** (Neoplasm, contiguous sites, Primary), **427.31** (Fibrillation, atrial), **492.8** (Emphysema)

Facility Services: This is an inpatient stay. The entire record would need to be reviewed before coding. We will not be assigning codes on inpatients.

CASE 9-11

9-11A OPERATIVE REPORT, THORACENTESIS

Professional Services: 32000 (Thoracentesis), **76942-26** (Ultrasound, Guidance); **511.9** (Effusion, pleura), **481** (Pneumonia, pneumococcal)

Facility Services: This is an inpatient stay. The entire record would need to be reviewed before coding. We will not be assigning codes on inpatients.

CASE 9-13

9-13A OPERATIVE REPORT, SEPTOPLASTY, TURBINOPLASTY, AND ETHMOIDECTOMY

Professional Services: 31255-LT (Ethmoidectomy, Endoscopy), **30520-51** (Septoplasty), **30140-51** and **30140-51-50** (Turbinate, Submucous Resection, Nose Excision); **470** (Deviation, septum, acquired), **478.0** (Hypertrophy, turbinate), **478.1** (Hypertrophy, nasal, ethmoid air cells)

Facility Services: 31255-LT (Ethmoidectomy, Endoscopy), **30520** (Septoplasty), **30140-50** (Turbinate, Submucous Resection, Nose Excision); **470** (Deviation, septum), **478.0** (Hypertrophy, Turbinate), **478.1** (Hypertrophy, nasal, ethmoid air cells).

CASE 9-15

9-15A THORACIC MEDICINE AND CRITICAL CARE CONSULTATION

Professional Services: 99252 (E/M, Consultation); **162.9** (Neoplasm, lung, Malignant, Primary)

Facility Services: This is an inpatient stay. The entire record would need to be reviewed before coding. We will not be assigning codes on inpatients.

9-15B THORACIC MEDICINE AND CRITICAL CARE PROGRESS REPORT

Professional Services: 99232 (E/M, Hospital); **786.05** (Shortness of breath)

Facility Services: This is an inpatient stay. The entire record would need to be reviewed before coding. We will not be assigning codes on inpatients.

9-15C THORACIC MEDICINE AND CRITICAL CARE PROGRESS REPORT

Professional Services: 99232 (E/M, Hospital); **511.9** (Effusion, pleura), **162.9** (Neoplasm, lung, Malignant, Primary)

Facility Services: This is an inpatient stay. The entire record would need to be reviewed before coding. We will not be assigning codes on inpatients.

9-15D RADIOLOGY REPORT, CHEST

Professional Services: 71020-26 (X-Ray, Chest); **511.9** (Effusion, pleura), **162.9** (Neoplasm, lung, Malignant, Primary)

Facility Services: This is an inpatient stay. The entire record would need to be reviewed before coding. We will not be assigning codes on inpatients.

9-15E OPERATIVE REPORT, ESOPHAGOGASTRODUODENOSCOPY

Professional Services: 43239 (Endoscopy, Gastrointestinal, Upper, Biopsy), **43450-59-51** (Dilation, Esophagus); **197.8** (Neoplasm, esophagus, upper [third], Secondary)

Facility Services: This is an inpatient stay. The entire record would need to be reviewed before coding. We will not be assigning codes on inpatients.

9-15F CT-GUIDED LUNG BIOPSY

Professional Services: 32405 (Biopsy, Lung), **76360-51-26** (CAT Scan Guidance, Needle Placement); **162.9** (Neoplasm, lung, Malignant, Primary)

Facility Services: This is an inpatient stay. The entire record would need to be reviewed before coding. We will not be assigning codes on inpatients.

9-15G PATHOLOGY REPORT

Professional Services: 88305 (Pathology, Surgical, Gross and Micro Exam, Level IV), **88104** (Cytopathology, Fluids); **162.9** (Neoplasm, lung, Primary)

Facility Services: This is an inpatient stay. The entire record would need to be reviewed before coding. We will not be assigning codes on inpatients.

9-15H ULTRASOUND MARKING FOR THORACENTESIS

Professional Services: 76942-26 (Ultrasound, Guidance, Thoracentesis); **511.9** (Effusion, pleura)

Facility Services: This is an inpatient stay. The entire record would need to be reviewed before coding. We will not be assigning codes on inpatients.

9-15I OPERATIVE REPORT, THORACENTESIS

Professional Services: 32002 (Thoracentesis), **32400** × **4** (Biopsy, Pleura, Needle); **162.9** (Neoplasm, lung, Primary)

Facility Services: This is an inpatient stay. The entire record would need to be reviewed before coding. We will not be assigning codes on inpatients.

9-15J PATHOLOGY REPORT

Professional Services: 88173 (Fine Needle Aspiration, Evaluation); **162.9** (Neoplasm, lung, Primary)

Facility Services: This is an inpatient stay. The entire record would need to be reviewed before coding. We will not be assigning codes on inpatients.

9-15K OXYGEN DESATURATION STUDY

Professional Services: 95807-26 (Oxygen, Sleep Study); **780.09** (Somnolence)

Facility Services: This is an inpatient stay. The entire record would need to be reviewed before coding. We will not be assigning codes on inpatients.

9-15L RADIOLOGY REPORT, CHEST

Professional Services: 71010-26 (X-Ray, Chest); **512.8** (Pneumothorax), **511.9** (Effusion, pleura)

Facility Services: This is an inpatient stay. The entire record would need to be reviewed before coding. We will not be assigning codes on inpatients.

9-15M OPERATIVE REPORT, THORACOSTOMY

Professional Services: 32020-LT (Thoracostomy, Tube); **511.9** (Effusion, pleura)

Facility Services: This is an inpatient stay. The entire record would need to be reviewed before coding. We will not be assigning codes on inpatients.

CASE 9-17

9-17A OPERATIVE REPORT, BRONCHOSCOPY

Professional Services: 31623 (Bronchoscopy, Brushing), **31624-51** (Bronchoscopy, Alveolar, Lavage); **793.1** (Abnormal radiological examination, lung), **V46.11** (Dependence, on, ventilator)

Facility Services: This is an inpatient stay. The entire record would need to be reviewed before coding. We will not be assigning codes on inpatients.

Chapter 10

Urinary, Male Genital, and Endocrine Systems

CASE 10-1

10-1A OPERATIVE REPORT, KIDNEY BIOPSY

Professional Services: 50200-RT (Biopsy, Kidney); **189.0** (Neoplasm, kidney, Malignant, Primary), **585.9** (Failure, chronic, renal)

Facility Services: 50200-RT (Biopsy, Kidney); **189.0** (Neoplasm, kidney, primary), **585.9** (Failure, renal, chronic).

CASE 10-3

10-3A OPERATIVE REPORT, NEPHRECTOMY

Professional Services: 50545 (Nephrectomy, Laparoscopic); **753.19** (Cyst, kidney, multiple)

Facility Services: This is an inpatient stay. The entire record would need to be reviewed before coding. We will not be assigning codes on inpatients.

CASE 10-5

10-5A URODYNAMIC ASSESSMENT

Professional Services: 51741-26 (Urodynamic Tests, Uroflowmetry), **51726-51-26** (Cystometrogram), **51784-51-26** (Electromyography, Sphincter Muscles, Anus), **51795-51-26** (Voiding Pressure Studies, Bladder); **585.9** (Failure, renal, chronic)

Facility Services: 51741 (Urodynamic Tests, Uroflowmetry), **51726** (Cystometrogram), **51784** (Electromyography, Sphincter Muscles, Anus), **51795** (Voiding Pressure Studies, Bladder); **585.9** (Failure, renal, chronic).

CASE 10-7

10-7A OPERATIVE REPORT, INTRAPERITONEAL BLADDER RUPTURE

Professional Services: 51865 (Repair, Bladder, Wound, Complicated); **867.1** (Injury, internal, bladder), **E881.0** (E code index, Fall, from, ladder)

Facility Services: This is an inpatient stay. The entire record would need to be reviewed before coding. We will not be assigning codes on inpatients.

CASE 10-9

10-9A OPERATIVE REPORT, URETEROSCOPIC STONE EXTRACTION

Professional Services: 52352 (Cystourethroscopy, Removal, Calculus), **52332-51** (Cystourethroscopy, Insertion, Indwelling Ureteral Stent), **76000** (Fluoroscopy, Ureter); **592.1** (Calculus, ureter)

Facility Services: 52352 (Cystourethroscopy, Removal, Calculus), **52332** (Cystourethroscopy, Insertion, Indwelling Ureteral Stent), **74480** (Fluoroscopic, Ureter); **592.1** (Calculus, ureter).

CASE 10-11

10-11A OPERATIVE REPORT, MEATOTOMY

Professional Services: 52281 (Cystourethroscopy, Meatotomy); **598.9** (Stenosis, urethra)

Facility Services: 52281 (Cystourethroscopy, Meatotomy); **598.9** (Stenosis, urethra).

CASE 10-13

10-13A OPERATIVE REPORT, CIRCUMCISION

Professional Services: 54152 (Circumcision, Surgical Excision, Other than Newborn); **605** (Phimosis), **607.1** (Balanitis), **112.2** (Balanitis, candidal)

Facility Services: 54152 (Circumcision, Surgical Excision, Other than Newborn); **605** (Phimosis), **607.1** (Balanitis), **112.2** (Balanitis, candidal).

CASE 10-15

10-15A OPERATIVE REPORT, VASECTOMY

Professional Services: 55250 (Vasectomy); **V25.2** (Sterilization)

Facility Services: 55250 (Vasectomy); **V25.2** (Sterilization).

CASE 10-17

10-17A TRANSRECTAL ULTRASOUND FOR PROSTATE VOLUME DETERMINATION AND BIOPSY

Professional Services: 55700 (Biopsy, Prostate), **76872-26** (Ultrasound, Prostate); **790.93** (Elevated, prostate specific antigen)

Facility Services: 55700 (Biopsy, Prostate), **76872** (Ultrasound, prostate); **790.93** (Elevated, prostate specific antigen).

CASE 10-19

10-19A OPERATIVE REPORT, LYMPHADENECTOMY, PROSTATECTOMY, AND PLASTIC REPAIR

Professional Services: 55845 (Prostatectomy, Retropubic, Radical), **51800-51** (Cystourethroplasty); **188.5** (Neoplasm, bladder, neck, Malignant, Primary), **196.6** (Neoplasm, lymph, pelvic, Malignant, Primary)

Facility Services: This is an inpatient stay. The entire record would need to be reviewed before coding. We will not be assigning codes on inpatients.

CASE 10-21

10-21A OPERATIVE REPORT, LEFT THYROID MASS

Professional Services: 60240 (Gland, Excision, Total); **241.0** (Nodule, thyroid)

Facility Services: This is an inpatient stay. The entire record would need to be reviewed before coding. We will not be assigning codes on inpatients.

Chapter 11

Female Genital System and Maternity Care/Delivery

CASE 11-1

11-1A EMERGENCY DEPARTMENT SERVICES

Professional Services: 99282 ([E/M] Emergency Department); **625.9** (Pains, adnexa)

Facility Services: A facility specific E/M level code would be assigned. These are different from one facility to the next. **625.9** (Pain, adnexa).

CASE 11-3

11-3A HISTORY AND PHYSICAL EXAMINATION

Professional Services: 99221-57 (E/M, Hospital, Initial); **625.0** (Dyspareunia), **625.3** (Dysmenorrhea), **617.9** (Endometriosis)

Facility Services: This is an inpatient stay. The entire record would need to be reviewed before coding. We will not be assigning codes on inpatients.

11-3B OPERATIVE REPORT, URETERAL STENTS

Professional Services: **52005** (Cystourethroscopy); **616.0** (Cervicitis), **617.0** (Adenomyosis, uterus), **617.1** (Endometriosis, ovary)

Facility Services: This is an inpatient stay. The entire record would need to be reviewed before coding. We will not be assigning codes on inpatients.

11-3C OPERATIVE REPORT, HYSTERECTOMY

Professional Services: **58150** (Hysterectomy, Abdominal, Total); **617.0** (Adenomyosis, uterus), **617.1** (Endometriosis, ovary), **616.0** (Cervicitis)

Facility Services: This is an inpatient stay. The entire record would need to be reviewed before coding. We will not be assigning codes on inpatients.

11-3D PATHOLOGY REPORT

Professional Services: **88307** (Pathology, Surgical, Gross and Micro Exam), **616.0** (Cervicitis), **617.0** (Endometriosis, uterus), **617.1** (Endometriosis, ovary)

Facility Services: This is an inpatient stay. The entire record would need to be reviewed before coding. We will not be assigning codes on inpatients.

11-3E DISCHARGE SUMMARY

Professional Services: **99238** (E/M, Hospital Discharge); **617.0** (Endometriosis, uterus), **617.1** (Endometriosis, ovary), **616.0** (Cervicitis)

Facility Services: This is an inpatient stay. The entire record would need to be reviewed before coding. We will not be assigning codes on inpatients.

CASE 11-5

11-5A OPERATIVE REPORT, DILATATION AND CURETTAGE

Professional Services: **58558** (Hysteroscopy, Surgical, with Biopsy); **182.0** (Neoplasm, uterus, endometrium, Primary)

Facility Services: This is an inpatient stay. The entire record would need to be reviewed before coding. We will not be assigning codes on inpatients.

CASE 11-7

11-7A REAL-TIME ULTRASOUND

Professional Services: **76815-26** (Echography, Pregnant Uterus); **656.73** (Malformation, placenta)

Facility Services: **76815** (Echography, Pregnant Uterus), **656.73** (Malformation, placenta).

11-7B SONOGRAM

Professional Services: **76816-26** (Echography, Pregnant Uterus); **656.73** (Malformation, placenta)

Facility Services: **76816** (Echography, Pregnant Uterus), **656.73** (Malformation, placenta).

11-7C OPERATIVE REPORT, CESAREAN SECTION

Professional Services: **59515** (Cesarean Delivery, Postpartum Care); **654.21** (Section, Cesarean, previous, in pregnancy or childbirth), **652.81** (Presentation, fetal, breech), **656.61** (Excess, fetus, affecting management of pregnancy), **216.5** (Neoplasm, skin, abdominal wall, Benign), **V27.0** (Outcome of delivery, single liveborn)

Facility Services: This is an inpatient stay. The entire record would need to be reviewed before coding. We will not be assigning codes on inpatients.

11-7D DISCHARGE SUMMARY

Professional Services: **99238** (E/M, Hospital Discharge Service); **654.21** (Section, Cesarean, previous, in pregnancy or childbirth), **652.81** (Presentation, fetal, breech), **656.61** (Excess, fetus, affecting management of pregnancy), **V27.0** (Outcome of delivery, single, liveborn), **216.5** (Neoplasm, skin, abdominal wall, Benign)

Facility Services: This is an inpatient stay. The entire record would need to be reviewed before coding. We will not be assigning codes on inpatients.

CASE 11-9

11-9A OB/GYN CONSULTATION

Professional Services: **99231** (E/M, Hospital Service, Subsequent), **643.83** (Pregnancy complicated by vomiting), **642.03** (Hypertension; complicating pregnancy, childbirth, or the puerperium; chronic), **648.03** (Pregnancy complicated by diabetes), **787.01** (Nausea, with vomiting), **787.91** (Diarrhea), **250.41** (Diabetic Nephropathy, type I), **583.81** (Nephropathy)

Facility Services: This is an inpatient stay. The entire record would need to be reviewed before coding. We will not be assigning codes on inpatients.

11-9B DUPLEX VENOUS EXAMINATION

Professional Services: **93970-26** (Duplex Scan, Venous Studies); **646.83** (Pregnancy, complicated, other specified condition), **729.81** (Swelling, leg)

Facility Services: This is an inpatient stay. The entire record would need to be reviewed before coding. We will not be assigning codes on inpatients.

11-9C ULTRASOUND

Professional Services: 76815-26 (Fetal Testing, Ultrasound); **V28.8** (Screening Antenatal, specified)

Facility Services: This is an inpatient stay. The entire record would need to be reviewed before coding. We will not be assigning codes on inpatients.

11-9D BIOPHYSICAL PROFILE

Professional Services: 76818-26 (Fetal Biophysical Profile); **648.03** (Diabetes, complicating pregnancy), **250.01** (Diabetes, type I)

Facility Services: This is an inpatient stay. The entire record would need to be reviewed before coding. We will not be assigning codes on inpatients.

11-9E DOPPLER UMBILICAL ARTERIAL

Professional Services: 76820-26 (Doppler, Arterial Study, Umbilical Artery); **648.03** (Pregnancy, complicated, diabetes), **642.03** (Hypertension, complicating pregnancy, with renal disease, unspecified), **250.41** (Diabetic Nephropathy, type 1), **583.81** (Nephropathy)

Facility Services: This is an inpatient stay. The entire record would need to be reviewed before coding. We will not be assigning codes on inpatients.

11-9F OB ULTRASOUND

Professional Services: 76815-26 (Fetal Testing, Ultrasound); **644.03** (Labor, preterm)

Facility Services: This is an inpatient stay. The entire record would need to be reviewed before coding. We will not be assigning codes on inpatients.

11-9G OB ULTRASOUND

Professional Services: 76946-26 (Ultrasound, Guidance, Amniocentesis); **V28.2** (Screening, antenatal, based on Amniocentesis)

Facility Services: This is an inpatient stay. The entire record would need to be reviewed before coding. We will not be assigning codes on inpatients.

11-9H OPERATIVE REPORT, AMNIOCENTESIS

Professional Services: 59000 (Amniocentesis); **648.03** (Diabetes, gestational, complicating pregnancy), **250.41** (Diabetic Nephropathy, type I), **583.81** (Nephropathy)

Facility Services: This is an inpatient stay. The entire record would need to be reviewed before coding. We will not be assigning codes on inpatients.

11-9I OB ULTRASOUND

Professional Services: 76816-26 (Fetal Testing, Ultrasound); **V28.8** (Screening, antenatal, specified condition)

Facility Services: This is an inpatient stay. The entire record would need to be reviewed before coding. We will not be assigning codes on inpatients.

11-9J OPERATIVE REPORT, CESAREAN SECTION

Professional Services: 59515 (Cesarean Delivery, Postpartum Care), **58611** (Cesarean Delivery, Tubal Ligation, at time of); **648.01** (Pregnancy, complicated by diabetes), **250.41** (Diabetic Nephropathy, type I), **583.81** (Nephropathy), **654.21** (Cesarean delivery, section), **V27.0** (Outcome of delivery, single liveborn), **V25.2** (Sterilization)

Facility Services: This is an inpatient stay. The entire record would need to be reviewed before coding. We will not be assigning codes on inpatients.

11-9K PATHOLOGY REPORT

Professional Services: 88307 (Pathology, Surgical, Gross and Micro Exam, Placenta), **88302 × 2** (Surgical Pathology, Gross and Micro Exam, Fallopian Tubes); **648.01** (Pregnancy, complicated by diabetes), **250.41** (Diabetic Nephropathy, type I), **583.81** (Nephropathy)

Facility Services: This is an inpatient stay. The entire record would need to be reviewed before coding. We will not be assigning codes on inpatients.

Chapter 12
Nervous System

CASE 12-1

12-1A OPERATIVE REPORT, VENTRICULOSTOMY

Professional Services: 61107 (Burr Hole); **331.4** (Hydrocephalus), **431** (Hemorrhage, intracerebral)

Facility Services: This is an inpatient stay. The entire record would need to be reviewed before coding. We will not be assigning codes on inpatients.

CASE 12-3

12-3A OPERATIVE REPORT, CRANIECTOMY

Professional Services: 61510 (Craniectomy, Surgical), **61795** (Stereotaxis, Computed Assisted, Brain Surgery); **225.0** (Neoplasm, brain, NEC, Benign), **434.00** (Clot, brain)

Facility Services: This is an inpatient stay. The entire record would need to be reviewed before coding. We will not be assigning codes on inpatients.

12-3B PATHOLOGY REPORT

Professional Services: 88307 (Pathology, Surgical, Gross and Micro Exam); **225.0** (Neoplasm, brain, NEC, Benign)

Facility Services: This is an inpatient stay. The entire record would need to be reviewed before coding. We will not be assigning codes on inpatients.

CASE 12-5

12-5A OPERATIVE REPORT, PTERYGOCRANIOTOMY AND CRANIOPLASTY

Professional Services: 61700 (Aneurysm Repair, Carotid Artery), **69990** (Operating Microscope); **437.3** (Aneurysm, brain), **430** (Hemorrhage, subarachnoid)

Facility Services: This is an inpatient stay. The entire record would need to be reviewed before coding. We will not be assigning codes on inpatients.

CASE 12-7

12-7A OPERATIVE REPORT, CRANIOPLASTY

Professional Services: 62141 (Cranioplasty, for Defect); **738.19** (Deformity, cranium)

Facility Services: This is an inpatient stay. The entire record would need to be reviewed before coding. We will not be assigning codes on inpatients.

CASE 12-9

12-9A OPERATIVE REPORT, LUMBAR PUNCTURE

Professional Services: 62270 (Spinal Tap, Lumbar); **784.0** (Headache, vascular)

Facility Services: This is an inpatient stay. The entire record would need to be reviewed before coding. We will not be assigning codes on inpatients.

CASE 12-11

12-11A PREOPERATIVE CONSULTATION

Professional Services: 99252 (E/M, Consultation); **343.9** (Palsy, cerebral)

Facility Services: This is an inpatient stay. The entire record would need to be reviewed before coding. We will not be assigning codes on inpatients.

12-11B OPERATIVE REPORT, INTRATHECAL CATHETER PLACEMENT

Professional Services: 62350 (Catheterization, Spinal Cord), **62361-51** (Pump, Insertion, Intra-Arterial); **333.7** (Dystonia, torsion, symptomatic)

Facility Services: This is an inpatient stay. The entire record would need to be reviewed before coding. We will not be assigning codes on inpatients.

12-11C OPERATIVE REPORT, REMOVAL OF BARD PORT

Professional Services: 62365-58 (Removal, Reservoir, Spinal Cord), **62362-51** (Replacement, Spinal Cord, Programmable Pump); **333.7** (Dystonia, torsion, symptomatic)

Facility Services: This is an inpatient stay. The entire record would need to be reviewed before coding. We will not be assigning codes on inpatients.

12-11D DISCHARGE SUMMARY

Professional Services: 99238 (E/M, Discharge Service); **343.9** (Palsy, cerebral), **333.7** (Dystonia, torsion, symptomatic)

Facility Services: This is an inpatient stay. The entire record would need to be reviewed before coding. We will not be assigning codes on inpatients.

CASE 12-13

12-13A OPERATIVE REPORT, HEMILAMINECTOMY AND FORAMINOTOMY

Professional Services: 63042-LT (Hemilaminectomy, L4-L5), **63044-LT** (Hemilaminectomy, L5-S1); **724.4** (Radiculitis, lumbar NEC)

Facility Services: This is an inpatient stay. The entire record would need to be reviewed before coding. We will not be assigning codes on inpatients.

CASE 12-15

12-15A OPERATIVE REPORT, CAGE FUSION

Professional Services: 22558 (Spine, Fusion, Anterior Approach), **22851** (Spine, Insertion, Instrumentation), **959527-26** (Evoked Potential, Somatosensory Testing); **722.52** (Degeneration, intervertebral disc, lumbar)

Facility Services: This is an inpatient stay. The entire record would need to be reviewed before coding. We will not be assigning codes on inpatients.

CASE 12-17

12-17A OPERATIVE REPORT, DISKECTOMY

Professional Services: 63075 (Diskectomy), **63076** (Diskectomy), **63081-51** (Decompression, Spinal Cord), **20931** (Allograft, Spine Surgery, Structural), **22554-51** (Spine, Fusion, Anterior Approach), **22845** (Fixation, Skeletal, Spinal Insertion), **22585** (Arthrodesis, Vertebra, Cervical), **95925-26** (Evoked Potentials, Upper Extremities); **723.0**

(Stenosis, spinal, cervical), **722.0** (Displacement, intervertebral disc, cervical)

Facility Services: This is an inpatient stay. The entire record would need to be reviewed before coding. We will not be assigning codes on inpatients.

CASE 12-19

12-19A ELECTROENCEPHALOGRAM REPORT

Professional Services: 95822-26 (Electroencephalography, Coma); **780.39** (Convulsion), **780.01** (Coma), **794.02** (Abnormal, EEG)

Facility Services: 95822 (Electroencephalography, coma), **780.39** (Convulsion), **780.01** (Coma), **794.02** (Abnormal, EEG)

Chapter 13

Eye and Auditory Systems

CASE 13-1

13-1A CLINIC PROGRESS NOTE, EYE EXAMINATION

Professional Services: 92002-57 (Ophthalmology, Diagnostic, Eye Examination, New Patient); **366.04** (Cataract, juvenile, nuclear)

Facility Services: No facility services were provided.

CASE 13-3

13-3A CLINIC PROGRESS NOTE, SENILE CATARACTS

Professional Services: 92012 (Ophthalmology, Diagnostic, Eye Examination, Established Patient); **366.10** (Cataracts, senile)

Facility Services: No facility services were provided.

CASE 13-5

13-5A CLINIC PROGRESS NOTE, EYE EXAMINATION

Professional Services: 92002 (Ophthalmology, Eye Exam, New Patient); **250.51, 362.01** (Diabetic, retinopathy)

Facility Services: No facility services were provided.

13-5B CLINIC PROGRESS NOTE, PHOTOCOAGULATION

Professional Services: 67228-LT (Destruction, Retina, Photocoagulation); **250.51, 362.01** (Diabetic, retinopathy)

Facility Services: No facility services were provided.

CASE 13-7

13-7A OPERATIVE REPORT, NASOLACRIMAL DUCT PROBING

Professional Services: 68811-RT and **68811-50-LT** or **68811-50** (Lacrimal Duct, Exploration, with Anesthesia); **743.65** (Obstruction, lacrimonasal)

Facility Services: 68811-50 (Bilateral Lacrimal Duct, Exploration, with Anesthesia); **743.65** (Obstruction, lacrimonasal duct, congenital).

CASE 13-9

13-9A OPERATIVE REPORT, PRESSURE EQUALIZATION TUBE REMOVAL

Professional Services: 69424-50 or **69424** and **69424-50** (Removal, Ventilating, Tube); **996.69** (Complication, infection and inflammation, due to, catheter, NEC)

Facility Services: 69424-50 (Removal, Ventilating Tube); **996.69** (Complication, infection and inflammation, due to, catheter, NEC).

CASE 13-11

13-11A OPERATIVE REPORT, TUBE REMOVAL

Professional Services: 69436-LT (Tympanotomy); **996.69** (Complication, infected and inflammation, due to, catheter, NEC)

Facility Services: 69436-LT (Tympanotomy); **996.69** (Complication, infected and inflammation, due to, catheter, NEC).

CASE 13-13

13-13A OPERATIVE REPORT, TYMPANOPLASTY

Professional Services: 69633-RT (Tympanoplasty, without Mastoidectomy, with Ossicular Chain Reconstruction); **389.03** (Loss, hearing, conductive), **385.23** (Discontinuity, ossicles, ossicular chain)

Facility Services: This is an inpatient stay. The entire record would need to be reviewed before coding. We will not be assigning codes on inpatients.

Chapter 14
Anesthesia

CASE 14-1

14-1A OPERATIVE REPORT, FLAPS AND GRAFTS

Professional Services: 01480-P3 (Anesthesia, Leg, Lower), **99100**

Facility Services: No CPT code assignment for anesthesia is made in the hospital setting.

CASE 14-3

14-3A OPERATIVE REPORT, FUSION WITH AUTOGRAFT

Professional Services: 01480-P1 (Anesthesia, foot)

Facility Services: No CPT code assignment for anesthesia is made in the hospital setting.

CASE 14-5

14-5A OPERATIVE REPORT, EXCISION OF RIGHT CAROTID BODY TUMOR

Professional Services: 00350-P2 (Anesthesia, neck), **99100** (Qualifying Circumstances)

Facility Services: No CPT code assignment for anesthesia is made in the hospital setting.

CASE 14-7

14-7A OPERATIVE REPORT, HYSTEROSCOPY, DILATATION, AND CURETTAGE

Professional Services: 00952-P1 (Anesthesia, uterus)

Facility Services: No CPT code assignment for anesthesia is made in the hospital setting.

CASE 14-9

14-9A OPERATIVE REPORT, NASOLACRIMAL DUCT PROBING

Professional Services: 00140-P1-QK-QX (Anesthesia, Eye)

Facility Services: No CPT code assignment for anesthesia is made in the hospital setting.

Glossary

A-mode one-dimensional ultrasonic display reflecting the time it takes a sound wave to reach a structure and reflect back; maps the structure's outline
active immunization injection that can either be a toxoid or a vaccine; causes an immune response to protect the patient from later infection by a specific disease
admission attention to an acute illness or injury resulting in admission to a hospital
amputation the removal of a limb or appendage that has been too damaged or diseased for treatment
analgesia absence of sensibility to pain
anesthesiologist a physician who specializes in the care of a patient before, during, and after surgery, including the evaluation and preparation of a patient for surgery
anesthetist a nurse or technician trained to administer anesthetics
angioplasty surgical or percutaneous procedure in a vessel to dilate the vessel opening; used in the treatment of atherosclerotic disease
anoscope instrument used in an examination of the anus
antepartum before childbirth
anteroposterior from front to back
artery vessel that carries oxygenated blood from the heart to body tissue
arthrocentesis puncture and aspiration of a joint
arthroscopy examination of the interior of a joint with an arthroscope (specialized endoscope)
atelectasis incomplete expansion of the lung or a portion of the lung
attending physician the physician with the primary responsibility for care of the patient
axial projection any projection that allows an x-ray beam to pass through a body part lengthwise

B-scan two-dimensional display of tissues and organs
balanitis inflammation of the glans penis
benign not progressive or recurrent
bilirubin orange-colored pigment in bile; accumulation leads to jaundice
biopsy removal of a small piece of living tissue for diagnostic purposes
brachytherapy therapy using radioactive sources that are placed inside the body
bronchospasm spasmodic contraction of the muscle of the bronchi causing constriction of the airway

cardioversion electrical shock to the heart to restore normal rhythm
cardioverter-defibrillator surgically placed device that directs an electric current shock to the heart to restore rhythm
cataract opaque covering on or in the lens
catheter tube placed into the body to put fluid in or take fluid out
cerebrovascular disease (CVD) blockage of arteries to the brain
cholecystectomy removal of the gallbladder
circumcision the removal of all or part of the foreskin
closed treatment procedure in which a fracture is repaired without exposure
colposcope scope used in colposcopy
colposcopy examination of the cervix and vagina by means of a colposcope
computed axial tomography (CAT or CT) procedure by which selected planes of tissue are pinpointed through computer enhancement, and images may be reconstructed by analysis of variance in absorption of the tissue
comminuted fracture one in which the bone is crushed or shattered
concurrent care the provision of similar services (e.g., hospital visits) to the same patient by more than one physician on the same day. Each physician provides services for a separate condition not reasonably expected to be managed by the attending physician. When concurrent care is provided, the diagnosis must reflect the medical necessity of different specialties
confirmatory consultation type of consultation requested by patients, insurance companies, and/or third party payers as an additional opinion and diagnosis
conscious sedation a decreased level of consciousness in which the patient is not completely asleep
consultant the physician providing a consultation to a requesting physician; a consultant is not an attending physician
consultation includes those services rendered by a physician whose opinion or advice is requested by another physician or agency concerning the evaluation and/or treatment of a patient
contributing factors counseling, coordination of care, nature of the presenting problem, and time of an E/M service
cranioplasty surgical correction of defects in the skull
craniotomy the surgical removal of (or an incision into) the cranium
cryoablation the removal of tissue by destroying it with extreme cold

cytopathology laboratory work done to determine whether any cellular changes are present

debridement cleansing or removal of dead tissue from a wound

decubitus recumbent positions where the x-ray beam is placed horizontally

dermis second layer of skin, holding blood vessels, nerve endings, sweat glands, and hair follicles

diagnostic ultrasound technique using high-frequency sound waves to determine the density of the outline of tissue to detect the cause of illness and disease

dialysis mechanical cleansing of the blood; can be temporary or permanent

differential actual count of the amount or number of blood constituents

direct face-to-face time the time a physician spends directly with a patient during an office visit, which can include obtaining a history, performing an examination, and/or discussing the results

discharge release from the hospital

distal farther from the point of attachment or origin

donor site the site from which tissue is taken to repair another site

Doppler ultrasound a diagnostic procedure using sound that can be standard black and white or color; can be transmitted only through solid or liquids

dosimetry scientific calculation of radiation emitted from various radioactive sources

duplex scan one method of vascular flow analysis using sound waves and real-time/color-flow Doppler imaging to produce a color picture of the blood flow within the vessels

dyspnea shortness of breath; difficult or painful breathing

echocardiography radiographic recording of the heart or heart walls or surrounding tissues

effusion the escape of fluid from blood vessels into a body part or tissue

ejection fraction the percentage of blood pumped with each contraction of the heart

endocrinologist a physician who specializes in the diagnosis and treatment of conditions of the endocrine system

endometrium the inner mucous membrane of the uterus

endoscopy inspection of body organs or cavities using a lighted scope that may be inserted through an existing opening or through a small incision

entropion a medical condition in which the lower eyelid and eyelashes roll inward toward the eye

epidermis outer layer of skin

epididymitis inflammation of the epididymis

epiphora abnormal overflow of tears, sometimes due to a blockage of the lacrimal passages

excision cutting or taking away (in reference to lesion removal, it is full-thickness removal of a lesion that may include simple closure)

excisional removal of an entire lesion for biopsy

external fixation application of a device that holds bones in place from outside the body

fistula abnormal opening from one area to another area or to the outside of the body

foramina a natural opening or passage

gastroenterologist a physician who specializes in the diagnoses and treatment of the digestive system

graft *autograft* is taken from the patient's own body; *allograft* is taken from another person's body, either alive or cadaver; *bilaminate graft* is made of artificial skin; *pinch graft* is a small, split-thickness repair; *split graft* is a repair that involves the epidermis and some of the dermis; *full-thickness graft* is a repair that involves the epidermis and all of the dermis; *xenograft* is one taken from another species

global surgical procedure a set amount of preoperative, intraoperative, and postoperative services bundled into a service code

gastrointestinal pertaining to the stomach and intestine

glucose blood sugar

gynecologist a physician specializing in the diagnosis, treatment, and management of female genital diseases and disorders

hemangioma benign tumor formed of blood vessels, common in infants and children

hematoma a localized collection of blood in any body space

hemodialysis cleansing of the blood outside of the body

hemoglobin protein found in red blood cells that transport oxygen through the bloodstream

hemogram graphic picture (or written record) of a detailed blood assessment

hemoptysis the expectoration of blood in sputum

hydrocele sac or accumulation of fluid

hypertrophy the enlargement or overgrowth of an organ due to the increase in size of its cells

hypotension abnormally low blood pressure

hypothermia low body temperature; sometimes induced during surgical procedures

hysterectomy surgical removal of the uterus

hysteroscope scope used in hysteroscopy

hysteroscopy visualization of the canal of the uterine cervix and uterine cavity using a scope placed through the vagina

incidental findings those findings that were not the reason a diagnostic test was performed; may be unrelated to the reason the test was ordered

incontinence inability to control excretory functions, such as urination

indicators written physician orders to a laboratory that set standards for any tests performed

infusion the administration of medicine over an extended period of time

inpatient one who has been formally admitted to a health care facility

internal fixation placement of hardware (rods, pins, etc.) onto or into the bone to hold it in place for repair

interstitial situated between body tissues
intracavitary within a body cavity
intralesional into a lesion
intramuscular into a muscle
intraventricular within a ventricle
ischemia deficiency of blood in a body part, usually due to constriction or obstruction of a blood vessel

ketones carbon-based compounds that are by-products of fatty acid metabolism; accumulation of ketone bodies in urine may indicate diabetes
key components the history, examination, and medical decision making complexity of an E/M service

lamina either of the pair of broad plates of bone flaring out from the pedicles of the vertebral arches
laminectomy surgical excision of the lamina
laparoscopy exploration of the abdomen and pelvic cavities using a scope placed through a small incision in the abdominal wall
lateral away from the midline of the body (to the side)
lesion abnormal or altered tissue (e.g., wound, cyst, abscess, boil)
leukocytes white blood cells

M-mode one-dimensional display of movement of structures
magnetic resonance imaging (MRI) procedure that uses nonionizing radiation to view the body in a cross-sectional view
malignant used to describe a cancerous tumor that grows worse over time
manipulation an attempt to maneuver a bone back into proper alignment
mastectomy excision (removal) of the breast
myocardial pertaining to the heart muscle
myocardial perfusion scan a radiologic procedure performed to assess the amount of blood reaching a given area
myringotomy the creation of a hole and/or incision in the tympanic membrane

nephrectomy excision of a kidney, either entirely or partially
nephrologist a physician who specializes in the diagnosis and treatment of conditions of the kidney
nephrons filtering units in the kidneys
neurologist a physician who specializes in the diagnosis and treatment of conditions of the nervous system
neurosurgeon a physician who specializes in surgical procedures of the nervous system
newborn care evaluation and determination of care management of a newborn infant

oblique view radiographic view in which the body or part is rotated so the projection is neither frontal nor lateral
observation the classification status of a patient that requires an inpatient stay for a short period to gather further information for diagnosis and treatment; the patient does not require acute inpatient care or intensive resources
occult blood test to detect the presence of blood in stool samples
odontoid position/view with the patient's mouth open
office visit a face-to-face encounter between a physician and a patient to allow for primary management of a patient's health care status
onychectomy excision (removal) of a nail or nail bed
open treatment a procedure in which a fracture site is surgically exposed and visualized
ophthalmologist physician specializing in medical and surgical care of the eye and visual system
orthopedist a physician who specializes in the diagnosis and treatment of musculoskeletal disorders
otolaryngologist physician specializing in the management and treatment of patients with diseases and disorders of the ear, nose, and throat; often referred to as an ENT physician
outpatient a patient who receives services in an ambulatory health care facility and is currently not an inpatient

panel groups of laboratory tests that are performed together
panniculectomy removal of abdominal fat and skin
parenchyma an essential element of an organ; functional element, such as the renal parenchyma, which is the tissue that contains the nephrons
permanent section a specimen of tissue obtained during an operative procedure that is mounted and analyzed by a pathologist for the most definitive diagnosis
passive immunization injection of antibodies into the body to protect the patient from a specific disease; does not cause an immune response
percutaneous through the skin
peritoneal cavity the space within the abdominal lining
pharyngitis inflammation of the pharynx (i.e., sore throat)
phimosis constriction of the preputial orifice that does not allow the foreskin to fold back over the glans
photocoagulation procedure that uses a controlled laser to treat leaky retinal blood vessels and destroy abnormal vessels or tissues at the back of the eye
physical status modifier period of time after a surgical procedure
pleural cavity the body cavity containing the organs and membranes of the thoracic region
position placement of the patient during an x-ray examination
posteroanterior from back to front
postoperative after a surgical procedure
postpartum after childbirth
presenting problem a disease, condition, illness, injury, symptom, sign, finding, complaint, or any other reason for a patient encounter, with or without a diagnosis being established at the time of the patient visit
professional component term used in describing radiology services provided by a radiologist
projection the path of the x-ray beam
prone (ventral) lying on the stomach

proximal closer to the point of attachment or origin
pulmonologist physician specializing in treatment of diseases and disorders of the respiratory system

Qualifying Circumstances five-digit CPT codes that describe situations or conditions that make the administration of anesthesia more difficult than is normal
qualitative only the presence of; not an exact amount
quantitative the exact amount present

radiologist physician who specializes in the use of radioactive materials in the diagnosis and treatment of disease and illnesses
radiology branch of medicine concerned with the use of radioactive substances for diagnosis and therapy
reagent a substance that changes color when exposed to another substance
recipient site the site that receives tissue for repair
reconstruction the three-dimensional image created by putting together several cross-sectional views (CT scans, MRIs, etc.)
recumbent lying down
requesting physician physician asking for advice or opinion on the treatment, diagnosis, or management of a patient from another physician
ribbons radioactive seeds embedded on a tape that is temporarily inserted into body tissues to deliver a radiation dose over time; can be cut to determine the amount of radiation the patient receives

septoplasty surgical repair of the nasal septum
shunt a device that diverts fluids the body cannot drain properly from one body area to another
skin graft transplantation of tissue to repair a defect
source a container holding a radioactive element; can be directly inserted into the body to deliver a the radiation dose over time
specific gravity weight of urine compared with an equal volume of water
sphincters circular bands of muscles that constrict a passage or close a natural orifice
spirometry measurement of breathing capacity
stent mold that holds a surgically placed graft in place
stress test a test that assesses cardiovascular health and function (by echocardiogram) after application of stress to the heart, usually exercise, but sometimes other such as atrial pacing, the cold pressor test, or specific drugs
subarachnoid within the membranes of the brain and spinal cord
subcutaneous tissue below the dermis, primarily fat cells that insulate the body
sulcus a groove, trench, or valley shape
superbill (encounter form) a form listing the most frequently used procedures and codes; the results of a patient's visit are checked off and used for billing purposes
supine (dorsal) lying on the back
swimmers position/view in which the arms are over the head

tangential patient position that allows the x-ray beam to skim a body part; produces a profile of the structure of the body
thoracentesis surgical puncture of the thoracic cavity, usually using a needle, to remove fluids
tissue expander a sac of fluid or air or a plastic implant that is placed under the skin to stretch the skin. The stretched skin is used for grafting purposes or stretched to place an implant beneath the newly expanded skin.
tissue transfer piece of skin for grafting that is still partially attached to the original blood supply and is used to cover an adjacent wound area
tomography procedure that allows viewing of a single plane of the body by blurring out all but that particular level
toxoids bacteria that cause a disease
transesophageal echocardiography (TEE) echocardiogram performed by placing a probe down the esophagus and sending out sound waves to obtain images of the heart and its movement
tympanostomy excision of the tympanic membrane to insert a pressure equalization tube for fluid drainage

unit/floor time the time a physician spends in the hospital setting dealing with a patient's case. This can include bedside face-to-face time with the patient or time spent working in other settings (e.g., the nursing station) on behalf of the patient.
ureter the tube that carries urine from the kidneys to the bladder
urinalysis the analysis of urine
urobilinogen a colorless compound formed in the intestines by the reduction of bilirubin
urodynamics pertaining to the flow and motion of liquids in the urinary tract
urologist a physician who specializes in the diagnosis and treatment of conditions of the urinary system

vaccine a small dose of a virus or bacteria that is injected into the body to produce an immune response to protect the patient from later infection by a specific disease
vasectomy a male sterilization procedure in which the vas deferens is cut, preventing the sperm from mixing with the seminal fluid
vein vessel that carries unoxygenated blood to the heart from body tissues

Index

D

O

Q

R